Nursing Interventions
Classification (NIC)

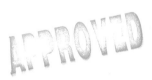

THE NIC LOGO

The NIC logo of a leaf and tree appears below and on the cover of this book. The leaf is an exact replica of one from a tree in the Linnaeus Botanical Garden in Uppsala, Sweden. The leaf was picked by an artist who lived next door to the garden for an imprint on a vase she was making. The vase was a present to a team member in 1990 just when the NIC Research team was looking for a logo. Because the leaf came from Linnaeus' garden, the team thought this was a meaningful logo. Carl Linnaeus (1701-1778) was the great classifier who brought order to the plant and animal kingdoms. In the logo, the leaf is joined with the tree, the universal symbol of taxonomy.

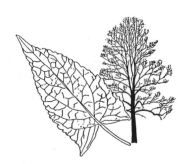

Nursing Interventions Classification (NIC)

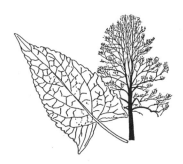

Sixth Edition

Editors

Gloria M. Bulechek, PhD, RN, FAAN
Professor Emerita
The University of Iowa
College of Nursing
Iowa City, Iowa

Joanne M. Dochterman, PhD
Professor Emerita
The University of Iowa
College of Nursing
Iowa City, Iowa

Howard K. Butcher, PhD, RN
Associate Professor
The University of Iowa
College of Nursing
Iowa City, Iowa

Cheryl M. Wagner, PhD, MBA/MSN, RN
Associate Dean
American Sentinel University
MSN Programs
Aurora, Colorado

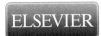

ELSEVIER
MOSBY

3251 Riverport Lane
St. Louis, Missouri 63043

Notices

Knowledge and best practice in this field are constantly changing. As new research and experience broaden our
understanding, changes in research methods, professional practices, or medical treatment may become necessary.

Practitioners and researchers must always rely on their own experience and knowledge in evaluating and
using any information, methods, compounds, or experiments described herein. In using such information
or methods they should be mindful of their own safety and the safety of others, including parties for whom
they have a professional responsibility.

With respect to any drug or pharmaceutical products identified, readers are advised to check the most
current information provided (i) on procedures featured or (ii) by the manufacturer of each product to be
administered, to verify the recommended dose or formula, the method and duration of administration, and
contraindications. It is the responsibility of practitioners, relying on their own experience and knowledge of
their patients, to make diagnoses, to determine dosages and the best treatment for each individual patient,
and to take all appropriate safety precautions.

To the fullest extent of the law, neither the Publisher nor the authors, contributors, or editors assume any liability
for any injury and/or damage to persons or property as a matter of products liability, negligence, or otherwise, or
from any use or operation of any methods, products, instructions, or ideas contained in the material herein.

Library of Congress Cataloging-in-Publication Data
Nursing interventions classification (NIC) / editors, Gloria M. Bulechek . . . [et al.].—6th ed.
  p. ; cm.
Includes bibliographical references and index.
ISBN 978-0-323-10011-3 (pbk. : alk. paper)
I. Bulechek, Gloria M.
[DNLM: 1. Nursing Process—classification. WY 15]

610.7301'2—dc23

         2012036567

Vice President and Publisher: Loren Wilson
Senior Content Strategist: Sandra Clark
Associate Content Development Specialist: Jennifer Palada
Publishing Service Manager: Julie Eddy
Project Manager: Jan Waters
Senior Book Designer: Amy Buxton

Printed in the United States of America

Last digit is the print number: 9   8   7   6   5   4   3   2   1

Preface

The NIC team was founded in 1987, so with this sixth edition, we are approaching 30 years of experience with standardized nursing language. Previous editions were published in 1992, 1996, 2000, 2004, and 2008. Joanne McCloskey Dochterman and Gloria M. Bulechek have served as editors on all six editions. Howard K. Butcher joined on the fifth edition and we welcome Cheryl M. Wagner as an editor with this edition.

NIC is a comprehensive standardized language that describes the treatments that nurses perform. We have expanded and revised the Classification with continued research efforts and input from the professional community. The features of this edition are as follows:

- Two updated chapters introduce the classification: Chapter One gives an overview of NIC and addresses 21 questions sometimes asked about NIC. Chapter Two focuses on implementation and use of NIC in practice, education, and research. Each of these chapters will be of interest to both the novice and experienced user of NIC. Material describing the beginning of NIC from 1987, and the research to develop the classification, appears in previous editions and has not been included in this edition. Appendix C contains a timeline with highlights of the evolution of NIC.
- There are a total of 554 interventions in this edition. Twenty-three of the interventions are new, and 128 of the previously included interventions have been revised for this edition. (See Appendix A for the list of new, revised, and deleted interventions.) The format for each of the interventions is the same as in previous editions. Each intervention has a label name, a definition, a list of activities that a nurse might do to carry out the intervention in the logical order that she or he might do these, a publication fact line, and a short list of background readings. The standardized language is the label name and the accompanying definition. The activities can be selected or modified as necessary to meet the specific needs of the population or individual. Thus NIC can be used to communicate a common meaning across settings but still provide a way for nurses to individualize care. The background readings for many of the interventions have been updated for this edition, with changes in activities made as indicated. The readings do not include, by any means, a complete reference list for any intervention. Effort was made to include

clinical guidelines when available and textbooks that are research based. They represent a few of the sources that were used in the development of the intervention's definition and activity list and provide support that this intervention is used by nurses. Each of the interventions has a unique code number to assist in computerization of NIC and facilitate reimbursement to nurses. The Front Matter contains a page with tips on approaches to finding an intervention.

- The NIC taxonomy, which was included for the first time in the second edition, has been updated to include all of the new interventions. The taxonomy in this edition, as in the previous three editions, includes 7 domains and 30 classes. The taxonomy, which appears in Part Two, helps nurses locate and choose an intervention and provides structure that can assist with curriculum design (See the overview of the NIC taxonomy on page 38 for more detail.)
- A feature continued since the third edition is specialty area core interventions that help to define the nature of the specialty. These lists of core interventions appear in Part Four and have been updated and expanded for this edition. The addition of 5 specialties, including Diabetes Nursing, HIV/AIDS Nursing, Home Health Nursing, Plastic Surgery Nursing, and Transplant Nursing, makes a total of 49 specialties with core interventions. (See the introduction to the core interventions on page 422 for more information.)
- Part Five of this edition contains the estimate of time to perform and minimum level of education that a provider needs to safely and competently administer the intervention. The time and education level are included for all 554 interventions in this edition. (See the introduction to the estimated time and education on page 448 for more information.)
- The linkages between NIC interventions and NANDA-I diagnoses have been updated for this edition and appear in Part Six. In the fifth edition, these linkages were moved to an electronic site, but due to user requests are being brought back into the book for this sixth edition.
- More than 60 nurses participated in reviewing and updating interventions to be sure current practice is reflected in this edition. The Recognition List in the Front Matter of the book lists these individuals. Interventions were sent

electronically for review, which included an update of background readings and additions to the list of activities and, in some cases, revision of definitions. We were pleased to receive suggestions for new interventions from several countries. Appendix B contains the guidelines for submission of a new or revised intervention.

- This edition contains a listing of all previous editions and translations of NIC. (See Appendix E.) Previous editions included a bibliography of publications about NIC; however, the growing number of publications from multiple countries has made the task of compiling a comprehensive bibliography difficult. Information about publications is being moved to the website for the Center for Nursing Classification and Clinical Effectiveness (www.nursing.uiowa.edu/cnc).

In summary, NIC captures the interventions performed by all nurses. As in the past, all of the interventions included in NIC are meant to be clinically useful, although some are more general than others. Because the interventions encompass a broad range of nursing practice, no nurse could be expected to perform all interventions listed here, or even a major portion. Many of the interventions require specialized training and some cannot be performed without appropriate certification. Other interventions describe basic hygiene and comfort measures that, in some instances, may be delegated to assistants, but still need to be planned and evaluated by nurses. The uses of NIC include the following:

- Helps demonstrate the impact that nurses have on the system of health care delivery
- Standardizes and defines the knowledge base for nursing curricula and practice
- Facilitates the appropriate selection of a nursing intervention
- Facilitates communication of nursing treatments to other nurses and other providers
- Enables researchers to examine the effectiveness and cost of nursing care
- Assists educators to develop curricula that better articulate with clinical practice
- Facilitates the teaching of clinical decision making to novice nurses
- Assists administrators in planning more effectively for staff and equipment needs
- Promotes the development of a reimbursement system for nursing services
- Facilitates the development and use of nursing information systems
- Communicates the nature of nursing to the public

When standardized language is used to document practice, we can compare and evaluate the effectiveness of care delivered in multiple settings by different providers. The use of standardized language does not inhibit our practice; rather, it communicates the essence of nursing care to others and helps us improve our practice through research. The development and use of this Classification helps to advance nursing knowledge by facilitating the clinical testing of nursing interventions. We believe the continued development and use of this Classification helps in the advancement of nursing knowledge and in the efforts of nursing to gain greater voice in the health policy arena. We continue to welcome your feedback and look forward to your continued input.

Gloria M. Bulechek
Howard K. Butcher
Joanne M. Dochterman
Cheryl M. Wagner

Strengths of the Nursing Intervention Classification

- *Comprehensive*—NIC includes the full range of nursing interventions for general practice as well as specialty areas. Interventions include physiological and psychosocial; illness treatment and prevention; health promotion; those for individuals, families, and communities; and indirect care. Both independent and collaborative interventions are included; they can be used in any practice setting regardless of philosophical orientation.
- *Research based*—The research to develop NIC used a multimethod approach; methods included content analysis, questionnaire survey to experts, focus group review, similarity analysis, hierarchical clustering, multidimensional scaling, and clinical field testing. The early research was partially funded by the National Institutes of Health, National Institute of Nursing Research. Ongoing work to update the classification builds on expert opinion and research based publications.
- *Developed inductively based on existing practice*—Original sources include current textbooks, care planning guides, and nursing information systems from clinical practice, augmented by clinical practice expertise of team members and experts in specialty areas of practice. The new additions and refinements are the result of suggestions from users and peer reviewers.
- *Reflects current clinical practice and research*—All interventions are accompanied by a list of background readings that support the development of the intervention. All interventions have been reviewed by experts in clinical practice and many by relevant clinical practice specialty organizations. A feedback process is used to incorporate suggestions from users in practice.
- *Has easy-to-use organizing structure* (domains, classes, interventions, and activities)—All domains, classes and interventions have definitions. Principles have been developed to maintain consistency and cohesion within the Classification; interventions are numerically coded.
- *Uses language that is clear and clinically meaningful*—Throughout the work, the language most useful in clinical practice has been selected. The language reflects clarity in conceptual issues, such as including only interventions and not diagnoses or outcomes.
- *Has established process and structure for continued refinement*—Suggestions for refinement are accepted from users around the world. The continued refinement of NIC is facilitated by the Center for Nursing Classification and Clinical Effectiveness, established in the College of Nursing at The University of Iowa in 1995 by the Iowa Board of Regents.
- *Has been field tested*—The process of implementation was initially studied in five field sites representing the various settings where nursing care takes place; hundreds of other clinical and educational agencies are also implementing the Classification. Steps for implementation have been developed to assist in the change process.
- *Accessible through numerous publications and media*—In addition to the classification itself, numerous articles and chapters have been published since 1990. Book and article reviews and publications about use and value of NIC attest to the significance of the work. A video was been made about the early development of NIC. Elsevier publishes a newsletter quarterly and maintains a Facebook page to keep people abreast of recent developments.
- *Linked to other nursing classifications*—Linkages of NIC to NANDA-I diagnoses are provided in Part 6 of this book to assist with clinical decision making. A third edition of a book linking the Nursing Outcomes Classification (NOC) outcomes and NIC interventions to NANDA-I diagnoses and other clinical conditions is available from Elsevier. Earlier editions of NIC were linked to Omaha system problems, NOC outcomes, RAP in long-term care, and OASIS for home health.
- *Recipient of national recognition*—NIC is recognized by the American Nurses Association, is included in the National Library of Medicine's *Metathesaurus for a Unified Medical Language*, is included in indexes of CINAHL, is mapped into SNOMED (Systemized Nomenclature of Medicine), and is registered in HL_7 (Health Level Seven International).
- *Developed at same site as outcomes classification*—The NOC of patient outcomes sensitive to nursing practice has also been developed at Iowa; both NIC and NOC are housed in the Center for Nursing Classification and Clinical Effectiveness (www.nursing.uiowa.edu/cnc).

- *Included in a growing number of vendor software clinical information systems*—The SNOMED has included NIC in its multidisciplinary record system. Several vendors have licensed NIC for inclusion in their software, targeted at both hospital and community settings, as well as practitioners in either general or specialty practice.

- *Global use*—NIC is an established classification of nursing interventions with 20 years of use in multiple countries. Translations are complete or in process for the following languages: Chinese, Dutch, French, German, Icelandic, Italian, Japanese, Korean, Norwegian, Portuguese, and Spanish.

Acknowledgments

Nothing of this magnitude is done alone. As with past editions, we wish to acknowledge help from a variety of sources:

The individuals and groups who submitted suggestions for new interventions or revised interventions and the individuals who reviewed submissions. This includes the "Center Fellows" who provide a variety of expertise and the peer reviewers who gave their time and expertise. This Classification is continuously improved to better reflect clinical practice and best practices through the participation of many. The names of individuals who assisted with changes to this edition are in the recognition list in the preliminary pages.

The University of Iowa College of Nursing, for support of the Center for Nursing Classification and Clinical Effectiveness, founded in 1995 to facilitate ongoing development of NIC and NOC. The support from individual contributors is creating an endowment at the University of Iowa Foundation that will provide permanent support for continued upkeep of the Classification.

Our editor, Sandra Clark, at Mosby/Elsevier who has guided this classification through two editions. We also thank her associates Michael Wisniewski, former Director of Licensing Sales, and Karen Delany, Licensing Specialist, for their thoughtful work with vendors and agencies who are moving nursing into the electronic world. We also thank Karen Delany for the production of the NIC/NOC Newsletter and maintenance of the Facebook page, which helps us to bring new information to the professional community.

The assistance of Sharon Sweeney, Coordinator, Center for Nursing Classification and Clinical Effectiveness at the College of Nursing, the University of Iowa, who assisted with meetings of the NIC team, the peer review process, and maintained the electronic documents. This was a complicated and time-consuming job that she managed well. The help of doctoral student Meghan McGonigal-Kenney and Tess Judge-Ellis, Associate Professor Clinical, in reviewing and revising interventions is also greatly appreciated.

NANDA International and the Nursing Outcomes Classification researchers for their ongoing cooperation through the NNN Alliance to work together to facilitate linkages between NANDA-I diagnoses, NIC interventions and NOC outcomes and to implement standardized language in practice.

The enthusiastic response to the Classification from many the nurses in the U.S. and around the world who are using NIC in a variety of ways — to document their practice, to help students to learn how to plan nursing care, to organize nursing text books, and to conduct research studies. The requests of practitioners and students is resulting in the inclusion of standardized language in clinical and educational software.

Recognition List, Sixth Edition

The following individuals contributed to this edition of NIC in multiple ways. Some submitted new interventions for consideration or suggested revisions to existing interventions. Some assisted in the review process of additions, revisions, or deletions to the classification. Others submitted examples of how they have implemented NIC in practice or education. All have made a valuable contribution to the users of NIC.

Deborah K. Bahe, Health Services Provider, University of Iowa Health Care, Iowa City, Iowa

Jessica Block, Nursing Instructor, Kirkwood Community College, Cedar Rapids, Iowa

Tom Blodgett, Lecturer, The University of Iowa College of Nursing, and Staff Nurse, University of Iowa Hospitals and Clinics, Iowa City, Iowa

Nicole Petsas Blodgett, Doctoral Student, The University of Iowa College of Nursing, Iowa City, Iowa

Jane Brokel, Assistant Professor, The University of Iowa College of Nursing, Iowa City, Iowa

Mary Clarke, Director, Nursing Practice, Research and Innovation Management, Genesis Medical Center, Davenport, Iowa

Rose Constantino, Associate Professor, University of Pittsburgh School of Nursing, Pittsburgh, Pennsylvania

Kennith Culp, Professor, The University of Iowa College of Nursing, Iowa City, Iowa

Sheri Cutler, Nursing Content Analyst, McKesson Provider Technologies, Westminster, Colorado

Jeanette Daly, Associate Research Scientist, University of Iowa Hospitals and Clinics Department of Family Medicine, Iowa City, Iowa

Martha Driessnack, Assistant Professor, The University of Iowa College of Nursing, Iowa City, Iowa

Kristi Febus, Graduate Student, The University of Iowa College of Nursing, Iowa City, Iowa

Susanna Funk, Graduate Student, The University of Iowa College of Nursing, Iowa City, Iowa

Vicente de la Osa Garcia, Supervising Nursing, Clinical Unit Department of Hematology and Hemotherapy, University Hospital Virgen del Rocio, Seville, Spain

Sue Gardner, Associate Professor, The University of Iowa College of Nursing, Iowa City, Iowa

Joe Greiner, Advanced Practice Nurse, University of Iowa Hospitals and Clinics, Iowa City, Iowa

Elem Kocaçal Güler, Research Assistant, Fundamentals of Nursing Department, Ege University School of Nursing, Bornova Izmir, Turkey

Andrew Hanson, Staff Nurse, Froedtert Hospital, Milwaukee, Wisconsin

Laura K. Hart, Associate Professor Emerita, The University of Iowa College of Nursing, Iowa City, Iowa

Helen Heiskell, Assistant Professor, South University College of Nursing, Savannah, Georgia

Deborah Hubbard, Nursing Clinical Specialist, University of Iowa Health Care, Iowa City, Iowa

Stacey Huynh, Graduate Student, The University of Iowa College of Nursing, Iowa City, Iowa

Todd Ingram, Assistant Professor Clinical, The University of Iowa College of Nursing, Iowa City, Iowa

Benjamin J. Jaggers, Staff Nurse, University of Iowa Hospitals and Clinics Geriatric Psychiatry, Iowa City, Iowa

Tess Judge-Ellis, Associate Professor Clinical, The University of Iowa College of Nursing, Iowa City, Iowa

Clare E. Kasse-Katuramu, Cambridge Health Alliance Whidden Memorial Hospital, Everett, Massachusetts

Teresa Kelechi, Associate Professor, Medical University of South Carolina College of Nursing, Charleston, South Carolina

María Rosario Jiménez León, Diplomado en enfermería, Hospitales Universitarios Virgen del Rocío, Seville, Spain

Ángela Cejudo López, Enfermera Gestora de Casos de Atención Primaria, Seville, Spain

Begoña López López, Associate Care Direction Liaison Nursing, Sanitary District of Primary Health Care of Seville, Seville, Spain

Rosairo López López, Nursing Staff, Bone Marrow Transplantation Unit, Department of Hematology and Hemotherapy, University Hospital Virgen del Rocio, Seville, Spain

Juan Mateu Lorenzo, Head of Nursing for Emergency and Radiology Services, Hospital ASEPEYO Sant Cugat del Vallès, Barcelona, Spain

Thomas J. Loveless, Coordinator of the Adult Nurse Practitioner Program, Thomas Jefferson University School of Nursing, Philadelphia, Pennsylvania

Der-Fa Lu, Assistant Professor, The University of Iowa College of Nursing, Iowa City, Iowa

Francisco José Márquez Malaver, Nursing Staff, Bone Marrow Transplantation Unit, Department of Hematology and Hemotherapy, University Hospital Virgen del Rocio, Seville, Spain

Ana Eva Granados Matute, Supervisora Unidad de Coordinación Cuidados Interniveles, Hospitales Universitarios Virgen del Rocío, Seville, Spain

Meghan McGonigal-Kenney, Student Research Assistant, The University of Iowa College of Nursing, Iowa City, Iowa

Dorothy Metz, Graduate Student, The University of Iowa College of Nursing, Iowa City, Iowa

Pamela Nelson, Clinical Nurse Specialist, Assistant Professor, Mayo School of Medicine, Rochester, Minnesota

David G. O'Dell, Graduate Program Director, South University, West Palm Beach, Florida

Abbey Pachter, Program Director, South University College of Nursing, Virginia Beach, Virginia

Montserrat Cordero Ponce, Diplomada en Enfermería, Hospital Duques Del Infantado Virgen del Rocío, Seville, Spain

Rebecca Porter, Doctoral Student, The University of Iowa College of Nursing, Iowa City, Iowa

Eugenio Coll del Rey, Nurse, University Hospital Virgen de las Nieves de Granada, Spain

Marcia E. Ring, Assistant Professor, University of Vermont College of Nursing and Health Sciences, Burlington Vermont

Cheryl Rodgers, Nursing Instructor, South University, Richmond, Virginia

Libby Rollinson, Director, Content Solutions, McKesson Provider Technologies, Westminster, Colorado

Serafín Fernández Salazar, Hospital de Alta Resolución Sierra de Segura, Empresa Pública Hospital Alto Guadalquivir, Jaén, Spain

Isabel María Romero Sánchez, Diplomada en Enfermería, Hospital Duques del Infantado, Hospitales Universitarios Virgen del Rocío, Seville, Spain

Lisa Segre, Assistant Professor, The University of Iowa College of Nursing, Iowa City, Iowa

Jamie Smith, Graduate Student, The University of Iowa College of Nursing, Iowa City, Iowa

Sashi Solomon, Graduate Student, The University of Iowa College of Nursing, Iowa City, Iowa

Victoria Steelman, Assistant Professor, The University of Iowa College of Nursing, Iowa City, Iowa

Elaine E. Steinke, Professor, Wichita State University, Wichita, Kansas

Ruth Swart, Instructor, Clinical Simulation Learning Center, University of Calgary Faculty of Nursing, Calgary, Alberta Canada

Mary P. Tarbox, Professor and Chair, Mount Mercy University Department of Nursing, Cedar Rapids, Iowa

Holly Toomey, Director, Nursing Solutions Product Management, McKesson Provider Technologies, Westminster, Colorado

Sharon Tucker, Director, Nursing Research & EBP, Department of Nursing & Patient Care Services, University of Iowa Hospitals & Clinics, Iowa City, Iowa

José Carlos Bellido Vallejo, Surgical Area Nurse, Jaén Hospital Complex, Jaén-Andalusia-Spain

Juan Carlos Quero Vallejo, Surgical Area Supervisor, Jaén Hospital Complex, Jaén-Andalusia-Spain

Mercedes Barroso Vázquez, Coordinación de Gestión Clínica de Cuidados, Unidad de Coordinación Asistencial, Hospitales Universitarios Virgen del Rocío, Seville, Spain

Bonnie J. Wakefield, Associate Research Professor, Sinclair School of Nursing, University of Missouri, Columbia, Missouri

Nancy Walker, Functional Analyst, Horizon Expert Plan, McKesson Provider Technologies, Westminster, Colorado

Fellows - Center for Nursing Classification & Clinical Effectiveness

The Center for Nursing Classification and Clinical Effectiveness at the College of Nursing, the University of Iowa has a fellows program. *Fellow, Center for Nursing Classification & Clinical Effectiveness* is designated for individuals who contribute significantly to the ongoing upkeep and implementation of NIC and NOC. These individuals are actively contributing to the Center and may include research team members, staff at cooperating agencies, retired professors, and visiting scholars. Students who are within a year of finishing doctoral dissertation and who have made substantial contributions to the work of the CNC are eligible.

Fellows donate a portion of their time to some work activity of the Center. They are available as resource persons for such activities as: ad hoc reviews of proposed new interventions and outcomes, participating in team or other meetings, serving on a planning committee for a conference, reviewing drafts of monographs, participating in grant writing activities, and advising the board of current developments related to classification work. An appointment of a fellow is for a 3-year period, or shorter time depending on need (e.g., Visiting Scholar).

The following individuals are serving as Fellows as of July 1, 2012:

Mary Ann Anderson, Associate Professor, University of Illinois, College of Nursing, Quad Cities Regional Program, Moline, IL

Ida Androwich, Professor, Loyola University, School of Nursing, Chicago, IL

Sandra Bellinger, Retired, Trinity College of Nursing & Health Sciences, Rock Island, IL

Sharon Eck Birmingham, Chief Nursing Executive, Clairvia Business Unit, Cerner Corporation, Durham, NC

Veronica Brighton, Assistant Professor Clinical, University of Iowa, College of Nursing

Jane Brokel, Assistant Professor, University of Iowa, College of Nursing

Gloria Bulechek, Professor Emerita, University of Iowa, College of Nursing

Lisa Burkhart, Associate Professor, Loyola University, School of Nursing, Chicago, IL

Howard Butcher, Associate Professor, University of Iowa, College of Nursing

Jill Scott-Cawiezell, Professor and Associate Dean for Academic Affairs, University of Iowa, College of Nursing

Teresa Clark, Advance Practice Nurse, Informatics, University of Iowa Hospitals and Clinics

Mary Clarke, Director of Nursing Practice, Research, and Innovation, Genesis Medical Center, Davenport, IA

Deborah Conley, Gerontological Clinical Nurse Specialist, Nebraska Methodist Hospital, Omaha, NE

Elaine Cook, Assistant Professor, Mount Mercy University, Cedar Rapids, IA

Sister Ruth Cox, Faculty, Kirkwood Community College, Cedar Rapids, IA

Martha Craft-Rosenberg, Professor Emerita, University of Iowa, College of Nursing

Jeanette Daly, Associate Research Scientist, University of Iowa Hospitals and Clinics

Connie Delaney, Dean and Professor, University of Minnesota, School of Nursing, Minneapolis, MN

Janice Denehy, Associate Professor Emerita, University of Iowa, College of Nursing

Joanne M. Dochterman, Professor Emerita, College of Nursing, University of Iowa

Gloria Dorr, Advance Practice Nurse, Informatics, University of Iowa Hospitals and Clinics

Mary Ann Fahrenkrug, Adjunct Faculty, Ambrose University, Davenport, IA

Joe Greiner, Advanced Practice Nurse, University of Iowa Hospitals and Clinics

Barbara Head, Assistant Professor Emerita, University of Nebraska Medical Center, College of Nursing, Omaha, NE

Todd Ingram, Assistant Professor Clinical, University of Iowa, College of Nursing

Gwenneth Jensen, Clinical Nurse Specialist, Sandford Health, Sioux Falls, SD

Marion Johnson, Professor Emerita, University of Iowa, College of Nursing

Tess Judge-Ellis, Associate Professor Clinical, University of Iowa, College of Nursing

Gail Keenan, Associate Professor, Director Nursing Informatics Initiative, University of Illinois, College of Nursing, Chicago, IL

Peg Kerr, Associate Professor, Nursing Department Head, University of Dubuque, Dubuque, IA

Cathy Konrad, Faculty, Trinity College of Nursing & Health Sciences, Rock Island, IL

Marie Kozel, CARE Project Lead, Methodist Health System, Omaha, NE

Mikyoung Lee, Assistant Professor, Indiana University, School of Nursing, Indianapolis, IN

Sue Lehmann, Assistant Professor Clinical, University of Iowa, College of Nursing

Der-Fa Lu, Assistant Professor, University of Iowa, College of Nursing

Meridean Maas, Professor Emerita, University of Iowa, College of Nursing

Paula Mobily, Associate Professor, University of Iowa, College of Nursing

Lou Ann Montgomery, Director Nursing Administration, Co-Director Nursing Clinical Education Center, University of Iowa Hospitals and Clinics

Sue Moorhead, Associate Professor & Director, Center for Nursing Classification & Clinical Effectiveness, University of Iowa, College of Nursing

Hye Jin Park, Assistant Professor, Florida State University, College of Nursing, Tallahassee, FL

Shelley-Rae Pehler, Associate Professor, University of Wisconsin- Eau Claire, Eau Claire, WI

Aleta Porcella, Clinical Nurse Specialist, Informatics, University of Iowa Hospitals and Clinics

Barb Rakel, Assistant Professor, College of Nursing, University of Iowa

David Reed, Research Associate, University of North Carolina, Cecil G. Sheps Center for Health Services Research, Chapel Hill, NC

K. Reeder, Assistant Professor, Goldfarb School of Nursing at Barnes-Jewish College, St. Louis, MO

Debra Schutte, Associate Professor, Michigan State University, College of Nursing

Cindy Scherb, Professor, Winona State University, Graduate Programs in Nursing University Center Rochester, Winona, MN

Lisa Segre, Assistant Professor, University of Iowa, College of Nursing

Margaret Simons, Diabetes Nurse Specialist, Iowa City VA Medical Center

Kelly Smith, Instructor Clinical, University of Iowa, College of Nursing

Janet Specht, Professor, College of Nursing, University of Iowa

Anita Stineman, Associate Professor Clinical, College of Nursing, University of Iowa

Elizabeth Swanson, Associate Professor, College of Nursing, University of Iowa

Mary Tarbox, Professor and Chair, Department of Nursing, Mt. Mercy University, Cedar Rapids, IA

Toni Tripp-Reimer, Professor, University of Iowa, College of Nursing

Hui-Chen Tseng, Postdoctoral Fellow, University of Utah, College of Nursing, Salt Lake City, UT

Sharon Tucker, Director, Nursing Research and Evidence-Based Practice, University of Iowa Hospitals and Clinics

Bonnie Wakefield, Associate Research Professor, University of Missouri, Sinclair School of Nursing, Columbia, MO

Cheryl M. Wagner, Associate Dean, American Sentinel University, MSN Programs, Aurora, CO

Ann Williamson, Associate Vice President for Nursing, UI Health Care and Chief Nursing Officer, University of Iowa Hospitals and Clinics,

Organizations that have Contributed to the Development of NIC

Nurses from a variety of specialty organizations have participated in the development and validation of NIC. These organizations include the following:

Academy of Medical-Surgical Nurses
Advocates for Child Psychiatric Nursing
American Academy of Ambulatory Care Nursing
American Association of Critical-Care Nurses
American Association of Diabetes Educators
American Association of Neuroscience Nurses
American Association of Nurse Anesthetists
American Association of Occupational Health Nurses
American Association of Spinal Cord Injury Nurses
American Board of Neuroscience Nurses
American College of Nurse-Midwives
American Holistic Nurses Association
American Nephrology Nurses Association
American Nurses Association
ANA Council on Gerontological Nursing
ANA Council on Maternal-Child Nursing
ANA Council on Psychiatric and Mental Health Nursing
American Psychiatric Nurses Association
American Radiological Nurses Association
American Society of Ophthalmic Registered Nurses, Inc.
American Society of Pain Management Nurses
American Society of Post-Anesthesia Nurses
American Urological Association Allied
Association for Practitioners in Infection Control
Association for Professionals in Infection Control and Epidemiology, Inc.
Association of Child and Adolescent Psychiatric Nurses, Inc.
Association of Community Health Nursing Educators
Association of Nurses in AIDS Care

Association of Operating Room Nurses, Inc.
Association of Pediatric Oncology Nurses
Association of Rehabilitation Nurses
Association of Women's Health, Obstetric and Neonatal Nurses
Dermatology Nurses Association
Developmental Disabilities Nurses Association
Drug and Alcohol Nursing Association, Inc.
Emergency Nurses Association
International Association for the Study of Pain
International Society of Nurses in Genetics
Intravenous Nurses Society
Midwest Nursing Research Society
NAACOG: The Organization for Obstetric, Gynecologic, Neonatal Nurses
National Association of Hispanic Nurses
National Association of Neonatal Nurses
National Association of School Nurses, Inc.
National Consortium of Chemical Dependency Nurses
National Flight Nurses Association
National Gerontological Nursing Association
National Nurses Society on Addictions
North American Nursing Diagnosis Association
Oncology Nursing Society
Society for Education and Research in Psychiatric-Mental Health Nursing
Society for Peripheral Vascular Nursing
Society for Vascular Nursing
Society of Gastroenterology Nurses and Associates, Inc.
Society of Otorhinolaryngology and Head-Neck Nurses, Inc.
Society of Pediatric Nurses
Society of Urologic Nurses and Associates

Definitions of Terms

CLASSIFICATION TERMS
Nursing Intervention

Any treatment, based upon clinical judgment and knowledge, that a nurse performs to enhance patient/client outcomes. Nursing interventions include both direct and indirect care; those aimed at individuals, families, and the community; and those for nurse-initiated, physician-initiated, and other provider-initiated treatments.

A *direct care intervention* is a treatment performed through interaction with the patient(s). Direct care interventions include both physiological and psychosocial nursing actions; both the "laying on of hands" actions and those that are more supportive and counseling in nature.

An *indirect care intervention* is a treatment performed away from the patient but on behalf of a patient or group of patients. Indirect care interventions include nursing actions aimed at management of the patient care environment and interdisciplinary collaboration. These actions support the effectiveness of the direct care interventions.

A *community (or public health) intervention* is targeted to promote and preserve the health of populations. Community interventions emphasize health promotion, health maintenance, and disease prevention of populations and include strategies to address the social and political climate in which the population resides.

A *nurse-initiated treatment* is an intervention initiated by the nurse in response to a nursing diagnosis. It is an autonomous action based on scientific rationale that is executed to benefit the client in a predicted way related to the nursing diagnosis and projected outcomes. These actions would include those treatments initiated by advanced nurse practitioners.

A *physician-initiated treatment* is an intervention initiated by a physician in response to a medical diagnosis but carried out by a nurse in response to a "doctor's order." Nurses may also carry out treatments initiated by other providers, such as pharmacists, respiratory therapists, or physician assistants.

Nursing Activities

The specific behaviors or actions that nurses do to implement an intervention and that assist patients/clients to move toward a desired outcome. Nursing activities are at the concrete level of action. A series of activities is necessary to implement an intervention.

Classification of Nursing Interventions

The ordering or arranging of nursing activities into groups or sets on the basis of their relationships and the assigning of intervention labels to these groups of activities.

Taxonomy of Nursing Interventions

Placement of the interventions based upon similarities into what can be considered a systematic organization. The NIC taxonomy structure has three levels: domains, classes, and interventions.

OTHER TERMS
Patient

A patient is any individual, group, family, or community who is the focus of nursing intervention. The terms *patient, individual,* and *person* are used in this book but, in some settings, *client* or another word may be the preferred term. Users should feel free to use the term that is most relevant to their care setting.

Family

Two or more individuals related by blood or by choice with shared responsibility to promote mutual development, health, and maintenance of relationships.

Community

A group of people and the relationships among them that develop as they share in common a physical environment and some agencies and institutions (e.g., school, fire department, voting place).

Parent

Mother, father, or other individual assuming the childrearing role.

Caregiver

Any person who provides health care or acts on behalf of someone else.

How to Find an Intervention

This edition of the Classification contains 554 interventions. There are several methods available for finding the desired intervention.

Alphabetically: If one knows the name of the intervention and desires to see the entire listing of activities and background readings (see Part Three)

NIC Taxonomy: If one wishes to identify related interventions in particular topic areas (see Part Two)

Linkages with NANDA-I Diagnoses: If one has a NANDA-I diagnosis and would like to have a list of suggested interventions (see Part Six)

Core Interventions by Specialty: If one is designing a course or information system for a particular specialty group, this is a good place to start (see Part Four)

Linkages with NANDA-I Diagnoses and NOC Outcomes: If one wants to review linkages between NANDA-I, NOC, and NIC refer to the companion book, *NOC and NIC Linkages to NANDA-I and Clinical Conditions: Supporting Critical Reasoning and Quality Care* (Johnson, et al., 2012)

An individual should not be overwhelmed by the size of the Classification that is intended to be comprehensive for all specialties and all disciplines. It does not take long to become familiar with the Classification and to locate the interventions most relevant to one's own practice. The selection of a nursing intervention for a particular patient is part of the clinical decision making of the nurse. Six factors should be considered when choosing an intervention: (1) desired patient outcomes, (2) characteristics of the nursing diagnosis, (3) research base for the intervention, (4) feasibility for doing the intervention, (5) acceptability to the patient, and (6) capability of the nurse. These are explained more fully in Chapter Two.

Contents

Detailed Contents

PART FOUR   Core Interventions for Nursing Specialty Areas, 421

PART FIVE Estimated Time and Education Level Necessary to Perform NIC Interventions, 447

PART SIX NIC Interventions Linked to NANDA-I Diagnoses, 461

PART SEVEN Appendixes, 565

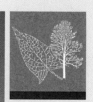

PART ONE

Overview of NIC

CHAPTER ONE

Understanding NIC

A DESCRIPTION OF NIC

The Nursing Interventions Classification (NIC) is a comprehensive standardized classification of interventions that nurses perform. It is useful for care planning, clinical documentation, communication of care across settings, integration of data across systems and settings, effectiveness research, productivity measurement, competency evaluation, reimbursement, teaching, and curricular design. The Classification includes the interventions that nurses do on behalf of patients, both independent and collaborative interventions, both direct and indirect care. An *intervention* is defined as *any treatment, based upon clinical judgment and knowledge, that a nurse performs to enhance patient/client outcomes*. Although an individual nurse will have expertise in only a limited number of interventions reflecting her or his specialty, the entire Classification captures the expertise of all nurses. NIC can be used in all settings (from acute care to intensive care units, to home care, to hospice care, to primary care) and all specialties (from critical care nursing to pediatric nursing and gerontological nursing). The entire Classification describes the domain of nursing; however, some of the interventions in the Classification are also done by other providers. Other health care providers are welcome to use NIC to describe their treatments.

NIC interventions include both the physiological (e.g., Acid-Base Management) and the psychosocial (e.g., Anxiety Reduction). Interventions are included for illness treatment (e.g., Hyperglycemia Management), illness prevention (e.g., Fall Prevention), and health promotion (e.g., Exercise Promotion). Most of the interventions are for use with individuals, but many are for use with families (e.g., Family Integrity Promotion) and some for entire communities (e.g., Environmental Management: Community). Indirect care interventions (e.g., Supply Management) are also included. Each intervention as it appears in the Classification is listed with a label name, a definition, a set of activities to carry out the intervention, and background readings. A notation that appears on each intervention just before the listing of background readings provides the edition(s) in which the intervention was developed and modified.

In this edition, there are 554 interventions and nearly 13,000 activities. The portions of the intervention that are standardized are the intervention labels and the definitions—these **should not** be changed when they are used. This allows for communication across settings and comparison of outcomes.

Care can be individualized, however, through the activities. From a list of approximately 10 to 30 activities per intervention, the provider selects the activities that are appropriate for the specific individual or family and then can add new activities if desired. All modifications or additions in activities should be congruent with the definition of the intervention. For each intervention, the activities are listed in logical order, from what a nurse would do first to what he or she would do last. For many activities the placement is not crucial, but for others, the time sequence is important. The lists of activities are fairly long because the Classification has to meet the needs of multiple users; students and novices need more concrete directions than experienced nurses. The activities are not standardized; this would be nearly impossible with so many of them and would defeat the purpose of using these to individualize care. The short lists of background readings at the end of each intervention are those that were found most helpful in developing the intervention or that support some of the activities in the intervention. They are a place to begin reading if one is new to the intervention, but they are by no means a complete reference list, nor are they inclusive of all the research on the intervention.

Although the lists of activities are very helpful for the teaching of an intervention and for implementation of the delivery of the intervention, they are not the essence of the Classification. The intervention label names and definitions are the key to the Classification; the names provide a summary label for the discrete activities and allow nurses to identify and communicate the nature of their work. Prior to NIC we only had long lists of discrete activities and no organizing structure; with NIC we can easily communicate our interventions with the label name that is defined with both a formal definition and a list of implementation activities.

The interventions are grouped into 30 classes and 7 domains for ease of use. The 7 domains are: (1) Physiological: Basic, (2) Physiological: Complex, (3) Behavioral, (4) Safety, (5) Family, (6) Health System, and (7) Community (see the Taxonomy beginning on p. 38). A few interventions are located in more than one class, but each has a unique number (code) that identifies the primary class and is not used for any other intervention. The NIC taxonomy was coded for several reasons: (1) to facilitate computer use, (2) to facilitate ease of data manipulation, (3) to enhance articulation with other coded systems, and (4) to allow for use in reimbursement. The codes for the 7 domains are 1 to 7; the codes for the 30 classes are A to Z, a, b, c, d. Each intervention has a unique number consisting of four spaces. If desired, activities can be coded sequentially after the decimal using two digits (numbers are not included in the text so as not to distract the reader). An example of a complete code is 4U-6140.02, which is Safety domain, Crisis Management class, Code Management intervention, second activity: "Ensure that patient's airway is open, artificial respirations are administered, and cardiac compressions are being delivered."

NIC interventions have been linked with NANDA International (NANDA-I) nursing diagnoses (included in this edition, see Part 6, p. 461), Omaha System problems,[13] resident assessment protocols (RAP) used in nursing homes,[7] and OASIS (Outcome and Assessment Information Set)[6] currently mandated for collection for Medicare/ Medicaid-covered patients receiving skilled home care. The linkages with Omaha, RAP, and OASIS are available from the Center for Nursing Classification and Clinical Effectiveness (CNC) at the University of Iowa, College of Nursing. NIC is linked to NANDA-I diagnoses, the Nursing Outcomes Classification (NOC), and 10 clinical conditions (e.g., hypertension, total joint replacement: hip/knee) in *NOC and NIC Linkages to NANDA-I and Clinical Conditions: Supporting Critical Reasoning and Quality Care* published by Elsevier in 2012.[14] This book, now in the third edition, unifies the NANDA-I, NOC, and NIC languages and serves as a valuable tool for developing care plans and nursing information systems.

The language used in the Classification is clear, consistently worded, and reflects language used in practice. Surveys to clinicians as well as 20 years of use of the Classification have demonstrated that all of the interventions are used in practice. Although the overall listing of more than 550 interventions may seem overwhelming at first to the practitioner or nursing student, we have seen that nurses soon discover those interventions that are used most often in their particular specialty or with their patient population. Other ways to locate the desired interventions are the taxonomy, the linkages with diagnoses, and the core interventions for specialties also contained in this edition.

The Classification is continually updated and has an ongoing process for feedback and review. In the back of this book are instructions for users to submit suggestions for modifications to existing interventions or propose a new intervention. Many of the changes in this edition have come about due to clinicians and researchers taking time to submit suggestions for modifications based upon their use in practice and research. These submissions are then put through a review process with editing and changes made as needed. All contributors whose changes are included in the next edition are acknowledged in the book. New editions of

the Classification are planned for approximately every five years. Work that is done between editions and other relevant publications that enhance the use of the Classification are available from the Center for Nursing Classification and Clinical Effectiveness at the University of Iowa.

The research to develop NIC began in 1987 and has progressed through four phases, each with some overlap in time:

Phase I: Construction of the Classification (1987-1992)
Phase II: Construction of the Taxonomy (1990-1995)
Phase III: Clinical Testing and Refinement (1993-1997)
Phase IV: Use and Maintenance (1996-ongoing)

Work conducted in each of these phases is described in previous editions of this book and in many other publications (e.g., see references [5,8,11,12,17]). The research was begun with seven years of funding from the National Institute of Nursing at the National Institutes of Health. Ongoing maintenance is supported by the Center for Nursing Classification and Clinical Effectiveness at the College of Nursing at the University of Iowa with financing largely through earnings from licenses and related products. NIC was developed by a large research team whose members represented multiple areas of clinical and methodological expertise. Members of this team as well as others who contribute to the continued development of NIC are appointed to three-year terms as *Fellows* in the Center. Fellows make significant contributions to the upkeep and implementation of NIC and NOC. These individuals include research team members, staff at collaborating agencies, retired professors, and visiting scholars. The current list of Fellows appears in the foreword matter of this book. For more information about the Center for Nursing Classification and Clinical Effectiveness, which houses NIC and NOC, please see the website: http://www.nursing.uiowa.edu/cnc.

Multiple research methods have been used in the development of NIC. An inductive approach was used in phase I to build the Classification based on existing practice. Original sources were current textbooks, care planning guides, and nursing information systems. Content analysis, focus group review, and questionnaires to experts in specialty areas of practice were used to augment the clinical practice expertise of team members. Phase II was characterized by deductive methods. Methods to construct the taxonomy included similarity analysis, hierarchical clustering, and multidimensional scaling. Through clinical field-testing, steps for implementation were developed and tested and the need for linkages between NANDA, NIC, and NOC were identified. Over time, more than 1000 nurses have completed questionnaires and approximately 50 professional associations have provided input about the Classification. More details are found in chapters in the earlier editions of NIC and in numerous articles and book chapters. A video made by the National League of Nursing and now available for rent from the Center for Nursing Classification and Clinical Effectiveness at the University of Iowa is a good historical resource of the early work.

Several tools are available that assist in the implementation of the Classification. Included in this book are the taxonomic structure to assist a user to find the intervention of choice, linkages with NANDA-I diagnoses to facilitate decision support with these diagnostic languages, the core intervention lists for areas of specialty practice, as well as the amount of time and level of education needed to perform each intervention. The next chapter contains information on use of NIC in practice, education, and research, including how to select an intervention, steps for implementation of NIC in a clinical or educational agency, as well as the use of NIC in effectiveness research. In addition, available from the Center for Nursing Classification and Clinical Effectiveness is an anthology of early publications and an education monograph to demonstrate one program's implementation and use of NIC and NOC in an undergraduate curriculum, as well as the linkage monographs described earlier. The publisher of NIC and NOC, Elsevier, maintains a Facebook page with current news about the classifications.

One indication of usefulness is national recognition. NIC is recognized by the American Nurses' Association (ANA) and is included as one data set that will meet the uniform guidelines for information system vendors in the ANA's Nursing Information and Data Set Evaluation Center (NIDSEC). NIC is included in the National Library of Medicine's Metathesaurus for a Unified Medical Language. The Cumulative Index to Nursing Literature (CINAHL) includes NIC interventions in its indexes. NIC was included in the Joint Commission on Accreditation for Health Care Organization's (JCAHO) accreditation requirements as one nursing classification system that can be used to meet the standard on uniform data. NIC is registered in HL 7 (Health Level 7), the U.S. standards organization for health care. NIC is also licensed for inclusion in SNOMED (Systematized Nomenclature of Medicine). Interest in NIC has been demonstrated in several other countries and translations into Chinese, Dutch, French, Icelandic, Italian, German, Japanese, Korean, Norwegian, Spanish, and Portuguese are completed or underway. Most of these translations are available in published book form (see Appendix E).

The best indication of usefulness, however, is the impressive list of individuals and health care agencies that use NIC. Many health care agencies have adopted NIC for use in standards, care plans, competency evaluation, and nursing information systems; nursing education programs are using NIC to structure curriculum and identify competencies for nursing students; vendors of information systems are incorporating NIC in their software; authors of major texts are using NIC to discuss nursing treatments; and researchers are using NIC to study the effectiveness of nursing

care. Permission to use NIC in publications, information systems, and web courses should be sought from Elsevier (see the inside front cover). Part of the money to purchase a license comes back to the Center to help with ongoing development of the Classification.

COMPANION CLASSIFICATION: NURSING OUTCOMES CLASSIFICATION

Following the development of NIC, we recognized that, in addition to diagnoses and interventions, a third classification, patient outcomes, was also needed to complete the requirements for documentation of a nursing clinical encounter. One of the NIC team members, Meridean Maas, sought out another colleague, Marion Johnson, who had long expressed interest in outcomes, and together they decided to form another research team to develop a classification of patient outcomes. They attempted to recruit different individuals so as not to dilute the strength of the NIC team, but some of the NOC team members were also NIC team members. This has been a strength, providing for continuity and understanding between the two groups. In the early years of NOC, Dochterman and Bulechek served as consultants to the new team. The NOC team researchers were able to use, or modify and use, many of the research approaches and methods that were developed by the NIC team. The NOC team was begun in 1991, and the first edition of NOC was published in 1997. The name of the classification and the acronym of NOC were deliberately selected so that there would be association with NIC.

Nursing Outcomes Classification (NOC) was first published by Mosby (now Elsevier) in 1997 with updated editions in 2000, 2004, and 2008.[18] New editions of NIC and NOC are on a concurrent publication cycle. Patient outcomes serve as the criteria against which to judge the success of a nursing intervention. Each outcome has a definition, a list of indicators that can be used to evaluate patient status in relation to the outcome, a five-point Likert scale to measure patient status, and a short list of references used in the development of the outcome. (See Chapter 2 for one example of a NOC outcome.) Examples of scales used with the outcomes are: 1, extremely compromised, to 5, not compromised; and 1, never demonstrated, to 5, consistently demonstrated. The outcomes are developed for use across the care continuum and therefore can be used to follow patient outcomes throughout an illness episode or over an extended period of care. The fifth edition of NOC is being published at the same time as this sixth edition of NIC. NOC, like NIC, is housed in the Center for Nursing Classification and Clinical Effectiveness at the University of Iowa, College of Nursing. As with NIC, NOC has also been translated into several other languages and has multiple adoptions in both education and practice.

CENTER FOR NURSING CLASSIFICATION AND CLINICAL EFFECTIVENESS

As stated previously, NIC and NOC are both housed in the Center for Nursing Classification and Clinical Effectiveness (CNC) at the University of Iowa, College of Nursing. The CNC was approved by the Iowa Board of Regents (the governing body that oversees the state's three public universities) in 1995 with the name of *Center for Nursing Classification*. In 2001 the name was expanded to the *Center for Nursing Classification and Clinical Effectiveness*. The purpose of the Center is to facilitate the continued development and use of NIC and NOC. The Center conducts the review processes and procedures for updating the Classifications, disseminates materials related to the Classifications, provides office support to assist faculty investigators to obtain funding, and offers research and education opportunities for students and visiting fellows. The Center provides a structure for the continued upkeep of the Classifications and for communication with the many nurses and others in education and health care facilities who are putting the languages in their curricula and documentation systems. The Center is physically located in three rooms on the fourth floor of the College of Nursing. One of the rooms is a conference room with a small library. Currently, Sue Moorhead is director and Sharon Sweeney is the coordinator. They are assisted in their decision-making by an Executive Board composed of the editors of the NIC and NOC books. The Fellows (see p. xii) assist with the work of the Center. Financial support for the Center comes from a variety of sources, including University and College funds, licensing, permission and product revenue from NIC, NOC, and related publications, grants, and income from Center initiatives. A substantial endowment for the support of the Center has been raised through donations over the past decade. The endowment helps to provide some permanent long-range security for the work of the Center. Information about the Center and products and happenings can be found on the website http://www.nursing.uiowa.edu/cnc. The Center receives visitors who come for a short period of study as well as national and international scholars who come for an extended period to work on a project. The Center co-sponsors the Institute for Informatics and Classification, which has been held at Iowa since 1998. This Institute provides an intensive experience in current information about the classifications and their use, as well as cutting edge issues in informatics.

QUESTIONS SOMETIMES ASKED ABOUT NIC

In this section we have tried to answer some of the common questions about NIC. Understanding the reasons why things have been done in a certain way (or not done) will assist in better use of the Classification. We began this section in the second edition of NIC and have continued to add to it. For this edition, we have grouped the questions under five related topics: (1) types of interventions, (2) choosing an intervention, (3) activities, (4) implementing/computerizing NIC, and (5) other. Questions 12 and 14 are new to this edition.

Types of Interventions

1. Does NIC cover treatments used by nurses practicing in specialty areas? Definitely yes. Many of the interventions in NIC require advanced education and experience in a clinical practice. For example, the following interventions may reflect the practice of a certified nurse working in obstetrics: Amnioinfusion, Birthing, Electronic Fetal Monitoring: Antepartum, Grief Work Facilitation: Perinatal Death, High-Risk Pregnancy Care, Labor Induction, Labor Suppression, Reproductive Technology Management, and Ultrasonography: Limited Obstetric. A similar list can be identified for most specialties.

The American Board of Neuroscience Nursing has incorporated NIC into their certification exam based upon role delineation surveys, which obtained information to define current neuroscience nursing practice.[4] The American Association of Neuroscience Nurses has incorporated NIC in the organizations' standards of practice and has identified the interventions core to neuroscience nursing, which appear in Part Four of this text. Susan Beyea[2] encourages specialty organizations to use the available standardized languages when developing standards and guidelines of nursing practice for the population of concern.

2. Does NIC include the important monitoring functions of the nurse? Very definitely yes. NIC includes many monitoring interventions (e.g., Electronic Fetal Monitoring: Antepartum, Health Policy Monitoring, Intracranial Pressure [ICP] Monitoring, Neurologic Monitoring, Surveillance, Surveillance: Late Pregnancy, Vital Signs Monitoring). These interventions consist mostly of monitoring activities but also include some activities to reflect the clinical judgment process, or what nurses are thinking and anticipating when they monitor. These interventions define what to look for and what to do when an anticipated event occurs. In addition, all interventions in NIC include monitoring activities when these are done as part of the intervention. We use the words *monitor* and *identify* to mean assessment activities that are part of an intervention. We have tried to use these words rather than the word *assess* in this intervention classification because *assessment* is the term used in the nursing process to refer to those activities that take place **before** diagnosis.

3. Does NIC include interventions that would be used by a primary care practitioner, especially interventions designed to promote health? Yes indeed. Although these are not grouped together in one class, NIC contains all of the interventions nurses use to promote health. Examples include: Anticipatory Guidance, Decision-Making Support, Developmental Enhancement: Adolescent, Developmental Enhancement: Child, Exercise Promotion, Health Education, Health Screening, Immunization/Vaccination, Management, Learning Facilitation, Nutrition Management, Weight Management, Oral Health Promotion, Parent Education: Adolescent, Parent Education: Childrearing Family, Parent Education: Infant, Risk Identification, Smoking Cessation Assistance, Substance Use Prevention, and Self-Responsibility Facilitation. Medication Prescribing is an intervention used by many advanced practice nurses working in primary care.

4. Does NIC include alternative therapies? We assume this question refers to treatments that are not part of mainstream medical practice in this country. Interventions in NIC that might be listed as alternative therapies include Aromatherapy, Autogenic Training, Biofeedback, Healing Touch, Hypnosis, Meditation Facilitation, Guided Imagery, Reiki, Relaxation Therapy, and Therapeutic Touch. Many of these interventions are located in the class "Psychological Comfort Promotion." Other alternative therapies will be added to NIC as they become part of accepted nursing practice.

5. Does the Classification include administrative interventions? The Classification includes indirect care interventions done by first-line staff or advance practice nurses but does not include, for the most part, those behaviors that are administrative in nature. An indirect care intervention is a treatment performed by a direct care provider away from the patient but on behalf of a patient or group of patients; an administrative intervention is an action performed by a nurse administrator (nurse manager or other nurse administrator) to enhance the performance of staff members to promote better patient outcomes. Some of the interventions in NIC, when used by an administrator to enhance staff performance, would then be administrative interventions. Most of these are located in the taxonomy in the Health System domain. It should be noted that the borders between direct, indirect, and administrative interventions are not firm and some NIC interventions may be used in various contexts. For example, the nurse in the hospital may provide Caregiver Support as an indirect intervention administered to a relative of the patient being cared for, but the nurse in the home, treating the whole family, may provide this intervention as direct care. With the addition of more interventions for communities, we have added interventions that are more administrative in nature, for example, Cost Containment and Fiscal Resource Management. These are, however, delivered by the primary care nurse in the community setting or by the case manager.

Choosing an Intervention

6. How do I find the interventions I use when there are so many interventions in NIC? At first glance, NIC, with over 550 interventions, may seem overwhelming. Remember, however, that NIC covers the practice domain of all nurses. An individual nurse will use only a portion of the interventions in NIC on a regular basis. These can be identified by reviewing the classes in the taxonomy that are most relevant to an individual's practice area or by reviewing the list of core interventions for one's specialty (see Part Four). In those agencies with nursing information systems, the interventions can be grouped by taxonomy class, nursing diagnosis, patient population (e.g., burn, cardiac, maternity), nursing specialty area, or unit. Many computer systems will also allow individual nurses to create and maintain a personal library of most used interventions. We have been told by nurses using the Classification that they quickly identify a relatively small number of interventions that reflect the core of their practice.

7. How do I decide which intervention to use when one intervention includes an activity that refers to another intervention? In some NIC interventions there is reference in the activity list to another intervention. For example, the intervention of Airway Management contains an activity that says "Perform endotracheal or nasotracheal suctioning, as appropriate." There is another intervention in NIC, Airway Suctioning, which is defined as "Removal of secretions by inserting a suction catheter into the patient's oral, nasopharyngeal, or tracheal airway" and has more than 20 activities listed under it. Another example is the intervention of Pain Management, which contains an activity that says "Teach the use of nonpharmacologic techniques (e.g., biofeedback, TENS, hypnosis, relaxation, guided imagery, music therapy, distraction, play therapy, activity therapy, acupressure, hot/cold application, and massage) before, after, and, if possible, during painful activities; before pain occurs or increases; and along with other pain relief measures." Nearly all of the techniques listed in the parentheses of this activity are listed in NIC as interventions, each with a definition and a set of defining activities. The two examples demonstrate that the more abstract, more global interventions sometimes refer to other interventions. Sometimes one needs the more global intervention, sometimes the more specific one, and sometimes both. The selection of nursing interventions for use with an individual patient is part of the clinical decision-making of the nurse. NIC reflects all possibilities. The nurse should choose the intervention(s) to use for a particular patient using the six factors discussed in the next chapter.

8. When is a new intervention developed? Why do

we believe that each of our interventions is different from others in the Classification? Maybe they are the same but are called something different? We developed the guiding principle that a new intervention is added if 50% or more of the activities are different from another related intervention. Thus, each time a new intervention is proposed, it is reviewed against other existing interventions. If 50% or more of the activities are not different, it is not viewed as significantly different and therefore is not added to the Classification.

With interventions that are types of a more general intervention (e.g., Sexual Counseling is a type of Counseling; Tube Care: Gastrointestinal is a type of Tube Care), the most pertinent activities are repeated in the more concrete intervention so that this intervention can stand alone. This should not be all the activities, rather just those that are essential to carrying out the intervention. In addition the intervention must have at least 50% new activities.

9. In a care plan, what's the structure for NIC and NOC? What do you choose and think about first? The answer to this reflects the clinical decision-

making of the provider planning and delivering the care. Individuals have different approaches to this, reflecting how they learned to do this in school refined by what they find works best for them and their typical patient population. As a general approach we suggest first making the diagnosis (or diagnoses), then select outcomes and indicators, rate the patient on these, then select the interventions and appropriate activities, implement these, and then rate the outcomes again. If you want to set goals, these can be derived from the NOC outcomes, for example, the patient is at 2 on X outcome and by discharge he should be at a level of 4. Sometimes, in some situations, this process is not possible or even desirable and one would want to use a different order. For example, in a crisis one would move immediately to the implementation of the intervention with the diagnosis and outcome left for later. The advantage of the standardized classifications is that they provide the language for the knowledge base of nursing. Educators and others can now focus on teaching and practice of skills in clinical decision-making; researchers can focus on examining the effects of interventions on patient outcomes in real practice situations. See the model in the next chapter that shows how standardized language can be used at the individual level, the unit/organizational level, and the network/state/country level.

Activities

10. Why are certain rather basic activities included in the activity list for some interventions but not others? For example, why should an activity related to

documentation be included in Discharge Planning and Referral and not in every intervention? Or, why should an activity related to evaluation of outcomes be included in Discharge Planning and not in all interventions? Or, why should an activity on establishing trust be included in Reminiscence Therapy or Support Group but not in other interventions?

Basic activities are included when they are critical for the implementation of that intervention (i.e., absolutely essential to communicate the essence of the intervention). They are not included when they are part of the routine but not a critical piece of the intervention. For example, hand washing is a routine part of many physical interventions but is not critical to interventions such as Bathing or Skin Care: Topical Treatments. (We are not saying that washing your hands should not be done for these interventions, just that this is not a critical activity.) Hand washing is a critical part, however, of such interventions as Infection Control and Contact Lens Care.

For the first time in this edition, we have included Patient Identification as an intervention. Although the identification of the patient is a critical activity for most interventions, the importance of doing this for current safety initiatives and the use of many new techniques and electronic devices have elevated this activity to intervention status.

11. Can I change the activities in an intervention when I use it with my patient? Yes. The standardized

language is the label name and the definition, and these should remain the same for all patients and all situations. The activities can be modified to better reflect the needs of the particular situation. These are advantages of NIC: it provides both a standardized language that will help us communicate across settings about our interventions and it allows for individualized care. The NIC activities use the modifiers *as appropriate, as needed,* and *as indicated* to reflect the fact that individuals are unique and may require different approaches. The NIC activities include all ages of patients, and, when used with adults, some of the activities directed at children may not be appropriate (and vice versa). In this case these can be omitted from an agency's list of activities. Also, the NIC interventions are not at the procedure level of specificity, and some agencies may wish to be more specific to reflect particular protocols developed for their populations. The activities can easily be modified to reflect this. At the same time that we believe that the activities can and should be modified to meet individual needs, we caution that activities should not be changed so much that the original NIC list is unrecognized. If this is done, then the intervention may in fact not be the same. Any modified or new activities should fit the definition of the intervention. In addition, when an activity is being added consistently for most patients and populations, then it may be needed in NIC's general listing of activities. In this case, we would urge the clinician to submit the proposed activity addition or change. In this way the activity list continues to reflect the best of current practice and is most useful in teaching the interventions to new practitioners.

Individualization of care is a core value of nurses. In fact, many standardized nursing interventions successfully tested in clinical trials have not been highly successful in improving outcomes in clinical practice, perhaps because they do not address individual characteristics or preferences for care.[1] Researchers at the University of Arkansas have established a Tailored Biobehavioral Intervention Center (NR009006) to develop methods for selecting critical characteristics on which to address the individual characteristics of persons when testing interventions. NIC activities help nurses to individualize care.

12. Why are the activities not standardized? Increasingly, as NIC is put into computer systems, we get asked this question. Those who design computer systems would like similar activities listed under different interventions to be worded the same so that it would be easier for them to create and use databases. So, we recently launched a project to systematically evaluate the feasibility of standardizing the activities. Two approaches were used. First, all of the nearly 13,000 activities in NIC were printed alphabetically using the first word (a verb) in the activities. One of the team members reviewed all of these and brought a sample to the NIC team for review. This approach revealed a small number of editorial concerns (e.g., missing commas before "as appropriate" or "as needed") and a very limited number of activities whose wording could be made identical to similar activities without changing the meaning. The second approach was to identify frequently addressed topics (nouns) such as: referral, medication side effects, environment, procedure or treatment, intake and output, privacy, approach, trust, listener, relationship, support, and vital signs. Using a computer search program, activities that included the identified topic (e.g., referral) were printed. These topic searches resulted in lists of anywhere from 100 to several hundred activities. One of the team members reviewed the topic listings and two of these were taken to the NIC team for discussion. Various approaches to standardization were proposed but team members agreed that rewording activities would result in loss of meaning and content. After this systematic review and deliberation, it was decided not to pursue standardization of activities any further.

The reasons that NIC activities are NOT standardized are:

1. As we have emphasized in the past, the focus and standardization of NIC is at the intervention label level. Activities can be added, deleted, or modified for each intervention as the situation requires. Further standardization of activities would defeat the nursing value of individualized care.
2. When one standardizes, one loses information. Each activity was written for a specific intervention and loss of information may be a detriment for both the caregiver (clinician or student) and the care recipient (patient).
3. The activities already have a standard format and follow rules for development (i.e., begin with a verb, list in order of doing, meet the definition of the intervention, use an already worded activity from a related intervention if the activity is one that also fits the new intervention). Indeed, many activities already are worded the same across similar interventions.
4. If the activity lists were standardized, the upkeep of such lists would be too time consuming, cumbersome, and expensive.

Implementing/Computerizing NIC

13. Does my health care agency need to be computerized to use NIC? No, NIC can be used in a manual care planning and documentation system. If the system is manual, nurses unfamiliar with NIC will need ready access to the NIC book. The book should also be available for nurses working in agencies that have computerized NIC (we think every unit should have a book and encourage individual nurses to have their own copies); with a computer, however, NIC can be stored and accessed electronically. Computers make it easy to access NIC interventions in a variety of ways (for now, by taxonomic classes and nursing diagnoses, but it is also possible by patient population, unit type, outcome, clinical path, etc.). Computers can easily accommodate a variety of clinical decision support screens for nurses. Documenting what we do for patients using a standardized language on computers makes it possible for nursing to build agency, state, regional, and national databases to do effectiveness research. If your agency is not computerized, help it to become computerized. But you do not have to wait for the computer to use NIC. NIC is helpful to communicate nursing care with or without a computer.

14. How should NIC be included in my computer system? We urge that computer systems be built using the standardized intervention labels. Nurses should plan, document, and communicate care at this level. Research should be done at this level, for example, comparing the use and outcomes of different interventions (e.g., see [10,19,20]). If one wishes to also document the activities, this, of course, can be done either by indicating those activities, that were implemented or by charting by exception for those activities not implemented. Some agencies only wish to document a short list of those activities that are essential for legal purposes or those that need further follow-up as "orders" for nursing assistants. Overall, however, we must begin to acknowledge that the standard of care for the delivery of a particular intervention involves the nurse doing the listed activities as they are appropriate for the particular patient and situation.

15. What is the best way to go about implementation of NIC in my agency? Other related questions include: Should I implement NIC and NOC together? Should I implement NIC at the same time I orient nurses to a new computer system? Should we do this on just a pilot unit first or put this up "live" for everyone at the same time? Chapter 2 lists helpful Steps for Implementation for practice agencies (Box 2-3) as well as Steps for Implementation for educational facilities (Box 2-8). There are also other materials in Chapter 2, such as examples of implementation forms used by practice agencies that have implemented NIC, to assist the beginning user. As for the questions related to how much to do at one time, there is no one right way; it truly does depend on the situation and the amount and nature of the changes, the resources and support available, and the time constraints. The companion NOC book has many helpful suggestions about implementation of NOC. We would caution not to make too many changes at once for this is often more than most can handle. On the other hand, don't drag a change out in small pieces for a long time. Duplicate charting (recording the same thing in more than one place) is discouraged. Piloting a change to work the bugs out (say, starting on one unit where the nurse manager and staff are supportive) is always a good idea. Providing time for training and having support staff available when the change is first made is important. Margaret Lunney has published an informative article on helping staff nurses use NANDA-I, NIC, and NOC as health care moves to the electronic health record.[16] It is important in the beginning to think about the uses of the data in the future, beyond the initial care planning or documentation purposes. Chapter 2 also covers the idea of setting up a comprehensive database for effectiveness research in the future.

16. When do I need to obtain a license? Other related questions include: Why do I need a license? Why isn't NIC in the public domain? Why is the copyright for NIC held by a publisher? A license is needed if you put NIC on a nursing information system or if you will use a substantial part of the Classification for commercial gain or advantage. NIC is published and copyrighted by Elsevier and this organization

processes requests for permissions to use the Classification. See the inside front cover for directions on who to contact for permission to use or licensing.

When we first began working on the NIC classification we had little idea of the magnitude of the work or its current widespread use or that it would be followed by NOC. We were looking for a way to get the work in print and disseminated quickly. As academics, we were familiar with the book publishing world, and, after some very serious review of alternative mechanisms and talks with other publishers, we selected Mosby (now Elsevier) as the publisher. Publication with Elsevier has several advantages. First, they have the resources and the contacts to produce a book, to market it, and to sell it. In addition, they have the legal staff and resources to process requests for permission and protect the copyright. This is especially important with standardized language, where alteration of terms will impede the goal of communication among nurses across specialties and between delivery sites. We view our relationship with Elsevier as a partnership.

Copyright does not restrict fair use. According to guidelines by the American Library Association, fair use allows materials to be copied if: (1) the portion copied is selective and sparing in comparison to the whole work; (2) the materials are not used repeatedly; (3) no more than one copy is made for each person; (4) the source and copyright notice is included on each copy; and (5) persons are not assessed a fee for the copy beyond the actual cost of reproduction. The determination of the amount that can be copied under fair use policies has to do with the effect of the copying on sales of the original material. The American Library Association says that no more than 10% of a work should be copied.

When someone puts NIC on an information system that will be used by multiple users, copyright is violated (a book is now being "copied" for use by hundreds of nurses) and so a licensing agreement is needed. Also, when someone uses large amounts of NIC in a book or software product that is then sold and makes money for that individual, then a permissions fee is necessary. Schools of nursing and health care agencies that want to use NIC in their own organizations and have no intention of selling a resulting product are free to do so. Fair use policies exist, however. For example, NIC and NOC should not be photocopied and used in syllabi semester after semester—the classification books should be adopted for use. Similarly, health care agencies should purchase a reasonable number of books (say, one per unit) rather than copy the interventions and place them in some procedure manual.

Requests for use of NIC and NOC should be sent to the permissions department of Elsevier. Many requests for permission to use do not violate copyright, and permission is given with no fee. Fees for use in a book depend on the amount of material used. Fees for use in information systems depend upon the number of users and average about

$5.00 per user per year. There is a flat fee for incorporating NIC into a vendor's database and then a sublicense fee for each sublicense undertaken based on the number of users. The fees are reasonable, and a substantial portion of the fees are being forwarded to the Center for Nursing Classification and Clinical Effectiveness to help support the ongoing development and use of NIC. The Classification is only useful if it reflects current practice; upkeep is time consuming and expensive and the fees generated from usage support this work.

17. How do I explain to the administrator at my institution that a license is needed? First, we want to repeat that only use in an information system requires a license and a fee; if you want to use NIC manually or for a particular project that does not violate copyright, please go ahead. In our experience, it is nurses and not health care administrators who are unfamiliar with licenses and fees. Most other health care classifications are copyrighted, and fees are required for use. For example, the Current Procedural Terminology (CPT) is copyrighted by the American Medical Association and the Diagnostic and Statistical Manual of Mental Disorders (DSM) is copyrighted by the American Psychiatric Association. Health care institutions regularly pay license fees now, but most nurses are not aware of these. Several years ago, at one Midwestern tertiary care hospital, 97 vendor software products were installed and more than $1,220,000 was spent annually on software license fees. No doubt the costs are more now.

License fees are often included as part of the software costs. NIC can be licensed from Elsevier (use of the language) for incorporation in an existing information system or purchased from a vendor with software (the vendor has purchased the license from Elsevier, and the software price includes the cost of the license). As more nurses understand the advantages of using standardized language and desire this in purchases of new information systems, more vendors will include NIC in their products.

In nursing, none of the professional organizations have the resources to maintain NIC, so another avenue was needed. We have been told by those in the medical field that having the Classification housed in a university setting has advantages over the professional organizational model, in which politics (what is in and what is out) may play a part. Ongoing development and maintenance, however, require resources. Classifications and other works in the public domain are often those for which there will be no upkeep—you can use what is there but do not expect it to be kept current. We have attempted to make NIC as accessible as possible but to also collect fees so that we can have a revenue stream to finance the maintenance work that must continue.

18. What is a reference terminology model? Why are these being developed? Will they make classifications such as NIC obsolete? A reference terminology (RT) model identifies the parts of a concept (i.e., the parts of any diagnosis or any intervention) that can be used behind the screens in computer systems to assist these systems to talk with each other. For example, an intervention might consist of an action, a recipient, and a route. When we went to high school in the 1950s, we were asked to diagram sentences to learn the parts of a sentence (e.g., the noun, verb, adverb); an RT model works to represent concepts in a similar way. Theoretically, an RT model enables differing vocabularies (e.g., NIC and Omaha) to be mapped to one RT model and, thus, compared with each other. We say theoretically because this approach has not yet been tested in practice. In the late 1990s and early 2000s, there was a mushrooming of terminology models, examples include HL7 (in the U.S. for all of health care), CEN (in Europe for all of health care), SNOMED (for use in the U.S. and Europe), and ISO-Nursing (for nursing internationally). We consider the International Classification of Nursing Practice (ICNP), with its axes, an RT model that is more helpful behind the screens than useful to practicing nurses as a front end terminology.

A second part of this question is whether the creation of an RT model will make classifications like NIC obsolete. No, NIC is a front end language designed for communication among nurses and between nurses and other providers. We want nurses to be able to write and talk NIC. On the other hand, RT models are for use behind the screens: if they do succeed, they will help vendors to build computer systems that can use and compare different front end languages. RT models are pretty hard to understand and not clinically useful. Even if they allow the user to document care in their own words (versus standardized language) this is not desirable (except in a free text notes section that supplements and elaborates on the standardized language) for the profession because we would still have the problem of lack of communication among ourselves and between ourselves and others as to what we do. We will always need a standardized language to communicate the work of nursing—NIC is intended to be just that.

19. Is there commercial software available with NIC in it? Are there vendors that have clinical nursing software with NIC? Yes. This is a growing area. When a licensing agreement for NIC is made with Elsevier, the user is sent a CD-Rom to make it easier to transfer the language to a computer system. A growing number of vendors are including NIC in their information systems and website information for them is listed in the next chapter (Box 2-2).

Additional licensing agreements are in process. We do not endorse any particular product; prospective users should contact the vendors directly for review of their products. Other software has been developed for specific purposes, for example the system built for research data collection by Gail Keenan and her colleagues in Michigan.[15] We believe that the inclusion of NIC in SNOMED-CT will facilitate and encourage the incorporation of NIC in vendor products. If your vendor does not include NIC, ask about future plans at their user meetings. Vendors will build their products according to user demand. Nurses need to speak up and ask for standardized language to be included in clinical information systems.

Other

20. How does NIC compare to other classifications?

The American Nurses Association recognizes 12 terminologies for nursing practice information infrastructure. Some are data element sets, some are interface terminologies, and some are multidisciplinary terminologies. Compared with the other classifications, NIC is the most comprehensive for interventions. Of all the classifications, only NANDA-I, NIC, and NOC are comprehensive and have ongoing efforts to keep them current. The relationships that link these classifications,[14] as well as a proposal for a common organizing structure,[9] present users with a comprehensive classification system that can be used to document care across settings and specialties.

21. Should we use a nursing classification when most of health care is being delivered by interdisciplinary teams?

Occasionally we hear something like "we can't use anything that is labeled nursing and comes from nursing when everything is now going to be interdisciplinary." We hear this, by the way, from nurses rather than from physicians or other power holders in the interdisciplinary arena. At the same time, it is assumed that using medical language does not violate this artificial interdisciplinary principle. We believe that nurses who are members of an interdisciplinary team addressing the development and implementation of a computerized integrated patient care record should be, in fact must be, the spokespersons for use of NIC and NOC. Yes, these have the nursing word in their titles because they were developed inductively through research based on the work of nurses by nurses. Taken as a whole, they reflect the discipline of nursing, but any one individual intervention may be done by other types of providers and any one outcome may be influenced by the treatments of other providers or by many other factors. This is a situation in which nursing has something of value that the other providers, for the most part, do not. NIC and NOC document the contributions of nurses and can be

used, or adapted and used, by others if they wish. Nurses should not shrink from talking about these nursing initiatives; rather they should assertively offer them as the nursing contribution to the interdisciplinary goal of a computerized patient record that can cross settings and specialties.

This is not inconsistent with being a good team member in an interdisciplinary environment. It is essential for successful outcomes to be achieved by interdisciplinary teams that nurse members communicate their unique perspective and knowledge. What is a good team member? There are three essential qualities: (1) the person has something that contributes to the overall functioning of the team, (2) the person is good at what he or she does, and (3) others understand what the person can do. Would a baseball team welcome a member who could not play any position and was a poor batter? Definitely not. Would they welcome someone who was eager to help but unable to say how he or she could help? Maybe, but this person would end up being water boy or girl rather than playing a position. Being a good team member means that the person has something to contribute and communicates ideas. Baseball teams emphasize the importance of specific and different roles and skills of members. No one suggests that because a team member is called a pitcher or a shortstop the member is not a team player. Players are not told that they are not good team members if they sharpen their individual knowledge and skills and are acknowledged for individual performance. A baseball team, or any team for that matter, improves effectiveness by maximizing and integrating the contributions of individual members. Baseball managers would undoubtedly get a good laugh from the notion that they should conceal and minimize the contributions of individual team members to increase the effectiveness of the team.

We have heard a few individuals say that there should be only one language that is shared by all health[1] disciplines. If this is possible, we believe that the one language should develop inductively through the sharing and adding on to the current languages that exist. Perhaps, over time, we will build one large common language whereby some intervention and outcome terms are shared by many providers. But even if we can build one large common language, it will always be used in parts because the whole is too great to learn, communicate, and study, and all interventions and outcomes are not the business of every discipline. The one very large language will be broken down and used in parts for the same reasons that there are disciplines—the whole is too large and complex to be mastered by any one individual, hence different disciplines represent different specialized perspectives.

22. How does NIC contribute to theory development in nursing? The intervention labels are the concepts, the names of the treatments provided by nurses. The definitions and activities that accompany the labels provide for definition and description of the interventions. Clarification of intervention concepts contributes to the development of nursing knowledge and facilitates communication within the discipline. As nursing's ability to link diagnoses, interventions, and outcomes grows, prescriptive theory for nursing practice will evolve. The NIC is a crucial development because it provides the lexical elements for middle-range theories in nursing that will link diagnoses, interventions, and outcomes. Interventions are the key element in nursing. All other aspects of nursing practice are contingent upon, and secondary to, the treatments that identify and delineate our discipline. This intervention-centric approach does not diminish the importance of the patient; but from a disciplinary perspective the phenomenon of interest of the patient is important because it can be affected by nursing action. We believe that use of standardized languages for nursing diagnoses, interventions, and outcomes heralds a new era in the development of nursing theory, moving from the past focus on grand theory to the development and use of nursing middle-range theories. (For more discussion, see [3] and [21].) Although we believe that, in the future, nursing grand theories will be replaced by nursing middle-range theories, for the present, NIC can be used with any existing grand theory. NIC can be used by any institution, nursing specialty, or care delivery model regardless of philosophical orientation.

SUMMARY

This chapter provides an overview of NIC, and brief overviews of NOC as well as the Center for Nursing Classification and Clinical Effectiveness at the College of Nursing, the University of Iowa, where the Classification is maintained. A series of 21 frequently asked questions about NIC are presented and answered. Overall, the chapter provides a convenient and quick way to become familiar with NIC.

References

1. Beck, C., McSweeney, J. C., Richards, D. C., Roberson, P. K., Tsai, P., & Souder, E. (2010). Challenges in tailored intervention research. *Nursing Outlook, 58*(2), 104–110.
2. Beyea, S. (2001). Nursing specialties: Structured vocabularies, synergy of efforts—A win-win for nursing. *International Journal of Nursing Terminologies and Classification, 12*(2), 63–65.
3. Blegen, M. A., & Tripp-Reimer, T. (1997). Implications of nursing taxonomies for middle-range theory development. *Advances in Nursing Science, 19*(3), 37–49.
4. Blissitt, P. A., Roberts, S., Hinkle, J. L., & Knopp, E. M. (2003). Defining neuroscience nursing practice: The 2001 role delineation study. *Journal of Neuroscience Nursing, 35*(1), 8–15.
5. Bulechek, G. M. & McCloskey, J. C. (Eds.). (1992). Symposium on nursing interventions. *Nursing clinics of North America, 27*(2). Philadelphia: W. B. Saunders.
6. Center for Nursing Classification. (2000). NIC interventions and NOC outcomes linked to the OASIS Information Set. Iowa City, IA: Author.
7. Center for Nursing Classification. (2000). *Standardized nursing language in long term care* (R. Cox, Preparer]. Iowa City, IA: Author.
8. Cohen, M. Z., Kruckeberg, T., McCloskey, J. C., Bulechek, G. M., Craft, J. J., Crossley, J. D., et al. (1992). Inductive methodology and a research team. *Nursing Outlook, 39*(4), 162–165.
9. Dochterman, J. M., & Jones, D. (Eds.). (2003). *Harmonization in nursing language classification.* Washington, DC: American Nurses Association.
10. Dochterman, J., Titler, M., Wang, J., Reed, D., Pettit, D., Mathew-Wilson, M., et al. (2005). Describing use of nursing interventions for three groups of patients. *Journal of Nursing Scholarship, 37*(1), 57–66.
11. Iowa Intervention Project. (1993). The NIC taxonomy structure. *Image, 25*(3), 187–192.
12. Iowa Intervention Project. (1995). Validation and coding of the NIC taxonomy structure. *Image, 27*(1), 43–49.
13. Iowa Intervention Project. (1996). *NIC interventions linked to Omaha System Problems.* Iowa City, IA: Center for Nursing Classification.
14. Johnson, M., Moorhead, S., Bulechek, G., Butcher, H., Maas, M., & Swanson, E. (Eds.). (2012). *NOC and NIC linkages to NANDA-I and clinical conditions: Supporting critical reasoning and quality care.* Maryland Heights, MO: Elsevier Mosby.
15. Keenan, G., Stocker, J., Geo-Thomas, A., Soparkar, N., Barkauskas, V., & Lee, J. (2002). The HANDS project: Studying and refining the automated collection of a cross-setting clinical data set. *Computers in Nursing, 20*(3), 89–100.
16. Lunney, M. (2006). Staff development: Helping nurses use NANDA, NIC, and NOC: Novice to expert. *Journal of Nursing Administration, 36*(3), 89–100.
17. McCloskey, J. C., Bulechek G. M., & Donahue W. (1998). Nursing interventions core to specialty practice. *Nursing Outlook, 46*(2), 67–76.
18. Moorhead, S., Johnson M., Maas M., & Swanson, E. (Eds.). (2008). *Nursing outcomes classification (NOC)* (4th ed.). St Louis: Mosby.
19. Titler, M., Dochterman, J., Kim, T., Kanak, M., Shever, L., Picone, et al. (2007). Cost of care for seniors hospitalized for hip fractures and related procedures. *Nursing Outlook, 55*(1), 5–14.
20. Titler, M., Dochterman, J., Xie, X., Kanak, M., Fei, Q., Picone, D., & Shever, L. (2006). Nursing interventions and other factors associated with discharge disposition in older patients after hip fractures. *Nursing Research, 55*(4), 231–242.
21. Tripp-Reimer, T., Woodworth, G., McCloskey, J., & Bulechek, G. (1996). The dimensional structure of nursing interventions. *Nursing Research, 45*(1), 10–17.

CHAPTER TWO

Use of NIC in Practice, Education, and Research

In his book, *The Information: A History, A Theory, A Flood*, James Gleick[23] asserts that information is the fuel and vital principle that our world runs on. Gleick describes in-depth how information pervades all the sciences and transforms every branch of knowledge. Similarly, the evolutionary theorist, Richard Dawkins[18] asserted "what lies at the heart of every living thing is not a fire, not warm breath, not a spark of life . . . rather if you want to understand life, you need to think in terms of information, words, instructions, and information technology." (p. 112) Gleick's and Dawkins' notions of the centrality of information apply to all fields of science, including nursing. Information lies at the heart of nursing.

Information *is* knowledge. Nursing is a scientific discipline, and like all disciplines, nursing has a unique body of knowledge. According to *Nursing's Social Policy Statement: The Essence of the Profession,*[3] nursing's purpose includes the application of scientific knowledge to the processes of diagnosis and treatment through the use of judgment and critical thinking within the context of a caring relationship that facilitates health and healing. As a branch of knowledge, nursing is comprised of information about the nature of health and illness, as well as the strategies and treatments to promote health and well-being.

Central to any scientific system of knowledge is having a means to classify and structure categories of information.[11,23,35] NIC identifies the treatments nurses perform, organizes this information into a coherent structure, and provides the language to communicate with individuals, families, communities, members of other disciplines, and the general public. When NIC is used to document the work of nurses in practice, then we have the beginning of a mechanism to determine the impact of nursing care on patient outcomes. Clark and Lang[16] reminded us of the importance of nursing languages and classifications when asserting, "If we cannot name it, we cannot control it, finance it, teach it, or put it into public policy." (p. 27)

This chapter has three major sections. The first section addresses the use of NIC in practice, including how to select an intervention for a particular patient, implementation of NIC in a clinical practice agency, and the implementation and uses of NIC in computerized database information systems. The second section addresses use in education, including integrating NIC into nursing education curricula and how NIC is used for clinical decision-making in the Outcome-Present State-Test (OPT) model of reflective clinical reasoning. The third section focuses on the use of NIC in research with an emphasis on how NIC can be used in efficacy and effectiveness research.

USE OF NIC IN PRACTICE
Selecting an Intervention

Nurses use clinical judgment with individuals, families, and communities to improve their health, to enhance their ability to cope with health problems, and to promote their quality of life. The selection of a nursing intervention for a particular patient is part of the clinical judgment of the nurse. Six factors should be considered when choosing an intervention: (1) desired patient outcomes, (2) characteristics of the nursing diagnosis, (3) research base for the intervention, (4) feasibility for doing the intervention, (5) acceptability to the patient, and (6) capability of the nurse.

Desired Patient Outcomes Patient outcomes should be specified before an intervention is chosen. They serve as the criteria against which to judge the success of a nursing intervention. Outcomes describe behaviors, responses, and feelings of the patient in response to the care provided. Many variables influence outcomes, including the clinical problem; interventions prescribed by the health care providers; the health care providers themselves; the environment in which care is received; the patient's own motivation, genetic structure, and pathophysiology; and the patient's significant others. There are many intervening or mediating variables in each situation, making it difficult to establish a causal relationship between nursing interventions and patient outcomes in some instances. The nurse must identify for each patient the outcomes that can be reasonably expected and can be attained as the result of nursing care.

The most effective way to specify outcomes is by use of the Nursing Outcomes Classification (NOC).[40] NOC contains 490 outcomes for individuals, families, and communities that are representative for all settings and clinical specialties. Each NOC outcome describes patient states at a conceptual level with indicators expected to be responsive to nursing intervention. The indicators for each outcome allow measurement of the outcomes at any point on a 5-point Likert scale from most negative to most positive. Repeated ratings over time provide identification of changes in the patient's condition. Thus, NOC outcomes are used to monitor the extent of progress, or lack of progress, throughout an episode of care. NOC outcomes have been developed to be used in all settings, all specialties, and across the continuum of care. The NOC outcome of Comfort Status is displayed in Box 2-1 to show the label, definition, indicators, and measurement scale. NOC outcomes have been linked to NANDA International (NANDA-I) diagnoses, and these linkages appear in the back of the NOC book. NIC interventions have also been linked to NOC outcomes, and to NANDA-I diagnoses and those linkages are available in a book titled *NOC and NIC Linkages to NANDA-I and Clinical Conditions: Supporting Critical Reasoning and Quality of Care.*[32]

Characteristics of the Nursing Diagnosis Outcomes and interventions are selected in relationship to particular nursing diagnoses. The use of standardized nursing language began in the early 1970s with the development of the NANDA nursing diagnosis classification. A nursing diagnosis according to NANDA-I is "a clinical judgment about individual, family, or community experiences/responses to actual or potential health problems/life processes" and "provides the basis for selection of nursing interventions to achieve outcomes for which the nurse has accountability."[41] (p. 515) The elements of an actual NANDA-I diagnosis statement are the label, the related factors (causes or associated factors), and the defining characteristics (signs and symptoms). Interventions are directed toward altering the etiological factors

---

Box 2-1

Sample NOC Outcome
Comfort Status—2008

Definition: Overall physical, psychospiritual, sociocultural, and environmental ease and safety of an individual

OUTCOME TARGET RATING: Maintain at_____ Increase to_____

	Severely compromised	Substantially compromised	Moderately compromised	Mildly compromised	Not compromised	
OUTCOME OVERALL RATING	1	2	3	4	5	
Indicators:						
200801 Physical well-being	1	2	3	4	5	NA
200802 Symptom control	1	2	3	4	5	NA
200803 Psychological well-being	1	2	3	4	5	NA
200804 Physical surroundings	1	2	3	4	5	NA
200805 Room temperature	1	2	3	4	5	NA
200806 Social support from family	1	2	3	4	5	NA
200807 Social support from friends	1	2	3	4	5	NA
200808 Social relationships	1	2	3	4	5	NA
200809 Spiritual life	1	2	3	4	5	NA
200810 Care consistent with cultural beliefs	1	2	3	4	5	NA
200811 Care consistent with needs	1	2	3	4	5	NA
200812 Ability to communicate needs	1	2	3	4	5	NA

Domain-Perceived Health (V)   **Class**-Health & Life Quality (U) 4th edition 2008

Outcome Content References:

Gropper, E. (1992). Promoting health by promoting comfort. *Nursing Forum, 27*(2), 5–8.

Hamilton, J. (1989). Comfort and the hospitalized chronically ill. *Journal of Gerontological Nursing, 15*(4), 28–33.

Kennedy, G. (1991). *A nursing investigation of comfort and comforting care of the acutely ill patient.* Unpublished doctoral dissertation, The University of Texas, Austin.

Kolcaba, K. (2003). *Comfort theory and practice: A vision for holistic health care and research.* New York: Springer.

Kolcaba, K., & DiMarco, M. (2005). Comfort theory and its application to pediatric nursing. *Pediatric Nursing, 31*(3), 187–194.

Kolcaba, K., Panno, J., & Holder, C. (2000). Acute care for elders (ACE): A holistic model for geriatric orthopaedic nursing care. *Journal of Orthopaedic Nursing, 19*(6), 53–60.

Tipton, L. (2001). A qualitative study of hope and the environment of persons living with cancer. *Dissertation Abstracts International, 62*(03), 1326B. (UMI No. 3008460).

From: Moorhead, S., Johnson, M., Maas, M., & Swanson, E. (Eds.). (2013). *Nursing outcomes classification (NOC)* (5th ed.). St. Louis: Elsevier.

(related factors) or causes of the diagnosis. If the intervention is successful in altering the etiology, the patient's status can be expected to improve. It may not always be possible to change the etiological factors and when this is the case, it is necessary to treat the defining characteristics (signs and symptoms).

To assist in selecting appropriate nursing interventions, Part Six in this book lists major and suggested interventions to treat NANDA-I nursing diagnoses. In addition, the recently published *NOC and NIC Linkages to NANDA-I and Clinical Conditions: Supporting Clinical Reasoning and Quality Care*[32] text is an invaluable resource for identifying outcomes and interventions for all NANDA-I nursing diagnoses as well as for 10 common clinical conditions of asthma, chronic obstructive pulmonary disease, colon and rectal cancer, depression, diabetes mellitus, heart failure, hypertension, pneumonia, stroke, and total joint replacement: hip/knee.

Research Base for the Intervention The Institute of Medicine (IOM) in the report *Health Professions Education: A Bridge to Quality*[25] outlined changes in the education of all health care professions that included employing evidence-based practice. The Agency for Healthcare Research and Quality (AHRQ), the IOM, and other government agencies that are clearinghouses for clinical guidelines have sanctioned the use of evidence-based practice as the basis for all health care delivery.[24] These agencies have emphasized that interventions supported by research evidence improve patient outcomes and clinical practice. It is essential now that nurses develop clinical inquiry skills, which requires nurses to continually question if the care being given is the best possible practice. To determine the best practice, evidence based on research needs to be known and used in choosing interventions. Thus, the nurse who uses an intervention needs to be familiar with its research base. The research will indicate the effectiveness of using the intervention with certain types of patients. Some interventions and their corresponding nursing activities have been widely tested for specific populations, whereas others need to be tested and are based on expert clinical knowledge. Nursing diagnosis handbooks such as Ackley and Ladwig[1] provide research references from case studies on a single client to systematic reviews that provide additional research evidence related to NIC interventions. Nurses learn about the research related to particular interventions through their education programs and also how to keep their knowledge current by finding and evaluating research studies. If there is no research base for an intervention to assist a nurse in the choosing of an intervention, then the nurse would use scientific principles (e.g., infection transmission) or would consult an expert about the specific populations for which the intervention might work.[49] In addition, agencies use models such as the *Iowa Model for Evidence-Based Practice*

to Promote Quality of Care to guide work on assembling evidence for treating a particular clinical problem and deciding on a practice protocol.[50]

Feasibility for Performing the Intervention Feasibility concerns include the ways in which the particular intervention interacts with other interventions, both those of the nurse and those of other health care providers. It is important that the nurse is involved in the total plan of care for the patient. Other feasibility concerns, critical in today's health care environment, are the cost of the intervention and the amount of time required for implementation. The nurse needs to consider the interventions of other providers, the cost of the intervention, and the time needed to adequately implement an intervention when choosing a course of action.

Acceptability to the Patient An intervention must be acceptable to the patient and family. The nurse is frequently able to recommend a choice of interventions to assist in reaching a particular outcome. To facilitate an informed choice, the patient should be given information about each intervention and how he or she is expected to participate. Most importantly, the patient's values, beliefs, and culture must all be considered when choosing an intervention.

Capability of the Nurse The nurse must be able to carry out the particular intervention. In order for the nurse to be competent to implement the intervention, the nurse must: (1) have knowledge of the scientific rationale for the intervention; (2) possess the necessary psychomotor and interpersonal skills; and (3) be able to function within the particular setting to effectively use health care resources.[9] It is clear from just glancing at the total list of 554 interventions that no one nurse has the capability of doing all of the interventions. Nursing, like other health disciplines, is specialized, and individual nurses perform within their specialty and refer or collaborate when other skills are needed.

After considering each of the above factors for a particular patient, the nurse would select the intervention(s). This is not as time consuming as it sounds when elaborated in writing. As Benner[7] has demonstrated, the student and beginning nurse should examine these things systematically, but with experience, the nurse synthesizes this information and is able to recognize patterns rapidly. One advantage of the classification is that it facilitates the teaching and learning of decision-making for the novice nurse. Using standardized language to communicate the nature of our interventions does not mean that we stop delivering individualized care. Interventions are tailored to individuals by selective choice of the activities and by modification of the activities as appropriate for the patient's age and the patient's and family's physical, social, emotional, and spiritual status. These modifications are made by the nurse, using sound clinical judgment.

Implementing NIC in a Clinical Practice Agency

Increasingly, a number of vendors who develop computerized clinical information systems (CIS) are including standardized nursing terminologies in hospital and health care settings. Anderson, Keenan, and Jones[5] compared five nursing terminologies that included nursing diagnoses, interventions, and outcomes. There were 879 publications on the NANDA, NIC, and NOC (NNN) terminologies, more than the total publications for the four other terminologies combined. NNN literature was found in 21 countries and in 28 states in the United States. Thus, it is not surprising that NIC is being implemented into a wide range of computer information systems in the United States as well as countries around the world including Belgium, Brazil, Canada, Denmark, England, France, Germany, Iceland, Japan, Spain, Switzerland, and The Netherlands. Box 2-2 lists some of the health care system computer vendors who have licensed NIC for incorporation into their software products. Computer documentation systems including NIC are currently being used in a large number of diverse health care settings. Including NIC along with other standardized nursing terminologies such as NANDA-I and NOC in computerized clinical information systems can be used not only to plan and document nursing care, but also provides a way to enhance clinical decision-making, share information, and track the achievement of patient outcomes.[15, 34, 37, 38] Figure 2-1 is one example of how NIC appears in an electronic information system.

According to the Institute of Medicine report *The Future of Nursing: Leading Change, Advancing Health,*[30] "there is no greater opportunity to transform practice than through technology." (p. 136). As Gleick[23] points out, the rise of placing information in mathematical and electronic form allows computers to rapidly process, store, and retrieve information. The IOM report *Crossing the Quality Chasm: A New Health System for the 21st Century*[28] cited numerous examples of how automated clinical information systems contribute to reduced errors, increased access to diagnostic tests and treatment results, and improved communication and coordination of care. Information systems also serve as an aid to clinical decision-making, documentation of care, and determination of the cost of care. The American Recovery and Reinvestment Act (ARRA) (Public Law 111-5) in 2009 included provisions to create incentives for the adoption and meaningful use of health information technology. In order for nursing to be included in this initiative, it is essential that "nursing elements" be included in all electronic health records. Nursing elements of electronic records refer to any information related to the nursing diagnosis, treatment, and outcomes relevant to nursing. Casey[14] points out that electronic health records will not benefit nursing until nurses are better able to describe their work, which will guide the design of information systems.

Box 2-2

Vendors Who Have Licenses for NIC

Healthland www.healthland.com	NIC and NOC Integrated with their Clinical Documentation software system for care planning. System is used by small to midsize hospitals.
DIPS ASA www.dips.com	NIC integrated within their Electronic Patient Record System for care planning. Company located in Norway.
DxR Development Group www.dxrgroup.com	Web-based system for teaching students nursing process. Product called DxR Nursing.
Clinical eNotes, LLC www.eclinicalnotes.com	NIC and NOC integrated within a nursing documentation section of an electronic documentation system for hospice providers.
McKesson Corporation www.mckesson.com	NIC and NOC integrated within Horizon Expert Plan for use in care planning.
Nurse's Aide, LLC www.nursesaide.net	Product for School Nurses to assist with their care plans for students.
Robin Technologies, Inc www.careplans.com	NIC and NOC are used within plans of care for use by students and nurses in long term care facilities.
SNOMED-CT www.snomed.com	NIC and NOC used within mapping tool. (Ownership of SNOMED has transferred to International Health Terminology Standards Development Organisation)
Typhon Group, LLC www.typhongroup.com	NIC and NOC integrated within their Registered Nurse Student Tracking (RNST) program used by nursing schools. Product helps student users develop patient care plans.

Provided October 2011 by Karen Delany at Licensing Department, Elsevier, 1600 JFK Blvd. Suite 1800, Philadelphia, PA 19103.

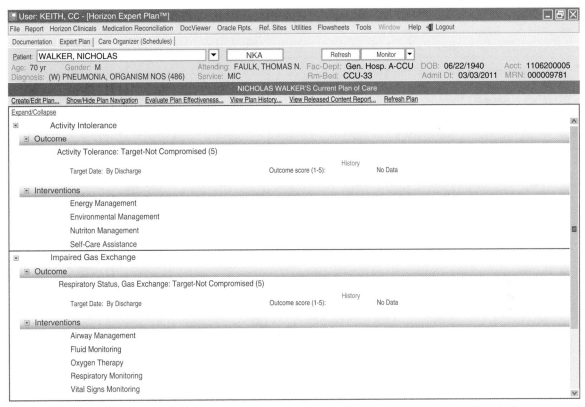

Fig. 2-1 Example of an Electronic Nursing Care Plan. *(Source: Horizon Expert Plan - patent pending, McKesson Provider Technologies, Westminster, Colorado, June 1, 2011.)*

Furthermore, nursing content in the electronic health record must be standardized and based on evidence-based practice. NIC is standardized and available in electronic form and ready to be integrated into health information systems. The use of NIC provides terms for clinical decision-making support, and enables the documentation, storage, and retrieval of clinical information about nursing treatments. Electronic implementation of standardized nursing languages facilitates the communication of nursing care provided to other nurses and health care providers; makes feasible a means for billing and the reimbursement for the provision of nursing care; and allows for the evaluation of the achievement of nursing outcomes and quality of nursing care. When electronic health record data, including NIC interventions, are stored in and retrievable from large data warehouses, nurses will be able to conduct large scale nursing effectiveness and cost effectiveness studies with comparisons among many different health care settings.[37, 48]

The time and cost for implementation of NIC into a nursing information system in a clinical practice agency depends on the agency's selection and use of a nursing information system, the computer competency of nurses, and the nurses' previous use and understanding of standardized nursing language. The change to use of nursing standardized language using a computer represents, for many, a major change in the way in which nurses have traditionally documented care, and effective change strategies need to be used. Complete implementation of NIC throughout an agency may take months to several years; the agency should devote resources for computer programming, education, and training. As major vendors design and update clinical nursing information systems that include NIC, implementation will be easier.

In this section we include tools for implementation. Box 2-3 provides steps for implementation of NIC in a clinical practice agency. Although not all of the steps must be done in every institution, the list is helpful in planning for implementation. We have found that successful implementation of the steps requires knowledge about change and nursing information systems. In addition, it is a good idea to have an evaluation process established. There are numerous publications that describe the processes of implementing NIC into a wide variety of practice settings, which can be located by a computer search of nursing literature.

Box 2-3

Steps for Implementation of NIC in a Clinical Practice Agency

A. Establish Organizational Commitment to NIC

- Identify the key person responsible for implementation (e.g., person in charge of nursing informatics).
- Create an implementation task force with representatives from key areas.
- Provide NIC materials to all members of the task force.
- Purchase copies of the NIC book and circulate readings about NIC to units.
- Have members of the task force begin to use the NIC language in every day discussion.
- Access the Center of Nursing Classification website at the University of Iowa, the NIC/NOC Elsevier Newsletter, and NIC on Facebook.

B. Prepare an Implementation Plan

- Write the specific goals to be accomplished.
- Do a force field analysis to determine driving and restraining forces.
- Determine if an in-house evaluation will be done and the nature of the evaluation effort.
- Identify which of NIC interventions are most appropriate for the agency/unit.
- Determine the extent to which NIC is to be implemented; for example, in standards, care planning, documentation, discharge summary, performance evaluation.
- Prioritize the implementation efforts.
- Choose 1-3 pilot units. Get members from these units involved in the planning.
- Develop a written timeline for implementation.
- Review current system and determine the logical sequence of actions to integrate NIC.
- Create work groups of expert clinical users to review NIC interventions and activities, determine how these will be used in the agency, and develop needed forms.

- Distribute the work of the expert clinicians to other users for evaluation and feedback before implementation.
- Encourage the development of a *NIC champion* on each of the units.
- Keep other key decision makers in the agency informed.
- Determine the nature of the total nursing data set. Work to ensure that all units are collecting data on all variables in a uniform manner so that future research can be done.
- Make plans to ensure that all nursing data are retrievable.
- Identify learning needs of staff and plan ways to address these.

C. Carry Out the Implementation Plan

- Develop the screens/forms for implementation. Review each NIC intervention and decide whether all parts (e.g., label, definition, activities, references) are to be used. Determine whether there are critical activities to document and whether further details are desired.
- Provide training time for staff.
- Implement NIC on the pilot unit(s) and obtain regular feedback.
- Update content or create new computer functions as needed.
- Use focus groups to clarify issues and address concerns/questions.
- Use data on positive aspects of implementation in house-wide presentations.
- Implement NIC house wide.
- Collect post-implementation evaluation data and make changes as needed.
- Identify key markers to use for ongoing evaluation and continue to monitor and maintain the system.
- Provide feedback to the Center for Nursing Classification.

Those leaders who are directing the implementation effort as well as administrators, computer information system designers, and practicing nurses will benefit from reading the literature describing the implementation process. Box 2-4 includes "rules of thumb" for using NIC in an information system. Following these will help ensure that data are captured in a consistent manner. In some computer systems, due to space restrictions, there is a need to shorten some of the NIC activities. Although this is becoming less of a necessity as computer space for nursing expands, Box 2-5 provides guidelines for shortening NIC activities to fit in a computer system.

There is a national agenda to move to electronic health records; however, there are many settings in which manual nursing care plans are still used. It is very feasible to use standardized language in a manual/paper or non-computer system. In fact, implementation is easier if the nursing staff can learn to use standardized language before introduction of an electronic system. Figure 2-2 illustrates a manual nursing care plan that incorporates NANDA-I, NOC, and NIC. This is one of 68 care plans developed and used at Genesis Health Care System in Davenport, Iowa. This agency has been a field testing site for NIC for many years. At one point, they were entirely computerized but due to hospital mergers and a change in computer vendors the nursing care plans are currently manual.

Use of a Standardized Language Model

The model depicted in Figure 2-3 illustrates the use of standardized language for documentation of actual care delivered by the nurse at the bedside that generates data for decision-making about cost and quality issues in the health care agency. The data is also useful for making health policy decisions. The three-level model indicates that use of standardized language for documentation of patient care not only assists the practicing nurse to communicate to others but also leads to several other important uses.

Box 2-4

Implementation Rules of Thumb for Using NIC in a Nursing Information System

1. The information system should clearly indicate that NIC is being used.
2. NIC intervention labels and definitions should appear in whole and should be clearly labeled as interventions and definitions.
3. Activities are not interventions and should not be labeled as such on the screens.
4. Documentation that the intervention was planned or delivered should be captured at the intervention label level. In addition, an agency may choose to have nurses identify specific activities within the intervention for patient care planning and documentation.
5. The number of activities required in an information system should be kept as few as possible for each intervention so as not to overburden the provider.
6. If activities are included on the information system, they should be written to the extent possible (given the constraints of the data structure) as they appear in NIC. Activities that must be rewritten to fit short field constraints should reflect the intended meaning.
7. All additional or modified activities should be consistent with the definition of the intervention.
8. Modification of NIC activities should be done sparingly and only as needed in the practice situation.
9. NIC interventions should be a permanent part of the patient's record with capability to retrieve this information.

Box 2-5

Guidelines for Shortening NIC Activities to Fit in a Computer System

Introduction: While things are changing, some computer systems still restrict space, thereby not allowing for the number of characters necessary for including the entire length of the NIC activities. If this is the case, we would advise requesting more space. However, if for whatever reason this is not possible, the following guidelines should be used to decrease the length of the activities. If these guidelines are followed, all activities should be less than 125 characters.

Guidelines:
1. Eliminate all "as appropriates" and "as needed" found after a comma at the end of some activities.
2. Remove all e.g.'s found inside of parentheses.
3. Delete words or dependent clauses that describe other parts of an activity.
4. Use the abbreviation pt for patient and nse for nurse.
5. Do NOT create new language and do not replace words.
   (Note: We have decided not to suggest word abbreviations in addition to what is already in NIC as most agencies have an agreed upon list of abbreviations that they are required to

use; these lists are not uniform across agencies and creating yet another list may lead to further confusion.)

Examples:
Monitor core body temperature, as appropriate.
   Perform and document the patient's health history and physical assessment evaluating preexisting conditions, allergies, and contraindications for specific anesthetic agents or techniques.
   Deliver anesthetic consistent with each patient's physiological needs, clinical judgment, patient's requests, and Standards for Nurse Anesthesia Practice.
   Obtain ordered specimen for laboratory analysis of acid-base balance (e.g. ABC, urine, and serum levels), as appropriate.
   Screen for symptoms of a history of domestic abuse (e.g., numerous accidental injuries, multiple somatic symptoms, chronic abdominal pain, chronic headaches, pelvic pain, anxiety, depression, posttraumatic stress syndrome, and other psychiatric disorders.

At the individual level, each nurse uses standardized language in the areas of diagnoses, interventions, and outcomes to communicate patient care plans and to document care delivered. We recommend the use of NANDA-I, NIC, and NOC as the classifications in the areas of diagnoses, interventions, and outcomes. Each of these classifications is comprehensive across specialty and practice setting, and each has ongoing research efforts to maintain the currency of the classifications. An individual nurse working with a patient or group of patients/clients asks herself several questions according to the steps of the nursing process. What are the patient's nursing

diagnoses? What are the patient outcomes that I am trying to achieve? What interventions do I use to obtain these outcomes? The identified diagnoses, outcomes, and interventions are then documented using the standardized language in these areas. A nurse working with an information system that contains the classification will document care provided by choosing the concept label for the intervention. Not all of the activities will be done for every patient. To indicate which activities were done, the nurse could either highlight those done or simply document the exceptions, depending on the existing documentation system. A nurse working with a

PATIENT PLAN OF CARE – CARDIAC OUTPUT, DECREASED

GENESIS HEALTH SYSTEM

☐ **GMC - Davenport, IA**   ☐ **GMC - DeWitt, IA**   ☐ **GMC - Silvis, IL**

Cardiac output, decreased: Inadequate blood pumped by the heart to meet metabolic demands of the body

Signs and symptoms: Observed or reported (select at least 2)

<u>Altered heart rate/rhythm</u>
☐ Arrhythmias (tachycardia/bradycardia)   ☐ Palpitations

<u>Altered Contractility</u>
☐ Restlessness
☐ Crackles   ☐ Orthopnea   ☐ Decreased cardiac index
☐ Cough   ☐ Paroxysmal nocturnal dyspnea   ☐ Decreased ejection fraction
                  ☐ Decreased stroke volume index   ☐ Decreased left ventricular stroke
                                                          work index

<u>Behavioral/emotional</u>
☐ Anxiety   ☐ Restlessness

<u>Altered preload</u>
☐ Jugular vein distention
☐ Murmurs   ☐ Fatigue   ☐ Edema
                  ☐ Decreased or increased   ☐ Decreased or increased pulmonary
                    central venous pressure (CVP)   artery wedge pressure (PAWP)

<u>Altered afterload</u>
☐ Clammy skin
☐ Prolonged capillary refill   ☐ Dyspnea   ☐ Oliguria
☐ Variations in blood pressure readings ☐ Increased or decreased pulmonary   ☐ Increased/decreased systemic
                  vascular resistance (PVR)   vascular resistance (SVR)
                  ☐ Decreased peripheral pulses

Related factors	Outcomes	Outcome scoring						Interventions
		Adm/ initial Date/ time/ initials	Date/ time/ initials	Date/ time/ initials	Date/ time/ initials	Date/ time/ initials	**DC/ final** Date/ time/ initials	
☐ Altered heart rate/rhythm ☐ Altered stroke volume ☐ Altered preload ☐ Altered afterload ☐ Altered contractility	☐ <u>Cardiac pump effectiveness</u> -BP -Peripheral pulses -Apical heart rate -Central venous pressure -Ejection fraction -Angina not present -Activity tolerance -Neck vein distention -Dysrhythmias -Peripheral edema -Dyspnea at rest -Weight -Impaired cognition -Urine output							☐ Dysrhythmia management ☐ Fluid monitoring ☐ Cardiac care: acute ☐ Cardiac care: rehabilitative ☐ Cardiac precautions ☐ Shock management: cardiac ☐ Shock prevention ☐ Cardiac care ☐ Hemodynamic regulation

Dev. 2.11   (Page 1 of 2)   0279 CF
                                         (Tab – Plan of Care)

Fig. 2-2 Example of a Manual Nursing Care Plan. *(Source: Genesis Health System, 1227 E. Rusholme Street, Davenport, IA.)*

-Diaphoresis
-Pulmonary edema
-Pallor
-Cyanosis
-Flushed
-Ascites

☐ Electrolyte monitoring

☐ Invasive hemodynamic monitoring

☐ <u>Tissue perfusion: cardiac</u>
-EKG findings
-Cardiac enzymes
-Nausea
-Angina
-Bradycardia
-Tachycardia

☐ Shock management: cardiac

☐ Fluid/electrolyte management

☐ Emotional support

☐ <u>Tissue perfusion: pulmonary</u>
-Partial pressure of CO2 (PaCO2)
-Oxygen saturation
-Unexplained anxiety

☐ Circulatory care: mechanical assist device

☐ (Other NIC) _____

☐ <u>Tissue perfusion: peripheral</u>
-Capillary refill: toes
-Capillary refill: fingers
-Extremity skin temperature
-Muscle cramps
-Parasthesia

☐ (Other NOC) _____

Definition of scoring scales	1	2	3	4	5
Cardiac pump effectiveness: Adequacy of blood volume ejected from the left ventricle to support systemic perfusion pressure	Severe deviation from normal range	Substantial deviation from normal range	Moderate deviation from normal range	Mild deviation from normal range	No deviation from normal range
Tissue perfusion: cardiac: Adequacy of blood flow through the coronary vasculature to maintain heart function	Severe	Substantial	Moderate	Moderate	None
Tissue perfusion: pulmonary: Adequacy of blood flow through pulmonary vasculature to perfuse alveoli/capillary unit					
Tissue perfusion: peripheral: Adequacy of blood flow through the small vessels of the extremities to maintain tissue function					

Fig. 2-2, cont'd

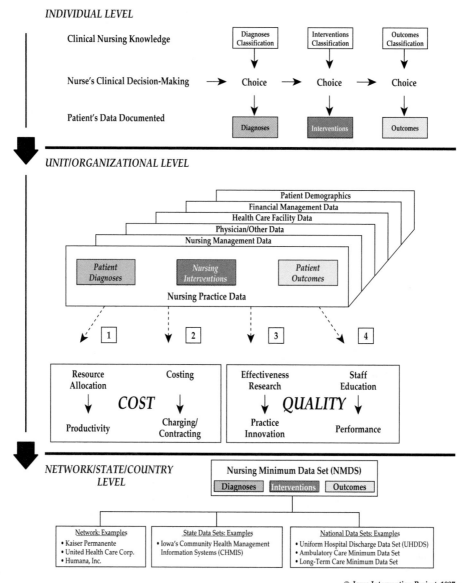

INDIVIDUAL LEVEL

Clinical Nursing Knowledge — Diagnoses Classification | Interventions Classification | Outcomes Classification

Nurse's Clinical Decision-Making → Choice → Choice → Choice

Patient's Data Documented — Diagnoses | Interventions | Outcomes

UNIT/ORGANIZATIONAL LEVEL

Patient Demographics
Financial Management Data
Health Care Facility Data
Physician/Other Data
Nursing Management Data

Patient Diagnoses | *Nursing Interventions* | *Patient Outcomes*

Nursing Practice Data

1   2   3   4

Resource Allocation   Costing
COST
Productivity   Charging/Contracting

Effectiveness Research   Staff Education
QUALITY
Practice Innovation   Performance

NETWORK/STATE/COUNTRY LEVEL

Nursing Minimum Data Set (NMDS)
Diagnoses | Interventions | Outcomes

Network: Examples
• Kaiser Permanente
• United Health Care Corp.
• Humana, Inc.

State Data Sets: Examples
• Iowa's Community Health Management Information Systems (CHMIS)

National Data Sets: Examples
• Uniform Hospital Discharge Data Set (UHDDS)
• Ambulatory Care Minimum Data Set
• Long-Term Care Minimum Data Set

© Iowa Intervention Project, 1997

Fig. 2-3 Nursing Practice Data: Three Levels

manual information system will write in the chosen NIC intervention labels as care planning and documentation are done. The activities can also be specified depending on the agency's documentation system. Although the activities may be important in communicating the care of an individual patient, the intervention label is the place to begin when planning care.

This part of the model can be thought of as documentation of the key decision points of the nursing process using standardized language. It makes apparent the importance of

nurses' skills in clinical decision-making. We have found that, even though NIC requires nurses to learn a new language and a different way to conceptualize what they do (naming the intervention concept rather than listing a series of discrete behaviors), they quickly adapt and in fact become the driving force to implement the language. With or without computerization, the adoption of NIC makes it easier for nurses to communicate what they do, with each other and with other providers. Care plans are much shorter, and interventions can be linked to diagnoses and outcomes. Because an individual nurse's decisions about diagnoses, interventions, and outcomes are collected in a uniform way, the information can be aggregated to the level of the unit or organization.

At the unit/organizational level, the information about individual patients is aggregated for all the patients in the unit (or other group) and, in turn, in the entire facility. This aggregated nursing practice data can then be linked to information contained in the nursing management database. The management database includes data about the nurses and others who provide care and the means of care delivery. In turn, the nursing practice and management data can be linked with data about the treatments made by physicians and other providers, facility information, patient information, and financial data. Most of these data, with the exception of data about treatments of providers other than physicians, are already collected in a uniform way and are available for use.

The model illustrates how the clinical practice data linked with other data in the agency's information system can be used to determine both cost and quality of nursing care. The cost side of the model addresses resource allocation and costing out of nursing services; the quality side of the model addresses effectiveness research and staff education. The use of standardized language to plan and document care does not automatically result in knowledge about cost and quality but provides the potential for data for decision-making in these areas. The steps to accomplish resource allocation, costing out of nursing service, effectiveness research, and staff education are briefly outlined below. Explanation of some managerial and financial terms is provided in parentheses for those not familiar with these areas.

Cost

Resource allocation—distributing staff and supplies
- Determine the interventions and related outcomes/type of population.
- Determine and apply the rules for staffing mix (ratio of professional to nonprofessional nursing care providers) per type of population.
- Allocate other resources (supplies and equipment) accordingly.
- Determine productivity (ratio of output to input or the ratio of work produced to people and supplies needed to produce the work) of the staff.

Costing—determining the cost of nursing services rendered to the patient
- Identify the interventions delivered to the patient.
- Affix a price per intervention, taking into account the level of provider and time spent.
- Determine an overhead charge (amount billed for business expenses that are not chargeable to a particular service but are essential to the production of services

such as heat, light, building, and repairs); allocate evenly to all patients and be able to provide justification.
- Determine the cost of care delivery per patient (direct care interventions plus overhead).
- Determine the charge per patient or use the information to contract for nursing services (establishing a business arrangement for the delivery of nursing services at a fixed price).

Quality

Effectiveness research—determining effects or outcomes of nursing interventions
- Identify the research questions (e.g., what combination of interventions gives the best outcomes for a particular type of patient?).
- Select the outcomes to be measured.
- Identify and collect the intervening variables (e.g., patient characteristics, physician treatments, staff mix, workload).
- Analyze the data.
- Make recommendations for practice innovations.

Staff education— ensuring competency to deliver the needed interventions
- Determine the level of competence of the nurses related to particular interventions.
- Provide education as needed and repeat measure of competence.
- Determine the nurse's level of accountability for the interventions and whether the intervention or part of the intervention is delegated.
- Provide education as needed related to decision-making, delegation, and team building.
- Evaluate performance in terms of achievement of patient outcomes.
- Use information in nurse's performance evaluation, taking into consideration the nurse's ability to competently perform the intervention and overall level of professional accountability.

The two sides of the model are interactive. Cost and quality should always be considered hand in hand. In addition, the four paths do not mean to imply that these are mutually exclusive. Research can be conducted on the cost side, and costs can be determined for research and education. The four distinct paths, however, are helpful to indicate the main areas of use of these data at an organizational level.

The *network/state/country level* of the model involves the "sending forward" of nursing data to be included in large databases that are used for bench marking for determination of quality and for health policy making. Werley and Lang[51] described the Nursing Minimum Data Set (NMDS) and identified 16 variables that should be included in large policy-making databases. These include the three clinical variables of diagnoses, interventions, and outcomes; nursing intensity (defined as staff mix and hours of care), which will be collected in the nursing management database, and 12 other variables, such as patient's age, sex, and race, and the expected payer of the bill, which are available from other parts of the clinical record. The model indicates that the nursing data on diagnoses, interventions, and outcomes are aggregated by facility and then included in the larger regional and national databases. A growing number of networks of care providers also are constructing databases. According to Jacox,[31] nursing has remained essentially invisible in these clinical and administrative databases. She listed the following ramifications of the invisibility of nursing and nursing care in the databases nearly two decades ago and they are still relevant today:

- We cannot describe the nursing care received by patients in most health care settings.
- Much of nursing practice is described as the practice of others, especially physicians.
- We cannot describe the effects of nursing practice on patient outcomes.
- We often cannot describe nursing care within a single setting, let alone across settings.
- We cannot identify what nurses do so that they may be reimbursed for it.

- We cannot tell the difference in patient care and costs when care is delivered by physicians as contrasted with nurses.
- This invisibility perpetuates the view of nursing as a part of medicine that does not need to be separately identified.

Estimating nursing care requirements for patients and projecting these requirements for determining staffing levels are a challenge for nurse managers. Many agencies have their own patient classification scale or use one from the literature, such as the Sunrise Patient Acuity (Van Slyck and Associates), Trend Care Systems (Trend Care Systems Pty Ltd.) or the Patient Classification Scale;[26] however, these typically are not usable across different settings. To fill this void, the acuity scale shown in Box 2-6 was developed with help from individuals in different settings as an easy-to-use patient acuity scale that can be used across settings. Although testing of the scale has been limited, its usefulness in all settings has been demonstrated. Nurse to patient ratios could also be determined by identifying the major interventions for patients at the unit level and identifying and calculating the estimated time and level of education required to safely implement the intervention as identified in Part Five of this book. There is strong evidence of a

---

Box 2-6

NIC Patient Acuity Scale

Instructions: Rate each patient on this scale once a day (or as appropriate in your practice).

Acuity level of patient (circle one):

1. A self-care patient who is primarily in contact with the health care system for assistance with health promotion activities. The patient may require some assistance to cope with the effects of disease or injury but the amount of treatment provided is not more than that which could be provided on a brief outpatient visit. *The patient in this category is often seeking routine health screening tests, such as mammograms, Pap smears, parenting instructions, weight loss and blood pressure checks, sports physicals, and well baby check-ups. The teaching aspects of care are usually brief and often limited to take home written instructions.*

2. A patient who is relatively independent as a self-care agent but may have some limitations in total self-care. The patient requires periodic nursing assessment and interventions for needs that may be simple or complex. Teaching activities form a good part of the care delivered and health care requirements include the need for education about prevention. *Examples of patients that may fit in this category include: women at high risk for a complicated pregnancy, individuals with hard-to-control diabetes or newly diagnosed diabetics, individuals who have a stable psychiatric illness, a family with a child with attention deficit disorder, and cardiac patients in the rehabilitation stage.*

3. The patient is unable to find enough resources or energies to meet his or her own needs and is dependent upon others for self-care requirements. This person requires continuing nursing intervention but the care is predictable and not in the nature of an emergency. *Examples of patients who fit this category are: someone with an unstable or energy draining chronic illness, a woman in active labor, a long term care patient, a hospice patient, a depressed psychiatric patient, and a stabilized post-operative patient.*

4. The patient is acutely ill and dependent upon others for self-care requirements with needs that may change quickly. The patient requires continuing nursing assessment and intervention and care requirements are not predictable. *Examples of patients in this category are: a post-operative patient recovering from major surgery during the first 24-36 hours, someone suffering from an acute psychiatric episode, and a woman in the high risk pregnancy category in active labor.*

5. The patient is critically ill and requires life-saving measures to maintain life. The patient has no ability to act as his own self-care agent and requires constant assessment and nursing intervention to maintain an existence. *Examples of patients in this category are: patients in intensive care receiving full life support, psychiatric patients in intensive care, low birth weight preemies, head injury accident victims, and, in general, those individuals with multisystem failures.*

relationship between nurse staffing, patient safety, and quality of care. According to the American Nurses Association (ANA),[4] 15 states and the District of Columbia have enacted legislation or adopted regulations to address nurse staffing. Seven states have mandated hospitals to establish a staffing committee.

USE OF NIC IN EDUCATION

Knowledge and skills in information and patient care technology are critical in preparing baccalaureate nursing graduates to deliver quality patient care in a variety of healthcare settings. The *Essentials of Baccalaureate Education for Professional Nursing Practice*[2] endorses the inclusion of information technology as foundational to nursing education and practice. Improvement of cost effectiveness and patient care safety depend on evidence-based practice, outcomes research, interprofessional care coordination, and electronic health records, all of which involve information management and technology. Thus, graduates of baccalaureate programs need to be competent in using both patient care technologies and information management systems. Furthermore, the American Association of Colleges of Nursing[2] calls for the use of standardized terminologies as foundational to the development of effective clinical information systems (CIS). Integration of standardized terminologies into the CIS not only supports day-to-day nursing practice but also the capacity to enhance interprofessional communication and automatically generate standardized data to continuously evaluate and improve practice.[2]

Nursing diagnoses have been included in most of the major care planning textbooks since the 1980s, and now NIC is increasingly being incorporated in a wide variety of nursing specialty textbooks as well as books that help students with the planning of care. Inclusion of standardized nursing language in a curriculum focuses the teaching on clinical decision-making (the selection of the appropriate nursing diagnoses, outcomes, and interventions for a particular patient/client). Some of the helpful books for the teaching of clinical decision-making to new students are listed in Box 2-7. These resources are rapidly expanding as more educational programs teach standardized nursing language as the knowledge base of nursing. Every major nursing publishing company is incorporating standardized nursing language in both printed and electronic resources.

More importantly, NIC can assist faculty in organizing the curricular content in all clinical courses. Specialty course content can be structured around the core interventions for specific clinical conditions and their associated nursing diagnoses. Teaching clinical reasoning and decision-making is enhanced when nurses are taught to use standardized nursing languages, including NIC.[41] In addition, texts that use case studies that incorporate NIC, such as Lunney's[36] *Critical Thinking to Achieve Positive Health Outcomes: Nursing Case*

Box 2-7

Selected Texts that Incorporate NIC

Ackley, B. & Ladwig, G. B. (2011). *Nursing diagnosis handbook: An evidence-based guide to planning care* (9th ed.). St. Louis: Elsevier Mosby.

Berman, A. J. & Snyder, S. (2012). *Kozier & Erb's fundamentals of nursing: Concepts, process, and practice* (9th ed.). Upper Saddle River, NJ: Prentice Hall.

Fortinash, K. M. & Worret, P. A. (2006). *Psychiatric nursing care plans* (5th ed.). St Louis: Mosby.

Hockenberry, M. J. & Wilson, D. (2011). *Wong's nursing care of infants and children* (9th ed.). St. Louis: Mosby Elsevier.

Johnson, M., Moorhead, S., Bulechek, G., Butcher, H., Mass, M., & Swanson, E. (Eds.). (2012). *NOC and NIC linkages to NANDA-I and clinical conditions: Supporting clinical reasoning and quality care* (3rd ed.). Maryland Heights, MO: Elsevier Mosby.

Lewis, S., Dirkse, S., Heitkemper, M., Bucher, L., & Camera, I. (2011). *Medical-surgical nursing: Assessment and management of clinical problems* (8th ed.). St. Louis: Elsevier Mosby.

London, M., Ladewig, P., Ball, J., Bindler, R., & Cowen, K. (2010). *Maternal & child nursing care* (3rd ed.). Upper Saddle River, NJ: Prentice Hall.

Lunney, M. (2009). *Critical thinking to achieve positive health outcomes: Nursing case studies and analyses.* Ames, IA: Wiley-Blackwell.

Pillitteri, A. (2009). *Maternal child health nursing: Care of the childbearing and childrearing family* (6th ed.). Philadelphia: Lippincott Williams & Wilkins.

Smeltzer, S., Bare, B., Hinkle, J., & Cheever, K. (2010). *Brunner & Suddarth's textbook of medical-surgical nursing* (12th ed.). Philadelphia: Lippincott Williams & Wilkins.

Wilkinson, J. M. & Ahern, N. R. (2008). *Prentice Hall nursing diagnosis handbook* (9th ed.). Upper Saddle River, NJ: Prentice Hall.

Studies and Analyses, can be used in both the teaching of clinical reasoning in didactic courses and teaching in clinical settings. Faculty and students can develop their own case studies incorporating standardized nursing languages and faculty can teach students to integrate NIC interventions into the plans of care developed for their assigned patients. Another useful resource to assist faculty members implementing standardized language in an undergraduate curriculum is a monograph written by Cynthia Finesilver and Debbie Metzler and their colleagues and students at Bellin College in Green Bay, Wisconsin, and available from the Center for Nursing Classification and Clinical Effectiveness at The University of Iowa.[20] Although change may sometimes be slower in academic settings, implementation of NIC in an educational setting can be easier than in a practice setting because fewer individuals are involved and there are usually no issues related to use in an information system. Nevertheless, changing a curriculum to incorporate standardized languages is a big change and some guidelines for making the change help. Box 2-8 lists Steps for Implementation of NIC in an Educational Setting. These are similar to

---

Box 2-8

Steps for Implementation of NIC in an Educational Setting

A. Establish Organizational Commitment to NIC

- Identify the key person responsible for implementation (e.g., head of curriculum committee).
- Create an implementation task force with representatives from key areas.
- Access the Center for Nursing Classification website, the NIC/NOC Elsevier Newsletter, and NIC on Facebook.
- Provide NIC materials to all members of the task force.
- Purchase and distribute copies of the latest edition of NIC.
- Circulate readings about NIC to faculty.
- Examine the philosophic issues regarding the centrality of nursing interventions in nursing.
- Have members of the task force and other key individuals begin to use the NIC language in everyday discussion.

B. Prepare an Implementation Plan

- Write specific goals to be accomplished.
- Do a force field analysis to determine driving and restraining forces.
- Determine if an in-house evaluation will be done and the nature of the evaluation.
- Determine the extent to which NIC is to be implemented; for example, in graduate as well as undergraduate programs, in philosophy statements, process recordings, care plans, case studies, orientation for new faculty.
- Prioritize the implementation efforts.
- Develop a written timeline for implementation.
- Create work groups of faculty and perhaps students to review NIC interventions and activities, determine where these will be taught in the curriculum and how they relate to current materials, and develop or redesign any needed forms.
- Identify which of NIC interventions should be taught at the graduate level and at the undergraduate level.
- Identify which interventions should be taught in which courses.
- Distribute the drafts of decisions to other faculty for evaluation and feedback.
- Encourage the development of a *NIC champion* in each department or course group.
- Keep other key decision makers informed of your plans.
- Identify learning needs of faculty and plan ways to address these.

C. Carry Out the Implementation Plan

- Revise the syllabi; order the NIC textbook for students; ask the library to order books.
- Provide time for discussion and feedback in course groups.
- Implement NIC one course at a time and obtain feedback from both faculty and students.
- Update course content as needed.
- Determine impact on and implications for supporting courses and prerequisites and restructure these as needed.
- Report progress on implementation regularly at faculty meetings.
- Collect post-implementation evaluation data and make changes in curriculum as needed.
- Identify key markers to use for ongoing evaluation and continue to monitor and maintain the system.
- Provide feedback to the Center for Nursing Classification.

Steps for Implementation of NIC in a Clinical Practice Agency (see Box 2-3), but the specific actions relate to the academic setting and course development. The central decision that must be made is that faculty adopts a nursing philosophical orientation and focus, rather than the more traditional medical orientation with nursing implications added on.

Not all interventions can or should be addressed at the undergraduate level; faculty must decide which interventions should be learned by all undergraduate students and which require advanced education and should be learned in a master's program. Some interventions are unique to specialty areas and perhaps are best taught only in specialty elective courses. Connie Delaney, while a professor at The University of Iowa, elaborated the steps to identify which interventions are taught in what courses. Delaney (personal communication, March 14, 1997) recommended the following steps, which we have expanded:

1. Identify the NIC interventions that are never taught in the curriculum (e.g., associate, baccalaureate, master's) and eliminate these from further action.

2. Using the remaining interventions, have each course group identify the interventions that are taught in their course or area of teaching responsibility. That is, identify what is currently taught with the NIC intervention terms.

3. Compile this information into a master grid (interventions on one axis and each course on the other axis) and distribute it to all faculty members.

4. Have a faculty discussion, noting the interventions that are unique to certain courses and those that are taught in more than one course. Clearly articulate the unique perspective offered by each course for each intervention that is taught in more than one place (e.g., is the intervention being delivered to a different population?). Should both courses continue to teach the intervention or should content be deleted in one course? Review interventions that are not located in any courses but that faculty believe should be taught at this level. Should content be added?

5. Affirm consensus of the faculty on what interventions are taught where.

The same process can, of course, be done with nursing diagnoses (using NANDA-I) and with patient outcomes (using NOC). Many educational programs already use NANDA-I diagnoses and can implement NIC by reviewing the NANDA-I to NIC linkages and determining the interventions that might be taught in relationship with NANDA-I diagnoses.

Using NIC in the Outcome-Present State-Test (OPT) Model of Reflective Clinical Reasoning

Decision-making models provide the structure and process that facilitate clinical reasoning. Clinical reasoning is the effective use of knowledge using reflective, creative, concurrent, and critical thinking processes to achieve desired patient outcomes. Since the 1950s, the nursing process has provided the structure facilitating clinical reasoning in the education of student nurses. The nursing process 5-step model (assessment, diagnosis, planning, intervention, and evaluation or *ADPIE*) is a standard of nursing practice. Standardized languages facilitate the teaching of the nursing process when they are fully integrated into each of the five steps. Assessment leads to the identification of NANDA-I diagnoses in the **D**iagnostic phase; **P**lanning care for each diagnosis involves choosing relevant NIC interventions and selected activities and selecting nursing sensitive NOC outcomes and indicators; the **I**ntervention phase is the process implementing NIC interventions and activities; and **E**valuation is the process of determining the changes in the NOC indicators.

Although the nursing process has demonstrated its usefulness as a clinical decision-making method, the traditional nursing process presents a number of limitations for contemporary nursing practice. Today, nursing practice calls for an emphasis on knowing the patient's "story" thereby placing the patient's situation in a meaningful context. Pesut and Herman[43] point out that the traditional nursing process does not explicitly focus on outcomes; de-emphasizes reflective and concurrent creative thinking; is more procedure orientated rather than focusing on the structures and processes of thinking; uses stepwise and linear thinking that limits relational thinking needed to understand the complex interconnections among the patient's presenting problems; and limits the development of practice relevant theory. In response to the need for a more contemporary model for clinical reasoning, Pesut and Herman developed the OPT model of reflective clinical reasoning.

The OPT model (see Figure 2-4) provides a major advancement in the teaching and practice of clinical decision-making by using a clinical reasoning structure. Pesut[42] asserts "clinical thinking and reasoning presupposes the use of a standardized nursing language . . . nursing knowledge classification systems provide the vocabulary for clinical thinking." (p. 3) Contrary to the traditional nursing process, the OPT model of reflective clinical reasoning provides a structure for clinical thinking with a focus on outcomes and is not a step-wise linear process. Clinical reasoning that focuses on outcomes enhances quality improvement by

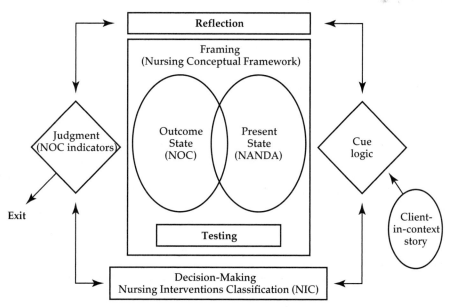

Fig. 2-4 Integrating Outcome Present State Test (OPT) Model with NANDA-I, NIC, and NOC (*Modified from* Clinical Reasoning: The Art and Science of Critical and Creative Thinking, *by Pesut, D. & Herman, J. 1999. Reprinted with permission of Delmar Learning, a division of Thomson Learning: wwwthomsonrights.com.*)

optimizing the evaluation of effectiveness rather than focusing primarily on problems. In the OPT model of clinical reasoning, the nurse simultaneously focuses on problems and outcomes by juxtapositions of both at the same time. The model requires that nurses simultaneously consider relationships among diagnoses, interventions, and outcomes with attention to the evidence. Rather than considering one problem at a time, the OPT requires one to consider several identified problems simultaneously and to discern which problem or issue is central and most important in relationship with all the other problems. The model's emphasis on: the patient's story, framing the story in a discipline specific conceptual framework, use of reflective thinking, emphasis on outcomes, mapping the web of relationships among the nursing diagnoses, and identifying the keystone issue provide a distinct advantage over the traditional nursing process. As an emerging clinical decision-making model, the OPT model provides a new process for teaching, learning, and practicing nursing.

The OPT model begins by listening to the *Client-in-Context Story* to gather important information regarding the context, major issues, and insights of the patient's situation. Pesut and Herman[43] suggest the use of a *clinical reasoning web* worksheet, which is a pictorial representation of the functional relationships among diagnoses describing the present state. Examining the relationships among the diagnoses using systems thinking and synthesis enables nurses to identify the *keystone issue*. The keystone issue is the one or more diagnoses that are central to the patient's story that support a majority of the other nursing diagnoses. Keystone issues guide clinical reasoning by identifying the central diagnosis that needs to be addressed first and also contributes to framing the reasoning process. *Framing* an event, problem, or situation is like using a lens through which one views and interprets the patient's story. The story may be framed by a specific nursing theory, a particular model, a developmental perspective, or a set of policies and procedures. Framing the patient's story by a particular nursing theory enables the nurse to "think nursing" rather than thinking medicine, psychology, sociology, or from some other non-nursing perspective.[12] The *Present State* is the description of the patient in context, or the initial condition. The present state will change with time as a result of both the nursing care and due to the changes in the nature of the patient's situation. The issues describing the present state may be organized by identifying the nursing diagnoses using the NANDA-I taxonomy.[41] NANDA-I diagnoses provide a structure and give meaning to the cues. Pesut and Herman[43] describe in detail how the nurse creates a clinical reasoning web to describe the present state by identifying the relationship among and between the NANDA-I diagnoses associated with the patient's health condition. Informed by nursing knowledge and/or by the direction the patient chooses to go, outcomes are identified that indicate the client's desired condition. NOC outcomes[40] provide the means to identify the *Outcome State* and are identified by juxtaposing or making a side-by-side comparison of a specified outcome state with present state data. NOC outcomes are a state, behavior, or perception that is measured along a continuum in response to a nursing intervention. *Testing* is thinking about how the gaps between the present state (NANDA-I diagnoses) and the desired state (NOC nursing sensitive outcomes) will be filled. While testing, the nurse juxtaposes the present state and outcome state while considering what NIC interventions can be used to bridge the gap. *Decision-Making* involves selecting and implementing the specific nursing interventions. The nurse identifies nursing interventions and the specific nursing actions that will help patients reach their desired outcomes. The taxonomy of NIC interventions will facilitate the identification of standardized nursing interventions that are chosen based on their ability to help transition patients from problem states to more desirable outcome states. *Judgment* is the process of drawing conclusions based on actions taken. Throughout all the process of the OPT model, the nurse uses *Reflection* by observing oneself while simultaneously thinking about client situations.

Within the OPT model, NIC can be used in conjunction with NANDA-I and NOC to assist students in developing the skills necessary for clinical decision-making. Kautz, Kuiper, Pesut, and Williams[33] have conducted extensive research into the teaching of clinical reasoning using standardized nursing languages with the OPT model. The findings noted "that students who consistently used NNN language with OPT models were the students who performed well in the clinical area and did better in completing their clinical reasoning webs and OPT model worksheets." (p. 137)

USE OF NIC IN RESEARCH

The provision of high quality, client-centered evidence-based care consists of delivering appropriate, acceptable, effective, safe, and efficient interventions.[46] Increasingly, health care finance is being driven by outcome-orientated health care delivery systems, quality of care, and cost effective health care dependent on the use of the interventions most effective in achieving desired outcomes. Providing and maintaining cost effective optimal quality care requires the designing and evaluating of interventions as a means to establish a sound knowledge base to guide clinical decision-making regarding the selecting and implementing of interventions that are most effective in improving the patient's condition. In general, evaluating nursing interventions is accomplished through efficacy research and effectiveness research. The use of standardized language opens up many exciting possibilities for nursing in conducting both efficacy and effectiveness research.

Efficacy Intervention Research Testing nursing treatments began with Rita Dumas' classic work in the 1960s. Although multiple studies have been conducted since then, there is no greater effort needed in nursing research today than conducting the research to establish which interventions achieve the best desired patient outcomes. Burns and Grove[10] offer an prospective approach to testing nursing interventions which consists of planning the project, gathering information, developing an intervention theory, designing the intervention, establishing an observation system, testing the intervention, collecting and analyzing data, and disseminating results. An essential aspect of efficacy research is when the project team begins to gather information about the intervention. The process of gathering information about the intervention is enhanced when the researchers begin examining the nursing intervention using a standardized taxonomy since a validated taxonomy describes and categorizes nursing interventions that represent the essence of nursing knowledge about care phenomena and their relationship to the overall concept of care. We believe that the NIC provides the concepts and language for identifying and defining interventions for nursing intervention testing research. Using a standardized language in nursing intervention-testing research assures that research findings by multiple research teams can be systematically compared. Furthermore, using NIC intervention concept labels as the basis of nursing intervention research enables researchers to work together, grounds the focus of the research in a primary source of knowledge on nursing interventions, and contributes to the development of discipline specific knowledge. For example, Gerdner[22] studied the use of music therapy as an intervention with patients with dementia and Butcher is conducting research on the effect of journaling in reducing stress in family caregivers (National Institute of Nursing Research/National Institutes of Health/R15NR8213).

Recent advances in nursing intervention research suggest the need to test interventions that are either targeted or tailored. Beck and colleagues[6] define targeted interventions as those designed to address a single characteristic of a group, such as age, gender, diagnosis, or ethnicity. Tailored interventions are those designed to address individual characteristics of persons within a sample, such as personality factors, goals, needs, preferences, and resources. The researchers point out some of the challenges and processes to conducting targeted or tailored intervention research, and point out the importance that the intervention be standardized. The NIC taxonomy offers researchers a source for identifying standardized nursing interventions that can be individualized for designing targeted and tailored

intervention-testing research. Even if standardized interventions are found to be effective, a tailored or targeted intervention may promote better adherence, achieve better outcomes, and be more cost efficient. There are a wide range of studies that can be conducted based on the use of NIC interventions to assist with targeting and tailoring of nursing interventions.

Determining the dose of an intervention is also important in determining the effect of an intervention in practice. In other words, it is essential that nurse researchers make well-grounded decisions about which nursing interventions to test as well as how much of each intervention should be provided to achieve a desired outcome. Reed, Titler, Dochterman, Shever, Kanak, and Picone[44] discuss dose in terms of the amount, frequency, and duration of the intervention. They suggest that counting the number of activities in a NIC intervention is a way of determining the amount. Duration can be determined by noting the total time spent on all activities. Further granularity can be achieved by weighting each activity as to its strength, so different activities can have their own assigned value and the values would then be summed to determine the dose of the intervention.[44] The authors conclude that measuring and reporting the dose of an intervention in research is essential to the development of an evidence base to support practice.

Maintaining the integrity of the intervention across participants and settings is also important because inconsistent intervention delivery may result in variability in the outcomes achieved.[13,46] Using NIC, this means that a substantial number of the activities listed for a particular intervention should be done and that all activities that are done should be consistent with the definition of the intervention. It is important that the activities be tailored for individual care, but they must not vary so much that the intervention is no longer the same. At present, there is no solution to the issue of dose of the intervention. A proxy measure, such as the amount of time a practitioner uses when doing the intervention, is helpful and may suffice as a measure of dose in some studies. Another solution is to know the number and extent of the specific activities that are done. Although we have not coded the nursing activities, some vendors and agencies have coded the activities, but others do not have the memory storage capacity required for large data sets and have chosen not to document this level of detail. Although the documentation of the intervention label is most important for comparison of data across sites, it is also important to have a way to ascertain the consistent implementation of the intervention. This can be done by an agency's adoption of a standard protocol for the delivery of the intervention, the collection of the time spent for intervention delivery, or by documentation of the activities related to the intervention.

Effectiveness Intervention Research In effectiveness research, nurse researchers use actual clinical data contained in the agency databases as the variables (e.g., interventions, outcomes, specific patient characteristics, specific provider characteristics, specific treatment setting characteristics) and their measures to evaluate the effectiveness of the intervention. Effectiveness research is often designed to study the effect of provider interventions on patient outcomes for the purpose of facilitating better clinical decision-making and to make better use of resources. To analyze data about the use and effectiveness of nursing interventions, it is necessary to also collect, in a systematic way, other information that can be used in conjunction with the NIC data about interventions to address a variety of questions. Early in the process of implementation, an institution should identify key research questions to be addressed with clinical data contained in an electronic documentation system. After the research questions are identified, the variables needed to address the questions and whether the data are currently collected or should be collected in the new system can be determined. The data that will be obtained from the identified variables must be linked with each other at the individual patient level. Address these concerns when setting up a nursing information system to prevent problems later. The following three questions are examples of types of questions that can be studied using actual clinical data:

- *What interventions typically occur together?* When information is systematically collected about the treatments nurses perform, clusters of interventions that typically occur together for certain types of patients can be identified. We need to identify interventions that are frequently used together for certain types of patients so we can study their interactive effects. This information will also be useful in the construction of critical paths, determining costs of services, and planning for resource allocation.

- *Which nurses use which interventions?* Systematic documentation of intervention use will allow us to study and compare the use rate of particular interventions by type of unit and facility. Implementation of NIC will allow us to learn which interventions are used by which nursing specialties. Determining the interventions used most frequently on a specific type of unit or in a certain type of agency will help to determine which interventions should be on that unit's/agency's nursing information system. It will also help in the selection of personnel to staff that unit and in the structuring of the continuing education provided to the personnel on these units.

- *What are the related diagnoses and outcomes for particular interventions?* Knowing which interventions work best for specific diagnoses and lead to certain outcomes can be used to assist nurses to make better clinical decisions. In addition, this information can help us to design treatment plans for patients that have the best chances of success.

The recommended data elements to address these questions are listed in Box 2-9 and include both a definition and the proposed measurement. Consistent definition and measurement are necessary to aggregate and compare data from different units in different settings. These variables and their measures have been discussed with representatives from several types of agencies and care settings in an attempt to make them meaningful in all settings. As can be seen from the list, more than clinical nursing data is needed. The patient's identity number is needed to link information; age, sex, race/ethnicity are included to provide some demographic information on the patient population; the physician's diagnoses and interventions, medications, and the work unit's type, staff mix, average patient acuity, and workload are included for controls. That is, for some analyses we may need to control one or more of these to determine if the nursing intervention was the cause of the effect on the patient outcome.

Our work with these variables demonstrates that the profession still must grapple with several issues related to the collection of standardized data. For example, the collection and coding of medications (Number 8) in easily retrievable form is not yet available in most facilities. Although nursing research can be done without the knowledge of medications, many of the outcomes that are achieved by nurses are also influenced by certain drugs, and so the control for medication effect is desirable. At the present time there is also no unique number that identifies the primary nurse (Number 13). Consequently, it is not currently possible to attribute clinical interventions or outcomes to particular nurses based on documentation data. Additionally, health care facilities do not collect the unit data (Numbers 20 through 24) in a standardized way. Thus, if one wished to compare these data across facilities, the data would need to be translated facility by facility to common measures such as those proposed in Box 2-9.

The method to conduct effectiveness research with actual clinical data is outlined in a monograph based on research conducted by a team at Iowa.[48] This publication outlines methods for retrieving clinical nursing data from electronic systems, storing it according to privacy requirements, applying risk adjustment techniques, and analyzing the impact of nursing treatments. The study evaluating the effectiveness of NIC interventions was a five year effectiveness grant funded by NINR and AHRQ, entitled "Nursing Interventions and Outcomes in Three Older Populations" (Titler, R01 NR 05331).

Box 2-9

Data Elements for Effectiveness Research in Nursing

Definitions and Measurement

Facility Data

1. Facility Identification Number—

Definition: a number that identifies the organization where the patient/client was provided nursing care
   Measurement: use Medicare identification number

Admission Data

2. Patient Identification Number—

Definition: the unique number, assigned to each patient/client within a health care facility that distinguishes and separates one patient record from another in that facility
   Measurement: use the facility's record number

3. Date of Birth—

Definition: the day of the patient's birth
   Measurement: month, day, and year of birth

4. Gender—

Definition: the patient's sex
   Measurement: male, female, unknown

5. Race—

Definition: a class or kind of people unified by community of interests, habits, or characteristics
   Measurement: use UHDDS codes: **1**. American Indian or Alaska Native; **2**. Asian/Pacific Islander; **3**. black, not Hispanic; **4**. Hispanic; **5**. white, not Hispanic; **6**. other (please specify); **7**. unknown

6. Marital Status—

Definition: legally recognized union of man and woman
   Measurement: **1**. married; **2**. widowed; **3**. divorced; **4**. separated; **5**. never married; **6**. unknown

7. Admission Date—

Definition: date of initiation of care
   Measurement: month, day, year

Medications

8. Medications —

Definition: a medicinal substance used to cure disease or relieve symptoms
   Measurement: **1**. name of drug; **2**. route of administration: 1. PO, 2. IM/SC, 3. IV, 4. aerosol, 5. rectal, 6. eye drops, 7. other; **3**. dose: amount of drug prescribed; **4**. frequency: number of times per day given; **5**. start date: date drug began this episode of care: month, day, year; **6**. stop date: date drug discontinued this episode of care: month, day, year

Physician Data

9. Physician Identification Number—

Definition: a number across settings that identifies the physician who is primarily responsible for the medical care of the patient/client during the care episode

   Measurement: unique number used by provider to bill for services (UHDDS uses attending and operating)

10. Medical Diagnosis—

Definition: the medical conditions that coexist at the time of admission, that develop subsequently, or that affect the treatment received and/or the length of stay; all diagnoses that affect the current episode of care
   Measurement: names of medical diagnoses as listed on the patient's bill using ICD-9-CM codes

11. Diagnosis Related Group (DRG)—

Definition: the U.S. prospective payment system used for reimbursement of Medicare patients; categorizes discharged patients into approximately 500 groups based upon medical diagnosis, age, treatment procedure, discharge status, and sex
   Measurement: the three digit number and name of the DRG which this patient was assigned

12. Medical Intervention—

Definition: a treatment prescribed by a physician; all significant procedures for the current episode of care
   Measurement: **1**. names of physician procedures listed on the patient bill using CPT codes; **2**. start date: date procedure began this episode of care: month, day, year; **3**. stop date: date procedure discontinued this episode of care: month, day, year

Nursing Data

13. Nurse Identification Number—

Definition: a number across settings that identifies the nurse who is primarily responsible for the nursing care of the patient or client during the care episode
   Measurement: number each nurse in facility; a national registry does not exist at the current time

14. Nursing Diagnosis—

Definition: a clinical judgment made by a nurse about the patient's response to an actual or potential health problem or life process during this episode of care that affects the treatments received and/or the length of stay
   Measurement: names of nursing diagnoses using NANDA-I terms and codes

15. Nursing Intervention—

Definition: a treatment performed by a nurse
   Measurement: **1**. names of treatments delivered to patient during episode of care using NIC terms and codes; **2**. start date: date intervention began this episode of care: month, day, year; **3**. stop date: date intervention discontinued for this episode of care: month, day, year

Outcomes

16. Patient Outcomes—

Definition: an aspect of patient/client health status that is influenced by nursing intervention during this episode of care
   Measurement: **1**. names of outcomes using NOC terms; **2**. date identified; **3**. date outcome is stopped; **4**. status of outcome at beginning and end of episode of care (use NOC scale)

Continued

Box 2-9

Data Elements for Effectiveness Research in Nursing—cont'd

17. Discharge Date—

Definition: date of termination of an episode of care
  Measurement: month, day, and year

18. Disposition—

Definition: plan for continuing health care made upon discharge
  Measurement: use NMDS with modification: **1.** discharged to home or self care (routine discharge); **2.** discharged to home with referral to organized community nursing service; **3.** discharged to home with arrangements to see nurse in ambulatory setting; **4.** transfer to a short term hospital; **5** transfer to a long term institution; **6.** died; **7.** left against medical advice; **8.** still a patient; **9.** other

19. Cost of Care—

Definition: provider's charges for the services rendered to the client incurred during the episode of care
  Measurement: total charges billed for episode of care (from patient's bill)

Unit Data

20. Unit Type—

Definition: name of type of unit or specialty area which best characterizes where majority of patient care is delivered
  Measurement: all units answer both parts *A* and *B*:
  A. Where is the location of nursing care? (Check only one site)
  ____Ambulatory care/Outpatient
  ____Community
  ____Home
  ____Hospital
  ____Long term care setting/Nursing home
  ____Occupational health
  ____Rehabilitation agency
  ____School
  ____Other (please describe):_____
  B. What is the specialty that best characterizes the type of care being delivered? (Choose only one)
  ____General medical
  ____General surgical
  ____General medical surgical
  ____Geriatric
  ____Intensive or emergency care (e.g. CCU, MICU, PICU, SICU, ER, OR, RR)
  ____Maternal-child
  ____Psychiatric (adult or child, including substance abuse)
  ____Specialty medicine (e.g. bone marrow, cardiology, dermatology, hematology, hemodialysis, neurology, oncology, pulmonary, radiology)
  ____Specialty surgery (e.g. EENT, neurosurgery, orthopedics, urology)
  ____Other (please describe):_____

21. Staff Mix—

Definition: ratio of professional to non-professional nursing care providers in the unit/clinic/group where care is being provided
  Measurement: number of RNs to non-professional staff who *worked* on unit/clinic/group each day of patient's stay (collect daily for patient's length/episode of care—if cannot get daily, take weekly average). Allocate 12 hour shifts or other irregular shifts to times actually worked, i.e. a person who works 12 hours 7:30 am to 7:30pm is allocated 8 hours (1 FTE) on days and 4 hours (.5 FTE) on evenings. Count only actual direct care hours, i.e. remove the head nurse and charge nurse unless they are providing direct care, remove the unit secretary and do not include non-productive hours (such as orientation, continuing education).
  # of FTE RNs days_____
  # of FTE RNs evenings_____
  # of FTE RNs nights _____
  # of FTE LPN/LVNs days_____
  # of FTE LPN/LVNs nights_____
  # of FTE LPN/LVNs evenings_____
  # of FTE aides days _____
  # of FTE aides evenings_____
  # of FTE aides nights_____
  # others days (please identify) _____
  # others evenings (please identify) _____
  # others nights (please identify) _____

22. Hours of Nursing Care—

Definition: hours of nursing care administered per patient day in unit/clinic/group where care is delivered
  Measurement: hours of care (actual staffing) by RNs, LPNs, and aides
  Days: RN hours _____LPN hours_____
  aide hours _____others hours _____
  Evenings: RN hours _____ LPN hours _____
  aide hours _____ others hours _____
  Nights: RN hours _____ LPN hours _____
  aide hours _____ others hours _____
  NOTE: These are the same people as in number 21.

23. Patient Acuity—

Definition: average illness level of patients cared for on the unit
  Measurement: patient is rated on agreed upon patient acuity scale

24. Workload—

Definition: the amount of nursing service provided on a unit
  Measurement: the average patient acuity (number 23) times the number of occupied beds per day (or number of patients seen in ambulatory) divided by the number of RNs working or number of total nursing personnel working (number 21)
  Midnight census or number of patients encountered per day

The study examined the use of interventions in three groups of elderly patients in one acute care facility that has a large, electronic system for the documentation of nursing care. The aims of the grant, as completed, were:

1. Identify the frequently used nursing interventions, pharmacological treatments, and medical treatments for the hospitalized elderly with heart failure, hip fracture, and for those who receive the Fall Prevention nursing intervention.
2. Describe the relationships among patient characteristics, patient clinical conditions (medical diagnoses, severity of illness), treatments (nursing interventions, medical treatments, pharmacological treatments), characteristics of nursing units, and outcomes of hospitalized elderly patients (heart failure, hip fracture, fall prevention).
3. The investigator should: A) Compare the length of stay of acute care for hospitalizations that received the nursing intervention of Pain Management with those hospitalizations that did not receive Pain Management in the Hip Procedure group. B) Compare the discharge disposition of hospitalizations that received the nursing intervention Fluid Management to the hospitalizations that did not receive Fluid Management in the Heart Failure group. C) Compare hospital costs for hospitalizations that received high use of the nursing intervention Surveillance to hospitalizations that received low use of Surveillance.
4. Develop a guideline for construction and use of a nursing effectiveness research database built from electronic data repositories.

Several publications that demonstrate the effect of NIC interventions on patient outcomes that resulted from this research are now available. For example:

Dochterman, J., Titler, M., Wang, J., Reed, D., Pettit, D., Mathew-Wilson, M., Budreau, G., Bulechek, G., Kraus, V., & Kanak, M. (2005). Describing use of nursing interventions for three groups of patients. *Journal of Nursing Scholarship, 37*(1), 57-66.

Kanak, M., Titler, M., Shever, L., Fei, Q., Dochterman, J., & Picone, D. (2008). The effects of hospitalization on multiple units. *Applied Nursing Research, 21*(1), 15-22.

Picone, D., Titler, M., Dochterman, J., Shever, L., Kim, T., Abramowitz, P., Kanak, M., & Qin, R. (2008). Predictors of medication errors among elderly hospitalized patients. *American Journal of Medical Quality, 23*(2), 115-127.

Reed, D., Titler, M., Dochterman, J., Shever, L., Kanak, M., & Picone, D. (2007). Measuring the dose of nursing intervention. *International Journal of Nursing Terminologies and Classifications, 18*(4), 121-130.

Shever, L., Titler, M., Dochterman, J., Fei, Q., & Picone, D. M. (2007). Patterns of nursing intervention use across six days of acute care hospitalization for three older patient populations. *International Journal of Nursing Terminologies and Classifications, 18*(1), 18-29.

Titler, M., Jensen, G., Dochterman, J., Xie, X., Kanak, M., Reed, D., & Shever, L. (2008). Cost of hospital care for older adults with heart failure: Medical, pharmaceutical, and nursing costs. *Health Services Research, 43*(2), 635-655.

Titler, M., Dochterman, J., Kim, T., Kanak, M., Shever, L., Picone, D., Everett, L., & Budreau, G. (2007). Costs of care for seniors hospitalized for hip fractures and related procedures. *Nursing Outlook, 55*(1), 5-14.

Titler, M., Dochterman, J., Picone, D., Everett, L., Xie, X., Kanak, M., & Fei, Q. (2005). Cost of hospital care for elderly at risk of falling. *Nursing Economic$, 23*(6), 290-306.

Titler, M., Dochterman, J., Xie, X., Kanak, M., Fei, Q., Picone, D., & Shever, L. (2006). Nursing interventions and other factors associated with discharge disposition in older patients after hip fractures. *Nursing Research, 55*(4), 231-242.

These articles demonstrate the benefits of effectiveness research using standardized nursing language. For example, in the publication examining patterns of nursing interventions in patients hospitalized with heart failure and hip procedures and who were at risk for falling,[45] the authors concluded that not only did the use of NIC allow for the extraction of data from the electronic medical record but found that Surveillance, Intravenous (IV) Therapy, Fluid Management, and Diet Staging were the four most frequent interventions implemented in all four groups of older adults in an acute care setting. The researchers also were able to identify what nursing interventions were unique and specific to each patient group and concluded that nursing intervention data using NIC provided administrators with information about the care provided that was useful for evaluating staffing, allocating resources, educating nursing staff, and evaluating nurse competency.

The article by Dochterman and colleagues[19] documented the use of NIC interventions for three patient populations: heart failure, hip fracture, and fall prevention. Findings showed that the mean number of interventions done at least once during a single hospitalization ranged from 18 to 22 for the three populations. Interventions used during 50% or more hospitalizations were identified for each population. Six interventions were used in all three populations: Cough Enhancement, Diet Staging, Fluid Management, Intravenous (IV) Therapy, Pain Management, and Tube Care. The authors conclude that knowledge of interventions used by patient population can help nurse managers plan for type and amount of staff needed on a unit.

In another analysis, Titler and colleagues[47] looked at the impact of nursing interventions on hospital cost for seniors who were hospitalized for a hip fracture or related procedure. An effectiveness model included multiple variables related to patient characteristics (e.g. age), clinical conditions (e.g. medical diagnosis), nursing unit characteristics (e.g. average RN/patient ratio) as well as the interventions of physicians, nurses, and pharmacists. Findings showed that most of the variables that impact cost are interventions, especially medical interventions and medications. A substantial number of nursing interventions did not increase cost. RN staffing below the unit average was associated with increased cost. The authors stated that this was the first study that looked at nursing interventions related to hospital cost, made possible by the use of NIC in a clinical information system.

Comparative effectiveness research (CER) is now being legislated as a priority for translational research. Translational research includes the process of applying discoveries generated during research in the laboratory and in preclinical studies to the development of trials and studies in humans as well as research aimed at enhancing the adoption of best practices in the community. As charged in the American Recovery and Reinvestment Act (ARRA), the Institute of Medicine defined comparative effectiveness research as "the generation and synthesis of evidence that compares the benefits and harms of alternative methods to prevent, diagnose, treat, and monitor a clinical condition or to improve the delivery of care . . . at both the individual and population level."[29] (p. 29) CER addresses whether an intervention works better than other interventions in a practice where patients are more heterogeneous than those recruited and accepted in clinical trials. Nurse researchers must also begin to engage in the methods of comparative effectiveness research because it provides the means to identify which interventions work for what patients under specific circumstances. Key elements in comparative effectiveness research are direct comparison of effective interventions, the study of patients in typical clinical care situations, and tailoring the intervention to the needs of individual patients. However, it is important to note, using standardized interventions, such as those provided in NIC, makes comparisons of interventions among patient populations and across settings possible when designing CER studies.

Translation of NIC into Evidence-Based Protocols
Translation involves the development of guidelines for implementing the intervention into day-to-day practice and the inclusion of the guidelines as a standard part of usual practice. Guidelines usually are created in the form of protocols or evidenced-based guidelines that convert scientific knowledge into clinical actions in a form that is available to clinicians. Guidelines describe a process of patient care management that has the potential to improve the quality of clinical and consumer decision-making. The nursing profession has focused on development and use of guidelines since the Agency for Health Care Policy and Research (AHCPR) national initiative throughout the 1990s. Because the focus of a guideline is management of a clinical condition, incorporating NIC into protocols is very useful in describing the nursing interventions contained in the guideline. To illustrate the relationship between NIC interventions and NOC outcomes in evidence-based protocols, we have worked with the Gerontological Nursing Interventions Research Center (GNIRC) at The University of Iowa College of Nursing to incorporate NIC in a number of protocols including those focusing on managing medication,[8] preventing elder abuse,[17] promoting spirituality,[21] managing relocation,[27] and managing pain.[39]

SUMMARY

Nurses are information and knowledge users, and NIC facilitates the use of knowledge about nursing interventions in practice, education, and research. NIC is a primary source for intervention knowledge development in nursing and provides the knowledge content for guiding nursing treatments. As the largest group of health care knowledge workers, nurses rely on extensive clinical information to implement and evaluate the processes and outcomes of their clinical decision-making care. Standardized NIC interventions facilitate the knowledge-user role by structuring nursing treatments designed to achieve desired patient outcomes. Furthermore, computerized mechanisms greatly assist nurse knowledge users by bringing knowledge resources to the point of care so they can be quickly accessible during the actual clinical decision-making process. NIC interventions are already in a wide variety of health care information systems that are used at the point of care for planning and documenting nursing care. When nursing care is documented and stored in data-warehouses, the data can be retrieved so that effectiveness and comparative effectiveness research can be done.

Nurses are committed to delivering high quality nursing interventions. The benefits of using NIC are clear and well established. Since NIC was first developed in 1992, there has been rapid movement incorporating NIC in nursing practice, education, and research. Each edition of NIC offers new advances, including new and revised interventions, new uses of NIC in nursing education, new applications of NIC in practice settings that enhance clinical decision-making and documentation of nursing care, and new knowledge generated through the use of NIC in effectiveness research. We continually work to improve NIC and look forward to your feedback and suggestions for improvement.

References

1. Ackley, B., & Ladwig, G. (2011). *Nursing diagnosis handbook: An evidence-based guide to planning care* (9th ed.). St. Louis: Mosby.
2. American Association of Colleges of Nursing. (2008). *The essentials of baccalaureate education for professional nursing practice*. Washington, DC: Author.
3. American Nurses Association. (2010). *Nursing's social policy statement: The essence of the profession*. Silver Spring, MD: Author.
4. American Nurses Association (ANA). (2011). *Staffing plans and ratios*. Retrieved from http://www.nursingworld.org/Main Menucategories/ANAPoliticalPower/State/StateLegislativeAgenda/StaffingPlansandRatios_1.aspx
5. Anderson, C. A., Keenan, G., & Jones, J. (2009). Using bibliometrics to support your selection of a nursing terminology set. *Computers, Informatics, Nursing, 27*(2), 82–90.
6. Beck, C., McSweeney, J. C., Richards, K. C., Robinson, P. K., Tsai, P-F., & Souder, E. (2010). Challenges in tailored intervention research. *Nursing Outlook, 58*(2), 10–110.
7. Benner, P. (Ed.). (1994). *Interpretive phenomenology: Embodiment, caring, and ethics in health and illness*. Thousand Oaks, CA: Sage.
8. Bergman-Evans, B. (2005). *Evidence-based protocol. Improving medication management for older adults*. Iowa City, IA: The University of Iowa, College of Nursing, Gerontological Nursing Interventions Research Center.
9. Bulechek, G. M., & McCloskey, J. C. (Eds.). (2000). *Nursing interventions: Effective nursing treatments* (3rd ed.). Philadelphia: W. B. Saunders.
10. Burns, N., & Grove, S. K. (2009). *The practice of nursing research: Appraisal, synthesis, and generation of evidence* (6th ed., pp. 317–338). St. Louis: Saunders Elsevier.
11. Butcher, H. (2011). Creating the nursing theory-research-practice nexus. In P. S. Cowen, & S. Moorhead (Eds.), *Current issues in nursing* (8th ed., pp. 123–135). St. Louis: Mosby.
12. Butcher, H., & Johnson, M. (2012). Use of linkages for clinical reasoning and quality improvement. In: M. Johnson, S. Moorhead, G. Bulechek, H. Butcher, M. Mass, & E. Swanson (Eds.), *NOC and NIC linkages to NANDA-I and clinical conditions: Supporting clinical reasoning and quality of care* (3rd ed., pp. 11–23). Maryland Heights: Elsevier Mosby.
13. Carter, J., Moorhead, S., McCloskey, J., & Bulechek, G. (1995). Using the nursing interventions classification to implement Agency for Health Care Policy and Research guidelines. *Journal of Nursing Care Quality, 9*(2), 76–86.
14. Casey, A. (2011). Global challenges of electronic records for nursing. In P. S. Cowen, & S. Moorhead (Eds.), *Current issues in nursing* (8th ed., pp. 340–347). St. Louis: Mosby Elsevier.
15. Clancy, T., Delaney, C., Morrison, B., & Gunn, J. (2006). The benefits of standardized nursing languages in complex adaptive systems such as hospitals. *The Journal of Nursing Administration, 36*(9), 426–434.
16. Clark, J., & Lang, N. (1992). Nursing's next advance: An international classification for nursing practice. *International Nursing Review, 39*(4), 109–112.
17. Daly, J. M. (2004). *Evidence-based protocol: Elder abuse prevention*. Iowa City, IA: The University of Iowa, College of Nursing, Gerontological Nursing Interventions Research Center.
18. Dawkins, R. (1986). *The blind watchmaker*. New York: Norton.
19. Dochterman, J., Titler, M., Wang, J., Reed, D., Pettit, D., Mathew-Wilson, M., et al. (2005). Describing use of nursing interventions for three groups of patients. *Journal of Nursing Scholarship, 37*(1), 57–66.
20. Finesilver, C., & Metzler, D. (Eds.). (2002). *Curriculum guide for implementation of NANDA, NIC, and NOC into an undergraduate nursing curriculum*. Iowa City, IA: College of Nursing, Center for Nursing Classification and Clinical Effectiveness.
21. Gaskamp, C. D., Meraviglia, M., & Sutter, R. (2005). *Evidence-based protocol: Promoting spirituality in the older adult*. Iowa City, IA: The University of Iowa, College of Nursing, Gerontological Nursing Interventions Research Center.
22. Gerdner, L. (2000). The effects of individualized vs. classical "relaxation" music on the frequency of agitation in elderly persons with Alzheimer's disease and related disorders. *International Psychogeriatrics, 12*(1), 49–65.
23. Gleick, J. (2011). *The information: A history, a theory, a flood*. New York: Pantheon.
24. Goode, C., Sanders, C., Del Monte, J., Chon, D., Dare, A., Merrifield, L., et al. (2011). Laying the foundation for evidence-based practice for nurse residents. In P. S. Cowen, & S. Moorhead (Eds.), *Current issues in nursing* (8th ed., pp. 385–390). St. Louis: Mosby Elsevier.
25. Greiner, A. C., & Knebel, E. (Eds.). (2003). *Health professions education: A bridge to quality*. Washington, DC: The National Academies Press.
26. Harper, K., & McCully, C. (2007). Acuity systems dialogue and patient classification system essentials. *Nursing Administration Quarterly, 31*(4), 284–299.
27. Hertz, J. E., Koren, M. E., Robertson, J. F., & Rossetti, J. (2005). *Evidence-based practice guideline: Management of relocation in cognitively intact older adults*. Iowa City, IA: The University of Iowa, College of Nursing, Gerontological Nursing Interventions Research Center.
28. Institute of Medicine (2001). *Crossing the quality chasm: A new health system for the 21st century*. Washington, DC: The National Academies Press.
29. Institute of Medicine (2009). *Initial national priorities for comparative effectiveness research*. Washington, DC: The National Academies Press.
30. Institute of Medicine (2011). *The future of nursing: Leading change, advancing health*. Washington, DC: The National Academies Press.
31. Jacox, A. (1995). Practice and policy implications of clinical and administrative databases. In N. M. Lang (Ed.), *Nursing data systems: The emerging framework*. Washington, DC: American Nurses Association.
32. Johnson, M., Moorhead, S., Bulechek, G., Butcher, H., Mass, M., & Swanson, E. (2012). *NOC and NIC linkages to NANDA-I and clinical conditions: Supporting clinical reasoning and quality of care* (3rd ed.). Maryland Heights: Elsevier Mosby.
33. Kautz, D. D., Kuiper, R., Pesut, D. J., & Williams, R. L. (2006). Using NANDA, NIC, and NOC (NNN) language for clinical reasoning with the Outcome-Present State (OPT) model. *International Journal of Nursing Terminologies and Classification, 17*(3), 129–138.
34. Lee, M. (2011). Personal health records as a tool for improving the delivery of health care. In P. S. Cowen, & S. Moorhead (Eds.), *Current issues in nursing* (8th ed., pp. 331–339). St. Louis: Mosby Elsevier.
35. Lunney, M. (2003). Theoretical explanations for combining NANDA, NIC, and NOC. In J. M. Dochterman, & D. A. Jones (Eds.), *Unifying nursing languages: The harmonization of NANDA, NIC, and NOC* (pp. 35–45). Washington, DC: American Nurses Association.

36. Lunney, M. (2009). *Critical thinking to achieve positive health outcomes: Nursing case studies and analyses.* Ames, IA: Wiley-Blackwell.

37. Maas, M., Scherb, C., & Head, B. (2012). Use of NNN in computerized information systems. In M. Johnson, S. Moorhead, G. Bulechek, H. Butcher, M. Mass, & E. Swanson (Eds.), *NOC and NIC linkages to NANDA-I and clinical conditions: Supporting clinical reasoning and quality of care* (3rd ed., pp. 24–34). Maryland Heights, MO: Elsevier Mosby.

38. McBride, A. B. (2006). Informatics and the future of nursing practice. In C. A. Weaver, C. W. Delaney, P. Weber, & R. L. Carr (Eds.), *Nursing informatics for the 21st century: An international look at practice, trends and the future* (pp. 8–12). Chicago: Healthcare Information and Management Systems Society.

39. McLennon, S. M. (2005). *Evidence-based protocol: Persistent pain management.* Iowa City, IA: The University of Iowa, College of Nursing, Gerontological Nursing Interventions Research Center.

40. Moorhead, S, Johnson, M., Maas, M., & Swanson, E. (Eds.). (2013). *Nursing outcomes classification (NOC)* (5th ed.). St. Louis: Elsevier.

41. NANDA International. (2012). *Nursing diagnoses: Definitions & classification 2012-2014* [T. H. Herdman (Ed.)]. West Sussex, United Kingdom: Wiley-Blackwell.

42. Pesut, D. (2002). Nursing nomenclatures and eye-roll anxiety control. *Journal of Professional Nursing, 18*(1), 3–4.

43. Pesut, D., & Herman, J. (1999). *Clinical reasoning: The art and science of critical and creative thinking.* Albany, NY: Delmar.

44. Reed, D., Titler, M. G., Dochterman, J., Shever, L., Kanak, M., & Picone, D. (2007). Measuring the dose of nursing intervention. *International Journal of Nursing Terminologies and Classifications, 18*(4), 121–130.

45. Shever, L., Titler, M., Dochterman, J., Fei, Q., & Picone, D. (2007). Patterns of nursing intervention use across six days of acute care hospitalization for three older patient populations. *International Journal of Nursing Terminologies and Classifications, 18*(1), 18–29.

46. Sidani, S., & Braden, C. J. (1998). *Evaluating nursing interventions: A theory-driven approach.* Thousand Oaks, CA: Sage.

47. Titler, M., Dochterman, J., Kim, T., Kanak, M., Shever, L., Picone, D., et al. (2007). Costs of care for seniors hospitalized for hip fractures and related procedures. *Nursing Outlook, 55*(1), 5–14.

48. Titler, M., Dochterman, J., & Reed, D. (2004). *Guideline for conducting effectiveness research in nursing and other healthcare services.* Iowa City, IA: The University of Iowa, College of Nursing, Center for Nursing Classification and Clinical Effectiveness.

49. Titler, M., Kleiber, C., Steelman, V., Goode, C., Rakel, B., Barry-Walker, J., et al. (1994). Infusing research into practice to promote quality care. *Nursing Research, 43*(5), 307–313.

50. Titler, M., Kleiber, C., Steelman, V., Rakel, B., Budreau, G., Everett, L., et al. (2001). The Iowa model of evidence-based practice to promote quality care. *Critical Care Clinics of North America, 13*(4), 497–509.

51. Werley, H. H., & Lang, N. M. (Eds.). (1988). *Identification of the nursing minimum data set.* New York: Springer.

PART TWO

Taxonomy of Nursing Interventions

Overview of the NIC Taxonomy

The 554 interventions in the *Nursing Interventions Classifications (NIC)* Sixth Edition have been organized, as in the last three editions, into 7 domains and 30 classes. This three-level taxonomic structure is included on the following pages. At the top, most abstract level are 7 *domains* (numbered 1 to 7). Each domain includes *classes* (assigned alphabetical letters) or groups of related interventions (each with a unique code of four numbers) that are at the third level of the taxonomy. Only intervention label names are used in the taxonomy. Refer to the alphabetical listing in the book for the definition and defining activities for each intervention. The taxonomy was constructed using the methods of similarity analysis, hierarchical clustering, clinical judgment, and expert review. Refer to previous editions for more details on the construction, validation, and coding of the taxonomy.

The taxonomy clusters relate interventions for ease of use. The groupings represent all areas of nursing practice. Nurses in any specialty should remember that they should use the whole taxonomy with a particular patient, not just interventions from one class or domain. The taxonomy is theory neutral; the interventions can be used with any nursing theory and in any of the various nursing settings and health care delivery systems. The interventions can also be used with various diagnostic classifications, including NANDA International, International Classification of Diseases (ICD), Diagnostic & Statistical Manual of Mental Disorders (DSM), and the Omaha System Problem List.

Each of the interventions has been assigned a unique number to facilitate computerization. If one wishes to identify the class and domain of the intervention, one would use six digits (e.g., 1A-0140 is Body Mechanics Promotion and is located in the Activity and Exercise Management class in the Physiological: Basic domain). Activity codes are not included in this book as we did not wish the classification to be dominated by numbers. If one wishes to assign codes, then each intervention's activities can be numbered using two spaces after a decimal (e.g., 1A-0140.01). Given the sheer number of activities and the amount of resources that would be needed to keep track of them and the changes in activities over time, there has been no attempt to assign unique codes to activities. If activities are coded in a particular facility, they need to be used together with the related intervention code.

Some interventions have been included in two classes but are coded according to the primary class. We have attempted to keep cross-referencing to a minimum because the taxonomy could easily become long and unwieldy. Interventions are listed in another class only if they were judged to be sufficiently related to the interventions in that class. No intervention is listed in more than two classes. Interventions that are more concrete (i.e., those with colons in the title) have been coded at the fourth digit (e.g., Exercise Therapy: Ambulation is coded 0221). Occasionally an intervention is located in only one class but has a code that is assigned to another class (e.g., Nutritional Counseling is located in class D, Nutrition Support, but is coded 5246 to indicate that it is a counseling intervention). The interventions in each class are listed alphabetically, but the numbers may not be sequential because of additions and deletions. The last two classes in the domain Health System (Health System Management, coded a, and Information Management, coded b) contain many of the indirect care interventions (those that would be included in overhead costs).

The taxonomy first appeared in the second edition of NIC in 1996 with 6 domains and 27 classes. The third edition, published in 2000, included one new domain (Community) and three new classes: Childrearing Care (coded Z) in the Family domain and Community Health Promotion and Community Risk Management in the Community domain (c and d). In this edition, no new domains or classes were added; the 23 new interventions were easily placed in the existing classes.

The coding guidelines used for this and previous editions are summarized as follows:
- Each intervention is assigned a unique four-digit code, which belongs to the intervention as long as the intervention exists, regardless of whether it should change class in some future edition.
- Codes are retired when interventions are deleted; no code is used more than once. Interventions that have a modification in label name only that does not change the nature of the intervention will keep the same code number. In this case the label name change does not affect the intervention, but the change was needed for a compelling reason (e.g., Abuse Protection was changed to Abuse Protection Support in the third edition to distinguish the intervention from an outcome in NOC that

had the same name; Conscious Sedation was changed in the fourth edition to Sedation Management to better reflect current practice).

- Interventions that have a modification in label name only that *does* change the nature of the intervention are assigned a new code, and the previous code is retired (e.g., in the third edition Triage became Triage: Disaster, indicating the more discrete nature of this intervention and distinguishing it from the new interventions of Triage: Emergency Center and Triage: Telephone).
- Cross-referencing is avoided if possible, and no intervention is cross-referenced in more than two classes; the number assigned is selected from the primary class.

- Interventions that are most concrete are coded using the fourth digit.
- Interventions are listed alphabetically within each class; the code numbers may not be sequential because of changes, additions, and deletions.
- Although the codes originally begun in the second edition were assigned logically and this logical order is being continued when possible, *codes are context free* and should not be interpreted to have any meaning except as a four-digit number.
- Activities are not coded, but if one desires to do this, use two (or more if indicated in your computer system) spaces to the right of a decimal and number the activities as they appear in each intervention (e.g., 0140.01, 0140.02).

NIC TAXONOMY

	Domain 1	Domain 2	Domain 3
Level 1 Domains	**1. Physiological: Basic** Care that supports physical functioning	**2. Physiological: Complex** Care that supports homeostatic regulation	**3. Behavioral** Care that supports psychosocial functioning and facilitates life style changes
Level 2 Classes	**A Activity and Exercise Management** Interventions to organize or assist with physical activity and energy conservation and expenditure **B Elimination Management** Interventions to establish and maintain regular bowel and urinary elimination patterns and manage complications due to altered patterns **C Immobility Management** Interventions to manage restricted body movement and the sequelae **D Nutrition Support** Interventions to modify or maintain nutritional status **E Physical Comfort Promotion** Interventions to promote comfort using physical techniques **F Self-Care Facilitation** Interventions to provide or assist with routine activities of daily living	**G Electrolyte and Acid-Base Management** Interventions to regulate electrolyte/acid base balance and prevent complications **H Drug Management** Interventions to facilitate desired effects of pharmacological agents **I Neurologic Management** Interventions to optimize neurologic function **J Perioperative Care** Interventions to provide care prior to, during, and immediately after surgery **K Respiratory Management** Interventions to promote airway patency and gas exchange **L Skin/Wound Management** Interventions to maintain or restore tissue integrity **M Thermoregulation** Interventions to maintain body temperature within a normal range **N Tissue Perfusion Management** Interventions to optimize circulation of blood and fluids to the tissue	**O Behavior Therapy** Interventions to reinforce or promote desirable behaviors or alter undesirable behaviors **P Cognitive Therapy** Interventions to reinforce or promote desirable cognitive functioning or alter undesirable cognitive functioning **Q Communication Enhancement** Interventions to facilitate delivering and receiving verbal and nonverbal messages **R Coping Assistance** Interventions to assist another to build on own strengths, to adapt to a change in function, or achieve a higher level of function **S Patient Education** Interventions to facilitate learning **T Psychological Comfort Promotion** Interventions to promote comfort using psychological techniques

Domain 4	Domain 5	Domain 6	Domain 7
4. Safety Care that supports protection against harm	**5. Family** Care that supports the family	**6. Health System** Care that supports effective use of the health care delivery system	**7. Community** Care that supports the health of the community
U *Crisis Management* Interventions to provide immediate short-term help in both psychological and physiological crises V *Risk Management* Interventions to initiate risk reduction activities and continue monitoring risks over time	W *Childbearing Care* Interventions to assist in the preparation for childbirth and management of the psychological and physiological changes before, during, and immediately following childbirth Z *Childrearing Care* Interventions to assist in raising children X *Lifespan Care* Interventions to facilitate family unit functioning and promote the health and welfare of family members throughout the lifespan	Y *Health System Mediation* Interventions to facilitate the interface between patient/family and the health care system a *Health System Management* Interventions to provide and enhance support services for the delivery of care b *Information Management* Interventions to facilitate communication about health care	c *Community Health Promotion* Interventions that promote the health of the whole community d *Community Risk Management* Interventions that assist in detecting or preventing health risks to the whole community

Level 1 Domains	1. PHYSIOLOGICAL: BASIC Care that supports physical functioning		
Level 2 Classes	**A Activity and Exercise Management** Interventions to organize or assist with physical activity and energy conservation and expenditure	**B Elimination Management** Interventions to establish and maintain regular bowel and urinary elimination patterns and manage complications due to altered patterns	**C Immobility Management** Interventions to manage restricted body movement and the sequelae
Level 3 Interventions	0140 Body Mechanics Promotion 0180 Energy Management 0200 Exercise Promotion 0201 Exercise Promotion: Strength Training 0202 Exercise Promotion: Stretching 0221 Exercise Therapy: Ambulation 0222 Exercise Therapy: Balance 0224 Exercise Therapy: Joint Mobility 0226 Exercise Therapy: Muscle Control 5612 Teaching: Prescribed Exercise **S***	0550 Bladder Irrigation 0410 Bowel Incontinence Care 0412 Bowel Incontinence Care: Encopresis **Z** 0430 Bowel Management 0440 Bowel Training 0450 Constipation/Impaction Management 0460 Diarrhea Management 0466 Enema Administration 0470 Flatulence Reduction 0480 Ostomy Care **L** 0490 Rectal Prolapse Management 0560 Pelvic Muscle Exercise 0630 Pessary Management 0640 Prompted Voiding 1804 Self-Care Assistance: Toileting **F** 1876 Tube Care: Urinary 0570 Urinary Bladder Training 0580 Urinary Catheterization 0582 Urinary Catheterization: Intermittent 0590 Urinary Elimination Management 0600 Urinary Habit Training 0610 Urinary Incontinence Care 0612 Urinary Incontinence Care: Enuresis **Z** 0620 Urinary Retention Care	0740 Bed Rest Care 0762 Cast Care: Maintenance 0764 Cast Care: Wet 6580 Physical Restraint **V** 0840 Positioning 0846 Positioning: Wheelchair 1806 Self-Care Assistance: Transfer **F** 0910 Splinting 0940 Traction/Immobilization Care 0970 Transfer
	0100 to 0399	**0400 to 0699**	**0700 to 0999**

* Letter indicates another class where the intervention is also included.

D Nutrition Support
Interventions to modify or maintain nutritional status

1020 Diet Staging
1024 Diet Staging: Weight Loss Surgery
1030 Eating Disorders Management
1056 Enteral Tube Feeding
1050 Feeding **F**
1080 Gastrointestinal Intubation
1100 Nutrition Management
1120 Nutrition Therapy
5246 Nutritional Counseling
1160 Nutritional Monitoring
1803 Self-Care Assistance: Feeding **F**
1860 Swallowing Therapy **F**
5614 Teaching: Prescribed Diet S
1200 Total Parenteral Nutrition (TPN) Administration **G**
1874 Tube Care: Gastrointestinal
1240 Weight Gain Assistance
1260 Weight Management
1280 Weight Reduction Assistance

1000 to 1299

E Physical Comfort Promotion
Interventions to promote comfort using physical techniques

1320 Acupressure
1330 Aromatherapy
1340 Cutaneous Stimulation
1350 Dry Eye Prevention
6482 Environmental Management: Comfort
1380 Heat/Cold Application
1390 Healing Touch
1480 Massage
1450 Nausea Management
1400 Pain Management
1440 Premenstrual Syndrome (PMS) Management
1460 Progressive Muscle Relaxation
3550 Pruritus Management **L**
1520 Reiki
5465 Therapeutic Touch
1540 Transcutaneous Electrical Nerve Stimulation (TENS)
1570 Vomiting Management

1300 to 1599

F Self-Care Facilitation
Interventions to provide or assist with routine activities of daily living

1610 Bathing
1620 Contact Lens Care
6462 Dementia Management: Bathing **V**
1630 Dressing
1640 Ear Care
1650 Eye Care
1050 Feeding **D**
1660 Foot Care
1670 Hair and Scalp Care
1680 Nail Care
1710 Oral Health Maintenance
1720 Oral Health Promotion
1730 Oral Health Restoration
1750 Perineal Care
1770 Postmortem Care
1800 Self-Care Assistance
1801 Self-Care Assistance: Bathing/Hygiene
1802 Self-Care Assistance: Dressing/Grooming
1803 Self-Care Assistance: Feeding **D**
1805 Self-Care Assistance: IADL
1804 Self-Care Assistance: Toileting **B**
1806 Self-Care Assistance: Transfer **C**
1850 Sleep Enhancement
1860 Swallowing Therapy **D**
5603 Teaching: Foot Care **S**
1870 Tube Care

1600 to 1899

Level 1 Domains	2. PHYSIOLOGICAL: COMPLEX Care that supports homeostatic regulation		
Level 2 Classes	**G. Electrolyte and Acid-Base Management** Interventions to regulate electrolyte/acid base balance and prevent complications	**H Drug Management** Interventions to facilitate desired effects of pharmacological agents	
Level 3 Interventions	1910 Acid-Base Management 1911 Acid-Base Management: Metabolic Acidosis 1912 Acid-Base Management: Metabolic Alkalosis 1913 Acid-Base Management: Respiratory Acidosis **K*** 1914 Acid-Base Management: Respiratory Alkalosis **K** 1920 Acid-Base Monitoring 2000 Electrolyte Management 2001 Electrolyte Management: Hypercalcemia 2002 Electrolyte Management: Hyperkalemia 2003 Electrolyte Management: Hypermagnesemia 2004 Electrolyte Management: Hypernatremia 2005 Electrolyte Management: Hyperphosphatemia 2006 Electrolyte Management: Hypocalcemia 2007 Electrolyte Management: Hypokalemia 2008 Electrolyte Management: Hypomagnesemia 2009 Electrolyte Management: Hyponatremia 2010 Electrolyte Management: Hypophosphatemia 2020 Electrolyte Monitoring 2080 Fluid/Electrolyte Management **N** 2100 Hemodialysis Therapy 2110 Hemofiltration Therapy 2120 Hyperglycemia Management 2130 Hypoglycemia Management 2150 Peritoneal Dialysis Therapy 4232 Phlebotomy: Arterial Blood Sample **N** 1200 Total Parenteral Nutrition (TPN) Administration **D**	2210 Analgesic Administration 2214 Analgesic Administration: Intraspinal 2840 Anesthesia Administration **J** 4054 Central Venous Access Device Management **N** 6430 Chemical Restraint **V** 2240 Chemotherapy Management **S** 2280 Hormone Replacement Therapy 2300 Medication Administration 2308 Medication Administration: Ear 2301 Medication Administration: Enteral 2310 Medication Administration: Eye 2311 Medication Administration: Inhalation 2302 Medication Administration: Interpleural 2312 Medication Administration: Intradermal 2313 Medication Administration: Intramuscular (IM) 2303 Medication Administration: Intraosseous 2319 Medication Administration: Intraspinal 2314 Medication Administration: Intravenous (IV)	2320 Medication Administration: Nasal 2304 Medication Administration: Oral 2315 Medication Administration: Rectal 2316 Medication Administration: Skin 2317 Medication Administration: Subcutaneous 2318 Medication Administration: Vaginal 2307 Medication Administration: Ventricular Reservoir 2380 Medication Management 2390 Medication Prescribing 2395 Medication Reconciliation **V** 2400 Patient-Controlled Analgesia (PCA) Assistance 2260 Sedation Management 5616 Teaching: Prescribed Medication **S** 4270 Thrombolytic Therapy Management **N**
	1900 to 2199	**2200 to 2499**	

* Letter indicates another class where the intervention is also included.

I. Neurologic Management
Interventions to optimize neurologic function

2540 Cerebral Edema Management
2550 Cerebral Perfusion Promotion
2560 Dysreflexia Management
2570 Electroconvulsive Therapy (ECT) Management
2590 Intracranial Pressure (ICP) Monitoring
2620 Neurologic Monitoring
2660 Peripheral Sensation
    Management
0844 Positioning: Neurologic
2680 Seizure Management **V**
2690 Seizure Precautions
2720 Subarachnoid Hemorrhage
    Precautions
1878 Tube Care: Ventriculostomy/Lumbar Drain
2760 Unilateral Neglect Management

J. Perioperative Care
Interventions to provide care before, during, and
  immediately after surgery

2840 Anesthesia Administration **H**
2860 Autotransfusion **N**
3000 Circumcision Care **W**
6545 Infection Control: Intraoperative
0842 Positioning: Intraoperative
2870 Postanesthesia Care
2880 Preoperative Coordination **Y**
3582 Skin Care: Donor Site **L**
3583 Skin Care: Graft Site **L**
2900 Surgical Assistance
2910 Surgical Instrumentation Management
2920 Surgical Precautions **V**
2930 Surgical Preparation
5610 Teaching: Preoperative **S**
3902 Temperature Regulation:
    Perioperative **M**

2500 to 2799 **2800 to 3099**

Level 1 Domains

2. PHYSIOLOGICAL: COMPLEX—CONT'D
Care that supports homeostatic regulation

Level 2 Classes

K. **Respiratory Management**	L. **Skin/Wound Management**
Interventions to promote airway patency and gas exchange	Interventions to maintain or restore tissue integrity

Level 3 Interventions

K	L
1913 Acid-Base Management: Respiratory Acidosis **G***	3420 Amputation Care
1914 Acid-Base Management: Respiratory Alkalosis **G**	3440 Incision Site Care
3120 Airway Insertion and Stabilization	3460 Leech Therapy
3140 Airway Management	3480 Lower Extremity Monitoring
3160 Airway Suctioning	0480 Ostomy Care **B**
6412 Anaphylaxis Management **V**	3500 Pressure Management
3180 Artificial Airway Management	3520 Pressure Ulcer Care
3200 Aspiration Precautions **V**	3540 Pressure Ulcer Prevention **V**
3210 Asthma Management	3550 Pruritus Management **E**
3230 Chest Physiotherapy	3582 Skin Care: Donor Site **J**
3250 Cough Enhancement	3583 Skin Care: Graft Site **J**
4106 Embolus Care: Pulmonary **N**	3584 Skin Care: Topical Treatments
3270 Endotracheal Extubation	3590 Skin Surveillance
3300 Mechanical Ventilation Management: Invasive	3620 Suturing
3302 Mechanical Ventilation Management: Noninvasive	3660 Wound Care
3304 Mechanical Ventilation Management: Pneumonia Prevention **V**	3661 Wound Care: Burns
3310 Mechanical Ventilatory Weaning	3662 Wound Care: Closed Drainage
3316 Nasal Irrigation	3664 Wound Care: Nonhealing
3320 Oxygen Therapy	3680 Wound Irrigation
3350 Respiratory Monitoring	
1872 Tube Care: Chest	
3390 Ventilation Assistance	

3100 to 3399   **3400 to 3699**

* Letter indicates another class where the intervention is also included.

M. Thermoregulation

Interventions to maintain body temperature within a normal range

3740 Fever Treatment
3786 Hyperthermia Treatment
3790 Hypothermia Induction Therapy
3800 Hypothermia Treatment
3840 Malignant Hyperthermia Precautions **U**
3900 Temperature Regulation
3902 Temperature Regulation: Perioperative **J**

N. Tissue Perfusion Management

Interventions to optimize circulation of blood and fluids to the tissue

2860 Autotransfusion **J**
4010 Bleeding Precautions
4020 Bleeding Reduction
4021 Bleeding Reduction: Antepartum Uterus **W**
4022 Bleeding Reduction: Gastrointestinal
4024 Bleeding Reduction: Nasal
4026 Bleeding Reduction: Postpartum Uterus **W**
4028 Bleeding Reduction: Wound
4030 Blood Products Administration
4035 Capillary Blood Sample
4040 Cardiac Care
4044 Cardiac Care: Acute
4046 Cardiac Care: Rehabilitative
4050 Cardiac Risk Management
4054 Central Venous Access Device Management **H**
4062 Circulatory Care: Arterial Insufficiency
4064 Circulatory Care: Mechanical Assist Device
4066 Circulatory Care: Venous Insufficiency
4070 Circulatory Precautions
4095 Defibrillator Management: External **U**
4096 Defibrillator Management: Internal
4240 Dialysis Access Maintenance
4090 Dysrhythmia Management
4104 Embolus Care: Peripheral
4106 Embolus Care: Pulmonary **K**
4110 Embolus Precautions
2080 Fluid/Electrolyte Management **G**

4120 Fluid Management
4130 Fluid Monitoring
4140 Fluid Resuscitation
4150 Hemodynamic Regulation
4170 Hypervolemia Management
4180 Hypovolemia Management
4190 Intravenous (IV) Insertion
4200 Intravenous (IV) Therapy
4210 Invasive Hemodynamic Monitoring
4091 Pacemaker Management: Permanent
4092 Pacemaker Management: Temporary
4220 Peripherally Inserted Central Catheter (PICC) Care
4232 Phlebotomy: Arterial Blood Sample **G**
4234 Phlebotomy: Blood Unit Acquisition
4235 Phlebotomy: Cannulated Vessel
4238 Phlebotomy: Venous Blood Sample
4250 Shock Management
4254 Shock Management: Cardiac
4256 Shock Management: Vasogenic
4258 Shock Management: Volume
4260 Shock Prevention
4266 Stem Cell Infusion
4270 Thrombolytic Therapy Management **H**

*Level 1
Domains*

*Level 2
Classes*

*Level 3
Interventions*

3. BEHAVIORAL
Care that supports psychosocial functioning and facilitates life style changes

O. Behavior Therapy	P. Cognitive Therapy
Interventions to reinforce or promote desirable behaviors or alter undesirable behaviors	Interventions to reinforce or promote desirable cognitive functioning or alter undesirable cognitive functioning

O. Behavior Therapy

4310 Activity Therapy
4320 Animal-Assisted Therapy **Q***
4330 Art Therapy **Q**
4340 Assertiveness Training
4350 Behavior Management
4352 Behavior Management: Overactivity/
    Inattention
4354 Behavior Management: Self-Harm
4356 Behavior Management: Sexual
4360 Behavior Modification
4362 Behavior Modification: Social Skills
4364 Commendation
4370 Impulse Control Training
4380 Limit Setting
4390 Milieu Therapy
4400 Music Therapy **Q**
4410 Mutual Goal Setting
4420 Patient Contracting
6926 Phototherapy: Mood/Sleep Regulation
4470 Self-Modification Assistance
4480 Self-Responsibility Facilitation
4490 Smoking Cessation Assistance
4500 Substance Use Prevention
4510 Substance Use Treatment
4512 Substance Use Treatment: Alcohol
    Withdrawal
4514 Substance Use Treatment: Drug
    Withdrawal
4516 Substance Use Treatment: Overdose
4430 Therapeutic Play **Q**

P. Cognitive Therapy

4640 Anger Control Assistance
4680 Bibliotherapy
4700 Cognitive Restructuring
4720 Cognitive Stimulation
4740 Journaling
5520 Learning Facilitation **S**
5540 Learning Readiness Enhancement **S**
4760 Memory Training
4820 Reality Orientation
4860 Reminiscence Therapy

4300 to 4599   **4600 to 4899**

* Letter indicates another class where the intervention is also included.

Q. Communication Enhancement
Interventions to facilitate delivering and receiving
verbal and nonverbal messages

4920 Active Listening
4320 Animal-Assisted Therapy **O**
4330 Art Therapy **O**
4974 Communication Enhancement: Hearing Deficit
4976 Communication Enhancement: Speech Deficit
4978 Communication Enhancement: Visual Deficit
5000 Complex Relationship Building
5020 Conflict Mediation
5328 Listening Visits **R**
4400 Music Therapy **O**
5100 Socialization Enhancement
4430 Therapeutic Play **O**

Level 1 Domains	3. BEHAVIORAL—CONT'D Care that supports psychosocial functioning and facilitates life style changes	
Level 2 Classes	**R. Coping Assistance** Interventions to assist another to build on own strengths, to adapt to a change in function, or achieve a higher level of function	**S. Patient Education** Interventions to facilitate learning
Level 3 Interventions	5210 Anticipatory Guidance **Z** 5220 Body Image Enhancement 5230 Coping Enhancement 5240 Counseling 6160 Crisis Intervention **U** 5250 Decision-Making Support **Y** 5260 Dying Care 5270 Emotional Support 5280 Forgiveness Facilitation 5242 Genetic Counseling **W** 5290 Grief Work Facilitation 5294 Grief Work Facilitation: Perinatal Death **W** 5300 Guilt Work Facilitation 5310 Hope Inspiration 5320 Humor 5326 Life Skills Enhancement 5328 Listening Visits **Q** 5330 Mood Management 5340 Presence 5360 Recreation Therapy 5422 Religious Addiction Prevention 5424 Religious Ritual Enhancement 5350 Relocation Stress Reduction 5370 Role Enhancement **X** 5380 Security Enhancement 5390 Self-Awareness Enhancement 5395 Self-Efficacy Enhancement 5400 Self-Esteem Enhancement 5248 Sexual Counseling 5426 Spiritual Growth Facilitation 5420 Spiritual Support 5430 Support Group 5440 Support System Enhancement 5450 Therapy Group 5460 Touch 5410 Trauma Therapy: Child 5470 Truth Telling 5480 Values Clarification	2240 Chemotherapy Management **H** 6784 Family Planning: Contraception **W** 5510 Health Education **c** 5515 Health Literacy Enhancement 5520 Learning Facilitation **P** 5540 Learning Readiness Enhancement **P** 5562 Parent Education: Adolescent **Z** 5566 Parent Education: Childrearing Family **Z** 5568 Parent Education: Infant **Z** 5580 Preparatory Sensory Information 5602 Teaching: Disease Process 5603 Teaching: Foot Care **F** 5604 Teaching: Group 5606 Teaching: Individual 5640 Teaching: Infant Nutrition 0–3 Months **Z** 5641 Teaching: Infant Nutrition 4–6 Months **Z** 5642 Teaching: Infant Nutrition 7–9 Months **Z** 5643 Teaching: Infant Nutrition 10–12 Months **Z** 5645 Teaching: Infant Safety 0-3 Months **Z** 5646 Teaching: Infant Safety 4–6 Months **Z** 5647 Teaching: Infant Safety 7-9 Months **Z** 5648 Teaching: Infant Safety 10-12 Months **Z** 5655 Teaching: Infant Stimulation 0-4 Months **Z** 5656 Teaching: Infant Stimulation 5-8 Months **Z** 5657 Teaching: Infant Stimulation 9-12 Months **Z** 5610 Teaching: Preoperative **J** 5614 Teaching: Prescribed Diet **D** 5612 Teaching: Prescribed Exercise **A** 5616 Teaching: Prescribed Medication **H** 5618 Teaching: Procedure/Treatment 5620 Teaching: Psychomotor Skill 5622 Teaching: Safe Sex 5624 Teaching: Sexuality 5660 Teaching: Toddler Nutrition 13–18 Months **Z** 5661 Teaching: Toddler Nutrition 19–24 Months **Z** 5662 Teaching: Toddler Nutrition 25–36 Months **Z** 5665 Teaching: Toddler Safety 13–18 Months **Z** 5666 Teaching: Toddler Safety 19–24 Months **Z** 5667 Teaching: Toddler Safety 25–36 Months **Z** 5634 Teaching: Toilet Training **Z**
	5200 to 5499	**5500 to 5799**

* Letter indicates another class where the intervention is also included.

T. Psychological Comfort Promotion
Interventions to promote comfort using psychological techniques

5820 Anxiety Reduction
5840 Autogenic Training
5860 Biofeedback
5880 Calming Technique
5900 Distraction
6000 Guided Imagery
5920 Hypnosis
5960 Meditation Facilitation
6040 Relaxation Therapy
5922 Self-Hypnosis Facilitation

Level 1
Domains

4. SAFETY
Care that supports protection against harm

Level 2
Classes

U. Crisis Management
Interventions to provide immediate short-term help in both psychological and physiological crises

Level 3
Interventions

6140 Code Management
6160 Crisis Intervention **R***
4095 Defibrillator Management: External **N**
6200 Emergency Care
7170 Family Presence Facilitation **X**
6240 First Aid
3840 Malignant Hyperthermia Precautions **M**
6260 Organ Procurement
6300 Rape-Trauma Treatment
6320 Resuscitation
6340 Suicide Prevention **V**
6362 Triage: Disaster
6364 Triage: Emergency Center
6366 Triage: Telephone

6100 to 6399

* Letter indicates another class where the intervention is also included.

V. Risk Management
Interventions to initiate risk reduction activities and continue monitoring risks over time

6400 Abuse Protection Support
6402 Abuse Protection Support: Child **Z**
6403 Abuse Protection Support: Domestic Partner
6404 Abuse Protection Support: Elder
6408 Abuse Protection Support: Religious
6410 Allergy Management
6412 Anaphylaxis Management **K**
6420 Area Restriction
3200 Aspiration Precautions **K**
6522 Breast Examination
6430 Chemical Restraint **H**
6440 Delirium Management
6450 Delusion Management
6460 Dementia Management
6462 Dementia Management: Bathing **F**
6466 Dementia Management: Wandering
6470 Elopement Precautions
6480 Environmental Management
6486 Environmental Management: Safety
6487 Environmental Management: Violence Prevention
6490 Fall Prevention
6500 Fire-Setting Precautions
6510 Hallucination Management
6520 Health Screening **d**
6530 Immunization/Vaccination Management **c**
6540 Infection Control
6550 Infection Protection
6560 Laser Precautions
6570 Latex Precautions
3304 Mechanical Ventilation Management: Pneumonia Prevention **K**
2395 Medication Reconciliation **H**
6574 Patient Identification
6580 Physical Restraint **C**
6590 Pneumatic Tourniquet Precautions
3540 Pressure Ulcer Prevention **L**
6600 Radiation Therapy Management
6610 Risk Identification **d**
6630 Seclusion
2680 Seizure Management **I**
6648 Sports-Injury Prevention: Youth **Z**
6340 Suicide Prevention **U**
2920 Surgical Precautions **J**
6650 Surveillance
6670 Validation Therapy
9050 Vehicle Safety Promotion **d**
6680 Vital Signs Monitoring

Level 1
Domains

Level 2
Classes

Level 3
Interventions

5. FAMILY
Care that supports the family

W. Childbearing Care
Interventions to assist in the preparation for childbirth and management of the psychological and physiological changes before, during, and immediately following childbirth

6700 Amnioinfusion
6720 Birthing
4021 Bleeding Reduction: Antepartum Uterus **N***
4026 Bleeding Reduction: Postpartum Uterus **N**
6750 Cesarean Birth Care
6760 Childbirth Preparation
3000 Circumcision Care **J**
6771 Electronic Fetal Monitoring: Antepartum
6772 Electronic Fetal Monitoring: Intrapartum
7104 Family Integrity Promotion: Childbearing Family
6784 Family Planning: Contraception **S**
6786 Family Planning: Infertility
6788 Family Planning: Unplanned Pregnancy
7160 Fertility Preservation
5242 Genetic Counseling **R**
5294 Grief Work Facilitation: Perinatal Death **R**
6800 High-Risk Pregnancy Care
6824 Infant Care: Newborn
6826 Infant Care: Preterm
6830 Intrapartal Care
6834 Intrapartal Care: High-Risk Delivery
6840 Kangaroo Care
6850 Labor Induction
6860 Labor Suppression
6870 Lactation Suppression
6900 Nonnutritive Sucking
6924 Phototherapy: Neonate
6930 Postpartal Care
5247 Preconception Counseling
6950 Pregnancy Termination Care
6960 Prenatal Care
7886 Reproductive Technology Management
6972 Resuscitation: Fetus
6974 Resuscitation: Neonate
6612 Risk Identification: Childbearing Family
6656 Surveillance: Late Pregnancy
1875 Tube Care: Umbilical Line
6982 Ultrasonography: Limited Obstetric

6700 to 6999

*Letter indicates another class where the intervention is also included.

Z. Childrearing Care
Interventions to assist in raising children

6402 Abuse Protection Support: Child **V**
5210 Anticipatory Guidance **R**
6710 Attachment Promotion
1052 Bottle Feeding
0412 Bowel Incontinence Care: Encopresis **B**
8240 Cup Feeding: Newborn
8272 Developmental Enhancement: Adolescent
8274 Developmental Enhancement: Child
8278 Developmental Enhancement: Infant
6820 Infant Care
5244 Lactation Counseling
7200 Normalization Promotion
5562 Parent Education: Adolescent **S**
5566 Parent Education: Childrearing Family **S**
5568 Parent Education: Infant **S**
8300 Parenting Promotion
8340 Resiliency Promotion
7280 Sibling Support
6648 Sports-Injury Prevention: Youth **V**
5640 Teaching: Infant Nutrition 0–3 Months **S**
5641 Teaching: Infant Nutrition 4–6 Months **S**
5642 Teaching: Infant Nutrition 7–9 Months **S**
5643 Teaching: Infant Nutrition 10–12 Months **S**
5645 Teaching: Infant Safety 0-3 Months **S**
5646 Teaching: Infant Safety 4–6 Months **S**
5647 Teaching: Infant Safety 7-9 Months **S**
5648 Teaching: Infant Safety 10-12 Months **S**
5655 Teaching: Infant Stimulation 0-4 Months **S**
5656 Teaching: Infant Stimulation 5-8 Months **S**
5657 Teaching: Infant Stimulation 9-12 Months **S**
5660 Teaching: Toddler Nutrition 13–18 Months **S**
5661 Teaching: Toddler Nutrition 19–24 Months **S**
5662 Teaching: Toddler Nutrition 25–36 Months **S**
5665 Teaching: Toddler Safety 13–18 Months **S**
5666 Teaching: Toddler Safety 19–24 Months **S**
5667 Teaching: Toddler Safety 25–36 Months **S**
5634 Teaching: Toilet Training **S**
0612 Urinary Incontinence Care: Enuresis **B**

X. Lifespan Care
Interventions to facilitate family unit functioning and promote the health and welfare of family members throughout the lifespan

7040 Caregiver Support
7100 Family Integrity Promotion
7110 Family Involvement Promotion
7120 Family Mobilization
7170 Family Presence Facilitation **U**
7130 Family Process Maintenance
7140 Family Support
7150 Family Therapy
7180 Home Maintenance Assistance
7260 Respite Care
6614 Risk Identification: Genetic
5370 Role Enhancement **R**

*Level 1
Domains*

6. HEALTH SYSTEM
Care that supports effective use of the health care delivery system

*Level 2
Classes*

Y. Health System Mediation
Interventions to facilitate the interface between patient/family and the health care system

*Level 3
Interventions*

7310 Admission Care
7320 Case Management **c***
7330 Culture Brokerage
5250 Decision-Making Support **R**
7370 Discharge Planning
6485 Environmental Management: Home Preparation
7380 Financial Resource Assistance
7400 Health System Guidance
7410 Insurance Authorization
7440 Pass Facilitation
7460 Patient Rights Protection
2880 Preoperative Coordination **J**
7500 Sustenance Support
7560 Visitation Facilitation

a. Health System Management
Interventions to provide and enhance support services for the delivery of care

7610 Bedside Laboratory Testing
7620 Controlled Substance Checking
7630 Cost Containment
7640 Critical Path Development
7650 Delegation
7660 Emergency Cart Checking
7680 Examination Assistance
8550 Fiscal Resource Management **c**
7690 Laboratory Data Interpretation
7700 Peer Review
7710 Physician Support
7722 Preceptor: Employee
7726 Preceptor: Student
7760 Product Evaluation
7800 Quality Monitoring
7820 Specimen Management
7850 Staff Development
7830 Staff Supervision
7840 Supply Management
7880 Technology Management
7890 Transport: Interfacility
7892 Transport: Intrafacility

b. Information Management
Interventions to facilitate communication about health care

7910 Consultation
7930 Deposition/Testimony
7920 Documentation
7940 Forensic Data Collection
7960 Health Care Information Exchange
7970 Health Policy Monitoring **c**
7980 Incident Reporting
8020 Multidisciplinary Care Conference
8060 Order Transcription
8080 Prescribing: Diagnostic Testing
8086 Prescribing: Non-Pharmalogic Treatment
8100 Referral
8120 Research Data Collection
8140 Shift Report
6658 Surveillance: Remote Electronic
8180 Telephone Consultation
8190 Telephone Follow-Up

Level 1
Domains

7. COMMUNITY
Care that supports the health of the community

Level 2
Classes

c. Community Health Promotion
Interventions that promote the health of the whole community

Level 3
Interventions

7320 Case Management **Y***
8500 Community Health Development
8550 Fiscal Resource Management **a**
5510 Health Education **S**
7970 Health Policy Monitoring **b**
6530 Immunization/Vaccination Management **V**
8700 Program Development
8750 Social Marketing

8500-8799

*Letter indicates another class where the intervention is also included.

d. Community Risk Management
Interventions that assist in detecting or preventing health risks to the whole community

8810 Bioterrorism Preparedness
8820 Communicable Disease Management
8840 Community Disaster Preparedness
6484 Environmental Management: Community
6489 Environmental Management: Worker Safety
8880 Environmental Risk Protection
6520 Health Screening **V**
6610 Risk Identification **V**
6652 Surveillance: Community
9050 Vehicle Safety Promotion **V**

PART THREE

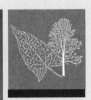

The Classification

A

Abuse Protection Support   6400

Definition: Identification of high-risk dependent relationships and actions to prevent further infliction of physical or emotional harm

Activities:
- Identify adult(s) with a history of unhappy childhoods associated with abuse, rejection, excessive criticism, or feelings of being worthless and unloved as children
- Identify adult(s) who have difficulty trusting others or feel disliked by others
- Identify whether individual feels asking for help is an indication of personal incompetence
- Identify level of social isolation present in family situation
- Determine whether family needs periodic relief from care responsibilities
- Identify whether adult at risk has close friends or family available to help with children, when needed
- Determine relationship between husband and wife
- Determine whether adults are able to take over for each other when one is too tense, tired, or angry to deal with a dependent family member
- Determine whether child/dependent adult is viewed differently by an adult based on sex, appearance, or behavior
- Identify crisis situations that may trigger abuse, such as poverty, unemployment, divorce, or death of a loved one
- Monitor for signs of neglect in high-risk families
- Observe a sick or injured child/dependent adult for signs of abuse
- Listen to the explanation of how the illness or injury happened
- Identify when the explanation of the cause of the injury is inconsistent between those involved
- Encourage admission of child/dependent adult for further observation and investigation, as appropriate
- Record times and duration of visits during hospitalization
- Monitor parent-child interactions and record observations, as appropriate
- Monitor for underreactions or overreactions on the part of an adult
- Monitor child/dependent adult for extreme compliance, such as passive submission to hospital procedures
- Monitor child for role reversal, such as comforting the parent, or overactive or aggressive behavior
- Listen attentively to adult who begins to talk about own problems
- Listen to pregnant woman's feelings about pregnancy and expectations about the unborn child
- Monitor new parent's reactions to infant, observing for feelings of disgust, fear, or unrealistic expectations
- Monitor for a parent who holds newborn at arm's length, handles him/her awkwardly, or asks for excessive assistance
- Monitor for repeated visits to a clinic, emergency room, or physician's office for minor problems
- Monitor for a progressive deterioration in the physical and emotional care provided to a child/dependent adult in the family
- Monitor child for signs of failure to thrive, depression, apathy, developmental delay, or malnutrition
- Determine expectations adult has for child to determine if expected behaviors are realistic
- Instruct parents on realistic expectations of child based on developmental level
- Establish rapport with families with a history of abuse for long-term evaluation and support
- Help families identify coping strategies for stressful situations
- Instruct adult family members on signs of abuse
- Refer adult(s) at risk to appropriate specialists
- Inform the physician of observations indicative of abuse
- Report any situations where abuse is suspected to the proper authorities
- Refer adult(s) to shelters for abused spouses, as appropriate
- Refer parents to Parents Anonymous for group support, as appropriate
- Encourage patient to contact police when physical safety is threatened
- Inform patient of laws and services relevant to abuse

1st edition 1992; revised 2000, 2004

Background Readings:

Bohn, D. K. (1990). Domestic violence and pregnancy: Implications for practice. *Journal of Nurse-Midwifery, 35*(2), 86–98.

Boyd, M. R. (2005). Caring for abused persons. In M. A. Boyd (Ed.), *Psychiatric nursing: Contemporary practice* (3rd ed., pp. 823–856). Philadelphia: Lippincott Williams & Wilkins.

Lancaster, J. & Kerschner, D. (1992). Violence and human abuse. In M. Stanhope, & J. Lancaster (Eds.), *Community health in nursing* (3rd ed., pp. 411–427). St. Louis: Mosby.

Roberts, C. & Quillan, J. (1992). Preventing violence through primary care intervention. *Nurse Practitioner, 17*(8), 62–70.

Vickrey, P. G. (2001). Protecting the older adult. *Nursing Management, 30*(7), 34–38.

Abuse Protection Support: Child   6402

Definition: Identification of high-risk, dependent child relationships and actions to prevent possible or further infliction of physical, sexual, or emotional harm or neglect of basic necessities of life

Activities:
- Identify mothers who have a history of no or late (4 months or later) prenatal care
- Identify parents who have had another child removed from the home or have placed previous children with relatives for extended periods
- Identify parents who have a history of substance abuse, depression, or major psychiatric illness
- Identify parents who demonstrate an increased need for parent education (e.g., parents with learning problems, parents who verbalize feelings of inadequacy, parents of a first child, teen parents)

- Identify parents with a history of domestic violence or a mother who has a history of numerous "accidental" injuries
- Identify parents with a history of unhappy childhoods associated with abuse, rejection, excessive criticism, or feelings of being worthless and unloved
- Identify crisis situations that may trigger abuse (e.g., poverty, unemployment, divorce, homelessness, domestic violence)
- Determine whether the family has an intact social support network to assist with family problems, respite child care, and crisis child care
- Identify infants and children with high-care needs (e.g., prematurity, low birth weight, colic, feeding intolerances, major health problems in the first year of life, developmental disabilities, hyperactivity, attention deficit disorders)
- Identify caretaker explanations of child's injuries that are improbable or inconsistent, allege self-injury, blame other children, or demonstrate a delay in seeking treatment
- Determine whether a child demonstrates signs of physical abuse (e.g., numerous injuries, unexplained bruises and welts, burns, fractures, unexplained facial lacerations and abrasions, human bite marks, whiplash, shaken infant syndrome)
- Determine whether the child demonstrates signs of neglect (e.g., failure to thrive, wasting of subcutaneous tissue, consistent hunger, poor hygiene, constant fatigue and listlessness, skin afflictions, apathy, unyielding body posture, inappropriate dress for weather conditions)
- Determine whether the child demonstrates signs of sexual abuse (e.g., difficulty walking or sitting, torn or bloody underclothing, reddened or traumatized genitals, vaginal or anal lacerations, recurrent urinary tract infections, poor sphincter tone, acquired sexually transmitted diseases, pregnancy, promiscuous behavior, history of running away)
- Determine whether the child demonstrates signs of emotional abuse (e.g., lags in physical development, habit disorders, conduct learning disorders, neurotic traits or psychoneurotic reactions, behavioral extremes, cognitive developmental lags, attempted suicide)
- Encourage admission of child for further observation and investigation, as appropriate
- Record times and durations of visits during hospitalizations
- Monitor parent-child interactions and record observations
- Determine whether acute symptoms in child abate when child is separated from family
- Determine whether parents have unrealistic expectations or negative attributions for their child's behavior
- Monitor child for extreme compliance, such as passive submission to invasive procedures
- Monitor child for role reversal, such as comforting the parent, or overactive or aggressive behavior
- Listen to pregnant woman's feelings about pregnancy and expectations about the unborn child
- Monitor new parents' reactions to their infant, observing for feelings of disgust, fear, or disappointment in gender
- Monitor for a parent who holds newborn at arm's length, handles newborn awkwardly, asks for excessive assistance, and verbalizes or demonstrates discomfort in caring for the child
- Monitor for repeated visits to clinics, emergency rooms, or physicians' offices for minor problems
- Establish a system to flag the records of children who are suspected victims of child abuse or neglect
- Monitor for a progressive deterioration in the physical and emotional state of the infant or child
- Determine parent's knowledge of basic care needs and provide appropriate child care information, as indicated

- Instruct parents on problem solving, decision making, and childrearing and parenting skills, or refer parents to programs where these skills can be learned
- Help families identify coping strategies for stressful situations
- Provide parents with information on how to cope with protracted infant crying, emphasizing that they should not shake the baby
- Provide the parents with noncorporal punishment methods for disciplining children
- Provide pregnant women and their families with information on the effects of smoking, poor nutrition, and substance abuse on the baby's and their health
- Engage parents and child in attachment-building exercises
- Provide parents and their adolescents with information on decision-making and communication skills and refer to youth services counseling, as appropriate
- Provide older children with concrete information on how to provide for the basic care needs of their younger siblings
- Provide children with positive affirmations of their worth, nurturing care, therapeutic communication, and developmental stimulation
- Provide children who have been sexually abused with reassurance that the abuse was not their fault and allow them to express their concerns through play therapy appropriate for age
- Refer at-risk pregnant women and parents of newborns to nurse home visitation services
- Provide at-risk families with a Public Health Nurse referral to ensure that the home environment is monitored, that siblings are assessed, and that families receive continued assistance
- Refer families to human services and counseling professionals, as needed
- Provide parents with community resource information (e.g., addresses and phone numbers of agencies that provide respite care, emergency child care, housing assistance, substance abuse treatment, sliding-fee counseling services, food pantries, clothing distribution centers, domestic abuse shelters)
- Inform physician of observations indicative of abuse or neglect
- Report suspected abuse or neglect to proper authorities
- Refer a parent who is being battered and at-risk children to a domestic violence shelter
- Refer parents to Parents Anonymous for group support, as appropriate

2nd edition 1996; revised 2000, 2013

Background Readings:

Asgeirsdottier, B. B., Sigfusdottir, I. D., Gudjonsson, G. H., & Sigurdsson, J. F. (2011). Associations between sexual abuse and family conflict/violence, self-injurious behavior, and substance use: The mediating role of depressed mood and anger. *Child Abuse and Neglect, 35*(3), 210–219.

Bylander, M. & Kydd, J. (2008). Violence to children, definition and prevention of. In L. Kurtz (Ed.), *Encyclopedia of violence, peace, and conflict* (2nd ed., pp. 2318–2330). St. Louis: Mosby.

Cowen, P. S. (2006). Child maltreatment: Developmental and health effects. In P. S. Cowen & S. Moorhead (Eds.), *Current issues in nursing* (7th ed., pp. 684–701). St. Louis: Mosby.

Cowen, P. S. (2006). Child neglect prevention: The pivotal role of nursing. In P. S. Cowen & S. Moorhead (Eds.), *Current issues in nursing* (7th ed., pp. 702–727). St. Louis: Mosby.

Dubowitz, H., Kim, J., Black, M. M., Weisbart, C., Semiatin, J., & Magder, L. S. (2011). Identifying children at high risk for a child maltreatment report. *Child Abuse and Neglect, 35*(2): 96–104.

Scannapieco, M. & Connell-Carrick, K. (2005). *Understanding child maltreatment: An ecological and developmental perspective.* New York: Oxford University Press.

Abuse Protection Support: Domestic Partner   6403

Definition: Identification of high-risk, dependent domestic relationships and actions to prevent possible or further infliction of physical, sexual, or emotional harm or exploitation of a domestic partner

Activities:
- Screen for risk factors associated with domestic abuse (e.g., history of domestic violence, abuse, rejection, excessive criticism, or feelings of being worthless and unloved; difficulty trusting others or feeling disliked by others; feeling that asking for help is an indication of personal incompetence; high physical care needs; intense family care responsibilities; substance abuse; depression; major psychiatric illness; social isolation; poor relationships between domestic partners; multiple marriages; pregnancy; poverty; unemployment; financial dependence; homelessness; infidelity; divorce; or death of a loved one)
- Screen for symptoms of a history of domestic abuse (e.g., numerous accidental injuries, multiple somatic symptoms, chronic abdominal pain, chronic headaches, pelvic pain, anxiety, depression, post-traumatic stress syndrome, and other psychiatric disorders)
- Monitor for signs and symptoms of physical abuse (e.g., numerous injuries in various stages of healing; unexplained lacerations, bruises, or welts; patches of missing hair; restraining marks on wrists or ankles; "defensive" bruises on forearms; human bite marks)
- Monitor for signs and symptoms of sexual abuse (e.g., presence of semen or dried blood, injury to external genital, acquired sexually transmitted diseases; or dramatic behavioral or health changes of an undetermined etiology)
- Monitor for signs and symptoms of emotional abuse (e.g., low self-esteem, depression, humiliation and defeat; overly cautious behavior around partner; aggression against self or suicidal gestures)
- Monitor for signs and symptoms of exploitation (e.g., inadequate provision for basic needs when adequate resources are available, deprivation of personal possessions, unexplained loss of social support checks, lack of knowledge of personal finances or legal matters)
- Document evidence of physical or sexual abuse using standardized assessment tools and photographs
- Listen attentively to individual who begins to talk about own problems
- Identify inconsistencies in explanation of cause of injury(ies)
- Determine congruence between the type of injury and the description of cause
- Interview patient or knowledgeable other about suspected abuse in the absence of partner
- Encourage admission to a hospital for further observation and investigation, as appropriate
- Monitor partner interactions and record observations, as appropriate (e.g., record times and duration of partner visits during hospitalization, under- or overreactions by partner)
- Monitor the individual for extreme compliance, such as passive submission to hospital procedures
- Monitor for progressive deterioration in the physical and emotional state of individuals
- Monitor for repeated visits to a clinic, emergency room, or physician's office for minor problems
- Establish a system to flag individual records where there is suspicion of abuse
- Provide positive affirmation of worth
- Encourage expression of concerns and feelings which may include fear, guilt, embarrassment, and self-blame
- Provide support to empower victims to take action and make changes to prevent further victimization
- Assist individuals and families in developing coping strategies for stressful situations
- Assist individuals and families to objectively evaluate strengths and weaknesses of relationships
- Refer individuals at risk for abuse or who have suffered abuse to appropriate specialists and services (e.g., public health nurse, human services, counseling, legal assistance)
- Refer abusive partner to appropriate specialists and services
- Provide confidential information regarding domestic violence shelters, as appropriate
- Initiate development of a safety plan for use in the event that violence escalates
- Report any situations where abuse is suspected in compliance with mandatory reporting laws
- Initiate community education programs designed to decrease violence
- Monitor use of community resources

3rd edition 2000; revised 2004, 2013

Background Readings:

Boursnell, M. & Prosser, S. (2010). Increasing identification of domestic violence in emergency departments: A collaborative contribution to increasing the quality of practice of emergency nurses. *Contemporary Nurse, 35*(1), 35–46.

Garcia-Moreno, C., Heise, L., Jansen, H., Ellsberg, M., & Watts, C. (2005). Violence against women. *Science, 310*(5752), 1282–1283.

Klein, A. R. (2009). *Practical implications of current domestic violence research: For law enforcement, prosecutors and judges.* Washington, DC: National Institute of Justice.

Pillitteri, A. (2007). *Maternal and child health nursing: Care of the childbearing and childrearing family* (5th ed.). Philadelphia: Lippincott Williams & Wilkins.

Smith, J. S., Rainey, S. L., Smith, K. R., Alamares, C., & Grogg, D. (2008). Barriers to the mandatory reporting of domestic violence encountered by nursing professionals. *Journal of Trauma Nursing, 15*(1), 9–11.

Taylor, J. Y. (2006). Care of African American women survivors of intimate partner violence. In P. S. Cowen & S. Moorhead (Eds.), *Current issues in nursing* (7th ed., pp. 727–731). St. Louis: Mosby.

Abuse Protection Support: Elder   6404

Definition: Identification of high-risk, dependent elder relationships and actions to prevent possible or further infliction of physical, sexual, or emotional harm; neglect of basic necessities of life; or exploitation

Activities:

- Identify elder patients who perceive themselves to be dependent on caretakers due to impaired health status, limited economic resources, depression, substance abuse, or lack of knowledge of available resources and alternatives for care
- Identify care arrangements that were made or continue under duress with only minimal consideration of the elder's care needs (e.g., the caregivers' abilities, characteristics, and competing responsibilities; need for environmental accommodations; and the history and quality of the relationships between the elder and the caregivers)
- Identify family crisis situations that may trigger abuse (e.g., poverty, unemployment, divorce, homelessness, death of a loved one)
- Determine whether the elder patient and their caretakers have a functional social support network to assist the patient in performing activities of daily living and in obtaining health care, transportation, therapy, medications, community resource information, financial advice, and assistance with personal problems
- Identify elder patients who rely on a single caretaker or family unit to provide extensive physical care assistance and monitoring
- Identify caretakers who demonstrate impaired physical or mental health (e.g., substance abuse, depression, fatigue, back injuries due to unassisted lifting, injuries that were inflicted by patient); financial problems or dependency; failure to understand patient's condition or needs; intolerant or hypercritical attitudes towards patient, burnout; or those who threaten patient with abandonment, hospitalization, institutionalization, or painful procedures
- Identify family caretakers who have a history of being abused or neglected in childhood
- Identify caretaker explanations of patient's injuries that are improbable, inconsistent, allege self injury, blame others, include activities beyond elder's physical abilities, or demonstrate a delay in seeking treatment
- Determine whether elder patient demonstrates signs of physical abuse (e.g., numerous injuries in various stages of healing, unexplained lacerations, abrasions, bruises, burns or fractures, patches of missing hair, human bite marks)
- Determine whether the elder patient demonstrates signs of neglect (e.g., poor hygiene, inadequate or inappropriate clothing, untreated skin lesions, contractures, malnutrition, inadequate aids to mobility and perception [canes, glasses, hearing aids], no dentures or decayed fractured teeth, vermin infestation, medication deprivation or oversedation, deprivation of social contacts)
- Determine whether the elder patient demonstrates signs of sexual abuse (e.g., presence of semen or dried blood, injury to external genital, acquired sexually transmitted diseases, dramatic behavioral or health changes of undetermined etiology)
- Determine whether the elder patient demonstrates signs of emotional abuse (e.g., low self esteem, depression, humiliation and defeat, overly cautious behavior around caretaker, aggression against self or suicidal gestures)
- Determine whether the elder patient demonstrates signs of exploitation (e.g., inadequate provision for basic needs when adequate resources are available, deprivation of personal possessions, unexplained loss of Social Security or pension checks, lack of knowledge of personal finances or legal matters)
- Encourage admission of patient for further observation and investigation, as appropriate
- Monitor patient-caretaker interactions and record observations
- Determine whether acute symptoms in patient abate when they are separated from caretakers
- Determine whether caretakers have unrealistic expectations for patient's behavior or if they have negative attributions for the behavior
- Monitor for extreme compliance to caretakers' demands or passive submission to invasive procedures
- Monitor for repeated visits to clinics, emergency rooms, or physicians' offices for injuries, inadequate health care monitoring, inadequate surveillance, or inadequate environmental adaptations
- Provide patients with positive affirmation of their worth and allow them to express their concerns and feelings, which may include fear, guilt, embarrassment, and self-blame
- Assist caretakers to explore their feelings about relatives or patients in their care and to identify factors that are disturbing and appear to contribute to abusive and neglectful behaviors
- Assist patients in identifying inadequate and harmful care arrangements and help them and their family members identify mechanisms for addressing these problems
- Discuss concerns about observations of at-risk indicators separately with the elder patient and the caretaker
- Determine the patient's and caretaker's knowledge and ability to meet the patient's care and safety needs and provide appropriate teaching
- Help patients and their families identify coping strategies for stressful situations, including the difficult decision to discontinue home care
- Determine deviations from normal aging and note early signs and symptoms of ill health through routine health screenings
- Promote maximum independence and self-care through innovative teaching strategies and the use of repetition, practice, reinforcement, and individualized pacing
- Provide environmental assessment and recommendations for adapting the home to promote physical self-reliance or refer to appropriate agencies for assistance
- Assist with restoration of full range of activities of daily living as possible
- Instruct on the benefits of a routine regimen of physical activity, provide tailored exercise regimens, and refer to physical therapy or exercise programs as appropriate in order to prevent dependency
- Implement strategies to enhance critical thinking, decision-making, and remembering
- Provide a public health nurse referral to ensure that the home environment is monitored and that the patient receives continued assistance
- Provide referrals for patients and their families to human services and counseling professionals
- Provide elder patients and their caretakers with community resource information (e.g., addresses and phone numbers of agencies that provide senior service assistance, home health

A

- care, residential care, respite care, emergency care, housing assistance, transportation, substance abuse treatment, sliding-fee counseling services, food pantries and Meals on Wheels, clothing distribution centers)
- Caution patients to have their Social Security or pension checks directly deposited, not to accept personal care in return for transfer of assets, and not to sign documents or make financial arrangements before seeking legal advice
- Encourage patients and their families to plan in advance for care needs, including who will assume responsibility if the patient becomes incapacitated, and how to explore abilities, preferences, and options for care
- Consult with community resources for information
- Inform physician of observations indicative of abuse or neglect
- Report suspected abuse or neglect to proper authorities

2nd edition 1996; revised 2000, 2004, 2013

Background Readings:

Brandl, G. (2007). *Elder abuse detection and intervention: A collaborative approach.* New York: Springer.

Cohen, M., Halevy-Levin, S., Gagin, R., Priltuzky, D., & Friedman, G. (2010). Elder abuse in long-term care residences and the risk indicators. *Ageing and Society, 30*(6), 1027–1040.

Fraser, A. (2010). Preventing abuse of older people. *Nursing Management, 17*(6), 26–29.

Gorbien, M. J. & Eisenstein, A. R. (2005). Elder abuse and neglect: An overview. *Clinics in Geriatric Medicine, 21*(2), 279–292.

Lemko, K. & Fulmer, T. (2006). Nursing care: Victims of violence—elder mistreatment. In P.S. Cowen & S. Moorhead (Eds.), *Current issues in nursing* (7th ed. pp. 732–737). St. Louis: Mosby.

Post, L., Page, C., Conner, T., Prokhorov, A., Fang, Y., & Biroscak, B. J. (2010). Elder abuse in long-term care: Types, patterns, and risk factors. *Research on Aging, 32*(3), 323–348.

Abuse Protection Support: Religious   6408

Definition: Identification of high-risk, controlling religious relationships and actions to prevent infliction of physical, sexual, or emotional harm and/or exploitation

Activities:
- Identify individuals who are dependent on the religious "leader" due to impaired or altered religious development, mental or emotional impairment, depression, substance abuse, lack of social resources, or financial issues
- Identify patterns of behavior, thinking, and feeling in which a person experiences "control over" his/her religious journey by another
- Identify church/family history for religious and/or ritual abuse, problem solving and coping methods, emotional stability, degree of persuasive and manipulative techniques used, and religious addiction
- Determine whether the individual demonstrates signs of physical abuse, emotional abuse, exploitation, or religious addiction
- Monitor individual and "leader" interactions noting level of obedience demanded, tolerance for differences, persuasive and manipulation techniques employed, maturationally appropriate methods, content, and sense of "love" principle/life force/deity
- Determine whether individual has a religious functional network to assist in meeting needs for belonging, care, and transcendence in a healthy manner
- Offer prayer and healing services for the person and for past generational healing of the family/congregation
- Help identify resources to meet the religious "safety" and support of the individual and group
- Provide interpersonal support on a regular basis as needed
- Refer for appropriate religious counseling
- Refer to professional specialist if occult and/or satanic ritual abuse is suspected
- Report suspected abuse to proper church and/or legal authorities

3rd edition 2000

Background Readings:

Linn, M., Linn, D., & Fabricant, S. (1985). *Healing the greatest hurt.* New York: Paulist Press.

Linn, M., Linn, S. F., & Linn, D. (1994). *Healing spiritual abuse and religious addiction.* New York: Paulist Press.

MacNutt, F. (1995). *Deliverance from evil spirits: A practical manual.* Grand Rapids, MI: Baker Book House.

McAll, K. (1982). *Healing the family tree.* London: Sheldon Press.

Acid-Base Management   1910

Definition: Promotion of acid-base balance and prevention of complications resulting from acid-base imbalance

Activities:
- Maintain a patent airway
- Position to facilitate adequate ventilation (e.g., open airway and elevate head of bed)
- Maintain patent IV access
- Monitor trends in arterial pH, $PaCO_2$, and HCO_3 to determine particular type of imbalance (e.g., respiratory or metabolic) and compensatory physiologic mechanisms present (e.g., pulmonary or renal compensation, physiological buffers)
- Maintain concurrent examination of arterial pH and plasma electrolytes for accurate treatment planning
- Monitor arterial blood gases (ABGs) and serum and urine electrolyte levels, as appropriate
- Obtain ordered specimen for laboratory analysis of acid-base balance (e.g., ABGs, urine, and serum), as appropriate
- Monitor for potential etiologies before attempting to treat acid-base imbalances as it is more effective to treat etiology than imbalance

- Determine pathologies needing direct intervention versus those requiring supportive care
- Monitor for complications of corrections of acid-base imbalances (e.g., rapid reduction in chronic respiratory alkalosis resulting in metabolic acidosis)
- Monitor for mixed acid-base derangements (e.g., primary respiratory alkalosis and primary metabolic acidosis)
- Monitor respiratory pattern
- Monitor determinants of tissue oxygen delivery (e.g., PaO_2, SaO_2, hemoglobin levels, and cardiac output), if available
- Monitor for symptoms of respiratory failure (e.g., low PaO_2 and elevated $PaCO_2$ levels, and respiratory muscle fatigue)
- Monitor determination of oxygen consumption (e.g., SvO_2 and $avDO_2$ levels), if available
- Monitor intake and output
- Monitor hemodynamic status, including CVP, MAP, PAP, and PCWP levels, if available
- Monitor for loss of acid (e.g., vomiting, nasogastric output, diarrhea, and diuresis), as appropriate
- Monitor for loss of bicarbonate (e.g., fistula drainage and diarrhea), as appropriate
- Monitor neurological status (e.g., level of consciousness and confusion)
- Provide mechanical ventilatory support, if necessary
- Provide for adequate hydration and restoration of normal fluid volumes, if necessary
- Provide for restoration of normal electrolyte levels (e.g., potassium and chloride), if necessary
- Administer prescribed medications as based on trends in arterial pH, $PaCO_2$, HCO_3, and serum electrolytes, as appropriate
- Instruct patient to avoid excessive use of medications containing HCO_3, as appropriate

- Sedate patient to reduce hyperventilation, if appropriate
- Treat fever, as appropriate
- Administer pain medication, as appropriate
- Administer oxygen therapy, as appropriate
- Administer microbial agents and bronchodilators, as appropriate
- Administer low flow oxygen and monitor for CO_2 narcosis, in case of chronic hypercapnia
- Instruct the patient and/or family on actions instituted to treat the acid-base imbalance

1st edition 1992; revised 2013

Background Readings:

American Association of Critical-Care Nurses. (2006). *Core curriculum for critical care nursing* (6th ed.). Philadelphia: Saunders.

Appel, S. J. & Downs, C. A. (2007). Steady a disturbed equilibrium. Accurately interpret the acid-base balance of acutely ill patients. *Nursing Critical Care 2*(4), 45–53.

Clancy, J. & McVicar, A. (2007). Intermediate and long-term regulation of acid-base homeostasis. *British Journal of Nursing, 16*(17), 1076–1079.

Isenhour, J. L. & Slovis, C. M. (2008). Arterial blood gas analysis: A 3-step approach to acid-base disorders. *The Journal of Respiratory Diseases, 29*(2), 74–82.

Kraut, J. A. & Madeas, N. E. (2001). Approach to patients with acid-base disorders. *Respiratory Care, 46*(4), 392–402.

Lian, J. X. (2010). Interpreting and using the arterial blood gas analysis. *Nursing Critical Care, 5*(3), 26–36.

Porth, C. M. (2007). *Essentials of pathophysiology* (2nd ed.). Philadelphia: Lippincott Williams & Wilkins.

Powers, F. (1999). The role of chloride in acid-base balance. *Journal of Intravenous Nursing, 22*(5), 286–290.

Smeltzer, S. C. & Bare, B. G. (2004). *Brunner & Suddarth's textbook of medical surgical nursing* (Vol. 1) (10th ed.). Philadelphia: Lippincott Williams & Wilkins.

Acid-Base Management: Metabolic Acidosis 1911

Definition: Promotion of acid-base balance and prevention of complications resulting from serum HCO_3 levels lower than desired or serum hydrogen ion levels higher than desired

Activities:
- Maintain a patent airway
- Monitor respiratory pattern
- Maintain patent IV access
- Monitor for potential etiologies before attempting to treat acid-base imbalances (i.e., it is more effective to treat etiology than imbalance)
- Determine pathologies needing direct intervention versus those requiring supportive care
- Monitor for causes of HCO_3 deficit or hydrogen ion excess (e.g., methanol or ethanol ingestion, uremia, diabetic ketoacidosis, alcoholic ketoacidosis, lactic acidosis, sepsis, hypotension, hypoxia, ischemia, isoniazid or iron ingestion, salicylate toxicity, diarrhea, hyperalimentation, hyperparathyroidism)
- Calculate anion gap to assist in determining causes of metabolic acidosis (e.g., non-anion gap indicates electrolyte influenced causes; anion gap indicates loss of bicarbonate causes)
- Use mnemonics to assist in determining causes of metabolic acidosis (e.g., MUDPILES: **M**ethanol ingestion, **U**remia, **D**iabetic, alcoholic, or starvation ketoacidosis, **P**araldehyde ingestion, **I**soniazid or iron poisoning, **L**actic acidosis, **E**thylene glycol ingestion, **S**alicylate ingestion; HARDUP: **H**yperalimentation,

Acetazolamide, **R**enal tubular acidosis, renal insufficiency, **D**iarrhea and diuretics, **U**teroenterostomy, **P**ancreatic fistula)
- Monitor for electrolyte imbalances associated with metabolic acidosis (e.g., hyponatremia, hyperkalemia or hypokalemia, hypocalcemia, hypophosphatemia, and hypomagnesemia), as appropriate
- Monitor for signs and symptoms of worsening HCO_3 deficit or hydrogen ion excess (e.g., Kussmaul-Kien respirations, weakness, disorientation, headache, anorexia, coma, urinary pH level less than 6, plasma HCO_3 level less than 22 mEq/L, plasma pH level less than 7.35, base excess less than -2 mEq/L, associated hyperkalemia, and possible CO_2 deficit)
- Administer fluids as indicated for excessive losses from underlying condition (e.g., diarrhea, diuretics, hyperalimention)
- Administer oral or parenteral HCO_3 agents, if appropriate
- Use parenteral HCO_3 agents cautiously in premature infants, neonates, and small children
- Avoid administration of medications resulting in lowered HCO_3 level (e.g., chloride-containing solutions and anion exchange resins), as appropriate
- Prevent complications from excessive HCO_3 administration (e.g., metabolic alkalosis, hypernatremia, volume overload,

A

- decreased oxygen delivery, decreased cardiac contractility, and enhanced lactic acid production)
- Administer prescribed insulin, fluid hydration (isotonic and hypotonic) and potassium for treatment of diabetic ketoacidosis, as appropriate
- Administer prescribed medications for treatment of inappropriate substance ingestion (e.g., alcohol, salicylate, ethylene glycol) or renal insufficiency
- Monitor intake and output
- Monitor determinants of tissue oxygen delivery (e.g., PaO_2, SaO_2, hemoglobin levels, and cardiac output), as appropriate
- Reduce oxygen consumption (e.g., promote comfort, control fever, and reduce anxiety), as appropriate
- Monitor loss of bicarbonate through the GI tract (e.g., diarrhea, pancreatic fistula, small bowel fistula, and ileal conduit), as appropriate
- Monitor for decreasing bicarbonate and acid buildup from excessive nonvolatile acids (e.g., renal failure, diabetic ketoacidosis, tissue hypoxia, and starvation), as appropriate
- Prepare renal failure patient for dialysis (i.e., assist with catheter placement for dialysis), as appropriate
- Assist with dialysis (e.g., hemodialysis or peritoneal dialysis), as appropriate
- Institute seizure precautions
- Provide frequent oral hygiene
- Maintain bed rest, as indicated
- Monitor for CNS manifestations of worsening metabolic acidosis (e.g., headache, drowsiness, decreased mentation, seizures, and coma), as appropriate
- Monitor for cardiopulmonary manifestations of worsening metabolic acidosis (e.g., hypotension, hypoxia, arrhythmias, and Kussmaul-Kien respiration), as appropriate
- Monitor for GI manifestations of worsening metabolic acidosis (e.g., anorexia, nausea, and vomiting), as appropriate
- Provide adequate nutrition for patients experiencing chronic metabolic acidosis

- Provide comfort measures to deal with the GI effects of metabolic acidosis
- Encourage diet low in carbohydrate to decrease CO_2 production (e.g., administration of hyperalimentation and total parenteral nutrition), as appropriate
- Monitor calcium and phosphate levels for patients experiencing chronic metabolic acidosis to prevent bone loss
- Instruct the patient and/or family on actions instituted to treat the metabolic acidosis

1st edition 1992; revised 2013

Background Readings:

Appel, S. J. & Downs, C. A. (2007). Steady a disturbed equilibrium. Accurately interpret the acid-base balance of acutely ill patients. *Nursing Critical Care, 2*(4), 45–53.

Aschner, J. L. & Poland, R. L. (2008). Sodium bicarbonate: Basically useless therapy. *Pediatrics, 122*(4), 831–835.

Clancy, J. & McVicar, A. (2007). Intermediate and long-term regulation of acid-base homeostasis. *British Journal of Nursing, 16*(17), 1076–1079.

Isenhour, J. L. & Slovis, C. M. (2008). Arterial blood gas analysis: A 3-step approach to acid-base disorders. *The Journal of Respiratory Diseases, 29*(2), 74–82.

Jones, M. B. (2010). Pediatric care: Basic interpretation of metabolic acidosis. *Critical Care Nurse, 30*(5), 63–70.

Kovacic, V., Roguljic, L., & Kovacic, V. (2003). Metabolic acidosis of chronically hemodialyzed patients. *American Journal of Nephrology, 23*(3), 158–164.

Lian, J. X. (2010). Interpreting and using the arterial blood gas analysis. *Nursing Critical Care, 5*(3), 26–36.

Porth, C. M. (2007). *Essentials of pathophysiology* (2nd ed.). Philadelphia: Lippincott Williams & Wilkins.

Powers, F. (1999). The role of chloride in acid-base balance. *Journal of Intravenous Nursing, 22*(5), 286–290.

Acid-Base Management: Metabolic Alkalosis   1912

Definition: Promotion of acid-base balance and prevention of complications resulting from serum HCO_3 levels higher than desired

Activities:
- Maintain a patent airway
- Monitor respiratory pattern
- Maintain patent IV access
- Monitor for potential etiologies before attempting to treat acid-base imbalances (i.e., it is more effective to treat etiology than imbalance)
- Determine pathologies needing direct intervention versus those requiring supportive care
- Monitor for causes of HCO_3 buildup or hydrogen ion loss (e.g., gastric fluid loss, vomiting, NG drainage, persistent diarrhea, loop or thiazide diuretics, cystic fibrosis, posthypercapnia syndrome in mechanically ventilated patients, primary aldosteronism, excessive ingestion of licorice)
- Calculate urine chloride concentration to assist in determining causes of metabolic alkalosis (e.g., saline responsive is indicated when urine chloride concentration is < 15mmol/L; non-saline responsive is indicated when urine chloride concentration is >25mmol/L)

- Use mnemonics to assist in determining causes of metabolic alkalosis (e.g., DAMPEN: **D**iuretics; **A**denoma secretor; **Mis**cellaneous including Bartter's syndrome, penicillin, potassium deficiency, bulimia; **P**osthypercapnia; **E**mesis; **N**asogastric tube; A BELCH: **A**lkali ingestion with decreased glomerular filtration rate, 11-**B**-hydroxylase deficiency, **E**xogenous steroids, **L**icorice ingestion, **C**ushing's syndrome and disease, **H**yperaldosteronism)
- Obtain ordered specimen for laboratory analysis of acid-base balance, as appropriate
- Monitor arterial blood gases (ABGs) and serum and urine electrolyte levels, as appropriate
- Administer dilute acid (e.g., isotonic hydrochloride, arginine monohydrochloride), as appropriate
- Administer H_2 receptor antagonist (e.g., ranitidine and cimetidine) to block hydrochloride secretion from the stomach, as appropriate

- Administer carbonic anhydrase-inhibiting diuretics (e.g., acetazolamide and metazolamide) to increase excretion of bicarbonate, as appropriate
- Administer chloride to replace deficient anion (e.g., ammonium chloride, arginine hydrochloride, normal saline), as appropriate
- Administer prescribed IV potassium chloride until underlying hypokalemia is corrected
- Administer potassium-sparing diuretics (e.g., spironolactone and triamterene), as appropriate
- Administer antiemetics to reduce loss of HCl in emesis, as appropriate
- Replace extracellular fluid deficit with IV saline, as appropriate
- Irrigate NG tube with isotonic saline to avoid electrolyte wash-out, as appropriate
- Monitor intake and output
- Monitor for complications of corrections of acid-base imbalances (i.e., rapid reduction in metabolic alkalosis results in metabolic acidosis)
- Monitor for mixed acid-base derangements (e.g., primary metabolic alkalosis and primary respiratory acidosis) presenting as inappropriate metabolic compensations shrouding a primary respiratory disorder
- Calculate differences in observed HCO_3 and expected change in HCO_3 to determine presence of mixed acid-base derangement
- Monitor determinants of tissue oxygen delivery (e.g., PaO_2, SaO_2, hemoglobin levels, cardiac output), if available
- Avoid administration of alkaline substances (e.g., IV sodium bicarbonate, PO or NG antacids), as appropriate
- Monitor for electrolyte imbalances associated with metabolic alkalosis (e.g., hypokalemia, hypercalcemia, hypochloremia), as appropriate
- Monitor for associated excesses of bicarbonate (e.g., hyperaldosteronism, glucocorticoid excess, licorice abuse), as appropriate
- Monitor for renal loss of acid (e.g., diuretic therapy), as appropriate
- Monitor for GI loss of acid (e.g., vomiting, NG suctioning, high chloride content diarrhea), as appropriate
- Monitor patient receiving digitalis for toxicity resulting from hypokalemia associated with metabolic alkalosis, as appropriate

- Monitor for neurological and/or neuromuscular manifestations of metabolic alkalosis (e.g., seizures, confusion, stupor, coma, tetany, hyperactive reflexes)
- Monitor for pulmonary manifestations of metabolic alkalosis (e.g., bronchospasm, hypoventilation)
- Monitor for cardiac manifestations of metabolic alkalosis (e.g., arrhythmias, reduced contractility, decreased cardiac output)
- Monitor for GI manifestations of metabolic alkalosis (e.g., nausea, vomiting, diarrhea)
- Instruct the patient and/or family on actions instituted to treat the metabolic alkalosis

1st edition 1992; revised 2004, 2013

Background Readings:

Appel, S. J. & Downs, C. A. (2007). Steady a disturbed equilibrium. Accurately interpret the acid-base balance of acutely ill patients. *Nursing Critical Care* 2(4), 45–53.

Clancy, J. & McVicar, A. (2007). Intermediate and long-term regulation of acid-base homeostasis. *British Journal of Nursing, 16*(17), 1076–1079.

Huang, L. H. & Priestley, M. A. (2008). Pediatric metabolic alkalosis. <http://emedicine.medscape.com/article/906819-overview/>

Isenhour, J. L. & Slovis, C. M. (2008). Arterial blood gas analysis: A 3-step approach to acid-base disorders. *The Journal of Respiratory Diseases, 29*(2), 74–82.

Khanna, A. & Kurtzman, N. A. (2001). Metabolic alkalosis. *Respiratory Care, 46*(4), 354–365.

Kraut, J. A. & Madeas, N. E. (2001). Approach to patients with acid-base disorders. *Respiratory Care, 46*(4), 392–402.

Lian, J. X. (2010). Interpreting and using the arterial blood gas analysis. *Nursing Critical Care, 5*(3), 26–36.

Lynch, F. (2009). Arterial blood gas analysis: Implications for nursing. *Pediatric Nursing, 21*(1), 41–44.

Porth, C. M. (2007). *Essentials of pathophysiology* (2nd ed.). Philadelphia: Lippincott Williams & Wilkins.

Ruholl, L. (2006). Arterial blood gases: Analysis and nursing responses. *MEDSURG Nursing, 15*(6), 343–351.

Acid-Base Management: Respiratory Acidosis   1913

Definition: Promotion of acid-base balance and prevention of complications resulting from serum $PaCO_2$ levels higher than desired or serum hydrogen ion levels higher than desired

Activities
- Maintain a patent airway
- Maintain airway clearance (e.g., suction, insert or maintain artificial airway, chest physiotherapy, and cough-deep breath), as appropriate
- Monitor respiratory pattern
- Maintain patent IV access
- Obtain ordered specimen for laboratory analysis of acid-base balance (e.g., ABG, urine, and serum levels), as appropriate
- Monitor for potential etiologies before attempting to treat acid-base imbalances (i.e., it is more effective to treat etiology than imbalance)
- Monitor for possible causes of carbonic acid excess and respiratory acidosis (e.g., airway obstruction, depressed ventilation, CNS depression, neurological disease, chronic lung disease, musculoskeletal disease, chest trauma, pneumothorax, respiratory infection, ARDS, cardiac failure, acute opioid

ingestion, use of respiratory depressant drugs, obesity hypoventilation syndrome)
- Determine pathologies needing direct intervention versus those requiring supportive care
- Monitor for signs and symptoms of carbonic acid excess and respiratory acidosis (e.g., hand tremor with extensions of arms, confusion, drowsiness progressing to coma, headache, slowed verbal response, nausea, vomiting, tachycardia, warm sweaty extremities, pH level less than 7.35, $PaCO_2$ level greater than 45 mm Hg, associated hypochloremia, and possible HCO_3 excess)
- Support ventilation and airway patency in the presence of respiratory acidosis and rising $PaCO_2$ level, as appropriate
- Administer oxygen therapy, as appropriate
- Administer microbial agents and bronchodilators, as appropriate

A

- Administer medication therapy aimed at reversing the effects of inappropriate sedative drugs (e.g., naloxone to reverse narcotics, flumazenil to reverse benzodiazepines), as appropriate
- Maintain caution when reversing the effects of benzodiazepines to avoid seizures if reversal is accomplished too vigorously
- Administer low flow oxygen and monitor for CO_2 narcosis in cases of chronic hypercapnia (e.g., COPD)
- Administer noninvasive positive-pressure ventilation techniques (e.g., nasal continuous positive-pressure ventilation, nasal bilevel ventilation) for hypercapnia related to obesity hypoventilation syndrome or musculoskeletal disease
- Monitor for hypoventilation and treat causes (e.g., inappropriate low-minute mechanical ventilation, chronic reduction in alveolar ventilation, COPD, acute opioid ingestion, obstructive or restrictive airway diseases)
- Monitor ABG levels for decreasing pH level, as appropriate
- Monitor for indications of chronic respiratory acidosis (e.g., barrel chest, clubbing of nails, pursed-lips breathing, and use of accessory muscles), as appropriate
- Monitor determinants of tissue oxygen delivery (e.g., PaO_2, SaO_2, hemoglobin levels, cardiac output) to determine the adequacy of arterial oxygenation
- Monitor for symptoms of respiratory failure (e.g., low PaO_2, elevated $PaCO_2$ levels, respiratory muscle fatigue)
- Position patient for optimum ventilation-perfusion matching (e.g., good lung down, prone, semi-Fowler's), as appropriate
- Monitor work of breathing (e.g., respiratory rate, heart rate, use of accessory muscles, diaphoresis)
- Provide mechanical ventilatory support, if necessary
- Provide low-carbohydrate, high-fat diet to reduce CO_2 production, if indicated
- Provide frequent oral hygiene
- Monitor GI functioning and distention to prevent reduced diaphragmatic movement, as appropriate
- Promote adequate rest periods (e.g., 90 minutes of undisturbed sleep, organize nursing care, limit visitors, coordinate consults), as appropriate
- Monitor neurological status (e.g., level of consciousness and confusion)
- Instruct the patient and/or family on actions instituted to treat the respiratory acidosis
- Contract with patient's visitors for limited visitation schedule to allow for adequate rest periods to reduce respiratory compromise, if indicated

1st edition 1992; revised 2004, 2013

Background Readings:

Appel, S. J. & Downs, C.A. (2007). Steady a disturbed equilibrium. Accurately interpret the acid-base balance of acutely ill patients. *Nursing Critical Care 2*(4), 45–53.

Clancy, J. & McVicar, A. (2007). Intermediate and long-term regulation of acid-base homeostasis. *British Journal of Nursing, 16*(17), 1076–1079.

Isenhour, J. L. & Slovis, C. M. (2008). Arterial blood gas analysis: A 3-step approach to acid-base disorders. *The Journal of Respiratory Diseases, 29*(2), 74–82.

Kraut, J. A. & Madeas, N. E. (2001). Approach to patients with acid-base disorders. *Respiratory Care, 46*(4), 392–402.

Lian, J. X. (2010). Interpreting and using the arterial blood gas analysis. *Nursing Critical Care, 5*(3), 26–36.

Lynch, F. (2009). Arterial blood gas analysis: Implications for nursing. *Pediatric Nursing, 21*(1), 41–44.

Porth, C. M. (2007). *Essentials of pathophysiology* (2nd ed.). Philadelphia: Lippincott Williams & Wilkins.

Ruholl, L. (2006). Arterial blood gases: Analysis and nursing responses. *MEDSURG Nursing, 15*(6), 343–351.

Acid-Base Management: Respiratory Alkalosis   1914

Definition: Promotion of acid-base balance and prevention of complications resulting from serum $PaCO_2$ levels lower than desired

Activities:
- Maintain a patent airway
- Monitor respiratory pattern
- Maintain patent IV access
- Monitor for potential etiologies before attempting to treat acid-base imbalances (i.e., it is more effective to treat etiology than imbalance)
- Determine pathologies needing direct intervention versus those requiring supportive care
- Monitor for hyperventilation and treat causes (e.g., inappropriate high-minute mechanical ventilation, anxiety, hypoxemia, lung lesions, severe anemia, salicylate toxicity, CNS injury, hypermetabolic states, GI distention, pain, high altitude, septicemia, stress)
- Reduce oxygen consumption by promoting comfort, controlling fever, and reducing anxiety to minimize hyperventilation, as appropriate
- Provide rebreather mask for hyperventilating patient, as appropriate
- Sedate patient to reduce hyperventilation, if appropriate
- Reduce high-minute ventilation (e.g., rate, mode, tidal volume) in mechanically overventilated patients, as appropriate
- Monitor end-tidal CO_2 level, as appropriate
- Promote adequate rest periods of at least 90 minutes of undisturbed sleep (e.g., organized nursing care, limited visitors, coordinated consults), as appropriate
- Administer parenteral chloride solutions to reduce HCO_3 while correcting the cause of respiratory alkalosis, as appropriate
- Monitor trends in arterial pH, $PaCO_2$, and HCO_3 to determine effectiveness of interventions
- Monitor for symptoms of worsening respiratory alkalosis (e.g., alternating periods of apnea and hyperventilation, increasing anxiety, increased heart rate without increased blood pressure, dyspnea, dizziness, tingling in extremities, hyperreflexia, frequent sighing and yawning, blurred vision, diaphoresis, dry mouth, pH level of greater than 7.45, $PaCO_2$ less than 35 mm Hg, associated hyperchloremia, HCO_3 deficit)
- Obtain ordered specimen for laboratory analysis of acid-base balance (e.g., ABGs, urine, serum), as appropriate
- Maintain concurrent examination of arterial pH and plasma electrolytes for accurate treatment planning
- Monitor arterial blood gases (ABGs) and serum and urine electrolyte levels, as appropriate

A

- Monitor for hypophosphatemia and hypokalemia associated with respiratory alkalosis, as appropriate
- Monitor for complications of corrections of acid-base imbalances (e.g., rapid reduction in chronic respiratory alkalosis resulting in metabolic acidosis)
- Monitor for mixed acid-base derangements (e.g., primary respiratory alkalosis and primary metabolic acidosis) presenting as inappropriate respiratory compensations shrouding a primary metabolic disorder
- Calculate differences in observed $PaCO_2$ and expected change in $PaCO_2$ to determine presence of mixed acid-base derangement
- Monitor for indications of impending respiratory failure (e.g., low PaO_2 level, respiratory muscle fatigue, low SaO_2/SvO_2 level)
- Provide oxygen therapy, if necessary
- Provide mechanical ventilatory support, if necessary
- Position to facilitate adequate ventilation (e.g., open airway, elevate head of bed)
- Monitor intake and output
- Monitor for neurological and/or neuromuscular manifestations of respiratory alkalosis (e.g., paresthesias, tetany, seizures), as appropriate
- Monitor for cardiopulmonary manifestations of respiratory alkalosis (e.g., arrhythmias, decreased cardiac output, hyperventilation)
- Administer sedatives, pain relief, antipyretics, as appropriate
- Administer neuromuscular-blocking agents only if patient is mechanically ventilated, if indicated
- Promote stress reduction
- Provide frequent oral hygiene

- Promote orientation
- Instruct the patient and/or family on actions instituted to treat the respiratory alkalosis
- Contract with patient's visitors for limited visitation schedule to allow for adequate rest periods to reduce respiratory compromise, if indicated

1st edition 1992; revised 2013

Background Readings:

Appel, S. J. & Downs, C. A. (2007). Steady a disturbed equilibrium. Accurately interpret the acid-base balance of acutely ill patients. *Nursing Critical Care 2*(4), 45–53.

Clancy, J. & McVicar, A. (2007). Intermediate and long-term regulation of acid-base homeostasis. *British Journal of Nursing, 16*(17), 1076–1079.

Foster, G. T., Vaziri, N. D., & Sassoon, C. S. (2001). Respiratory alkalosis. *Respiratory Care, 46*(4), 384–391.

Isenhour, J. L. & Slovis, C. M. (2008). Arterial blood gas analysis: A 3-step approach to acid-base disorders. *The Journal of Respiratory Diseases, 29*(2), 74–82.

Kraut, J. A. & Madeas, N. E. (2001). Approach to patients with acid-base disorders. *Respiratory Care, 46*(4), 392–402.

Lian, J. X. (2010). Interpreting and using the arterial blood gas analysis. *Nursing Critical Care, 5*(3), 26–36.

Lynch, F. (2009). Arterial blood gas analysis: Implications for nursing. *Pediatric Nursing, 21*(1), 41–44.

Ruholl, L. (2006). Arterial blood gases: Analysis and nursing responses. *MEDSURG Nursing, 15*(6), 343–351.

Acid-Base Monitoring   1920

Definition: Collection and analysis of patient data to regulate acid-base balance

Activities:
- Obtain ordered specimen for laboratory analysis of acid-base balance (e.g., ABGs, urine, and serum) in at-risk populations, as appropriate
- Obtain sequential specimens to determine trends
- Analyze trends in serum pH in the patient experiencing conditions with escalating effects on pH levels (e.g., hyperventilating patients, diabetic or alcoholic ketoacidotic patients, septic patients)
- Analyze trends in serum pH in at risk populations (e.g., patients with compromised respiratory status, renal impairment, diabetes mellitus, prolonged diarrhea or vomiting, Cushing's syndrome)
- Note if arterial pH level is on the alkaline or acidotic side of the mean (7.35–7.45)
- Note if $PaCO_2$ level shows respiratory acidosis, respiratory alkalosis, or normalcy
- Note if the HCO_3 level shows metabolic acidosis, metabolic alkalosis, or normalcy
- Examine trends in serum pH in conjunction with $PaCO_2$ and HCO_3 trends to determine whether the acidosis or alkalosis is compensated or uncompensated
- Note if the compensation is pulmonary, metabolic, or is physiologically buffered
- Identify potential etiologies before attempting to treat acid-base imbalances as it is more effective to treat etiology than imbalance

- Identify the presence or absence of an anion gap (greater than 14 mEq/L), signaling an increased production or decreased excretion of acid products
- Monitor for signs and symptoms of HCO_3 deficit and metabolic acidosis (e.g., Kussmaul-Kien respirations, weakness, disorientation, headache, anorexia, coma, urinary pH level less than 6, plasma HCO_3 level less than 22 mEq/L, plasma pH level less than 7.35, base excess less than -2 mEq/L, associated hyperkalemia, and possible CO_2 deficit)
- Monitor for causes of metabolic acidosis (e.g., methanol or ethanol ingestion, uremia, diabetic ketoacidosis, alcoholic ketoacidosis, paraldehyde ingestion, lactic acidosis, sepsis, hypotension, hypoxia, ischemia, malnutrition, diarrhea, renal failure, hyperalimentation, hyperparathyroidism, salicylate toxicity, ethylene glycol ingestion)
- Monitor for signs and symptoms of HCO_3 excess and metabolic alkalosis (e.g., numbness and tingling of the extremities, muscular hypertonicity, shallow respirations with pause, bradycardia, tetany, urinary pH level greater than 7, plasma HCO_3 level greater than 26 mEq/L, plasma pH level greater than 7.45, BE greater than 2 mEq/L, associated hypokalemia, and possible CO_2 =retention)
- Monitor for causes of metabolic alkalosis (e.g., diuretics, emesis, nasogastric tube, posthypercapnia, potassium deficiency; alkali ingestion, Cushing's syndrome, hyperaldosteronism, hypochloremia, excessive ingestion of medications containing HCO_3)

A

- Monitor for signs and symptoms of $PaCO_2$ level deficit and respiratory alkalosis (e.g., frequent sighing and yawning, tetany, paresthesia, muscular twitching, palpitations, tingling and numbness, dizziness, blurred vision, diaphoresis, dry mouth, convulsions, pH level greater than 7.45, $PaCO_2$ less than 35 mm Hg, associated hyperchloremia, and possible HCO_3 deficit)
- Monitor for causes of respiratory alkalosis (e.g., hyperventilation, mechanical over-ventilation, hepatic disease, pregnancy, septicemia, pain, CNS lesions, and fever)
- Monitor for signs and symptoms of $PaCO_2$ level excess and respiratory acidosis (e.g., hand tremor with extensions of arms, confusion, drowsiness progressing to coma, headache, slowed verbal response, nausea, vomiting, tachycardia, warm sweaty extremities, pH level less than 7.35, $PaCO_2$ level greater than 45 mm Hg, associated hypochloremia, and possible HCO_3 excess)
- Monitor for possible causes of respiratory acidosis (e.g., airway obstruction, depressed ventilation, CNS depression, neurological disease, chronic lung disease, musculoskeletal disease, chest trauma, infection, ARDS, cardiac failure, acute opioid ingestion, and use of respiratory depressant drugs)
- Compare current status with previous status to detect improvements and deterioration in patient's condition

- Initiate and/or change medical treatment to maintain patient parameters within limits ordered by the physician, using established protocols

1st edition 1992; revised 2013

Background Readings:

Appel, S. J. & Downs, C. A. (2007). Steady a disturbed equilibrium: Accurately interpret the acid-base balance of acutely ill patients. *Nursing Critical Care 2*(4), 45-53.

Clancy, J. & McVicar, A. (2007). Intermediate and long-term regulation of acid-base homeostasis. *British Journal of Nursing, 16*(17), 1076-1079.

Coombs, M. (2001). Making sense of arterial blood gases. *Nursing Times, 97*(27), 36-38.

Isenhour, J. L. & Slovis, C. M. (2008). Arterial blood gas analysis: A 3-step approach to acid-base disorders. *The Journal of Respiratory Diseases, 29*(2), 74-82.

Lian, J. X. (2010). Interpreting and using the arterial blood gas analysis. *Nursing Critical Care, 5*(3), 26-36.

Powers, F. (1999). The role of chloride in acid-base balance. *Journal of Intravenous Nursing, 22*(5), 286-290.

Smeltzer, S. C. & Bare, B. G. (2004). *Brunner & Suddarth's textbook of medical surgical nursing* (Vol. 1) (10th ed.). Philadelphia: Lippincott Williams & Wilkins.

Active Listening   4920

Definition: Attending closely to and attaching significance to a patient's verbal and nonverbal messages

Activities:
- Establish the purpose for the interaction
- Display interest in the patient
- Use questions or statements to encourage expression of thoughts, feelings, and concerns
- Focus completely on the interaction by suppressing prejudice, bias, assumptions, preoccupying personal concerns, and other distractions
- Display an awareness of and sensitivity to emotions
- Use nonverbal behavior to facilitate communication (e.g., be aware of physical stance conveying nonverbal messages)
- Listen for the unexpressed message and feeling, as well as content, of the conversation
- Be aware of which words are avoided, as well as the nonverbal message that accompanies the expressed words
- Be aware of the tone, tempo, volume, pitch, and inflection of the voice
- Identify the predominant themes
- Determine the meaning of the message by reflecting on attitudes, past experiences, and the current situation
- Time a response so that it reflects understanding of the received message
- Clarify the message through the use of questions and feedback
- Verify understanding of messages through use of questions or feedback

- Use a series of interactions to discover the meaning of behavior
- Avoid barriers to active listening (e.g., minimizing feelings, offering easy solutions, interrupting, talking about self, and premature closure)
- Use silence/listening to encourage the expression of feelings, thoughts, and concerns

1st edition 1992; revised 1996, 2004

Background Readings:

Audio Visual Campus. (1993). *Active listening* [Video]. San Diego: Levitz Sommer Productions.

Craven, R. F. & Hirnle, C. J. (2000). *Fundamentals of nursing: Human health and function* (3rd ed., pp. 336-338). Philadelphia: Lippincott Williams & Wilkins.

Deering, C. (2006). Therapeutic relationships and communication. In W. K. Mohr (Ed.), *Psychiatric-mental health nursing* (6th ed., pp. 53–58). Philadelphia: Lippincott Williams & Wilkins.

Helms, J. (1985). Active listening. In G. M. Bulechek & J. C. McCloskey (Eds.), *Nursing interventions: Treatments for nursing diagnosis* (pp. 328–337). Philadelphia: Saunders.

Johnson, B. S. (1993). *Psychiatric–mental health nursing: Adaptation and growth/pocket guide to psychiatric nursing interventions* (3rd ed., pp. 65–68). Philadelphia: Lippincott Williams & Wilkins.

Activity Therapy 4310

Definition: Prescription of and assistance with specific physical, cognitive, social, and spiritual activities to increase the range, frequency, or duration of an individual's or group's activity

Activities:
- Determine patient ability to participate in specific activities
- Collaborate with occupational, physical, or recreational therapists in planning and monitoring an activity program, as appropriate
- Determine patient's commitment to increasing frequency and range of activity
- Assist patient to explore the personal meaning of usual activity (e.g., work) and favorite leisure activities
- Assist patient to choose activities and achievement goals for activities consistent with physical, psychological, and social capabilities
- Assist patient to focus on abilities, rather than on deficits
- Assist patient to identify and obtain resources required for the desired activity
- Encourage creative activities, as appropriate
- Assist patient to obtain transportation to activities, as appropriate
- Assist patient to identify preferences for activities
- Assist patient to identify meaningful activities
- Assist patient to schedule specific periods for activities into daily routine
- Assist patient and family to identify deficits in activity level
- Identify strategies to promote patient participation in desired activities
- Instruct patient and family regarding the role of physical, social, spiritual, and cognitive activity in maintaining function and health
- Instruct patient and family how to perform desired or prescribed activity
- Coordinate patient selection of age appropriate activities
- Assist patient and family to adapt environment to accommodate desired activity
- Provide activities to increase attention span in consultation with occupational therapist
- Facilitate activity substitution when patient has limitations in time, energy, or movement, in consultation with occupational, physical, or recreational therapists
- Encourage involvement in group activities or therapies, as appropriate
- Refer to community centers or activity programs, as appropriate
- Assist with regular physical activities (e.g., ambulation, transfers, turning, and personal care), as needed
- Provide gross motor activities for hyperactive patient
- Promote a physically active lifestyle to avoid unneeded weight gain, as appropriate
- Suggest methods of increasing daily physical activity, as appropriate
- Make environment safe for continuous large muscle movement, as indicated

- Provide motor activity to relieve muscle tension
- Provide activities with implicit and emotional memory components (e.g., specially selected religious activities) for dementia patients, as appropriate
- Provide noncompetitive, structured, and active group games
- Promote engagement in recreational and diversional activities aimed at reducing anxiety (e.g., group singing; volleyball; table tennis; walking; swimming; simple, concrete tasks; simple games; routine tasks; housekeeping chores; grooming; and puzzles and cards)
- Employ animal-assisted activity programs, as appropriate
- Provide positive reinforcement for participation in activities
- Instruct family to provide positive reinforcement for participation in activities
- Allow for family participation in activities, as appropriate
- Assist patient to develop self-motivation and reinforcement
- Monitor emotional, physical, social, and spiritual response to activity
- Assist patient and family to monitor own progress toward goal achievement

1st edition 1992; revised 2013

Background Readings:

Chilvers, R., Corr, S. & Singlehurst, H. (2010). Investigation into the occupational lives of healthy older people through their use of time. *Australian Occupational Therapy Journal, 57*(1), 24–33.

Chu, C., Liu, C., Sun, C., & Lin, J. (2009). The effect of animal-assisted activity on inpatients with schizophrenia. *Journal of Psychosocial Nursing & Mental Health Services, 47*(12), 42–48.

Dorrestein, M. (2006). Leisure activity assessment in residential care: Improving occupational outcomes for residents. *New Zealand Journal of Occupational Therapy, 53*(2), 20–26.

Griffiths, S. (2008). The experience of creative activity as a treatment medium. *Journal of Mental Health, 17*(1), 49–63.

Ketteridge, A. & Boshoff, K. (2008). Exploring the reasons why adolescents participate in physical activity and identifying strategies that facilitate their involvement in such activity. *Australian Occupational Therapy Journal, 55*(4), 273–282.

Lloyd, C., Williams, P. L., Simpson, A., Wright, D., Fortune, T., & Lal, S. (2010). Occupational therapy in the modern adult acute mental health setting: A review of current practice. *International Journal of Therapy & Rehabilitation, 17*(9), 483–493.

Shirley, D., van der Ploeg, H. P., & Bauman, A. E. (2010). Physical activity promotion in the physical therapy setting: Perspectives from practitioners and students. *Physical Therapy, 90*(9), 1311–1322.

Vance, D. E., Eaves, Y. D., Keltner, N. L., & Struzick, T. S. (2010). Practical implications of procedural and emotional religious activity therapy for nursing. *Journal of Gerontological Nursing, 36*(8), 22–29.

Acupressure 1320

Definition: Application of firm, sustained pressure to special points on the body to decrease pain, produce relaxation, and prevent or reduce nausea

Activities:
- Screen for contraindications, such as contusions, scar tissue, infection, serious cardiac conditions (also contraindicated for young children)
- Decide on applicability of acupressure for treatment of a particular individual
- Determine individual's degree of psychological comfort with touch
- Determine desired outcomes
- Refer to acupressure text to match the etiology, location, and symptomology to appropriate acupoint after advanced training in the techniques of acupressure
- Determine which acupoint(s) to stimulate, depending on desired outcome
- Explain to individual that you will be searching for a tender area(s)
- Encourage individual to relax during the stimulation
- Probe deeply with finger, thumb, or knuckle for a very pressure-sensitive spot in the general location of the acupoint
- Observe verbal or postural cues to identify desired point or location (such as wincing, "ouch")
- Stimulate acupoint by pressing in with finger, thumb, or knuckle and using one's body weight to lean into the point to which pressure is applied
- Use finger pressure or wristbands to apply pressure to selected acupoint for treating nausea
- Apply steady pressure over hypertonic muscle tissue for pain until relaxation is felt or pain is reported to have decreased, usually 15 to 20 seconds
- Repeat procedure over same point on opposite side of body
- Treat the contralateral points first when there is extreme tenderness at any one point
- Apply steady pressure until the nausea subsides or maintain wristbands indefinitely during actual or anticipated nausea
- Observe for relaxation and verbalizations of decreases in discomfort or nausea
- Use daily acupressure applications during the first week of treatment for pain
- Recommend use of progressive relaxation techniques and/or stretching exercises between treatments
- Teach family/significant other to provide acupressure treatments
- Document action and individual response to acupressure

2nd edition 1996

Background Readings:

Dibble, S. L., Chapman, J., Mack, K. A., & Shih, A. (2000). Acupressure for nausea: Results of a pilot study. *Oncology Nursing Forum, 27*(1), 41–47.
Lorenzi, E. A. (1999). Complementary/alternative therapies. So many choices. *Geriatric Nursing, 20*(3), 125–133.
Mann, E. (1999). Using acupuncture and acupressure to treat postoperative emesis. *Professional Nurse, 14*(10), 691–694.
Windle, P. E., Borromeo, A., Robles, H., & Ilacio-Uy, V. (2001). The effects of acupressure on the incidence of postoperative nausea and vomiting in postsurgical patients. *Journal of PeriAnesthesia Nursing, 16*(3), 158–162.

Admission Care 7310

Definition: Facilitating entry of a patient into a health care facility

Activities:
- Introduce yourself and your role in providing care
- Orient patient/family/significant others to expectations of care
- Provide appropriate privacy for the patient/family/significant others
- Orient patient/family/significant others to immediate environment
- Orient patient/family/significant others to agency facilities
- Obtain admission history including past medical illnesses, medications, and allergies
- Perform admission physical assessment, as appropriate
- Perform admission financial assessment, as appropriate
- Perform admission psychosocial assessment, as appropriate
- Perform admission religious assessment, as appropriate
- Perform admission risk assessment (e.g., risk for falls, tuberculosis screening, skin assessment)
- Provide patient with "Patient's Bill of Rights"
- Obtain advance care directive information (i.e., Living Will and Durable Power of Attorney for Healthcare)
- Document pertinent information
- Maintain confidentiality of patient data
- Identify patient at risk for readmission
- Establish patient plan of care, nursing diagnoses, outcomes, and interventions
- Begin discharge planning
- Implement safety precautions, as appropriate
- Label patient's chart, room door, and/or head of bed, as indicated
- Notify physician of admission and patient status
- Obtain physician's orders for patient care

1st edition 1992; revised 2004

Background Readings:

Perry, A. & Potter, P. A. (2002). *Clinical nursing skill and techniques* (5th ed.). St. Louis: Mosby.

Airway Insertion and Stabilization   3120

A

Definition: Insertion or assistance with insertion and stabilization of an artificial airway

Activities:

- Perform hand hygiene
- Use personal protective equipment (PPE) (gloves, goggles, and mask), as appropriate
- Select the correct size and type of oropharyngeal or nasopharyngeal airway
- Position patient and head, as appropriate
- Suction mouth and oropharynx
- Insert oro/nasopharyngeal airway, ensuring that it reaches to the base of the tongue, supporting the tongue in a forward position
- Tape the oro/nasopharyngeal airway in place
- Monitor for dyspnea, snoring, or inspiratory crowing when oro/nasopharyngeal airway is in place
- Change the oro/nasopharyngeal airway daily and inspect mucosa
- Insert a laryngeal mask airway (LMA), as appropriate
- Insert an esophageal obturator airway (EOA), as appropriate
- Auscultate for breath sounds bilaterally before inflating the esophageal cuff of the EOA
- Collaborate with the physician to select the correct size and type of endotracheal tube (ET) or tracheostomy tube
- Select artificial airways with high-volume, low-pressure cuffs
- Limit insertion of endotracheal tubes and tracheostomies to qualified and credentialed personnel
- Encourage physicians to place ETs via the oropharyngeal route, as appropriate
- Assist with insertion of an endotracheal tube by gathering necessary intubation and emergency equipment, positioning patient, administering medications as ordered, and monitoring the patient for complications during insertion
- Assist with emergent tracheostomy by setting up appropriate support equipment, administering medications, providing a sterile environment, and monitoring for changes in the patient's condition
- Instruct patient and family about the intubation procedure
- Hyperoxygenate with 100% oxygen for 3-5 minutes, as appropriate
- Auscultate the chest after intubation
- Observe for systematic chest wall movement
- Monitor oxygen saturation (SpO_2) by noninvasive pulse oximetry and CO_2 detection
- Monitor respiratory status, as appropriate
- Inflate endotracheal/tracheostomy cuff, using minimal occlusive volume technique or minimal leak technique
- Stabilize endotracheal/tracheostomy tube with adhesive tape, twill tape, or commercially available stabilizing device
- Mark endotracheal tube at the position of the lips or nares, using the centimeter markings on the ET, and document
- Verify tube placement with a chest radiograph, ensuring cannulation of the trachea 2 to 4 cm above the carina
- Minimize leverage and traction of the artificial airway by suspending ventilator tubing from overhead supports, using flexible catheter mounts and swivels, and supporting tubes during turning, suctioning, and ventilator disconnection/reconnection

1st edition 1992; revised 2013

Background Readings:

Day, M. W. (2005). Laryngeal mask airway. In D. L. Wiegand, & K. Carlson, (Eds.), *AACN procedure manual for critical care* (5th ed., p. 4252). St. Louis: Saunders.

Evans-Smith, P. (2005). *Taylor's clinical nursing skills.* Philadelphia: Lippincott Williams & Wilkins.

Goodrich, C. & Carlson, K. K. (2005). Endotracheal intubation (perform). In D. L. Wiegand, & K. Carlson, (Eds.), *AACN procedure manual for critical care* (5th ed., pp. 9–20). St. Louis: Saunders.

Scott, J. M. (2005). Endotracheal intubation (assist). In D. L. Wiegand, & K. Carlson, (Eds.), *AACN procedure manual for critical care* (5th ed., pp. 20–27). St. Louis: Saunders.

Skillings, K. N. & Curtis, B. L. (2005). Nasopharyngeal airway insertion. In D. L. Wiegand, & K. Carlson, (Eds.), *AACN procedure manual for critical care* (5th ed., pp. 53–56). St. Louis: Saunders.

Skillings, K. N. & Curtis, B. L. (2005). Oropharyngeal airway insertion. In D. L. Wiegand, & K. Carlson, (Eds.), *AACN procedure manual for critical care* (5th ed., pp. 57–61). St. Louis: Saunders.

A

Airway Management 3140

Definition: Facilitation of patency of air passages

Activities:
- Open the airway, using the chin lift or jaw thrust technique, as appropriate
- Position patient to maximize ventilation potential
- Identify patient requiring actual/potential airway insertion
- Insert oral or nasopharyngeal airway, as appropriate
- Perform chest physical therapy, as appropriate
- Remove secretions by encouraging coughing or suctioning
- Encourage slow, deep breathing; turning; and coughing
- Use fun techniques to encourage deep breathing for children (e.g., blow bubbles with bubble blower; blow on pinwheel, whistle, harmonica, balloons, party blowers; have blowing contest using ping-pong balls, feathers)
- Instruct how to cough effectively
- Assist with incentive spirometer, as appropriate
- Auscultate breath sounds, noting areas of decreased or absent ventilation and presence of adventitious sounds
- Perform endotracheal or nasotracheal suctioning, as appropriate
- Administer bronchodilators, as appropriate
- Teach patient how to use prescribed inhalers, as appropriate
- Administer aerosol treatments, as appropriate
- Administer ultrasonic nebulizer treatments, as appropriate
- Administer humidified air or oxygen, as appropriate
- Remove foreign bodies with McGill forceps, as appropriate
- Regulate fluid intake to optimize fluid balance
- Position to alleviate dyspnea
- Monitor respiratory and oxygenation status, as appropriate

1st edition 1992; revised 2000, 2004

Background Readings:

American Association of Critical-Care Nurses. (1998). *Core curriculum for critical care nursing* (5th ed.). Philadelphia: Saunders.

Perry, A. G. & Potter, P. A. (2002). *Clinical nursing skills and techniques* (5th ed.). St. Louis: Mosby.

Racht, E. M. (2002). 10 pitfalls in airway management: How to avoid common airway management complications. *Journal of Emergency Medical Services, 27*(3), 28–34, 36–38, 40–42.

Airway Suctioning 3160

Definition: Removal of secretions by inserting a suction catheter into the patient's oral, nasopharyngeal, or tracheal airway

Activities:
- Perform hand hygiene
- Use universal precautions
- Use personal protective equipment (e.g., gloves, goggles, and mask), as appropriate
- Determine the need for oral and/or tracheal suctioning
- Auscultate breath sounds before and after suctioning
- Inform the patient and family about suctioning
- Aspirate the nasopharynx with a bulb syringe or suction device, as appropriate
- Provide sedation, as appropriate
- Insert a nasal airway to facilitate nasotracheal suctioning, as appropriate
- Instruct the patient to take several deep breaths before nasotracheal suctioning and use supplemental oxygen, as appropriate
- Hyperoxygenate with 100% oxygen for at least 30 seconds, using the ventilator or manual resuscitation bag before and after each pass
- Hyperinflate using tidal volumes that are indexed to the size of the patient, as appropriate
- Use closed-system suctioning, as indicated
- Use sterile disposable equipment for each tracheal suction procedure
- Select a suction catheter that is one half the internal diameter of the endotracheal tube, tracheostomy tube, or patient's airway
- Instruct the patient to take slow, deep breaths during insertion of the suction catheter via the nasotracheal route
- Leave the patient connected to the ventilator during suctioning if a closed tracheal suction system or an oxygen insufflation device adaptor is being used
- Use the lowest amount of wall suction necessary to remove secretions (e.g., 80 to 120 mm Hg for adults)
- Monitor for presence of pain
- Monitor patient's oxygen status (SaO_2 and SvO_2 levels), neurological status (e.g., mental status, ICP, cerebral perfusion pressure [CPP]), and hemodynamic status (e.g., MAP level and cardiac rhythms) immediately before, during, and after suctioning
- Base the duration of each tracheal suction pass on the necessity to remove secretions and the patient's response to suctioning
- Suction the oropharynx after completion of tracheal suctioning
- Clean area around tracheal stoma after completion of tracheal suctioning, as appropriate
- Stop tracheal suctioning and provide supplemental oxygen if patient experiences bradycardia, an increase in ventricular ectopy, and/or desaturation
- Vary suctioning techniques, based on the clinical response of the patient
- Monitor and note secretion color, amount, and consistency
- Send secretions for culture and sensitivity tests, as appropriate
- Instruct the patient and/or family how to suction the airway, as appropriate

1st edition 1992; revised 2013

Background Readings:

Chulay, M. (2005). Suctioning: Endotracheal or tracheostomy tube. In D. L. Wiegand, & K. Carlson, (Eds.), *AACN procedure manual for critical care* (5th ed., pp. 63–70). St. Louis: Saunders.

Evans-Smith, P. (2005). *Taylor's clinical nursing skills.* Philadelphia: Lippincott Williams & Wilkins.

Sole, M. L., Byers, J. F., Ludy, J. E., Zhang, Y., Banta, C. M., & Brummel, K. (2003). A multisite survey of suctioning techniques and airway management practices. *American Journal of Critical Care, 12*(3), 220–230.

Stone, K. S., Preusser, B. A., Groch, K. F., Karl, J. I., & Gronyon, D. S. (1991). The effect of lung hyperinflation and endotracheal suctioning on cardiopulmonary hemodynamics. *Nursing Research, 40*(2), 76–79.

Thompson, L. (2000). Tracheal suctioning of adults with an artificial airway. *Best Practice. 4*(4), 1329–1874.

Allergy Management 6410

Definition: Identification, treatment, and prevention of allergic responses to food, medications, insect bites, contrast material, blood, and other substances

Activities:
- Identify known allergies (e.g., medication, food, insect, environmental) and usual reaction
- Notify caregivers and health care providers of known allergies
- Document all allergies in clinical record, according to protocol
- Place an allergy band on patient, as appropriate
- Monitor patient for allergic reactions to new medications, formulas, foods, latex, and/or test dyes
- Monitor the patient following exposures to agents known to cause allergic responses for signs of generalized flush, angioedema, urticaria, paroxysmal coughing, severe anxiety, dyspnea, wheezing, orthopnea, vomiting, cyanosis, or shock
- Keep patient under observation for 30 minutes following administration of an agent known to be capable of inducing an allergic response
- Instruct the patient with medication allergies to question all new prescriptions for potential allergic reactions
- Encourage patient to wear a medical alert tab, as appropriate
- Identify immediately the level of threat an allergic reaction presents to patient's health status
- Monitor for reoccurrence of anaphylaxis within 24 hours
- Provide life-saving measures during anaphylactic shock or severe reactions
- Provide medication to reduce or minimize an allergic response
- Assist with allergy testing, as appropriate
- Administer allergy injections, as needed
- Watch for allergic responses during immunizations
- Instruct patient/parent to avoid allergic substances, as appropriate
- Instruct patient/parent in how to treat rashes, vomiting, diarrhea, or respiratory problems associated with exposure to allergy-producing substance
- Instruct patient to avoid further use of substances causing allergic responses
- Discuss methods to control environmental allergens (e.g., dust, mold, and pollen)
- Instruct patient and caregiver(s) on how to avoid situations that put them at risk and how to respond if an anaphylactic reaction should occur
- Instruct patient and caregiver on use of epinephrine pen

1st edition 1992; revised 1996, 2000

Background Readings:

Hendry, C. & Farley, A. H. (2001). Understanding allergies and their treatment. *Nursing Standard, 15*(35), 47–53.

Hoole, A., Pickard, C., Ouimette, R., Lohr, J., & Greenberg, R. (1995). *Patient care guidelines for nurse practitioners* (4th ed.). Philadelphia: Lippincott.

Lemone, P. & Burke, K. (1996). *Medical surgical nursing: Critical thinking in client care.* Menlo Park, CA: Addison-Wesley.

Trzcinski, K. M. (1993). Update on common allergic diseases. *Pediatric Nursing, 19*(4), 410–415.

Amnioinfusion 6700

Definition: Infusion of fluid into the uterus during labor to relieve umbilical cord compression or to dilute meconium-stained fluid

Activities:
- Observe for signs of inadequate amniotic fluid volume (e.g., oligohydramnios, asymmetric intrauterine growth retardation, postdatism, known fetal urinary tract abnormalities, and prolonged rupture of membranes)
- Recognize potential contraindications for amnioinfusion (e.g., amnionitis, polyhydramnios, multiple gestation, severe fetal distress, fetal scalp pH < 7.20, known fetal anomaly, known uterine anomaly)
- Observe for variable or prolonged fetal heart decelerations during intrapartal electronic monitoring
- Document presence of thick meconium fluid with rupture of membranes
- Ensure informed consent
- Prepare equipment needed for amnioinfusion
- Flush intrauterine catheter with infusate
- Use universal precautions
- Place intrauterine catheter using sterile technique
- Calibrate and flush catheter after placement using universal precautions
- Infuse 500 to 1000 cc of isotonic IV solution rapidly into the uterine cavity per protocol or physician order
- Place patient in Trendelenburg position, as appropriate
- Maintain continuous infusion at prescribed rates
- Monitor intrauterine pressure readings
- Observe characteristics of return fluid
- Change perineal pads, as appropriate
- Document changes in intrapartal electronic monitor tracings
- Observe for signs of adverse reaction (e.g., uterine overdistension, umbilical cord prolapse, and amniotic fluid embolism)
- Obtain cord blood gas levels at the time of delivery to evaluate effectiveness of intervention

2nd edition 1996; revised 2004

Background Readings:

Longobucco, D. & Winkler, E. (1999). Amnioinfusion: Intrapartum indications and administration. *Mother Baby Journal, 4*(2), 13–18.

Pillitteri, A. (2007). *Maternal and child health nursing: Care of the childbearing and childrearing family* (5th ed.). Philadelphia: Lippincott Williams & Wilkins.

Snell, B. J. (1993). The use of amnioinfusion in nurse-midwifery practice. *Journal of Nurse-Midwifery, 39*(2), 62S–70S.

Weismiller, D. G. (1998). Transcervical amnioinfusion. *American Family Physician, 57*(3), 504–510.

A

Amputation Care 3420

Definition: Promotion of physical and psychological healing before and after amputation of a body part

Activities:

- Encourage the patient to participate in the decision to amputate when possible
- Review informed consent with patient
- Provide information and support before and after surgery
- Facilitate use of a pressure-relieving mattress
- Position stump in proper body alignment
- Place a below-the-knee stump in an extended position
- Avoid putting stump in a dependent position to decrease edema and vascular stasis
- Avoid disturbing stump dressing immediately after surgery as long as there is no leakage or sign of infection
- Wrap the stump, as required
- Promote a smooth, conical-shaped stump through wrapping for a proper prosthesis fit
- Monitor amount of edema present in stump
- Monitor for phantom limb pain (i.e., check for burning, cramping, throbbing, crushing, or tingling pain where the limb was)
- Explain that phantom limb pain may start several weeks after surgery and may be triggered by pressure on other areas
- Administer pharmacologic and non-pharmacologic (e.g., TENS, phonophoresis, and massage) pain control, as needed
- Monitor for psychological concerns (e.g., depression and anxiety) and adjustment related to change in body image
- Monitor wound healing at incision site
- Place affected area in whirlpool bath, as appropriate
- Monitor tissue for skin integrity (e.g., fungal infection, contact dermatitis, and scar management)
- Instruct patient how to correctly perform post-surgical exercises (e.g., range of motion, endurance, and strengthening)
- Encourage patient to perform range-of motion, endurance, and strengthening exercises after surgery, providing assistance when necessary
- Instruct patient to avoid sitting for long periods
- Instruct in transfer techniques and assistive devices (e.g., trapeze)
- Assist patient with grieving process associated with the loss of the body part (e.g., accept initial need for concealment of stump)
- Provide gentle persuasion and support to view and handle altered body part
- Facilitate the identification of needed modifications in lifestyle and assistive devices (e.g., home and car)
- Identify modifications in clothing required
- Set mutual goals for progressive self-care
- Encourage patient to practice self-care of stump
- Provide appropriate education for self-care after discharge
- Instruct patient on signs and symptoms to be reported to health care provider (e.g., chronic pain, skin breakdown, tingling, absent peripheral pulse, cool skin temperature, and changes in functional needs or goals)
- Discuss potential long-term goals for rehabilitation (e.g., walking without a support device)
- Encourage and facilitate interaction with persons with similar amputations, as appropriate
- Supervise initial use and care of the prosthesis
- Cleanse the prosthesis
- Instruct patient and family how to care for and apply the prosthesis
- Assess prosthesis regularly for stability, ease of movement, energy efficiency, and gait appearance
- Remove prosthesis prior to surgery, as appropriate
- Secure prosthesis when not in use
- Refer to specialist for modification of prosthesis or treatment of complications related to its use

1st edition 1992; revised 2004, 2013

Background Readings:

Bloomquist, T. (2001). Amputation and phantom limb pain: A pain-prevention model. *American Association of Nurse Anesthetists Journal, 69*(3), 211–217.

Bryant, G. (2001). Stump care. *American Journal of Nursing, 101*(2), 67–71.

Department of Veterans Affairs, Department of Defense. (2007). *VA/DoD Clinical practice guideline for rehabilitation of lower limb amputation.* Washington, DC: Author.

Esquenazi, A. & DiGiacomo, R. (2001). Rehabilitation after amputation. *Journal of the American Podiatric Association, 91*(1), 13–22.

Gibson, J. (2001). Lower limb amputation. *Nursing Standard, 15*(28), 47–52.

Perry, A. G. & Potter, P. A. (2010). *Clinical nursing skills and techniques* (7th ed., pp. 1028–1032). St. Louis: Mosby.

Sjodahl, C., Jarnlo, G. B., & Persson, B. (2001). Gait improvement in unilateral transfemoral amputees by a combined psychological and physiotherapeutic treatment. *Journal of Rehabilitation Medicine, 33*(3), 114–118.

Analgesic Administration   2210   **A**

Definition: Use of pharmacologic agents to reduce or eliminate pain

Activities:

- Determine pain location, characteristics, quality, and severity before medicating patient
- Check medical order for drug, dose, and frequency of analgesic prescribed
- Check history for drug allergies
- Evaluate the patient's ability to participate in selection of analgesic, route, and dose, and involve the patient, as appropriate
- Choose the appropriate analgesic or combination of analgesics when more than one is prescribed
- Determine analgesic selections (narcotic, nonnarcotic, or NSAID), based on type and severity of pain
- Determine the preferred analgesic, route of administration, and dosage to achieve optimal analgesia
- Choose the IV route, rather than IM, for frequent pain medication injections, when possible
- Sign out narcotics and other restricted drugs, according to agency protocol
- Monitor vital signs before and after administering narcotic analgesics with first-time dose or if unusual signs are noted
- Attend to comfort needs and other activities that assist relaxation to facilitate response to analgesia
- Administer analgesics around the clock to prevent peaks and troughs of analgesia, especially with severe pain
- Set positive expectations regarding the effectiveness of analgesics to optimize patient response
- Administer adjuvant analgesics and/or medications when needed to potentiate analgesia
- Consider use of continuous infusion, either alone or in conjunction with bolus opioids, to maintain serum levels
- Institute safety precautions for those receiving narcotic analgesics, as appropriate
- Instruct to request PRN pain medication before the pain is severe
- Inform the individual that with narcotic administration, drowsiness sometimes occurs during the first 2 to 3 days and then subsides

- Correct misconceptions/myths patient or family members may hold regarding analgesics, particularly opioids (e.g., addiction and risks of overdose)
- Evaluate the effectiveness of analgesic at regular frequent intervals after each administration, but especially after the initial doses, also observing for any signs and symptoms of untoward effects (e.g., respiratory depression, nausea and vomiting, dry mouth, and constipation)
- Document response to analgesic and any untoward effects
- Evaluate and document level of sedation for patients receiving opioids
- Implement actions to decrease untoward effects of analgesics (e.g., constipation and gastric irritation)
- Collaborate with the physician if drug, dose, route of administration, or interval changes are indicated, making specific recommendations based on equianalgesic principles
- Teach about the use of analgesics, strategies to decrease side effects, and expectations for involvement in decisions about pain relief

1st edition 1992; revised 1996

Background Readings:

Clinton, P. & Eland, J. A. (1991). Pain. In M. Maas, K. Buckwalter, & M. Hardy (Eds.), *Nursing diagnoses and interventions for the elderly* (pp. 348–368). Redwood City, CA: Addison-Wesley.

Craven, R. F. & Hirnle, C. J. (2000). *Fundamentals of nursing: Human health and function* (3rd ed., pp. 1161–1168). Philadelphia: Lippincott Williams & Wilkins.

Herr, K. A. & Mobily, P. R. (1992). Interventions related to pain. *Nursing Clinics of North America, 27*(2), 347–370.

McCaffery, M. & Beebe, A. (1989). *Pain: Clinical manual for nursing practice* (pp. 42–123). St. Louis: Mosby.

Perry, A. G. & Potter, P. A. (1990). *Clinical nursing skills and techniques* (pp. 96–101). St. Louis: Mosby.

Smeltzer, S. C. & Bare, B. G. (2004). *Brunner & Suddarth's textbook of medical surgical nursing* (Vol. 1) (10th ed.). Philadelphia: Lippincott Williams & Wilkins.

Analgesic Administration: Intraspinal   2214

Definition: Administration of pharmacologic agents into the epidural or intrathecal space to reduce or eliminate pain

Activities:

- Check patency and function of catheter, port, and/or pump
- Ensure that IV access is in place at all times during therapy
- Label the catheter and secure it appropriately
- Ensure that the proper formulation of the drug is used (e.g., high concentrating and preservation free)
- Ensure narcotic antagonist availability for emergency administration and administer per physician order, as necessary

- Start continuous infusion of analgesic agent after correct catheter placement has been verified, and monitor rate to ensure delivery of prescribed dosage of medication
- Monitor temperature, blood pressure, respirations, pulse, and level of consciousness at appropriate intervals and record on flow sheet
- Monitor level of sensory blockade at appropriate intervals and record on flow sheet

A

- Monitor catheter site and dressings to check for a loose catheter or wet dressing, and notify appropriate personnel per agency protocol
- Administer catheter site care according to agency protocol
- Secure needle in place with tape and apply appropriate dressing according to agency protocol
- Monitor for adverse reactions, including respiratory depression, urinary retention, undue somnolence, itching, seizures, nausea, and vomiting
- Monitor orthostatic blood pressure and pulse before the first attempt at ambulation
- Instruct patient to report side effects, alterations in pain relief, numbness of extremities, and need for assistance with ambulation if weak
- Follow institutional policies for injection of intermittent analgesic agents into the injection port
- Provide adjunct medications as appropriate (e.g., antidepressants, anticonvulsants, and nonsteroidal antiinflammatory agents)
- Increase intraspinal dose, based on pain intensity score
- Instruct and guide patient through nonpharmalogic measures (e.g., relaxation therapy, guided imagery, and biofeedback) to enhance pharmacological effectiveness

- Instruct patient about proper home care for external or implanted delivery systems, as appropriate
- Remove or assist with removal of catheter according to agency protocol

2nd edition 1996

Background Readings:

American Nurses Association. (1992). ANA position statement: The role of the registered nurse in the management of analgesia by catheter techniques. *SCI Nursing, 9*(2), 54–55.

El-Baz, N. & Goldin, M. (1987). Continuous epidural infusion of morphine for pain relief after cardiac operations. *Journal of Cardiovascular Surgery, 93*(6), 878–883.

Keeney, S. (1993). Nursing care of the postoperative patient receiving epidural analgesia. *MEDSURG Nursing, 2*(3), 191–196.

Paice, J. & Magolan, J. (1991). Intraspinal drug therapy. *Nursing Clinics of North America, 26*(2), 477–498.

Smeltzer, S. C. & Bare, B. G. (2004). *Brunner & Suddarth's textbook of medical surgical nursing* (Vol. 1) (10th ed.). Philadelphia: Lippincott Williams & Wilkins.

Wild, L. & Coyne, C. (1992). The basics and beyond: Epidural analgesia. *American Journal of Nursing, 92*(4), 26–34.

Anaphylaxis Management   6412

Definition: Promotion of adequate ventilation and tissue perfusion for an individual with a severe allergic (antigen-antibody) reaction

Activities:
- Identify and remove source of allergen, if possible
- Administer aqueous epinephrine 1:1000 subcutaneously dosing appropriate for age
- Place individual in a comfortable position
- Apply tourniquet per protocol immediately proximal to the allergen point of entry (e.g., injection site, IV site, insect bite), when possible, as appropriate
- Establish and maintain a patent airway
- Administer oxygen at high flow rate (10-15 L/min)
- Monitor vital signs
- Start an IV infusion of normal saline, lactated Ringer's, or a plasma volume expander, as appropriate
- Reassure the individual and the family members
- Monitor for signs of shock (e.g., respiratory difficulty, cardiac arrhythmias, seizures, and hypotension)
- Monitor for self-reports of impending doom
- Maintain flow sheet of activities, including vital signs and medication administration
- Administer IV fluids rapidly (1000 ml/hr) to support blood pressure, per physician order or protocol
- Administer spasmolytics, antihistamines, or corticosteroids as indicated if urticaria, angioedema, or bronchospasm present

- Consult with other healthcare providers and refer, as needed
- Monitor for recurrence of anaphylaxis within 24 hours
- Instruct the individual and family on the use of an epinephrine injection pen
- Instruct the individual and family on prevention of future episodes

3rd edition 2000; revised 2004

Background Readings:

Hoole, A., Pickard, C., Ouimette, R., Lohr, J. H., & Greenberg, R. (1996). *Individual care guidelines for nurse practitioners* (4th ed.). Philadelphia: Lippincott.

Jevon, P. (2001). Anaphylaxis: Emergency treatments. *Nursing Times, 96*(14), 39–40.

Lemone, P. & Burke, K. (1996). *Medical surgical nursing: Critical care thinking in client care.* Redwood City, CA: Addison-Wesley.

Project Team of the Resuscitation Council (UK). (1999). Emergency medical treatment of anaphylactic reaction. *Journal of Accidental Emergency Medicine, 16*(4), 243–247.

Anesthesia Administration   2840   **A**

Definition: Preparation for and administration of anesthetic agents and monitoring of patient responsiveness during administration

Activities:
- Verify patient identification
- Perform and document the patient's health history and physical assessment, evaluating preexisting conditions, allergies, and contraindications for specific anesthetic agents or techniques
- Request appropriate consultations, as well as diagnostic and laboratory studies, based on the patient's health status and proposed surgery
- Implement indicated preoperative activities to prepare patient physiologically for surgery and anesthesia
- Develop and document an anesthetic plan appropriate for the patient and procedure
- Collaborate with involved health care providers throughout all phases of anesthesia care
- Inform the patient what to expect from anesthesia, answering any questions and concerns
- Obtain informed consent
- Perform a safety check on all anesthesia equipment before each anesthetic is administered
- Ensure availability of essential emergency and resuscitation equipment
- Start appropriate intravenous and invasive monitoring lines and initiate noninvasive monitoring modalities
- Administer appropriate preanesthetic medications and fluids
- Assist in the transfer of the patient from the stretcher to the operating room table
- Position patient to prevent peripheral nerve damage and pressure injuries
- Ensure proper placement of safety strap and continuous patient safety throughout all phases of anesthesia care
- Deliver anesthetic consistent with each patient's physiological needs, patient's requests, clinical judgment, and Standards for Nurse Anesthesia Practice
- Assess and maintain an adequate airway, ensuring adequate oxygenation during all phases of anesthesia care
- Determine acceptable blood loss and administer blood, if needed
- Calculate appropriate fluid needs and administer intravenous fluids, as indicated
- Monitor vital signs, respiratory and circulatory adequacy, response to anesthesia, and other physiological parameters; measure and evaluate appropriate lab values
- Administer adjunct drugs and fluids necessary to manage the anesthetic, maintain physiological homeostasis, and correct adverse or unfavorable responses to anesthesia and surgery
- Provide eye protection
- Assess and clinically manage emergence from anesthesia by administering indicated medications, fluids, and ventilatory support
- Transfer patient to the postanesthesia or intensive care unit with appropriate monitoring and oxygen therapy
- Provide comprehensive patient report to nursing staff on arrival in unit
- Manage postoperative pain and anesthetic side effects
- Ascertain patient recovery and stability in the immediate postoperative period before transfer of care
- Provide postanesthesia follow-up evaluation and care related to anesthesia side effects and complications after discharge from postanesthesia care area

1st edition 1992; revised 1996

Background Readings:

American Association of Nurse Anesthetists. (2006). *Professional practice manual for the certified registered nurse anesthetist.* Park Ridge, IL: Author.
Barash, P. G., Cullen, B. F., & Stoeling, R. K. (1989). *Handbook of clinical anesthesia.* Philadelphia: Lippincott.
Waugaman, W. R., Foster, S. D., & Rigor, B. M. (1992). *Principles and practice of nurse anesthesia.* Norwalk, CT: Appleton & Lange.

Anger Control Assistance   4640

Definition: Facilitation of the expression of anger in an adaptive, nonviolent manner

Activities:
- Establish basic trust and rapport with patient
- Use a calm, reassuring approach
- Determine appropriate behavioral expectations for expression of anger, given patient's level of cognitive and physical functioning
- Limit access to frustrating situations until patient is able to express anger in an adaptive manner
- Encourage patient to seek assistance of nursing staff or responsible others during periods of increasing tension
- Monitor potential for inappropriate aggression and intervene before its expression
- Prevent physical harm if anger is directed at self or others (e.g., restrain and remove potential weapons)
- Discourage intense activities (e.g., punching bag, pacing, excessive exercise)
- Educate on methods to modulate experience of intense emotion (e.g., assertiveness training, relaxation techniques, writing in a journal, distraction)
- Provide reassurance to patient that nursing staff will intervene to prevent patient from losing control
- Encourage use of collaboration to solve problems
- Offer PRN medications, as appropriate
- Use external controls (e.g., physical or manual restraint, time outs, and seclusion) as needed (as last resort) to calm patient who is expressing anger in a maladaptive manner
- Provide feedback on behavior to help patient identify anger
- Assist patient in identifying the source of anger

A

- Identify the function that anger, frustration, and rage serve for the patient
- Identify consequences of inappropriate expression of anger
- Assist patient in planning strategies to prevent the inappropriate expression of anger
- Identify with patient the benefits of expressing anger in an adaptive, nonviolent manner
- Establish expectation that patient can control his/her behavior
- Instruct on use of calming measures (e.g., time outs and deep breaths)
- Assist in developing appropriate methods of expressing anger to others (e.g., assertiveness and use of feeling statements)
- Provide role models who express anger appropriately
- Support patient in implementing anger control strategies and in the appropriate expression of anger
- Provide reinforcement for appropriate expression of anger

1st edition 1992; revised 2008

Background Readings:

Bushman, B. J. (2002). Does venting anger feed or extinguish the flame? Catharsis, rumination, distraction, and aggressive responding. *Personality and Social Psychology Bulletin, 28*(6), 724–731.

Carpenito, L. J. (2004). *Nursing diagnosis: Application to clinical practice* (10th ed.). Philadelphia: Lippincott Williams & Wilkins.

Harris, D. & Morrison, E. F. (1995). Managing violence without coercion. *Archives of Psychiatric Nursing, 9*(4), 203–210.

Kanak, M. F. (1992). Interventions related to safety. *Nursing Clinics of North America, 27*(2), 371–395.

Morrison, E. F. (1993). Toward a better understanding of violence in psychiatric settings: Debunking the myths. *Archives of Psychiatric Nursing, 7*(6), 328–335.

Schultz, J. M. & Videbeck, S. L. (2005). *Lippincott's manual of psychiatric nursing careplans* (7th ed.). Philadelphia: Lippincott Williams & Wilkins.

Stuart, G. & Laraia, M. T. (2005). *Principles and practice of psychiatric nursing* (8th ed.). St. Louis: Mosby.

Animal-Assisted Therapy   4320

Definition: Purposeful use of animals to provide affection, attention, diversion, and relaxation

Activities:

- Determine patient's acceptance of animals as therapeutic agents
- Determine if any allergies to animals
- Teach patient/family purpose and rationale for having animals in a care environment
- Enforce standards for screening, training, and grooming of animals in therapy program
- Enforce standards for health maintenance of animals in the therapy program
- Fulfill health inspector's rules concerning animals in an institution
- Develop/have protocol that outlines appropriate response to accident or injury as result of animal contact
- Provide therapy animals for patient such as dogs, cats, horses, snakes, turtles, gerbils, guinea pigs, and birds
- Avoid animal visits with unpredictable or violent patients
- Monitor closely animal visits with patients with special conditions (e.g., open wounds, delicate skin, multiple IV lines, or other equipment)
- Facilitate patient holding and petting therapy animals
- Encourage repeated stroking of the therapy animal
- Facilitate patient watching therapy animals
- Encourage patient expression of emotions to animals
- Arrange for patient to exercise, as appropriate
- Encourage patient to play with therapy animals
- Encourage patient to feed/groom animals
- Have patient and others who pet or contact an animal wash hands
- Provide an opportunity to reminisce and share about previous experiences with pets/other animals

1st edition 1992; revised 2000

Background Readings:

Barba, B. E. (1995). The positive influence of animals: Animal assisted therapy in acute care. *Clinical Nurse Specialist, 9*(4), 199–202.

Cole, K. M. (1999). Animal-assisted therapy. In G. M. Bulechek & J. C. Dochterman (Eds.), *Nursing interventions: Effective nursing treatments* (3rd ed., pp. 508–519). Philadelphia: Saunders.

Giuliano, K., Bloniasz, E., & Bell, J. (1999). Implementation of a pet visitation program in critical care. *Critical Care Nurse, 19*(3), 43–50.

Johnson, R. A. (2002). Commentary: Human-animal interaction research as an area of inquiry in nursing. *Western Journal of Nursing Research, 24*(6), 713–715.

Jorgenson, J. (1997). Therapeutic use of companion animals in health care. *Image: The Journal of Nursing Scholarship, 29*(3), 249–254.

Owen, O. G. (2001). Paws for thought. *Nursing Times, 97*(9), 28–29.

Anticipatory Guidance   5210

Definition: Preparation of patient for an anticipated developmental or situational crisis

Activities:
- Assist the patient to identify possible upcoming, developmental or situational crisis, and the effects the crisis may have on personal and family life
- Instruct about normal development and behavior, as appropriate
- Provide information on realistic expectations related to the patient's behavior
- Determine the patient's usual methods of problem solving
- Assist the patient to decide how the problem will be solved
- Assist the patient to decide who will solve the problem
- Use case examples to enhance the patient's problem-solving skills, as appropriate
- Assist the patient to identify available resources and options for course of action, as appropriate
- Rehearse techniques needed to cope with upcoming developmental milestone or situational crisis with the patient, as appropriate
- Assist the patient to adapt to anticipated role changes
- Provide a ready reference for the patient (e.g., educational materials, pamphlets), as appropriate
- Suggest printed literature and electronic sources for the patient to read, as appropriate
- Refer the patient to community agencies, as appropriate
- Schedule visits at strategic developmental or situational points
- Schedule extra visits for patient with concerns or difficulties
- Schedule follow-up phone calls to evaluate success or reinforcement needs
- Provide the patient with a phone number to call for assistance, if necessary
- Include the family and significant others, when possible

1st edition 1992; revised 2013

Background Readings:

Craft-Rosenberg, M. & Krajicek, M. (2006). *Nursing excellence for children and families.* New York: Springer.

Hagan, J., Shaw, J., & Duncan, P. (2007). *Bright futures: Guidelines for health supervision of infants, children, and adolescents* (3rd ed.). Elk Grove Village, IL: American Academy of Pediatrics.

Rancour, P. (2008). Using archetypes and transitions theory to help patients move from active treatment to survivorship. *Clinical Journal of Oncology Nursing, 12*(6), 935–940.

Rosen, L. (2008). Infant sleep and feeding. *Journal of Obstetric, Gynecologic & Neonatal Nursing, 37*(6), 706–714.

Sattler, B. & Davis, A. (2008). Nurses' role in children's environmental health protection. *Pediatric Nursing, 34*(4) 329–339.

Skybo, T. & Policka, B. (2006). Health promotion model for childhood violence prevention and exposure. *Journal of Clinical Nursing, 16*(1), 38–45.

Anxiety Reduction   5820

Definition: Minimizing apprehension, dread, foreboding, or uneasiness related to an unidentified source of anticipated danger

Activities:
- Use a calm, reassuring approach
- Clearly state expectations for patient's behavior
- Explain all procedures, including sensations likely to be experienced during the procedure
- Seek to understand the patient's perspective of a stressful situation
- Provide factual information concerning diagnosis, treatment, and prognosis
- Stay with patient to promote safety and reduce fear
- Encourage family to stay with patient, as appropriate
- Provide objects that symbolize safeness
- Administer back rub/neck rub, as appropriate
- Encourage noncompetitive activities, as appropriate
- Keep treatment equipment out of sight
- Listen attentively
- Reinforce behavior, as appropriate
- Create an atmosphere to facilitate trust
- Encourage verbalization of feelings, perceptions, and fears
- Identify when level of anxiety changes
- Provide diversional activities geared toward the reduction of tension
- Help patient identify situations that precipitate anxiety
- Control stimuli, as appropriate, for patient needs
- Support the use of appropriate defense mechanisms
- Assist patient to articulate a realistic description of an upcoming event
- Determine patient's decision-making ability
- Instruct patient on the use of relaxation techniques
- Administer medications to reduce anxiety, as appropriate
- Assess for verbal and nonverbal signs of anxiety

1st edition 1992; revised 2004

Background Readings:

Badger, J. M. (1994). Calming the anxious patient. *American Journal of Nursing, 94*(5), 46–50.

Noud, R. B. & Lee, K. (2005). Anxiety disorders. In M. A. Boyd (Ed.), *Psychiatric nursing: Contemporary practice* (3rd ed., pp. 374–419). Philadelphia: Lippincott Williams & Wilkins.

Perry, A. G. & Potter, P. A. (2002). *Clinical nursing skills and techniques* (5th ed.). St. Louis: Mosby.

A

Area Restriction 6420

Definition: Use of least restrictive limitation of patient mobility to a specified area for purposes of safety or behavior management

Activities:
- Establish that the least restrictive measure is being initiated (if a lower level was used, establish that it was deemed ineffective before advancing to the next level of restriction)
- Obtain a licensed independent practitioner (LIP) order as required by selection of measure based on institutional policy and state, federal, and regulatory agencies (e.g., Centers for Medicare & Medicaid Services, The Joint Commission)
- Identify for patient and significant others those behaviors which necessitated the intervention
- Explain the procedure, purpose, and time period of the intervention to patient and significant others in understandable and nonpunitive terms
- Identify for the patient and significant others the appropriate behaviors necessary for termination of the intervention, repeat as needed
- Restrict to designated area that is appropriate
- Modulate human and environmental sensory stimuli (e.g., visiting sessions, sights, sounds, lighting, temperature, etc.) in the designated area, as needed
- Use protective devices and measures (e.g., motion detectors, alarms, fences, gates, side rails, mitts, closed chairs, locked doors, restraints)
- Provide appropriate level of supervision/surveillance to monitor patient and allow for therapeutic actions, as needed
- Administer PRN medications, as appropriate (e.g., anxiolytics, antipsychotics, sedatives)
- Monitor patient's response to the procedure
- Provide for the patient's physical needs and safety (e.g., cardiovascular, respiratory, neurological, elimination and nutrition, and skin integrity), as appropriate
- Provide for the patient's psychological comfort and safety
- Offer structured activities within the designated area, as appropriate
- Give immediate feedback about inappropriate behavior the patient can control and that contributes to need for continued restrictive measure
- Provide verbal reminders, as necessary, to remain in designated area
- Assist patient to modify inappropriate behavior, when possible
- Provide positive reinforcement for appropriate behavior
- Monitor the need for changes (i.e., lower/higher level measure, continue, or discontinue) to the restrictive measure at regular intervals
- Involve patient, when appropriate, in decision to change a restrictive measure (i.e., lower/higher level measure, continue, or discontinue)
- Hold a debriefing session (i.e., covering behaviors leading to the measures, and patient concerns about the intervention) with patient and staff following termination of the intervention
- Document (e.g., rationale for the restrictive measure, patient's physical and psychological condition, nursing care provided, and the rationale for terminating the intervention) at appropriate points in care according to institutional policy, state, federal, and/or regulatory agency requirements

1st edition 1992; revised 2008

Background Readings:

American Psychiatric Nurses Association. (2000). *Position statement on the use of seclusion and restraint.* Arlington, VA: Author.

Clark, M. A. (2005). Involuntary admission and the medical inpatient: Judicious use of physical restraint. *MEDSURG Nursing, 14*(4), 213–218.

Gillies, J., Moriarty, H., Short, T., Pesnell, P., Fox, C., & Cooney, A. (2005). An innovative model for restraint use at the Philadelphia Veterans Affairs Medical Center. *Nursing Administration Quarterly, 29*(1), 45–56.

Harper-Jaques, S. & Reimer, M. (2005). Management of aggression and violence. In M. A. Boyd (Ed.), *Psychiatric nursing: Contemporary practice* (3rd ed., pp. 802–822). Philadelphia: Lippincott Williams & Wilkins.

McCloskey, R. M. (2004). Caring for patients with dementia in an acute care environment. *Geriatric Nursing, 25*(3), 139–44.

Park, M., Hsiao-Chen, T. J., & Ledford, L. (2005). *Changing the practice of physical restraint use in acute care.* Iowa City, IA: The University of Iowa, College of Nursing, Gerontological Nursing Interventions Research Center.

Rickelman, B. L. (2006). The client who displays angry, aggressive, or violent behavior. In W. K. Mohr (Ed.), *Psychiatric mental health nursing* (6th ed., pp. 659–686). Philadelphia: Lippincott Williams & Wilkins.

Aromatherapy 1330

Definition: Administration of essential oils through massage, topical ointments or lotions, baths, inhalation, douches, or compresses (hot or cold) to calm and soothe, provide pain relief, and enhance relaxation and comfort

Activities:
- Obtain verbal consent for use of aromatherapy
- Select appropriate essential oil or blend of essential oils to obtain desired outcome
- Determine individual response to the selected aroma (e.g., like vs. dislike) prior to use
- Use education and training in the background and philosophy in the use of essential oils, mode of action, and any contraindications
- Monitor individual for discomfort and nausea before and after administration
- Dilute essential oils with appropriate carrier oils prior to topical use
- Monitor for contact dermatitis associated with possible allergy to essential oils
- Monitor for exacerbation of asthma in conjunction with use of essential oils, as appropriate
- Instruct individual on purposes and application of aromatherapy, as appropriate

- Monitor baseline and follow-up vital signs, as appropriate
- Monitor individual for preadmission and postadministration report of level of stress, mood, and anxiety, as appropriate
- Administer essential oil using appropriate methods (e.g., massage, inhalation) and to appropriate areas of the body (e.g., feet, back)
- Document physiological responses to aromatherapy, as appropriate
- Evaluate and document response to aromatherapy

4th edition 2004

Background Readings:

Bryan-Brown, C. W. & Dracup, K. (1995). Alternative therapies. *American Journal of Critical Care, 4*(6), 416–418.

Buckle, J. (1998). Clinical aromatherapy and touch: Complementary therapies for nursing practice. *Critical Care Nurse, 18*(5), 54–61.

Buckle, J. (2001). The role of aromatherapy in nursing care. *Nursing Clinics of North America, 36*(1), 57–72.

Cooke, B. & Ernst, E. (2000). Aromatherapy: A systematic review. *British Journal of General Practice, 50*(455), 493–496.

Dunn, C., Sleep, J., & Collett, D. (1995). Sensing an improvement: An experimental study to evaluate the use of aromatherapy, massage and periods of rest in an intensive care unit. *Journal of Advanced Nursing, 21*(1), 34–40.

Petersen, D. (1997). Aromatherapy: Psychological effects of essential oils. *Alternative Therapies in Clinical Practice, 4*(5), 165–167.

Stevensen, C. J. (1994). The psychophysiological effects of aromatherapy massage following cardiac surgery. *Complementary Therapies in Medicine, 2*(1), 27–35.

Tate, S. (1997). Peppermint oil: A treatment for postoperative nausea. *Journal of Advanced Nursing, 26*(3), 543–549.

Wheeler Robins, J. L. (1999). The science and art of aromatherapy. *Journal of Holistic Nursing, 17*(1), 5–17.

Art Therapy   4330

Definition: Facilitation of communication through drawings or other art forms

Activities:
- Identify form of art-based activity (e.g., pre-existing, impromptu, directed, spontaneous)
- Identify art medium to be used, such as drawings (e.g., self portrait, human figure drawings, family kinetic drawings), photos and other media (e.g., photo journal, media journal), graphics (e.g., timeline, body maps), or artifacts (e.g., masks, sculpture)
- Discuss with patient what to make, using direct or nondirect approach, as appropriate
- Provide art supplies appropriate for developmental level and goals for therapy
- Provide a quiet environment that is free from interruptions
- Monitor patient's engagement during the art-making process, including verbal comments and behaviors
- Encourage patient to describe drawing or artistic creation
- Discuss description of drawing or artistic creation with patient
- Record patient interpretation of drawings or artistic creation
- Identify themes in artwork collected over a period of time
- Copy patient's artwork for files, as needed and as appropriate
- Use human figure drawings to determine patient's self-concept
- Use drawings to determine the effects of stress events (e.g., hospitalization, divorce, or abuse) on patient
- Encourage patient to describe and talk about the art product and the art-making process
- Incorporate patient's description and interpretation of the art activity into patient assessment data
- Compare art product and art-making process to patient's developmental level and prior art making activities
- Interpret meaning of significant aspects of the drawings, incorporating patient assessment data and literature on art therapy
- Avoid reading meaning into drawings before having a complete history, baseline drawings, and a collection of drawings done over a period
- Provide referral, as indicated (e.g., social work, art therapy)

1st edition 1992; revised 2013

Background Readings:

Cox, M. (2005). *The pictorial world of the child*. New York: Cambridge Press.

Darley, S. (2008). *The expressive arts activity book: A resource for professionals*. Philadelphia: Jessica Kingsley.

Dixon, S. D. & Stein, M. T. (2006). *Encounters with children: Pediatric behavior and development* (4th ed.). St. Louis: Mosby.

Driessnack, M. (2006). 'Draw-and-tell conversations' with children. *Qualitative Health Research, 16*(10), 1414–1435.

Driessnack, M. (2009). Using the Colored Eco-Genetic Relationship Map (CEGRM) with children. *Nursing Research, 58*(5), 304–311.

Malchiodi, C. A. (2002). *The soul's palette: Drawing on art's transformative power*. Boston: Shambhala.

McNiff, S. (2004). *Art heals: How creativity cures the soul*. Boston: Shambhala.

Seiden, D. (2001). *Mind over matter: The uses of materials in art, education, and therapy*. Chicago: Magnolia Street.

Artificial Airway Management 3180

Definition: Maintenance of endotracheal and tracheostomy tubes and prevention of complications associated with their use

Activities:
- Perform hand hygiene
- Use universal precautions
- Use personal protective equipment (e.g., gloves, goggles, and mask), as appropriate
- Provide an oropharyngeal airway or bite block to prevent biting on the endotracheal tube, as appropriate
- Provide 100% humidification of inspired air, oxygen, or gas
- Provide adequate systemic hydration via oral or intravenous fluid administration
- Inflate endotracheal/tracheostoma cuff using minimal occlusive volume (MOV) technique or minimal leak technique (MLT)
- Maintain inflation of the endotracheal/tracheostoma cuff at 15 to 25 mm Hg during mechanical ventilation and during and after feeding
- Monitor cuff pressures every 4 to 8 hours during expiration using a three-way stopcock, calibrated syringe, and manometer
- Check cuff pressure immediately after delivery of any general anesthesia or manipulation of endotracheal tube
- Institute endotracheal suctioning, as appropriate
- Suction the oropharynx and secretions from the top of the tube cuff before deflating the cuff
- Change endotracheal tapes/ties every 24 hours, inspect the skin and oral mucosa, and reposition ET to the other side of the mouth
- Loosen commercial endotracheal tube holders at least once a day, and provide skin care
- Auscultate for presence of lung sounds bilaterally after insertion and after changing endotracheal/tracheostomy ties
- Note the centimeter reference marking on endotracheal tube to monitor for possible displacement
- Assist with chest x-ray examination, as needed, to monitor position of tube
- Minimize leverage and traction on the artificial airway by suspending ventilator tubing from overhead supports, using flexible catheter mounts and swivels, and supporting tubes during turning, suctioning, and ventilator disconnection and reconnection
- Monitor for presence of crackles and rhonchi over large airways
- Monitor secretions color, amount, and consistency
- Perform oral care (i.e., use toothbrush, swabs, mouth and lip moisturizer), as needed
- Monitor for decrease in exhale volume and increase in inspiratory pressure in patients receiving mechanical ventilation
- Institute measures to prevent spontaneous decannulation (i.e., secure artificial airway with tape or ties, administer sedation and muscle paralyzing agent, use arm restraints), as appropriate
- Provide additional intubation equipment and ambu bag in a readily available location
- Provide trachea care every 4 to 8 hours as appropriate: Clean the inner cannula, clean and dry the area around the stoma, and change tracheostomy ties
- Inspect skin around tracheal stoma for drainage, redness, irritation, and bleeding
- Inspect and palpate for air under skin every 8 hours
- Monitor for presence of pain
- Maintain sterile technique when suctioning and providing tracheostomy care
- Shield the tracheostomy from water
- Tape the tracheostomy obturator to head of bed
- Tape a second tracheostomy (same type and size) and forceps to head of bed
- Institute chest physiotherapy, as appropriate
- Ensure that endotracheal/tracheostomy cuff is inflated during feedings, as appropriate
- Elevate head of the bed equal to or greater than 30 degrees or assist patient to a sitting position in a chair during feedings, as appropriate

1st edition 1992; revised 2013

Background Readings:

Chulay, M. (2005). Suctioning: Endotracheal or tracheostomy tube. In D. Wielaned, & K. Carlson, (Eds.), *AACN procedure manual for critical care*, (5th ed., pp.63–70). St. Louis: Saunders.

Evans-Smith, P. (2005). *Taylor's clinical nursing skills*. Philadelphia: Lippincott Williams & Wilkins.

Schleder, B., Stott, K., & Lloyd, R. (2002). The effect of a comprehensive oral care protocol on patients at risk for ventilator-associated pneumonia. *Journal of Advocate Health Care*, 4(1), 27–30.

Simmons-Trau, D., Cenek, P., Counterman, J., Hockenbury, D., & Litwiller, L. (2004). Reducing VAP with 6 Sigma. *Nurse Manager*, 35(6), 41–45.

Skillings, K. N. & Curtis, B. L. (2005). Tracheal tube cuff care. In D. Wielaned, & K. Carlson, (Eds.), *AACN procedure manual for critical care*, (5th ed., pp. 71–86). St. Louis: Saunders.

Sole, M. L., Byers, J. F., Ludy, J. E., Zhang, Y., Banta, C. M., & Brummel, K. (2003). A multisite survey of suctioning techniques and airway management practices. *American Journal of Critical Care*, 12(3), 220–230.

Tablan, O., Anderson, L., Besser, R., Bridges, C., & Hajjeh, R. (2004). Guidelines for preventing health-care—associated pneumonia, 2003. *Morbidity & Mortality Weekly Report*, 53(RR-3), 1–36.

Aspiration Precautions 3200

A

Definition: Prevention or minimization of risk factors in the patient at risk for aspiration

Activities:
- Monitor level of consciousness, cough reflex, gag reflex, and swallowing ability
- Screen for dysphagia, as appropriate
- Maintain an airway
- Minimize use of narcotics and sedatives
- Minimize use of medications known to delay gastric emptying, as appropriate
- Monitor pulmonary status
- Monitor bowel care needs
- Position upright equal to or greater than 30 (NG feedings) to 90 degrees or as far as possible
- Keep head of bed elevated 30 to 45 minutes after feeding
- Keep tracheal cuff inflated, as appropriate
- Keep suction setup available
- Supervise eating or assist as necessary
- Feed in small amounts
- Check NG or gastrostomy placement before feeding
- Check NG or gastrostomy residual before feeding
- Avoid feeding, if residuals are high (e.g., greater than 250 cc for feeding tubes or greater than 100 cc for PEG tubes)
- Use continuous NG pump feedings in place of gravity or bolus, if appropriate
- Use prokinetic agents, as appropriate
- Avoid liquids or use thickening agent
- Offer foods or liquids that can be formed into a bolus before swallowing
- Cut food into small pieces
- Request medication in elixir form
- Break or crush pills before administration
- Inspect oral cavity for retained food or medications
- Provide oral care
- Suggest speech pathology consult, as appropriate
- Suggest barium cookie swallow or video fluoroscopy, as appropriate

1st edition 1992; revised 2013

Background Readings:

Bowman, A., Greiner, J. E., Doerschug, K. C., Little, S. B., Bombei, C. L., & Comried, L. M. (2005). Implementation of an evidence-based feeding protocol and aspiration risk reduction algorithm. *Critical Care Nursing Quarterly, 28*(4), 324–333.
Eisenstadt, E. S. (2010). Dysphagia and aspiration pneumonia in older adults. *Journal of the American Academy of Nurse Practitioners, 22*(1), 17–22
Evans-Smith, P. (2005). *Taylor's clinical nursing skills.* Philadelphia: Lippincott Williams & Wilkins.
Maas, M. L., Buckwalter, K. C., Hardy, M. D., Tripp-Reimer, T., Titler, M. G., & Specht, J. P. (Eds.). (2001). *Nursing care of older adults: Diagnoses, outcomes, and interventions* (pp. 167–168). St. Louis: Mosby.
Perry, L. & Love, C. P. (2001) Screening for dysphagia and aspiration in acute stroke: A systematic review. *Dysphagia, 16*(1), 7–18.

Assertiveness Training 4340

Definition: Assistance with the effective expression of feelings, needs, and ideas while respecting the rights of others

Activities:
- Determine barriers to assertiveness (e.g., developmental stage, chronic medical or psychiatric condition, and female socialization)
- Help patient recognize and reduce cognitive distortions that block assertion
- Differentiate between assertive, aggressive, and passive-aggressive behaviors
- Help to identify personal rights, responsibilities, and conflicting norms
- Help clarify problem areas in interpersonal relationships
- Promote expression of thoughts and feelings, both positive and negative
- Help identify self-defeating thoughts
- Assist patient to distinguish between thought and reality
- Instruct patient in the different ways to act assertively
- Instruct patient about strategies for practicing assertive behavior (e.g., making requests, saying no to unreasonable requests, and initiating and concluding conversation)
- Facilitate practice opportunities, using discussion, modeling, and role playing
- Help practice conversational and social skills (e.g., use of "I" statements, nonverbal behaviors, openness, and accepting compliments)
- Praise efforts to express feelings and ideas
- Monitor anxiety level and discomfort related to behavioral change

1st edition 1992; revised 1996

Background Readings:

Barker, P. (1990). Breaking the shell. *Nursing Times, 86*(46), 36–38.
Chitty, K. K. (2004). Mood disorders. In C. R. Kneisl, H. S. Wilson, & E. Trigoboff (Eds.), *Contemporary psychiatric-mental health nursing* (pp. 334–365). Upper Saddle River, NJ: Pearson Prentice Hall.
Craven, R. F. & Hirnle, C. J. (2000). *Fundamentals of nursing: Human health and function* (3rd ed., p. 1311). Philadelphia: Lippincott Williams & Wilkins.
Pointer, P. & Lancaster, J. (1988). Assertiveness. In M. Stanhope & J. Lancaster (Eds.), *Community health nursing* (2nd ed., pp. 609–625). St. Louis: Mosby.
Sadler, A. G. (1985). Assertiveness training. In G. M. Bulechek & J. C. McCloskey (Eds.), *Nursing interventions: Treatments for nursing diagnoses* (pp. 234–254). Philadelphia: Saunders.
Smith, K. E., Schreiner, B., Jackson, C., & Travis, L. B. (1993). Teaching assertive communication skills to adolescents with diabetes: Evaluation of a camp curriculum. *The Diabetes Educator, 19*(2), 136–141.

Asthma Management 3210

Definition: Identification, treatment, and prevention of reactions to inflammation/constriction in the airway passages

Activities:
- Determine baseline respiratory status to use as a comparison point
- Document baseline measurements in clinical record
- Compare current status with previous status to detect changes in respiratory status
- Obtain spirometry measurements (FEV_1, FVC, FEV_1/FVC ratio) before and after the use of a short-acting bronchodilator
- Monitor peak expiratory flow rate (PERF), as appropriate
- Educate patient on the use of the PERF meter at home
- Monitor for asthmatic reactions
- Determine client/family understanding of disease and management
- Instruct client/family on antiinflammatory and bronchodilator medications and their appropriate usage
- Teach proper techniques for using medication and equipment (e.g., inhaler, nebulizer, peak flow meter)
- Determine compliance with prescribed treatments
- Encourage verbalization of feelings about diagnosis, treatment, and impact on lifestyle
- Identify known triggers and usual reaction
- Teach client to identify and avoid triggers, as possible
- Establish a written plan with the client for managing exacerbations
- Assist in the recognition of signs/symptoms of impending asthmatic reaction and implementation of appropriate response measures
- Monitor rate, rhythm, depth, and effort of respiration
- Note onset, characteristics, and duration of cough
- Observe chest movement, including symmetry, use of accessory muscles, and supraclavicular and intercostal muscle retractions
- Auscultate breath sounds, noting areas of decreased/absent ventilation and adventitious sounds
- Administer medication as appropriate and/or per policy and procedural guidelines
- Auscultate lung sounds after treatment to determine results
- Offer warm fluids to drink, as appropriate
- Coach in breathing/relaxation techniques
- Use a calm, reassuring approach during asthma attack
- Inform client/family about the policy and procedures for carrying and administration of asthma medications at school
- Inform parent/guardian when child has needed/used PRN medication in school, as appropriate
- Refer for medical assessment, as appropriate
- Establish a regular schedule of follow-up care
- Instruct and monitor pertinent school staff in emergency procedures
- Prescribe and/or renew asthma medications, as appropriate

4th edition 2004

Background Readings:

American Academy of Allergy, Asthma, & Immunology. (1999). *Pediatric asthma: Promoting best practice. Guide for managing asthma in children.* Milwaukee, WI: Author.

Pillitteri, A. (2007). *Maternal and child health nursing: Care of the childbearing and childrearing family* (5th ed.). Philadelphia: Lippincott Williams & Wilkins.

Silkworth, C. K. (1993). IHP: Asthma. In M. K. Haas (Ed.), *The school nurse's source book of individualized healthcare plans, Volume 1.* (pp. 133–150). North Branch, MN: Sunrise River Press.

Szilagyi, P. & Kemper, K. (1999). Management of chronic childhood asthma in the primary care office. *Pediatric Annals, 28*(1), 43–52.

University of Michigan Health System. (2000). *Asthma: Guidelines for clinical care.* http://cme.med.umich.edu/pdf/guideline/asthma05.pdf/

Yoos, H. L. & McMullen, A. (1999). Symptom monitoring in childhood asthma: How to use a peak flow meter. *Pediatric Annals, 28*(1), 31–39.

Attachment Promotion 6710

Definition: Facilitating the development of an affective, enduring relationship between infant and parent

Activities:
- Discuss with patient culture-based expressions of attachment prior to and after birth
- Discuss patient's reaction to pregnancy
- Determine patient's image of unborn child
- Discuss patient's experience of hearing fetal heart tones
- Discuss patient's experience of viewing fetal ultrasound image
- Discuss patient's experience of fetal movements
- Encourage patient to attend prenatal classes
- Instruct patient's partner on ways to participate during labor and delivery
- Place newborn skin-to-skin with parent immediately after birth
- Provide opportunity for parent to see, hold, and examine newborn immediately after birth (i.e., delay unnecessary procedures and provide privacy)
- Facilitate eye contact between parent and newborn immediately after birth (i.e., demonstrate en face positioning, dim room lights, and provide a quiet, private environment)
- Complete maternal and newborn assessments while allowing parent to hold newborn
- Share information gained from physical assessments of infant with parent
- Inform parent of care being given to infant
- Provide pain relief to mother
- Encourage mother to breastfeed, if appropriate
- Provide adequate breastfeeding education and support, if appropriate
- Instruct parent on infant cues for feeding (e.g., rooting, sucking on fingers, crying)

- Instruct parent on importance of feeding as nurturing activity, as it provides opportunity for extended eye contact and physical closeness
- Assist parent in identifying infant's need when crying (e.g., hunger, pain, fatigue, fussiness)
- Encourage consistent, prompt response to infant crying
- Demonstrate infant soothing techniques to parent
- Discuss infant behavioral characteristics with parent
- Point out infant cues that show responsiveness to parent
- Instruct parent on signs of overstimulation
- Encourage frequent, sustained physical closeness between infant and parent (e.g., skin-to-skin contact, breastfeeding, child carrying, and sleeping in close proximity to infant)
- Instruct parent on various ways of providing skin-to-skin contact (e.g., kangaroo care, massaging, and co-bathing)
- Instruct parent on infant cares (e.g., diaper changing, feeding, holding, massaging)
- Encourage use of family members and friends for infant caregiving
- Reinforce caregiver role behaviors
- Encourage parent to identify family characteristics observed in infant
- Provide assistance in self-care to maximize focus on infant
- Assist parent of multiples in recognizing individuality of each infant
- Facilitate parent's complete access to and care of hospitalized infant
- Explain equipment used to monitor hospitalized infant
- Instruct parent how to transfer infant from incubator, warmer bed, or bassinet while managing equipment and tubing
- Demonstrate ways to touch infant confined to isolette
- Provide visual objects depicting infant (e.g., photograph of infant, infant footprint) to parent of hospitalized infant
- Update parent frequently on status of hospitalized infant
- Instruct parent on attachment development, emphasizing its complexity, ongoing nature, and opportunities

- Provide anticipatory guidance on developmental milestones that will occur
- Determine how family is coping with transitions
- Provide opportunity for parent to discuss topics of concern (e.g., fears, questions pertaining to infant care, feelings of exhaustion, pain management, and ways to interact with and respond to infant)
- Monitor factors that may interfere with optimal attachment (e.g., mental health disturbance in parent, financial strain, parent and child separation due to medical or surgical intervention, difficulties with breastfeeding, providing foster care, and adopting)
- Provide referral to services (i.e., financial, pastoral care, and counseling), if appropriate

1st edition 1992; revised 2013

Background Readings:

Denehy, J. A. (1992). Interventions related to parent-infant attachment. In G. M. Bulechek & J. C. McCloskey (Eds.), Symposium on nursing interventions. *Nursing Clinics of North America, 27*(2), 425–444.

Gribble, K. D. (2007). A model for caregiving of adopted children after institutionalization. *Journal of Child & Adolescent Psychiatric Nursing, 20*(1), 14–26.

Moore, E. R., Anderson, G. C., & Bergman, N. (2007). Early skin-to-skin contact for mothers and their healthy newborn infants. *Cochrane Database of Systematic Reviews*, Issue 3. Art. No.: CD003519. doi: 10.1002/14651858. CD003519.pub2.

Murphy, N. L. (2009). Facilitating attachment after international adoption. *The American Journal of Maternal Child Nursing, 34*(4), 210–215.

Ward, S. L. & Hisley, S. M. (2009). *Maternal-child nursing care: Optimizing outcomes for mothers, children, & families.* Philadelphia: F. A. Davis.

Wheeler, B. & Wilson, D. (2007). Health promotion of the newborn and family. In M. J. Hockenberry & D. Wilson (Eds.), *Wong's nursing care of infants and children* (8th ed., pp. 257–309). St. Louis: Mosby.

Autogenic Training   5840

Definition: Assisting with self-suggestions about feelings of heaviness and warmth for the purpose of inducing relaxation

Activities:
- Choose a quiet, comfortable setting
- Prepare a quiet environment
- Take precautions to prevent interruptions
- Instruct patient on purpose for the intervention
- Seat patient in a reclining chair or place in recumbent position
- Have patient wear comfortable, unrestricted clothing
- Read a prepared script to patient, pausing for enough time for the statement to be internally repeated
- Use statements in the script which elicit feelings of heaviness, lightness, or floating of specific body parts
- Instruct patient to repeat statements to self and to elicit the feeling within the body part being directed
- Rehearse with the script for about 15 to 20 minutes
- Encourage patient to remain relaxed for another 15 to 20 minutes
- Proceed to elicit feelings of warmth after heaviness sensations have been mastered
- Follow the procedure for eliciting heaviness using a prepared script or audiotape for eliciting warmth

- Provide home instructions with a script or audiotape for patient to use
- Encourage patient to practice session three times a day
- Instruct patient to keep a diary to document progress made with each session

1st edition 1992; revised 2008

Background Readings:

Crowther, D. (2001). Autogenic therapy. In D. Rankin-Box (Ed.), *The nurse's handbook of complementary therapies* (2nd ed., pp. 139–144). London: Bailliere Tindall.

Kanji, N. & Ernst, E. (2000). Autogenic training for stress and anxiety: A systematic review. *Complementary Therapies in Medicine, 8*, 106–110.

Linden, W. (1990). *Autogenic training: A clinical guide.* New York: Guilford.

Linden, W. (1994). Autogenic training: A narrative and quantitative review of clinical outcome. *Biofeedback Self-Regulation, 19*(3), 227–264.

Autotransfusion   2860

Definition: Collecting and reinfusing blood that has been lost intraoperatively or postoperatively from clean wounds

Activities:

- Screen for appropriateness of salvage (contraindications include sepsis, infection, tumor at the site, blood containing an irrigant that is not injectable, hemostatic agents, or microcrystalline collagen)
- Obtain patient's informed consent
- Instruct patient regarding procedure
- Use appropriate blood retrieval system
- Label collection device with the patient's name, hospital number, date, and time that collection was begun
- Monitor patient and system frequently during retrieval
- Maintain integrity of the system before, during, and after blood retrieval
- Screen blood for appropriateness of reinfusion
- Maintain integrity of blood between salvage and reinfusion
- Prepare blood for reinfusion
- Document time of initiation of collecting, condition of blood, type and amount of anticoagulants, and retrieval volume
- Reinfuse transfusion within 6 hours of retrieval
- Maintain universal precautions

2nd edition 1996; revised 2008

Background Readings:

American Association of Blood Banks. (1990). *Guidelines for blood salvage and reinfusion in surgery and trauma.* Arlington, VA: Author.

Arlington, R. G., Costigan, K. A., & Aievoli, C. P. (1992). Postoperative orthopaedic blood salvage and reinfusion. *Orthopaedic Nursing, 11*(3), 30–38.

Failla, S. D. & Radaslovich, N. (1993). Ask the OR. *American Journal of Nursing, 93*(6), 74.

LeMone, P. & Burke, K. M. (2000). *Medical–surgical nursing: Critical thinking in client care* (2nd ed., p. 281). Upper Saddle River, NJ: Prentice Hall.

Peterson, K. J. (1992). Nursing management of autologous blood transfusion. *Journal of Intravenous Nursing, 15*(3), 128–34.

Smeltzer, S. C. & Bare, B. G. (2004). *Brunner & Suddarth's textbook of medical surgical nursing* (Vol. 1) (10th ed.). Philadelphia: Lippincott Williams & Wilkins.

Bathing 1610

Definition: Cleaning of the body for the purposes of relaxation, cleanliness, and healing

Activities:
- Assist with chair shower, tub bath, bedside bath, standing shower, or sitz bath, as appropriate or desired
- Wash hair, as needed and desired
- Bathe in water of a comfortable temperature
- Use fun bathing techniques with children (e.g., wash dolls or toys; pretend a boat is a submarine; punch holes in bottom of plastic cup, fill with water, and let it "rain" on child)
- Assist with perineal care, as needed
- Assist with hygiene measures (e.g., use of deodorant or perfume)
- Administer foot soaks, as needed
- Shave patient, as indicated
- Apply lubricating ointment and cream to dry skin areas
- Offer hand washing after toileting and before meals
- Apply drying powders to deep skin folds
- Monitor skin condition while bathing
- Monitor functional ability while bathing

1st edition 1992, revised 2000

Background Readings:

Perry, A. G. & Potter, P. A. (2002). *Clinical nursing skills and techniques* (5th ed.). St. Louis: Mosby.

Sloane, P. D., Rader, J., Barrick, A. L., Hoeffer, B., Dwyer, D., McKenzie, D., et al. (1995). Bathing persons with dementia. *The Gerontologist, 35*(5), 672–678.

Wong, D. L. (1995). *Whaley & Wong's nursing care of infants and children* (5th ed.). St. Louis: Mosby.

Bed Rest Care 0740

Definition: Promotion of comfort and safety and prevention of complications for a patient unable to get out of bed

Activities:
- Explain reasons for requiring bed rest
- Place on an appropriate therapeutic mattress or bed
- Position in proper body alignment
- Avoid using rough-textured bed linens
- Keep bed linen clean, dry, and wrinkle free
- Apply a footboard to the bed
- Use devices on the bed that protect the patient
- Apply appliances to prevent footdrop
- Raise siderails, as appropriate
- Place bed-positioning switch within easy reach
- Place the call light within reach
- Place bedside table within patient's reach
- Attach trapeze to the bed, as appropriate
- Turn, as indicated by skin condition
- Turn the immobilized patient at least every 2 hours, according to a specific schedule
- Monitor skin condition
- Teach bed exercises, as appropriate
- Facilitate small shifts of body weight
- Perform passive and active range-of-motion exercises
- Assist with hygiene measures (e.g., use of deodorant or perfume)
- Assist with activities of daily living
- Apply antiembolism stockings
- Monitor for complications of bedrest (e.g., loss of muscle tone, back pain, constipation, increased stress, depression, confusion, sleep cycle changes, urinary tract infections, difficulty with urination, pneumonia)
- Place in upright posture intermittently for patients unable to be out of bed every day to protect against orthostatic intolerance

1st edition 1992, revised 2013

Background Readings:

Cheng, K. (2010). Prolonged bed rest duration after percutaneous coronary intervention. *CONNECT: The World of Critical Care Nursing, 7*(2), 111–114.

Dunn, L.L., Handley, M. C., & Carter, M. R. (2006). Antepartal bed rest: Conflicts, costs, controversies, and ethical considerations. *Online Journal of Health Ethics, 3*(1).

Fox, M. T., Sidani, S., & Brooks, D. (2010). The relationship between bed rest and sitting orthostatic intolerance in adults residing in chronic care facilities, *Journal of Nursing and Healthcare of Chronic Illness, 2*(3), 187–196.

Norton, L., Coutts, P., Fraser, C., Nicholson, T., & Sibbald, R.G. (2007). Is bed rest an effective treatment modality for pressure ulcers? In D. L. Kesner, G. Rodeheaver, & R. G. Sibbald (Eds.), *Chronic wound care: A clinical source book for healthcare professionals* (4th ed., chap. 12). Malvern, PA: HMP Communications.

Sprague, A. E. (2004). The evolution of bed rest as a clinical intervention. *Journal of Obstetrics, Gynecologic & Neonatal Nursing, 33*(5), 542–561.

B

Bedside Laboratory Testing   7610

Definition: Performance of laboratory tests at the bedside or point of care

Activities:
- Obtain adequate training/orientation before performing testing
- Participate in color blindness testing, as needed for particular test and as required by institution
- Participate in proficiency testing programs, as required by institution
- Follow institutional procedures for specimen collection and preservation, as appropriate
- Label specimens immediately to minimize sample mix-ups, as appropriate
- Use appropriate specimen for the bedside test being performed
- Perform bedside testing on collected specimens in a timely manner
- Use universal precautions when handling specimens for testing
- Store reagents according to manufacturer's requirements or as stated in your institution's procedure manual
- Check expiration date of any reagent preparation, including test strips and contents of commercial kits to avoid using expired reagents
- Follow manufacturer guidelines and institutional procedures for instrument calibration
- Document instrument calibration, as required
- Perform quality control checks according to manufacturer recommendation or as stated in institution procedure
- Document quality control checks, as required
- Perform test according to manufacturer directions or as stated in institutional procedures
- Ensure accurate timing with testing that requires prescribed times
- Document results of tests, according to institutional procedure
- Report abnormal or critical results to physician, as appropriate
- Perform cleaning and maintenance of instruments according to manufacturer guidelines or as stated in institutional procedure
- Document cleaning and maintenance, as required
- Report test results to patient, as appropriate

2nd edition 1996

Background Readings:

College of American Pathologists, Commission on Laboratory Accreditation. (1993). *Inspection checklist: Ancillary testing.* Northfield, IL: Author.

Corbett, J. V. (1992). *Laboratory tests & diagnostic procedures with nursing diagnoses* (3rd ed.). Norwalk, CT: Appleton & Lange.

Fischbach, F. & Dunning, M. B. (2006). *Nurses' quick reference to common laboratory and diagnostic tests* (4th ed.). Philadelphia: Lippincott Williams & Wilkins.

Kee, J. L. (1991). *Laboratory and diagnostic tests with nursing implications* (3rd ed.). Norwalk, CT: Appleton & Lange.

Perry, A. C. & Potter, P. A. (1998). *Clinical nursing skills & techniques* (4th ed.). St. Louis: Mosby.

Behavior Management   4350

Definition: Helping a patient to manage negative behavior

Activities:
- Hold the patient responsible for his/her behavior
- Communicate expectation that patient will retain control
- Consult with family to establish patient's cognitive baseline
- Set limits with patient
- Refrain from arguing or bargaining about the established limits with the patient
- Establish routines
- Establish shift-to-shift consistency in environment and care routine
- Use consistent repetition of health routines as a means of establishing them
- Avoid interruptions
- Increase physical activity, as appropriate
- Limit number of caregivers
- Utilize a soft, low speaking voice
- Avoid cornering the patient
- Redirect attention away from agitation source
- Avoid projecting a threatening image
- Avoid arguing with patient
- Ignore inappropriate behavior
- Discourage passive-aggressive behavior
- Praise efforts at self-control
- Medicate as needed
- Apply wrist/leg/chest restraints, as necessary

Background Readings:

Ackerman, L. L. (1992). Interventions related to neurological care. In G. M. Bulechek & J. C. McCloskey (Eds.), Symposium on nursing interventions. *Nursing Clinics of North America, 27*(2), 325–346.

American Nurses' Association Council in Medical-Surgical Nursing Practice & American Association of Neuroscience Nurses. (1985). *Neuroscience nursing practice: Process and outcome for selected diagnoses.* Kansas City, MO: American Nurse's Association.

Boyd, M. A. (2005). Psychiatric-mental health nursing interventions. In. M. A. Boyd (Ed.) *Psychiatric nursing: Contemporary practice* (3rd ed., pp. 218–232). Philadelphia: Lippincott Williams & Wilkins.

Coucouvanis, J. A. (1990). Behavior management. In M. J. Craft & J. A. Denehy (Eds.), *Nursing interventions for infants and children* (pp. 151–165). Philadelphia: Saunders.

Hinkle, J. (1988). Nursing care of patients with minor head injury. *Journal of Neuroscience Nursing, 20*(1), 8–14.

Phylar, P. A. (1989). Management of the agitated and aggressive head injury patient in an acute hospital setting. *Journal of Neuroscience Nursing, 21*(6), 353–356.

Woody, S. (1988). Episodic dyscontrol syndrome and head injury: A case presentation. *Journal of Neuroscience Nursing, 20*(3), 180–184.

1st edition 1992; revised 2000

Behavior Management: Overactivity/Inattention   4352

B

Definition: Provision of a therapeutic milieu that safely accommodates the patient's attention deficit and/or overactivity while promoting optimal function

Activities:

- Provide a structured and physically safe environment, as necessary
- Use a calm, matter-of-fact, reassuring approach
- Determine appropriate behavioral expectations and consequences given the patient's level of cognitive functioning and capacity for self-control
- Develop a behavioral management plan that is carried out consistently by all care providers
- Communicate rules, behavioral expectations, and consequences using simple language with visual cues, as necessary
- Refrain from arguing or bargaining about established limits
- Provide reassurance that staff will assist patient with managing his/her behavior, as necessary
- Praise desired behaviors and efforts at self-control
- Provide consistent consequences for both desired and undesired behavior(s)
- Obtain patient's attention before initiating verbal interactions (e.g., call by name and obtain eye contact)
- Give any instructions/explanations slowly, using simple and concrete language
- Ask patient to repeat instructions before beginning tasks
- Break multiple-step instructions into simple steps
- Allow patient to carry out one instruction before being given another
- Provide assistance, as necessary, to complete task(s)
- Provide positive feedback for completion of each step
- Provide aides that will increase environmental structure, concentration, and attention to tasks (e.g., watches, calendars, signs, and step-by-step written instructions)
- Decrease or withdraw verbal and physical cues as they become unnecessary
- Monitor and regulate level of activity and stimulation in environment
- Maintain a routine schedule that includes a balance of structured time (e.g., physical and nonphysical activities) and quiet time
- Limit choices, as necessary
- Redirect or remove patient from source of overstimulation (e.g., a peer or a problem situation)
- Use external controls, as necessary, to calm patient (e.g., time out, seclusion, and physical restraint)
- Monitor physical status of overactive patient (e.g., body weight, hydration, and condition of feet in patient who paces)
- Monitor fluid and nutritional intake
- Provide high-protein, high-calorie finger foods and fluids that can be consumed "on the run"
- Limit excessive intake of food and fluids
- Limit intake of caffeinated food and fluids
- Instruct in problem-solving skills
- Encourage the expression of feelings in an appropriate manner
- Teach/reinforce appropriate social skills
- Set limits on intrusive, interruptive behavior(s)
- Provide illness teaching to patient/significant others if the overactivity or inattention is illness-based (e.g., attention deficit disorder, hyperactivity, mania, and schizophrenia)
- Administer medications (e.g., stimulants and antipsychotics) to promote desired behavior changes
- Monitor patient for medication side effects and desired behavioral outcomes
- Provide medication teaching to patient/significant others
- Discuss reasonable behavioral expectations for patient with family/significant others
- Teach behavioral management techniques to significant others
- Assist patient and involved others (family, employers, and teachers) to adapt the home, work, or school environment(s) to accommodate limitations imposed by chronic inattention and overactivity
- Facilitate family coping through support groups, respite care, and family counseling, as appropriate

2nd edition 1996

Background Readings:

Cipkala-Gaffin, J. A. & Cipkala-Gaffin, G. L. (1989). Developmental disabilities and nursing interventions. In L. M. Birckhead (Ed.), *Psychiatric mental health nursing. The therapeutic use of self* (pp. 349–379). Philadelphia: Lippincott.

Fortinash, K. M. & Holoday-Worret, P. A. (1991). *Psychiatric nursing care plans.* St. Louis: Mosby.

Kendall, P. C. & Braswell, L. (1985). *Cognitive-behavioral therapy for impulsive children.* New York: The Guilford Press.

Scahill, L., Hamrin, V., & Deering, C. G. (2005). Psychiatric disorders diagnosed in childhood and adolescence. In M. A. Boyd (Ed.), *Psychiatric nursing: Contemporary practice* (3rd ed., pp. 603–639). Philadelphia: Lippincott Williams & Wilkins.

Stockard, S. (1987). Disorders of childhood. In J. Norris, M. Kunes-Connell, S. Stockard, P. M. Ehrhart, & G. R. Newton (Eds.), *Mental health-psychiatric nursing. A continuum of care* (pp. 657–691). New York: John Wiley & Sons.

Townsend, M. C. (1988). *Nursing diagnoses in psychiatric nursing: A pocket guide for care plan construction.* Philadelphia: F. A. Davis.

Behavior Management: Self-Harm   4354

Definition: Assisting the patient to decrease or eliminate self-mutilating or self-abusive behaviors

Activities:
- Determine the motive/reason for the behavior(s)
- Develop appropriate behavioral expectations and consequences, given the patient's level of cognitive functioning and capacity for self-control
- Communicate behavioral expectations and consequences to patient
- Remove dangerous items from the patient's environment
- Apply, as appropriate, mitts, splints, helmets, or restraints to limit mobility and ability to initiate self-harm
- Provide ongoing surveillance of patient and environment
- Communicate risk to other care providers
- Instruct patient in coping strategies (e.g., assertiveness training, impulse control training, and progressive muscle relaxation), as appropriate
- Anticipate trigger situations that may prompt self-harm and intervene to prevent it
- Assist patient to identify situations and/or feelings that may prompt self-harm
- Contract with patient, as appropriate, for "no self-harm"
- Encourage patient to seek out care providers to talk as the urge to harm self occurs
- Teach and reinforce patient effective coping behaviors and appropriate expression of feelings
- Administer medications, as appropriate, to decrease anxiety, stabilize mood, and decrease self-stimulation
- Use a calm, nonpunitive approach when dealing with self-harmful behavior(s)
- Avoid giving positive reinforcement to self-harmful behavior(s)
- Provide the predetermined consequences if patient is engaging in self-harmful behaviors
- Place patient in a more protective environment (e.g., area restriction and seclusion) if self-harmful impulses/behaviors escalate
- Assist patient, as appropriate, to level of cognitive functioning to identify and assume responsibility for the consequences of behavior (e.g., dress own self-inflicted wound)
- Assist patient to identify trigger situations and feelings that prompted self-harmful behavior
- Assist patient to identify more appropriate coping strategies that could have been used and their consequences
- Monitor patient for medication side effects and desired outcomes
- Provide medication teaching to patient/significant others
- Provide family/significant other with guidelines as to how self-harmful behavior can be managed outside the care environment
- Provide illness teaching to patient/significant others if self-harmful behavior is illness-based (e.g., borderline personality disorder, or autism)
- Monitor patient for self-harmful impulses that may progress to suicidal thoughts/gestures

2nd edition 1996

Background Readings:
Fortinash, K. M. & Holoday-Worret, P. A. (1989). *Psychiatric nursing care plans*. St. Louis: Mosby.
Limandri, B. J. & Boyd, M. A. (2005). Personality and impulse-control disorder. In M. A. Boyd (Ed.), *Psychiatric nursing: Contemporary practice* (3rd ed., pp. 420–469). Philadelphia: Lippincott Williams & Wilkins.
Linehan, M., Armstrong, H., Suarez, A., Allmon, D., & Heard, H. (1991). Cognitive-behavioral treatment of chronically parasuicidal borderline patients. *Archives of General Psychiatry, 48*(12), 1060–1064.
Pawlicki, C. M. & Gaumer, C. (1993). Nursing care of the self-mutilating patient. *Bulletin of the Menninger Clinic, 57*(3), 380–389.
Spillers, G. (1991). Suicide potential. In G. K. McFarland & M. D. Thomas (Eds.), *Psychiatric mental health nursing. Application of the nursing process* (pp. 475–482). Philadelphia: Lippincott.
Stockard, S. (1987). Disorders of childhood. In J. Norris, M. Kunes-Connell, S. Stockard, P. M. Ehrhart, & G. R. Newton (Eds.), *Mental health-psychiatric nursing. A continuum of care* (pp. 657–691). New York: John Wiley & Sons.
Townsend, M. C. (1988). *Nursing diagnoses in psychiatric nursing: A pocket guide for care plan construction*. Philadelphia: F. A. Davis.
Valente, S. M. (1991). Deliberate self injury: Management in a psychiatric setting. *Journal of Psychosocial Nursing and Mental Health Services, 29*(12), 19–25.

Behavior Management: Sexual   4356

Definition: Delineation and prevention of socially unacceptable sexual behaviors

Activities:
- Identify sexual behaviors that are unacceptable, given the particular setting and patient population
- Specify explicit expectations (based on level of cognitive functioning and capacity for self-control) related to sexual behavior or verbalizations that might be directed toward others or objects in the environment
- Discuss with patient the consequences of socially unacceptable sexual behavior and verbalizations
- Discuss the negative impact that socially unacceptable sexual behavior may have on others
- Avoid assigning roommates with communication difficulties, history of inappropriate sexual activity, or heightened vulnerabilities (e.g., younger children)
- Assign patient to a private room if assessed to be at high risk for socially unacceptable sexual behavior
- Limit patient's physical mobility (e.g., area restriction), as needed, to decrease opportunity for socially unacceptable sexual behavior(s)
- Communicate risk to other care providers
- Provide appropriate level of supervision/surveillance to monitor patient

B

- Use a calm, matter-of-fact approach when responding to socially unacceptable sexual remarks and behavior
- Redirect from any socially unacceptable sexual behavior/ verbalizations
- Discuss with patient why the sexual behavior or verbalization is unacceptable
- Provide the predetermined consequences for undesirable sexual behavior
- Teach/reinforce appropriate social skills
- Provide sex education, as appropriate, to developmental level
- Discuss with patient acceptable ways to fulfill individual sexual needs in privacy
- Discourage initiation of sexual or intimate relationships while under severe stress
- Encourage appropriate expression of feelings about past situational or traumatic crises
- Provide counseling, as needed, for patient who has been sexually abused

- Assist family with understanding of and management of unacceptable sexual behaviors(s)
- Provide opportunities for staff to process their feelings about patient sexual behavior that is socially unacceptable

2nd edition 1996

Background Readings:

Fontaine, K. L. (2004). Gender identity and sexual disorder. In C. R. Kneisl, H. S. Wilson, & E. Trigoboff (Eds.), *Contemporary psychiatric-mental health nursing* (pp. 400–424). Upper Saddle River, NJ: Prentice Hall.

Stockard, S. & Cullen, S. (1987). Personality disorders. In J. Norris, M. Kunes-Connell, S. Stockard, P. M. Ehrhart, & G. R. Newton (Eds.), *Mental health–psychiatric nursing: A continuum of care* (pp. 571–603). New York: John Wiley & Sons.

Thompson, J. M., McFarland, G. K., Hirsch, J. E., Tucker, S. M., & Bowers, A. C. (1989). *Mosby's manual of clinical nursing* (2nd ed.). St. Louis: Mosby.

Behavior Modification 4360

Definition: Promotion of a behavior change

Activities:
- Determine patient's motivation to change
- Assist patient to identify strengths, and reinforce these
- Encourage substitution of undesirable habits with desirable habits
- Introduce patient to persons (or groups) who have successfully undergone the same experience
- Ensure that the intervention is implemented consistently by all staff
- Reinforce constructive decisions concerning health needs
- Give feedback in terms of feelings when patient is noted to be free of symptoms and looks relaxed
- Avoid showing rejection or belittlement as patient struggles with changing behavior
- Offer positive reinforcement for patient's independently made decisions
- Encourage patient to examine own behavior
- Assist the patient in identifying even small successes
- Identify the patient's problem in behavioral terms
- Identify the behavior to be changed (target behavior) in specific, concrete terms
- Break down behavior to be changed into smaller, measurable units of behavior (e.g., stopping smoking: number of cigarettes smoked)
- Use specific time periods when measuring units of behavior (e.g., number of cigarettes smoked per day)
- Determine whether the identified target behavior needs to be increased, decreased, or learned
- Consider that it is easier to increase a behavior than to decrease a behavior
- Establish behavioral objectives in written form
- Develop a behavior change program
- Establish a baseline occurrence of the behavior before initiating change

- Develop a method (e.g., a graph or chart) for recording behavior and its changes
- Encourage the patient to participate in monitoring and recording behaviors
- Discuss the behavior modification process with the patient/ significant other
- Facilitate the involvement of other health care providers in the modification process, as appropriate
- Facilitate family involvement in the modification process, as appropriate
- Administer positive reinforcers on a predetermined schedule (continuous or intermittent) for desired behaviors
- Withdraw positive reinforcers from undesired behaviors, and attach reinforcers to a more desirable replacement behavior
- Encourage the patient to participate in the selection of meaningful reinforcers
- Choose reinforcers that can be controlled (e.g., used only when behavior to be changed occurs)
- Coordinate a token or point system of reinforcement for complex or multiple behaviors
- Develop a treatment contract with the patient to support implementation of the token/point system
- Foster skills acquisition by systematically reinforcing simple components of the skill or task
- Promote learning of desired behavior by using modeling techniques
- Determine changes in behavior by comparing baseline occurrences with postintervention occurrences of behavior
- Document and communicate modification process, to treatment team, as necessary
- Follow up reinforcement over longer term (phone or personal contact)

1st edition 1992; revised 2013

B

Background Readings:

Boyd, M. A. (2005). Psychiatric-mental health nursing interventions. In M. A. Boyd (Ed.), *Psychiatric nursing: Contemporary practice* (3rd ed., pp. 218–232). Philadelphia: Lippincott Williams & Wilkins.

Coucouvanis, J. A. & McCarthy, A. M. (2001). Behavior modification. In M. Craft-Rosenberg & J. Denehy (Eds), *Nursing interventions for infants, children, and families* (pp. 427–444). Thousand Oaks, CA: Sage.

Nelson, P. J. (2008). Behavior modification. In B. J. Ackley, G. B. Ladwig, B. A. Swan, & S. J. Tucker (Eds.), *Evidence-based nursing care guidelines: Medical-surgical interventions* (pp. 99–105). St. Louis: Mosby.

Stuart, G. W. (2009). Cognitive and behavior change interventions. In G. W. Stuart (Ed.), *Principles and practice of psychiatric nursing* (9th ed., pp. 559–572). St. Louis: Mosby.

Townsend, M. C. (2009). Behavior therapy. *Psychiatric mental health nursing: Concepts of care in evidence-based practice.* (6th ed., pp. 279–288). Philadelphia: F. A. Davis.

Behavior Modification: Social Skills   4362

Definition: Assisting the patient to develop or improve interpersonal social skills

Activities:

- Assist patient to identify interpersonal problems resulting from social skill deficits
- Encourage patient to verbalize feelings associated with interpersonal problems
- Assist patient to identify desired outcomes for problematic interpersonal relationships or situations
- Assist patient to identify possible courses of action and their social/interpersonal consequences
- Identify a specific social skill(s) that will be the focus of training
- Assist patient to identify the behavioral steps for the targeted social skill(s)
- Provide models who demonstrate the behavioral steps in the context of situations that are meaningful to the patient
- Assist patient to role play the behavioral steps
- Provide feedback (e.g., praise or rewards) to patient about performance of targeted social skill(s)
- Educate patient's significant others (e.g., family, peers, employers), as appropriate, about the purpose and process of social skills training
- Involve significant others in social skills training sessions (e.g., role play) with patient, as appropriate
- Provide feedback to patient and significant others about the appropriateness of their social responses in training situations
- Encourage patients/significant others to self-evaluate outcomes of their social interactions, self-reward for positive outcomes, and problem solve less desirable outcomes

Background Readings:

Boyd, M. A. (2005). Psychiatric-mental health nursing interventions. In M. A. Boyd (Ed.), *Psychiatric nursing: Contemporary practice* (3rd ed., pp. 218–232). Philadelphia: Lippincott Williams & Wilkins.

Halford, W. K. & Hayes, R. (1991). Psychological rehabilitation of chronic schizophrenic patients: Recent findings on social skills training and family psychoeducation. *Clinical Psychology Review, 11*(1), 23–44.

Hartley, R. & Robinson, C. (1987). Mental retardation. In J. Norris, M. Kunes-Connell, S. Stockard, P. M. Ehrhart, & G. R. Newton (Eds.), *Mental health-psychiatric nursing: A continuum of care* (pp. 495–525). New York: John Wiley & Sons.

Hollinger, J. D. (1987). Social skills for behaviorally disordered children as preparation for mainstreaming: Theory, practice, and new directions. *Remedial and Special Education, 8*(4), 17–27.

Liberman, R. P., DeRisi, W. J., & Mueser, K. T. (1989). *Social skills training with psychiatric patients.* New York: Pergamon Press.

McGinnis, E., Goldstein, A. P., Sprafkin, R. P., & Gershaw, N. J. (1984). *Skillstreaming the elementary school child: A structured learning approach to teaching prosocial skills.* Champaign, IL: Research Press.

Westwell, J. & Martin, M. L. (1991). Social interaction, impaired. In G. K. McFarland & M. D. Thomas (Eds.), *Psychiatric mental health nursing: Application of the nursing process* (pp. 437–443). Philadelphia: Lippincott.

2nd edition 1996

Bibliotherapy   4680

Definition: Therapeutic use of literature to enhance expression of feelings, active problem solving, coping, or insight

Activities:

- Identify the patient's emotional, cognitive, developmental, and situational needs
- Determine ability for reading independently
- Set therapy goals (e.g., emotional change; personality development; learn new values and attitudes)
- Consult with a librarian who is skilled in book finding
- Consult sources to recommend literature for therapy
- Make selections appropriate for reading level
- Select stories, poems, essays, articles, self-help books, or novels that reflect the situation or feelings the patient is experiencing
- Read aloud, if needed or feasible
- Use pictures and illustrations
- Encourage reading and rereading
- Assist in helping the patient identify with the characters and emotional content in the literature
- Examine and talk about the feelings expressed by the characters

- Facilitate dialogue to help the patient compare and contrast the image, character, situation, or concept in the literature with his/her situation
- Assist in helping the patient recognize how the situation in the literature can help with making desired changes
- Follow up reading sessions with play sessions or role modeling work, either individually or in therapy groups
- Evaluate goal attainment

1st edition 1992; revised 2008

Background Readings:

Abdullah, M. H. (2002). *Bibliotherapy*. Bloomington, IN: ERIC Digest: Education Resources Information Center Clearing House on Reading English and Communication.

Cohen, L. J. (1992). Bibliotherapy: The therapeutic use of books for women. *Journal of Nurse-Midwifery, 37*(2), 91–95.

Cohen, L. J. (1993). Discover the healing power of books. *American Journal of Nursing, 93*(10), 70–74.

Hynes, A. M. & Hynes-Berry, M. (1986). *Bibliotherapy, the interactive process: A handbook*. Boulder, CO: Westview Press.

Marrs, R. W. (1995). A meta-analysis of bibliotherapy studies. *American Journal of Community Psychology, 23*(6), 843–870.

McArdle, S. & Byrt, R. (2001). Fiction, poetry and mental health: Expressive and therapeutic uses of literature. *Journal of Psychiatric and Mental Health Nursing, 8*, 517–524.

Silverberg, L. I. (2003). Bibliotherapy: The therapeutic use of didactic and literary texts in treatment, diagnosis, prevention, and training. *Journal of the American Osteopathic Association, 103*(3), 131–135.

Biofeedback   5860

Definition: Assisting the patient to gain voluntary control over physiological responses using feedback from electronic equipment that monitor physiologic processes

Activities:

- Interview patient to obtain a health history
- Analyze nature of the specific health condition to be treated
- Determine abilities and willingness for using the biobehavioral treatment
- Discuss rationale for using biofeedback and type of feedback
- Determine patient's acceptance of this type of treatment
- Decide on the specific monitoring device to be used (e.g., thermal feedback; electrodermal response or galvanic skin response; electromyography feedback; finger pulse feedback; breathing biofeedback; electroencephalograph biofeedback)
- Construct treatment plan to treat the problem
- Explain the procedure concerning the specific monitoring equipment used
- Arrange therapy room so that patient cannot touch any conductive object
- Connect patient to the instrumentation device, as needed
- Operate the biofeedback device according to instructions
- Establish an appropriate baseline against which to compare treatment effect
- Assist patient to learn to modify bodily responses to equipment cues
- Instruct patient to check instrumentation before use to ensure proper functioning
- Answer fears and concerns related to the instrumentation
- Discuss timing, frequency, length, and setting for sessions with patient/family
- Identify appropriate criteria for reinforcement of patient's responses
- Provide feedback of progress after each session
- Set conditions with patient to evaluate therapeutic outcome

1st edition 1992; revised 2008

Background Readings:

Andrasik, F. & Lords, A. O. (2004). Biofeedback. In L. Freeman (Ed.), *Mosby's complementary & alternative medicine: A research-based approach* (2nd ed., pp. 207–235). St. Louis: Mosby.

Anselmo, J. (2005). Relaxation: The first step to restore, renew, and self-heal. In B. M. Dossey, L. Keegan, & C. E. Guzzetta (Eds.), *Holistic nursing: A handbook for practice* (4th ed., pp. 523–566). Sudbury, MA: Jones and Bartlett.

Bray, D. (2001). Biofeedback. In D. Rankin-Box (Ed.), *The nurse's handbook of complementary therapies* (pp. 145–152). London: Bailliere Tindall.

Fontaine, K. L. (2005). *Complementary & alternative therapies for nursing practice* (2nd ed.). Upper Saddle River, NJ: Prentice Hall.

Good, M. (2006). Biofeedback. In M. Snyder & R. Lindquist, (Eds.), *Complementary/alternative therapies in nursing* (5th ed., pp. 117–128). New York: Springer.

Micozzi, M. S. (2006). *Fundamentals of complementary and integrative medicine* (3rd ed.). Philadelphia: Saunders.

Bioterrorism Preparedness   8810

Definition: Preparing for an effective response to bioterrorism events or disaster

Activities:

- Identify potential types of chemical agents that are likely terrorism agents (e.g., nerve agents, mustard agents, cyanide)
- Identify potential types of biological agents that are likely terrorism agents (e.g., anthrax, smallpox, botulism, plague)
- Follow instructions regarding involvement in screening clients during a bioterrorism event
- Integrate biological and chemical terrorism into agency disaster preparedness planning and evaluation
- Identify all community medical, emergency, and social agency resources available (e.g., World Health Organization [WHO],

Federal Emergency Management Agency [FEMA], National Disaster Medical System [NDMS], Centers for Disease Control and Prevention [CDC], state and local public health agencies)
- Consider current WHO and CDC recommended strategies to contain natural or deliberate disease and chemical events
- Become familiar with signs and symptoms and common onset presentations of clients exposed to bioterrorism agents
- Modify initial client assessment questions and history to be inclusive of exposure risk and physical symptoms of exposure
- Monitor clients with vague flu-like symptoms
- Report suspicious symptoms to appropriate triage officers and health agencies
- Consult appropriate epidemiology and infection control professionals, as necessary
- Consider the reliability of information, especially in emergencies, potential disasters, or mass exposures
- Maintain current knowledge of protective equipment, protective procedures, and isolation techniques
- Ensure that protective equipment (e.g., hazmat suits, headgear, gloves, respirators) are available and in good working order
- Be familiar with and follow all decontamination policies, procedures, and protocols
- Participate in continuing education to maintain up-to-date knowledge

4th edition 2004

Background Readings:

Federal Emergency Management Agency (FEMA). (2002). *Managing the emergency consequences of terrorist incidents*. Washington, DC: Author.

Gebbie, K. M. & Qureshi, K. (2002). Emergency and disaster preparedness: Core competency for nurses. *American Journal of Nursing, 102*(1), 46–51.

Rebmann, T. (2006). Bioterrorism and emerging infections: Emergency preparedness for nurses. In P. S. Cowen & S. Moorhead (Eds.), *Current issues in nursing* (7th ed., pp. 768–776). St. Louis: Mosby.

Reilly, C. M. & Dleason, D. (2002). Smallpox. *American Journal of Nursing, 102*(2), 51–55.

Smeltzer, S. C. & Bare, B. G. (Eds.). (2004). Terrorism, mass casualty, and disaster nursing. In *Brunner & Suddarth's textbook of medical surgical nursing* (Vol. 2) (10th ed., pp. 2183–2198). Philadelphia: Lippincott Williams & Wilkins.

Veenema, T. G. (2002). Chemical and biological terrorism: Current updates for nurse educators. *Nursing Education Perspectives, 23*(2), 62–71.

World Health Organization. (2006). *Frequently asked questions regarding the deliberate use of biological agents and chemicals as weapons*. <http://www.who.int/csr/delibepidemics/faqbioagents/en/>

Birthing   6720

Definition: Delivery of a baby

Activities:
- Provide anticipatory guidance for delivery
- Include support person(s) in birth experience, as appropriate
- Perform vaginal exam to determine fetal position and station
- Maintain patient modesty and privacy in a quiet environment during delivery
- Adhere to patient's requests for management of delivery, when these requests are consistent with standards of perinatal care
- Obtain permission of patient and partner when other health care personnel enter delivery area
- Assist patient with position for delivery
- Stretch perineal tissue, as appropriate, to minimize lacerations or episiotomy
- Inform patient about the need for an episiotomy
- Administer local anesthetic before delivery or episiotomy, as indicated
- Perform episiotomy, as appropriate
- Instruct patient on shallow breathing (e.g., "panting") with delivery of head
- Deliver fetal head slowly, maintaining flexion until parietal bones are born
- Support perineum during delivery
- Check for the presence of a nuchal cord
- Reduce nuchal cord, as appropriate (e.g., clamp and cut cord or slip over head)
- Suction secretions from nares and mouth of infant with a bulb syringe after delivery of head
- Suction for meconium-stained fluid, as appropriate
- Cleanse and dry infant's head after delivery
- Assist delivery of shoulders
- Use maneuvers to release shoulder dystocia (e.g., suprapubic pressure or McRobert's maneuver), as appropriate
- Deliver the body of infant slowly
- Support infant body
- Clamp and cut umbilical cord after pulsations have ceased, when not contraindicated
- Obtain cord blood, if Rh negative or as needed for cord blood gas evaluation
- Anticipate spontaneous expulsion of the placenta
- Assign the 1-minute Apgar score
- Apply controlled umbilical cord traction, while guarding the fundus of uterus
- Inspect cervix for lacerations after delivery of placenta
- Administer local anesthetic before surgical repair, when indicated
- Suture episiotomy or lacerations, as appropriate
- Perform rectal exam to ensure tissue integrity
- Inspect placenta, membranes, and cord after delivery
- Estimate blood loss after parturition
- Cleanse perineum
- Apply perineal pad
- Praise maternal and support person efforts
- Provide information about infant's appearance and condition

- Encourage verbalization of questions or concerns about birth experience and newborn
- Consult with attending physician about indicators of actual or potential complications
- Document events of birth
- Sign birth certificate, as appropriate

1st edition 1992; revised 1996

Background Readings:

Adams, C. J. (Ed.). (1983). *Nurse-midwifery: Health care for women and newborns.* New York: Grune & Stratton.

Mattson, S. & Smith, J. E. (Eds.). (1993). *Core curriculum for maternal-newborn nursing.* Philadelphia: Saunders.

Scott-Ricci, S. (2007). *Essentials of maternity, newborn and women's health nursing.* Philadelphia: Lippincott Williams & Wilkins.

Varney, H. (1987). *Nurse-midwifery* (2nd ed.). St. Louis: Mosby.

Bladder Irrigation 0550

Definition: Instillation of a solution into the bladder to provide cleansing or medication

Activities:

- Determine whether the irrigation will be continuous or intermittent
- Observe universal precautions
- Explain the procedure to the client
- Set up sterile irrigating supplies, maintaining sterile technique per agency protocol
- Cleanse site of entry or end of Y-connector with alcohol wipe
- Instill irrigating fluid, per agency protocol
- Monitor and maintain correct flow rate, as necessary
- Record amount of fluid used, characteristics of fluid, amount returned, and patient responsiveness, according to agency protocol

2nd edition 1996

Background Readings:

Ellis, J. R., Nowlis, E. A., & Bentz, P. M. (1988). *Modules for basic nursing skills* (4th ed.). Boston: Houghton Mifflin.

Evans-Smith, P. (2005). *Taylor's clinical nursing skills.* Philadelphia: Lippincott Williams & Wilkins.

Gilbert, V. & Gobbi, M. (1989). Making sense of bladder irrigation. *Nursing Times, 85*(16), 40–42.

Potter, P. & Perry, A. (1998). *Fundamentals of nursing: Concepts, process, and practice* (4th ed.). St. Louis: Mosby.

Bleeding Precautions 4010

Definition: Reduction of stimuli that may induce bleeding or hemorrhage in at-risk patients

Activities:

- Monitor the patient closely for hemorrhage
- Note hemoglobin/hematocrit levels before and after blood loss, as indicated
- Monitor for signs and symptoms of persistent bleeding (e.g., check all secretions for frank or occult blood)
- Monitor coagulation studies, including prothrombin time (PT), partial thromboplastin time (PTT), fibrinogen, fibrin degradation/split products, and platelet counts, as appropriate
- Monitor orthostatic vital signs, including blood pressure
- Maintain bed rest during active bleeding
- Administer blood products (e.g., platelets and fresh frozen plasma), as appropriate
- Protect the patient from trauma, which may cause bleeding
- Avoid injections (IV, IM, or SQ), as appropriate
- Instruct the ambulating patient to wear shoes
- Use soft toothbrush or toothettes for oral care
- Use electric razor, instead of straight-edge, for shaving
- Tell patient to avoid invasive procedures; if they are necessary, monitor closely for bleeding
- Coordinate timing of invasive procedures with platelet or fresh frozen plasma transfusions, if appropriate
- Refrain from inserting objects into a bleeding orifice
- Avoid taking rectal temperatures
- Avoid lifting heavy objects
- Administer medications (e.g., antacids), as appropriate
- Instruct patient to avoid aspirin or other anticoagulants
- Instruct patient to increase intake of foods rich in vitamin K
- Use therapeutic mattress to minimize skin trauma
- Avoid constipation (e.g., encourage fluid intake and stool softeners), as appropriate
- Instruct the patient and/or family on signs of bleeding and appropriate actions (e.g., notify the nurse) should bleeding occur

1st edition 1992; revised 1996

Background Readings:

Cullen, L. M. (1992). Interventions related to circulatory care. In G. M. Bulechek & J. C. McCloskey (Eds.), Symposium on nursing interventions. *Nursing Clinics of North America, 27*(2), 445–476.

Jennings, B. (1991). The hematologic system. In J. Alspach (Ed.), *AACN's core curriculum for critical care nursing* (4th ed., pp. 675–747). Philadelphia: Saunders.

Smeltzer, S. C. & Bare, B. G. (2004). *Brunner & Suddarth's textbook of medical surgical nursing* (Vol. 1) (10th ed.). Philadelphia: Lippincott Williams & Wilkins.

Smeltzer, S. C. & Bare, B. G. (2004). *Brunner & Suddarth's textbook of medical surgical nursing* (Vol. 2) (10th ed.). Philadelphia: Lippincott Williams & Wilkins.

Thompson, J. M., McFarland, G. K., Hirsch, J. E., & Tucker, S. M. (1998). *Mosby's clinical nursing* (4th ed.). St. Louis: Mosby.

B

Bleeding Reduction 4020

Definition: Limitation of the loss of blood volume during an episode of bleeding

Activities:

- Identify the cause of the bleeding
- Monitor the patient closely for hemorrhage
- Apply direct pressure or pressure dressing, if appropriate
- Apply ice pack to affected area, as appropriate
- Monitor the amount and nature of blood loss
- Monitor size and character of hematoma, if present
- Note hemoglobin/hematocrit levels before and after blood loss
- Monitor trends in blood pressure and hemodynamic parameters, if available (e.g., central venous pressure and pulmonary capillary/artery wedge pressure)
- Monitor fluid status, including intake and output
- Monitor coagulation studies, including prothrombin time (PT), partial thromboplastin time (PTT), fibrinogen, fibrin degradation/split products, and platelet counts, as appropriate
- Monitor determinants of tissue oxygen delivery (e.g., PaO_2, SaO_2, and hemoglobin levels and cardiac output), if available
- Monitor neurological functioning
- Inspect for bleeding from mucous membranes, bruising after minimal trauma, oozing from puncture sites, and presence of petechiae
- Monitor for signs and symptoms of persistent bleeding (i.e., check all secretions for frank or occult blood)
- Arrange availability of blood products for transfusion, if necessary
- Maintain patent IV access
- Administer blood products (e.g., platelets and fresh frozen plasma), as appropriate
- Hematest all excretions and observe for blood in emesis, sputum, feces, urine, NG drainage, and wound drainage, as appropriate
- Perform proper precautions in handling blood products or bloody secretions
- Evaluate patient's psychological response to hemorrhage and perception of events
- Instruct the patient and family on signs of bleeding and appropriate actions (i.e., notify the nurse), should further bleeding occur
- Instruct the patient on activity restrictions
- Instruct patient and family on severity of blood loss and appropriate actions being performed

1st edition 1992; revised 2008; 2013

Background Readings:

American Association of Critical Care Nurses. (2006). *Core curriculum for critical care nursing* (6th ed.) [J. G. Alspach, Ed.]. Philadelphia: Saunders.

Berman, A., Snyder, S., Kozier, B., & Erb, G. (2008). *Kozier & Erb's fundamentals of nursing: Concepts, processes, and practice.* (8th ed.). Upper Saddle River, NJ: Prentice Hall.

Monahan, F., Sands, J., Neighbors, M., Marek, J., & Green, C. (2007). *Phipps' medical-surgical nursing: Health and illness perspectives* (8th ed.). St. Louis: Mosby.

Smeltzer, S., Bare, B., Hinkle, J., & Cheever, K. (2010). Emergency nursing. In *Brunner & Suddarth's textbook of medical-surgical nursing* (12th ed., pp. 2153–2190). Philadelphia: Lippincott Williams & Wilkins.

Bleeding Reduction: Antepartum Uterus 4021

Definition: Limitation of the amount of blood loss from the pregnant uterus during third trimester of pregnancy

Activities:

- Obtain client history of blood loss (e.g., onset, amount, presence of pain, and presence of clots)
- Review for risk factors related to late pregnancy bleeding (e.g., abruptio, smoking, cocaine use, pregnancy-induced hypertension, and placenta previa)
- Obtain an accurate estimate of fetal age by last menstrual period report, prior ultrasound dating reports, or obstetrical history, if available
- Inspect perineum for amount and characteristic of bleeding
- Monitor maternal vital signs, as needed, based on amount of blood loss
- Monitor fetal heart rate electronically
- Palpate for uterine contractions or increased uterine tone
- Observe electronic fetal tracing for evidence of uteroplacental insufficiency (e.g., late decelerations, decreased long-term variability, and absent accelerations)
- Initiate fetal resuscitation, as appropriate, for abnormal (nonreassuring) signs of uteroplacental insufficiency
- Delay digital cervical exam until location of placenta has been verified (e.g., ultrasound report)
- Perform ultrasound for placental location
- Perform or assist with speculum exam to visualize blood loss and cervical status
- Weigh Chux or pads to accurately estimate blood loss
- Inspect clothing, sheets, or mattress pad in the event of hemorrhage
- Initiate emergency procedures for antepartum hemorrhage, as appropriate (e.g., oxygen therapy, IV therapy, and type and cross)
- Draw blood for diagnostic tests, as appropriate (e.g., Kleihauer-Betke, ABO, Rh, CBC, and clotting studies)
- Administer Rho(D) immune globulin, as appropriate
- Record intake and output
- Elevate lower extremities to increase perfusion to vital organs and fetus
- Administer blood products, as appropriate
- Initiate safety measures (e.g., strict bed rest and lateral position)
- Instruct patient to report increases in vaginal bleeding (e.g., gushes, clots, and trickles) during hospitalization
- Teach patient to differentiate between old and fresh bleeding
- Instruct client on life-style changes to reduce the chance of further bleeding, as appropriate (e.g., smoking cessation assistance, sexual abstinence, bed rest care, constipation management, nutrition management, and coping enhancement)

- Provide discharge planning, including referral to home care nurses
- Schedule follow-up antepartum fetal surveillance
- Discuss reasons to return to the hospital
- Discuss use of emergency medical system for transportation, as appropriate

2nd edition 1996

Background Readings:

Littleton, L. Y. & Engebretson, J. C. (2002). *Maternal, neonatal, and women's health nursing* (pp. 510–514). Albany, NY: Delmar.

Mattson, S. & Smith, J. E. (Eds.). (1993). *Core curriculum for maternal-newborn nursing*. Philadelphia: Saunders.

B

Bleeding Reduction: Gastrointestinal   4022

Definition: Limitation of the amount of blood loss from the upper and lower gastrointestinal tract and related complications

Activities:

- Evaluate patient's psychological response to hemorrhage and perception of events
- Maintain a patent airway, if necessary
- Monitor determinants of tissue oxygen delivery (e.g., PaO_2, SaO_2, and hemoglobin levels and cardiac output), if available
- Monitor for signs and symptoms of persistent bleeding (e.g., check all secretions for frank or occult blood)
- Monitor fluid status, including intake and output, as appropriate
- Administer IV fluids, as appropriate
- Monitor for signs of hypovolemic shock (e.g., decreased blood pressure, rapid thready pulse, increased respiratory rate, diaphoresis, restlessness, cool clammy skin)
- Measure abdominal girth, as appropriate
- Hematest all excretions and observe for blood in emesis, sputum, feces, urine, NG drainage, and wound drainage, as appropriate
- Document color, amount, and character of stools
- Monitor coagulation studies and complete blood count (CBC) with white blood count (WBC) differential, as appropriate
- Avoid administration of anticoagulants
- Monitor coagulation studies, including prothrombin time (PT), partial thromboplastin time (PTT), fibrinogen, fibrin degradation/split products, and platelet counts, as appropriate
- Administer medications (e.g., lactulose or vasopressin), as appropriate
- Avoid extremes in gastric pH level by administration of appropriate medication (e.g., antacids or histamine-2 blocking agent), as appropriate
- Insert nasogastric tube to suction and monitor secretions, if appropriate
- Maintain pressure in cuffed/balloon nasogastric tube, if appropriate
- Perform nasogastric lavage, as appropriate
- Promote stress reduction
- Assess the patient's nutritional status
- Establish a supportive relationship with the patient and family
- Instruct the patient and family on activity restriction and progression
- Instruct the patient and/or family on procedures (e.g., endoscopy, sclerosis, and surgery), if appropriate
- Instruct the patient and/or family on the need for blood replacement, as appropriate
- Instruct the patient and/or family to avoid the use of anti-inflammatory medications (e.g., aspirin and ibuprofen)
- Coordinate counseling for the patient and/or family (e.g., clergy, Alcoholics Anonymous), if appropriate

1st edition 1992; revised 2008

Background Readings:

Cullen, L. M. (1992). Interventions related to circulatory care. In G. M. Bulechek & J. C. McCloskey (Eds.), Symposium on nursing interventions. *Nursing Clinics of North America, 27*(2), 445–476.

Delaune, S. & Ladner, P. (2006). *Fundamentals of nursing: Standards & practice* (3rd ed.). Clifton Park, NY: Thomson Delmar Learning.

Kozier, B., Erb, G., Berman, A., & Snyder, S. (2004). *Fundamentals of nursing: Concepts, process, and practice* (7th ed.). Upper Saddle River, NJ: Prentice Hall.

Monahan, F., Sands, J., Neighbors, M., Marek, J., & Green, C. (2007). *Phipps' medical-surgical nursing: Health and illness perspectives* (8th ed.). St. Louis: Mosby.

Bleeding Reduction: Nasal   4024

Definition: Limitation of the amount of blood loss from the nasal cavity

Activities:

- Apply manual pressure over the bridge of the nose
- Identify the cause of the bleeding
- Monitor the amount and nature of blood loss
- Monitor the amount of bleeding into the oropharynx
- Apply ice pack to affected area
- Place packing in nasal cavity, if appropriate
- Administer blood products (e.g., platelets and fresh frozen plasma), as appropriate
- Note hemoglobin/hematocrit levels before and after blood loss, as indicated
- Promote stress reduction

B

- Provide pain relief/comfort measures
- Maintain a patent airway
- Assist patient with oral care, as appropriate
- Administer humidified oxygen, if appropriate
- Monitor vital signs, as appropriate
- Place patient in mid-Fowler's position, as appropriate
- Instruct the patient on activity restrictions, if appropriate
- Instruct patient to avoid traumatizing nares (e.g., avoid scratching, blowing, or touching nose)
- Instruct the patient and/or family on signs of bleeding and appropriate actions (e.g., notify the nurse), should further bleeding occur

1st edition 1992; revised 2008

Background Readings:

American Association of Critical Care Nurses. (2006). *Core curriculum for critical care nursing* (6th ed.) [J. G. Alspach, Ed.]. Philadelphia: Saunders.

Cullen, L. M. (1992). Interventions related to circulatory care. In G. M. Bulechek & J. C. McCloskey (Eds.), Symposium on nursing interventions. *Nursing Clinics of North America, 27*(2), 445–476.

Kozier, B., Erb, G., Berman, A., & Snyder, S. (2004). *Fundamentals of nursing: Concepts, process, and practice* (7th ed.). Upper Saddle River, NJ: Prentice Hall.

Monahan, F., Sands, J., Neighbors, M., Marek, J., & Green, C. (2007). *Phipps' medical-surgical nursing: Health and illness perspectives* (8th ed.). St. Louis: Mosby.

Bleeding Reduction: Postpartum Uterus 4026

Definition: Limitation of the amount of blood loss from the postpartum uterus

Activities:

- Review obstetrical history and labor record for risk factors for postpartum hemorrhage (e.g., prior history of postpartum hemorrhage, long labor, induction, preeclampsia, prolonged second stage, assisted delivery, multiple birth, cesarean birth, or precipitous birth)
- Apply ice to fundus
- Increase frequency of fundal massage
- Evaluate for bladder distention
- Encourage voiding or catheterize distended bladder
- Observe characteristics of lochia (e.g., color, clots, and volume)
- Weigh amount of blood loss
- Request additional nurses to help with emergency procedures and to assume care for newborn
- Elevate legs
- Initiate IV infusion
- Start second IV line, as appropriate
- Administer IV or IM oxytocics, per protocol or order
- Notify primary practitioner of patient status
- Monitor maternal vital signs every 15 minutes or more frequently, as appropriate
- Cover with warm blankets
- Monitor maternal color, level of consciousness, and pain
- Initiate oxygen therapy at 6 to 8 L per face mask
- Insert Foley catheter with urometer to monitor urine output
- Order emergency laboratory or blood
- Administer blood products, as appropriate
- Assist primary practitioner with packing uterus, evacuating hematoma, or suturing lacerations, as appropriate
- Keep patient and family informed of clinical condition and management
- Provide perineal care, as needed
- Prepare for emergency hysterectomy, as needed
- Discuss events with nursing team for provision of adequate postpartum surveillance of maternal status

2nd edition 1996

Background Readings:

Littleton, L. Y. & Engbertson, J. C. (2002). *Maternal, neonatal, and women's health nursing* (pp. 908–911). Albany, NY: Delmar.

Mattson, S. & Smith, J. E. (Eds.). (1993). *Core curriculum for maternal-newborn nursing.* Philadelphia: Saunders.

Bleeding Reduction: Wound 4028

Definition: Limitation of the blood loss from a wound that may be a result of trauma, incisions, or placement of a tube or catheter

Activities:

- Apply manual pressure over the bleeding or the potential bleeding area
- Apply ice pack to affected area
- Apply pressure dressing to site of bleeding
- Use mechanical device (e.g., C-type clamp) for applying pressure for longer periods, if appropriate
- Replace or reinforce pressure dressing, as appropriate
- Monitor vital signs, as appropriate
- Monitor accurate intake and output
- Place bleeding extremity in an elevated position
- Maintain continuous bladder irrigation, if appropriate
- Monitor size and character of hematoma, if present
- Monitor pulses distal to bleeding site
- Instruct patient to apply pressure to site when sneezing, coughing, and so on

B

- Instruct the patient on activity restrictions, if appropriate
- Instruct the patient and/or family on signs of bleeding and appropriate actions (e.g., notify the nurse), should further bleeding occur

1st edition 1992; revised 2008

Background Readings:
American Association of Critical Care Nurses. (2006). *Core curriculum for critical care nursing* (6th ed.) [J. G. Alspach, Ed.]. Philadelphia: Saunders.

Cullen, L. M. (1992). Interventions related to circulatory care. In G. M. Bulechek & J. C. McCloskey (Eds.), Symposium on nursing interventions. *Nursing Clinics of North America, 27*(2), 445–476.

Kozier, B., Erb, G., Berman, A., & Snyder, S. (2004). *Fundamentals of nursing: Concepts, process, and practice* (7th ed.). Upper Saddle River, NJ: Prentice Hall.

Monahan, F., Sands, J., Neighbors, M., Marek, J., & Green, C. (2007). *Phipps' medical-surgical nursing: Health and illness perspectives* (8th ed.). St. Louis: Mosby.

Blood Products Administration 4030

Definition: Administration of blood or blood products and monitoring of patient's response

Activities:
- Verify physician's orders
- Obtain patient's transfusion history
- Obtain or verify patient's informed consent
- Verify that blood product has been prepared, typed, and cross-matched (if applicable) for the recipient
- Verify correct patient, blood type, Rh type, unit number, and expiration date, and record per agency protocol
- Instruct patient about signs and symptoms of transfusion reactions (itching, dizziness, shortness of breath, and/or chest pain)
- Assemble administration system with filter appropriate for blood product and recipient's immune status
- Prime administration system with isotonic saline
- Prepare an IV pump approved for blood product administration, if indicated
- Perform venipuncture, using appropriate technique
- Avoid transfusion of more than one unit of blood or blood product at a time, unless necessitated by recipient's condition
- Monitor IV site for signs and symptoms of infiltration, phlebitis, and local infection
- Monitor vital signs (e.g., baseline, throughout, and after transfusion)
- Monitor for transfusion reactions
- Monitor for fluid overload
- Monitor and regulate flow rate during transfusion
- Refrain from administering IV medications or fluids, other than isotonic saline, into blood or blood product lines
- Refrain from transfusing product removed from controlled refrigeration for more than 4 hours
- Change filter and administration set at least every 4 hours
- Administer saline when transfusion is complete
- Document time frame of transfusion
- Document volume infused
- Stop transfusion if blood reaction occurs and keep veins open with saline
- Obtain blood sample and first voided urine specimen after a transfusion reaction
- Coordinate the return of the blood container to the lab after a blood reaction
- Notify laboratory immediately in the event of a blood reaction
- Maintain universal precautions

1st edition 1992; revised 1996, 2004

Background Readings:
Alexander, M. (2000). Editorial: Infusion nursing standards of practice. *Journal of Intravenous Nursing, 23*(6S), 1.

American Association of Blood Banks. (1994). *Standards for blood banks and transfusion services* (12th ed.). Bethesda, MD: Author.

American Red Cross, Council of Community Blood Centers, and American Association of Blood Banks. (1994). *Circular of information for the use of human blood and blood components.* Bethesda, MD: Author

Perry, A. G. & Potter, P. A. (2002). *Clinical nursing skills and techniques* (5th ed.). St. Louis: Mosby.

Body Image Enhancement 5220

Definition: Improving a patient's conscious and unconscious perceptions and attitudes toward his/her body

Activities:
- Determine patient's body image expectations based on developmental stage
- Use anticipatory guidance to prepare patient for predictable changes in body image
- Determine if perceived dislike for certain physical characteristics creates a dysfunctional social paralysis for teenagers and other high-risk groups
- Assist patient to discuss changes caused by illness or surgery, as appropriate
- Help patient determine the extent of actual changes in the body or its level of functioning
- Determine if a recent physical change has been incorporated into patient's body image
- Assist patient to separate physical appearance from feelings of personal worth, as appropriate

B

- Assist patient to determine the influence of a peer group on the patient's perception of present body image
- Assist patient to discuss changes caused by puberty, as appropriate
- Assist patient to discuss changes caused by a normal pregnancy, as appropriate
- Assist patient to discuss changes caused by aging, as appropriate
- Teach the patient the normal changes in the body associated with various stages of aging, as appropriate
- Assist the patient to discuss stressors affecting body image due to congenital condition, injury, disease, or surgery
- Identify the effects of the patient's culture, religion, race, sex, and age in terms of body image
- Monitor frequency of statements of self-criticism
- Monitor whether patient can look at the changed body part
- Monitor for statements that identify body image perceptions concerned with body shape and body weight
- Use self-picture drawing as a mechanism of evaluating a child's body image perceptions
- Instruct children about the functions of the various body parts, as appropriate
- Determine patient's and family's perceptions of the alteration in body image versus reality
- Identify coping strategies used by parents in response to changes in child's appearance
- Determine how child responds to parent's reactions, as appropriate
- Teach parents the importance of their responses to the child's body changes and future adjustment, as appropriate
- Assist parents to identify feelings prior to intervening with child, as appropriate
- Determine if a change in body image has contributed to increased social isolation
- Assist patient in identifying parts of his/her body that have positive perceptions associated with them

- Identify means of reducing the impact of any disfigurement through clothing, wigs, or cosmetics, as appropriate
- Assist patient to identify actions that will enhance appearance
- Assist the hospitalized patient to apply cosmetics prior to seeing visitors, as appropriate
- Facilitate contact with individuals with similar changes in body image
- Identify support groups available to patient
- Assist patient at risk for anorexia or bulimia to develop more realistic body image expectations
- Use self-disclosure exercises with groups of teenagers or others distraught over normal physical attributes

1st edition 1992; revised 2000

Background Readings:

Blaesing, S. & Brockhaus, J. (1972). The development of body image in the child. *Nursing Clinics of North America, 7*(4), 597–607.

Haber, J., McMahon, A. L., Price-Hoskins, P., & Sideleau, B. F. (1997). *Comprehensive psychiatric nursing* (5th ed.). St. Louis: Mosby.

Janelli, L. M. (1986). Body image in older adults: A review of the literature. *Rehabilitation Nursing, 11*(4), 6–8.

McBride, L. G. (1986). Teaching about body image: A technique for improving body satisfaction. *Journal of School Health, 56*(2), 76–77.

Nichols, P. (1996). *Clear thinking: Clearing dark thought with new words and images.* Iowa City, IA: River Lights.

Williams, M. L. (1987). The nursing diagnosis of body image disturbance in adolescents dissatisfied with their physical characteristics. *Holistic Nursing Practice, 1*(4), 52–59.

Wilson, H. S. & Kneisl, C. R. (1992). *Psychiatric nursing* (4th ed.). Menlo Park, CA: Addison-Wesley.

Vernon, A. (1989). *Thinking, feeling, behaving: An emotional education curriculum for adolescents (grades 1–6).* Champaign, IL: Research Press.

Vernon, A. (1989). *Thinking, feeling, behaving: An emotional education curriculum for adolescents (grades 7–12).* Champaign, IL: Research Press.

Body Mechanics Promotion   0140

Definition: Facilitating the use of posture and movement in daily activities to prevent fatigue and musculoskeletal strain or injury

Activities:
- Determine patient's commitment to learning and using correct posture
- Collaborate with physical therapy in developing a body mechanics promotion plan, as indicated
- Determine patient's understanding of body mechanics and exercises (e.g., return demonstration of correct techniques while performing activities/exercises)
- Instruct patient on structure and function of spine and optimal posture for moving and using the body
- Instruct patient about need for correct posture to prevent fatigue, strain, or injury
- Instruct patient how to use posture and body mechanics to prevent injury while performing any physical activities
- Determine patient awareness of own musculoskeletal abnormalities and the potential effects of posture and muscle tissue
- Instruct to use a firm mattress/chair or pillow, if appropriate
- Instruct to avoid sleeping prone
- Assist to demonstrate appropriate sleeping positions

- Assist to avoid sitting in the same position for prolonged periods
- Demonstrate how to shift weight from one foot to another while standing
- Instruct patient to move feet first and then body when turning to walk from a standing position
- Use the principles of body mechanics in conjunction with safe patient handling and movement aids
- Assist patient/family to identify appropriate posture exercises
- Assist patient to select warm-up activities before beginning exercise or work not done routinely
- Assist patient to perform flexion exercises to facilitate back mobility, as indicated
- Instruct patient/family regarding frequency and number of repetitions for each exercise
- Monitor improvement in patient's posture/body mechanics
- Provide information about possible positional causes of muscle or joint pain

1st edition 1992; revised 2008

Background Readings:

Kozier, B., Erb, G., Berman, A., & Snyder, S. J. (2004). *Fundamentals of nursing: Concepts, process, and practice* (7th ed.). Upper Saddle River, NJ: Prentice Hall.

Patient Safety Center of Inquiry, Veterans Health Administration and Department of Defense. (2005). *Patient care ergonomics resource guide: Safe patient handling and movement.* <http://www.visn8.va.gov/visn8/patientsafetycenter/resguide/ErgoGuidePtOne.pdf/>

Perry, A. G. & Potter, P. A. (2006). *Clinical nursing skills and techniques* (6th ed.). St. Louis: Mosby.

Smith, S. F., Duell, D. J., & Martin, B. C. (2004). *Clinical nursing skills: Basic to advanced skills* (6th ed.). Upper Saddle River, NJ: Prentice Hall.

B

Bottle Feeding   1052

Definition: Preparation and administration of fluids to an infant via a bottle

Activities:
- Determine infant state prior to initiating feeding
- Warm formula to room temperature before feeding
- Hold infant during feeding
- Position infant in a semi-Fowler's position for feeding
- Burp the infant frequently during and after the feeding
- Place nipple on top of tongue
- Control fluid intake by regulating softness of nipple, size of the hole, and size of the bottle
- Increase infant alertness by loosening infant's clothes, rubbing hands and feet, or talking to infant
- Encourage sucking by stimulating the rooting reflex, if appropriate
- Increase effectiveness of suck by compressing cheeks in unison with suck, if appropriate
- Provide chin support to decrease leaking of formula and improve lip closure
- Monitor fluid intake
- Monitor/evaluate suck reflex during feeding
- Monitor infant weight, as appropriate
- Boil unpasteurized milk
- Boil water used for preparing formula, if indicated
- Instruct parent or caregiver on sterilization techniques for feeding equipment
- Instruct parent or caregiver on proper dilution of concentrated formula
- Instruct parent on proper storage of formula
- Determine water source used to dilute concentrated or powdered formula
- Determine fluoride content of water used to dilute concentrated or powdered formula and refer for flouride supplementation, if indicated
- Caution parent or caregiver about using microwave oven to warm formula
- Instruct and demonstrate to parent oral hygiene techniques appropriate to infant's dentition to be used after each feeding

1st edition 1992; revised 2000

Background Readings:

May, K. A. & Mahlmeister, L. R. (1994). *Maternal and neonatal nursing: Family-centered care* (3rd ed.). Philadelphia: Lippincott.

Olds, S. B., London, M. L., & Ladewig, P. A. (1992). *Maternal-newborn nursing: A family centered approach* (4th ed.). Menlo Park, CA: Addison-Wesley.

Pillitteri, A. (2007). *Maternal and child health nursing: Care of the childbearing and childrearing family* (5th ed.). Philadelphia: Lippincott Williams & Wilkins.

Bowel Incontinence Care   0410

Definition: Promotion of bowel continence and maintenance of perianal skin integrity

Activities:
- Determine physical or psychological cause of fecal incontinence
- Determine onset and type of incontinence, frequency of episodes, and any related change in bowel function or stool consistency
- Explain etiology of problem and rationale for actions
- Eliminate the cause of the incontinence (e.g., medication, infection, fecal impaction), if possible
- Determine goals of bowel management program with patient/family
- Discuss procedures and expected outcomes with patient
- Instruct patient or family to record fecal output, as appropriate
- Wash perianal area with soap and water and dry it thoroughly after each stool
- Use nonionic detergent preparation (e.g., Peri-Wash) for cleansing, as appropriate
- Protect the skin from excess moisture of urine, stool, or perspiration with a moisture barrier cream (e.g., petrolatum, lanolin, dimethicone), as needed
- Use powder and creams on perianal area with caution
- Monitor perianal skin for development of pressure ulcer and for infection
- Keep bed and clothing clean
- Implement bowel training program, as appropriate
- Schedule toileting with a commode at bedside or a bedpan, as appropriate
- Monitor for adequate bowel evacuation
- Monitor diet and fluid requirements
- Avoid foods that cause diarrhea
- Administer prescribed medication for diarrhea (e.g., loperamide, atropine)
- Monitor for side effects of medication administration

B

- Use rectal tube, anal plug device, or fecal collection device (e.g., FlexiSeal Fecal Management System, Zossi Bowel Management System) with persons with intact skin, as appropriate
- Empty rectal device as needed
- Change external device frequently
- Provide incontinent pads, as needed
- Provide protective pants, as needed

1st edition 1992; revised 2013

Background Readings:

Leung, F. W., Schnelle, J., & Rao, S. S. (2008). Fecal incontinence. In E. A. Capezuti, E. L. Siegler, & M. D. Mezey, (Eds.), *Encyclopedia of elder care* (2nd ed., pp. 303–305). New York: Springer.

Padmanabhan, A., Stern, M., Wishin, J., Mangino, M., Richey, K., & DeSane, M. (2007). Clinical evaluation of a flexible fecal incontinence management system. *American Journal of Critical Care, 16*(4), 384–393.

Rao, S. S. (2004). Diagnosis and management of fecal incontinence. *American Journal of Gastroenterology, 99*(8), 1584–1604.

Shamliyan, T., Wyman, J., Bliss, D.Z., Kane, R.L., & Wilt, T. J. (2007). *Prevention of fecal and urinary incontinence in adults.* Evidence Report/Technology Assessment No. 161. AHRQ Publication No. 08-E003. Rockville, MD: Agency for Healthcare Research and Quality.

Slater, W. (2003). Management of fecal incontinence of a patient with spinal cord injury. *British Journal of Nursing, 12*(12), 727–734.

Wishin, J., Gallagher, T. J., & McCann, E. (2008). Emerging options for the management of fecal incontinence in hospitalized patients. *Journal of Wound, Ostomy, and Continence Nursing 35*(1), 104–110.

Bowel Incontinence Care: Encopresis 0412

Definition: Promotion of bowel continence in children

Activities:

- Gather information about toilet training history, duration of encopresis, and attempts made to eliminate the problem
- Determine cause of soiling (e.g., constipation and fecal impaction), as appropriate
- Order tests for physical causes (e.g., endoscopy, radiographic procedures, and stool analysis)
- Prepare child and family for diagnostic tests
- Perform rectal exam, as appropriate
- Instruct family about physiology of normal defecation and toilet training
- Recommend dietary changes or behavioral therapy, as appropriate
- Conduct family psychosocial assessment, including responses of caregivers and self-esteem of child
- Use play therapy to assist the child with working through feelings
- Investigate family communication patterns, strengths, and coping abilities
- Encourage parents to foster security by removing anxiety associated with toileting
- Encourage parents to demonstrate love and acceptance at home to counteract peer ridicule
- Discuss psychosocial dynamics of encopresis with parents (e.g., familial patterns, family disruption, self-esteem issues, and self-limiting characteristic)
- Discuss ways to reward toileting behavior
- Refer for family therapy, as appropriate

2nd edition 1996

Background Readings:

Gleeson, R. M. (1990). Bowel continence for the child with a neurogenic bowel. *Rehabilitation Nursing, 15*(6), 319–321.

Mott, S. R., James, S. R., & Sperhac, A. M. (1990). *Nursing care of children and families* (2nd ed.). Redwood City: Addison-Wesley.

Poulton, S. (2001). Bowel incontinence care: Encopresis. In M. Craft-Rosenberg & J. Denehy (Eds.), *Nursing interventions for infants, children, and families* (pp. 407–426). Thousand Oaks, CA: Sage.

Sprague-McRae, J. M., Lamb, W., & Homer, D. (1993). Encopresis: A study of treatment alternatives and historical behavioral characteristics. *Nurse Practitioner, 18*(10), 52–63.

Wong, D. L. (1997). *Whaley & Wong's essentials of pediatric nursing* (5th ed.). St. Louis: Mosby.

Bowel Management 0430

Definition: Establishment and maintenance of a regular pattern of bowel elimination

Activities:

- Note date of last bowel movement
- Monitor bowel movements including frequency, consistency, shape, volume, and color, as appropriate
- Monitor bowel sounds
- Report an increase in frequency of and/or high-pitched bowel sounds
- Report diminished bowel sounds
- Monitor for signs and symptoms of diarrhea, constipation, and impaction
- Evaluate for fecal incontinence, as necessary
- Note preexisting bowel problems, bowel routine, and use of laxatives
- Teach patient about specific foods that are assistive in promoting bowel regularity
- Instruct patient/family members to record color, volume, frequency, and consistency of stools
- Insert rectal suppository, as needed
- Initiate a bowel training program, as appropriate
- Encourage decreased gas-forming food intake, as appropriate
- Instruct patient on foods high in fiber, as appropriate
- Give warm liquids after meals, as appropriate
- Evaluate medication profile for gastrointestinal side effects
- Obtain a guaiac for stools, as appropriate
- Refrain from doing rectal/vaginal examination if medical condition warrants

Background Readings:

Craft, M. J. & Denehy, J. A. (Eds.). (1990). *Nursing interventions for infants and children.* Philadelphia: Saunders.

Craven, R. F. & Hirnle, C. J. (2000). *Fundamentals of nursing: Human health and function* (3rd ed., pp. 1077–1114). Philadelphia: Lippincott Williams & Wilkins.

Goetz, L. L., Hurvitz, E. A., Nelson, V. S., & Waring, W. (1998). Bowel management in children and adolescents with spinal cord injury. *The Journal of Spinal Cord Medicine, 21*(4), 335–341.

Hardy, M. A. (1991). Normal changes with aging. In M. Maas, K. C. Buckwalter, & M. Hardy (Eds.), *Nursing diagnoses and interventions for the elderly* (pp. 145–146). Redwood City, CA: Addison-Wesley.

McLane, A. M. & McShane, R. E. (1991). Constipation. In M. Maas, K. Buckwalter & M. Hardy (Eds.), *Nursing diagnoses and interventions for the elderly* (pp. 147–158). Redwood City, CA: Addison-Wesley.

Mangan, P. & Thomas, L. (1988). Preserving dignity. *Geriatric Nursing and Home Care, 8*(9), 14.

Smeltzer, S. C. & Bare, B. G. (2004). *Brunner & Suddarth's textbook of medical surgical nursing* (Vol. 1) (10th ed.). Philadelphia: Lippincott Williams & Wilkins.

Smeltzer, S. C. & Bare, B. G. (2004). *Brunner & Suddarth's textbook of medical surgical nursing* (Vol. 2) (10th ed.). Philadelphia: Lippincott Williams & Wilkins.

1st edition 1992; revised 2000

Bowel Training 0440

Definition: Assisting the patient to train the bowel to evacuate at specific intervals

Activities:

- Individualize the bowel program with patient and appropriate others
- Consult with physician and patient regarding use of suppositories
- Instruct patient/family about the principles of bowel training
- Instruct patient about which foods are high in bulk
- Provide foods high in bulk and/or that have been identified as assistive by the patient
- Ensure adequate fluid intake
- Ensure adequate exercise
- Initiate an uninterrupted, consistent scheduled time for defecation
- Ensure privacy
- Administer suppository, as appropriate
- Use a bisacodyl suppository based in polyethylene glycol, if tolerable
- Use a small enema, as appropriate
- Instruct patient about digital rectal dilatation, as appropriate
- Perform digital rectal dilatation as necessary
- Determine bowel status regularly
- Modify bowel program, as needed

Background Readings:

Heitkemper, M. M., Dirksen, S. R., O'Brien, P. G., & Bucher, L. (2007). *Medical-surgical nursing: Assessment and management of clinical problems.* St. Louis: Mosby.

Frisbie, J. H. (1997). Improved bowel care with a polyethylene glycol based bisacadyl suppository. *Journal of Spinal Cord Medicine, 20*(2), 227–229.

Maas, M. & Specht, J. (2001). Bowel incontinence. In M. Maas, K. Buckwalter, M. Hardy, T. Tripp-Reimer, M. Titler, & J. Specht (Eds.), *Nursing care of older adults: Diagnoses, outcomes, & interventions* (pp. 238–251). St. Louis: Mosby.

McLane, A. M. & McShane, R. E. (1992). Bowel management. In G. M. Bulechek & J. C. McCloskey (Eds.), *Nursing interventions: Essential nursing treatments* (2nd ed., pp. 73–85). Philadelphia: Saunders.

Smeltzer, S. C. & Bare, B. G. (2004). *Brunner & Suddarth's textbook of medical surgical nursing* (Vol. 1) (10th ed.). Philadelphia: Lippincott Williams & Wilkins.

Smeltzer, S. C. & Bare, B. G. (2004). *Brunner & Suddarth's textbook of medical surgical nursing* (Vol. 2) (10th ed.). Philadelphia: Lippincott Williams & Wilkins.

1st edition 1992; revised 2013

Breast Examination 6522

B

Definition: Inspection and palpation of the breasts and related areas

Activities:
- Assess possible risk factors for the development of breast cancer, including age, age at first pregnancy, age at menarche, age at menopause, family history, history of breast disease, parity status, and history of breastfeeding
- Ascertain whether or not patient has noticed any pain, lump, thickening, or tenderness of the breast, discharge, distortion, retraction, or scaling of the nipple
- Assist patient to positions of comfort as exam proceeds, always allowing privacy and sensitivity, as needed
- Explain specific steps of exam as you proceed
- Conduct exam while patient is in upright then supine position
- Instruct patient to remove gown
- Inspect the breasts for size, shape, changes in skin texture or color, including any redness, dimpling, puckering, scaling, or retraction of the skin
- Note symmetry and contour of the breasts and the position of the nipples bilaterally for any deviation or abnormality
- Instruct patient to utilize four different positions for visual inspection—arms at side, hands at waist and push inward toward hips, hands behind the head, and arms across waist with chest falling forward
- Assess for nipple discharge by gently squeezing each nipple
- Inspect and palpate lymph node chains, including the supraclavicular, infraclavicular, lateral, central, subscapular, and anterior nodes for any abnormalities
- Note the number, size, location, consistency, and mobility of nodes
- Place a small pillow or towel under the shoulder blade of the breast to be examined, abduct the arm on the same side of that breast, and place the patient's hand behind her head
- Using a systematic approach, palpate breast tissue with the palmar surface of the first three fingers of the examiner's dominant hand
- Move in a rotary fashion and compress the breast tissue against the chest wall

- Examine all four quadrants of the breast, including the axillary tail
- Note any masses, including location, shape, size (in cm), tenderness, mobility, and consistency
- Observe mastectomy scar site for presence of a rash, edema, thickening, and erythema, as appropriate
- Repeat same process with other breast
- Document all findings
- Report abnormalities to physician or nurse in charge, as appropriate
- Encourage patient to demonstrate self-palpation during and after clinical breast examination
- Instruct the patient about the importance of regular breast self-examination
- Advise regular mammograms as appropriate for age, condition, and risk

3rd edition 2000

Background Readings:

American Nurses Foundation. (1994). *Clinician's handbook of preventive services.* Waldorf, MD: American Nurses Publishing.

Champion, V. L. (1995). Results of a nurse-delivered intervention on proficiency and nodule detection with breast self-examination. *Oncology Nursing Forum, 22*(5), 819–824.

Edge, V. & Miller, M. (1994). *Women's health care.* St. Louis: Mosby.

Mettlin, C. & Dodd, G. D. (1991). The American Cancer Society guidelines for the cancer-related checkup: An update. *CA: A Cancer Journal for Clinicians. 41*(5), 279–282.

Perry, A. G. & Potter, P. A. (1998). *Clinical nursing skills and techniques* (4th ed.). St. Louis: Mosby.

Shaw, S. L. (1994). The role of the nurse in a comprehensive breast center. *Journal of Oncology Management, 3*(6), 49–51.

Calming Technique   5880

Definition: Reducing anxiety in patient experiencing acute distress

Activities:
- Maintain calm, deliberate manner
- Maintain eye contact with patient
- Reduce or eliminate stimuli creating fear or anxiety
- Stay with patient
- Reassure patient of personal safety or security
- Identify significant others whose presence can assist patient
- Hold and comfort an infant or child
- Rock an infant, as appropriate
- Speak softly or sing to an infant or child
- Offer pacifier to infant, as appropriate
- Instruct patient on techniques to use to calm an infant (e.g., speak to infant, hand on belly, restraining arms, picking up, and holding and rocking)
- Provide time and space to be alone, as appropriate
- Sit and talk with patient
- Facilitate the patient's expression of anger in a constructive manner
- Rub forehead, as appropriate
- Offer warm fluids or milk
- Offer back rub, as appropriate
- Offer warm bath or shower
- Instruct patient on methods to decrease anxiety (e.g., slow breathing techniques, distraction, visualization, meditation, progressive muscle relaxation, listening to soothing music), as appropriate
- Provide antianxiety medications, as needed

1st edition 1992, revised 2013

Background Readings:

Badger, J. M. (1994). Calming the anxious patient. *American Journal of Nursing, 94*(5), 46–50.

Hopkins, G. (2005). Calming presence. *Community Care, 1596,* 42–43.

Kneisl, C. R., Wilson, H. S., & Trigoboff, E. (2004). *Contemporary psychiatric-mental health nursing.* Upper Saddle River, NJ: Prentice Hall.

Miller, T. (2003). Treating anxiety: A calming influence. *Healthcare Traveler, 11*(5), 42–47.

Stuart. G. W. (2009). Anxiety responses and anxiety disorders. In G. W. Stuart (Ed.), *Principles and practice of psychiatric nursing* (9th ed.). (pp. 218–240). St. Louis: Mosby.

Ward, S. L. & Hisley, S. M. (2009). *Maternal-child nursing care: Optimizing outcomes for mothers, children, & families.* Philadelphia: F. A. Davis.

Capillary Blood Sample   4035

Definition: Obtaining an arteriovenous sample from a peripheral body site, such as the heel, finger, or other transcutaneous site

Activities:
- Verify correct patient identification
- Minimize anxiety for the patient using age-appropriate procedures
- Maintain standard precautions
- Select puncture site (e.g., outer lower aspect of heel, sides of distal phalanges of the fingers or toes, alternative sites such as the forearm)
- Puncture outer aspect of heel no deeper than 2.4 mm on infants
- Warm the site for approximately 5 minutes if specimen is to be an arterialized sample, according to agency protocol
- Use aseptic technique during skin puncture
- Puncture skin manually with a lancet or an approved penetration device according to manufacturer's specifications
- Wipe off first drop of blood with dry gauze, as per manufacturer's specifications or agency protocol
- Collect blood in manner appropriate to test being performed (e.g., allow a drop of blood to fall onto manufacturer's specified area of filter paper or test strips, draw blood into tubes by capillary action as droplets form)
- Apply intermittent pressure as far away from the puncture site as possible to promote blood flow
- Avoid hemolysis caused by excessive squeezing or "milking" of puncture site
- Follow manufacturer's guidelines regarding timing on tests and preservation of blood sample (e.g., sealing blood tubes), as necessary
- Label specimen as necessary, according to agency protocol
- Send specimen to laboratory, as necessary
- Bandage site, as necessary
- Teach and monitor self-sampling capillary blood, as appropriate
- Dispose of equipment properly
- Document completion of capillary blood sampling

4th edition 2004

Background Readings:

Escalante-Kanashiro, R. & Tatalean-Da-Fieno, J. (2000). Capillary blood gases in a pediatric intensive care unit. *Critical Care Medicine, 28*(1), 224–226.

Fletcher, M. & MacDonald, M. G. (1993). *Atlas of procedures in neonatology* (2nd ed.). Philadelphia: Lippincott.

Meehan, R. M. (1998). Heel sticks in neonates for capillary blood sampling [corrected]. *Neonatal Network—Journal of Neonatal Nursing, 17*(1), 12–27.

Perry, A. G. & Potter, P. A. (2002). *Clinical nursing skills and techniques* (5th ed.). St. Louis: Mosby.

Pettersen, M. D., Driscoll, D. J., Moyer, T. P., Dearani, J. A., & McGregor, C. G. (1999). Measurement of blood serum cyclosporine levels using capillary "fingerstick" sampling: A validation study. *Transplant International, 12*(6), 429–432.

Wong, D. L., Perry, S. E., & Hockenberry, M. J. (2002). *Maternal child nursing care.* St. Louis: Mosby.

Yum, S. I. & Roe, J. (1999). Capillary blood sampling for self-monitoring of blood glucose. *Diabetes Technology and Therapeutics, 1*(1), 29–37.

C

C

Cardiac Care   4040

Definition: Limitation of complications resulting from an imbalance between myocardial oxygen supply and demand for a patient with symptoms of impaired cardiac function

Activities:

- Routinely monitor patient physically and psychologically per agency policy
- Ensure activity level that does not compromise cardiac output or provoke cardiac events
- Encourage gradual increase in activity when condition is stabilized (i.e., encourage slower paced activities or shorter periods of activity with frequent rest periods following exercise)
- Instruct the patient on the importance of immediately reporting any chest discomfort
- Evaluate any episodes of chest pain (e.g., intensity, location, radiation, duration, and precipitating and alleviating factors)
- Monitor ECG for ST changes, as appropriate
- Perform a comprehensive appraisal of peripheral circulation (i.e., check peripheral pulses, edema, capillary refill, color, and temperature of extremity) routinely per agency policy
- Monitor vital signs frequently
- Monitor cardiovascular status
- Monitor for cardiac dysrhythmias, including disturbances of both rhythm and conduction
- Document cardiac dysrhythmias
- Note signs and symptoms of decreased cardiac output
- Monitor respiratory status for symptoms of heart failure
- Monitor abdomen for indications of decreased perfusion
- Monitor fluid balance (e.g., intake/output and daily weight)
- Monitor appropriate laboratory values (e.g., cardiac enzymes, electrolyte levels)
- Monitor pacemaker functioning, if appropriate
- Evaluate blood pressure alterations
- Evaluate the patient's response to ectopy or dysrhythmias
- Provide antiarrhythmic therapy according to unit policy (e.g., antiarrhythmic medication, cardioversion, or defibrillation), as appropriate
- Monitor patient's response to antiarrhythmic medications
- Instruct the patient and family on treatment modalities, activity restriction, and progression
- Arrange exercise and rest periods to avoid fatigue
- Restrict smoking
- Monitor the patient's activity tolerance
- Monitor for dyspnea, fatigue, tachypnea, and orthopnea
- Establish a supportive relationship with the patient and family
- Identify the patient's methods of handling stress
- Promote effective techniques for reducing stress
- Perform relaxation therapy, if appropriate
- Recognize psychological effects of underlying condition
- Screen patients for anxiety and depression, encouraging treatment with suitable antidepressants, as indicated
- Encourage noncompetitive activities for patients at risk for impaired cardiac function
- Discuss modifications in sexual activity with patient and significant other, if appropriate
- Instruct patient and family on the aims of care and how progress will be measured
- Ensure that all staff are aware of these goals and are working together to provide consistent care
- Refer to heart failure program or cardiac rehabilitation program for education, evaluation, and guided support to increase activity and rebuild life, as appropriate
- Offer spiritual support to the patient and family (i.e., contact a member of the clergy), as appropriate

1st edition 1992; revised 2000, 2013

Background Readings:

American Association of Critical Care Nurses. (2006). *Core curriculum for critical care nursing* (6th ed.) [J. G. Alspach, Ed.]. Philadelphia: Saunders.

Chummun, H., Gopaul, K., & Lutchman, A. (2009). Current guidance on the management of acute coronary syndrome. *British Journal of Nursing,18*(21), 1292–1298.

Clancy, J., McVicar, A., & Hubbard, J. (2011). Homeostasis 4: Nurses as agents of control in myocardial infarction. *British Journal of Nursing, 20*(6), 373–378.

Marshall, K. (2011). Acute coronary syndrome: Diagnosis, risk assessment and management. *Nursing Standard, 25*(23), 47–57.

LeMone, P., Burke, K. & Bauldoff, G. (2011). Nursing care of patient with coronary heart disease. *Medical-surgical nursing: Critical thinking in patient care* (5th ed., pp. 908–969). Boston: Pearson.

Smith, S. Jr., Allen, J., Blair, S., Bonow, R., Brass, L., Fonarow, G., et al. (2006). AHA/ACC guidelines for secondary prevention for patients with coronary and other atherosclerotic vascular disease: 2006 update. *Circulation, 113*(19), 2363–2372.

Thomas, S. A., Chapa, D. W., Friedmann, E., Durden, C., Ross, A., Lee, M. C., et al. (2008). Depression in patients with heart failure: Prevalence, pathophysiological mechanisms, and treatment. *Critical Care Nurse, 28*(2), 40–55.

Cardiac Care: Acute   4044

Definition: Limitation of complications for a patient recently experiencing an episode of an imbalance between myocardial oxygen supply and demand resulting in impaired cardiac function

Activities:

- Evaluate chest pain (e.g., intensity, location, radiation, duration, and precipitating and alleviating factors)
- Instruct the patient on the importance of immediately reporting any chest discomfort
- Provide immediate and continuous means to summon nurse, and let the patient and family know calls will be answered immediately
- Monitor ECG for ST changes, as appropriate
- Perform a comprehensive appraisal of cardiac status including peripheral circulation

- Monitor cardiac rhythm and rate
- Auscultate heart sounds
- Recognize the frustration and fright caused by inability to communicate and exposure to strange machinery and environment
- Auscultate lungs for crackles or other adventitious sounds
- Monitor the effectiveness of oxygen therapy, if appropriate
- Monitor determinants of oxygen delivery (e.g., PaO_2 and hemoglobin levels and cardiac output), if appropriate
- Monitor neurological status
- Monitor intake and output, urine output, and daily weight, as appropriate
- Select best EKG lead for continuous monitoring, as appropriate
- Obtain 12-lead EKG, as appropriate
- Draw serum, CK, LDH, and AST levels, as appropriate
- Monitor renal function (e.g., BUN and Cr levels), as appropriate
- Monitor liver function tests, if appropriate
- Monitor lab values for electrolytes that may increase the risk of dysrhythmias (e.g., serum potassium and magnesium), as appropriate
- Obtain chest x-ray, as appropriate
- Monitor trends in blood pressure and hemodynamic parameters, if available (e.g., central venous pressure and pulmonary capillary or artery wedge pressure)
- Provide small, frequent meals
- Provide appropriate cardiac diet (i.e., limit intake of caffeine, sodium, cholesterol, and food high in fat)
- Refrain from giving oral stimulants
- Substitute artificial salt, if appropriate
- Limit environmental stimuli
- Maintain an environment conducive to rest and healing
- Avoid causing intense emotional situations
- Identify the patient's methods of handling stress
- Promote effective techniques for reducing stress
- Perform relaxation therapy, if appropriate
- Refrain from arguing
- Discourage decision making when the patient is under severe stress
- Avoid overheating or chilling the patient
- Refrain from inserting a rectal tube
- Refrain from taking rectal temperatures
- Refrain from doing a rectal or vaginal examination
- Delay bathing, if appropriate
- Instruct the patient to avoid activities that result in the Valsalva maneuver (e.g., straining during bowel movement)
- Administer medications that will prevent episodes of the Valsalva maneuver (e.g., stool softeners, antiemetics), as appropriate
- Prevent peripheral thrombus formation (i.e., turn every 2 hours and administer low-dose anticoagulants)
- Administer medications to relieve or prevent pain and ischemia, as needed
- Monitor effectiveness of medication
- Instruct patient and family on the aims of care and how progress will be measured
- Ensure that all staff are aware of these goals and are working together to provide consistent care
- Offer spiritual support to the patient and family (i.e., contact a member of the clergy), as appropriate

1st edition 1992; revised 2000, 2013

Background Readings:

American Association of Critical Care Nurses. (2006). *Core curriculum for critical care nursing* (6th ed.) [J. G. Alspach, Ed.]. Philadelphia: Saunders.

Chummun, H., Gopaul, K., & Lutchman, A. (2009). Current guidance on the management of acute coronary syndrome. *British Journal of Nursing, 18*(21), 1292–1298.

Clancy, J., McVicar, A., & Hubbard, J. (2011). Homeostasis 4: Nurses as agents of control in myocardial infarction. *British Journal of Nursing, 20*(6), 373–378.

Kushner, F., Hand, M., Smith, S. Jr., King, S. III, Anderson, J., Antman, E., et al. (2009). 2009 focused updates: ACC/AHA guidelines for the management of patients with ST-elevation myocardial infarction (updating the 2004 guideline and 2007 focused update) and ACC/AHA/SCAI guidelines on percutaneous coronary intervention (updating the 2005 guideline and 2007 focused update). *Journal of the American College of Cardiology, 54*(23), 2205–2241.

LeMone, P., Burke, K. & Bauldoff, G. (2011). Nursing care of patient with coronary heart disease. *Medical-surgical nursing: Critical thinking in patient care* (5th ed., pp. 908–969). Boston: Pearson.

Marshall, K. (2011). Acute coronary syndrome: Diagnosis, risk assessment and management. *Nursing Standard, 25*(23), 47–57

Wright, R., Anderson, J., Adams, C., Bridges, C., Casey, D. Jr, Ettinger, S., Fesmire, F., et al. (2011). 2011 ACCF/AHA focused update of the guidelines for the management of patients with unstable angina/non–ST-elevation myocardial infarction (updating the 2007 guideline). *Journal of the American College of Cardiology, 57*(19), 1920–1959.

Cardiac Care: Rehabilitative   4046

Definition: Promotion of maximum functional activity level for a patient who has experienced an episode of impaired cardiac function that resulted from an imbalance between myocardial oxygen supply and demand

Activities:
- Monitor the patient's activity tolerance
- Maintain ambulation schedule, as tolerated
- Encourage realistic expectations for the patient and family
- Instruct the patient and family on appropriate prescribed and over-the-counter medications
- Instruct the patient and family on cardiac risk factor modification (e.g., smoking cessation, diet, and exercise), as appropriate
- Instruct the patient on self-care of chest pain (i.e., take sublingual nitroglycerine every 5 minutes three times; if chest pain is unrelieved, seek emergency medical care)

- Instruct the patient and family on the exercise regimen, including warm-up, endurance, and cool-down, as appropriate
- Instruct the patient and family on any lifting/pushing weight limitations, if appropriate
- Instruct the patient and family on any special considerations with activities of daily living (i.e., isolate activities and allow rest periods), if appropriate
- Instruct the patient and family on wound care and precautions (e.g., sternal incision or catheterization site), if appropriate
- Instruct the patient and family on follow-up care
- Coordinate patient referrals (e.g., dietary, social services, and physical therapy)
- Instruct the patient and family on access of emergency services available in their community, as appropriate
- Screen patient for anxiety and depression, as appropriate

1st edition 1992; revised 2000, 2013

Background Readings:

LeMone, P., Burke, K. & Bauldoff, G. (2011). Nursing care of patient with coronary heart disease. *Medical-surgical nursing: Critical thinking in patient care* (5th ed., pp. 908–969). Boston: Pearson.

Nazarko, L. (2008). Cardiology: Cardiac rehabilitation. *Nursing & Residential Care, 10*(9), 439–442.

Smith, S. Jr., Allen, J., Blair, S., Bonow, R., Brass, L., Fonarow, G., et al. (2006). AHA/ACC guidelines for secondary prevention for patients with coronary and other atherosclerotic vascular disease: 2006 update. *Circulation, 113*(19), 2363–2372.

Thomas, S., Chapa, D., Friedmann, E., Durden, C., Ross, A., Lee, M., et al. (2008). Depression in patients with heart failure: Prevalence, pathophysiological mechanisms, and treatment. *Critical Care Nurse, 28*(2), 40–55.

Cardiac Risk Management   4050

Definition: Prevention of an acute episode of impaired cardiac function by minimizing contributing events and risk behaviors

Activities:

- Screen patient for risk behaviors associated with adverse cardiac events (e.g., smoking, obesity, sedentary lifestyle, high blood pressure, history of previous cardiac events, family history of cardiac events)
- Identify patient's readiness to learn lifestyle modification (e.g., diet, smoking, alcohol intake, exercise, and cholesterol levels)
- Instruct patient and family on signs and symptoms of early cardiac disease and worsening cardiac disease, as appropriate
- Instruct patient and family on cardiac risk factor modification, as appropriate
- Prioritize areas for risk reduction in collaboration with patient and family
- Instruct patient and family to monitor blood pressure and heart rate routinely and with exercise, as appropriate
- Encourage exercise as indicated by patient cardiac risk factor
- Instruct the patient on regular and progressive exercise, as appropriate
- Encourage 30 minutes of exercise daily, as appropriate
- Instruct patient on need to achieve exercise goals in incremental periods of 10 minutes multiple times daily, if intolerant to sustained 30 minute activities
- Instruct patient and family on symptoms of cardiac compromise indicating need for rest
- Instruct patient and family on strategies for restricting or eliminating smoking
- Instruct patient and family on strategies for a heart healthy diet (e.g., low sodium, low fat, low cholesterol, high fiber, adequate fluid, appropriate caloric intake)
- Encourage patient to keep caloric intake at a level that achieves desired weight
- Instruct patient and family on therapies to reduce cardiac risk (e.g., medication therapies, blood pressure monitoring, fluid restrictions, alcohol restrictions, cardiac rehabilitation)
- Provide both verbal and written information to patient, family, and caregivers for all pertinent cares, as indicated
- Focus care and treatment goals to enable the patient to maintain weight control, to remain a nonsmoker, and to remain as active as possible
- Refer to heart failure program or cardiac rehabilitation program for lifestyle changes, as appropriate
- Alleviate patient's anxieties by providing accurate information and correcting any misconceptions
- Screen patient for anxiety and depression, as appropriate
- Identify the patient's methods of handling stress
- Promote effective techniques for reducing stress
- Perform relaxation therapy, if appropriate
- Monitor patient's progress at regular intervals

1st edition 1992; revised 2013

Background Readings:

American Association of Critical Care Nurses. (2006). *Core curriculum for critical care nursing* (6th ed.) [J. G. Alspach, Ed.]. Philadelphia: Saunders.

Chummun, H., Gopaul, K., & Lutchman, A. (2009). Current guidance on the management of acute coronary syndrome. *British Journal of Nursing, 18*(21), 1292–1298.

Greenland, P., Alpert, J., Beller, G., Benjamin, E., Budoff, M., Fayad, Z., et al. (2010). 2010 ACCF/AHA guideline for assessment of cardiovascular risk in asymptomatic adults: A report of the American College of Cardiology Foundation/American Heart Association Task Force on Practice Guidelines. *Journal of the American College of Cardiology, 56*(25), 2182–2199.

LeMone, P., Burke, K. & Bauldoff, G. (2011). Nursing care of patient with coronary heart disease. *Medical-surgical nursing: Critical thinking in patient care* (5th ed., pp. 908–969). Boston: Pearson.

Nazarko, L. (2008). Cardiology: Cardiac rehabilitation. *Nursing & Residential Care, 10*(9), 439–442.

Smith, S. Jr., Allen, J., Blair, S., Bonow, R., Brass, L., Fonarow, G., et al. (2006). AHA/ACC guidelines for secondary prevention for patients with coronary and other atherosclerotic vascular disease: 2006 update. *Circulation, 113*(19), 2363–2372.

Thomas, S., Chapa, D., Friedmann, E., Durden, C., Ross, A., Lee, M. C., et al. (2008). Depression in patients with heart failure: Prevalence, pathophysiological mechanisms, and treatment. *Critical Care Nurse, 28*(2), 40–55.

Caregiver Support   7040

Definition: Provision of the necessary information, advocacy, and support to facilitate primary patient care by someone other than a health care professional

Activities:
- Determine caregiver's level of knowledge
- Determine caregiver's acceptance of role
- Accept expressions of negative emotion
- Acknowledge difficulties of caregiving role
- Explore strengths and weaknesses with the caregiver
- Acknowledge dependency of patient on caregiver, as appropriate
- Make positive statements about caregiver's efforts
- Encourage caregiver to assume responsibility, as appropriate
- Provide support for decisions made by caregiver
- Encourage the acceptance of interdependency among family members
- Monitor family interaction problems related to care of patient
- Provide information about patient's condition in accordance with patient preferences
- Teach caregiver the patient's therapy in accordance with patient preferences
- Teach caregiver techniques to improve security of patient
- Provide for follow-up health caregiver assistance through phone calls and/or community nurse care
- Monitor for indicators of stress
- Explore with caregiver how she/he is coping
- Teach caregiver stress management techniques
- Educate caregiver about the grieving process
- Support caregiver through grieving process
- Encourage caregiver participation in support groups
- Teach caregiver health care maintenance strategies to sustain own physical and mental health
- Foster caregiver social networking
- Identify sources of respite care
- Inform caregiver of health care and community resources
- Teach caregiver strategies to access and maximize health care and community resources
- Act for caregiver if overburdening becomes apparent
- Notify emergency services agency/personnel about the patient's stay at home, health status, and technologies in use with consent of patient and family
- Discuss caregiver limits with patient
- Provide encouragement to caregiver during times of setback for patient
- Support caregiver in setting limits and taking care of self

1st edition 1992; revised 2004

Background Readings:
Craft, M. J. & Denehy, J. A. (1990). *Nursing interventions for infants and children*. Philadelphia: Saunders.
Craft, M. J. & Willadsen, J. A. (1992). Interventions related to family. In G. M. Bulechek & J. C. McCloskey (Eds.), Symposium on nursing interventions. *Nursing Clinics of North America, 27*(2), 517–540.
Maas, M. L., Buckwalter, K. C., Hardy, M. D., Tripp-Reimer, T., Titler, M. G., & Specht, J. P. (Eds.). (2001). *Nursing care of older adults: Diagnoses, outcomes, & interventions* (pp. 686–693). St. Louis: Mosby.
Moore, L. W., Marocco, G., Schmidt, S. M., Guo, L., & Estes, J. (2002) Perspectives of caregivers of stroke survivors: Implications for nursing, *MEDSURG Nursing, 11*(6), 289–295.

Case Management   7320

Definition: Coordinating care and advocating for specified individuals and patient populations across settings to reduce cost, reduce resource use, improve quality of health care, and achieve desired outcomes

Activities:
- Identify individuals or patient populations who would benefit from case management (e.g., high cost, high volume, and/or high risk)
- Identify payment source for case management service
- Explain the role of the case manager to patient and family
- Explain the cost of service to patient and/or family before rendering care
- Obtain patient or family's permission to be enrolled in a case management program, as appropriate
- Develop relationships with patient, family, and other health care providers, as needed
- Use effective communication skills with patient, family, and other health care providers
- Treat patient and family with dignity and respect
- Maintain patient and family confidentiality and privacy
- Assess patient's physical health status, mental status, functional capability, formal and informal support systems, financial resources, and environmental conditions, as needed
- Determine treatment plan with input from patient and/or family
- Explain critical paths to patient and family
- Individualize critical path for patient
- Determine outcomes to be obtained with input from patient and/or family
- Discuss plan of care and intended outcomes with patient's physician
- Negotiate work schedule with the nurse manager (head nurse) to attend weekly group practice meetings, as needed
- Integrate care management information and revised interventions (processes) into intershift report and group practice meetings, as needed
- Evaluate progress toward established goals on a continual basis
- Revise interventions and goals as necessary to meet patient's needs
- Identify resources and/or services needed
- Coordinate provision of needed resources or services
- Coordinate care with other pertinent health care providers (e.g., other nurses, physicians, social workers, third-party payers, physical therapists)

C

- Provide direct care as necessary
- Educate patient and/or family on importance of self-care
- Encourage appropriate patient and/or family decision-making activities
- Document all case management activities
- Monitor plan for quality, quantity, timeliness, and effectiveness of services
- Facilitate access to necessary health and social services
- Assist patient and/or family with access to the health care delivery system
- Guide patient and/or family through the health care delivery system
- Assist patient and/or family in making informed decisions regarding health care
- Advocate for patient as necessary
- Recognize need to merge patient, clinical, and financial concerns
- Notify patient and/or family of change in service, termination of service, and discharge from case management program
- Promote efficient use of resources
- Monitor cost effectiveness of care
- Modify care to increase cost effectiveness, as needed
- Establish quality improvement program to evaluate case management activities
- Document cost effectiveness of case management
- Report outcomes to insurers and other third-party payers
- Market services to individuals, families, insurers, and employers

3rd edition 2000

Background Readings:

Bahe, D. K. (2001). Case management. In M. Craft-Rosenberg & J. Denehy (Eds.), *Nursing interventions for infants, children, and families* (pp. 259–280). Thousand Oaks, CA: Sage.

Bower, K. (1988). *Case management by nurses.* Washington, DC: American Nurses Publishing.

Crummer, M. B. & Carter, V. (1993). Critical pathways—the pivotal tool. *Journal of Cardiovascular Nursing, 7*(4), 30–37.

Davis, V. (1996). Staff development for nurse case management. In E. L. Cohen (Ed.), *Nurse case management in the 21st century* (pp. 189–196). St. Louis: Mosby.

Flarey, D. L. & Blancett, S. S. (1996). *Handbook of nursing case management: Health care delivery in a world of managed care.* Gaithersburg, MD: Aspen.

Newell, M. (1996). *Using case management to improve health outcomes.* Gaithersburg, MD: Aspen.

Zander, K. (1993). The impact of managing care on the role of a nurse. *Series on Nursing Administration, 5,* 65–82.

Cast Care: Maintenance 0762

Definition: Care of a cast after the drying period

Activities:

- Monitor for signs of infection (foul-smelling cast, erythema, fever)
- Monitor for signs of cast impairment of circulation or neurological function (e.g., pain, pallor, pulselessness, paresthesias, paralysis, and pressure) on affected extremity
- Monitor circulation and neurological function of tissues above and below cast
- Address compromised circulation and pain symptoms immediately (e.g., reposition cast, perform range of motion [ROM] to extremity, immediate cast pressure-relieving action)
- Inspect cast for signs of drainage from wounds under the cast
- Mark the circumference of any drainage as a gauge for future assessments
- Protect the cast if close to groin
- Instruct patient not to scratch skin under the cast with any objects
- Offer alternatives to scratching (e.g., cold air from a hair dryer)
- Avoid getting a plaster cast wet (e.g., use appropriate protection for bathing or toileting, protective socks or gloves)
- Position cast on pillows to lessen strain on other body parts with cast heel off pillow
- Apply ice for first 24 to 36 hours to reduce swelling or inflammation
- Elevate casted extremity at or above heart level to reduce swelling or inflammation
- Check for cracking or breaks in the cast
- Apply an arm sling for support, if appropriate
- Pad rough cast edges and traction connections
- Teach patient and family care of cast
- Document cast care instructions given to patient and family
- Document observations of patient ability to perform cast care

1st edition 1992; revised 2008

Background Readings:

McCance, K. L. & Huether, S. E. (2006). *Pathophysiology: The biologic basis for disease in adults and children* (5th ed.). St. Louis: Mosby.

Perry, A. G. & Potter, P. A. (2006). *Clinical nursing skills and techniques* (6th ed.). St. Louis: Mosby.

Potter, P. A. & Perry, A. G. (2005). *Fundamentals of nursing* (6th ed.). St. Louis: Mosby.

Smeltzer, S. C. & Bare, B. G. (2004). *Brunner & Suddarth's textbook of medical-surgical nursing* (10th ed.). Philadelphia: Lippincott Williams & Wilkins.

Cast Care: Wet   0764

Definition: Care of a new cast during the drying period

Activities:
- Monitor for signs of cast impairment of circulation or neurological function (e.g., pain, pallor, pulselessness, paresthesias, paralysis, and pressure) on affected extremity
- Monitor circulation and neurological function of tissues above and below cast
- Address compromised circulation and pain symptoms immediately to avoid permanent damage in neurovascular status (e.g., reposition cast, report unresolved symptoms as needing immediate cast pressure relieving action)
- Support the cast with pillows during the drying period
- Handle the casted extremity with palms only until the cast is dry to avoid cau sing finger indentations that can lead to pressure sores
- Inform the patient that the cast will feel warm as the cast dries
- Protect cast if close to groin
- Maintain the angles of the cast during the drying period
- Inspect cast for signs of drainage from wounds under the cast
- Mark the circumference of any drainage as a gauge for future assessments
- Explain the need for limited activity while cast dries

- Identify any change in sensation or increased pain at the fracture site
- Apply ice for first 24 to 35 hours to reduce swelling or inflammation, as indicated
- Elevate casted extremity at or above heart level to reduce swelling or inflammation, as indicated
- Teach patient and family care of cast
- Document cast care instructions given to patient and family

1st edition 1992; revised 2008

Background Readings:

Perry, A. G. & Potter, P. A. (2006). *Clinical nursing skills and techniques* (6th ed.). St. Louis: Mosby.

Potter, P. A. & Perry, A. G. (2005). *Fundamentals of nursing* (6th ed.). St. Louis: Mosby.

Smeltzer, S. C. & Bare, B.G. (2004). *Brunner & Suddarth's textbook of medical-surgical nursing* (10th ed.). Philadelphia: Lippincott Williams & Wilkins.

Smith, S. & Duell, D. (1992). *Clinical nursing skills* (3rd ed.). Los Altos, CA: National Nursing Review.

Central Venous Access Device Management   4054

Definition: Care of the patient with prolonged venous access through the use of a device inserted into the central circulation

Activities:
- Determine the type of Central Venous Access Device (CVAD) in place
- Determine manufacturer and agency recommendations, guidelines, protocols, policies, and procedures related to the particular device
- Determine patient's and/or family's understanding of the purpose, care, and maintenance of the CVAD
- Provide information to patient and family related to the device (e.g., indications, functions, type of device to be used, care of device, potential complications) to reduce patient uncertainty, fear and anxiety
- Explain the entire procedure to patient when inserting, providing care for, accessing for medication or fluid therapy, or removing a device
- Avoid use of the line until confirmation of tip placement post-implantation with baseline chest x-ray
- Assure subclavian and jugular vein tips located within the lower third of the superior vena cava
- Report catheter tips positioned within the heart as they have an increased risk of mortality
- Report catheter tips positioned perpendicular to the vein wall as there is an increased risk of vessel erosion, hydrothorax, hydromediastinum, tamponade, and extravasation
- Employ strict aseptic technique whenever device is handled, accessed, or used to administer medications, to reduce potential for catheter-related bloodstream infections
- Maintain universal precautions

- Adapt care to the type of device (i.e., use clamp at all times with open-ended or midline CVADs, use Huber needles for port access, use saline flushes with non-return valves, use clear transparent dressing to anchor non-tunneled, midline, and PICC CVADs)
- Check patency of the CVAD immediately before administering prescribed medications/infusions
- Aspirate blood from the device to check patency before administering prescribed therapy, as indicated per device type
- Employ further actions to ensure patency if difficulty encountered with aspiration or no blood return, per manufacturer and agency protocol for occluded devices
- Administer saline flush for valved catheter maintenance as valve prevents blood reflux into the lumen of the catheter, thus preventing thrombotic occlusion
- Flush non-valved (or open-ended) CVADs with heparinized saline weekly, with the strength of heparin per agency policy
- Flush implanted ports with heparinized saline monthly, with the strength of heparin per agency policy
- Flush PICCs weekly with heparinized saline if not in use, with the strength of heparin per agency policy
- Employ needle-free devices to promote a closed system
- Employ 10 cc syringes for access of CVADs as smaller gauge silastic catheters appear to create greater pressure of pounds per square inch, which may result in the rupture of the catheter and clots forced into bloodstream
- Assure that intravenous tubing line is securely taped into position

- Assure tubing is laying on the bed or arm of the treatment chair; do not allow intravenous tubing to dangle or pull
- Use self-adhesive anchoring devices where appropriate, or per agency policy
- Change clear fluid administration sets every 72 hours, blood sets every 12 hours, and parenteral nutrition administration sets every 24 hours, or per agency policy
- Use new IV solutions and administration sets for new CVADs
- Discard existing infusion sets assuring that infusion sets from old devices to new devices are not exchanged
- Maintain accurate record of infusate(s)
- Do not allow the CVAD to be inserted near a stoma or areas such as diapers in children, where contact with fecal material may occur
- Apply gauze dressing for the first 24 hours following operative insertion
- Apply a clear dressing under strict aseptic technique weekly thereafter or sooner if soiled, perforated, or the dressing is lifting off
- Use transparent semi-permeable dressings with non-tunneled devices and change every 7 days or sooner if wet or dirty, or per agency policy
- Use 2% chlorhexidine in 70% isopropyl alcohol solution for cleansing the exit wound and catheter at all dressing changes, and to decontaminate the skin prior to CVAD insertion, unless patient has a known allergy to chlorhexidine
- Decontaminate CVADs with 2% chlorhexidine gluconate in 70% isopropyl and allow to dry prior to accessing, unless contraindicated by the manufacturer
- Obtain chest x-ray immediately in the event of suspected line infiltration, compromise, or migration
- Monitor for arm swelling or increased warmth on side ipsilateral to implanted device
- Monitor for complications of CVADs (e.g., pneumothorax, cardiac tamponade, arterial puncture, hemorrhage, hemothorax, hydrothorax, air embolus, brachial nerve plexus injury, thoracic duct injury, infection, misplacement)
- Inspect entry site daily for redness, pain, tenderness, warmth, or swelling as devices are associated with increased risk of infection
- Remove device if any signs of inflammation, leakage, or discharge from the entry site
- Ensure any infusions attached to the CVAD have been switched off prior to removing a device
- Position patient supine, head down if possible, for insertion and removal of non-tunneled CVADs
- Place gauze over the entry site and apply light to moderate pressure to remove CVAD to avoid catheter fracture, tearing, and/or embolization
- Place CVAD tip in sterile container and send for culture if infection is suspected
- Apply firm pressure to the puncture site after removing the CVAD for at least 2 minutes until hemostasis is achieved

- Apply an airtight transparent dressing immediately after CVAD removal ensuring a good seal is achieved, and keep in place for 72 hours
- Monitor x-rays for pinch-off sign in catheters that are occluded or prior to removal as pinch-off catheters are more likely to tear or fracture
- Use an antimicrobial-impregnated catheter for patients considered to be at-risk for catheter related sepsis
- Consider length of time device is needed before recommending device (e.g., less than 7 days use peripheral IV; 1 to 4 weeks use midline catheter or PICC line; 1 month to 1 year use PICC, tunneled CVAD, implantable port; longer than 1 year use tunneled CVAD, implantable port)
- Document pertinent data in patient permanent record for initial insertion of CVAD (e.g., manufacturer, model number, serial number, implant date)
- Instruct patient of the signs and symptoms of dysfunctional CVAD (e.g., tachycardia, hypotension, dyspnea, agitation, independent filling of access needle with fluid or blood, shoulder or back pain, cardiac arrest)
- Instruct patient to carry CVAD manufacturer identification card at all times
- Instruct patient to wear a medical alert bracelet or necklace that identifies patient as a CVAD patient

6th edition 2013

Background Readings:

Cummings-Winfield, C. & Mushani-Kanji, T. (2008). Restoring patency to central venous access devices. *Clinical Journal of Oncology Nursing, 12*(6), 925–934.

Douglas, L., Aspin, A., Jimmeson, N., & Lawrance, V. (2009). Central venous access devices: Review of practice. *Pediatric Nursing, 21*(5), 19–22.

Gabriel, J. (2010). Vascular access devices: Securement and dressings. *Nursing Standard, 24*(52), 41–46.

Gabriel, J., Bravery, K., Dougherty, L., Kayley, J., & Malster, M. (2005). Vascular access: Indications and implications for patient care. *Nursing Standard, 19*(26), 45–52, 54, 56.

Hamilton, H. (2006). Complications associated with venous access devices: Part 1 of 2. *Nursing Standard, 20*(26), 43–51, 53.

Mitchell, M. D., Anderson, B. J., Williams, K., & Umscheid, C.A. (2009). Heparin flushing and other interventions to maintain patency of central venous catheters: A systematic review. *Journal of Advanced Nursing, 65*(10), 2007–2021.

Scales, K. (2010). Central venous access devices: Part 1: Devices for acute care. *British Journal of Nursing, 19*(2), 88–92.

Scales, K. (2010). Central venous access devices: Part 2: For intermediate and long-term use. *British Journal of Nursing, 19*(5), S20–S25.

Schulmeister, L. (2010). Management of non-infectious central venous access device complications. *Seminars in Oncology Nursing, 26*(2), 132–134.

Cerebral Edema Management 2540

Definition: Limitation of secondary cerebral injury resulting from swelling of brain tissue

Activities:
- Monitor for confusion, changes in mentation, complaints of dizziness, syncope
- Monitor neurologic status closely and compare to baseline
- Monitor vital signs
- Monitor CSF drainage characteristics: color, clarity, consistency
- Record CSF drainage
- Monitor CVP, PAWP, and PAP, as appropriate
- Monitor ICP and CPP
- Analyze ICP waveform
- Monitor respiratory status: rate, rhythm, depth of respirations; PaO_2, pCO_2, pH, bicarbonate
- Allow ICP to return to baseline between nursing activities
- Monitor patient's ICP and neurologic response to care activities
- Decrease stimuli in patient's environment
- Plan nursing care to provide rest periods
- Give sedation, as needed
- Note patient's change in response to stimuli
- Screen conversation within patient's hearing
- Administer anticonvulsants, as appropriate
- Avoid neck flexion, or extreme hip/knee flexion
- Avoid Valsalva maneuvers
- Administer stool softeners
- Position with head of bed up 30 degrees or greater
- Avoid use of PEEP
- Administer paralyzing agent, as appropriate
- Encourage family/significant other to talk to patient
- Restrict fluids
- Avoid hypotonic IV fluids
- Adjust ventilator settings to keep $PaCO_2$ at prescribed level
- Limit suction passes to less than 15 seconds
- Monitor lab values: serum and urine osmolality, sodium, potassium
- Monitor volume pressure indices
- Perform passive range-of-motion exercises
- Monitor intake and output
- Maintain normothermia
- Administer loop-active or osmotic diuretics
- Implement seizure precautions
- Titrate barbiturate to achieve suppression or burst-suppression of EEG as ordered
- Establish means of communication: ask yes or no questions; provide magic slate, paper and pencil, picture board, flashcards, VOCAID device

1st edition 1992; revised 2004

Background Readings:

American Association of Critical-Care Nurses. (1998). *Core curriculum for critical care nursing* (5th ed.). Philadelphia: Saunders.

American Academy of Pediatrics. (1999). The management of minor closed head injury in children. *Pediatrics, 104*(6), 1407–1415.

Orfanelli, L. (2001). Neurologic examination of the toddler. *American Journal of Nursing, 101*(12), 24CC–24FF.

Yanko, J. R. & Mitcho, K. (2001). Acute care management of severe traumatic brain injuries. *Critical Care Nursing Quarterly, 23*(4), 1–23.

Cerebral Perfusion Promotion 2550

Definition: Promotion of adequate perfusion and limitation of complications for a patient experiencing or at risk for inadequate cerebral perfusion

Activities:
- Consult with physician to determine hemodynamic parameters, and maintain hemodynamic parameters within this range
- Induce hypertension with volume expansion or inotropic or vasoconstrictive agents, as ordered, to maintain hemodynamic parameters and maintain/optimize cerebral perfusion pressure (CPP)
- Administer and titrate vasoactive drugs, as ordered, to maintain hemodynamic parameters
- Administer agents to expand intravascular volume, as appropriate (e.g., colloid, blood products, and crystalloid)
- Administer volume expanders to maintain hemodynamic parameters, as ordered
- Monitor prothrombin time (PT) and partial thromboplastin time (PTT), if using hetastarch as a volume expander
- Administer rheologic agents (e.g., low-dose mannitol or low molecular weight dextrans), as ordered
- Keep hematocrit level around 33% for hypervolemic hemodilution therapy
- Phlebotomize patient, as appropriate, to maintain hematocrit level in desired range
- Maintain serum glucose level within normal range
- Consult with physician to determine optimal head of bed (HOB) placement (e.g., 0, 15, or 30 degrees) and monitor patient's responses to head positioning
- Avoid neck flexion or extreme hip/knee flexion
- Keep pCO_2 level at 25 mm Hg or greater
- Administer calcium channel blockers, as ordered
- Administer vasopressin, as ordered
- Administer and monitor effects of osmotic and loop-active diuretics and corticosteroids
- Administer pain medication, as appropriate
- Administer anticoagulant medication, as ordered
- Administer antiplatelet medications, as ordered
- Administer thrombolytic medications, as ordered
- Monitor patient's PT and PTT to keep one to two times normal, as appropriate
- Monitor for anticoagulant therapy side effects
- Monitor for signs of bleeding (e.g., test stool and NG drainage for blood)
- Monitor neurological status

- Calculate and monitor CPP
- Monitor patient's ICP and neurological response to care activities
- Monitor mean arterial pressure (MAP)
- Monitor CVP
- Monitor PAWP and PAP
- Monitor respiratory status (e.g., rate, rhythm, and depth of respirations; partial oxygen pressure, pCO_2, pH, and bicarbonate levels)
- Auscultate lung sounds for crackles or other adventitious sounds
- Monitor for signs of fluid overload (e.g., rhonchi, jugular venous distention (JVD), edema, and increase in pulmonary secretions)
- Monitor determinants of tissue oxygen delivery (e.g., $PaCO_2$, SaO_2, and hemoglobin levels and cardiac output), if available
- Monitor lab values for changes in oxygenation or acid-base balance, as appropriate
- Monitor intake and output

2nd edition 1996

Background Readings:

Bronstein, K. S., Popovich, J. M., & Stewart-Amidei, C. (1991). *Promoting stroke recovery: A research based approach for nurses*. St. Louis: Mosby.

Hickey, J. V. (1992). *The clinical practice of neurological and neurosurgical nursing*. Philadelphia: Lippincott.

Hummel, S. K. (1989). Cerebral vasospasm: Current concepts of pathogenesis and treatment. *Journal of Neuroscience Nursing, 21*(4), 216–224.

Mitchell, S. K. & Yates, R. R. (1986). Cerebral vasospasm: Theoretical causes, medical management and nursing implications. *Journal of Neuroscience Nursing, 18*(6), 315–323.

Smeltzer, S. C. & Bare, B. G. (2004). *Brunner & Suddarth's textbook of medical surgical nursing* (Vol. 2) (10th ed.). Philadelphia: Lippincott Williams & Wilkins.

Stewart-Amidei, C. (1989). Hypervolemic hemodilution: A new approach to subarachnoid hemorrhage. *Heart & Lung, 18*(6), 590–598.

Cesarean Birth Care   6750

Definition: Provision of care to a patient delivering a baby through an abdominal incision into the uterus

Activities:
- Orient patient to unit
- Review prenatal history
- Explain reasons for surgery
- Discuss feelings, questions, and concerns patient has about surgery
- Obtain or confirm informed consent
- Obtain necessary blood work and document results
- Monitor vital signs
- Monitor fetal heart rate
- Prepare abdomen for surgery
- Place intravenous line
- Insert indwelling urinary catheter
- Administer medications
- Encourage intimate partner or support person to be present during delivery
- Give information about events taking place and sensations patient may be experiencing during surgery
- Give information about infant
- Transfer patient to recovery room or labor room
- Monitor physiological aspects of recovery (e.g., pain, uterine changes, airway patency, and lochia)
- Inspect condition of surgical incision and dressing
- Assist in performing leg exercises, turning, coughing, and deep breathing
- Encourage mother to breastfeed, if appropriate
- Provide adequate breastfeeding education and support, if appropriate (i.e., demonstrate infant positioning adaptations according to mobility limitations)
- Facilitate family bonding and attachment by minimizing maternal-infant separation (e.g., present infant en face to mother, provide unobstructed view of infant, facilitate skin-to-skin contact, and transfer mother and infant together)

1st edition 1992; revised 2013

Background Readings:

Chertok, I. R. (2006). Breast-feeding initiation among post-caesarean women of the Negev, Israel. *British Journal of Nursing, 15*(4), 205–208.

Nolan, A. & Lawrence, C. (2009). A pilot study of a nursing intervention protocol to minimize maternal-infant separation after cesarean birth. *Journal of Obstetric, Gynecologic, & Neonatal Nursing, 38*(4), 430–442.

Ward, S. L. & Hisley, S. M. (2009). Caring for the woman experiencing complications during labor and birth. *Maternal-child nursing care: Optimizing outcomes for mothers, children, & families.* (pp. 427–465). Philadelphia: F. A. Davis.

Chemical Restraint   6430

Definition: Administration, monitoring, and discontinuation of psychotropic agents used to control an individual's extreme behavior

Activities:
- Implement alternative interventions to attempt to eliminate the need for restraint
- Provide divisional activities prior to the use of restraints (e.g., television, visitors)
- Identify for the patient and significant others those behaviors that necessitated the intervention (e.g., agitation, violence)
- Explain the procedure, purpose, and duration of the intervention to patient and significant other in understandable terms
- Follow the five rights of medication administration
- Note patient's medical history and history of allergies
- Monitor the patient's response to the medication
- Monitor level of consciousness
- Monitor vital signs
- Provide appropriate level of supervision/surveillance to monitor patient and to allow for therapeutic actions, as needed
- Provide for patient's psychological comfort, as needed
- Monitor skin color, temperature, sensation, and condition
- Provide for movement and exercise, according to patient's level of self-control, condition, and abilities
- Position patient to facilitate comfort and prevent aspiration and skin breakdown
- Assist with periodic changes in body position
- Assist with needs related to nutrition, elimination, hydration, and personal hygiene
- Evaluate, at regular intervals, patient's need for continued restrictive intervention
- Involve patient, when appropriate, in making decisions to move to a more/less restrictive form of intervention

4th edition 2004

Background Readings:
Kow, J. V. & Hogan, D. B. (2000). Use of physical and chemical restraints in medical teaching units. *Canadian Medical Association Journal, 162*(3), 339–340.

Middleton, H., Keene, R. G., Johnson, C., Elkins, A. D., & Keem A. E. (1999). Physical and pharmacologic restraints in long-term care facilities. *Journal of Gerontological Nursing, 25*(7), 26–33.

Pearson, G. (2006). Psychopharmacology. In W. K. Mohr (Ed.), *Psychiatric-mental health nursing* (6th ed., pp. 243–286). Philadelphia: Lippincott Williams & Wilkins.

Chemotherapy Management   2240

Definition: Assisting the patient and family to understand the action and minimize side effects of antineoplastic agents

Activities:
- Monitor pretreatment screening work-ups for patients at risk for earlier onset, longer duration, and more distressing side effects
- Promote activities to modify the identified risk factors
- Monitor for side effects and toxic effects of treatment
- Provide information to patient and family on antineoplastic drug effect on malignant cells
- Teach patient and family about the effects of therapy on bone marrow functioning
- Instruct patient and family on ways to prevent infection, such as avoiding crowds, using good hygiene and handwashing techniques
- Instruct patient to promptly report fevers, chills, nosebleeds, excessive bruising, and tarry stools
- Instruct patient and family to avoid the use of aspirin products
- Institute neutropenic and bleeding precautions
- Determine the patient's previous experience with chemotherapy-related nausea and vomiting
- Administer medications as needed to control side effects (e.g., antiemetics for nausea and vomiting)
- Minimize stimuli from noises, light, and odors (especially food odors)
- Teach the patient relaxation and imagery techniques to use before, during, and after treatments, as appropriate
- Offer the patient a bland and easily digested diet
- Administer chemotherapeutic drugs in the late evening, so the patient may sleep at the time emetic effects are greatest
- Ensure adequate fluid intake to prevent dehydration and electrolyte imbalance
- Monitor the effectiveness of measures to control nausea and vomiting
- Offer six small feedings daily, as tolerated
- Instruct patient to avoid hot, spicy foods
- Provide nutritious, appetizing foods of patient's choice
- Monitor nutritional status and weight
- Monitor for indications of infection of oral mucous membranes
- Encourage good oral hygiene with use of dental cleansing devices, such as unwaxed, non-shredding floss, sonic toothbrushes, or water Pik, as appropriate
- Initiate oral health restoration activities, such as use of artificial saliva, saliva stimulants, non-alcohol-based mouth sprays, sugarless mints, and fluoride treatments, as appropriate
- Teach patient on self-assessment of oral cavity including signs and symptoms to report for further evaluation (e.g., burning, pain, tenderness)
- Teach patient need for frequent dental follow-up care as dental caries form rapidly
- Teach patient to use oral nystatin suspension to control fungal infection, as appropriate
- Teach patient to avoid temperature extremes and chemical treatments of the hair while receiving treatment
- Inform patient that hair loss is expected, as determined by type of therapy

- Assist patient in planning for hair loss, as appropriate, by teaching about available alternatives such as wigs, scarves, hats, and turbans
- Teach patient to gently wash and comb hair and to sleep on a silk pillowcase to prevent further hair loss, as appropriate
- Reassure patient that hair will grow back after treatment is terminated, as appropriate
- Teach patient and family to monitor for organ toxicity, as determined by type of therapy
- Discuss potential aspects of sexual dysfunction, as appropriate
- Teach implications of therapy on sexual function, including the time frame for contraceptive use, as appropriate
- Monitor fatigue level by soliciting the patient's description of fatigue
- Teach patient and family techniques of energy management, as appropriate
- Assist patient in managing fatigue by planning frequent rest periods, spacing of activities, and limiting daily demands, as appropriate
- Facilitate expression of fears about prognosis or success of treatments
- Provide concrete objective information related to the effects of therapy to reduce patient uncertainty, fear, and anxiety about treatment-related symptoms
- Instruct long-term survivors and their families of the possibility of second malignancies and the importance of reporting increased susceptibility to infection, fatigue, or bleeding
- Follow recommended guidelines for safe handling of parenteral antineoplastic drugs during drug preparation and administration

1st edition, 1992; revised 2008

Background Readings:

Barsevick, A. M., Whitmer, K., Sweeney, C., & Nail, L. M. (2002). A pilot study examining energy conservation for cancer treatment-related fatigue. *Cancer Nursing, 25*(5), 333–341.

Brown, K. A., Esper, P., Kelleher, L. O., Brace O'Neill, J. E., Polovich, M., & White, J. M. (Eds.), (2001). *Chemotherapy and biotherapy guidelines and recommendations for practice*. Pittsburgh, PA: Oncology Nursing Society.

LeMone, P. & Burke, K. M. (2000). *Medical-surgical nursing: Critical thinking in client care* (2nd ed., pp. 338–344). Upper Saddle River, NJ: Prentice Hall.

Nail, L. M. (2002). Fatigue in patients with cancer. *Oncology Nursing Forum, 29*(3), 537–546.

Oncology Nursing Society. (2004). *Statement on the scope and standards of oncology nursing practice*. Pittsburgh, PA: Author.

Oncology Nursing Society, Itano, J., & Taoka, K. N. (2005). *Core curriculum for oncology nursing practice* (4th ed.). Philadelphia: Saunders.

Wegeneka, M. H. (1999). Chemotherapy management. In G. Bulechek & J. McCloskey (Eds.), *Nursing interventions: Effective nursing treatments* (3rd ed., pp. 285–296). Philadelphia: Saunders.

Yarbro, C. H., Frogge, M. H., & Goodman, M. (2005). *Cancer nursing: Principles and practice*. Sudbury, MA: Jones & Bartlett.

Chest Physiotherapy 3230

Definition: Assisting the patient to mobilize airway secretions via percussion, vibration, and postural drainage

Activities:

- Determine presence of contraindications for use of chest physiotherapy (e.g., acute exacerbation of COPD, pneumonia without evidence of excess sputum production, osteoporosis, lung cancer, and cerebral edema)
- Perform chest physiotherapy at least two hours after eating
- Explain purpose and procedures used during chest physiotherapy to patient
- Position any necessary equipment nearby (e.g., suctioning equipment, sputum container, and tissues)
- Monitor respiratory and cardiac status (e.g., rate, rhythm, breath sounds, and depth of breath)
- Monitor amount and character of secretions
- Determine lung segment(s) containing excessive secretions
- Position patient with the lung segment to be drained in uppermost position, making modifications for patients unable to tolerate prescribed position (i.e., avoid placing patient with COPD, acute head injury, and cardiac problems in Trendelenburg position as it can increase shortness of breath, intracranial pressure, and stress, respectively)
- Use pillows to support patient in designated position
- Strike chest rhythmically and in rapid succession using cupped hands over area(s) to be drained for 3-5 minutes, avoiding percussion over spine, kidneys, female breasts, incisions, and broken ribs
- Apply pneumatic, acoustical, or electrical chest percussors
- Rapidly and vigorously vibrate hands, keeping shoulders and arms straight and wrists stiff, on area(s) to be drained while patient exhales or coughs 3-4 times
- Instruct patient to expectorate loosened secretions via deep breathing
- Encourage coughing during and after procedure
- Suction loosened secretions
- Monitor patient tolerance during and after procedure (e.g., pulse oximetry, vital signs, and reported comfort level)

1st edition 1992; revised 2013

Background Readings:

Cantin, A. M., Bacon, M., & Berthiaume, Y. (2006). Mechanical airway clearance using the frequencer electro-acoustical transducer in cystic fibrosis. *Clinical & Investigative Medicine, 29*(3), 159–65.

Craven, R. F. & Hirnle, C. J. (2009). Oxygenation: Respiratory function. In *Fundamentals of nursing: Human health and function* (6th ed., pp. 816–876). Philadelphia: Lippincott Williams & Wilkins.

Nelson, D. M. (1992). Interventions related to respiratory care. In G. M. Bulechek & J. C. McCloskey (Eds.), Symposium on nursing interventions. *Nursing Clinics of North America, 27*(2), 301–324.

Smith, S.F., Duell, D.J., & Martin, B.C. (2008). Respiratory care. *Clinical nursing skills: Basic to advanced skills* (7th ed., pp. 939–1002). Upper Saddle River, New Jersey: Pearson Prentice Hall.

Workman, M. L. (2010). Care of patients with noninfectious lower respiratory problems. In D. D. Ignatavicius, & M. L. Workman (Eds.), *Medical-surgical nursing: Patient-centered collaborative care* (6th ed., pp. 609–652). St. Louis: Saunders.

Yang, M., Yan, Y., Yin, X., Wang, B. Y., Wu, T., Liu, G. J., et al. (2010). Chest physiotherapy for pneumonia in adults. *Cochrane Database of Systematic Reviews*, Issue 2. Art. No.: CD006338. doi: 10.1002/14651858.CD006338. pub2.

Childbirth Preparation   6760

Definition: Providing information and support to facilitate childbirth and to enhance the ability of an individual to develop and perform the parental role

Activities:

- Teach the mother and partner about the physiology of labor and delivery
- Explore childbirth plan for labor and delivery (e.g., the birthing environment, who will assist mother, who will be in attendance, what technology will be used, who will cut the cord, feeding preferences, and discharge plans)
- Educate mother and partner about signs of labor
- Inform mother about when to come to the hospital in preparation for delivery
- Discuss pain control options with mother
- Instruct mother on steps to be taken if desire is to avoid episiotomy, such as perineal massage, Kegel exercises, optimal nutrition, and prompt treatment of vaginitis
- Inform mother about delivery options if complications arise
- Explain routine monitoring that may occur during labor and delivery
- Teach mother and partner breathing and relaxation techniques to be used during labor and delivery
- Teach partner measures to comfort mother during labor (e.g., back rub, back pressure, and positioning)
- Prepare partner to coach mother during labor and delivery
- Review American Academy of Pediatrics recommendations for breastfeeding
- Discuss advantages and disadvantages of breastfeeding and bottle feeding
- Instruct mother to prepare nipples for breastfeeding, as indicated
- Encourage mother to put the infant to breast after delivery
- Provide opportunity for mother to be in close proximity to infant during postpartum hospitalization to facilitate bonding and breastfeeding
- Determine parent's knowledge and attitudes about parenting
- Promote parent's self-efficacy in taking on parental role
- Provide anticipatory guidance for parenthood
- Discuss arrangements for sibling care during hospitalization
- Determine how parent(s) prepared sibling(s) for coming of new baby, as appropriate
- Assist parent(s) in planning strategies to prepare siblings for newborn
- Refer parent(s) to sibling preparation class
- Assist parent to select a physician or clinic to receive child health supervision for newborn
- Encourage mother to obtain an approved infant car safety seat to transport newborn home from hospital

1st edition 1992; revised 2008

Background Readings:

American Academy of Pediatrics. (2005). Policy statement: Breastfeeding and the use of human milk. *Pediatrics, 115*(2), 496–506.

Bradley, L., Horan, M. J, & Molloy, P. (2004). Pregnancy and childbearing. In M. C. Condon (Ed.), *Women's health: Body, mind, sprit: An integrated approach to wellness and illness* (pp. 463–499). Upper Saddle River, NJ: Prentice Hall.

Kirkham, C., Harris, S., & Grzybowski, S. (2005). Evidence-based prenatal care: Part l. General prenatal care and counseling issues. *American Family Physician, 71*(7), 1307–1316, 1321–1322.

Littleton, L. Y. & Engebertson, J. C. (2002). *Maternal, neonatal, and women's health nursing* (pp. 477–489). Albany, NY: Delmar.

Institute for Clinical Systems Improvement (ICSI). (2005). *Health care guideline: Routine prenatal care.* Bloomington, MN: Author.

Wong, D. L., Perry, S. E., & Hockenberry, J. J. (2004). *Maternal child nursing care.* St. Louis: Mosby.

Circulatory Care: Arterial Insufficiency   4062

Definition: Promotion of arterial circulation

Activities:

- Perform a comprehensive appraisal of peripheral circulation (e.g., check peripheral pulses, edema, capillary refill, color, and temperature)
- Determine the ankle-brachial index (ABI), as appropriate
- Evaluate peripheral edema and pulses
- Inspect skin for arterial ulcers or tissue breakdown
- Monitor degree of discomfort or pain with exercise, at night, or while resting
- Place extremity in a dependent position, as appropriate
- Administer antiplatelet or anticoagulant medications, as appropriate
- Change the patient's position at least every 2 hours, as appropriate
- Encourage the patient to exercise, as tolerated
- Protect the extremity from injury (e.g., sheepskin under feet and lower legs, footboard/bed cradle at foot of bed, well-fitted shoes)
- Provide warmth (e.g., additional bed clothes, increasing the room temperature), as appropriate
- Instruct the patient on factors that interfere with circulation (e.g., smoking, restrictive clothing, exposure to cold temperatures, and crossing of legs and feet)
- Instruct the patient on proper foot care
- Avoid applying direct heat to the extremity
- Maintain adequate hydration to decrease blood viscosity
- Monitor fluid status, including intake and output
- Implement wound care, as appropriate

3rd edition 2000; revised 2004

Background Readings:

Anonymous. (2001). Arterial vs. venous ulcers: Diagnosis and treatment. *Advances in Skin & Wound Care, 14*(3), 146–149.

Hayward, L. (2002). Wound care. Patient-centered leg ulcer care. *Nursing Times, 98*(2), 59, 61.

Hiatt, W. R. & Regensteiner, J. G. (1993). Nonsurgical management of peripheral arterial disease. *Hospital Practice, 28*(2), 59–70.

Circulatory Care: Mechanical Assist Device   4064

Definition: Temporary support of the circulation through the use of mechanical devices or pumps

Activities:
- Perform a comprehensive appraisal of peripheral circulation (e.g., check peripheral pulses, edema, capillary refill, color, and temperature of extremity)
- Monitor sensorium and cognitive abilities
- Monitor degree of chest discomfort or pain
- Evaluate pulmonary artery pressures, systemic pressures, cardiac output, and systemic vascular resistance, as indicated
- Assist with insertion or implantation of the device
- Observe for hemolysis as indicated by blood in the urine, hemolyzed blood specimens, increase in daily serum hemoglobin, frank bleeding, and hyperkalemia
- Observe cannulas for kinks or disconnections
- Determine activated clotting times every hour, as appropriate
- Administer anticoagulants or antithrombolytics, as ordered
- Monitor the device regularly to ensure proper functioning
- Have back-up equipment available at all times
- Administer positive inotropic agents, as appropriate
- Monitor coagulation profiles every six hours, as appropriate
- Administer blood products, as appropriate
- Monitor urine output every hour
- Monitor electrolytes, BUN, and creatinine daily
- Monitor weight daily
- Monitor intake and output
- Obtain chest x-ray daily
- Use strict aseptic technique in changing dressings
- Administer prophylactic antibiotics
- Monitor for fever and leukocytosis
- Collect blood, urine, sputum, and wound cultures for temperatures greater than 38 degrees C, as appropriate
- Administer antifungal oral solutions
- Administer total parenteral nutrition, as appropriate
- Administer pain medications, as needed
- Teach patient and family about the device
- Provide emotional support for the patient and family

2nd edition 1996; revised 2000

Background Readings:

LeMone, P. & Burke, K. M. (2000). *Medical-surgical nursing: Critical thinking in client care* (2nd ed., pp. 1110–1112). Upper Saddle River, NJ: Prentice Hall.

Ruzevich, S. (1993). Cardiac assist devices. In J. M. Clochesy, C. Breu, S. Cardin, E. B. Rudy, & A. A. Whittaker (Eds.), *Critical care nursing* (pp. 183–192). Philadelphia: Saunders.

Circulatory Care: Venous Insufficiency   4066

Definition: Promotion of venous circulation

Activities:
- Perform a comprehensive appraisal of peripheral circulation (e.g., check peripheral pulses, edema, capillary refill, color, and temperature)
- Evaluate peripheral edema and pulses
- Inspect skin for stasis ulcers and tissue breakdown
- Implement wound care (debridement, antimicrobial therapy), as needed
- Apply dressing appropriate for wound size and type, as appropriate
- Monitor degree of discomfort or pain
- Instruct the patient on the importance of compression therapy
- Apply compression therapy modalities (short-stretch or long-stretch bandages), as appropriate
- Elevate affected limb 20 degrees or greater above the level of the heart, as appropriate
- Change the patient's position at least every 2 hours, as appropriate
- Encourage passive or active range-of-motion exercises, especially of the lower extremities exercises, during bed rest
- Administer antiplatelet or anticoagulant medications, as appropriate
- Protect the extremity from injury (e.g., sheepskin under feet and lower legs, footboard/bed cradle at foot of bed, well-fitted shoes)
- Instruct the patient on proper foot care
- Maintain adequate hydration to decrease blood viscosity
- Monitor fluid status, including intake and output

3rd edition 2000; revised 2004

Background Readings:

Anonymous. (2001). Arterial vs. venous ulcers: Diagnosis and treatment. *Advances in Skin & Wound Care, 14*(3), 146–149.

Hayward, L. (2002). Wound care. Patient-centered leg ulcer care. *Nursing Times, 98*(2), 59, 61.

Hess, C. T. (2001). Clinical management extra: Management of a venous ulcer: A case study approach. *Advances in Skin & Wound Care, 14*(3), 148–149.

Kunimoto, B. T. (2001). Management and prevention of venous leg ulcers: A literature-guided approach. *Ostomy/Wound Management, 47*(6), 36–49.

Circulatory Precautions   4070

Definition: Protection of a localized area with limited perfusion

Activities:
- Perform a comprehensive appraisal of peripheral circulation (i.e., check peripheral pulses, edema, capillary refill, color, temperature of extremity, and ankle brachial index, if indicated)
- Target at risk patients (e.g., diabetics, smokers, elderly, hypertensive patients and those with elevated cholesterol levels) for comprehensive peripheral assessments and modification of risk factors
- Do not start an IV or draw blood in the affected extremity
- Refrain from taking blood pressure in affected extremity
- Refrain from applying pressure or tourniquet to affected extremity
- Maintain adequate hydration to prevent increased blood viscosity
- Avoid injury to affected area
- Prevent infection in wounds
- Instruct the patient to test bath water before entering to avoid burning skin
- Instruct patient on foot and nail care
- Instruct patient and family on protection from injury of affected area
- Encourage smoking cessation and regular exercise in patients with claudication
- Encourage walking to the point of claudication and a little bit more each time to assist in the development of collateral circulation in the lower extremities
- Instruct patient and family on medication therapies for blood pressure control, anticoagulation, and reduction of cholesterol levels
- Instruct patient on avoidance of beta blockers for blood pressure control (i.e., causes constriction of peripheral vessels and worsens claudication)
- Instruct patient on diet measures to improve circulation (e.g., diet low in saturated fat and good intake of omega 3 fish oils)
- Instruct diabetic patients on the need for proper management of blood sugar
- Instruct patient on proper skin care (e.g., moisturizing dry skin on legs, prompt attention to wounds and potential ulcers)
- Provide patient and family with smoking cessation information, if applicable
- Monitor extremities for areas of heat, redness, pain, or swelling
- Instruct patient on signs and symptoms indicating a need for emergent care (e.g., pain that does not go away upon rest, wound complications, loss of feeling)
- Encourage patient participation in vascular rehabilitation programs

1st edition 1992; revised 2013

Background Readings:

Bonham, P. A., Flemister, B. G., Goldberg, M., Crawford, P. E., Johnson, J. J., & Varnado, M. F. (2009). What's new in lower-extremity arterial disease? WOCN's 2008 clinical practice guideline. *Journal of Wound, Ostomy & Continence Nursing, 36*(1), 37–44.

Conen, D., Everett, B., Kurth, T., Creager, M. A., Buring, J. E., Ridker, P. M., et al. (2011). Smoking, smoking status, and risk for symptomatic peripheral artery disease in women: A cohort study. *Annals of Internal Medicine, 154*(11), 719–726.

Lawson, G. (2010). The importance of obtaining ankle-branchial indexes in older adults: The other vital sign. *Journal of Vascular Nursing, 23*(2), 46–51.

Selby, M. (2008). Peripheral arterial disease. *Practice Nurse, 36*(7), 33–34, 36–37.

Sieggreen, M. (2008). Understanding critical limb ischemia. *Nursing, 38*(10), 50–56.

Ward, C. (2010). Peripheral arterial disease. *MEDSURG Nursing, 19*(4), 247–248.

Circumcision Care   3000

Definition: Preprocedural and post procedural support to males undergoing circumcision

Activities:
- Verify that the surgical consent is properly signed
- Verify correct patient identification
- Administer preprocedure pain control approximately 1 hour prior to the procedure (i.e., acetaminophen)
- Position the patient in a comfortable position during the procedure
- Use a padded circumcision seat for infants
- Use a radiant warmer to maintain body temperature during the procedure
- Shield infant's eyes from direct light
- Use a pacifier dipped in sucrose during the procedure and until the next feeding with permission from parent/guardian
- Swaddle the infant's upper body during the circumcision
- Play soft, appropriate music during the procedure
- Monitor vital signs
- Administer a topical local analgesia agent (e.g., eutectic mixture of local anesthetics [EMLA]), as ordered
- Assist the physician with the dorsal penile nerve block, as appropriate
- Apply white petroleum jelly and/or dressing, as appropriate
- Monitor for bleeding every 30 minutes for a least 2 hours post procedure
- Provide post procedure pain control every 4 to 6 hours for 24 hours (i.e., acetaminophen)
- Instruct the patient/parent of signs and symptoms to report to the physician (e.g., increased temperature, bleeding, swelling, inability to urinate)
- Arrange for cultural accommodations

4th edition 2004

Background Readings:

Alkalay, A. L. & Sola, A. (2000). Analgesia and local anesthesia for non-ritual circumcision in stable healthy newborns. *Neonatal Intensive Care, 13*(2), 19–22.

Joyce, B. A., Keck, J. F., & Gerkensmeyer, J. (2001). Evaluation of pain management interventions for neonatal circumcision pain. *Journal of Pediatric Health Care, 15*(3), 105–114.

Williamson, M. L. (1997). Circumcision anesthesia: A study of nursing implications for dorsal penile nerve block. *Pediatric Nursing, 12*(1), 59–63.

University of Iowa Hospital and Clinics, Children's and Women's Services, Department of Nursing. (2000). *Circumcision standard of practice.* Iowa City, Iowa: Author.

Definition: Coordination of emergency measures to sustain life

Activities:
- Evaluate patient's responsiveness to determine appropriate action
- Call for help if no breathing or no normal breathing and no response
- Call a code according to agency standard while obtaining the automated external defibrillator (AED) or assuring that someone is obtaining the automated external defibrillator
- Assure patient's airway is open
- Perform cardiopulmonary resuscitation that focuses on chest compressions in adults and compressions with breathing efforts for children, as appropriate
- Deliver cardioversion or defibrillation as soon as possible
- Minimize the interval between stopping chest compressions and delivering a shock, if indicated
- Bring the code cart to the bedside
- Monitor the quality of CPR provided
- Attach the cardiac monitor and determine the rhythm, assuring defibrillations will not be interrupted
- Assure that someone is oxygenating the patient and assisting with intubation, as indicated
- Initiate an IV line and administer IV fluids, as indicated
- Ensure that someone is (1) setting up medications, (2) delivering medications, (3) interpreting EKG and delivering cardioversion/ defibrillation, as needed, and (4) documenting care
- Remind personnel of current Advanced Cardiac Life Support protocols, as appropriate
- Ensure that special resuscitation protocols (e.g. asthma, anaphylaxis, pregnancy, morbid obesity, pulmonary embolism, electrolyte imbalance, ingestion of toxic substances, trauma, accidental hypothermia, avalanche, drowning, electric shock or lightning strikes, percutaneous coronary interventions, cardiac tamponade, cardiac surgery) are instituted, where appropriate
- Offer family members and significant others opportunities to be present during resuscitation when in the best interests of the patient
- Support family members who are present during resuscitation (i.e. ensure safe environment, provide explanations and commentary, allow appropriate communication with patient, continually assess needs, provide opportunities to reflect on resuscitation efforts after event)
- Ensure that someone is coordinating care of other patients on the nursing unit
- Terminate code as indicated by patient condition
- Assure organized post cardiac arrest care (e.g. cardiopulmonary and neurological support, therapeutic hypothermia, tapering of inspired oxygen concentration to avoid harmful hyperoxia, avoidance of hyperventilation)
- Implement appropriate procedures for possible tissue and organ donation that are timely, effective, and supportive of the family members' and patient's desires
- Review actions after code to identify areas of strength and those which need to be improved
- Provide opportunities for team members to be involved in team debriefings or reflect on resuscitation efforts after event
- Perform emergency cart check per agency protocol

1st edition 1992; revised 2008; 2013

Background Readings:

American Association of Critical Care Nurses. (2006). *Core curriculum for critical care nursing* (6th ed.) [J. G. Alspach, Ed.]. Philadelphia: Saunders.

Boucher, M. (2010). Family-witnessed resuscitation. *Emergency Nurse, 18*(5), 10–14.

Carlson, K. (Ed.). (2009). *Advanced critical care nursing*. Philadelphia: Saunders Elsevier.

Field, J. M., Hazinski, M. F., Sayre, M. R., Chameides, L., Schexnayder, S. M., Hemphill, R., Samson, R. A., et al. (2010). Part 1: Executive summary: 2010 American Heart Association guidelines for cardiopulmonary resuscitation and emergency cardiovascular care. *Circulation, 122*(18 Suppl. 3), S640-S656.

Hazinski, M. F. (Ed.). (2010). *Highlights of the 2010 American Heart Association guidelines for CPR and ECC*. Dallas, TX: American Heart Association.

Urden, L., Stacy, K. M., & Lough, M. E. (2010). *Critical care nursing: Diagnosis and management* (6th ed.). St. Louis: Mosby Elsevier.

Wiegand, D. J. (Ed.). (2011). *AACN procedure manual for critical care* (6th ed.). St. Louis: Saunders Elsevier.

Cognitive Restructuring 4700

Definition: Challenging a patient to alter distorted thought patterns and view self and the world more realistically

Activities:
- Help the patient accept the fact that self-statements mediate emotional arousal
- Help patient understand the inability to attain desirable behaviors frequently results from irrational self-statements
- Assist patient in changing irrational self-statements to rational self-statements
- Point out styles of dysfunctional thinking (e.g., polarized thinking, overgeneralization, magnification, personalization)
- Assist patient in labeling the painful emotion (e.g., anger, anxiety, hopelessness) that he/she is feeling
- Assist patient in identifying the perceived stressors (e.g., situations, events, interactions with other people) that contributed to his/her stress
- Assist patient to identify own faulty interpretations about the perceived stressors
- Assist patient in recognizing the irrationality of certain beliefs compared with actual reality
- Assist patient to replace faulty interpretations with more reality-based interpretations of stressful situations, events, interactions
- Make statement/ask question that challenges patient's perception/ behavior, as appropriate
- Make statement that describes alternative way of looking at situation
- Assist patient to identify belief system that affects health status
- Make use of patient's usual belief system to see situation in different way

1st edition 1992; revised 2000, 2004

Background Readings:

McKay, M., Davis, M., & Fanning, P. (1981). *Thoughts and feelings: The art of cognitive stress intervention*. Richmond, CA: New Harbenger Publication.

Mohr, W. K. (2006). Neuroscience: Biology and behavior. In W. K. Mohr (Ed.), *Psychiatric-mental health nursing* (6th ed., pp. 37–54). Philadelphia: Lippincott Williams & Wilkins.

Pender, N. (1996). *Health promotion in nursing practice* (3rd ed.). Stanford, CT: Appleton & Lange.

Scandrett-Hibdon, S. (1992). Cognitive reappraisal. In G. M. Bulechek & J. C. McCloskey (Eds.), *Nursing interventions: Essential nursing treatments* (2nd ed., pp. 462–471). Philadelphia: Saunders.

Cognitive Stimulation   4720

Definition: Promotion of awareness and comprehension of surroundings by utilization of planned stimuli

Activities:
- Consult with family to establish patient's cognitive baseline
- Inform patient of recent nonthreatening news events
- Offer environmental stimulation through contact with varied personnel
- Present change gradually
- Provide a calendar
- Stimulate memory by repeating patient's last expressed thought
- Orient to time, place, and person
- Talk to patient
- Demonstrate caregiver sensitivity by responding promptly and appropriately to cues
- Stimulate development by engaging in activities to enhance achievement and learning by being attuned to the patient's needs
- Offer cognitive stimulation at work such as training opportunities, cognitive richness to work content, opportunities for growth, and multitasking
- Encourage cognitive stimulation outside of work such as reading or active participation in cultural and artistic activities
- Encourage the use of a multistimulation program (e.g., singing and listening to music, creative activities, exercise, conversation, social interactions, or problem solving) to promote and protect cognitive capacity
- Ask for opinions and views rather than factual answers
- Provide planned sensory stimulation
- Use television, radio, or music as part of planned stimuli program
- Allow for rest periods
- Place familiar objects and photographs in patient's environment
- Use repetition to present new material
- Vary methods of presentation of material
- Use memory aids: checklists, schedules, and reminder notices
- Reinforce or repeat information

- Present information in small, concrete portions
- Ask patient to repeat information
- Use touch purposefully, as appropriate
- Provide verbal and written instructions

1st edition 1992; revised 2013

Background Readings:

Albers, E. M., Riksen-Walraven, J. M., & Weerth, C. D. (2010). Developmental stimulation in child care centers contributes to young infants' cognitive development. *Infant Behavior and Development, 33*(4), 401–408.

Karatay, G. & Akkus, Y. (2010). The effectiveness of a stimulation program on cognitive capacity among individuals older than 60. *Western Journal of Nursing Research, 33*(1), 26–44

Livingston, G., Johnston, K., Katona, C., Paton, J., & Lyketsos, C. G. (2005). Systematic review of psychological approaches to the management of neuropsychiatric symptoms of dementia. *American Journal of Psychiatry, 162*(11), 1996–2021.

Marquié, J. C., Duarte, L. R., Bessières, P., Dalm, C., Gentil, C., & Ruidavets, J. B. (2010). Higher mental stimulation at work is associated with improved cognitive functioning in both young and older workers. *Ergonomics, 53*(11), 1287–1301.

Pearson, G. (2006). Psychopharmacology. In W. K. Mohr (Ed.), *Psychiatric-mental health nursing* (6th ed., pp. 243–286). Philadelphia: Lippincott Williams & Wilkins.

Spector, A., Orrell, M., & Woods, B. (2010). Cognitive stimulation therapy (CST): Effects on different areas of cognitive function for people with dementia. *International Journal of Geriatric Psychiatry, 25*(12), 1253–1258.

Niu, Y. X., Tan, J. P., Guan, J. Q., Zhang, Z. Q., & Wang, L. N. (2010). Cognitive stimulation therapy in the treatment of neuropsychiatric symptoms of Alzheimer's disease: A randomized controlled trial. *Clinical Rehabilitation, 24,* 1102–1111.

Commendation   4364

Definition: Offering statements of praise and admiration to identify and emphasize the strengths and capabilities evident in the individual, family, or community

Activities:
- Recognize resourcefulness in coping with present situation
- Assist individuals to realize their personal strengths, potential, and capacity
- Demonstrate your valuing of individual or family
- Build collaborative relationship with individual or family
- Support and encourage learning
- Recognize individual's strength in modifying behavior to address the situation
- Provide positive feedback to encourage and sustain new behavior
- Acknowledge the capacity to live with chronic, long-term health issue or illness, as appropriate
- Congratulate one in achieving improved outcome
- Reinforce a behavior or outcome to increase the probability that it will be sustained

- Facilitate motivation to continue with improved behavioral changes to attain the main goal
- Apply strategies to reinforce learning, and promote confidence and worth in learner
- Write up statements of praise and send to individual or other persons (e.g., supervisor, award program), as appropriate

6th edition 2013

Background Readings:

Abualrub, R. F. & Al-Zaree, I. M. (2008). Job stress, recognition, job performance, and intention to stay at work among Jordanian hospital nurses. *Journal of Nursing Administration, 16*(3), 227–236.

C

Day, R. A., Paul, P., Williams, B., Smeltzer, S. C., & Bare, B. (2010). *Brunner and Suddarth's textbook of Canadian medical-surgical nursing* (2nd ed.). Philadelphia: Lippincott Williams & Wilkins.

Kozier, B., Erb, G., Berman, A., Snyder, S. J., Bouchal, S. R., Hirst, S., et al. (2010). *Fundamentals of Canadian nursing: Concepts, process and practice* (2nd ed.). Toronto: Pearson Education Canada.

McElheran, N. G. & Harper-Jacques, S. R. (1994). Commendations: A resource intervention for clinical practice. *Clinical Nurse Specialist, 8*(1), 7–10.

Psychological Associates and Diseases Attacking the Immune System Foundation. (2009). *Literature review on meaningful recognition in nursing* (pp. 1–32). St. Louis: Psychological Associates.

Stone, C. L. & Rowles, C. J. (2002). What rewards do clinical preceptors in nursing think are important? *Journal for Nurses in Staff Development, 18*(3), 162–166.

Tourangeau, A. E. & Cranley, L. A. (2006). Nurse intention to remain employed: Understanding and strengthening determinants. *Journal of Advanced Nursing, 55*(4), 497–509.

Communicable Disease Management 8820

Definition: Working with a community to decrease and manage the incidence and prevalence of contagious diseases in a specific population

Activities:

- Monitor at-risk populations for compliance with prevention and treatment regimen
- Monitor adequate continuation of immunization in targeted populations
- Provide vaccine to targeted populations, as available
- Monitor incidence of exposure to communicable diseases during known outbreak
- Monitor sanitation
- Monitor environmental factors that influence the transmission of communicable diseases
- Provide information about adequate preparation and storage of food, as needed
- Provide information about adequate control of vectors and animal reservoir hosts, as needed
- Inform the public regarding disease and activities associated with management, as needed
- Promote access to adequate health education related to prevention and treatment of communicable diseases and prevention of recurrence
- Improve surveillance systems for communicable diseases, as needed
- Promote legislation that ensures appropriate monitoring and treatment for communicable diseases
- Report activities to appropriate agencies, as required

3rd edition 2000

Background Readings:

Beneson, A. (Ed.). (1995). *Control of communicable diseases manual* (16th ed.). Washington DC: American Public Health Association.

McEwen, M. (1998). *Community based nursing*. Philadelphia: Saunders.

Stanhope, M. & Lancaster, J. (1996). *Community health nursing: Promoting health aggregates, families and individuals* (4th ed.). St. Louis: Mosby.

Communication Enhancement: Hearing Deficit 4974

Definition: Use of strategies augmenting communication capabilities for a person with diminished hearing

Activities:

- Perform or arrange for routine hearing assessments and screenings
- Monitor for excessive accumulation of cerumen
- Instruct patient not to use foreign objects smaller than patient's fingertip (e.g., cotton-tipped applicators, bobby pins, toothpicks, and other sharp objects) for cerumen removal
- Remove excessive cerumen with twisted end of washcloth while pulling down the auricle
- Consider ear irrigation for the removal of excessive cerumen if watchful waiting, manual removal, and ceruminolytic agents are ineffective
- Note and document patient's preferred method of communication (e.g., verbal, written, lip reading, or American Sign Language) in plan of care
- Gain patient's attention prior to speaking (i.e., obtain attention through touch)
- Avoid noisy backgrounds while communicating
- Avoid communicating more than 2-3 feet from patient
- Use gestures when necessary
- Listen attentively, allowing patient adequate time to process communication and respond
- Refrain from shouting at patient
- Facilitate lip reading by facing patient directly in good lighting
- Ask patient to suggest strategies for improved communication (e.g., speaking toward better ear and moving to well-lit area)
- Face the patient directly, establishing eye contact and avoiding turning away mid-sentence
- Simplify language, as appropriate (i.e., do not use slang and use short, simple sentences)
- Use a lower, deeper voice when speaking
- Avoid "baby talk" and exaggerated expressions
- Avoid smoking, chewing food or gum, and covering mouth when speaking
- Verify what was said or written using patient's response before continuing
- Facilitate use of hearing aids and assistive listening devices (e.g., phone amplifier, hardwire device, personal frequency modulation, and computers)
- Remove and insert hearing aid properly

- Remove hearing aid battery when hearing aid is not in use for several days
- Clean detachable earmold using a mild soapy solution, removing moisture or debris with soft cloth, and avoiding isopropyl alcohol, solvents, and oil
- Clean non-detachable earmold using a damp cloth, removing moisture or debris with soft cloth, and avoiding isopropyl alcohol, solvents, and oil
- Check hearing aid batteries routinely, replacing when necessary
- Refer to manufacturer's guidelines on proper use of, care for, and maintenance of hearing aids and assistive listening devices
- Instruct patient, nursing personnel, and family on use of, care for, and maintenance of hearing aids and assistive listening devices
- Assist patient or family in acquiring hearing aid and assistive listening device
- Refer to primary care provider or specialist for evaluation, treatment, and hearing rehabilitation

1st edition 1992; revised 2000, 2013

Background Readings:

Adams-Wendling, L. & Pimple, C. (2008). Nursing management of hearing impairment in nursing facility residents [S. Adams & M. G. Titler, Eds.]. *Journal of Gerontological Nursing, 34*(11), 9–17.

Lindblade, D. & McDonald, M. (1995). Removing communication barriers for the hearing-impaired elderly. *MEDSURG Nursing, 4*(5), 377–385.

Maas, M. L., Buckwalter, K. C., Hardy, M. D., Tripp-Reimer, T., Titler, M. G., & Specht, J. P. (Eds.). (2001). *Nursing care of older adults: Diagnoses, outcomes, & interventions* (p. 485). St. Louis: Mosby.

Smeltzer, S. C. & Bare, B. G. (2004). *Brunner & Suddarth's textbook of medical surgical nursing* (Vol. 2) (10th ed.). Philadelphia: Lippincott Williams & Wilkins.

Communication Enhancement: Speech Deficit   4976

Definition: Use of strategies augmenting communication capabilities for a person with impaired speech

Activities:

- Monitor speech speed, pressure, pace, quantity, volume, and diction
- Monitor cognitive, anatomical, and physiological processes associated with speech capabilities (e.g., memory, hearing, and language)
- Instruct patient or family on cognitive, anatomical, and physiological processes involved in speech capabilities
- Monitor patient for frustration, anger, depression, or other responses to impaired speech capabilities
- Recognize emotional and physical behaviors as forms of communication
- Provide alternative methods of speech communication (e.g., writing tablet, flash cards, eye blinking, communication board with pictures and letters, hand signals or other gestures, and computer)
- Provide alternative methods of writing or reading, as appropriate
- Adjust communication style to meet needs of client (i.e., stand in front of patient when speaking, listen attentively, present one idea or thought at a time, speak slowly while avoiding shouting, use written communication, or solicit family's assistance in understanding patient's speech)
- Maintain structured environment and routines (i.e., ensure consistent daily schedules, provide frequent reminders, and provide calendars and other environmental cues)
- Modify environment to minimize excess noise and decrease emotional distress (i.e., limit visitors and excessive equipment noise)
- Ensure call light is within reach and central call light system is marked to indicate patient cannot speak
- Repeat what patient said to ensure accuracy
- Instruct patient to speak slowly
- Phrase questions so patient can answer using a simple yes or no, being aware that patient with expressive aphasia may provide automatic responses that are incorrect
- Collaborate with family and speech language pathologist or therapist to develop a plan for effective communication
- Provide one-way valve for patient with tracheostomy, replacing need for finger occlusion over tube
- Instruct patient or family on use of speech aids after laryngectomy (e.g., esophageal speech, electrolarynges, tracheoesophageal fistulas)
- Allow patient to hear spoken language frequently, as appropriate
- Provide positive reinforcement, as appropriate
- Use interpreter, as necessary
- Refer patient to community support systems (e.g., The International Association of Laryngectomees and American Cancer Society)
- Provide referral to speech language pathologist or therapist
- Coordinate rehabilitation team activities

2nd edition 1996; revised 2013

Background Readings:

Craven, R. F. & Hirnle, C. J. (2009). Cognitive processes. *Fundamentals of nursing: Human health and function* (6th ed., pp. 1237–1268). Philadelphia: Lippincott Williams & Wilkins.

Ignatavicius, D. D. & Workman, M. L. (2010). *Medical-surgical nursing: Patient-centered collaborative care* (6th ed.). St. Louis: Saunders.

Kelly, H., Brady, M. C., & Enderby, P. (2010). Speech and language therapy for aphasia following stroke. *Cochrane Database of Systematic Reviews*, Issue 5. Art. No.: CD000425. doi: 10.1002/14651858. CD000425.pub2.

Law, J., Garrett, Z., & Nye, C. (2003). Speech and language therapy interventions for children with primary speech and language delay or disorder. *Cochrane Database of Systematic Reviews*, Issue 3. Art. No: CD004110. doi: 10.1002/14651858.CD004110.

C

Communication Enhancement: Visual Deficit 4978

Definition: Use of strategies augmenting communication capabilities for a person with diminished vision

Activities:
- Perform or arrange for routine vision assessments and screenings
- Monitor functional implications of diminished vision (e.g., risk of injury, depression, anxiety, and ability to perform activities of daily living and valued activities)
- Identify yourself when entering the patient's space
- Assist patient in enhancing stimulation of other senses (e.g., savoring aroma, taste, and texture of food)
- Ensure that patient's eyeglasses or contact lens have current prescription, are cleaned, and stored properly when not in use
- Provide adequate room lighting
- Minimize glare (i.e., offer sunglasses or draw window covering)
- Provide literature with large print
- Describe environment to patient
- Maintain uncluttered environment
- Avoid rearranging items in patient's environment without notifying patient
- Provide daily living aids (e.g., clock and telephone with large numbers)
- Apply labels to distinguish frequently-used items (i.e., color-code dials on appliances, mark medication bottles using high-contrasting colors or rubber bands, and safety-pin labels on similar-colored clothing)
- Use bright, contrasting colors in environment
- Read mail, newspaper, and other pertinent information to patient
- Identify items on food tray in relation to numbers on a clock
- Fold paper money in different ways for easy identification
- Provide magnifying devices (e.g., handheld, stand, and video magnifier)
- Provide sight substitutes (e.g., Braille materials, audio books, talking watches, and tactile markers)
- Assist parents, family, educators, and caretakers involved with a child with diminished vision in meeting informational needs (e.g., how to teach child, anticipatory guidance, and developmental considerations)
- Instruct parents, family, educators, and caretakers to recognize and respond to nontraditional expressive forms of communication (e.g., movements and facial expressions)
- Assist parents, family, educators, and caretakers in developing reliable, functional communication systems (e.g., microswitches or speech-output devices)
- Assist patient or family in identifying available resources for vision rehabilitation
- Provide referral for the patient in need of surgical or other medical treatment
- Provide referral for supportive services (e.g., social, occupational, and psychological)

1st edition 1992; revised 2013

Background Readings:

American Academy of Ophthalmology Vision Rehabilitation Committee. (2007). *Preferred practice pattern guidelines: Vision rehabilitation for adults.* San Francisco, CA: Author.

Craven, R. F. & Hirnle, C. J. (2009). *Fundamentals of nursing: Human health and function* (6th ed.). Philadelphia: Lippincott Williams & Wilkins.

Maas, M. L., Buckwalter, K. C., Hardy, M. D., Tripp-Reimer, T., Titler, M. G., & Specht, J. P. (Eds.). (2001). *Nursing care of older adults: Diagnoses, outcomes, & interventions* (pp. 483–485). St. Louis: Mosby.

Parker, A. T., Grimmett, E. S., & Summers, S. (2008). Evidence-based communication practices for children with visual impairments and additional disabilities: An examination of single-subject design studies. *Journal of Visual Impairment & Blindness, 102*(9), 540–552.

Community Disaster Preparedness 8840

Definition: Preparing for an effective response to a large-scale disaster

Activities:
- Identify potential types of disasters for area (e.g., weather-related, industrial, environmental)
- Work with other agencies in planning for a disaster (e.g., law enforcement, fire department, Red Cross, Salvation Army, ambulance services, social service agencies)
- Develop plans for specific types of disasters (e.g., multiple-casualty incident, bomb, tornado, hurricane, flood, chemical spill), as appropriate
- Identify all community medical and social agency resources available to respond to a disaster
- Develop a disaster notification network to alert personnel
- Develop triage procedures
- Establish prearranged roles during a disaster
- Identify rendezvous site for assisting disaster victims
- Identify alternate rendezvous sites for health care personnel
- Know where disaster equipment and supplies are stored
- Conduct periodic checks of equipment
- Check and restock supplies routinely
- Educate health care personnel on disaster plan(s) on a routine basis
- Encourage community preparation for disaster events
- Educate community members on safety, self-help, and first aid measures
- Encourage community members to have a personal preparedness plan (e.g., emergency telephone numbers, battery-operated radio, working flashlight, first aid kit, medical information, physician information, persons to be notified in an emergency)
- Assist to prepare shelters and emergency aid stations
- Conduct mock disaster drills annually or as appropriate
- Evaluate performance of disaster personnel after a disaster or mock disaster drill

- Identify mechanism for debriefing for health care personnel after a disaster
- Sensitize health care personnel to the potential psychological effects (e.g., depression, sadness, fear, anger, phobias, guilt, irritability, anxiety) of a disaster
- Identify postdisaster referral resources (e.g., rehabilitation, convalescence, counseling)
- Identify postdisaster needs (e.g., ongoing disaster-related health care needs, collection of epidemiological data, assessment of cause of disaster, steps for prevention of reoccurrence)
- Update disaster plans, as needed

3rd edition 2000

Background Readings:

Grant, H. D., Murray, R. H., & Bergeron, J. D. (1994). *Emergency care* (6th ed.). Upper Saddle River, NJ: Prentice-Hall

Ossler, C. C. (1992). The community health nurse in occupational health. In M. Stanhope & J. Lancaster (Eds.), *Community health nursing: Process and practice for promoting health* (pp. 731–746). St. Louis: Mosby.

Santamaria, B. (1995). Nursing in a disaster. In C. M. Smith & F. A. Maurer (Eds.), *Community health nursing: Theory and practice* (pp. 382–400). Philadelphia: Saunders.

Community Health Development | 8500

Definition: Assisting members of a community to identify a community's health concerns, mobilize resources, and implement solutions

Activities:

- Identify health concerns, strengths, and priorities with community partners
- Provide opportunities for participation by all segments of the community
- Assist community members in raising awareness of health problems and concerns
- Engage in dialogue to define community health concerns and develop action plans
- Facilitate implementation and revision of community plans
- Assist community members with resource development and procurement
- Enhance community support networks
- Identify and develop potential community leaders
- Maintain open communication with community members and agencies
- Strengthen contacts between individuals and groups to discuss common and competing interests
- Provide an organizational framework through which people can enhance communication and negotiation skills
- Provide an environment, creating situations in which individuals and groups feel safe expressing their views
- Develop strategies for managing conflict
- Unify community members behind a common mission
- Assure that community members maintain control of decision making
- Build commitment to the community by demonstrating how participation will influence individual lives and improve outcomes
- Develop mechanisms for member involvement in local, state, and national activities related to community health concerns

3rd edition 2000

Background Readings:

Denhan, A., Quinn, S., & Gamble, D. (1998). Community organizing for health promotion in the rural south: An exploration of community competence. *Family and Community Health, 2*(1), 1–21.

Eng, E. & Parker, E. (1994). Measuring community competence in the Mississippi Delta: The interface between program evaluation and empowerment. *Health Education Quarterly, 21*(2), 119–120.

May, K., Mendelson, C., & Ferketich, S. (1995). Community empowerment in rural health care. *Public Health Nursing, 12*(1), 25–30.

Spradley, B. & Allender, J. (1996). *Community health nursing: Concepts and practice* (4th ed.). Philadelphia: Lippincott.

Stanhope, M. & Lancaster, J. (1996). *Community health nursing: Promoting health of aggregates, families and individuals* (4th ed.). St. Louis: Mosby.

Complex Relationship Building | 5000

Definition: Establishing a therapeutic relationship with a patient to promote insight and behavioral change

Activities:

- Identify own attitude toward the patient and situation, repeat as needed
- Determine the ethical boundaries of the relationship, as needed
- Deal with personal feelings evoked by the patient that may interfere with the effectiveness of therapeutic interactions
- Provide for physical comfort before interactions
- Discuss confidentiality of information shared
- Create climate of warmth and acceptance
- Reassure patient of your interest in him/her as a person, as appropriate
- Use self-disclosure, as appropriate
- Return at established time to demonstrate trustworthiness and interest in the patient
- Maintain open body posture
- Adjust physical distance between nurse and patient, as appropriate
- Monitor patient's nonverbal messages
- Seek clarification of nonverbal messages, as appropriate

- Respond to patient's nonverbal messages, as appropriate
- Reflect the main ideas back to the patient in your own words
- Return conversation to main subject, as needed
- Develop special ways of communicating (e.g., images, other words), as needed
- Establish mutually acceptable agreement on time and length of meetings, as appropriate
- Discuss responsibilities of patient in the one-to-one, nurse-patient relationship
- Assist patient to identify areas of need to be addressed during meetings
- Set limits of acceptable behavior during therapeutic sessions, as appropriate
- Establish time of next interaction before ending the meeting each time
- Summarize conversation at end of the discussion
- Use summary as a starting point for future conversations
- Identify patient's readiness to explore identified problems and develop strategies for change
- Encourage patient to take the time needed to express himself/herself
- Assist the patient to identify feelings that impede ability to interact with others (e.g., anger, anxiety, hostility, or sadness)
- Support patient's efforts to interact with others in a positive manner

- Prepare for termination of relationship, as appropriate
- Facilitate patient's attempts to review therapeutic relationship experiences
- Convey recognition of accomplishments during relationship

2nd edition 1996; revised 2004, 2008

Background Readings

Deering, C. (2006). Therapeutic relationships and communication. In W. K. Mohr (Ed.), *Psychiatric mental health nursing* (6th ed., pp. 55–78). Philadelphia: Lippincott Williams & Wilkins.

Forchuk, C. & Boyd, M. A. (2005). Communication and the therapeutic relationship. In M. A. Boyd (Ed.), *Psychiatric nursing: Contemporary practice* (3rd ed., pp. 173–188). Philadelphia: Lippincott Williams & Wilkins.

Hagerty, B. M. & Patusky, K. I. (2003). Reconceptualizing the nurse-patient relationship. *Journal of Nursing Scholarship, 35*(2), 145–150.

Peplau, H. (1952). *Interpersonal relations in nursing*. New York: G. P. Putnam's Sons.

Peplau, H. (1997). Peplau's theory of interpersonal relations. *Nursing Science Quarterly, 10*(4), 162–167.

Stockmann, C. (2005). A literature review of the progress of the psychiatric nurse-patient relationship as described by Peplau. *Issues in Mental Health Nursing, 26*(9), 911–919.

Conflict Mediation   **5020**

Definition: Facilitation of constructive dialogue between opposing parties with a goal of resolving disputes in a mutually acceptable manner

Activities:

- Provide a private, neutral setting for conversation
- Allow parties to voice personal concerns
- Offer guidance through the process
- Maintain own neutrality throughout the process
- Employ a variety of communication techniques (e.g., active listening, questioning, paraphrasing, reflecting)
- Facilitate defining the issues
- Assist parties to identify possible solutions to the issues
- Facilitate search for outcomes acceptable to both parties
- Support the efforts of the participants to foster resolution
- Monitor flow of mediation process

3rd edition 2000

Background Readings:

Arnold, E. & Boggs, K. U. (1995). *Interpersonal relationships: Professional communication skills for nurses* (2nd ed.). Philadelphia: Saunders.

Schwebel, A. I. & Clement, J. A. (1996). Mediation as a mental health service: Consumer's and family members' perceptions. *Psychiatric Rehabilitation Journal, 20*(1), 55–58.

Severson, M. M. (1995). Social work and the pursuit of justice through mediation. *National Association of Social Workers, 40*(5), 683–691.

Sullivan, E. J. & Decker, P. J. (1992). *Effective management in nursing*. Redwood City, CA: Addison-Wesley.

Constipation/Impaction Management   **0450**

Definition: Prevention and alleviation of constipation/impaction

Activities:
- Monitor for signs and symptoms of constipation
- Monitor for signs and symptoms of impaction
- Monitor bowel movements, including frequency, consistency, shape, volume, and color, as appropriate
- Monitor bowel sounds
- Consult with physician about a decrease/increase in frequency of bowel sounds
- Monitor for signs and symptoms of bowel rupture and/or peritonitis
- Explain etiology of problem and rationale for actions to patient
- Identify factors (e.g., medications, bed rest, and diet) that may cause or contribute to constipation
- Institute a toileting schedule, as appropriate
- Encourage increased fluid intake, unless contraindicated
- Evaluate medication profile for gastrointestinal side effects
- Instruct patient/family to record color, volume, frequency, and consistency of stools
- Teach patient/family how to keep a food diary
- Instruct patient/family on high-fiber diet, as appropriate
- Instruct patient/family on appropriate use of laxatives
- Instruct patient/family on the relationship of diet, exercise, and fluid intake to constipation/impaction
- Evaluate recorded intake for nutritional content
- Advise patient to consult physician if constipation or impaction persists
- Suggest use of laxative/stool softener, as appropriate
- Inform patient of procedure for manual removal of stool, if necessary
- Remove the fecal impaction manually, if necessary
- Administer enema or irrigation, as appropriate
- Weigh patient regularly
- Teach patient or family about normal digestive processes
- Teach patient/family about time frame for resolution of constipation

1st edition 1992; revised 2000, 2004

Background Readings:

Battle, E. & Hanna, C. (1980). Evaluation of a dietary regimen for chronic constipation: Report of a pilot study. *Journal of Gerontological Nursing, 6*(9), 527–532.

Craven, R. F. & Hirnle, C. J. (2000). *Fundamentals of nursing: Human health and function* (3rd ed., pp. 1084–1085). Philadelphia: Lippincott Williams & Wilkins.

McLane, A. M. & McShane, R. E. (2001). Constipation. In M. L. Maas, K. C. Buckwalter, M. D. Hardy, T. Tripp-Reimer, M. G. Titler, & J. P. Specht (Eds.), *Nursing care of older adults: Diagnoses, outcomes, & interventions* (pp. 220–237). Redwood City, CA: Addison-Wesley.

Taylor, C. M. (1987). *Nursing diagnosis cards.* Springhouse, PA: Springhouse.

Yakabowich, M. (1990). Prescribe with care: The role of laxatives in treatment of constipation. *Journal of Gerontological Nursing, 16*(7), 4–11.

Consultation   **7910**

Definition: Using expert knowledge to work with those who seek help in problem solving to enable individuals, families, groups, or agencies to achieve identified goals

Activities:
- Identify the purpose for consultation
- Collect data and identify problem which is focus of consultation
- Identify and clarify expectations of all parties involved
- Provide expert knowledge for those seeking help
- Involve those who are seeking help throughout the consulting process
- Identify accountability structure
- Determine the appropriate model of consultation to be used (e.g., purchase of expertise model, process consultation model)
- Identify fee expectations, as appropriate
- Develop a written contract to define agreement and avoid misunderstandings
- Promote ability of those seeking help to progress with more self-direction and responsibility
- Prepare a final report of recommendations
- Respond professionally to acceptance or rejection of ideas

3rd edition 2000

Background Readings:

Clemen-Stone, S., McGuire, S., & Eigisti, D. (1997). *Comprehensive community health nursing: Family, aggregate, and community practice.* St. Louis: Mosby.

Hau, M. L. (1997). Ten common mistakes to avoid as an independent consultant. *American Association of Occupational Health Nurses Journal, 45*(1), 17–24.

Hoffman, S. (1998). Professional practice consultation – opportunity or opportunism. *Journal of Professional Nursing, 14*(2), 67.

Iglesias, G. H. (1998). Role evolution of the mental health clinical nurse specialist in home care. *Clinical Nurse Specialist, 12*(1), 38–44.

Mastroianni, I. & Machles, D. (1997). What are consulting services worth? Applying cost analysis techniques to evaluate effectiveness. *American Association of Occupational Health Nurses Journal, 45*(1), 35–45.

Stackhouse, J. (1998). *Into the community: Nursing in ambulatory and home care.* Philadelphia: Lippincott Williams & Wilkins.

Stanhope, M. & Lancaster, J. (1996). *Community health nursing: Promoting health of aggregates, families and individuals* (4th ed.). St. Louis: Mosby.

C

Contact Lens Care 1620

Definition: Assisting patient in the proper use of contact lenses

Activities:
- Monitor eyes and surrounding area for open lesions and ecchymosis
- Determine patient's understanding of required lens care
- Determine patient's physical and emotional capability to learn and perform required lens care
- Instruct patient to perform hand hygiene before touching lenses
- Instruct patient on proper care of contact lenses, depending on type (e.g., hard or soft)
- Instruct patient to remove lenses at appropriate interval (e.g., remove daily-wear lenses at night and do not wear disposable lenses more than once)
- Instruct patient wearing extended-wear contacts of increased risks (e.g., corneal ulcers and infection-caused eruptions)
- Instruct patient wearing hard contacts of increased risks (e.g., corneal edema and corneal abrasions)
- Instruct patient on symptoms to report to health care professional (e.g., eye and conjunctiva redness, discomfort or pain, excessive tearing, and visual changes)
- Instruct patient to use recommended solutions to clean, moisten, rinse, and disinfect lenses
- Instruct patient to rub and rinse lenses with recommended solution prior to and following storage
- Instruct patient on importance of monitoring for and discontinuing use of recalled contact lens care products
- Instruct patient not to use saliva, tap water, or sterile saline found in healthcare agencies for rinsing or storing lenses
- Instruct patient to avoid exposing eyes to tap water, swimming pool or spa water when wearing lenses
- Instruct patient to store lenses in lens container with recommended solution
- Instruct on care of lens container (e.g., clean daily, leave open to air, and replace regularly)
- Instruct patient how to examine lenses for damage
- Instruct the patient who wears eye cosmetics to use caution in their selection and application (i.e., choose cosmetics without irritating properties and apply prior to lens insertion)
- Instruct patient to avoid exposure to or use of damaging or irritating environmental contaminants (e.g., dust, smoke, soaps, lotions, creams, and sprays)
- Instruct patient to carry appropriate identification on type and care for lenses
- Provide lens care for the patient unable to do so for self (e.g., removal, cleaning, storing, and insertion)
- Make referral to eye specialist, as appropriate

1st edition 1992; revised 2013

Background Readings

Craven, R. F. & Hirnle, C. J. (2009). Self-care and hygiene. *Fundamentals of nursing: Human health and function* (6th ed., pp. 703–755). Philadelphia: Lippincott Williams & Wilkins.

Craven, R. F. & Hirnle, C. J. (2009). Sensory perception. *Fundamentals of nursing: Human health and function* (6th ed., pp. 1216–1236). Philadelphia: Lippincott Williams & Wilkins.

Smith, S. F., Duell, D.J., & Martin, B.C. (2008). Personal hygiene. *Clinical nursing skills: Basic to advanced skills* (7th ed., pp. 208–248). Upper Saddle River, New Jersey: Pearson Prentice Hall.

Sweeney, D., Holden, B., Evans, K., Ng, V., & Cho, P. (2009). Best practice contact lens care: A review of the Asia Pacific Contact Lens Care Summit. *Clinical & Experimental Optometry, 92*(2), 78–89.

Workman, M. L. (2010). Care of patients with eye and vision problems. In D. D. Ignatavicius, & M. L. Workman (Eds.), *Medical-surgical nursing: Patient-centered collaborative care* (6th ed., pp. 1084–1108). St. Louis: Saunders.

Controlled Substance Checking 7620

Definition: Promoting appropriate use and maintaining security of controlled substances

Activities:
- Account for controlled substance cabinet keys at all times
- Follow agency protocol for dispensing and administering controlled substances
- Count all controlled substances with an RN on opposite shift
- Inspect packaging of controlled substances for signs of tampering
- Report discrepancy(ies) immediately, per agency policy
- Follow agency protocol for resolving discrepancy(ies)
- Lock controlled substances cabinet after count is finished
- Document accuracy of count on appropriate form
- Count controlled substances received from pharmacy
- Return controlled substances not in routine use to pharmacy
- Document wasting of controlled substances
- Monitor for evidence of misadministration or diversion of controlled substances
- Report suspected misadministration or diversion of controlled substances, according to agency policy

2nd edition 1996

Background Readings:

Carlson, G. M., Castile, J. A., & Janousek, J. P. (1988). Guidelines for the prevention and detection of controlled substance diversion. *Hospital Pharmacy, 23*(12), 1057–1059.

Craven, R. F. & Hirnle, C. J. (2000). *Fundamentals of nursing: Human health and function* (3rd ed., pp. 503–505). Philadelphia: Lippincott Williams & Wilkins.

Karch, A. M. (2006). Introduction to drugs. *Focus on nursing pharmacology* (3rd ed., pp. 3–16). Philadelphia: Lippincott Williams & Wilkins.

Coping Enhancement   5230

Definition: Facilitation of cognitive and behavioral efforts to manage perceived stressors, changes, or threats that interfere with meeting life demands and roles

Activities:

- Assist the patient in identifying appropriate short- and long-term goals
- Assist the patient in examining available resources to meet the goals
- Assist the patient in breaking down complex goals into small, manageable steps
- Encourage relationships with persons who have common interests and goals
- Assist the patient to solve problems in a constructive manner
- Appraise a patient's adjustment to changes in body image, as indicated
- Appraise the impact of the patient's life situation on roles and relationships
- Encourage patient to identify a realistic description of change in role
- Appraise the patient's understanding of the disease process
- Appraise and discuss alternative responses to situation
- Use a calm, reassuring approach
- Provide an atmosphere of acceptance
- Assist the patient in developing an objective appraisal of the event
- Help patient to identify the information he/she is most interested in obtaining
- Provide factual information concerning diagnosis, treatment, and prognosis
- Provide the patient with realistic choices about certain aspects of care
- Encourage an attitude of realistic hope as a way of dealing with feelings of helplessness
- Evaluate the patient's decision-making ability
- Seek to understand the patient's perspective of a stressful situation
- Discourage decision making when the patient is under severe stress
- Encourage gradual mastery of the situation
- Encourage patience in developing relationships
- Encourage social and community activities
- Encourage the acceptance of limitations of others
- Acknowledge the patient's spiritual/cultural background
- Encourage the use of spiritual resources, if desired
- Explore patient's previous achievements
- Explore patient's reasons for self-criticism
- Confront patient's ambivalent (angry or depressed) feelings
- Foster constructive outlets for anger and hostility
- Arrange situations that encourage patient's autonomy
- Assist patient in identifying positive responses from others
- Encourage the identification of specific life values
- Explore with the patient previous methods of dealing with life problems
- Introduce patient to persons (or groups) who have successfully undergone the same experience
- Support the use of appropriate defense mechanisms
- Encourage verbalization of feelings, perceptions, and fears
- Discuss consequences of not dealing with guilt and shame
- Encourage the patient to identify own strengths and abilities
- Reduce stimuli in the environment that could be misinterpreted as threatening
- Appraise patient needs/desires for social support
- Assist the patient to identify available support systems
- Determine the risk of the patient inflicting self-harm
- Encourage family involvement, as appropriate
- Encourage the family to verbalize feelings about ill family member
- Provide appropriate social skills training
- Assist the patient to identify positive strategies to deal with limitations and manage needed lifestyle or role changes
- Instruct the patient on the use of relaxation techniques, as needed
- Assist the patient to grieve and work through the losses of chronic illness and/or disability, if appropriate
- Assist the patient to clarify misconceptions
- Encourage the patient to evaluate own behavior

1st edition 1992; revised 2013

Background Readings:

Boyd, M. A. (Ed.). (2009). *Psychiatric nursing: Contemporary practice* (4th ed.). Philadelphia: Lippincott Williams & Wilkins.

Carroll-Johnson, R., Gorman, L., & Bush, N. (Eds.). (2006) *Psychosocial nursing care along the concern continuum* (2nd ed.) Pittsburgh, PA: Oncology Nursing Society.

Clarke, P. & Black, S. E. (2005). Quality of life following stroke: Negotiating disability, identity, and resources. *Journal of Applied Gerontology, 24*(4), 319–336.

Garcia, C. (2009) Conceptualization and measurement of coping during adolescence: A review of the literature. *Journal of Nursing Scholarship, 42*(2), 166–185.

Lorenz, R. (2010). Coping with preclinical disability: Older women's experiences of everyday activities. *Journal of Nursing Scholarship, 42*(4), 439–447.

Meadus, F. (2007). Adolescents coping with mood disorder: A grounded theory study. *Journal of Psychiatric and Mental Health Nursing, 14*(2), 209–217.

Pavlish, C. & Ceronsky, L. (2009). Oncology nurses' perceptions of nursing roles and professional attribute in palliative care. *Clinical Journal of Oncology Nursing, 13*(4), 404–412.

Peek, G. & Melnyk, B. (2010). Coping interventions for parents of children newly diagnosed with cancer: An evidence review with implications for clinical practice and future research. *Pediatric Nursing, 36*(6), 306–313.

Stuart, G. W. (2009). *Principles and practice of psychiatric nursing* (9th ed.). St. Louis: Mosby.

Cost Containment 7630

Definition: Management and facilitation of efficient and effective use of resources

Activities:
- Use supplies and equipment efficiently and effectively
- Document current or previously utilized resources
- Determine the appropriate health care setting (e.g., home care, urgent care, emergency department, clinic, acute care, long-term care) needed to provide services
- Assign personnel within budget according to patient acuity
- Communicate and coordinate patient care needs with other departments so care is delivered in a timely manner
- Evaluate necessity of health care (e.g., procedures, laboratory tests, specialty care)
- Consult and negotiate with other disciplines to prevent unnecessary/duplicative tests and procedures
- Discharge patients as soon as appropriate
- Investigate competitive prices for supplies and equipment
- Determine if supplies should be disposable or reusable
- Determine if supplies should be purchased or leased
- Secure supplies and equipment at competitive prices
- Use standardized documentation (i.e., critical paths) to contain costs and maintain quality, as appropriate
- Collaborate with interdisciplinary teams to contain costs and maintain quality, as appropriate
- Use/refer to quality improvement programs to monitor delivery of quality patient care in a cost-effective manner
- Evaluate services and programs for cost effectiveness on an ongoing basis
- Identify mechanisms to reduce costs
- Inform patient of the cost and alternatives of when and where to acquire health care services
- Inform patient of the cost, time, and alternatives involved in a specific test or procedure
- Encourage patient/family to ask questions about services and charges
- Discuss patient's financial situation
- Explore with patient creative options to secure needed resources

3rd edition 2000

Background Readings:

DeBour, L. M. (1990). Organizations as financial systems. In J. Dienemann (Ed.), *Nursing administration: Strategic perspectives and application* (pp. 263–297). Norwalk, CT: Appleton & Lange.

Gillies, D. A. (1994). *Nursing management: A systems approach* (3rd ed.). Philadelphia: Saunders.

Lound, J. L. (1994). Managing fiscal resources. In L. M. Simms, S. A. Price, & N. E. Ervin (Eds.), *The professional practice of nursing administration* (pp. 173–184). Albany, NY: Delmar.

Marquis, B. L. & Huston, C. J. (1992). *Leadership roles and management functions in nursing: Theory and application.* Philadelphia: Lippincott.

Swansburg, R. C. (1993). *Introductory management and leadership for clinical nurses: A text-workbook.* Sudbury, MA: Jones and Bartlett.

Tappen, R. M. (1995). *Nursing leadership and management: Concepts and practice* (3rd ed.). Philadelphia: F. A. Davis.

Cough Enhancement 3250

Definition: Promotion of deep inhalation by the patient with subsequent generation of high intrathoracic pressures and compression of underlying lung parenchyma for the forceful expulsion of air

Activities:
- Monitor results of pulmonary function tests, particularly vital capacity, maximal inspiratory force, forced expiratory volume in 1 second (FEV_1), and FEV_1/FVC, as appropriate
- Assist patient to a sitting position with head slightly flexed, shoulders relaxed, and knees flexed
- Encourage patient to take several deep breaths
- Encourage patient to take a deep breath, hold it for 2 seconds, and cough two or three times in succession
- Instruct patient to inhale deeply, bend forward slightly, and perform three or four huffs (against an open glottis)
- Instruct patient to inhale deeply several times, to exhale slowly, and to cough at the end of exhalation
- Initiate lateral chest wall rib spring techniques during the expiration phase of the cough maneuver, as appropriate
- Compress abdomen below the xiphoid with the flat hand, while assisting the patient to flex forward as the patient coughs
- Instruct patient to follow coughing with several maximal inhalation breaths
- Encourage use of incentive spirometry, as appropriate
- Promote systemic fluid hydration, as appropriate
- Assist patient to use a pillow or rolled blanket as a splint against incision when coughing

1st edition 1992; revised 2004

Background Readings

Perry, A. G. & Potter, P. A. (2002). *Clinical nursing skills and techniques* (5th ed.). St. Louis: Mosby.

Thelan, L. A. & Urden, L. D. (1993). *Critical care nursing: Diagnosis and management* (2nd ed.). St. Louis: Mosby.

Counseling   5240

Definition: Use of an interactive helping process focusing on the needs, problems, or feelings of the patient and significant others to enhance or support coping, problem solving, and interpersonal relationships

Activities:
- Establish a therapeutic relationship based on trust and respect
- Demonstrate empathy, warmth, and genuineness
- Establish the length of the counseling relationship
- Establish goals
- Provide privacy and ensure confidentiality
- Provide factual information as necessary and appropriate
- Encourage expression of feelings
- Assist patient to identify the problem or situation that is causing the distress
- Use techniques of reflection and clarification to facilitate expression of concerns
- Ask patient/significant others to identify what they can/cannot do about what is happening
- Assist patient to list and prioritize all possible alternatives to a problem
- Identify any differences between patient's view of the situation and the view of the health care team
- Determine how family behavior affects patient
- Verbalize the discrepancy between the patient's feelings and behaviors
- Use assessment tools (e.g., paper and pencil measures, audiotape, videotape, interactional exercises with other people) to help increase patient's self-awareness and counselor's knowledge of situation, as appropriate
- Reveal selected aspects of one's own experiences or personality to foster genuineness and trust, as appropriate
- Assist patient to identify strengths, and reinforce these
- Encourage new skill development, as appropriate
- Encourage substitution of undesirable habits with desirable habits
- Reinforce new skills
- Discourage decision-making when the patient is under severe stress, when possible

1st edition 1992; revised 2000

Background Readings:
Banks, L. J. (1992). Counseling. In G. M. Bulechek & J. C. McCloskey (Eds.), *Nursing interventions: Essentials nursing treatments* (pp. 279–291). Philadelphia: Saunders.

Boyd, M. A. (Ed.). (2005). *Psychiatric nursing: Contemporary practice* (3rd ed.). Philadelphia: Lippincott Williams & Wilkins.

Corey, G. (1991). *Theory and practice of counseling and psychotherapy* (4th ed.). Pacific Grove, CA: Brooks/Cole.

Crisis Intervention   6160

Definition: Use of short-term counseling to help the patient cope with a crisis and resume a state of functioning comparable to or better than the precrisis state

Activities:
- Provide atmosphere of support
- Avoid giving false reassurances
- Provide a safe haven
- Determine whether patient presents safety risk to self or others
- Initiate necessary precautions to safeguard the patient or others at risk for physical harm
- Encourage expression of feelings in a nondestructive manner
- Assist in identification of the precipitants and dynamics of the crisis
- Encourage patient to focus on one implication at a time
- Assist in identification of personal strengths and abilities that can be used in resolving the crisis
- Assist in identification of past/present coping skills and their effectiveness
- Assist in development of new coping and problem-solving skills, as needed
- Assist in identification of available support systems
- Link the patient and family with community resources, as needed
- Provide guidance about how to develop and maintain support system(s)
- Introduce patient to persons (or groups) who have successfully undergone the same experience
- Assist in identification of alternative courses of action to resolve the crisis
- Assist in evaluation of the possible consequences of the various courses of action
- Assist patient to decide on a particular course of action
- Assist in formulating a time frame for implementation of chosen course of action
- Evaluate with patient whether crisis has been resolved by chosen course of action
- Plan with patient how adaptive coping skills can be used to deal with crises in the future

1st edition 1992; revised 2008

Background Readings:
Aguilera, D. C. (1998). *Crisis intervention: Theory and methodology* (8th ed.). St. Louis: Mosby.

Barry, P. D. & Farmer, S. (2002). *Mental health & mental illness* (7th ed.). Philadelphia: Lippincott Williams & Wilkins.

Burgess, A. W. (1998). *Advanced practice psychiatric nursing*. Stamford, CT: Appleton & Lange.

Harkavy-Friedman, J. M. & Nelson, E. (1997). Management of the suicidal patient with schizophrenia. *Psychiatric Clinics of North America, 20*(3), 625–640.

Kanak, M. F. (1992). Interventions related to patient safety. In G. M. Bulechek & J. C. McCloskey (Eds.), Symposium on nursing interventions. *Nursing Clinics of North America, 27*(2), 371–396.

Kneisl, C. R. & Riley, E. A. (2004). Crisis intervention. In C. R. Kneisl, H. S. Wilson, & E. Trigoboff (Eds.), *Contemporary psychiatric-mental health nursing.* Upper Saddle River, NJ: Prentice Hall.

Kus, R. J. (1992). Crisis intervention. In G. M. Bulechek & J. C. McCloskey (Eds.), *Nursing interventions: Essential nursing treatments* (2nd ed., pp. 179–190). Philadelphia: Saunders.

Roberts, A. R. (Ed.). (2000). *Crisis intervention handbook: Assessment, treatment, and research* (2nd ed.). New York: Oxford University Press.

C

Critical Path Development 7640

Definition: Constructing and using a timed sequence of patient care activities to enhance desired patient outcomes in a cost-efficient manner

Activities:
- Conduct chart audit to determine current patterns of care for patient population
- Review current standards of practice related to patient population
- Collaborate with other health professionals to develop the critical path
- Identify appropriate intermediate and final outcomes with time frames
- Identify appropriate interventions with time frames
- Share critical path with patient and family, as appropriate
- Evaluate patient progress toward identified outcomes at defined intervals
- Calculate variances and report through appropriate channels
- Document patient progress toward identified outcomes, per agency policy
- Document reason for variances from planned interventions and expected outcomes
- Implement corrective action(s) for variance(s), as appropriate
- Revise critical path, as appropriate

2nd edition 1996

Background Readings:
Huber, D. (1996). *Leadership & nursing core management* (pp. 321–322). Philadelphia: Saunders.

Mosher, C., Cronk, P., Kidd, A., McCormick, P., Stockton, S., & Sulla, C. (1992). Upgrading practice with critical pathways. *American Journal of Nursing, 92*(1), 41–44.

Spath, P. L. (1994). *Clinical paths: Tools for outcomes management.* Chicago: American Hospital Association.

Thompson, K. S., Caddick, K., Mathie, J., & Abraham, T. (1991). Building a critical path for ventilator dependent patients. *American Journal of Nursing, 91*(7), 28–31.

Culture Brokerage 7330

Definition: The deliberate use of culturally competent strategies to bridge or mediate between the patient's culture and the biomedical health care system

Activities:
- Determine the nature of the conceptual differences that the patient and nurse have of the health problem or treatment plan
- Promote open discussion of cultural differences and similarities
- Identify, with the patient, cultural practices that may negatively impact health so the patient can make informed choices
- Discuss discrepancies openly and clarify conflicts
- Negotiate, when conflicts cannot be resolved, an acceptable compromise of treatment based on biomedical knowledge, knowledge of the patient's belief systems, and ethical standards
- Allow more than the usual time to process the information and work through a decision
- Appear relaxed and unhurried in interactions with the patient
- Use nontechnical language
- Arrange for cultural accommodation (e.g., late kitchen during Ramadan)
- Include the family, when appropriate, in the plan for adherence with the prescribed regimen
- Accommodate involvement of family to give support or direct care
- Translate the patient's symptom terminology into health care language that other professionals can more easily understand
- Facilitate intercultural communication (e.g., use of a translator, bilingual written materials/media, accurate nonverbal communication, avoid stereotyping)
- Provide information to the patient about the health care system
- Provide information to the health care providers about the patient's culture
- Assist other health care providers to understand and accept patient's reasons for nonadherence
- Alter the therapeutic environment by incorporating appropriate cultural elements
- Modify typical interventions (e.g., patient teaching) in culturally competent ways

1st edition 1992; revised 2000

Background Readings:
Caudle, P. (1993). Providing culturally sensitive health care to Hispanic clients. *Nurse Practitioner, 18*(12), 40–51.

Gorman, D. (1995). Multiculturalism and transcultural nursing in Australia. *Journal of Transcultural Nursing, 6*(2), 27–33.

Jackson, L. E. (1993). Understanding, eliciting, and negotiating clients' multicultural health beliefs. *Nurse Practitioner, 18*(4), 36–42.

Leininger, M. (1994). Culturally competent care: Visible and invisible. *Journal of Transcultural Nursing, 6*(1), 23–25.

Pillitteri, A. (2007). Sociocultural aspects of maternal and child health nursing. In A. Pillitteri (Ed.), *Maternal and child health nursing: Care of the childbearing and childrearing family* (5th ed., pp. 49–62). Philadelphia: Lippincott Williams & Wilkins.

Rairdan, B. & Higgs, Z. R. (1992). When your patient is a Hmong refugee. *American Journal of Nursing, 92*(3), 52–55.

Sloat, A. R. & Matsuura, W. (1990). Intercultural communication. In M. J. Craft & J. A. Denehy (Eds.), *Nursing interventions for infants and children* (pp. 166–180). Philadelphia: Saunders.

Tripp-Reimer, T., Brink, P. J., & Pinkam, C. (1999). Culture brokerage. In G. M. Bulechek & J. C. McCloskey (Eds.), *Nursing interventions: Effective nursing treatments* (3rd ed., pp. 637–649). Philadelphia: Saunders.

C

Cup Feeding: Newborn   8240

Definition: Preparation and administration of fluid to a newborn using a cup

Activities:
- Determine newborn state prior to initiating feeding
- Use clean cup without lid, spout, or lip
- Pour expressed milk at room temperature, or formula into cup
- Hold swaddled newborn upright or semi upright while supporting newborn's back, neck, and head
- Hold cup to newborn's lip resting slightly on the lower lip with cup's edges touching outer parts of upper lip
- Monitor for newborn signs of feeding readiness (e.g., increased alertness, open mouth and eyes, movements with mouth and face)
- Tip cup so that milk touches newborn's lips
- Avoid pouring milk too fast
- Monitor newborn's intake mechanism (i.e., preterm/low birth weight newborn tends to lap milk while full term/older infant tends to sip or suck milk)
- Monitor milk flow
- Burp the newborn frequently during and after the feeding
- Monitor for newborn signs of fullness (e.g., closing mouth, not taking in more milk, change in infant state, infant not responding to verbal or tactile stimulation)
- Discontinue feeding upon newborn sign of distress or infant sign of fullness
- Measure newborn's milk intake over 24 hours
- Instruct parent on cup feeding procedures
- Instruct parent about feeding readiness, distress, and feeding termination signs

6th edition 2013

Background Readings:
Abouelfettoh, A. M., Dowling, D. A., Dabash, S. A., Elguindy, S. R., & Seoud, I. A. (2008). Cup versus bottle feeding for hospitalized late preterm infants in Egypt: A quasi-experimental study. *International Breastfeeding Journal, 3*(27), 11.

Collins, C. T., Makrides, M., Gillis, J., & McPhee, A. J. (2008). Avoidance of bottles during the establishment of breast feeds in preterm infants. *Cochrane Database of Systematic Reviews*, Issue 4 Art. No.: CD005252. DOI:10.1002/14651858.CD005252.pub2.

Dowling, D. A., Meier, P. P., DiFiore, J. M., Blatz, M. A., & Martin, R. J. (2002). Cup-feeding for preterm infants: Mechanics and safety. *Journal of Human Lactation, 18*(1), 13–20.

Howard, C. R., de Blieck, E. A., ten Hoopen, C. B., Howard, F. M., Lanphear, B. P., & Lawrence, R. A. (1999). Physiologic stability of newborns during cup- and bottle-feeding. *Pediatrics, 104*(5), 1204–1207.

Lang, S., Lawrence, C. J., & Orme, R. L. (1994). Cup feeding: An alternative method of infant feeding. *Archives of Disease in Childhood, 71*(4), 365–369.

Marinelli, K. A., Burke, G. S., & Dodd, V. L. (2001). A comparison of the safety of cupfeedings and bottlefeedings in premature infants whose mothers intend to breastfeed. *Journal of Perinatology, 21*(6), 350–355.

Rocha, N. M., Martinez, F. E., & Jorge, S. M. (2002). Cup or bottle for preterm infants: Effects on oxygen saturation, weight gain and breastfeeding. *Journal of Human Lactation, 18*(2), 132–138.

World Health Organization. (1993). *Breastfeeding counseling: A training course*. Geneva, Switzerland: Author.

C

Cutaneous Stimulation 1340

Definition: Stimulation of the skin and underlying tissues for the purpose of decreasing undesirable signs and symptoms such as pain, muscle spasm, inflammation, or nausea

Activities:

- Discuss various methods of skin stimulation, their effects on sensation, and expectations of patient during activity
- Select a specific cutaneous stimulation strategy based on the individual's willingness to participate, ability to participate, preference, support of significant others, and contraindications
- Select the most appropriate type of cutaneous stimulation for the patient and the condition (e.g., massage, cold, ice, heat, menthol, vibration, or TENS)
- Instruct on indications for, frequency of, and procedure for application
- Select stimulation site, considering alternate sites when direct application is not possible (e.g., adjacent to, distal to, between affected areas and the brain)
- Consider acupressure points as sites of stimulation, as appropriate
- Determine the duration and frequency of stimulation based on method chosen
- Ensure that the electrical stimulation device is in good working order, as appropriate
- Apply stimulation directly on or around the affected site, as appropriate
- Encourage the use of an intermittent method of stimulation, as appropriate
- Allow the family to participate as much as possible
- Select alternate method or site of stimulation if altered sensation is not achieved
- Discontinue stimulation if increased pain or skin irritation occurs
- Evaluate and document response to stimulation

1st edition 1992, revised 2013

Background Readings:

Konno, R. (2010). Cochrane review summary for cancer nursing: Acupuncture-point stimulation for chemotherapy-induced nausea or vomiting. *Cancer Nursing 33*(6), 479–480.

Kubsch, S. M., Neveau, T., & Vandertie, K. (2001). Effect of cutaneous stimulation on pain reduction in emergency department patients. *Accident and Emergency Nursing, 9*(3), 143–151.

Smith, T. J., Coyne, P. J., Parker, G. L., Dodson, P., & Ramakrishnan, V. (2010). Pilot trial of a patient-specific cutaneous electrostimulation device (MC5-A Calmare) for chemotherapy-induced peripheral neuropathy. *Journal of Pain and Symptom Management, 40*(6), 883–891.

Timby, B. K. & Smith, N. E. (2007). Caring for clients with pain. *Introductory medical-surgical nursing* (9th ed., pp. 175–188). Philadelphia: Lippincott Williams & Wilkins.

Decision-Making Support 5250

Definition: Providing information and support for a patient who is making a decision regarding health care

Activities:
- Determine whether there are differences between the patient's view of own condition and the view of health care providers
- Assist patient to clarify values and expectations that may assist in making critical life choices
- Inform patient of alternative views or solutions in a clear and supportive manner
- Help patient identify the advantages and disadvantages of each alternative
- Establish communication with patient early in admission
- Facilitate patient's articulation of goals for care
- Obtain informed consent, when appropriate
- Facilitate collaborative decision making
- Be familiar with institution's policies and procedures
- Respect patient's right to receive or not to receive information
- Provide information requested by patient
- Help patient explain decision to others, as needed
- Serve as a liaison between patient and family
- Serve as a liaison between patient and other health care providers
- Use interactive computer software or web-based decision aides as an adjunct to professional support
- Refer to legal aid, as appropriate
- Refer to support groups, as appropriate

1st edition 1992; revised 2008

Background Readings:

Donahue, M. P. (1985). Advocacy. In G. M. Bulechek & J. C. McCloskey (Eds.), *Nursing interventions: Treatments for nursing diagnosis* (pp. 338–351). Philadelphia: Saunders.

Edwards, A. & Elwyn, G. (2001). *Evidence-based patient choice.* New York: Oxford University Press.

Edwards, A., Evans, R., & Elwyn, G. (2003). Manufactured but not imported: New directions for research in shared decision making support and skills. *Patient Education and Counseling, 50*(1), 33–38.

Marcus, P. E. (2004). Anxiety and related disorders. In K. M. Fortinash & P. A. Holoday-Worret (Eds.), *Psychiatric mental health nursing* (pp. 171–194). St. Louis: Mosby.

Moeller, M. D. (2005). Neurobiological responses and schizophrenia and psychotic disorders. In G. W. Stuart & M. T. Laraia (Eds.), *Principles and practice of psychiatric nursing* (8th ed., pp. 390–391). St. Louis: Mosby.

Sime, M. (1992). Decisional control. In M. Snyder (Ed.), *Independent nursing interventions* (2nd ed., pp. 110–114). Albany, NY: Delmar.

Defibrillator Management: External 4095

Definition: Care of the patient receiving defibrillation for termination of life-threatening cardiac rhythm disturbances

Activities:
- Initiate cardiopulmonary resuscitation, as indicated
- Prepare for immediate defibrillation of pulseless, unresponsive patient in conjunction with cardiopulmonary resuscitation
- Maintain cardiopulmonary resuscitation when not administering external defibrillation
- Determine type and operation techniques for available defibrillator
- Apply pads or paddles according to machine recommendations (e.g., paddles need conduction agent; pads are ready-made with conduction agent)
- Place appropriate monitoring devices on patients (automated external defibrillator pads or monitor leads)
- Place paddles or pads to avoid clothing or bed linens, as appropriate
- Determine need for shock per defibrillator instructions or interpretation of arrhythmia
- Charge machine to appropriate joules
- Use safety precautions before discharging (e.g., call "clear" three times, ensure no one is touching the patient including self)
- Monitor results and repeat as indicated
- Minimize interruptions to chest compressions in unresponsive patients
- Record events appropriately
- Assist in patient recovery as indicated (e.g., activate emergency medical systems when out of hospital for transport of patient to emergency care institution; arrange for transport within hospital to appropriate nursing unit for intensive cardiac care as indicated)
- Instruct new nursing staff on type and operation techniques for available defibrillator
- Assist in education of public related to proper use and indications of external defibrillation in cardiopulmonary arrest

5th edition 2008

Background Readings:

American Association of Critical Care Nurses. (2006). *Core curriculum for critical care nursing* (6th ed.) [J. G. Alspach, Ed.]. Philadelphia: Saunders.

American College of Cardiology Foundation and the American Heart Association. (2002). *Guideline update for implantation of cardiac pacemakers and antiarrhythmia devices.* Bethesda, MD: Author.

American Heart Association. (2005). Electric therapies: Automated external defibrillators, defibrillation, cardioversion, and pacing. *Circulation, 112*(24), 35–46.

American Heart Association. (2005). Guidelines for cardiopulmonary resuscitation and emergency cardiovascular care. *Circulation, 112*(24 Suppl. 1), IV1–IV211.

Lynn-McHale, D. J. & Carlson, K. K. (2005). *AACN procedure manual for critical care* (5th ed.). Philadelphia: Saunders.

Smeltzer, S. C. & Bare, B. G. (2004). *Brunner & Suddarth's textbook of medical-surgical nursing* (Vol. 1) (10th ed.). Philadelphia: Lippincott Williams & Wilkins.

Urden, L. D., Stacy, K. M., & Lough, M. E. (2006). *Thelan's critical care nursing: Diagnosis and management* (5th ed.). St. Louis: Mosby.

D

Defibrillator Management: Internal 4096

Definition: Care of the patient receiving permanent detection and termination of life-threatening cardiac rhythm disturbances through the insertion and use of an internal cardiac defibrillator

Activities:
- Provide information to patient and family related to defibrillator implantation (e.g., indications, functions, cardioversion experience, required lifestyle changes, potential complications)
- Provide concrete, objective information related to the effects of defibrillator therapy to reduce patient uncertainty, fear, and anxiety about treatment-related symptoms
- Document pertinent data in patient's permanent record regarding initial insertion of defibrillator (e.g., manufacturer, model number, serial number, implant date, mode of operation, capability for pacing and/or shock delivery, delivery system for shocks, upper and lower rate limits for rate-responsive devices)
- Confirm defibrillator placement post-implantation with baseline chest x-ray
- Monitor for potential complications associated with defibrillator insertion (e.g., pneumothorax, hemothorax, myocardial perforation, cardiac tamponade, hematoma, PVCs, infections, hiccups, muscle twitches)
- Observe for changes in cardiac or hemodynamic status, which indicate a need for modifications of defibrillator parameters
- Monitor for conditions that potentially influence sensing (e.g., fluid status changes, pericardial effusion, electrolyte or metabolic abnormalities, certain medications, tissue inflammation, tissue fibrosis, tissue necrosis)
- Monitor for arm swelling or increased warmth on side ipsilateral to implanted device and leads
- Monitor for redness or swelling at the device site
- Instruct to avoid tight or restrictive clothing that might cause friction at insertion site
- Instruct patient on activity restrictions (e.g., initial arm movement restrictions for pectoral implantations, avoidance of heavy lifting, avoid contact sports, adhere to driving restrictions)
- Monitor for symptoms of arrhythmias, ischemia, or heart failure (e.g., dizziness, syncope, palpitations, chest pain, shortness of breath) particularly with each outpatient contact
- Instruct patient and family member(s) regarding symptoms to report (e.g., dizziness, fainting, prolonged weakness, nausea, palpitations, chest pain, difficulty breathing, discomfort at insertion or external electrode site, electrical shocks)
- Instruct patient about emergent symptoms and what to do if symptoms occur (e.g., call emergency responders if dizzy)
- Monitor drug and electrolyte levels for patients receiving concurrent antiarrhythmic medications
- Monitor for metabolic conditions with adverse effects on defibrillators (acid-base disturbances, myocardial ischemia, hyperkalemia, severe hyperglycemia [greater than 600 mg/dl], renal failure, hypothyroidism)
- Instruct patient about potential defibrillator complications from electromagnetic interference (inappropriate discharges, potential proarrhythmic effects of defibrillator, decreased defibrillator generator life, cardiac arrhythmia, and cardiac arrest)
- Instruct patient about basic safety in avoidance of electromagnetic interference (e.g., keep at least 6 inches away from sources of interference, do not leave cell phones in the "on" mode in a shirt pocket over the defibrillator)
- Instruct patient about sources of highest electromagnetic interference (e.g., arc welding equipment, electronic muscle stimulators, radio transmitters, concert speakers, large motor-generator

systems, electric drills, handheld metal detectors, magnetic resonance imaging, radiation treatments)
- Instruct patient regarding special considerations at airport or government building security gates (e.g., always inform security guard of implantable defibrillator, walk through security gates, DO NOT allow handheld metal detectors near the device site, always walk quickly through metal detection devices or ask to be searched by hand, do not lean on or stand near detection devices for long periods)
- Instruct patient that handheld metal detectors contain magnets that can reset the defibrillator and cause malfunction
- Instruct patient to check manufacturer warnings when in doubt about household appliances
- Instruct patient to carry manufacturer identification card at all times
- Instruct patient to wear a medical alert bracelet or necklace that identifies defibrillator
- Instruct patient about the need for regular checkups with primary cardiologist
- Monitor for defibrillator problems that have occurred between scheduled checkup visits (e.g., inappropriate discharges, frequent discharges)
- Instruct patient to keep a detailed log of all discharges (e.g., time, location, and activity of patient when discharge occurred, physical symptoms before and after discharge) to review with the physician
- Instruct patient to consult primary cardiologist for all changes in medications
- Instruct patient with new defibrillator to refrain from operating motor vehicles until permitted per primary cardiologist (usually 3 to 6 months after the last symptomatic arrhythmic event)
- Instruct patient about the need for regular interrogation of defibrillator by cardiologist for routine maintenance
- Instruct patient about the need to obtain chest x-ray annually for defibrillator placement confirmation
- Avoid frightening family or friends about unexpected shocks
- Instruct patient's family (particularly sexual partners) that no harm comes to a person touching a patient who is receiving a defibrillator discharge (e.g., may feel the shock, but it is not harmful)
- Teach patient and family member(s) precautions and restrictions required
- Explore psychological responses (e.g., changes in self-image, depression due to driving restrictions, fear of shocks, increased anxiety, concerns related to sexual activities, changes in partner relationships)
- Encourage patient and family members to attend CPR classes
- Encourage attendance at support group meetings

5th edition 2008

Background Readings:
American Association of Critical Care Nurses. (2006). *Core curriculum for critical care nursing* (6th ed.) [J. G. Alspach, Ed.]. Philadelphia: Saunders.
American College of Cardiology Foundation and the American Heart Association. (2002). *Guideline update for implantation of cardiac pacemakers and antiarrhythmia devices.* Bethesda, MD: Author.

Burke, L. J. (1996). Securing life through technology acceptance: The first six months after transvenous internal cardioverter defibrillator implantation. *Heart & Lung, 25*(5), 352–366.

Dougherty, C. M., Benoliel, J. Q., & Bellin, C. (2000). Domains of nursing intervention after sudden cardiac arrest and automatic internal cardioverter defibrillator implantation. *Heart & Lung, 29*(2), 79–86.

Finch, N. J., Sneed, N. V., Leman, R. B., & Watson, J. (1997). Driving with an internal defibrillator: Legal, ethical and quality of life issues. *Journal of Cardiovascular Nursing, 11*(2), 58–67.

James, J. E. (1997). The psychological and emotional impact of living with an automated internal cardiverter defibrillator: How can nurses help? *Intensive and Critical Care Nursing, 13*(6), 316–323.

Lynn-McHale, D. J. & Carlson, K. K. (2005). *AACN procedure manual for critical care* (5th ed.). Philadelphia: Saunders.

Overbay, D. & Criddle, L. (2004). Mastering temporary invasive cardiac pacing. *Critical Care Nurse, 24*(3), 25–32.

Smeltzer, S. C. & Bare, B. G. (2004). *Brunner & Suddarth's textbook of medical-surgical nursing* (10th ed.). Philadelphia: Lippincott Williams & Wilkins.

Yeo, T. P. & Berg, N. C. (2005). Counseling patients with implanted cardiac devices. *The Nurse Practitioner, 29*(12), 58–65.

D

Delegation   7650

Definition: Transfer of responsibility for the performance of patient care while retaining accountability for the outcome

Activities:

- Determine the patient care that needs to be completed
- Identify the potential for harm
- Evaluate the complexity of the care to be delegated
- Determine the problem-solving and innovative skills required
- Consider the predictability of the outcome
- Evaluate the competency and training of the health care worker
- Explain the task to the health care worker
- Determine the level of supervision needed for the specific delegated intervention or activity (e.g., physically present or immediately available)
- Institute controls, so that the nurse can review the interventions or activities of the health care worker and intervene, as necessary
- Follow up with health care workers on a regular basis to evaluate their progress in completing the specific tasks
- Evaluate the outcome of the delegated intervention or activity and the performance of the health care worker
- Monitor patient's and family's satisfaction with care

2nd edition 1996

Background Readings:

American Association of Critical-Care Nurses. (1991). Consider this: Delegation. *Journal of Nursing Administration, 21*(7/8), 11, 13.

Blegen, M., Gardner, D., & McCloskey, J. C. (1992). Who helps you with your work? *American Journal of Nursing, 92*(1), 26–31.

Brown, S. T. (1985). Don't hesitate to delegate! *Nursing Success Today, 2*(12), 27–29.

Cronenwett, L. & Sanders, E. M. (1992). *Progress report on unlicensed assistive personnel.* Informational Report No. CNP-CNE-B. Washington, DC: American Nurses Association.

Hansten, R. & Washburn, M. (1992). Working with people: What do you say when you delegate work to others? *American Journal of Nursing, 92*(7), 48, 50.

Jung, F. (1991). Teaching registered nurses how to supervise nursing assistants. *Journal of Nursing Administration, 21*(4), 32–36.

Whitman, M. M. (2005). Return and report: Establishing accountability in delegation. *American Journal of Nursing, 105*(3), 97.

Delirium Management   6440

Definition: Provision of a safe and therapeutic environment for the patient who is experiencing an acute confusional state

Activities:

- Identify etiological factors causing delirium (e.g., check hemoglobin oxygen saturation)
- Initiate therapies to reduce or eliminate factors causing the delirium
- Recognize and document the motor subtype of the delirium (e.g., hypoactive, hyperactive, and mixed)
- Monitor neurological status on an ongoing basis
- Increase surveillance with a delirium rating scale universally understood by nursing staff when confusion first appears so that acute changes can be easily tracked
- Use family members or friendly hospital volunteers for surveillance of agitated patients instead of restraints
- Acknowledge the patient's fears and feelings
- Provide optimistic but realistic reassurance

- Allow the patient to maintain rituals that limit anxiety
- Provide patient with information about what is happening and what can be expected to occur in the future
- Avoid demands for abstract thinking if patient can think only in concrete terms
- Limit need for decision making if frustrating or confusing to patient
- Administer PRN medications for anxiety or agitation, but limit those with anticholinergic side effects
- Reduce sedation in general, but do control pain with analgesics, as indicated
- Encourage visitation by significant others, as appropriate
- Do not validate a delirium patient's misperceptions or inaccurate interpretations of reality (e.g., hallucinations or delusions)

D

- State your perception in a calm, reassuring, and nonargumentative manner
- Respond to the tone, rather than the content, of the hallucination or delusion
- Remove stimuli, when possible, that create excessive sensory stimuli (e.g., television or broadcast intercom announcements)
- Maintain a well-lit environment that reduces sharp contrasts and shadows
- Assist with needs related to nutrition, elimination, hydration, and personal hygiene
- Maintain a hazard-free environment
- Place identification bracelet on patient
- Provide appropriate level of supervision and surveillance to monitor patient and to allow for therapeutic actions, as needed
- Use physical restraints, as needed
- Avoid frustrating patient by quizzing with orientation questions that cannot be answered
- Inform patient of person, place, and time, as needed
- Provide a consistent physical environment and daily routine
- Provide caregivers who are familiar to the patient
- Use environmental cues (e.g., signs, pictures, clocks, calendars, and color coding of environment) to stimulate memory, reorient, and promote appropriate behavior
- Provide a low-stimulation environment for patient in whom disorientation is increased by overstimulation
- Encourage use of aids that increase sensory input (e.g., eyeglasses, hearing aids, and dentures)
- Approach patient slowly and from the front
- Address the patient by name when initiating interaction
- Reorient the patient to the health care provider with each contact
- Communicate with simple, direct, descriptive statements
- Prepare patient for upcoming changes in usual routine and environment before their occurrence

- Provide new information slowly and in small doses, with frequent rest periods
- Focus interpersonal interactions on what is familiar and meaningful to the patient

1st edition 1992; revised 2013

Background Readings:

Culp, K. R. & Cacchione, P. Z. (2008). Nutritional status and delirium in long-term care elderly individuals. *Applied Nursing Research, 21*(2), 66–74.

Lemiengre, J., Nelis, T., Joosten, E., Braes, T., Foreman, M., Gastmans, C., et al. (2006). Detection of delirium by bedside nurses using the confusion assessment method. *Journal of the American Geriatric Society, 54*(4), 685–689.

Meagher, D. (2009). Motor subtypes of delirium: Past, present and future. *International Review of Psychiatry, 21*(1), 59–73.

McCaffrey, R. (2009). The effect of music on acute confusion in older adults after hip or knee surgery. *Applied Nursing Research, 22*(2), 107–112.

Moyer, D. D. (2011). Review article: Terminal delirium in geriatric patients with cancer at end of life. *American Journal of Hospice and Palliative Medicine, 28*(1), 44–51.

Nelson, L. S. (2009). Teaching staff nurses the CAM-ICU for delirium screening. *Critical Care Nursing Quarterly, 32*(2), 137–143.

Wang, J. & Mentes, J. C. (2009). Factors determining nurses' clinical judgments about hospitalized elderly patients with acute confusion. *Issues in Mental Health Nursing, 30*(6), 399–405.

Yang, F. M., Marcantonio, E. R., Inouye, S. K., Kiely, D. K., Rudolph, J. L., Fearing, M. A., et al. (2009). Phenomenological subtypes of delirium in older persons: Patterns, prevalence, and prognosis. *Psychosomatics, 50*(3), 248–254.

Delusion Management   6450

Definition: Promoting the comfort, safety, and reality orientation of a patient experiencing false, fixed beliefs that have little or no basis in reality

Activities:
- Establish a trusting, interpersonal relationship with patient
- Provide patient with opportunities to discuss delusions with caregivers
- Avoid arguing about false beliefs; state doubt matter-of-factly
- Avoid reinforcing delusional ideas
- Focus discussion on the underlying feelings, rather than the content of the delusion ("It appears as if you may be feeling frightened.")
- Provide comfort and reassurance
- Encourage patient to validate delusional beliefs with trusted others (e.g., reality testing)
- Encourage patient to verbalize delusions to caregivers before acting on them
- Assist patient to identify situations where it is socially unacceptable to discuss delusions
- Provide recreational, diversional activities that require attention or skill
- Monitor self-care ability
- Assist with self-care, as needed
- Monitor physical status of patient
- Provide for adequate rest and nutrition

- Monitor delusions for presence of content that is self-harmful or violent
- Protect the patient and others from delusionally-based behaviors that might be harmful
- Maintain a safe environment
- Provide appropriate level of surveillance/supervision to monitor patient
- Reassure the patient of safety
- Provide for the safety and comfort of patient and others when patient is unable to control behavior (e.g., limit setting, area restriction, physical restraint, or seclusion)
- Decrease excessive environmental stimuli, as needed
- Assist patient to avoid or eliminate stressors that precipitate delusions
- Maintain a consistent daily routine
- Assign consistent caregivers on a daily basis
- Administer antipsychotic and antianxiety medications on a routine and as needed basis
- Provide medication teaching to patient/significant others
- Monitor patient for medication side effects and desired therapeutic effects
- Educate family and significant others about ways to deal with patient who is experiencing delusions

- Provide illness teaching to patient/significant others, if delusions are illness-based (e.g., delirium, schizophrenia, or depression)

2nd edition 1996

Background Readings:

Aromando, L. (1989). *Mental health and psychiatric nursing*. Springhouse, PA: Springhouse.

Beck, C. K., Rawlins, R. P., & Williams, S. R. (1988). *Mental health psychiatric nursing* (2nd ed.). St. Louis: Mosby.

Birckhead, L. M. (1989). Thought disorder and nursing interventions. In L. M. Birckhead (Ed.), *Psychiatric-mental health nursing: The therapeutic use of self* (pp. 311–347). Philadelphia: Lippincott.

Eklund, E. S. (1991). Perception/cognition, altered. In G. K. McFarland & M. D. Thomas (Eds.), *Psychiatric mental health nursing: Application to the nursing process* (pp. 332–357). Philadelphia: Lippincott.

Norris, J. (1987). Schizophrenia and schizophreniform disorders. In J. Norris, M. Kunes-Connell, S. Stockard, P. M. Ehrhart, & G. R. Newton (Eds.), *Mental health—psychiatric nursing: A continuum of care* (pp. 785–811). New York: John Wiley & Sons.

Varcarolis, E. M. (2000). *Psychiatric nursing clinical guide* (pp. 234–235). Philadelphia: Saunders.

D

Dementia Management   6460

Definition: Provision of a modified environment for the patient who is experiencing a chronic confusional state

Activities:

- Include family members in planning, providing, and evaluating care, to the extent desired
- Identify usual patterns of behavior for such activities as sleep, medication use, elimination, food intake, and self-care
- Determine physical, social, and psychological history of patient, usual habits, and routines
- Determine type and extent of cognitive deficit(s) using standardized assessment tool
- Monitor cognitive functioning, using a standardized assessment tool
- Determine behavioral expectations appropriate for patient's cognitive status
- Provide a low-stimulation environment (e.g., quiet, soothing music; nonvivid, simple, familiar patterns in decor; performance expectations that do not exceed cognitive processing ability; and dining in small groups)
- Provide adequate nonglare lighting
- Identify and remove potential dangers in environment for patient
- Place identification bracelet on patient
- Provide a consistent physical environment and daily routine
- Prepare for interaction with eye contact and touch, as appropriate
- Introduce self when initiating contact
- Address the patient distinctly by name when initiating interaction, and speak slowly
- Give one simple direction at a time
- Speak in a clear, low, warm, respectful tone of voice
- Use distraction, rather than confrontation, to manage behavior
- Provide unconditional positive regard
- Avoid touch and proximity if this causes stress or anxiety
- Provide caregivers that are familiar to the patient (e.g., avoid frequent rotations of staff assignments)
- Avoid unfamiliar situations when possible (e.g., room changes and appointments without familiar people present)
- Provide rest periods to prevent fatigue and reduce stress
- Monitor nutrition and weight
- Provide space for safe pacing and wandering
- Avoid frustrating patient by quizzing with orientation questions that cannot be answered
- Provide cues—such as current events, seasons, location, and names—to assist orientation
- Seat patient at small table in groups of three to five for meals, as appropriate
- Allow to eat alone, if appropriate
- Provide finger foods to maintain nutrition for patient who will not sit and eat
- Provide patient a general orientation to the season of the year by using appropriate cues (e.g., holiday decorations; seasonal decorations and activities; and access to contained, out-of-doors area)
- Decrease noise levels by avoiding paging systems and call lights that ring or buzz
- Select television or radio activities based on cognitive processing abilities and interests
- Select one-to-one and group activities geared to the patient's cognitive abilities and interests
- Label familiar photos with names of the individuals in photos
- Select artwork for patient rooms featuring landscapes, scenery, or other familiar images
- Ask family members and friends to see the patient one or two at a time, if needed, to reduce stimulation
- Discuss with family members and friends how best to interact with the patient
- Assist family to understand it may be impossible for patient to learn new material
- Limit number of choices patient has to make, so not to cause anxiety
- Provide boundaries, such as red or yellow tape on the floor, when low-stimulus units are not available
- Place patient's name in large block letters in room and on clothing, as needed
- Use symbols, other than written signs, to assist patient to locate room, bathroom, or other areas
- Monitor carefully for physiological causes of increased confusion that may be acute and reversible
- Remove or cover mirrors, if patient is frightened or agitated by them
- Discuss home safety issues and interventions

2nd edition 1996; revised 2004

Background Readings:

Aronson, M. K. (Ed.). (1994). *Reshaping dementia care*. Thousand Oaks, CA: Sage.

Burgener, S. C. & Twigg, P. (2002). Interventions for persons with irreversible dementia. *Annual Review of Nursing Research, 20*(1), 89–124.

Perry, A. G. & Potter, P. A. (2002). *Clinical nursing skills and techniques* (5th ed.). St. Louis: Mosby.

Stolley, J. M., Gerdner, L. A., & Buckwalter, K. C. (1999). Dementia management. In G. M. Bulechek & J. C. McCloskey (Eds.), *Nursing interventions: Effective nursing treatments* (3rd ed., pp. 533–548). Philadelphia: Saunders.

D

Dementia Management: Bathing   6462

Definition: Reduction of aggressive behavior during cleaning of the body

Activities:
- Personalize bath according to patient's usual bathing preferences and/or cultural traditions
- Use a flexible approach by providing choices and control over time of day and type of bath (shower, tub, or sponge bath)
- Avoid terms "bath" and "shower," if possible to reduce anxiety
- Ensure privacy and safety while undressing and bathing
- Simulate homelike environment as much as possible (e.g., wall treatment, soft music, aromatherapy, soft lighting)
- Provide comfortable environment (e.g., temperature, lighting, reduced noise)
- Give a reason for the bath (e.g., "Let's get your bath done before your daughter comes")
- Avoid rapid transportation to the bathroom
- Introduce to bath slowly by first letting water trickle on hand
- Allow time to perform care in an unrushed fashion
- Undress patient gradually in the bathroom while discussing something of interest other than the bath
- Use familiar bath products to promote relaxation
- Ensure water is appropriate temperature
- Reduce feelings of being cold by providing warm towels, washing face and hair last, wash feet first, or have beautician shampoo hair
- Place warm towel over head and shoulders while washing lower extremities
- Massage a soothing lotion into skin following bath
- View the patient as a whole person by focusing on the person rather than the task
- Assign a trusted caregiver with a friendly attitude
- Respond accordingly to patient's perceptions (e.g., temperature, pain, and fear of drowning)
- Use gentle persuasion, not coercion
- Use soft, reassuring tone of voice

- Discuss topics of interest to patient with a pleasant, calm approach
- Use gentle touch
- Give short, simple directions
- Encourage patient to assist with bath as able
- Use distraction rather than confrontation to manage behavior
- Maintain a quiet, peaceful environment
- Assign caregiver of same sex, if available
- Identify antecedents or "triggers" if aggressive behavior occurs
- Monitor for verbal and nonverbal warning signs of increasing agitation
- Give pain medication prior to bath if movement is painful
- Offer sponge bath if other methods produce agitation
- Remove dentures or offer something to eat to prevent biting during the bath
- Provide a washcloth or something to hold for grabbing during the bath
- Use comfortable bathing equipment

4th edition 2004

Background Readings:
Anderson, M. A., Wendler, M. C., & Congdon, J. (1998). Entering the world of dementia: CNA interventions for nursing home residents. *Journal of Gerontological Nursing, 24*(11), 31–37.
Farrell, M. M. (1997). Physically aggressive resident behavior during hygienic care. *Journal of Gerontological Nursing, 23*(5), 24–39.
Hoeffer, B., Rader, J., McKenzie, D., Lavelle, M., & Stewart, B. (1997). Reducing aggressive behavior during bathing cognitively impaired nursing home residents. *Journal of Gerontological Nursing, 23*(5), 16–23.
Sloane, P. D., Rader, J., Barrick, A. L., Hoeffer, B., Dwyer, D., McKenzie, D., et al. (1995). Bathing persons with dementia. *The Gerontologist, 35*(5), 672–678.

Dementia Management: Wandering   6466

Definition: Provision of care for a patient experiencing pacing patterns, elopement attempts, or getting lost unless accompanied

Activities:
- Include family members in planning, providing, and evaluating care, to the extent desired
- Identify usual patterns of wandering behavior
- Identify and remove potential dangers in environment for patient
- Modify unsafe aspects of patient's home (i.e., remove throw rugs, label rooms, and keep the house well lighted)
- Alert neighbors about the patient's wandering behavior
- Alert police and have current pictures taken
- Provide patient with a medical alert bracelet or necklace
- Provide a low-stimulation environment (e.g., quiet, soothing music; nonvivid and simple, familiar patterns in decor; performance expectations that do not exceed cognitive processing ability; and dining in small groups)

- Monitor carefully for physiological causes of increased confusion that may be acute and reversible
- Monitor nutrition and weight
- Monitor medication interactions, side effects, and desired therapeutic effects
- Recommend medication adjustments, as needed
- Assure the patient has adequate hydration
- Place patient's name in large block letters in room and on clothing, as needed
- Discuss home safety issues and interventions
- Install complex safety locks on doors to outside or basement
- Install alarm and sensor devices on doors.
- Use technological electronic devices to locate and monitor wandering (e.g., GPS [Global Position Satellite], RFID [Radio Frequency Identification])

- Provide boundaries, such as red or yellow tape on the floor, when low-stimulus units are not available
- Use symbols, other than written signs, to assist patient to locate room, bathroom, or other areas
- Install safety bars in bathroom
- Provide a consistent physical environment and daily routine
- Provide a secure and safe place for wandering
- Encourage physical activity during the daytime
- Avoid unfamiliar situations, when possible (e.g., room changes and appointments without familiar people present)
- Give patient a card with simple instructions (address and phone number) should the patient get lost
- Use night-lights
- Provide adequate nonglare lighting
- Remove or cover mirrors, if patient is frightened or agitated by them
- Prepare for interaction with eye contact and touch, as appropriate
- Introduce self when initiating contact
- Address the patient distinctly by name when initiating interaction, and speak slowly
- Give one simple direction at a time
- Speak in a clear, low, warm, respectful tone of voice
- Use distraction, rather than confrontation, to manage behavior
- Provide unconditional positive regard
- Avoid touch and proximity if this causes stress or anxiety
- Provide caregivers that are familiar to the patient
- Provide rest periods to prevent fatigue and reduce stress

6th edition 2013

D

Background Readings:

Algase, D. L. (2006). What's new about wandering behaviour? An assessment of recent studies. *International Journal of Older People Nursing, 1*(4), 226–234.

Beattie, E. R., Algase, D. L., & Song, J. (2004). Keeping wandering nursing home residents at the table: Improving food intake using a behavioral communication intervention. *Aging & Mental Health, 8*(2), 109–116.

Futrell, M., Melillo, K.D., & Remington, R. (2008). *Wandering: Evidence-based practice guideline*. Iowa City, IA: The University of Iowa College of Nursing Gerontological Nursing Interventions Research Center, Research Translation and Dissemination Core.

Hermans, D. G., Htay, U. H., & McShane, R. (2007). Non-pharmacological interventions for wandering of people with dementia in the domestic setting. *Cochrane Database of Systematic Reviews 2007,* Issue 1. Art. No: CD005994. doi: 10.1002/14651858.CD005994.pub2

McGonigal-Kenney, M. L. & Schutte, D. L. (2004). *Evidence-based practice guideline: Non-pharmacologic management of agitated behaviors in persons with Alzheimer disease and other chronic dementing conditions*. Iowa City, IA: The University of Iowa College of Nursing Gerontological Nursing Interventions Research Center, Research Translation and Dissemination Core.

Miskelly, F. (2004). A novel system of electronic tagging in patients with dementia and wandering. *Age and Ageing, 33*(3), 304–306.

Peatfield, J., Futrell, M., & Cox, C. (2002). Wandering: An integrative review. *Journal of Gerontological Nursing, 28*(4), 44–50.

Schonfeld, L., King-Kallimanis, B., Brown, L. M., Davis, D. M., Kearns, W. D., Molinari, V. A., et al. (2007). Wanderers with cognitive impairment in Department of Veterans Affairs nursing home care units. *Journal of the American Geriatrics Society, 55*(5), 692–699.

Deposition/Testimony 7930

Definition: Provision of recorded sworn testimony for legal proceedings based upon knowledge of the case

Activities:
- Contact your employer and malpractice carrier, as appropriate, when notice of deposition or subpoena for testimony is received
- Retain an attorney to represent you individually, as necessary
- Discuss the case only with the attorney(s) representing you at the deposition
- Avoid discussing the case with co-workers, physicians, and others involved without your attorney present
- Request that your attorney explain the deposition process
- Prepare by reviewing the clinical chart and reading or rereading any documents to be presented during the deposition
- Avoid taking any notes, documents, or reports into the deposition unless instructed by your attorney
- Prepare to admit mistakes that occurred
- Listen carefully to the entire question and understand it before you attempt to answer
- Listen to the questions asked and answer the questions directly and truthfully
- Ask for clarification if the question is unclear
- Avoid second-guessing a question or looking for traps
- Answer a question only if the person asking is finished; do not interject words while a question is being asked
- Answer questions based only on personal and professional knowledge; do not guess or speculate
- Answer "I do not remember" or "I don't recall", if you do not remember a fact
- Answer only the questions asked and do not volunteer any unsolicited information
- Answer questions with a "yes" or "no" answer, if possible
- Provide an explanation only if your attorney asks you for it
- Testify only about documents you have read
- Avoid answering a question to which your attorney objects
- Correct the opposing lawyer, particularly if facts are misstated
- Be respectful, courteous, and polite and do not argue with the other attorney
- Speak calmly, clearly, and with confidence, but do not be pompous or self-satisfied
- Spell unusual words after clearly enunciating them, if requested
- Ask to talk with your attorney privately, if needed
- Avoid offering to produce documents, let your attorney take the lead
- Communicate with the opposing counsel or the opposing party only with your attorney present
- Speak up and talk clearly so that all can be heard
- If tired, ask to get up to take a break
- Avoid taking any documents marked as exhibits

4th edition 2004

Background Readings:

Buppert, C. (1999). *Nurse practitioner's business practice & legal guide.* Gaithersburg, MD: Aspen.

Cady, R. (1999). Preparing to give a deposition. *American Journal of Maternal Child Nursing, 24*(2), 108.

Cady, R. (2000). Testifying at a trial: What you need to know. *American Journal of Maternal Child Nursing, 25*(4), 219.

Cohn, S. (1993). Glossary of legal terms. In *The complete lawyer* (pp. 41–43). Seattle, WA: Law Seminars International.

Dempski, K. (2000). If you have to give a deposition. *RN, 63*(1), 59–60.

Johnson, L. G. (1992). *The deposition guide: A practical handbook for witnesses* (pp. 17–21). Seattle, WA: Law Seminars International.

Maggiore, W. A. (1999). 9 tips for surviving a deposition. *Journal of Emergency Medical Services, 24*(12), 84–85.

Riffle, S. H. (1993). Going to court. In *The complete lawyer* (pp. 22–26). Seattle, WA: Law Seminars International.

Scott, R. W. (1999). *Health care malpractice: A primer on legal issues for professionals.* New York: McGraw-Hill.

Sullivan, G. H. (1995). Giving a deposition. *RN, 58*(9), 57–61.

D

Developmental Enhancement: Adolescent   8272

Definition: Facilitating optimal physical, cognitive, social, and emotional growth of individuals during the transition from childhood to adulthood

Activities:
- Build a trusting relationship with adolescent and adolescent caregiver(s)
- Encourage adolescent to be actively involved in decisions regarding his/her own health care
- Discuss normal developmental milestones and associated behaviors with adolescent and caregiver(s)
- Screen for health problems relevant to the adolescent and/or suggested by patient history (e.g., anemia; hypertension; hearing and vision disorders; hyperlipidemia; oral health problems; abnormal sexual maturation; abnormal physical growth; body image disturbances; eating disorders; poor nutrition; alcohol, tobacco, or drug use; unhealthy sexual behavior; infectious disease; poor self-concept; low self-esteem; depression; difficult relationships; abuse; learning problems; or work problems)
- Provide appropriate immunizations (e.g., measles, mumps, rubella, diphtheria, tetanus, hepatitis B)
- Provide health counseling and guidance to adolescent and adolescent caregiver(s)
- Promote personal hygiene and grooming
- Encourage participation in safe exercise on a regular basis
- Promote a healthy diet
- Facilitate development of sexual identity
- Encourage responsible sexual behavior
- Provide contraceptives with instruction for use, if needed
- Promote avoidance of alcohol, tobacco, and drugs
- Promote vehicle safety
- Facilitate decision-making ability
- Enhance communication skills
- Enhance assertiveness skills
- Facilitate a sense of responsibility for self and others
- Encourage nonviolent responses to conflict resolution
- Encourage adolescents to set goals
- Encourage development and maintenance of social relationships
- Encourage participation in school, extracurricular, and community activities
- Enhance parental effectiveness of adolescents
- Refer for counseling, as needed

3rd edition 2000

Background Readings:

Aquilino, M. L. (2001). Teen pregnancy: Primary prevention. In M. Craft-Rosenberg & J. Denehy (Eds.), *Nursing interventions for infants, children, and families* (pp. 659–676). Thousand Oaks, CA: Sage.

Archer, S. (Ed.). (1994). *Interventions for adolescent identity development.* Thousand Oaks, CA: Sage.

Papalia, D. & Olds, S. (1995). *Human development* (6th ed.). New York: McGraw-Hill.

Pillitteri, A. (2007). *Maternal and child health nursing: Care of the childbearing and childrearing family* (5th ed.). Philadelphia: Lippincott Williams & Wilkins.

Rice, F. (1997). *Child and adolescent development.* Upper Saddle River, NJ: Prentice Hall.

Ross-Alaolmolki, K. (2001). Teaching conflict resolution. In M. Craft-Rosenberg & J. Denehy (Eds.), *Nursing interventions for infants, children, and families* (pp. 691–706). Thousand Oaks, CA: Sage.

Developmental Enhancement: Child   8274

Definition: Facilitating or teaching parents/caregivers to facilitate the optimal gross motor, fine motor, language, cognitive, social, and emotional growth of preschool and school-aged children

Activities:
- Build a trusting relationship with child
- Establish one-on-one interaction with child
- Assist each child to become aware he/she is important as an individual
- Identify special needs of child and adaptations required as appropriate
- Build a trusting relationship with caregivers
- Teach caregivers about normal developmental milestones and associated behaviors
- Demonstrate activities that promote development to caregivers
- Facilitate caregiver's contact with community resources, as appropriate
- Refer caregivers to support group, as appropriate

- Facilitate integration of child with peers
- Make sure body language agrees with verbal communication
- Encourage child to interact with others by role modeling inter-action skills
- Provide activities that encourage interaction among children
- Assist child with sharing and taking turns
- Encourage child to express self through positive rewards or feedback for attempts
- Hold or rock and comfort child, especially when upset
- Foster cooperation, not competition, among children
- Create a safe, well-defined space for child to explore and learn
- Teach child how to seek help from others, when needed
- Encourage dreaming or fantasy, when appropriate
- Offer age-appropriate toys or materials
- Help child learn self-help skills (e.g., feeding, toileting, brushing teeth, washing hands, dressing)
- Listen to and discuss music
- Sing and talk to child
- Encourage child to sing and dance
- Teach child to follow directions
- Facilitate role playing of daily activities of adults in child's world (e.g., playing store, etc.)
- Be consistent and structured with behavior management/modification strategies
- Redirect attention, when needed
- Have child who is misbehaving "take breaks" or "time outs"
- Provide opportunity and materials for building, drawing, clay modeling, painting, and coloring
- Assist with cutting out and gluing various shapes
- Provide opportunity for doing puzzles and mazes
- Teach child to recognize and manipulate shapes
- Teach child to write name/recognize first letter/recognize name, as appropriate

- Name objects in environment
- Tell or read stories to child
- Work on ordering and sequencing of letters, numbers, and objects
- Assist with spatial organization
- Teach planning by encouraging child to guess what will happen next and have child list other possible choices, and so on
- Provide opportunities for and encourage exercise, large motor activities
- Teach child to jump over objects
- Teach child to perform somersaults
- Provide opportunity to play on playground
- Go on walks with child
- Monitor prescribed medication regime, as appropriate
- Assure that medical tests and/or treatments are done in a timely manner, as appropriate

3rd edition 2000

Background Readings:

American Public Health Association and the American Academy of Pediatrics. (1992). *Caring for our children – National health and safety performance standards: Guidelines for out-of-home child care programs.* Washington, DC: Author.

Kane, M. (1984). Cognitive styles of thinking and learning: Part 1. *Academic Therapy, 19*(5), 527–536.

Peck, J. (1989). Using storytelling to promote language and literacy development. *The Reading Teacher, 43*(2), 138–141.

Phillips, S. & Hartley, J. T. (1988). Developmental differences and interventions for blind children. *Pediatric Nursing, 14*(3), 201–204.

Pillitteri, A. (2007). *Maternal and child health nursing: Care of the childbearing and childrearing family* (5th ed.). Philadelphia: Lippincott Williams & Wilkins.

Developmental Enhancement: Infant   8278

Definition: Facilitating optimal physical, cognitive, social, and emotional growth of child under 1 year of age

Activities:

- Instruct parent on what constitutes appropriate infant nutrition and nutritional habits
- Discuss and support decision to breastfeed or bottle feed
- Instruct on proper storage, preparation, and handling of breast milk or prepared infant formula
- Introduce solid foods at approximately 6 months of age, instructing parent on the selection and preparation of foods, methods of introduction, and food storage
- Instruct parent to avoid offering the infant a bottle containing juice or milk while in bed
- Provide anticipatory guidance for infant weaning, including signs of readiness
- Encourage establishment of bedtime rituals that reduce or eliminate disturbances in sleep-wake cycle
- Assist parent in identifying presence of sleep disturbance or disorder
- Determine appropriate management technique for sleep disturbance or disorder
- Discuss the risks and benefits of infant and caregiver co-sleeping
- Provide visual, auditory, tactile, and kinetic stimulation during play

- Structure play and care around infant's behavioral style and temperament patterns
- Provide developmentally-appropriate safe toys and activities
- Explain the need for fluoride supplementation beginning at 6 months of age
- Instruct parent to begin cleaning infant's oral cavity with damp cloth upon eruption of first tooth
- Use soft-bristled toothbrush with water or non-fluoridated toothpaste once several teeth have erupted
- Determine appropriate scheduling for initial and subsequent dental exams
- Perform recommended screenings (e.g., anemia, lead exposure, and vision)
- Provide accurate information pertaining to risks, benefits, contraindications, and side effects of scheduled immunizations
- Identify need for additional immunizations for selected groups of children
- Provide anticipatory guidance concerning discipline, dependency, increased mobility, and safety
- Discuss timeout versus corporal punishment strategies for discipline, encouraging the former
- Instruct parent on injury prevention strategies tailored to child's specific developmental stage and curiosity level

- Encourage provision of safe space for infant exploration
- Discuss injury prevention strategies for fire and electrical burns, suffocation and aspiration, poisoning, falls, bodily injury, drowning, and motor vehicle injury
- Instruct parent on SIDS (Sudden Infant Death Syndrome) prevention strategies
- Instruct parent about child temperament and its association with infant's interaction type with others
- Promote and facilitate family bonding and attachment with infant
- Support and praise parent skills and efforts
- Discuss parent return to work and childcare options
- Identify and address presence of family strife, lack of support, and pathology
- Provide information to parent about child development and child rearing
- Refer for parenting education, as needed

6th edition 2013

Background Readings:

Ball, J. W. & Bindler, R. C. (2008). Health promotion and health maintenance for the newborn and infant. In *Pediatric nursing: Caring for children* (4th ed., pp. 281–308). Upper Saddle River, NJ: Pearson Prentice Hall.

Levine, D. A. (2006). Evaluation of the well child. In R. M. Kliegman, K. J. Marcdante, H. B. Jenson, & R. E. Behrman (Eds.), *Nelson essentials of pediatrics* (5th ed., pp. 34–43). Philadelphia: Saunders.

Wilson, D. (2007). Health promotion of the infant and family. In M. J. Hockenberry & D. Wilson (Eds.), *Wong's nursing care of infants and children* (8th ed., pp. 499–565). St. Louis: Mosby.

Wong, D. L., Hockenberry, M. J., Wilson, D., Perry, S. E., & Lowdermilk, D. L. (2006). The infant and family. *Maternal child nursing care.* (3rd ed., pp. 1027–1088). St. Louis: Mosby.

Dialysis Access Maintenance   4240

Definition: Preservation of vascular (arterial-venous) access sites

Activities:

- Monitor catheter exit site for migration
- Monitor access site for redness, edema, heat, drainage, bleeding hematoma, and decreased sensation
- Apply sterile gauze, ointment, and dressing to central venous dialysis catheter site with each treatment
- Monitor for AV fistula patency at frequent intervals (e.g., palpate for thrill and auscultate for bruit)
- Heparinize newly inserted central venous dialysis catheters
- Reheparinize central venous dialysis catheters after dialysis or every 72 hours
- Avoid mechanical compression of peripheral access sites
- Avoid mechanical compression of patient's limbs near central dialysis catheter
- Teach patient to avoid mechanical compression of peripheral access site
- Teach patient about how to care for dialysis access site
- Avoid venipuncture and blood pressures in peripheral access extremity

4th edition 2004

Background Readings:

Eisenbud, M. D. (1996). *The handbook of dialysis access.* Columbus, OH: Anadem.

Gutch, C. F., Stoner, M. H., & Carea, A. L. (1993). *Review of hemodialysis for nurses and dialysis personnel* (5th ed.). St. Louis: Mosby.

Lancaster, L. E. (Ed.). (1995). *ANNA's core curriculum for nephrology nurses* (3rd ed., Section X). Pitman, NJ: Anthony J. Jannetti.

Levine, D. Z. (1997). *Caring for the renal patient* (3rd ed.). Philadelphia: Saunders

Diarrhea Management   0460

Definition: Management and alleviation of diarrhea

Activities:

- Determine history of diarrhea
- Obtain stool for culture and sensitivity if diarrhea continues
- Evaluate medication profile for gastrointestinal side effects
- Teach patient appropriate use of antidiarrheal medications
- Instruct patient/family members to record color, volume, frequency, and consistency of stools
- Evaluate recorded intake for nutritional content
- Encourage frequent, small feedings, adding bulk gradually
- Teach patient to eliminate gas-forming and spicy foods from diet
- Suggest trial elimination of foods containing lactose
- Identify factors (e.g., medications, bacteria, tube feedings) that may cause or contribute to diarrhea
- Monitor for signs and symptoms of diarrhea
- Instruct patient to notify staff of each episode of diarrhea
- Observe skin turgor regularly
- Monitor skin in perianal area for irritation and ulceration
- Measure diarrhea/bowel output
- Weigh patient regularly
- Notify physician of an increase in frequency or pitch of bowel sounds
- Consult physician if signs and symptoms of diarrhea persist

- Instruct in low-fiber, high-protein, high-calorie diet, as appropriate
- Instruct in avoidance of laxatives
- Teach patient/family how to keep a food diary
- Teach patient stress-reduction techniques, as appropriate
- Assist patient in performing stress-reduction techniques
- Monitor safe food preparation
- Perform actions to rest the bowel (e.g., NPO, liquid diet)

1st edition 1992; revised 2000, 2004

Background Readings:

Hogan, C. M. (1998). The nurse's role in diarrhea management. *Oncology Nurse Forum, 25*(5), 879–886.

Taylor, C. M. (1987). *Nursing diagnosis cards*. Springhouse, PA: Springhouse.

Wadle, K. (2001). Diarrhea. In M. L. Maas, K. C. Buckwalter, M. D. Hardy, T. Tripp-Reimer, M. G. Titler, & J. P. Specht (Eds.), *Nursing care of older adults: Diagnoses, outcomes, & interventions* (pp. 227–237). St. Louis: Mosby.

Williams, M. S., Harper, R., Magnuson, B., Loan, T., & Kearney, P. (1998). Diarrhea management in enterally fed patients. *Nutrition in Clinical Problems, 13*(5), 225–229.

D

Diet Staging   1020

Definition: Instituting required diet restrictions with subsequent progression of diet as tolerated

Activities:
- Determine presence of bowel sounds
- Institute NPO, as needed
- Clamp nasogastric tube and monitor tolerance, as appropriate
- Monitor for alertness and presence of gag reflex, as appropriate
- Monitor tolerance to ingestion of ice chips and water
- Determine if patient is passing flatus
- Collaborate with other health care team members to progress diet as rapidly as possible without complications
- Progress diet from clear liquid, full liquid, soft, to regular or special diet, as tolerated, for adults and children
- Progress from glucose water or oral electrolyte solution, half-strength formula, to full-strength formula for babies
- Monitor tolerance to diet progression
- Offer six small feedings, rather than three meals, as appropriate
- Find ways to include patient preferences in the prescribed diet
- Make the environment in which the meal is offered as pleasant as possible
- Post the diet restrictions at bedside, on chart, and in care plan

1st edition 1992, revised 2013

Background Readings:

Dudek, S. G. (2007). Feeding patients: Hospital food and enteral and parenteral nutrition. In *Nutrition essentials for nursing practice* (5th rev. ed., pp. 417–456). Philadelphia: Lippincott Williams & Wilkins.

Holloway, N. M. (2003). *Medical-surgical care planning* (4th ed., p. 689). Ambler, PA: Lippincott, Williams & Wilkins

Nyberg, M. & Olsen, T. D. (2010). Meals at work: Integrating social and architectural aspects. *International Journal of Workplace Health Management, 3*(3), 222–232.

Stanfield, P. & Hui, Y. H. (2009). *Nutrition and diet therapy: Self-instructional approaches* (5th ed., p. 266). Sudbury, MA: Jones & Bartlett.

Diet Staging: Weight Loss Surgery   1024

Definition: Instituting required diet changes in progressive phases following bariatric surgery

Activities:
- Institute NPO or sips of water only for the first 24-48 hours following surgery, according to agency policy
- Administer solutions of dextrose, saline, or lactated ringers to provide adequate nutrition in first 24 hours and until patient can tolerate a full liquid diet
- Progress to a liquid diet that lasts 2-3 weeks
- Instruct patient to sip room-temperature liquids (e.g., broth, unsweetened juice, milk) slowly, consuming between two to three ounces at a time
- Instruct patients to carry with them sugar-free beverages and drink often
- Incorporate pureed foods (e.g., broth blended with well-cooked beans, fish or ground meats; yogurt, blended fruits) in diet once the patient's body has adjusted to liquids
- Add mashed solid foods (e.g., finely diced meats, canned fruits, oatmeal, eggs) between 6-8 weeks post surgery
- Instruct patient to eat the protein foods on the plate first
- Progress to firmer foods that are low in sugar, saturated and trans fat, and contain high quality protein, maintaining this diet for life
- Encourage patients to eat breakfast and at least 4 to 5 small meals daily
- Instruct patients to take small bites, eat slowly, and chew solids that are well-cooked
- Instruct patients to incorporate fresh fruit and vegetables in their fluid and food intake
- Monitor for lactose intolerance as a possible post surgical complication
- Work with a dietitian following surgery to ensure that protein nutrition is optimal and to modify the diet as required
- Find ways to include patient preferences in the prescribed diet
- Make the environment in which the meal is offered as pleasant as possible
- Post the diet restrictions at bedside, on chart, and in care plan
- Instruct patient to avoid foods and beverages with large amounts of sugar (e.g., soda, juice drinks, milk shakes, regular ice cream) as these may cause a dumping syndrome
- Instruct patient to avoid drinking approximately half an hour before eating, during the meal, and half an hour after the meal to reduce vomiting and diarrhea

- Instruct patient about need to take an adult strength multivitamin with iron, a B-complex supplement, and added calcium
- Monitor tolerance to diet progression
- Encourage patients to keep a record of types and quantities of foods that cause discomfort, distress, or intolerance
- Encourage patients to do at least 35 minutes of daily aerobic exercise with strength training three times per week to maintain a good metabolic rate
- Encourage attendance at a support group for several months post surgery

6th edition 2013

Background Readings:

Dowd, J. (2005). Nutrition management after gastric bypass surgery. *Diabetes Spectrum, 18*(2), 82–84.

Elliot, K. (2003). Nutritional considerations after bariatric surgery. *Critical Care Nursing Quarterly, 26*(2), 133–138.

Farraye, F. A. & Forse, A. (Eds.). (2005). *Bariatric surgery: A primer for your medical practice* (pp. 148–153). Thorofare, NJ: Slack.

Strohmayer, E., Via, M. A., & Yanagisawa, R. (2010). Metabolic management following bariatric surgery. *Mount Sinai Journal of Medicine, 77*(5), 431–445.

D

Discharge Planning 7370

Definition: Preparation for moving a patient from one level of care to another within or outside the current health care agency

Activities:

- Assist patient/family/significant others to prepare for discharge
- Determine the patient's abilities for discharge
- Collaborate with the physician, patient/family/significant others, and other health team members in planning for continuity of health care
- Coordinate efforts of different health care providers to ensure a timely discharge
- Identify patient's and primary caregiver's understanding of knowledge or skills required after discharge
- Identify patient teaching needed for post-discharge care
- Monitor readiness for discharge
- Communicate patient's discharge plans, as appropriate
- Document patient's discharge plans on chart
- Formulate a maintenance plan for post-discharge follow-up
- Assist patient/family/significant others in planning for the supportive environment necessary to provide the patient's post-hospital care
- Develop a plan that considers the health care, social, and financial needs of patient
- Arrange for post-discharge evaluation, as appropriate
- Encourage self-care, as appropriate
- Arrange discharge to next level of care
- Arrange for caregiver support, as appropriate
- Discuss financial resources if arrangements for health care are needed after discharge
- Coordinate referrals relevant to linkages among health care providers

1st edition 1992; revised 2008

Background Readings:

Hastings, S. N. & Heflin, M. T. (2005). A systematic review of interventions to improve outcomes for elders discharged from the emergency department. *Academic Emergency Medicine, 12*(10), 978–986.

Lowenstein, A. J. & Hoff, P. S. (1994). Discharge planning: A study of nursing staff involvement. *Journal of Nursing Administration, 24*(4), 45–50.

Luckmann, J. & Sorensen, K. C. (1987). *Medical-surgical nursing* (3rd ed.). Philadelphia: Saunders.

McClelland, E., Kelly, K., & Buckwalter, K. C. (1985). *Continuity of care: Advancing the concept of discharge planning.* New York: Harcourt Brace Jovanovich.

McKeehan, K. M. (1981). *Continuing care.* St. Louis: Mosby.

Meijer, R., van Limbeek, J., Peusens, G., Rulkens, M., Dankoor, K., Vermeulen, M., et al. (2005). The stroke unit discharge guideline, a prognostic framework for the discharge outcome from the hospital stroke unit: A prospective cohort study. *Clinical Rehabilitation, 19*(7), 770–778.

Remer, D., Buckwalter, K. C., & Maas, M. L. (1991). Translocation syndrome. In M. L. Maas, K. C. Buckwalter, & M. A. Hardy (Eds.), *Nursing diagnoses and interventions for the elderly* (pp. 493–504). Redwood City, CA: Addison-Wesley.

Distraction 5900

Definition: Purposeful diverting of attention or temporarily suppressing negative emotions and thoughts away from undesirable sensations

Activities:

- Encourage the individual to choose the distraction technique(s) desired (e.g., music, engaging in conversation or telling a detailed account of event or story, recalling positive event, focusing on photo or neutral object, guided imagery, humor, or deep breathing exercises)
- Instruct the patient on the benefits of stimulating a variety of senses (e.g., music, counting, television, reading, video/hand-held games, or virtual reality)
- Use distraction techniques for children (e.g., play, activity therapy, reading stories, singing songs, or rhythm activities) that are novel, appeal to more than one sense, and do not require literacy or thinking ability

- Suggest techniques consistent with energy level, ability, age appropriateness, developmental level, and effective use in the past
- Identify with the patient a list of pleasurable activities (e.g., exercise, going for walks, bubble baths, talking to friends or family)
- Individualize the content of the distraction technique, based on those used successfully in the past and age or developmental level
- Advise patient to practice the distraction technique before the time needed, if possible
- Instruct patient how to engage in the distraction (e.g., prompting neutral word, equipment, or materials) prior to the time needed, if possible
- Encourage participation of family and significant others and provide teaching, as necessary
- Use distraction alone or in conjunction with other measures or distractions, as appropriate
- Evaluate and document response to distraction

1st edition 1992; revised 2013

Background Readings:

Huffziger, S. & Kuehner, C. (2008). Rumination, distraction, and mindful self-focus in depressed patients. *Behaviour Research and Therapy, 47*(3), 224–230.

Kleiber, C. (2001). Distraction. In M. Craft-Rosenberg & J. Denehy (Eds.), *Nursing interventions for infants, children, and families* (pp. 315–328). Thousand Oaks, CA: Sage.

Kleiber, C., McCarthy, A. M., Hanrahan, K., Myers, L., & Weathers, N. (2007). Development of the distraction coaching index. *Children's Healthcare, 36*(3), 219–235.

Lemoult, J., Hertel, P. T., & Joormann, J. (2010). Training the forgetting of negative words: The role of direct suppression and the relation to stress reactivity. *Applied Cognitive Psychology, 24*(3), 365–375.

Malloy, K. M. & Milling, L. S. (2010). The effectiveness of virtual reality distraction for pain reduction: A systematic review. *Clinical Psychology Review, 30*(8), 1011–1018.

Masuda, A., Feinstein, A. B., Wendell, J. W., & Sheehan, S. T. (2010). Cognitive defusion versus thought distraction: A clinical rationale, training, and experiential exercise in altering psychological impacts of negative self-referential thoughts. *Behavior Modification, 34*(6), 520–538.

Schneider, S. M. & Workman, M. L. (2000). Virtual reality as a distraction intervention for older children receiving chemotherapy. *Pediatric Nursing, 26*(6), 593–597.

D

Documentation   7920

Definition: Recording of pertinent patient data in a clinical record

Activities:
- Record complete assessment findings in initial record
- Document nursing assessments, nursing diagnoses, nursing interventions, and outcomes of care provided
- Use guidelines as provided by the standards of practice for documentation in the setting
- Use standardized, systematic, and prescribed format needed/required by setting
- Use standardized forms, as indicated, for federal and state regulations and reimbursement
- Chart baseline assessments and care activities using agency specific forms/flow sheets
- Record all entries as promptly as possible
- Avoid duplication of information in record
- Record precise date and time of procedures or consultations by other health care providers
- Describe patient behaviors objectively and accurately
- Document evidence of client's specific claims (e.g., Medicare, workers' compensation, insurance, or litigation-related claims)
- Document and report situations, as mandated by law, for adult or child abuse
- Document use of major equipment or supplies, as appropriate
- Record ongoing assessments, as appropriate
- Record patient's response to nursing interventions
- Document that physician was notified of change in patient status
- Chart deviations from expected outcomes, as appropriate
- Record use of safety measures such as side rails, as appropriate
- Record specific patient behavior using patient's exact words
- Record involvement of significant others, as appropriate
- Record observations of family interactions and home environment, as appropriate
- Record resolution/status of identified problems
- Ensure that record is complete at time of discharge, as appropriate
- Summarize patient status at the conclusion of nursing services
- Sign record, using legal signature and title
- Maintain confidentiality of record
- Use documentation data in quality assurance and accreditation

2nd edition 1996; revised 2000

Background Readings:

Brent, N. J. (1998). Legalities in home care. Home care fraud & abuse: Dishonest documentation. *Home Healthcare Nurse, 16*(3), 196–198.

Cline, A. (1989). Streamlined documentation through exceptional charting. *Nursing Management, 20*(2), 62–64.

Coles, M. C. & Fullenwider, S. D. (1988). Documentation: Managing the dilemma. *Nursing Management, 19*(12), 65–66, 70, 72.

Edelstein, J. (1990). A study of nursing documentation. *Nursing Management, 21*(11), 40–43, 46.

Mandell, M. S. (1987). Charting: How it can keep you out of court. *Nursing Life, 7*(5), 46–48.

Miller, P. & Pastorino, C. (1990). Daily nursing documentation can be quick and thorough. *Nursing Management, 21*(11), 47-49.

Southard, P. & Frankel, P. (1989). Trauma care documentation: A comprehensive guide. *Journal of Emergency Nursing, 15*(5), 393–398.

Weber, J. & Kelley, J. H. (2006). Validating and documenting data. In *Health assessment in nursing* (3rd ed., pp 63–74). Philadelphia: Lippincott Williams, & Wilkins.

D

Dressing 1630

Definition: Choosing, putting on, and removing clothes for a person who cannot do this for self

Activities:
- Identify areas where patient needs assistance in dressing
- Monitor patient's ability to dress self
- Dress patient after personal hygiene completed
- Encourage participation in selection of clothing
- Encourage use of self-care devices, as appropriate
- Dress affected extremity first, as appropriate
- Dress in nonrestrictive clothing, as appropriate
- Dress in personal clothing, as appropriate
- Change patient's clothing at bedtime
- Select shoes/slippers conducive to walking and safe ambulation
- Offer to launder clothing, as necessary
- Give assistance until the patient is fully able to assume responsibility for dressing self

1st edition 1992; revised 2000

Background Readings:

Craven, R. F. & Hirnle, C. J. (2003). Self-care hygiene. In *Fundamentals of nursing: Human health and function* (4th ed., pp. 703–752). Philadelphia: Lippincott Williams, & Wilkins.

Engleman, K. K., Mathews, R. M., & Altus, D. E. (2002). Restoring dressing independence in persons with Alzheimer's disease: A pilot study. *American Journal of Alzheimer's Disease & Other Dementias, 17*(1), 37–43.

Sorensen, K. & Luckmann, J. (1986). *Basic nursing: A psychophysiologic approach* (2nd ed.). Philadelphia: Saunders.

Stryker, R. (1977). *Rehabilitative aspects of acute and chronic nursing care.* Philadelphia: Saunders.

Dry Eye Prevention 1350

Definition: Prevention and early detection of dry eye in an individual at risk

Activities:
- Monitor signs and symptoms (e.g., redness, burning, itching, drainage, pain around and in the eye, difficulty in opening eyes on waking and moving lids, blurred vision) of dry eye
- Identify personal characteristics (e.g., age, gender, hormones, autoimmune diseases, chemical burn) and environmental factors (e.g., dry air, air conditioning, sunlight) that may increase potential of dry eye
- Monitor blink reflex
- Identify eyelid position
- Monitor amount of tearing using tear strips
- Screen the corneal epithelial damage using a standard test
- Monitor patient's ability to wear, remove, and clean contact lenses, as appropriate
- Instruct patient to avoid prolonged reading and lengthy computer use
- Ensure the endotracheal bandages are not too tight in patients ventilated via endotracheal tube
- Monitor the mode and the pressure of the ventilator in mechanically ventilated patients
- Identify the frequency and the type of the care according to the eyelid position in lagophthalmos (e.g., in comatose, under deep sedation and neuromuscular blockage, facial paralysis, Bell's palsy, thyrotoxic exophthalmos, paralytic ectropion)
- Administer eye care at least twice a day, as appropriate
- Apply lubricants (e.g., eye drops, ointments) to support tear production, as appropriate
- Cover the eyes with effective devices (e.g., polyethylene cover, polyacrylamide gel, hypoallergenic tape), as appropriate
- Ensure the eyelids are closed
- Prepare the patient for a tarsorrhaphy to protect the cornea
- Inspect ocular surface and the cornea for effects of care and prophylactic treatment
- Report abnormal signs and symptoms to the physician

6th edition 2013

Background Readings:

Germano, E. M., Mello, M. J., Sena, D. F., Correia, J. B., & Amorim, M. M. (2009). Incidence and risk factors of corneal epithelial defects in mechanically ventilated children. *Critical Care Medicine, 37*(3), 1097–1100.

Kanski, J. J. (2007). *Clinical ophthalmology: A systemic approach* (6th ed.). Oxford: Butterworth-Heinemann.

Latkany, R. (2008). Dry eyes: Etiology and management. *Current Opinion in Ophthalmology, 19*(4), 287–291.

Rosenberg, J. B. & Eisen, L. A. (2008). Eye care in the intensive care unit: Narrative review and meta-analysis. *Critical Care Medicine, 36*(12), 3151–3155.

Stollery, R., Shaw, M., & Lee, A. (2005). *Ophthalmic nursing* (3rd ed.). Oxford: Blackwell.

Dying Care 5260

Definition: Promotion of physical comfort and psychological peace in the final phase of life

Activities:
- Identify the patient's care priorities
- Communicate willingness to discuss death
- Encourage patient and family to share feelings about death
- Assist patient and family to identify a shared meaning of death
- Seek to understand patient's actions, feelings, and attitudes
- Monitor patient for anxiety
- Stay physically close to frightened patient
- Monitor deterioration of physical and/or mental capabilities
- Reduce demand for cognitive functioning when patient is ill or fatigued
- Monitor mood changes
- Respect the patient's and family's specific care requests
- Include the family in care decisions and activities, as desired
- Support patient and family through stages of grief
- Monitor pain
- Minimize discomfort, when possible
- Medicate by alternate route when swallowing problems develop
- Postpone feeding when patient is fatigued
- Offer fluids and soft foods frequently
- Offer culturally appropriate foods
- Provide frequent rest periods
- Assist with basic care, as needed
- Respect the need for privacy
- Modify the environment, based on patient's needs and desires
- Support the family's efforts to remain at the bedside
- Facilitate obtaining spiritual support for patient and family
- Facilitate care by others, as appropriate
- Facilitate referral to hospice, as desired
- Facilitate discussion of funeral arrangements

1st edition 1992; revised 2013

Background Readings:

Adams, C. (2010). Dying with dignity in America: The transformational leadership of Florence Wald. *Journal of Professional Nursing. 26*(2), 125–132.

Cartwright, J. C., Miller, L, & Volpin, M. (2009). Hospice in assisted living: Promoting good quality care at end of life. *The Gerontologist, 49*(4), 508–516.

Klossner, N. J. & Hatfield, N. (2005). The dying child. In *Introductory maternity and pediatric nursing*. Philadelphia: Lippincott Williams & Wilkins.

LeGrand, S. B. & Walsh, D. W. (2010). Comfort measures: Practical care of the dying cancer patient. *American Journal of Hospice & Palliative Medicine, 27*(7), 488–493.

Law, R. (2009). Bridging worlds: Meeting the emotional needs of dying patients. *Journal of Advanced Nursing, 65*(12), 2630–2641.

Timby, B. K. & Smith, N. E. (2006). Caring for dying clients. In *Introductory medical-surgical nursing* (9th ed., pp. 102–111). Philadelphia: Lippincott Williams & Wilkins.

Dysreflexia Management 2560

Definition: Prevention and elimination of stimuli which cause hyperactive reflexes and inappropriate autonomic responses in a patient with a cervical or high thoracic cord lesion

Activities:
- Identify and minimize stimuli that may precipitate dysreflexia (e.g., bladder distention, renal calculi, infection, fecal impaction, rectal examination, suppository insertion, skin breakdown, and constrictive clothing or bed linen)
- Monitor for signs and symptoms of autonomic dysreflexia (e.g., paroxysmal hypertension, bradycardia, tachycardia, diaphoresis above the level of injury, facial flushing, pallor below the level of injury, headache, nasal congestion, engorgement of temporal and neck vessels, conjuctival congestion, chills without fever, pilomotor erection, and chest pain)
- Investigate and remove offending cause (e.g., distended bladder, fecal impaction, skin lesions, constricting bed clothes, supportive stockings, and abdominal binders)
- Place head of bed in upright position, as appropriate, to decrease blood pressure and promote cerebral venous return
- Stay with patient and monitor status every 3-5 minutes if hyperreflexia occurs
- Administer antihypertensive agents intravenously, as ordered
- Instruct patient and family about causes, symptoms, treatment, and prevention of dysreflexia

1st edition 1992; revised 2008

Background Readings:

McCance, K. L. & Huether, S. E. (2006). *Pathophysiology: The biologic basis for disease in adults and children* (5th ed.). St. Louis: Mosby.

Smeltzer, S. C. & Bare, B. G. (2004). *Brunner & Suddarth's textbook of medical-surgical nursing* (Vol. 2) (10th ed.). Philadelphia: Lippincott Williams & Wilkins.

Urden, L. D., Stacy, K. M., & Lough, M. E. (2006). *Thelan's critical care nursing: Diagnosis and management* (5th ed.). St. Louis: Mosby.

D

Dysrhythmia Management 4090

Definition: Preventing, recognizing, and facilitating treatment of abnormal cardiac rhythms

Activities:

- Ascertain patient and family history of heart disease and dysrhythmias
- Monitor for and correct oxygen deficits, acid-base imbalances, and electrolyte imbalances, which may precipitate dysrhythmias
- Apply electrocardiograhic (ECG) "wireless" telemetry or "hardwired" electrodes and connect to a cardiac monitor, as indicated
- Ensure appropriate lead selection in relation to patient needs
- Ensure proper lead placement and signal quality
- Set alarm parameters on the ECG monitor
- Ensure ongoing monitoring of bedside ECG by qualified individuals
- Monitor ECG changes that increase risk of dysrhythmia development (e.g., arrhythmia, ST-segment, ischemia, and QT-interval monitoring)
- Facilitate acquisition of a 12-lead ECG, as appropriate
- Note activities associated with the onset of dysrhythmias
- Note frequency and duration of dysrhythmia
- Monitor hemodynamic response to the dysrhythmia
- Determine whether patient has chest pain or syncope associated with the dysrhythmia
- Ensure ready access of emergency dysrhythmia medications
- Initiate and maintain IV access, as appropriate
- Administer Basic or Advanced Cardiac Life Support, if indicated
- Administer prescribed IV fluids and vasoconstrictor agents, as indicated, to facilitate tissue perfusion
- Assist with insertion of temporary transvenous or external pacemaker, as appropriate
- Instruct patient and family about the risks associated with the dysrhythmia(s)
- Prepare patient and family for diagnostic studies (e.g., cardiac catheterization or electrical physiological studies)
- Assist patient and family in understanding treatment options
- Instruct patient and family about actions and side effects of prescribed medications
- Instruct patient and family self-care behaviors associated with use of permanent pacemakers and AICD devices, as indicated
- Instruct patient and family measures to decrease the risk of recurrence of the dysrhythmia(s)
- Instruct patient and family how to access the emergency medical system
- Instruct a family member CPR, as appropriate

1st edition 1992; revised 2013

Background Readings:

American Association of Critical Care Nurses. (2006). *Core curriculum for critical care nursing* (6th ed.) [J. G. Alspach, Ed.]. Philadelphia: Saunders.

American Heart Association. (2005). Electric therapies: Automated external defibrillators, defibrillation, cardioversion, and pacing. *Circulation, 112* (24), 35–46.

American Heart Association. (2005). Guidelines for cardiopulmonary resuscitation and emergency cardiovascular care. *Circulation, 112*(24 Suppl. 1), IV1–IV211.

Drew, B., Califf, R., Funk, M., Kaufman, E. S., Krucoff, M. W., Laks, M. M., et al. (2004). Practice standards for electrocardiographic monitoring in hospital settings, An American Heart Association Scientific Statement from the Councils on Cardiovascular Nursing, Clinical Cardiology and Cardiovascular Disease in the Young. *Circulation, 110*(17), 2721–2746.

Funk, M., Winkler, C. G., May, J.L., Stephens, K., Fennie, K. P., Rose, L. L, et al. (2010). Unnecessary arrhythmia monitoring and underutilization of ischemia and QT interval monitoring in current clinical practice: Baseline results of the practical use of the latest standards for electrocardiography trial. *Journal of Electrocardiology, 43*(6):542–547.

Mckinley, M. G. (2011). Electrocardiographic leads and cardiac monitoring. In D. Wiegand, (Ed.), *AACN procedure manual for critical care* (6th ed., pp. 490–501). St. Louis: Saunders.

Urden, L. D., Stacy, K. M., & Lough, M. E. (2006). *Thelan's critical care nursing: Diagnosis and management* (5th ed.). St. Louis: Mosby.

Ear Care 1640

Definition: Prevention or minimization of threats to ear or hearing

Activities:
- Monitor auditory function
- Monitor anatomical structures for signs and symptoms of infection (e.g., inflamed tissue and drainage)
- Instruct patient on the ear's anatomical structures and their function
- Monitor for patient-reported signs and symptoms of dysfunction (e.g., pain, tenderness, itching, change in hearing, tinnitus, and vertigo)
- Monitor episodes of chronic otitis media (i.e., ensure appropriate preventative measures and treatments are employed)
- Instruct parent how to observe for signs and symptoms of auditory dysfunction or infection in child
- Administer hearing test, as appropriate
- Instruct patient on importance of annual hearing testing
- Instruct women of childbearing age on importance of prenatal care (e.g., avoidance of ototoxic medications, adequate dietary intake, and strict control of alcoholism)
- Inform parent about vaccinations which eliminate the possibility of sensorineural hearing loss (e.g., vaccination against rubella, measles, and mumps)
- Cleanse external ear using washcloth-covered finger
- Instruct patient how to cleanse ears
- Monitor for an excessive accumulation of cerumen
- Instruct patient not to use foreign objects smaller than patient's fingertip (e.g., cotton-tipped applicators, bobby pins, toothpicks, and other sharp objects) for cerumen removal
- Remove excessive cerumen with twisted end of washcloth while pulling down the auricle
- Consider ear irrigation for the removal of excessive cerumen if watchful waiting, manual removal, and ceruminolytic agents are ineffective

- Instruct parent to ensure child does not place foreign objects into ear
- Administer eardrops, as needed
- Instruct patient on proper eardrop administration
- Instruct patient how to monitor for persistent exposure to loud noise
- Instruct patient on importance of hearing protection during persistent exposure to loud noise
- Instruct parent to avoid bottle-feeding or allowing infant to bottle-feed while in supine position
- Instruct patient with pierced ears how to avoid infection at the insertion site
- Encourage use of earplugs for swimming, if patient is susceptible to ear infections
- Instruct patient on appropriate use of and care for assistive devices or treatments (e.g., hearing aids, medication regimen, and ear tubes)
- Instruct patient on signs and symptoms warranting reporting to health care provider
- Refer patient to ear care specialist, as needed

1st edition 1992; revised 2013

Background Readings:

Bryant, R. (2007). The child with cognitive, sensory, or communication impairment. In M. J. Hockenberry & D. Wilson (Eds.), *Wong's nursing care of infants and children* (8th ed., pp. 989–1027). St. Louis: Mosby.

Craven, R. F. & Hirnle, C. J. (2009). *Fundamentals of nursing: Human health and function* (6th ed.). Philadelphia: Lippincott Williams & Wilkins.

Russek, J. A. (2010). Care of patients with ear and hearing problems. In D. D. Ignatavicius & M. L. Workman (Eds.), *Medical-surgical nursing: Patient-centered collaborative care* (6th ed., pp. 1120–1137). St. Louis: Saunders.

Eating Disorders Management 1030

Definition: Prevention and treatment of severe diet restriction and overexercising or binging and purging of food and fluids

Activities:
- Collaborate with other members of health care team to develop a treatment plan; involve patient and/or significant others, as appropriate
- Confer with team and patient to set a target weight if patient is not within a recommended weight range for age and body frame
- Establish the amount of daily weight gain that is desired
- Confer with dietician to determine daily caloric intake necessary to attain and/or maintain target weight
- Teach and reinforce concepts of good nutrition with patient (and significant others as appropriate)
- Encourage patient to discuss food preferences with dietician
- Develop a supportive relationship with patient
- Monitor physiological parameters (vital signs, electrolytes), as needed
- Weigh on a routine basis (e.g., at same time of day and after voiding)

- Monitor intake and output of fluids, as appropriate
- Monitor daily caloric food intake
- Encourage patient self-monitoring of daily food intake and weight gain/maintenance, as appropriate
- Establish expectations for appropriate eating behaviors, intake of food/fluid, and amount of physical activity
- Use behavioral contracting with patient to elicit desired weight gain or maintenance behaviors
- Restrict food availability to scheduled, pre-served meals and snacks
- Observe patient during and after meals/snacks to ensure that adequate intake is achieved and maintained
- Accompany patient to bathroom during designated observation times following meals/snacks
- Limit time spent in bathroom during periods when not under observation
- Monitor patient for behaviors related to eating, weight loss, and weight gain

- Use behavior modification techniques to promote behaviors that contribute to weight gain and to limit weight loss behaviors, as appropriate
- Provide reinforcement for weight gain and behaviors that promote weight gain
- Provide remedial consequences in response to weight loss, weight loss behaviors, or lack of weight gain
- Provide support (e.g., relaxation therapy, desensitization exercises, opportunities to talk about feelings) as patient integrates new eating behaviors, changing body image, and lifestyle changes
- Encourage patient use of daily logs to record feelings, as well as circumstances surrounding urge to purge, vomit, overexercise
- Limit physical activity as needed to promote weight gain
- Provide a supervised exercise program, when appropriate
- Allow opportunity to make limited choices about eating and exercise as weight gain progresses in desirable manner
- Assist patient (and significant others as appropriate) to examine and resolve personal issues that may contribute to the eating disorder
- Assist patient to develop a self-esteem that is compatible with a healthy body weight
- Confer with health care team on routine basis about patient's progress
- Initiate maintenance phase of treatment when patient has achieved target weight and has consistently shown desired eating behaviors for designated period of time
- Monitor patient weight on routine basis
- Determine acceptable range of weight variation in relation to target range
- Place responsibility for choices about eating and physical activity with patient, as appropriate
- Provide support and guidance, as needed

- Assist patient to evaluate the appropriateness/consequences of choices about eating and physical activity
- Reinstitute weight gain protocol if patient is unable to remain in target weight range
- Institute a treatment program and follow-up care (medical, counseling) for home management

1st edition 1992; revised 2000

Background Readings:

Crisp, A. H. (1990). *Anorexia nervosa*. Philadelphia: Saunders.

Dudek, S. G. (2006). Obesity and eating disorders. In *Nutrition essentials for nursing practice* (5th rev. ed., pp. 375–416). Philadelphia: Lippincott Williams & Wilkins.

Garner, D. M., Rockert, W., Olmstead, M. P., Johnson, C., & Cosina, D. V. (1985). Psychoeducational principles in the treatment of bulimia and anorexia nervosa. In D. M. Garner & P. E. Garfinkel (Eds.), *Handbook of psychotherapy for anorexia nervosa and bulimia* (pp. 513–572). New York: Guilford Press.

Halmi, K. (1985). Behavioral management for anorexia nervosa. In D. M. Garner & P. E. Garfinkel (Eds.), *Handbook of psychotherapy for anorexia nervosa and bulimia* (pp. 147–159). New York: Guilford Press.

Love, C. C. & Seaton, H. (1991). Eating disorders: Highlights of nursing assessment and therapeutics. *Nursing Clinics of North America, 26*(3), 677–698.

Mohr, W. K. (2006). *Psychiatric-mental health nursing* (6th ed.). Philadelphia: Lippincott Williams & Wilkins.

Palmer, T. A. (1990). Anorexia nervosa, bulimia nervosa: Causal theories and treatment. *Nurse Practitioner, 15*(4), 13–21.

Plehn, K. W. (1990). Anorexia nervosa and bulimia: Incidence and diagnosis. *Nurse Practitioner, 15*(4), 22–31.

Electroconvulsive Therapy (ECT) Management   2570

Definition: Assisting with the safe and efficient provision of electroconvulsive (ECT) therapy in the treatment of psychiatric illness

Activities:
- Encourage patient (and significant others, as appropriate) to express feelings regarding the prospect of ECT treatment
- Instruct patient and/or significant others about the treatment
- Provide emotional support to patient and/or significant others, as needed
- Ensure that the patient (or the legal designee if the patient is unable to give informed consent) has adequate understanding of ECT when the physician seeks informed consent to administer ECT treatments
- Confirm there is a written order and signed consent for ECT treatment
- Record patient's height and weight in the medical record
- Discontinue or taper medications contraindicated for ECT as per physician order
- Review medication instructions with the outpatient who will be receiving ECT
- Inform the physician of any laboratory abnormalities for the patient
- Ensure that the patient receiving ECT has complied with the NPO requirement and medication instructions as ordered by the physician

- Assist patient to dress in loose fitting clothing (i.e., preferably hospital pajamas) that can be opened in front to allow placement of monitoring equipment
- Perform routine preoperative preparation (e.g., removal of dentures, jewelry, glasses, contact lenses; obtain vital signs; have patient void)
- Ensure that patient's hair is clean, dry, and devoid of hair ornaments in preparation for electrode placement
- Obtain a fasting blood glucose reading preprocedure and postprocedure for those patients who have insulin-dependent diabetes
- Ensure that patient is wearing an identification band
- Administer medications prior to and throughout the treatment as ordered by the physician
- Document the specifics of pretreatment preparation
- Verbally communicate unusual vital signs, physical complaints/symptoms, or unusual occurrences to the ECT nurse or ECT psychiatrist prior to the treatment
- Assist the treatment team in placing leads for various monitors (e.g., EEG, ECG) and monitoring equipment (e.g., pulse oximeter, blood pressure cuff, peripheral nerve stimulator) on to the patient
- Place a bite block in patient's mouth, and support chin allowing for airway patency during delivery of the electrical stimulus

- Document the time elapsed, as well as the type and amount of movement, during the seizure
- Document treatment-related data (e.g., medications given, patient response)
- Position the unconscious patient on his/her side on the stretcher with side rails raised
- Perform routine postoperative assessments (e.g., monitor vital signs, mental status, pulse oximeter, ECG)
- Administer oxygen, as ordered
- Suction oropharyngeal secretions, as needed
- Administer intravenous fluids, as ordered
- Provide supportive care and behavior management for postictal disorientation and agitation
- Notify the anesthesia provider or ECT psychiatrist if patient is destabilizing or failing to recover as expected
- Document care provided and patient response
- Observe patient in recovery area until fully awake, oriented to time/place, and can independently perform self-care activities
- Assist patient, when adequately alert, oriented, and physically stable to return to the inpatient nursing unit or another recovery area
- Provide the nursing staff that receive the post-ECT patient with a report on the treatment and patient's response to the treatment
- Determine level of observation needed by patient upon return to the unit or recovery area
- Provide that level of observation on the inpatient nursing unit or recovery area
- Place patient on fall precautions, as needed
- Observe the patient the first time that he/she attempts to ambulate independently to ensure that full muscle control has returned since receiving a muscle relaxant during the ECT treatment
- Ensure that the patient's gag reflex has returned prior to offering oral medications, food, or fluids
- Monitor patient for potential side effects of ECT (e.g., muscle soreness, headache, nausea, confusion, disorientation)
- Administer medications (e.g., analgesics, antiemetics) as ordered for the treatment of side effects
- Treat disorientation by restricting environmental stimulation and frequently reorienting patient

- Encourage patient to verbalize feelings about the experience of ECT
- Remind the amnesic patient that he/she had an ECT treatment
- Provide emotional support to the patient, as needed
- Reinforce teaching on ECT with patient and significant others, as appropriate
- Update significant others on patient's status, as appropriate
- Discharge the outpatient recipient of ECT to a responsible adult when patient had adequately recovered from the treatment per agency protocol
- Collaborate with treatment team to evaluate the effectiveness of the ECT (e.g., mood, cognitive status) and modify patient's treatment plan, as needed

4th edition 2004

Background Readings:

American Psychiatric Association. (2001). *The practice of electroconvulsive therapy. Recommendations for treatment, training, and privileging: A task force report of the American Psychiatric Association* (2nd ed.). Washington, DC: Author.

Frisch, N. C. (2001). Complementary and somatic therapies. In N. C. Frisch & L. E. Frisch (Eds.), *Psychiatric mental health nursing* (2nd ed., pp. 743–757). Clifton Park, NY: Delmar.

Scott, C. M. (2000). Mood disorders. In V. B. Carson (Ed.), *Mental health nursing: The nurse-patient journey* (pp. 679–720). Philadelphia: Saunders.

Sherr, J. (2000). Psychopharmacology and other biologic therapies. In K. M. Fortinash & P. A. Holoday-Worret (Eds.), *Psychiatric mental health nursing* (pp. 536–571). St. Louis: Mosby.

Stuart, G. (1998). Somatic therapies. In G. W. Stuart & M. T. Laraia (Eds.), *Principles and practice of psychiatric nursing* (6th ed., pp. 604–617). St. Louis: Mosby.

Townsend, M. C. (2000). *Psychiatric mental health nursing: Concepts of care* (3rd ed., pp. 283–290). Philadelphia: F. A. Davis.

University of Iowa Hospital & Clinics, Department of Nursing. (2001). *Electroconvulsive therapy – Pre-treatment.* Behavioral Health Service (BHS) – Psychiatric. Section II (7–10, 12).

Electrolyte Management   2000

Definition: Promotion of electrolyte balance and prevention of complications resulting from abnormal or undesired serum electrolyte levels

Activities:
- Monitor for abnormal serum electrolytes, as available
- Monitor for manifestations of electrolyte imbalance
- Maintain patent IV access
- Administer fluids, as prescribed, if appropriate
- Maintain accurate intake and output record
- Maintain intravenous solution containing electrolyte(s) at constant flow rate, as appropriate
- Administer supplemental electrolytes (e.g., oral, NG, and IV) as prescribed, if appropriate
- Consult physician on administration of electrolyte-sparing medications (e.g., spiranolactone), as appropriate
- Administer electrolyte-binding or electrolyte-excreting resins (e.g., sodium polystyrene sulfonate [Kayexalate]) as prescribed, if appropriate
- Obtain ordered specimens for laboratory analysis of electrolyte levels (e.g., ABG, urine, and serum levels), as appropriate

- Monitor for loss of electrolyte-rich fluids (e.g., nasogastric suction, ileostomy drainage, diarrhea, wound drainage, and diaphoresis)
- Institute measures to control excessive electrolyte loss (e.g., by resting the gut, changing type of diuretic, or administering antipyretics), as appropriate
- Irrigate nasogastric tubes with normal saline
- Minimize the amount of ice chips or oral intake consumed by patients with gastric tubes connected to suction
- Provide diet appropriate for patient's electrolyte imbalance (e.g., potassium-rich, low-sodium, and low-carbohydrate foods)
- Instruct the patient and/or family on specific dietary modifications, as appropriate
- Provide a safe environment for the patient with neurological and/or neuromuscular manifestations of electrolyte imbalance
- Promote orientation

- Teach patient and family about the type, cause, and treatments for electrolyte imbalance, as appropriate
- Consult physician if signs and symptoms of fluid and/or electrolyte imbalance persist or worsen
- Monitor patient's response to prescribed electrolyte therapy
- Monitor for side effects of prescribed supplemental electrolytes (e.g., GI irritation)
- Monitor closely the serum potassium levels of patients taking digitalis and diuretics
- Place on cardiac monitor, as appropriate
- Treat cardiac arrhythmias according to policy
- Prepare patient for dialysis (e.g., assist with catheter placement for dialysis), as appropriate

1st edition 1992; revised 2008

Background Readings:

American Association of Critical Care Nurses. (2006). *Core curriculum for critical care nursing* (6th ed.) [J. G. Alspach, Ed.]. Philadelphia: Saunders.

Banker, D., Whittier, G. C., & Rutecki, G. (2003). Acid-base disturbances: 5 rules that can simplify diagnosis. *Consultant, 43*(3), 381–384, 399–400.

McCance, K. L. & Huether, S. E. (2002). *Pathophysiology: The biologic basis for disease in adults and children.* St. Louis: Mosby.

Price, S. A. & Wilson, L. M. (2003). *Pathophysiology: Clinical concepts of disease processes* (6th ed.). St. Louis: Mosby.

Electrolyte Management: Hypercalcemia 2001

Definition: Promotion of calcium balance and prevention of complications resulting from serum calcium levels higher than desired

Activities:

- Monitor trends in serum levels of calcium (e.g., ionized calcium) in at risk populations (e.g., patients with malignancies, hyperparathyroidism, prolonged immobilization in severe or multiple fractures or spinal cord injuries)
- Estimate the concentration of the ionized fraction of calcium when total calcium levels only are reported (e.g., use serum albumin and appropriate formulas)
- Monitor patients receiving medication therapies that contribute to continued calcium elevation (e.g., thiazide diuretics, milk-alkali syndrome in peptic ulcer patients, Vitamin A and D intoxication, lithium)
- Monitor intake and output
- Monitor renal function (e.g., BUN and Cr levels)
- Monitor for digitalis toxicity (e.g., report serum levels above therapeutic range, monitor heart rate and rhythm before administering dose, and monitor for side effects)
- Observe for clinical manifestations of hypercalcemia (e.g., excessive urination, excessive thirst, muscle weakness, poor coordination, anorexia, intractable nausea [late sign], abdominal cramps, obstipation [late sign], confusion)
- Monitor for psychosocial manifestations of hypercalcemia (e.g., confusion, impaired memory, slurred speech, lethargy, acute psychotic behavior, coma, depression, and personality changes)
- Monitor for cardiovascular manifestations of hypercalcemia (e.g., dysrhythmias, prolonged PR interval, shortening of QT interval and ST segments, cone-shaped T wave, sinus bradycardia, heart blocks, hypertension, and cardiac arrest)
- Monitor for GI manifestations of hypercalcemia (e.g., anorexia, nausea, vomiting, constipation, peptic ulcer symptoms, abdominal pain, abdominal distension, paralytic ileus)
- Monitor for neuromuscular manifestations of hypercalcemia (e.g., weakness, malaise, paresthesias, myalgia, headache, hypotonia, decreased deep tendon reflexes, and poor coordination)
- Monitor for bone pain
- Monitor for electrolyte imbalances associated with hypercalcemia (e.g., hypophosphatemia or hyperphosphatemia, hyperchloremic acidosis, and hypokalemia from diuresis), as appropriate
- Provide therapies to promote renal excretion of calcium and limit further buildup of excess calcium (e.g., IV fluid hydration with normal saline or half-normal saline and diuretics, mobilizing the patient, restricting dietary calcium intake), as appropriate
- Administer prescribed medications to reduce serum ionized calcium levels (e.g., calcitonin, indomethacin, pilcamycin, phosphate, sodium bicarbonate, and glucocorticoids), as appropriate
- Monitor for systemic allergic reactions to calcitonin
- Monitor for fluid overload resulting from hydration therapy (e.g., daily weight, urine output, jugular vein distention, lung sounds, and right atrial pressure), as appropriate
- Avoid administration of vitamin D (e.g., calcifediol or ergocalciferol), which facilitates GI absorption of calcium, as appropriate
- Discourage intake of calcium (e.g., dairy products, seafood, nuts, broccoli, spinach, and supplements), as appropriate
- Avoid medications that prevent renal calcium excretion (e.g., lithium carbonate and thiazide diuretics), as appropriate
- Monitor for indications of kidney stone formation (e.g., intermittent pain, nausea, vomiting, and hematuria) resulting from calcium accumulation, as appropriate
- Encourage diet rich in fruits (e.g., cranberries, prunes, or plums) to increase urine acidity and reduce the risk of calcium stone formation, as appropriate
- Monitor for causes of increasing calcium levels (e.g., indications of severe dehydration and renal failure), as appropriate
- Encourage mobilization to prevent bone resorption
- Instruct patient and/or family in medications to avoid in hypercalcemia (e.g., certain antacids)
- Instruct the patient and/or family on measures instituted to treat the hypercalcemia
- Monitor for rebound hypocalcemia resulting from aggressive treatment of hypercalcemia
- Monitor for recurring hypercalcemia 1 to 3 days after cessation of therapeutic measures

1st edition 1992; revised 2008

Background Readings:

American Association of Critical Care Nurses. (2006). *Core curriculum for critical care nursing* (6th ed.) [J. G. Alspach, Ed.]. Philadelphia: Saunders.

American Heart Association. (2002). *ACLS Provider Manual.* Dallas, TX: Author.

American Nephrology Nurses' Association. (2005). *Nephrology nursing standards of practice and guidelines for care*. Pitman, NJ: Anthony J. Jannetti.

Cullen, L. M. (1992). Interventions related to fluid and electrolyte balance. In G. M. Bulechek & J. C. McCloskey (Eds.), Symposium on nursing interventions. *Nursing Clinics of North America, 27*(2), 569–597.

Oncology Nursing Society. (1996). *Statement on the scope and standards of oncology nursing practice*. Washington, DC: American Nurses Publishing.

Parker, J. (1998). *Contemporary nephrology nursing*. Pitman, NJ: Anthony J. Jannetti.

Smeltzer, S. C. & Bare, B. G. (2004). *Brunner & Suddarth's textbook of medical-surgical nursing* (10th ed.). Philadelphia: Lippincott Williams & Wilkins.

Springhouse Corporation. (2004). *Just the facts: Fluids and electrolytes*. Philadelphia: Lippincott Williams & Wilkins.

Electrolyte Management: Hyperkalemia   2002

E

Definition: Promotion of potassium balance and prevention of complications resulting from serum potassium levels higher than desired

Activities:

- Obtain specimens for laboratory analysis of potassium levels and associated electrolyte imbalances (e.g., ABG, urine, and serum levels), as appropriate
- Avoid false reports of hyperkalemia resulting from improper collection methodology (e.g., prolonged use of tourniquets during venous access, unusual exercise of extremity prior to venous access, delay in delivery of sample to laboratory)
- Verify all highly abnormal elevations of potassium
- Monitor cause(s) of increasing serum potassium levels (e.g., renal failure, excessive intake, and acidosis), as appropriate
- Monitor neurological manifestations of hyperkalemia (e.g., muscle weakness, reduced sensation, hyporeflexia, and paresthesias)
- Monitor cardiac manifestations of hyperkalemia (e.g., decreased cardiac output, heart blocks, peaked T waves, fibrillation, or asystole)
- Monitor gastrointestinal manifestations of hyperkalemia (e.g., nausea, intestinal colic)
- Monitor for hyperkalemia associated with a blood reaction, if appropriate
- Monitor lab values for changes in oxygenation or acid-base balance, as appropriate
- Monitor for symptoms of inadequate tissue oxygenation (e.g., pallor, cyanosis, and sluggish capillary refill)
- Administer electrolyte-binding and electrolyte-excreting resins (e.g., sodium polystyrene sulfonate [Kayexalate]) as prescribed, if appropriate
- Administer prescribed medications to shift potassium into the cell (e.g., 50% dextrose and insulin, sodium bicarbonate, calcium chloride, and calcium gluconate), as appropriate
- Insert rectal catheter for administration of cation-exchanging or binding resins (e.g., sodium polystyrene sulfonate [Kayexalate] per rectum), as appropriate
- Maintain potassium restrictions
- Maintain IV access
- Administer prescribed diuretics, as appropriate
- Avoid potassium-sparing diuretics (e.g., spironolactone [Aldactone] and triamterene [Dyrenium]), as appropriate
- Monitor for therapeutic effect of diuretic (e.g., increased urine output, decreased CVP/PCWP, and decreased adventitious breath sounds)
- Monitor renal function (e.g., BUN and Cr levels), if appropriate
- Monitor fluid status (e.g., intake and output, weight, adventitious breath sounds, shortness of breath), as appropriate
- Insert urinary catheter, if appropriate
- Prepare patient for dialysis (e.g., assist with catheter placement for dialysis), as appropriate
- Monitor patient's hemodynamic response to dialysis, as appropriate
- Monitor infused and returned volume of peritoneal dialysate, as appropriate
- Encourage adherence to dietary regimens (e.g., avoiding high-potassium foods, meeting dietary needs with salt substitutes and low-potassium foods), as appropriate
- Monitor for digitalis toxicity (e.g., report serum levels above therapeutic range, monitor heart rate and rhythm before administering dose, and monitor for side effects), as appropriate
- Monitor for unintentional potassium intake (e.g., penicillin G potassium or dietary), as appropriate
- Monitor potassium levels after therapeutic interventions (e.g., diuresis, dialysis, electrolyte-binding and electrolyte-excreting resins)
- Monitor for rebound hypokalemia (e.g., excessive diuresis, excessive use of cation-exchanging resins, and postdialysis)
- Monitor for cardiac instability and/or arrest and be prepared to institute ACLS, as appropriate
- Instruct patient about the rationale for use of diuretic therapy
- Instruct patient and/or family on measures instituted to treat the hyperkalemia

1st edition 1992; revised 2008

Background Readings:

American Association of Critical Care Nurses. (2006). *Core curriculum for critical care nursing* (6th ed.) [J. G. Alspach, Ed.]. Philadelphia: Saunders.

American Heart Association. (2002). *ACLS Provider Manual*. Dallas, TX: Author.

American Nephrology Nurses' Association. (2005). *Nephrology nursing standards of practice and guidelines for care*. Pitman, NJ: Anthony J. Jannetti.

Cullen, L. M. (1992). Interventions related to fluid and electrolyte balance. In G. M. Bulechek & J. C. McCloskey (Eds.), Symposium on nursing interventions. *Nursing Clinics of North America, 27*(2), 569–597.

Oncology Nursing Society. (1996). *Statement on the scope and standards of oncology nursing practice*. Washington, DC: American Nurses Publishing.

Parker, J. (1998). *Contemporary nephrology nursing*. Pitman, NJ: Anthony J. Jannetti.

Smeltzer, S. C. & Bare, B. G. (2004). *Brunner & Suddarth's textbook of medical-surgical nursing* (10th ed.). Philadelphia: Lippincott Williams & Wilkins.

Springhouse Corporation. (2004). *Just the facts: Fluids and electrolytes*. Philadelphia: Lippincott Williams & Wilkins.

E

Electrolyte Management: Hypermagnesemia   2003

Definition: Promotion of magnesium balance and prevention of complications resulting from serum magnesium levels higher than desired

Activities:
- Obtain specimens for laboratory analysis of magnesium level, as appropriate
- Monitor trends in magnesium levels, as available
- Monitor for electrolyte imbalances associated with hypermagnesemia (e.g., elevated BUN and Cr levels), as appropriate
- Assess dietary and pharmaceutical intake of magnesium
- Monitor for causes of increased magnesium levels (e.g., magnesium infusions, parenteral nutrition, magnesium rich dialysate solutions, antacids, laxatives, frequent magnesium sulfate enemas, lithium therapy, and renal insufficiency or failure)
- Monitor for causes of impaired magnesium excretion (e.g., renal insufficiency, advanced age)
- Monitor urinary output in patients on magnesium therapy
- Monitor for cardiovascular manifestations of hypermagnesemia (e.g., hypotension, flushing, bradycardia, heart blocks, widened QRS, prolonged QT, and peaked T waves)
- Monitor for CNS manifestations of hypermagnesemia (e.g., drowsiness, lethargy, confusion, and coma)
- Monitor for neuromuscular manifestations of hypermagnesemia (e.g., weak-to-absent deep tendon reflexes, muscle paralysis, and respiratory depression)
- Administer prescribed calcium chloride or calcium gluconate IV to antagonize neuromuscular effects of hypermagnesemia, as appropriate
- Increase fluid intake to promote dilution of serum magnesium levels and urine output, as indicated
- Maintain bed rest and limit activities, as appropriate
- Position patient to facilitate ventilation, as indicated
- Prepare patient for dialysis (e.g., assist with catheter placement for dialysis), as indicated
- Instruct patient and/or family on measures instituted to treat the hypermagnesemia

1st edition 1992; revised 2008

Background Readings:

American Association of Critical Care Nurses. (2006). *Core curriculum for critical care nursing* (6th ed.) [J. G. Alspach, Ed.]. Philadelphia: Saunders.

Cullen, L. M. (1992). Interventions related to fluid and electrolyte balance. In G. M. Bulechek & J. C. McCloskey (Eds.), Symposium on nursing interventions. *Nursing Clinics of North America, 27*(2), 569–598.

Luckey, A. & Parsa, C. (2003). Fluid and electrolytes in the aged. *Archives of Surgery, 138*(10), 1055–1060.

Metheny, N. M. (2000). *Fluid and electrolyte balance nursing considerations* (4th ed.). Philadelphia: Lippincott.

Springhouse Corporation. (2004). *Just the facts: Fluids and electrolytes.* Philadelphia: Lippincott Williams & Wilkins.

Topk, J. M. & Murray, P. T. (2003). Hypomagnesemia and hypermagnesemia. *Reviews in Endocrine & Metabolic Disorders, 4*(2), 195–206.

Electrolyte Management: Hypernatremia   2004

Definition: Promotion of sodium balance and prevention of complications resulting from serum sodium levels higher than desired

Activities:
- Monitor trends in serum levels of sodium in at-risk populations (e.g., unconscious patients, very old or very young patients, cognitively impaired patients, patients receiving hypertonic intravenous infusions)
- Monitor sodium levels closely in the patient experiencing conditions with escalating effects on sodium levels (e.g., diabetes insipidus, ADH deficiency, heatstroke, near drowning in sea water, dialysis)
- Monitor for neurological or musculoskeletal manifestations of hyponatremia (e.g., restlessness, irritability, weakness, disorientation, delusions, hallucinations, increased muscle tone or rigidity, tremors and hyperreflexia, seizures, coma [late signs])
- Monitor for cardiovascular manifestations of hyponatremia (e.g., orthostatic hypotension, flushed skin, peripheral and pulmonary edema, mild elevations in body temperature, tachycardia, flat neck veins)
- Monitor for GI manifestations of hyponatremia (e.g., dry swollen tongue and sticky mucous membranes)
- Obtain appropriate lab specimens for analysis of altered sodium levels (e.g., serum and urine sodium, serum and urine chloride, urine osmolality, and urine specific gravity)
- Monitor for electrolyte imbalances associated with hypernatremia (e.g., hyperchloremia and hyperglycemia), as appropriate
- Monitor for indications of dehydration (e.g., decreased sweating, decreased urine, decreased skin turgor, and dry mucous membranes)
- Monitor for insensible fluid loss (e.g., diaphoresis and respiratory infection)
- Monitor intake and output
- Weigh daily and monitor trends
- Maintain patent IV access
- Offer fluids at regular intervals for debilitated patients
- Administer adequate water intake for patients receiving enteral feeding therapy
- Collaborate for alternate routes of intake when oral intake is inadequate
- Administer isotonic (0.9%) saline, hypotonic (0.45% or 0.3%) saline, hypotonic (5%) dextrose, or diuretics based on fluid status and urine osmolality
- Administer prescribed antidiuretic agents (e.g., desmopressin [DDAVP] or vasopressin [Pitressin]) in the presence of diabetes insipidus
- Avoid administration/intake of high-sodium medications (e.g., sodium polystyrene sulfonate [Kayexalate], sodium bicarbonate, hypertonic saline)
- Maintain sodium restrictions, including monitoring medications with high-sodium content

- Administer prescribed diuretics in conjunction with hypertonic fluids for hypernatremia associated with hypervolemia
- Monitor for side effects resulting from rapid or over-corrections of hypernatremia (e.g., cerebral edema and seizures)
- Monitor renal function (e.g., BUN and Cr levels), if appropriate
- Monitor hemodynamic status, including CVP, MAP, PAP, and PCWP, if available
- Provide frequent oral hygiene
- Provide comfort measures to decrease thirst
- Promote skin integrity (e.g., monitor areas at risk for breakdown, promote frequent weight shifts, prevent shearing, and promote adequate nutrition), as appropriate
- Instruct patient on appropriate use of salt substitutes, as appropriate
- Instruct the patient/family about foods and over-the-counter medications that are high in sodium (e.g., canned foods and selected antacids)
- Institute seizure precautions, if indicated, in severe cases of hypernatremia
- Instruct the patient and/or family on measures instituted to treat the hypernatremia
- Instruct the family or significant other on signs and symptoms of hypovolemia (if hypernatremia is related to abnormal fluid intake or output)

1st edition 1992; revised 2008

Background Readings:

American Association of Critical Care Nurses. (2006). *Core curriculum for critical care nursing* (6th ed.) [J. G. Alspach, Ed.]. Philadelphia: Saunders.

American Heart Association. (2002). *ACLS provider manual.* Dallas, TX: Author.

American Nephrology Nurses' Association. (2005). *Nephrology nursing standards of practice and guidelines for care.* Pitman, NJ: Anthony J. Jannetti.

Cullen, L. M. (1992). Interventions related to fluid and electrolyte balance. In G. M. Bulechek & J. C. McCloskey (Eds.), Symposium on nursing interventions. *Nursing Clinics of North America, 27*(2), 569–597.

Oncology Nursing Society. (1996). *Statement on the scope and standards of oncology nursing practice.* Washington, DC: American Nurses Publishing.

Parker, J. (1998). *Contemporary nephrology nursing.* Pitman, NJ: Anthony J. Jannetti.

Smeltzer, S. C. & Bare, B. G. (2004). *Brunner & Suddarth's textbook of medical-surgical nursing* (10th ed.). Philadelphia: Lippincott Williams & Wilkins.

Springhouse Corporation. (2004). *Just the facts: Fluids and electrolytes.* Philadelphia: Lippincott Williams & Wilkins.

E

Electrolyte Management: Hyperphosphatemia   2005

Definition: Promotion of phosphate balance and prevention of complications resulting from serum phosphate levels higher than desired

Activities:
- Monitor trends in serum levels of phosphorus (e.g., inorganic phosphorus) in at risk-populations (e.g., patients receiving chemotherapy, patients with high phosphate intake, patients with high vitamin D intake)
- Monitor phosphate levels closely in the patient experiencing conditions with escalating effects on phosphate levels (e.g., acute and chronic renal failure, hypoparathyroidism, diabetic ketoacidosis, respiratory acidosis, profound muscle necrosis, rhabdomyolysis)
- Obtain specimens for laboratory analysis of phosphate and associated electrolyte levels (e.g., ABG, urine, and serum levels), as appropriate
- Monitor for electrolyte imbalances associated with hyperphosphatemia
- Monitor for manifestations of hyperphosphatemia (e.g., tingling sensations in fingertips and around mouth, anorexia, nausea, vomiting, muscle weakness, hyperreflexia, tetany, tachycardia)
- Monitor for symptoms of soft tissue, joint, and artery calcifications (e.g., decreased urine output, impaired vision, palpitations)
- Administer prescribed phosphate-binding and diuretic medications with food to decrease absorption of dietary phosphate
- Provide comfort measures for the GI effects of hyperphosphatemia
- Prevent constipation resulting from phosphate-binding medications
- Avoid laxatives and enemas that contain phosphate
- Administer prescribed calcium and vitamin D supplements to reduce phosphate levels
- Avoid phosphate-rich foods (e.g., dairy products, whole-grain cereal, nuts, dried fruits or vegetables, and organ meats)
- Prepare patient for dialysis (e.g., assist with catheter placement for dialysis), as appropriate
- Institute seizure precautions
- Instruct the patient and/or family on measures instituted to treat the hyperphosphatemia
- Instruct patient and/or family on signs and symptoms of impending hypocalcemia (e.g., changes in urine output)

1st edition 1992; revised 2008

Background Readings:

American Association of Critical Care Nurses. (2006). *Core curriculum for critical care nursing* (6th ed.) [J. G. Alspach, Ed.]. Philadelphia: Saunders.

American Heart Association. (2002). *ACLS provider manual.* Dallas, TX: Author.

American Nephrology Nurses' Association. (2005). *Nephrology nursing standards of practice and guidelines for care.* Pitman, NJ: Anthony J. Jannetti.

Cullen, L. M. (1992). Interventions related to fluid and electrolyte balance. In G. M. Bulechek & J. C. McCloskey (Eds.), Symposium on nursing interventions. *Nursing Clinics of North America, 27*(2), 569–597.

Oncology Nursing Society. (1996). *Statement on the scope and standards of oncology nursing practice.* Washington, DC: American Nurses Publishing.

Parker, J. (1998). *Contemporary nephrology nursing.* Pitman, NJ: Anthony J. Jannetti.

Smeltzer, S. C. & Bare, B. G. (2004). *Brunner & Suddarth's textbook of medical-surgical nursing* (10th ed.). Philadelphia: Lippincott Williams & Wilkins.

Springhouse Corporation. (2004). *Just the facts: Fluids and electrolytes.* Philadelphia: Lippincott Williams & Wilkins.

Electrolyte Management: Hypocalcemia   2006

Definition: Promotion of calcium balance and prevention of complications resulting from serum calcium levels lower than desired

Activities:

- Monitor trends in serum levels of calcium (e.g., ionized calcium) in at-risk populations (e.g., primary or surgically induced hypoparathyroidism, radical neck dissection [particularly first 24 to 48 hours postoperatively] any thyroid or parathyroid surgery, patients receiving massive transfusions of citrated blood, cardiopulmonary bypass)
- Monitor calcium levels closely in the patient experiencing conditions with depleting effects on calcium levels (e.g., osteoporosis, pancreatitis, renal failure, inadequate vitamin D consumption, hemodilution, chronic diarrhea, small bowel disease, medullary thyroid cancer, low serum albumin, alcohol abuse, renal tubular dysfunction, severe burns or infections, prolonged bedrest)
- Estimate the concentration of the ionized fraction of calcium when total calcium levels only are reported (e.g., use serum albumin and appropriate formulas)
- Observe for clinical manifestations of hypocalcemia (e.g., tetany [classic sign]; tingling in tips of fingers, feet, or mouth; spasms of muscles in face or extremities; Trousseau's sign; Chvostek's sign; altered deep tendon reflexes; seizures [late sign]).
- Monitor for psychosocial manifestations of hypocalcemia (e.g., personality disturbances, impaired memory, confusion, anxiety, irritability, depression, delirium, hallucinations, and psychosis)
- Monitor for cardiovascular manifestations of hypocalcemia (e.g., decreased contractility, decreased cardiac output, hypotension, lengthened ST segment, and prolonged QT interval, torsades de pointes)
- Monitor for GI manifestations of hypocalcemia (e.g., nausea, vomiting, constipation, and abdominal pain from muscle spasm)
- Monitor for integument manifestations of hypocalcemia (e.g., scaling, eczema, alopecia, and hyperpigmentation)
- Monitor for electrolyte imbalances associated with hypocalcemia (e.g., hyperphosphatemia, hypomagnesemia, and alkalosis)
- Monitor patients receiving medications that contribute to continued calcium loss (e.g., loop diuretics, aluminum-containing antacids, aminoglycosides, caffeine, cisplatin, corticosteroids, mithramycin, phosphates, isoniazid)
- Monitor fluid status, including intake and output
- Monitor renal function (e.g., BUN and Cr levels)
- Maintain patent IV access
- Administer appropriate prescribed calcium salt (e.g., calcium carbonate, calcium chloride, and calcium gluconate) using only calcium diluted in D_5W, administered slowly with a volumetric infusion pump, as indicated
- Maintain bedrest for patients receiving parenteral calcium replacement therapy to control side effect of postural hypotension
- Monitor blood pressure in patients receiving parenteral calcium replacement therapy
- Monitor infusions of calcium chloride closely for adverse effects (higher incidence of tissue sloughing with IV infiltration; not usually initial medication of choice in treatment plans)
- Monitor for side effects of IV administration of ionized calcium (e.g., calcium chloride), such as increased effects of digitalis, digitalis toxicity, bradycardia, postural hypotension, cardiac arrest, thrombophlebitis, soft tissue damage with extravasation, clotting, and thrombus formation, as appropriate

- Avoid administration of medications decreasing serum ionized calcium (e.g., bicarbonate and citrated blood), as appropriate
- Avoid administration of calcium salts with phosphates or bicarbonates to prevent precipitation
- Monitor for acute laryngeal spasm and tetany requiring emergency airway management
- Monitor for exacerbation of tetany resulting from hyperventilation or pressure on efferent nerves (e.g., by crossing legs), as appropriate
- Initiate seizure precautions in patients with severe hypocalcemia
- Initiate safety precautions in patients with potentially harmful psychosocial manifestations (e.g., confusion)
- Encourage increased oral intake of calcium (e.g., at least 1000 to 1500 mg/day from dairy products, canned salmon, sardines, fresh oysters, nuts, broccoli, spinach, and supplements), as appropriate
- Provide adequate intake of vitamin D (e.g., vitamin supplement and organ meats) to facilitate GI absorption of calcium, as appropriate
- Administer phosphate-decreasing medications (e.g., aluminum hydroxide, calcium acetate or calcium carbonate) as indicated in chronic renal failure patients
- Provide pain relief/comfort measures
- Monitor for over-correction and hypercalcemia
- Instruct the patient and/or family on measures instituted to treat hypocalcemia
- Instruct the patient on need for life-style changes to control hypocalcemia (regular weight-bearing exercises, decreased alcohol and caffeine intake, decreased cigarette smoking, strategies to reduce risks for falls)
- Instruct patient on medications which decrease the rate of bone loss (e.g., calcitonin, alendronate, raloxifene, risedronate)

1st edition 1992; revised 2008

Background Readings:

American Association of Critical Care Nurses. (2006). *Core curriculum for critical care nursing* (6th ed.) [J. G. Alspach, Ed.]. Philadelphia: Saunders.

American Heart Association. (2002). *ACLS Provider Manual.* Dallas, TX: Author.

American Nephrology Nurses' Association. (2005). *Nephrology nursing standards of practice and guidelines for care.* Pitman, NJ: Anthony J. Jannetti.

Cullen, L. M. (1992). Interventions related to fluid and electrolyte balance. In G. M. Bulechek & J. C. McCloskey (Eds.), Symposium on nursing interventions. *Nursing Clinics of North America, 27*(2), 569–597.

Oncology Nursing Society. (1996). *Statement on the scope and standards of oncology nursing practice.* Washington, DC: American Nurses Publishing.

Parker, J. (1998). *Contemporary nephrology nursing.* Pitman, NJ: Anthony J. Jannetti.

Smeltzer, S. C. & Bare, B. G. (2004). *Brunner & Suddarth's textbook of medical-surgical nursing* (10th ed.). Philadelphia, PA: Lippincott Williams & Wilkins.

Springhouse Corporation. (2004). *Just the facts: Fluids and electrolytes.* Philadelphia: Lippincott Williams & Wilkins.

Electrolyte Management: Hypokalemia 2007

Definition: Promotion of potassium balance and prevention of complications resulting from serum potassium levels lower than desired

Activities:

- Obtain specimens for laboratory analysis of potassium levels and associated electrolyte imbalances (e.g., ABG, urine, and serum levels), as appropriate
- Monitor for early presence of hypokalemia to prevent life-threatening sequelae in at-risk patients (e.g., fatigue, anorexia, muscle weakness, decreased bowel motility, paresthesias, dysrhythmias)
- Monitor lab values associated with hypokalemia (e.g., elevated glucose, metabolic alkalosis, reduced urine osmolality, urine potassium, hypochloremia, and hypocalcemia), as appropriate
- Monitor intracellular shifts causing decreasing serum potassium levels (e.g., metabolic alkalosis; dietary [especially carbohydrate] intake; and administration of insulin), as appropriate
- Monitor renal cause(s) of decreasing serum potassium levels (e.g., diuretics, diuresis, metabolic alkalosis, and potassium-losing nephritis), as appropriate
- Monitor GI cause(s) of decreasing serum potassium levels (e.g., diarrhea, fistulas, vomiting, and continuous NG suction), as appropriate
- Monitor dilutional cause(s) of decreasing serum potassium levels (e.g., administration of hypotonic solutions and increased water retention, secondary to inappropriate ADH), as appropriate
- Administer supplemental potassium, as prescribed
- Collaborate with physician and pharmacist for appropriate potassium preparations when supplementing potassium (e.g., IV potassium supplements only for severe or symptomatic hypokalemia or when the GI tract cannot be used)
- Monitor renal functions, EKG, and serum potassium levels during replacement, as appropriate
- Prevent/reduce irritation from oral potassium supplement (e.g., administer PO or NG potassium supplements during or after meals to minimize GI irritation, controlled-release microencapsulated tablets are preferred to decrease GI irritation and erosion, divide larger daily oral doses)
- Prevent/reduce irritation from intravenous potassium supplement (e.g., consider infusion via central line for concentrations greater than 10 mEq/L, dilute IV potassium adequately, administer IV supplement slowly, apply topical anesthetic to IV site), as appropriate
- Maintain patent IV access
- Provide continuous cardiac monitoring if potassium replacement rate exceeds 10 mEq/hour
- Administer potassium-sparing diuretics (e.g., spironolactone [Aldactone] or triamterene [Dyrenium]), as appropriate
- Monitor for digitalis toxicity (e.g., report serum levels above therapeutic range, monitor heart rate and rhythm before administering dose, and monitor for side effects), as appropriate
- Avoid administration of alkaline substances (e.g., IV sodium bicarbonate and PO or NG antacids), as appropriate
- Monitor neurological manifestations of hypokalemia (e.g., muscle weakness, altered level of consciousness, drowsiness, apathy, lethargy, confusion, and depression)
- Monitor cardiac manifestations of hypokalemia (e.g., hypotension, T wave flattening, T wave inversion, presence of U wave, ectopy, tachycardia, and weak pulse)
- Monitor renal manifestations of hypokalemia (e.g., acidic urine, reduced urine osmolality, nocturia, polyuria, and polydipsia)
- Monitor GI manifestations of hypokalemia (e.g., anorexia, nausea, cramps, constipation, distention, and paralytic ileus)
- Monitor pulmonary manifestations of hypokalemia (e.g., hypoventilation and respiratory muscle weakness)
- Position patient to facilitate ventilation
- Monitor for symptoms of respiratory failure (e.g., low PaO_2 and elevated $PaCO_2$ levels and respiratory muscle fatigue)
- Monitor for rebound hyperkalemia
- Monitor for excessive diuresis
- Monitor fluid status, including intake and output, as appropriate
- Provide foods rich in potassium (e.g., salt substitutes, dried fruits, bananas, green vegetables, tomatoes, yellow vegetables, chocolate, and dairy products), as appropriate
- Instruct patient and/or family on measures instituted to treat the hypokalemia
- Provide patient education related to hypokalemia resulting from laxative or diuretic abuse

1st edition 1992; revised 2008

Background Readings:

American Association of Critical Care Nurses. (2006). *Core curriculum for critical care nursing* (6th ed.) [J. G. Alspach, Ed.]. Philadelphia: Saunders.

American Heart Association. (2002). *ACLS provider manual.* Dallas, TX: Author.

American Nephrology Nurses' Association. (2005). *Nephrology nursing standards of practice and guidelines for care.* Pitman, NJ: Anthony J. Jannetti.

Cullen, L. M. (1992). Interventions related to fluid and electrolyte balance. In G. M. Bulechek & J. C. McCloskey (Eds.), Symposium on nursing interventions. *Nursing Clinics of North America, 27*(2), 569–597.

Infusion Nursing Society. (2006). Infusion nursing standards of practice. *Journal of Infusion Nursing, 29*(1S).

Kraft, M., Btaiche, I., Sacks, G., & Kudsk, K. (2005). Treatment of electrolyte disorders in adult patients in the intensive care unit. *American Journal Health-System Pharmacists, 62*(16), 1663–1682.

Oncology Nursing Society. (1996). *Statement on the scope and standards of oncology nursing practice.* Washington, DC: American Nurses Publishing.

Parker, J. (1998). *Contemporary nephrology nursing.* Pitman, NJ: Anthony J. Jannetti.

Pestana, C. (2000). *Fluids and electrolytes in the surgical patient.* Philadelphia: Lippincott Williams & Wilkins.

Smeltzer, S. C. & Bare, B. G. (2004). *Brunner & Suddarth's textbook of medical-surgical nursing* (10th ed.). Philadelphia: Lippincott Williams & Wilkins.

Springhouse Corporation. (2002). *Fluids & electrolytes made incredibly easy* (2nd ed.). Philadelphia: Lippincott Williams & Wilkins.

Springhouse Corporation. (2004). *Just the facts: Fluids and electrolytes.* Philadelphia: Lippincott Williams & Wilkins.

E

Electrolyte Management: Hypomagnesemia   2008

Definition: Promotion of magnesium balance and prevention of complications resulting from serum magnesium levels lower than desired

Activities:

- Obtain specimens for laboratory analysis of magnesium level, as appropriate
- Monitor trends in magnesium levels, as available
- Monitor for electrolyte imbalances associated with hypomagnesemia (e.g., hypokalemia, hypocalcemia), as appropriate
- Monitor for reduced intake due to malnutrition, prolonged IV fluid therapy, or use of enteral or parenteral nutrition containing insufficient amounts of magnesium, as appropriate
- Monitor for decreased levels of magnesium resulting from inadequate absorption of magnesium (e.g., surgical resection of bowel, pancreatic insufficiency, inflammatory bowel disease, and excess dietary intake of calcium), as appropriate
- Monitor for increased urinary excretion of magnesium (e.g., diuretics, renal disorders, renal excretion after transplant, diabetic ketoacidosis, hyper/hypoparathyroidism), as appropriate
- Monitor for increased GI loss of magnesium (e.g., NG suctioning, diarrhea, fistula drainage, acute pancreatitis), as appropriate
- Monitor renal sufficiency in patients receiving magnesium replacement
- Offer foods rich in magnesium (e.g., unmilled grains, green leafy vegetables, nuts, and legumes), as appropriate
- Administer prescribed oral supplements as indicated, continuing for several days after magnesium level returns to normal
- Administer prescribed IV magnesium for symptomatic hypomagnesemia, as appropriate
- Monitor for side effects of IV magnesium replacement (e.g., flushing, sweating, sensation of heat, and hypocalcemia), as appropriate
- Keep calcium gluconate available during rapid magnesium replacement in case of associated hypocalcemic tetany or apnea, as appropriate
- Avoid administration of magnesium-depleting medications (e.g., loop and thiazide diuretics, aminoglycoside antibiotics, amphotericin B, digoxin, and cisplatin), as appropriate

- Monitor for CNS manifestations of hypomagnesemia (e.g., lethargy, insomnia, auditory and visual hallucinations, agitation, and personality change)
- Monitor for neuromuscular manifestations of hypomagnesemia (e.g., weakness, muscle twitching, foot or leg cramps, paresthesias, hyperactive deep tendon reflexes, Chvostek's sign, Trousseau's sign, dysphagia, nystagmus, seizures, and tetany)
- Monitor for GI manifestations of hypomagnesemia (e.g., nausea, vomiting, anorexia, diarrhea, and abdominal distention)
- Monitor for cardiovascular manifestations of hypomagnesemia (e.g., widened QRS complexes, torsades de pointes, ventricular tachycardia, flattened T waves, depressed ST segments, prolonged QT, ectopy, tachycardia, elevated serum digoxin level)
- Instruct patient and/or family on measures instituted to treat the hypomagnesemia

1st edition 1992; revised 2008

Background Readings:

American Association of Critical Care Nurses. (2006). *Core curriculum for critical care nursing* (6th ed.) [J. G. Alspach, Ed.]. Philadelphia: Saunders.

Cullen, L. M. (1992). Interventions related to fluid and electrolyte balance. In G. M. Bulechek & J. C. McCloskey (Eds.), Symposium on nursing interventions. *Nursing Clinics of North America, 27*(2), 569–598.

Luckey, A. & Parsa, C. (2003). Fluid and electrolytes in the aged. *Archives of Surgery, 138*(10), 1055–1060.

Metheny, N. M. (2000). *Fluid and electrolyte balance: Nursing considerations* (4th ed.). Philadelphia: Lippincott Williams & Wilkins.

Saris, N., Mervaala, E., Karppanen, H., Khawaja, J. & Lewenstam, A. (2000). Magnesium: An update on physiology, clinical and analytical aspects. *Clinica Chimica Acta, 294*(1-2), pp. 1–26.

Springhouse Corporation. (2004). *Just the facts: Fluids and electrolytes.* Philadelphia: Lippincott Williams & Wilkins.

Topk, J. M. & Murray, P. T. (2003). Hypomagnesemia and hypermagnesemia. *Reviews in Endocrine & Metabolic Disorders, 4*(2), 195–206.

Electrolyte Management: Hyponatremia   2009

Definition: Promotion of sodium balance and prevention of complications resulting from serum sodium levels lower than desired

Activities:

- Monitor trends in serum levels of sodium in-at risk populations (e.g., confused elderly, patients on low-salt diet or diuretics)
- Monitor sodium levels closely in the patient experiencing conditions with depleting effects on sodium levels (e.g., oat-cell lung cancer, aldosterone deficiency, adrenal insufficiency, syndrome of inappropriate antidiuretic hormone [SIADH], hyperglycemia, vomiting, diarrhea, water intoxication, fistulas, excessive sweating)
- Monitor for neurological or musculoskeletal manifestations of hyponatremia (e.g., lethargy, increased ICP, altered mental status, headache, apprehension, fatigue, tremors, muscle weakness or cramping, hyperreflexia, seizures, coma [late signs])

- Monitor for cardiovascular manifestations of hyponatremia (e.g., orthostatic hypotension, elevated blood pressure, cold and clammy skin, poor skin turgor, hypovolemia, hypervolemia)
- Monitor for GI manifestations of hyponatremia (e.g., dry mucosa, decreased saliva production, anorexia, nausea, vomiting, abdominal cramps, and diarrhea)
- Obtain appropriate lab specimens for analysis of altered sodium levels (e.g., serum and urine sodium, serum and urine chloride, urine osmolality, and urine specific gravity)
- Monitor for electrolyte imbalances associated with hyponatremia (e.g., hypokalemia, metabolic acidosis, and hyperglycemia)
- Monitor for renal loss of sodium (oliguria)
- Monitor renal function (e.g., BUN and Cr levels)

- Monitor intake and output
- Weigh daily and monitor trends
- Monitor for indications of fluid overload/retention (e.g., crackles, elevated CVP or pulmonary capillary wedge pressure, edema, neck vein distention, and ascites), as appropriate
- Monitor hemodynamic status, including CVP, MAP, PAP, and PCWP, as available
- Restrict water intake as safest first line treatment of hyponatremia in patients with normal or excess fluid volume (800ml/24 hours)
- Maintain fluid restriction, as appropriate
- Encourage foods/fluids high in sodium, as appropriate
- Monitor all parenteral fluids for sodium content
- Administer hypertonic (3% to 5%) saline at 3 ml/kg/hr or per policy for cautious correction of hyponatremia in intensive care settings under close observation only, as appropriate
- Prevent rapid or over-correction of hyponatremia (e.g., serum Na level of greater than 125 mEq/L and hypokalemia)
- Administer plasma expanders cautiously and only in the presence of hypovolemia
- Avoid excessive administration of hypotonic IV fluids, especially in the presence of SIADH
- Administer diuretics only as indicated (e.g., thiazides, loop diuretics similar to furosemide, or ethacrynic acid)
- Limit patient activities to conserve energy, as appropriate
- Institute seizure precautions, if indicated, in severe cases of hyponatremia
- Instruct the patient and/or family on all therapies instituted to treat the hyponatremia

1st edition 1992; revised 2008

Background Readings:

American Association of Critical Care Nurses. (2006). *Core curriculum for critical care nursing* (6th ed.) [J. G. Alspach, Ed.]. Philadelphia: Saunders.

American Heart Association. (2002). *ACLS provider manual.* Dallas, TX: Author.

American Nephrology Nurses' Association. (2005). *Nephrology nursing standards of practice and guidelines for care.* Pitman, NJ: Anthony J. Jannetti.

Cullen, L. M. (1992). Interventions related to fluid and electrolyte balance. In G. M. Bulechek & J. C. McCloskey (Eds.), Symposium on nursing interventions. *Nursing Clinics of North America, 27*(2), 569–597.

Oncology Nursing Society. (1996). *Statement on the scope and standards of oncology nursing practice.* Washington, DC: American Nurses.

Parker, J. (1998). *Contemporary nephrology nursing.* Pitman, NJ: Anthony J. Jannetti.

Smeltzer, S. C. & Bare, B. G. (2004). *Brunner & Suddarth's textbook of medical-surgical nursing* (10th ed.). Philadelphia: Lippincott Williams & Wilkins.

Springhouse Corporation. (2004). *Just the facts: Fluids and electrolytes.* Philadelphia: Lippincott Williams & Wilkins.

E

Electrolyte Management: Hypophosphatemia   2010

Definition: Promotion of phosphate balance and prevention of complications resulting from serum phosphate levels lower than desired

Activities:

- Monitor trends in serum levels of inorganic phosphorus in at-risk populations (e.g., alcoholics, anorexia nervosa patients, severely debilitated elderly)
- Monitor phosphate levels closely in the patient experiencing conditions with depleting effects on phosphate levels (e.g., hyperparathyroidism, diabetic ketoacidosis, major thermal burns, prolonged intense hyperventilation, overzealous administration of simple carbohydrates in severe protein-calorie malnutrition)
- Obtain specimens for laboratory analysis of phosphate and associated electrolyte levels (e.g., ABG, urine, and serum levels), as appropriate
- Monitor for electrolyte imbalances associated with hypophosphatemia (e.g., hypokalemia; hypomagnesemia; respiratory alkalosis; metabolic acidosis)
- Monitor for decreasing levels of phosphate resulting from reduced intake and absorption (e.g., starvation, hyperalimentation without phosphate, vomiting, small bowel or pancreatic disease, diarrhea, and ingestion of aluminum or magnesium hydroxide antacids)
- Monitor for decreasing phosphate levels resulting from renal loss (e.g., hypokalemia, hypomagnesemia, heavy metal poisoning, alcohol, hemodialysis with phosphate-poor dialysate, thiazide diuretics, and vitamin D deficiency)
- Monitor for decreasing phosphate levels resulting from extracellular to intracellular shifts (e.g., glucose administration, insulin administration, alkalosis, and hyperalimentation)
- Monitor for neuromuscular manifestations of hypophosphatemia (e.g., weakness, lassitude, malaise, tremors, paresthesias, ataxia, muscle pain, increased creatinine phosphokinase, abnormal EMG, and rhabdomyolysis)
- Monitor for CNS manifestations of hypophosphatemia (e.g., irritability, fatigue, memory loss, reduced attention span, confusion, convulsions, coma, abnormal EEG, numbness, decreased reflexes, impaired sensory function, and cranial nerve palsies)
- Monitor for skeletal manifestations of hypophosphatemia (e.g., aching bone pain, fractures, and joint stiffness)
- Monitor for cardiovascular manifestations of hypophosphatemia (e.g., decreased contractility, decreased cardiac output, heart failure, and ectopy)
- Monitor for pulmonary manifestations of hypophosphatemia (e.g., rapid, shallow respirations; decreased tidal volume; and decreased minute ventilation)
- Monitor for GI manifestations of hypophosphatemia (e.g., nausea, vomiting, anorexia, impaired liver function, and portal hypertension)
- Monitor for hematological manifestations of hypophosphatemia (e.g., anemia, increased hemoglobin affinity with oxygen leading to increased SaO_2, increased risk of infection resulting from impaired WBC functioning, thrombocytopenia, bruising and hemorrhage resulting from platelet dysfunction)
- Administer prescribed phosphate supplements IV (replacement rate not to exceed 10 mEq/hr), as appropriate
- Administer PO phosphate replacement therapy when possible (preferred route)

- Monitor IV sites carefully for extravasation (tissue sloughing and necrosis occur with infiltration of phosphate supplements)
- Monitor for rapid or over-correction of hypophosphatemia (e.g., hyperphosphatemia, hypocalcemia, hypotension, hyperkalemia, hypernatremia, tetany, metastatic calcifications)
- Monitor renal function during parental phosphate supplementations, as appropriate
- Avoid phosphate-binding and diuretic medications (e.g., Amphojel, Phos-Lo cookie, and Basaljel)
- Encourage increased oral intake of phosphate (e.g., dairy products, whole-grain cereal, nuts, dried fruits or vegetables, and organ meats), as appropriate
- Conserve muscle strength (e.g., assist with passive or active range-of-motion exercises)
- Institute preventive care for infection avoidance (hypophosphatemia causes severe depletion of granulocytes)
- Instruct the patient and/or family on all measures instituted to treat the hypophosphatemia

1st edition 1992; revised 2008

Background Readings:

American Association of Critical Care Nurses. (2006). *Core curriculum for critical care nursing* (6th ed.) [J. G. Alspach, Ed.]. Philadelphia: Saunders.

American Heart Association. (2002). *ACLS provider manual.* Dallas, TX: Author.

American Nephrology Nurses' Association. (2005). *Nephrology nursing standards of practice and guidelines for care.* Pitman, NJ: Anthony J. Jannetti.

Cullen, L. M. (1992). Interventions related to fluid and electrolyte balance. In G. M. Bulechek & J. C. McCloskey (Eds.), Symposium on nursing interventions. *Nursing Clinics of North America, 27*(2), 569–597.

Oncology Nursing Society. (1996). *Statement on the scope and standards of oncology nursing practice.* Washington, DC: American Nurses.

Parker, J. (1998). *Contemporary nephrology nursing.* Pitman, NJ: Anthony J. Jannetti.

Smeltzer, S. C. & Bare, B. G. (2004). *Brunner & Suddarth's textbook of medical-surgical nursing* (Vol. 1) (10th ed.). Philadelphia: Lippincott Williams & Wilkins.

Springhouse Corporation. (2004). *Just the facts: Fluids and electrolytes.* Philadelphia: Lippincott Williams & Wilkins.

Electrolyte Monitoring   2020

Definition: Collection and analysis of patient data to regulate electrolyte balance

Activities:

- Monitor the serum level of electrolytes
- Monitor serum albumin and total protein levels, as indicated
- Monitor for associated acid-base imbalances
- Identify possible causes of electrolyte imbalances
- Recognize and report presence of electrolyte imbalances
- Monitor for fluid loss and associated loss of electrolytes, as appropriate
- Monitor for Chvostek and/or Trousseau sign
- Monitor for neurological manifestation of electrolyte imbalance (e.g., altered sensorium and weakness)
- Monitor adequacy of ventilation
- Monitor serum and urine osmolality levels
- Monitor EKG tracings for changes related to abnormal potassium, calcium, and magnesium levels
- Note changes in peripheral sensation, such as numbness and tremors
- Note muscle strength
- Monitor for nausea, vomiting, and diarrhea
- Identify treatments that can alter electrolyte status, such as GI suctioning, diuretics, antihypertensives, and calcium channel blockers
- Monitor for underlying medical disease that can lead to electrolyte imbalance
- Monitor for signs and symptoms of hypokalemia: muscular weakness, cardiac irregularities (PVC), prolonged QT interval, flattened or depressed T wave, depressed ST segment, presence of U wave, fatigue, paresthesia, decreased reflexes, anorexia, constipation, decreased GI motility, dizziness, confusion, increased sensitivity to digitalis, and depressed respirations
- Monitor for signs/symptoms of hyperkalemia: irritability, restlessness, anxiety, nausea, vomiting, abdominal cramps, weakness, flaccid paralysis, circumoral numbness and tingling, tachycardia progressing to bradycardia, ventricular tachycardia/fibrillation, tall peaked T waves, flattened P wave, broad slurred QRS complex, and heart block progressing to asystole
- Monitor for signs/symptoms of hyponatremia: disorientation, muscle twitching, nausea and vomiting, abdominal cramps, headaches, personality changes, seizures, lethargy, fatigue, withdrawal, and coma
- Monitor for signs and symptoms of hypernatremia: extreme thirst; fever; dry, sticky mucous membranes; tachycardia; hypotension; lethargy; confusion; altered mentation; and seizures
- Monitor for signs and symptoms of hypocalcemia: irritability, muscle tetany, Chvostek's sign (facial muscle spasm), Trousseau's sign (carpal spasm), peripheral numbness and tingling, muscle cramps, decreased cardiac output, prolonged ST segment and QT interval, bleeding, and fractures
- Monitor for signs and symptoms of hypercalcemia: deep bone pain, excessive thirst, anorexia, lethargy, weakened muscles, shortened QT segment, wide T wave, widened QRS complex, and prolonged P-R interval
- Monitor for signs and symptoms of hypomagnesemia: respiratory muscle depression, mental apathy, Chvostek's sign (facial muscle spasm), Trousseau's sign (carpal spasm), confusion, facial tics, spasticity, and cardiac dysrthmias
- Monitor for signs and symptoms of hypermagnesemia: muscle weakness, inability to swallow, hyporeflexia, hypotension, bradycardia, CNS depression, respiratory depression, lethargy, coma, and depression
- Monitor for signs and symptoms of hypophosphatemia: bleeding tendencies, muscular weakness, paresthesia, hemolytic anemia, depressed white cell function, nausea, vomiting, anorexia, and bone demineralization
- Monitor for signs and symptoms of hyperphosphatemia: tachycardia, nausea, diarrhea, abdominal cramps, muscle weakness, flaccid paralysis, and increased reflexes
- Monitor for signs and symptoms of hypochloremia: hyperirritability, tetany, muscular excitability, slow respirations, and hypotension
- Monitor for signs and symptoms of hyperchloremia: weakness; lethargy; deep, rapid breathing; and coma

- Administer prescribed supplemental electrolytes, as appropriate
- Provide diet appropriate for patient's electrolyte imbalance (e.g., potassium-rich foods or low-sodium diet)
- Teach patient ways to prevent or minimize electrolyte imbalance
- Instruct patient and/or family on specific dietary modifications, as appropriate
- Consult physician if signs and symptoms of fluid and/or electrolyte imbalance persist or worsen

1st edition1992; revised 2008

Background Readings:

American Association of Critical Care Nurses. (2006). *Core curriculum for critical care nursing* (6th ed.) [J. G. Alspach, Ed.]. Philadelphia: Saunders.

Elgart, H. N. (2004). Assessment of fluids and electrolytes. *AACN Clinical Issues, 15*(4), 607–621.

McCance, K. L. & Huether, S. E. (2002). *Pathophysiology: The biologic basis for disease in adults and children.* St. Louis: Mosby.

Price, S. A. & Wilson, L. M, (2003). *Pathophysiology: Clinical concepts of disease processes* (6th ed.). St. Louis: Mosby.

Sheppard, M. (2000). Monitoring fluid balance in acutely ill patients. *Nursing Times, 96*(21), 39–40.

E

Electronic Fetal Monitoring: Antepartum   6771

Definition: Electronic evaluation of fetal heart rate response to movement, external stimuli, or uterine contractions during antepartal testing

Activities:

- Review obstetrical history, if available, to determine obstetrical or medical risk factors requiring antepartum testing of fetal status
- Determine patient knowledge about reasons for antepartum testing
- Provide written patient education material for antepartum tests (e.g., nonstress, oxytocin challenge, and biophysical profile tests), as well as electronic fetal monitor
- Take maternal vital signs
- Inquire about oral intake, including diet, cigarette smoking, and medication use
- Label monitor strip per protocol
- Review prior antepartum tests
- Verify maternal and fetal heart rates before initiation of electronic fetal monitoring
- Instruct patient about the reason for electronic monitoring, as well as the types of information obtainable
- Perform Leopold maneuver to determine fetal position(s), as appropriate
- Apply tocotransducer snugly to observe contraction frequency and duration
- Apply ultrasound transducer(s) to area of uterus where fetal heart sounds are audible and trace clearly
- Differentiate among multiple fetuses by documenting on the tracing when simultaneous tracings are conducted, using one electronic fetal monitor
- Distinguish among multiple fetuses by comparing data when simultaneous tracings are conducted, using two different fetal monitors
- Discuss appearance of rhythm strip with mother and support person
- Reassure about normal fetal heart rate signs, including such typical features as artifact, loss of signal with fetal movement, high rate, and irregular appearance
- Adjust monitors to achieve and maintain clarity of the tracing(s)
- Obtain baseline tracing of fetal heart rate(s) per protocol for specific testing procedure
- Interpret electronic monitor strip for baseline heart rate(s), long-term variability, and presence of spontaneous accelerations, decelerations, or contractions
- Provide vibroacoustic stimulation, per protocol or physician or midwife order
- Initiate IV infusion, per protocol, to begin oxytocin challenge test, as appropriate, per physician or midwife order

- Increase oxytocin infusion, per protocol, until the appropriate number of contractions are achieved (e.g., usually 3 contractions in 10 minutes)
- Observe monitor strip for the presence or absence of late decelerations
- Interpret tracing based on protocol for nonstress or oxytocin challenge test criteria
- Perform ultrasound for biophysical profile testing, per protocol or physician or midwife order
- Score ultrasound based on protocol for biophysical profile criteria
- Communicate test results to primary practitioner or midwife
- Provide anticipatory guidance for abnormal test results (e.g., nonreassuring nonstress test, positive oxytocin challenge test, or low biophysical profile score)
- Reschedule antepartum testing, per protocol or physician or midwife order
- Provide written discharge instructions to remind patient of future testing times and other reasons to return for care (e.g., labor onset, spontaneous leaking of the bag of waters, bleeding, and decreased fetal movement)
- Clean equipment, including abdominal belts

2nd edition 1996

Background Readings:

Chez, B. F., Skurnick, J. H., Chez, R. A., Verklan, M. T., Biggs, S., & Hage, M. L.. (1990). Interpretations of nonstress tests by obstetric nurses. *Journal of Obstetric, Gynecologic and Neonatal Nursing, 19*(3), 227–232.

Eganhouse, D. J. (1992). Fetal monitoring of twins. *Journal of Obstetric, Gynecologic and Neonatal Nursing, 21*(1), 16–22.

Fresquez, M. L. & Collins, D. E. (1992). Advancement of the nursing role in antepartum fetal evaluation. *Journal of Perinatal and Neonatal Nursing, 5*(4), 16–22.

Gregor, C. L., Paine, L. L., & Johnson, T. R. B. (1991). Antepartum fetal assessment: A nurse-midwifery perspective. *Journal of Nurse-Midwifery, 36*(3), 153–167.

Nurses Association of the American College of Obstetricians and Gynecologists. (1991). *Nursing practice competencies and educational guidelines: Antepartum fetal surveillance and intrapartum fetal heart monitoring* (2nd ed.). Washington, DC: Author.

Pillitteri, A. (2007). *Maternal and child health nursing: Care of the childbearing and childrearing family* (5th ed.). Philadelphia: Lippincott Williams & Wilkins.

Sabey, P. L. & Clark, S. L. (1992). Establishing an antepartum testing unit: The nurse's role. *Journal of Perinatal and Neonatal Nursing, 5*(4), 23–32.

Electronic Fetal Monitoring: Intrapartum   6772

Definition: Electronic evaluation of fetal heart rate response to uterine contractions during intrapartal care

Activities:
- Verify maternal and fetal heart rates before initiation of electronic fetal monitoring
- Instruct woman and support person(s) about the reason for electronic monitoring, as well as information to be obtained
- Perform Leopold maneuver to determine fetal position(s)
- Apply tocotransducer snugly to observe contraction frequency and duration
- Palpate to determine contraction intensity with tocotransducer use
- Apply ultrasound transducer(s) to area of uterus where fetal heart sounds are audible and trace clearly
- Differentiate among multiple fetuses by documenting on the tracing when simultaneous tracings are conducted, using one electronic fetal monitor (e.g., baby A, baby B)
- Distinguish among multiple fetuses by comparing data when simultaneous tracings are conducted, using two separate fetal monitors
- Discuss appearance of rhythm strip with mother and support person
- Reassure about normal fetal heart rate signs, including such typical features as artifact, loss of signal with fetal movement, high rate, and irregular appearance
- Adjust monitors to achieve and maintain clarity of the tracing
- Interpret strip when at least a 10-minute tracing has been obtained of the fetal heart and uterine activity signals
- Document elements of the external tracing, including baseline heart rate(s), oscillatory patterns, long-term variability, accelerations, decelerations, and contraction frequency and duration
- Document relevant intrapartal care (e.g., vaginal exams, medication administration, and maternal vital signs) directly on the monitor strip, as appropriate
- Remove electronic monitors, as needed for ambulation, after verifying that the tracing is normal (e.g., reassuring)
- Use intermittent or telemetry fetal monitoring, if available, to facilitate maternal ambulation and comfort
- Initiate fetal resuscitation interventions to treat abnormal (e.g., nonreassuring) fetal heart patterns, as appropriate
- Document changes in fetal heart patterns after resuscitation
- Calibrate equipment, as appropriate, for internal monitoring with a spiral electrode and/or intrauterine pressure catheter
- Use universal precautions
- Apply internal fetal electrode after rupture of membranes, when necessary for reducing artifact or for evaluation of short-term variability

- Apply internal uterine pressure catheter after rupture of membranes when necessary for obtaining pressure data for uterine contractions and resting tone
- Document maternal response to application of internal monitors, including degree of discomfort or pain, appearance of amniotic fluid, and presence of bleeding
- Document fetal response to internal monitor placement, including short-term variability, accelerations, or decelerations of the fetal heart rate
- Keep physician informed of pertinent changes in the fetal heart rate, interventions for nonreassuring patterns, subsequent fetal response, labor progress, and maternal response to labor
- Continue electronic monitoring through second-stage labor or up to the time of cesarean delivery
- Remove internal monitors before cesarean delivery to prevent maternal infection
- Document monitor interpretation, according to institutional policy
- Provide safekeeping of intrapartal strip as part of the permanent patient record

2nd edition 1996

Background Readings:
Association of Women's Health, Obstetric, and Neonatal Nurses. (1993). *Fetal heart monitoring principles & practices.* Washington, DC: Author.
Carlton, L. L. (1990). Module 6: Basic intrapartum fetal monitoring. In E. J. Martin (Ed.), *Intrapartum management modules* (pp. 151–234). Baltimore: Williams & Wilkins.
Eganhouse, D. J. (1991). Electronic fetal monitoring: Education and quality assurance. *Journal of Obstetric, Gynecologic, and Neonatal Nursing, 20*(1), 16–22.
Eganhouse, D. J. (1992). Fetal monitoring of twins. *Journal of Obstetric, Gynecologic, and Neonatal Nursing, 21*(1), 16–22.
Gilbert, E. S. & Harmon, J. S. (1998). *Manual of high risk pregnancy & delivery* (2nd ed.). St. Louis: Mosby.
Murray, M. (1988). *Essentials of electronic fetal monitoring: Antepartal and intrapartal fetal monitoring.* Philadelphia: Lippincott.
Pillitteri, A. (2007). *Maternal and child health nursing: Care of the childbearing and childrearing family* (5th ed.). Philadelphia: Lippincott Williams & Wilkins.
Tucker, S. M. (1992). *Pocket guide to fetal monitoring* (3rd ed.). St. Louis: Mosby.

Elopement Precautions   6470

Definition: Minimizing the risk of a patient leaving a treatment setting without authorization when departure presents a threat to the safety of patient or others

Activities:
- Monitor patient for indicators of elopement potential (e.g., verbal indicators, loitering near exits, multiple layers of clothing, disorientation, separation anxiety, and homesickness)
- Clarify the legal status of patient (e.g., minor or adult and voluntary or court-ordered treatment)

- Communicate risk to other care providers
- Familiarize patient with environment and routine to decrease anxiety
- Limit patient to a physically-secure environment (e.g., locked or alarmed doors at exits and locked windows), as needed

- Provide adaptive devices to limit mobility, as needed (e.g., cribs, gates, Dutch doors, and physical restraint)
- Provide appropriate level of supervision/surveillance to monitor patient
- Increase supervision/surveillance when patient is outside secure environment (e.g., hold hands and increase staff-to-patient ratio)
- Provide adaptive devices that monitor patient's physical location (e.g., electronic sensors placed on patient that trigger alarms or locks)
- Record physical description (e.g., height, weight, eye/hair/skin color, and any distinguishing characteristics) for reference, should patient elope
- Provide patient with identification band
- Assign consistent caregivers on a daily basis
- Encourage patient to seek out care providers for assistance when experiencing feelings (e.g., anxiety, anger, and fear) that may lead to elopement
- Provide reassurance and comfort
- Discuss with patient why he/she desires to leave the treatment setting

- Identify with patient, when appropriate, the positive and negative consequences of leaving treatment
- Identify with patient, when possible, any variables that may be altered to make the patient feel more comfortable with remaining in the treatment setting
- Encourage patient, when appropriate, to make a commitment to continue treatment (e.g., contracting)

2nd edition 1996

Background Readings:

Cipkala-Gaffin, J. A. & Cipkala-Gaffin, G. L. (1989). Developmental disabilities and nursing interventions. In L. M. Birckhead (Ed.), *Psychiatric mental health nursing. The therapeutic use of self* (pp. 349-379). Philadelphia: Lippincott.

Holnsteiner, M. G. (1991). Elopement, potential for. In G. K. McFarland & M. D. Thomas (Eds.), *Psychiatric mental health nursing: Application of the nursing process* (pp. 222–227). Philadelphia: Lippincott.

McIndoe, K. I. (1986). Elope: Why psychiatric patients go AWOL. *Journal of Psychosocial Nursing, 26*(1), 16–20.

E

Embolus Care: Peripheral   4104

Definition: Management of a patient experiencing occlusion of peripheral circulation

Activities:
- Elicit a detailed patient health history in order to plan current and future preventative care
- Evaluate changes in respiratory and cardiac status (e.g., new-onset wheezing, hemoptysis, dyspnea, tachypnea, tachycardia, syncope) as patients who experience DVT are at a higher risk of recurrence and PE
- Evaluate all chest, shoulder, back or pleuritic pain (i.e., check for intensity, location, radiation, duration, and precipitating and alleviating factors)
- Perform a comprehensive appraisal of peripheral circulation (i.e., check peripheral pulses, edema, capillary refill, color, and temperature of extremity)
- Monitor for pain in affected area
- Monitor for signs of decreased venous circulation in affected extremity (e.g., increased extremity circumference, painful swelling and tenderness, pain worsening in dependent position, pain persisting with extremity use, palpable hard vein, enlargement of the superficial veins, severe cramping, redness and warmth, numbness and tingling, discoloration of skin, fever)
- Administer anticoagulant medication
- Elevate any suspected affected limb 20 degrees or greater above the level of the heart to improve venous return
- Apply the Well's Prediction Rule to assist with diagnosing DVT
- Instruct the patient and family regarding diagnostic procedures (e.g., plethysmography, computerized strain gauze, venography, D-dimer assay, multidetector spiral computerized tomography, magnetic resonance imaging, ultrasonography), as appropriate
- Apply graduated elastic compression stockings or sleeves to reduce the risk of postthrombotic syndrome or recurrence of DVT
- Remove graduated elastic compression stockings or sleeves for 15 to 20 minutes every 8 hours or per organizational policy and protocol
- Avoid antecubital intravenous access and instruct radiology and laboratory personnel to limit access of antecubital veins for tests, if possible

- Administer intravenous promethazine only in a 25cc to 50cc saline solution at a slow rate and avoid giving in less than 10cc saline dilution
- Assist patient with passive or active range of motion, as appropriate
- Maintain patient on bedrest and change position every 2 hours
- Provide for early ambulation and exercise under the direction and supervision of a physiotherapist
- Monitor neurological status
- Provide pain relief and comfort measures
- Elevate bed sheets by using bed cradle over the affected extremity, if appropriate
- Refrain from massaging or compressing affected limb muscles
- Instruct the patient not to massage or compress the affected area
- Monitor patient's prothrombin time (PT) and partial thromboplastin time (PTT) to keep one to two times normal, as appropriate
- Monitor for side effects from anticoagulant medications
- Keep protamine sulfate and vitamin K available in case of emergency
- Administer antacids and analgesics, as appropriate
- Instruct patient not to cross legs and to avoid sitting for long periods with legs dependent
- Instruct the patient to avoid activities that result in the Valsalva maneuver (e.g., straining during bowel movement)
- Administer medications that will prevent episodes of the Valsalva maneuver (e.g., stool softeners and antiemetics), as appropriate
- Instruct the patient and family on appropriate precautions (e.g., walking; drinking plenty of fluids; avoiding alcohol; avoiding long periods of immobility, especially with legs dependently positioned, such as in air travel or long automobile trips)
- Instruct the patient and family on all prophylactic low-dose anticoagulant and/or antiplatelet medication
- Instruct the patient to report excessive bleeding (e.g., unusual nosebleeds, vomiting blood, blood in the urine, bleeding gums,

unexpected vaginal bleeding, unusually heavy menstrual bleeding, bloody or tarry bowel movements), unusual bruising, unusual pain or swelling, blue or purple color of the toes, pain in the toes, ulcers or white spots in the mouth or throat
- Instruct the patient to wear a medical-alert bracelet
- Instruct patient to maintain a consistent diet (i.e., eat a consistent amount of green leafy vegetables, which are high in vitamin K and can interfere with anticoagulants, as the medication dosage will be adjusted to dietary intake)
- Administer prophylactic low-dose anticoagulant and/or anti-platelet medication (e.g., heparin, clopidogrel, warfarin, aspirin, dipyridamole, dextran) per organizational policy and protocol
- Instruct patient to take anticoagulant medication at the same time each day and not to double up the next day if a dose is missed
- Instruct patient to check with healthcare provider before taking any medication or herbal preparations (including over-the-counter products) before changing brands of medication, and before discontinuing a medication
- Instruct the patient and family on graduated elastic compression stockings
- Encourage smoking cessation

1st edition 1992; revised 2013

Background Readings:

American Association of Critical Care Nurses. (2006). *Core curriculum for critical care nursing* (6th ed.) [J. G. Alspach, Ed.]. Philadelphia: Saunders.

Agnelli, G. & Becattini, C. (2008). Treatment of DVT: How long is enough and how do you predict recurrence. *Journal of Thrombosis and Thrombolysis, 25*(1), 37–44.

Findlay, J., Keogh, M., & Cooper, L. (2010). Venous thromboembolism prophylaxis: The role of the nurse. *British Journal of Nursing (BJN), 19*(16), 1028–1032.

Fitzgerald, J. (2010). Venous thromboembolism: Have we made headway? *Orthopaedic Nursing, 29*(4), 226–234.

Houman Fekrazad, M., Lopes, R. D., Stashenko, G. J., Alexander, J. H., & Garcia, D. (2009). Treatment of venous thromboembolism: Guidelines translated for the clinician. *Journal of Thrombosis and Thrombolysis, 28*(3), 270–275.

Kearon, C., Kahn, S. R., Agnelli, G., Goldhaber, S., Raskob, G. E., & Comerota, A. J. (2008) Antithrombotic therapy for venous thromboembolic disease: American College of Chest Physicians evidence-based clinical practice guidelines (8th ed.). *Chest, 133*(Suppl. 6), 454S–545S.

Lancaster, S. L., Owens, A., Bryant, A. S., Ramey, L. S., Nicholson, J., Gossett, K., et al. (2010). Emergency: Upper-extremity deep vein thrombosis. *AJN: American Journal of Nursing, 110*(5), 48–52.

Lankshear, A., Harden, J., & Simms, J. (2010). Safe practice for patients receiving anticoagulant therapy. *Nursing Standard, 24*(20), 47–56.

Meetoo, D. (2010). In too deep: Understanding, detecting and managing DVT. *British Journal of Nursing (BJN), 19*(16), 1021–1022, 1024–1027.

Embolus Care: Pulmonary   4106

Definition: Management of a patient experiencing occlusion of pulmonary circulation

Activities:
- Prepare for thrombolytic therapy, as indicated (e.g., streptokinase, urokinase, activase)
- Elicit a detailed patient health history in order to plan current and future preventative care
- Evaluate changes in respiratory and cardiac status (e.g., new-onset wheezing, hemoptysis, dyspnea, tachypnea, tachycardia, syncope) as patients who experience PE or DVT are at a higher risk of recurrence
- Evaluate all chest, shoulder, back or pleuritic pain (i.e., check for intensity, location, radiation, duration, and precipitating and alleviating factors)
- Assist with diagnostic tests and assessments to rule out conditions with similar signs and symptoms (e.g., acute myocardial infarction; pericarditis; aortic dissection; pneumonia; pneumothorax; anxiety with hyperventilation; asthma; heart failure; pericardial tamponade; and gastrointestinal abnormalities, such as peptic ulcer, esophageal rupture, gastritis)
- Instruct the patient and/or family regarding diagnostic procedures (e.g., V/Q scan, D-dimer assay, multidetector spiral CT, ultrasonographies), as appropriate
- Auscultate lung sounds for crackles or other adventitious sounds
- Obtain arterial blood gas levels, as indicated
- Monitor determinants of tissue oxygen delivery (e.g., PaO_2, SaO_2, hemoglobin levels, and cardiac output)
- Monitor for symptoms of inadequate tissue oxygenation (e.g., pallor, cyanosis, and sluggish capillary refill)
- Monitor for symptoms of respiratory failure (e.g., low PaO_2 and elevated $PaCO_2$ levels and respiratory muscle fatigue)
- Initiate appropriate thromboprophylaxis regimen immediately, per organizational policy and protocol
- Administer prophylactic low-dose anticoagulant and/or anti-platelet medication (e.g., heparin, clopidogrel, warfarin, aspirin, dipyridamole, dextran), per organizational policy and protocol
- Elevate any suspected affected limb 20 degrees or greater above the level of the heart to improve venous return
- Apply graduated elastic compression stockings or sleeves (GECS) to reduce the risk of DVT or recurrence of DVT, per organizational policy and protocol
- Maintain graduated elastic compression stockings or sleeves to avoid development of post thrombotic syndrome (PTS)
- Apply intermittent pneumatic compression device stockings, per organizational policy and protocol
- Remove graduated elastic compression stockings or sleeves and intermittent pneumatic compression device stockings for 15 to 20 minutes every 8 hours or per organizational policy and protocol
- Avoid antecubital intravenous access and instruct radiology and laboratory personnel to limit access of antecubital veins for tests, if possible
- Assist patient with passive or active range of motion as appropriate
- Encourage flexion and extension of feet and legs at least ten times every hour
- Change patient position every 2 hours, encourage early mobilization or ambulate as tolerated
- Encourage good ventilation (e.g., incentive spirometry, cough and deep breath every 2 hours)

E

- Monitor lab values for changes in oxygenation or acid-base balance, as appropriate
- Instruct the patient and/or family regarding any planned treatments to remove the embolus (e.g., fibrinolysis, catheter embolectomy, or surgical pulmonary embolectomy)
- Encourage the patient to relax
- Monitor side effects of anticoagulant medications
- Avoid overwedging of pulmonary artery catheter to prevent pulmonary artery rupture, if appropriate
- Monitor pulmonary artery tracing for spontaneous wedge of catheter, if appropriate
- Reposition spontaneously wedged pulmonary artery catheter, if appropriate
- Maintain thromboprophylaxis following an embolus
- Instruct patient and family on need for anticoagulation following an embolus for a minimum of 3 months
- Provide detailed education to patient and family regarding prevention of future emboli and thrombi

1st edition 1992; revised 2013

Background Readings:

American Association of Critical Care Nurses. (2006). *Core curriculum for critical care nursing* (6th ed.) [J. G. Alspach, Ed.]. Philadelphia: Saunders.

Findlay, J., Keogh, M., & Cooper, L. (2010). Venous thromboembolism prophylaxis: The role of the nurse. *British Journal of Nursing (BJN)*, *19*(16), 1028–1032.

Fitzgerald, J. (2010). Venous thromboembolism: Have we made headway? *Orthopaedic Nursing*, *29*(4), 226–234.

Headley, C. M. & Melander, S. (2011). When it may be a pulmonary embolism. *Nephrology Nursing Journal*, *38*(2), 127–152.

Lancaster, S. L., Owens, A., Bryant, A. S., Ramey, L. S., Nicholson, J., Gossett, K., et al. (2010). Emergency: Upper-extremity deep vein thrombosis. *AJN: American Journal of Nursing*, *110*(5), 48–52.

Lankshear, A., Harden, J., & Simms, J. (2010). Safe practice for patients receiving anticoagulant therapy. *Nursing Standard*, *24*(20), 47–56.

Meetoo, D. (2010). In too deep: Understanding, detecting and managing DVT. *British Journal of Nursing (BJN)*, *19*(16), 1021–1022, 1024–1027.

Shaughnessy, K. (2007). Massive pulmonary embolism. *Critical Care Nurse*, *27*(1), 39–40, 42–51.

Yee, C.A. (2010). Conquering pulmonary embolism. *OR Nurse*, *4*(5), 18–24.

Embolus Precautions   4110

Definition: Reduction of the risk of an embolus in a patient with thrombi or at risk for thrombus formation

Activities:
- Elicit a detailed patient health history to determine risk level of patient (e.g., recent surgery, bone fractures, current cancer treatment, pregnancy, postpartum, immobility, paralysis, edematous extremities, COPD, stroke, CVAD, history of previous DVT or PE, or obesity put patients at high risk)
- Implement agency protocol for patients who are found at risk
- Critically evaluate any reports of new-onset wheezing, hemoptysis, or pain with inspiration; chest, shoulder, back, or pleuritic pain; dyspnea, tachypnea, tachycardia, or syncope
- Evaluate for the presence of Virchow's triad: venous stasis, hypercoagulability, and trauma resulting in intimal damage
- Perform a comprehensive appraisal of pulmonary status
- Perform a comprehensive appraisal of peripheral circulation (i.e., check peripheral pulses, edema, capillary refill, color, presence of pain in the affected extremity, and temperature of extremity)
- Initiate appropriate thromboprophylaxis regimen in at risk patients immediately per organizational policy and protocol
- Administer prophylactic low-dose anticoagulant and/or antiplatelet medication (e.g., heparin, clopidogrel, warfarin, aspirin, dipyridamole, dextran), per organizational policy and protocol
- Elevate any suspected affected limb 20 degrees or greater above the level of the heart to improve venous return
- Apply graduated elastic compression stockings or sleeves (GECS) to reduce the risk of DVT or recurrence of DVT, per organizational policy and protocol
- Maintain graduated elastic compression stockings or sleeves to avoid development of postthrombotic syndrome (PTS), which is precipitated by long-term clots in the affected extremity and poor venous flow
- Apply intermittent pneumatic compression device stockings, per organizational policy and protocol
- Remove graduated elastic compression stockings or sleeves and intermittent pneumatic compression device stockings for 15 to 20 minutes every 8 hours or per organizational policy and protocol
- Avoid antecubital intravenous access and instruct radiology and laboratory personnel to limit access of antecubital veins for tests, if possible
- Administer intravenous promethazine in a 25cc to 50cc saline solution at a slow rate and avoid giving in less than 10cc saline dilution
- Assist patient with passive or active range of motion, as appropriate
- Encourage flexion and extension of feet and legs at least ten times every hour
- Change patient position every 2 hours, encourage early mobilization or ambulate as tolerated
- Prevent injury to vessel lumen by preventing local pressure, trauma, infection, or sepsis
- Refrain from massaging or compressing affected limb muscles
- Instruct patient not to cross legs and to avoid sitting for long periods with legs dependent
- Instruct the patient to avoid activities that result in the Valsalva maneuver (e.g., straining during bowel movement)
- Administer medications that will prevent episodes of the Valsalva maneuver (e.g., stool softeners, antiemetics), as appropriate
- Instruct the patient and/or family on appropriate precautions (e.g., walking; drinking plenty of fluids; avoiding alcohol; avoiding long periods of immobility, especially with legs dependently positioned, such as in air travel or long automobile trips)
- Instruct the patient and/or family on all prophylactic low-dose anticoagulant and/or antiplatelet medication new
- Instruct the patient to report excessive bleeding (e.g., unusual nosebleeds, vomiting blood, blood in the urine, bleeding gums, unexpected vaginal bleeding, unusually heavy menstrual bleeding, bloody or tarry bowel movements), unusual bruising, unusual pain or swelling, blue or purple color of the toes, pain in the toes, ulcers or white spots in the mouth or throat
- Instruct the patient to wear a medical-alert bracelet
- Instruct patient to maintain a consistent diet (i.e., eat a consistent amount of green leafy vegetables, which are high in vitamin K and can interfere with anticoagulants, as the medication dosage will be adjusted to dietary intake)

- Instruct patient to take anticoagulant medication at the same time each day and not to double up the next day if a dose is missed
- Instruct patient to check with healthcare provider before taking any medication or herbal preparations, including over-the-counter products, before changing brands of medication, and before discontinuing a medication
- Instruct the patient and family on graduated elastic compression stockings
- Encourage smoking cessation

1st edition 1992; revised 2013

Background Readings:

American Association of Critical Care Nurses. (2006). *Core curriculum for critical care nursing* (6th ed.) [J. G. Alspach, Ed.]. Philadelphia: Saunders.

Findlay, J., Keogh, M., & Cooper, L. (2010). Venous thromboembolism prophylaxis: The role of the nurse. *British Journal of Nursing (BJN), 19*(16), 1028–1032.

Fitzgerald, J. (2010). Venous thromboembolism: Have we made headway? *Orthopaedic Nursing, 29*(4), 226–234.

Headley, C.M. & Melander, S. (2011). When it may be a pulmonary embolism. *Nephrology Nursing Journal, 38*(2), 127–152.

Lancaster, S.L., Owens, A., Bryant, A.S., Ramey, L.S., Nicholson, J., Gossett, K., et al. (2010). Emergency: Upper-extremity deep vein thrombosis. *AJN: American Journal of Nursing, 110*(5), 48–52.

Lankshear, A., Harden, J., & Simms, J. (2010). Safe practice for patients receiving anticoagulant therapy. *Nursing Standard, 24*(20), 47–56.

Meetoo, D. (2010). In too deep: Understanding, detecting and managing DVT. *British Journal of Nursing (BJN), 19*(16), 1021–1022, 1024–1027.

Shaughnessy, K. (2007). Massive pulmonary embolism. *Critical Care Nurse, 27*(1), 39–40, 42–51.

Yee, C.A. (2010). Conquering pulmonary embolism. *OR Nurse, 4*(5), 18–24.

Emergency Care   6200

Definition: Providing evaluation and treatment measures in urgent situations

Activities:

- Activate the emergency medical system
- Obtain the automated external defibrillator (AED) or assure that someone is obtaining the AED, if possible and appropriate
- Initiate rescue actions to the most critically ill patients in the case of multiple victims
- Evaluate any unresponsive patient to determine appropriate action
- Check for signs and symptoms of cardiac arrest
- Call for help if no breathing or no normal breathing and no response
- Instruct others to call for help, if needed
- Employ precautionary measures to reduce risk of infection while giving care
- Attach the AED and implement specified actions, as appropriate
- Assure rapid defibrillation, as appropriate
- Perform cardiopulmonary resuscitation that focuses on chest compressions in adults and compressions with breathing efforts for children, as appropriate
- Initiate 30 chest compressions at specified rate and depth, allowing for complete chest recoil between compressions, minimizing interruptions in compressions, and avoiding excessive ventilation, as appropriate
- Minimize the interval between stopping chest compressions and delivering a shock, if indicated
- Tailor rescue actions to the most likely cause of arrest (e.g., cardiac or respiratory)
- Create or maintain an open airway
- Check for signs and symptoms of severely compromised breathing (e.g., pneumothorax or flailing chest)
- Provide 2 rescue breaths after initial 30 chest compressions completed, as appropriate
- Perform the Heimlich maneuver, as appropriate
- Provide age appropriate care for elderly and children

- Check for signs and symptoms of severely compromised hemodynamic status (e.g., arterial trauma or rupture)
- Institute measures (e.g., pressure, pressure dressing, positioning) to reduce or minimize bleeding
- Institute measures for management of shock (e.g., positioning for optimal perfusion, MAST trousers), as needed
- Monitor the amount and nature of blood loss
- Monitor vital signs if possible and appropriate
- Check for signs and symptoms of compromised neurological status (e.g., paralysis, paresthesia, bowel or bladder incontinence)
- Immobilize patient with suspected head or spine injury using appropriate devices and techniques (i.e., apply cervical collar, move patient as a unit, and transport patient in supine position on backboard)
- Position patient's body part or body-as-unit in appropriate position (e.g., body part affected with insect sting lower than heart level, and left-side lying for poison ingestion or alcohol and drug intoxication)
- Immobilize fractures, large wounds, and any injured part
- Move patient only when necessary using appropriate technique and body mechanics
- Monitor for signs and symptoms of hypoglycemia (e.g., shakiness, tachycardia, chills, clamminess, drowsiness, dizziness, blurred vision, confusion)
- Monitor level of consciousness
- Remove patient from cold environment
- Remove patient's wet clothing
- Remove overheated patient from direct sunlight and heat source
- Fan the patient and give cool oral fluids, as needed
- Check for medical alert tags
- Administer medication (e.g., nitroglycerin, bronchodilator, activated charcoal, insulin, epinephrine, and antivenin), as needed

- Determine the history of the accident from the patient or others in the area
- Determine type of motor vehicle accident and use of restraining devices, if appropriate
- Determine the exact nature of trauma involved, if appropriate
- Determine whether an overdose of a drug or other substance is involved
- Determine whether toxic or poisonous substances are involved
- Send suspected drugs involved with patient to treatment facility, as appropriate
- Contact poison control center, proceeding with treatment as directed
- Do not leave suicidal patient alone
- Provide reassurance and emotional support to patient or family
- Assist with ongoing treatment, providing pertinent information surrounding life-threatening situation to other healthcare providers
- Coordinate medical transport, as appropriate
- Transport using a back board, as appropriate

1st edition 1992; revised 2013

Background Readings:

Carlson, K. (2009). *Advanced critical care nursing.* Philadelphia: Saunders.

Emergency Nurses Association. (2005). *Sheehy's manual of emergency care* (6th ed.) St. Louis: Mosby.

Emergency Nurses Association. (2007). *Emergency nursing core curriculum* (6th ed.). St. Louis: Saunders.

Field, J. M., Hazinski, M. F., Sayre, M. R., Chameides, L., Schexnayder, S. M., Hemphill, R., et al. (2010). Part 1: Executive summary: 2010 American Heart Association guidelines for cardiopulmonary resuscitation and emergency cardiovascular care. *Circulation, 122*(18 Suppl. 3), S640–S656.

Hazinski, M. F. (Ed.). (2010). *Highlights of the 2010 American Heart Association guidelines for CPR and ECC.* Dallas, TX: American Heart Association.

Hickey, J. V. (2009). *The clinical practice of neurological and neurosurgical nursing* (6th ed.). Philadelphia: Lippincott Williams & Wilkins.

Lynn-McHale Wiegand, D. J. (Ed.). (2011). *AACN procedure manual for critical care* (6th ed.). St. Louis: Saunders.

McQuillan, K. A., Flynn Makic, M. B., & Whalen, E. (2009). *Trauma nursing: From resuscitation through rehabilitation* (4th ed.). St. Louis: Saunders Elsevier.

Emergency Cart Checking   7660

Definition: Systematic review and maintenance of the contents of an emergency cart at established time intervals

Activities:

- Ensure ease of usability of equipment and supplies per proper cart design and location of supplies during initial cart setup and with all checks
- Compare equipment on cart with list of designated equipment
- Locate all designated equipment and supplies on cart
- Replace missing or outdated supplies and equipment
- Ensure that latex-free products are stocked where available, per agency protocol
- Ensure that equipment is operational via trial run (i.e., assemble laryngoscope and check light bulb function), as indicated
- Ensure that defibrillator remains plugged in and charging between all uses
- Test defibrillator per machine and agency protocol, including a trial discharge of low energy joules (less than 200)
- Clean equipment, as needed
- Verify current expiration date on all supplies and medications
- Document cart check, per agency policy
- Replace equipment, supplies, and medications as technology and guidelines are updated
- Ensure safeguarding of cart supplies, equipment, and patient information per agency protocol and governmental regulations (e.g., Health Insurance Portability and Accountability Act [HIPAA])
- Instruct new nursing staff on proper emergency cart checking procedures

2nd edition 1996; revised 2008

Background Readings:

American Association of Critical Care Nurses. (2006). *Core curriculum for critical care nursing* (6th ed.) [J. G. Alspach, Ed.]. Philadelphia: Saunders.

American Heart Association. (2005). Electric therapies: Automated external defibrillators, defibrillation, cardioversion, and pacing. *Circulation, 112*(24), 35–46.

American Heart Association. (2005). Guidelines for cardiopulmonary resuscitation and emergency cardiovascular care. *Circulation, 112*(24 Suppl. 1), IV1–IV211.

Bernstein, M. L. (1997). Latex-safe emergency cart products list. *Journal of Emergency Nursing, 24*(1), 58–61.

DeVita, M. A., Schaefer, J., Lutz, J., Dongilli, T., & Wang, H. (2004). Improving medical crisis team performance. *Critical Care Medicine, 32*(2), S61–S65.

Lynn-McHale, D. J., & Carlson, K. K. (2005). *AACN procedure manual for critical care* (5th ed.). Philadelphia: Saunders.

McLaughlin, R. C. (2003). Redesigning the crash cart: Usability testing improves one facility's medication drawers. *American Journal of Nursing, 103*(4), Hospital Extra: 64A, 64D, 64G–H.

Misko, L. & Molle, E. (2003). Teaching staff to manage cardiac arrest situations. *Journal for Nurses in Staff Development, 19*(6), 292–296.

Shanaberger, C. J. (1988). Equipment failure is often human failure. *Journal of Emergency Medical Services, 13*(1), 124–125.

E

Emotional Support   5270

Definition: Provision of reassurance, acceptance, and encouragement during times of stress

Activities:
- Discuss with the patient the emotional experience(s)
- Explore with patient what has triggered emotions
- Make supportive or empathetic statements
- Embrace or touch patient supportively
- Support the use of appropriate defense mechanisms
- Assist patient in recognizing feelings, such as anxiety, anger, or sadness
- Encourage the patient to express feelings of anxiety, anger, or sadness
- Discuss consequences of not dealing with guilt and shame
- Listen to/encourage expressions of feelings and beliefs
- Facilitate patient's identification of usual response pattern in coping with fears
- Provide support during denial, anger, bargaining, and acceptance phases of grieving
- Identify the function that anger, frustration, and rage serve for the patient
- Encourage talking or crying as means to decrease the emotional response
- Stay with the patient and provide assurance of safety and security during periods of anxiety
- Provide assistance in decision making
- Reduce demand for cognitive functioning when patient is ill or fatigued
- Refer for counseling, as appropriate

1st edition 1992; revised 2004

Background Readings:
Ahrens, J. (2002). Giving care and comfort in the aftermath of tragedy. *Caring Magazine, 21*(1), 10–11.
Arnold, E. & Boggs, K. (1989). *Interpersonal relationships: Professional communication skills for nurses.* Philadelphia: Saunders.
Boyle, K., Moddeman, G., & Mann, B. (1989). The importance of selected nursing activities to patients and their nurses. *Applied Nursing Research, 2*(4), 173–177.
Deering, C. (2006). Therapeutic relationships and communication. In W. K. Mohr (Ed.), *Psychiatric-mental health nursing* (6th ed., pp. 55–78). Philadelphia: Lippincott Williams & Wilkins.
Moore, J. C. & Hartman, C. R. (1988). Developing a therapeutic relationship. In C. K. Beck, R. P. Rawlins, & W. R. Williams (Eds.), *Mental health-psychiatric nursing: A holistic life-cycle approach* (2nd ed., pp. 92–117). St. Louis: Mosby.

Endotracheal Extubation   3270

Definition: Purposeful removal of the endotracheal tube from the nasopharyngeal or oropharyngeal airway

Activities:
- Position the patient for best use of ventilatory muscles, usually with the head of the bed elevated 75 degrees
- Instruct patient about the procedure
- Hyperoxygenate the patient and suction the endotracheal airway
- Suction the oral airway
- Deflate the endotracheal cuff and remove the endotracheal tube
- Encourage the patient to cough and expectorate sputum
- Administer oxygen as ordered
- Encourage coughing and deep breathing
- Suction the airway, as needed
- Monitor for respiratory distress
- Observe for signs of airway occlusion
- Monitor vital signs
- Encourage voice rest for 4 to 8 hours, as appropriate
- Monitor ability to swallow and talk

2nd edition 1996

Background Readings:
American Association of Critical Care Nurses. (2006). Core curriculum for critical care nursing (6th ed.) [J. G. Alspach, Ed.]. Philadelphia: Saunders.
Boggs, R. L. (1993). Airway management. In R. L. Boggs & M. Woodridge-King (Eds.), *AACN procedure manual for critical care* (3rd ed., pp. 1–65). Philadelphia: Saunders.
Elmquist, L. (1992). Decision-making for extubation of the post-anesthetic patient. *Critical Care Nursing Quarterly, 15*(1), 82–86.

Enema Administration   0466

Definition: Instillation of a solution into the lower gastrointestinal tract

Activities:
- Determine reason for enema (e.g., gastrointestinal cleansing; medication administration, distention reduction)
- Verify practitioner order for enema and absence of any contra-indications (e.g., glaucoma and increased intracranial pressure)
- Explain procedure to patient or family, including expected sensations during and after procedure (e.g., distention and urge to defecate)
- Gather and assemble equipment specific to type of enema
- Provide privacy
- Assist patient into appropriate position (e.g., left side-lying position with right knee flexed for adults and dorsal recumbent for children)
- Place waterproof or absorbent pad under hips and buttocks
- Cover patient with bath blanket leaving only rectal area uncovered

- Ascertain appropriate temperature of irrigating solution
- Instruct patient to exhale prior to inserting solution
- Insert lubricated tip of solution container or tubing into rectum, angling tip towards umbilicus and inserting appropriate length based on patient's age
- Squeeze bottle until all solution has entered rectum and colon
- Determine appropriate height of enema bag, solution volume, instillation rate, and handling of tubing
- Encourage patient to retain fluid until urge to defecate, assisting by squeezing buttocks if necessary
- Provide bedpan, commode, or easy access to toilet
- Monitor character of feces and solution (e.g., color, amount, and appearance)
- Monitor patient response to procedure, including signs of intolerance (e.g., rectal bleeding, distention, and abdominal pain), diarrhea, constipation, and impaction
- Assist patient in perineal cleansing

- Provide instruction to patient, caregiver, or unlicensed assistive personnel on enema administration
- Instruct on signs that warrant ending the procedure and reporting to health care practitioner (e.g., palpitations, diaphoresis, pallor, and shortness of breath)

6th edition 2013

Background Readings:

Craven, R. F. & Hirnle, C. J. (2009). Bowel elimination. In *Fundamentals of nursing: Human health and function* (6th ed., pp. 1116–1158). Philadelphia: Lippincott Williams & Wilkins.

Elkin, M. K., Perry, A. G., & Potter, P. A. (2007). Assisting with elimination. In *Nursing interventions & clinical skills* (4th ed., pp. 176–198). St. Louis: Mosby.

Smith, S. F., Duell, D. J., & Martin, B. C. (2008). Bowel elimination. In *Clinical nursing skills: Basic to advanced skills* (7th ed., pp. 811–847). Upper Saddle River, NJ: Pearson Prentice Hall.

E

Energy Management   0180

Definition: Regulating energy use to treat or prevent fatigue and optimize function

Activities:
- Assess patient's physiologic status for deficits resulting in fatigue within the context of age and development
- Encourage verbalization of feelings about limitations
- Use valid instruments to measure fatigue, as indicated
- Determine patient/significant other's perception of causes of fatigue
- Correct physiologic status deficits (e.g., chemotherapy-induced anemia) as priority items
- Select interventions for fatigue reduction using combinations of pharmacologic and non-pharmocologic categories, as appropriate
- Determine what and how much activity is required to build endurance
- Monitor nutritional intake to ensure adequate energy resources
- Consult with dietitian about ways to increase intake of high-energy foods
- Negotiate desired mealtimes which may or may not coincide with standard hospital schedules
- Monitor patient for evidence of excess physical and emotional fatigue
- Monitor cardiorespiratory response to activity (e.g., tachycardia, other dysrhythmias, dyspnea, diaphoresis, pallor, hemodynamic pressures, respiratory rate)
- Encourage aerobic workouts as tolerated
- Monitor/record patient's sleep pattern and number of sleep hours
- Monitor location and nature of discomfort or pain during movement/activity
- Reduce physical discomforts that could interfere with cognitive function and self-monitoring/regulation of activity
- Set limits with hyperactivity when it interferes with others or with the patient
- Assist the patient to understand energy conservation principles (e.g., the requirement for restricted activity or bedrest)
- Teach activity organization and time management techniques to prevent fatigue
- Assist the patient in assigning priority to activities to accommodate energy levels

- Assist the patient/significant other to establish realistic activity goals
- Assist the patient to identify preferences for activity
- Encourage the patient to choose activities that gradually build endurance
- Assist the patient to identify tasks that family and friends can perform in the home to prevent/relieve fatigue
- Consider electronic communication (e.g., email or instant messaging) to maintain contact with friends when visits are not practical or advisable
- Assist the patient to limit daytime sleep by providing activity that promotes wakefulness, as appropriate
- Limit environmental stimuli (e.g., light and noise) to facilitate relaxation
- Limit number of and interruptions by visitors, as appropriate
- Promote bedrest/activity limitation (e.g., increase number of rest periods) with protected rest times of choice
- Encourage alternate rest and activity periods
- Arrange physical activities to reduce competition for oxygen supply to vital body functions (e.g., avoid activity immediately after meals)
- Use passive and/or active range-of-motion exercises to relieve muscle tension
- Provide calming diversional activities to promote relaxation
- Offer aids to promote sleep (e.g., music or medications)
- Encourage an afternoon nap, if appropriate
- Assist patient to schedule rest periods
- Avoid care activities during scheduled rest periods
- Plan activities for periods when the patient has the most energy
- Assist patient to sit on side of bed ("dangle"), if unable to transfer or walk
- Assist with regular physical activities (e.g., ambulation, transfers, turning, and personal care), as needed
- Monitor administration and effect of stimulants and depressants
- Encourage physical activity (e.g., ambulation, performance of activities of daily living) consistent with patient's energy resources
- Evaluate programmed increases in levels of activities

- Monitor patient's oxygen response (e.g., pulse rate, cardiac rhythm, respiratory rate) to self-care or nursing activities
- Assist patient to self-monitor by developing and using a written record of calorie intake and energy expenditure, as appropriate
- Instruct the patient and/or significant other on fatigue, its common symptoms, and latent recurrences
- Instruct patient and significant other techniques of self-care that will minimize oxygen consumption (e.g., self-monitoring and pacing techniques for performance of activities of daily living)
- Instruct patient/significant other to recognize signs and symptoms of fatigue that require reduction in activity
- Instruct the patient/significant other on stress and coping interventions to decrease fatigue
- Instruct patient/significant other to notify health care provider if signs and symptoms of fatigue persist

1st edition 1992; revised 2008

Background Readings:

Erickson, J. M. (2004). Fatigue in adolescents with cancer: A review of the literature. *Clinical Journal of Oncology Nursing, 8*(2), 139–145.

Gelinas, C. & Fillion, L. (2004). Factors related to persistent fatigue following completion of breast cancer treatment. *Oncology Nursing Forum, 31*(2), 269–278.

Glick, O. (1992). Interventions related to activity and movement. In G. M. Bulechek & J. C. McCloskey (Eds.), Symposium on nursing interventions. *Nursing Clinics of North America, 27*(2), 541–569.

McFarland, G. K. & McFarlane, E. A. (1997). *Nursing diagnosis and intervention, planning for patient care* (3rd ed.). St. Louis: Mosby.

Nail, L. M. (2002). Fatigue in patients with cancer. *Oncology Nursing Forum, 29*(3), 537–544.

Oncology Nursing Society. (2005). *Core curriculum for oncology nursing* (4th ed.) [J. K. Itano & K. Taoka, Eds.]. Philadelphia: Saunders.

Piper, B. (1997). Measuring fatigue. In M. Frank-Stromborg & S. Olsen (Eds.), *Pathophysiological phenomena in nursing: Human response to illness* (pp. 219–234). Philadelphia: Saunders.

Enteral Tube Feeding   1056

Definition: Delivering nutrients and water through a gastrointestinal tube

Activities:

- Explain the procedure to the patient
- Insert a nasogastric, nasoduodenal, or nasojejunal tube, according to agency protocol
- Apply anchoring substance to skin and secure feeding tube with tape
- Monitor for proper placement of the tube by inspecting oral cavity, checking for gastric residual, or listening while air is injected and withdrawn, according to agency protocol
- Mark the tubing at the point of exit to maintain proper placement
- Confirming tube placement by x-ray examination is preferable prior to administering feedings or medications via the tube, per agency protocol
- Monitor for presence of bowel sounds every 4 to 8 hours, as appropriate
- Monitor fluid and electrolyte status
- Consult with other health care team members in selecting the type and strength of enteral feeding
- Elevate head of the bed 30 to 45 degrees during feedings
- Offer pacifier to infant during feeding, as appropriate
- Hold and talk to infant during feeding to simulate usual feeding activities
- Discontinue feedings 30 to 60 minutes before putting in a head down position
- Turn off the tube feeding 1 hour prior to a procedure or transport if the patient needs to be less than 30 degrees
- Irrigate the tube every 4 to 6 hours as appropriate during continuous feedings and after every intermittent feeding
- Use clean technique in administering tube feedings
- Check gravity drip rate or pump rate every hour
- Slow tube feeding rate and/or decrease strength to control diarrhea
- Monitor for sensation of fullness, nausea, and vomiting
- Check residual every 4 to 6 hours for the first 24 hours, then every 8 hours during continuous feedings
- Check residual before each intermittent feeding
- Hold tube feedings if residual is greater than 150 cc or more than 110% to 120% of the hourly rate in adults
- Keep cuff of endotracheal or tracheostomy tube inflated during feeding, as appropriate
- Keep open containers of enteral feeding refrigerated
- Change insertion site and infusion tubing according to agency protocol
- Wash skin around skin level device daily with mild soap and dry thoroughly
- Check water level in skin level device balloon, according to equipment protocol
- Discard enteral feeding containers and administration sets every 24 hours
- Refill feeding bag every 4 hours, as appropriate
- Monitor for presence of bowel sounds every 4 to 8 hours, as appropriate
- Monitor fluid and electrolyte status
- Monitor for growth height/weight changes monthly, as appropriate
- Monitor weight 3 times weekly initially, decreasing to once a month
- Monitor for signs of edema or dehydration
- Monitor fluid intake and output
- Monitor calorie, fat, carbohydrate, vitamin, and mineral intake for adequacy (or refer to dietitian) two times per week initially, decreasing to once a month
- Monitor for mood changes
- Prepare individual and family for home tube feedings, as appropriate
- Monitor weight at least three times a week, as appropriate for age

1st edition 1992; revised 1996, 2000, 2004

Background Readings:

Fellows, L. S., Miller, E. H., Frederickson, M., Bly, B., & Felt, P. (2000). Evidence-based practice for enteral feedings and aspiration prevention: Strategies, bedside detection and practice change. *MEDSURG Nursing, 9*(1), 27–31.

Mahan, K. L. & Escott-Stump, S. (2000). *In Krause's food, nutrition & diet therapy* (9th ed.). Philadelphia: Saunders.

Methany, N. A. & Titler, M. G. (2001). Assessing placement of feeding tubes. *American Journal of Nursing, 101*(5), 6–45.

Perry, A. G. & Potter, P. A. (2002). *Clinical nursing skills and techniques* (5th ed., pp. 559–616). St. Louis: Mosby.

Environmental Management 6480

Definition: Manipulation of the patient's surroundings for therapeutic benefit, sensory appeal, and psychological well-being

Activities:
- Create a safe environment for the patient
- Identify the safety needs of patient, based on level of physical and cognitive function and past history of behavior
- Remove environmental hazards (e.g., loose rugs and small, movable furniture)
- Remove harmful objects from the environment
- Safeguard with side rails/side-rail padding, as appropriate
- Escort patient during off-ward activities, as appropriate
- Provide low-height bed, as appropriate
- Provide adaptive devices (e.g., step stools or handrails), as appropriate
- Place furniture in room in an appropriate arrangement that best accommodates patient or family disabilities
- Provide sufficiently long tubing to allow freedom of movement, as appropriate
- Place frequently used objects within reach
- Provide single room, as indicated
- Consider the aesthetics of the environment when selecting roommates
- Provide a clean, comfortable bed and environment
- Provide a firm mattress
- Provide linens and gown in good repair, free of residual stains
- Place bed-positioning switch within easy reach
- Neatly arrange supplies and linens that must remain in the patient's view
- Block the patient's view of the bathroom, commode, or other equipment used for elimination
- Remove materials used during dressing changes and elimination, as well as any residual odors, prior to visitation and meals
- Reduce environmental stimuli, as appropriate
- Avoid unnecessary exposure, drafts, overheating, or chilling
- Adjust environmental temperature to meet patient's needs, if body temperature is altered
- Control or prevent undesirable or excessive noise, when possible
- Provide music of choice
- Provide headphones for private listening when music may disturb others
- Manipulate lighting for therapeutic benefit
- Provide attractively arranged meals and snacks
- Clean areas and utensils used for eating and drinking prior to patient use
- Limit visitors

- Individualize visiting restrictions to meet patient's and/or family's/significant other's needs
- Individualize daily routine to meet patient's needs
- Bring familiar objects from home
- Facilitate use of personal items such as pajamas, robes, and toiletries
- Maintain consistency of staff assignment over time
- Provide immediate and continuous means to summon nurse, and let the patient and family know they will be answered immediately
- Allow family/significant other to stay with patient
- Educate patient and visitors about the changes/precautions, so they will not inadvertently disrupt the planned environment
- Provide family/significant other with information about making home environment safe for patient
- Promote fire safety, as appropriate
- Control environmental pests, as appropriate
- Provide room deodorizers, as needed
- Provide care for flowers/plants
- Assist patient or patient's family to arrange cards, flowers, and gifts to enhance the patient's visual appreciation

1st edition 1992; revised 1996, 2000, 2004

Background Readings:

Ackerman, L. L. (1992). Interventions related to neurological care. In G. M. Bulechek & J. C. McCloskey (Eds.), Symposium on nursing interventions. *Nursing Clinics of North America, 27*(2), 325–346.

Drury, J. & Akins, J. (1991). Sensory/perceptual alterations. In M. Maas, K. Buckwalter, & M. Hardy (Eds.), *Nursing diagnoses and interventions for the elderly* (pp. 369–389). Redwood City, CA: Addison-Wesley.

Gerdner, L. & Buckwalter, K. (1999). Music therapy. In G. Bulechek & J. McCloskey (Eds.), *Nursing interventions: Effective nursing treatments* (3rd ed., pp. 451–468). Philadelphia: Saunders.

Phylar, P. A. (1989). Management of the agitated and aggressive head injury patient in an acute hospital setting. *Journal of Neuroscience Nursing, 21*(6), 353–356.

Schuster, E. & Keegan, L. (2000). Environment. In B. Dossey, L. Keegan, & C. Guzzetta (Eds.), *Holistic nursing: A handbook for practice* (3rd ed., pp. 249–282). Gaithersburg, MD: Aspen.

Stoner, N. (1999). Feeding. In G. Bulechek & J. McCloskey (Eds.), *Nursing interventions: Effective nursing treatments* (3rd ed., pp. 31–46). Philadelphia: Saunders.

Environmental Management: Comfort 6482

Definition: Manipulation of the patient's surroundings for promotion of optimal comfort

Activities:
- Determine patient's and family's goals for the management of the environment and optimum comfort
- Ease patient's and family's transition by warmly welcoming them to the new environment
- Give consideration to the placement of patients in multiple-bedded rooms (roommates with similar environmental concerns when possible)

- Provide single room if it is the patient's (and family's) preference and need is for quiet and rest, if possible
- Provide prompt attention to call bells, which should always be within reach
- Prevent unnecessary interruptions and allow for rest period
- Create a calm and supportive environment
- Provide a safe and clean environment
- Provide choice wherever possible for social activities and visitation

- Determine sources of discomfort, such as damp dressings, positioning of tubing, constrictive dressings, wrinkled bed linens, and environmental irritants
- Adjust room temperature to that most comfortable for the individual, if possible
- Provide or remove blankets to promote temperature comfort, as indicated
- Avoid unnecessary exposure, drafts, overheating, or chilling
- Adjust lighting to meet needs of individual activities, avoiding direct light in eyes
- Facilitate hygiene measures to keep the individual comfortable (e.g., wiping brow, applying skin creams, or cleaning body, hair, and oral cavity)
- Position patient to facilitate comfort (e.g., using principles of body alignment, support with pillows, support joints during movement, splint over incisions, and immobilize painful body part)
- Monitor skin, especially over body prominences, for signs of pressure or irritation
- Avoid exposing skin or mucous membranes to irritants (e.g., diarrheal stool and wound drainage)

- Provide relevant and useful educational resources concerning the management of illnesses and injuries to patients and their families, if appropriate

1st edition 1992; revised 2008

Background Readings:

Herr, K. A. & Mobily, P. R. (1992). Interventions related to pain. In G. M. Bulechek & J. C. McCloskey (Eds.), Symposium on nursing interventions. *Nursing Clinics of North America, 27*(2), 347–370.

Edvardsson, J. D., Sandman, P. O., & Rasmussen, B. H. (2005). Sensing an atmosphere of ease: A tentative theory of supportive care settings. *Scandinavian Journal of Caring Science, 19*(4), 344–353.

Roush, C. & Cox, J. (2000). The meaning of home: How it shapes the practice of home and hospice care. *Home Healthcare Nurse, 18*(6), 388–394.

Williams, A. & Irurita, V. (2005). Enhancing the therapeutic potential of hospital environments by increasing the personal control and emotional comfort of hospitalized patients. *Applied Nursing Research, 18*(1), 22–28.

Environmental Management: Community 6484

Definition: Monitoring and influencing of the physical, social, cultural, economic, and political conditions that affect the health of groups and communities

Activities:

- Initiate screening for health risks from the environment
- Participate in multidisciplinary teams to identify threats to safety in the community
- Monitor status of known health risks
- Participate in community programs to deal with known risks
- Collaborate in the development of community action programs
- Promote governmental policy to reduce specified risks
- Encourage neighborhoods to become active participants in community safety
- Coordinate services to at-risk groups and communities
- Conduct educational programs for targeted risk groups
- Work with environmental groups to secure appropriate governmental regulations

Background Readings:

Bracht, N. (1990). *Health promotion at the community level.* Newbury Park, CA: Sage.

Dever, G. (1991). *Community health analysis.* Gaithersburg, MD: Aspen.

Salazar, M. K. & Primomo, J. (1994). Taking the lead in environmental health. *American Association of Occupational Health Nurses (AAOHN), 42*(7), 317–324.

Stevens, P. & Hall, J. (1993). Environmental health in community health nursing. In J. F. Swanson & M. Albrecht (Eds.), *Community health nursing: Promoting the health of aggregates* (pp. 567–596). Philadelphia: Saunders.

2nd edition 1996; revised 2000

Environmental Management: Home Preparation 6485

Definition: Preparing the home for safe and effective delivery of care

Activities:

- Consult with patient and caregivers concerning preparation for care delivery at home
- Monitor the home environment to receive the patient
- Order and validate operation of any equipment needed
- Order and confirm delivery of any medication and supplies needed

- Prepare teaching plans for use in the home to coincide with any earlier teaching already accomplished
- Arrange scheduling of support personnel
- Confirm that emergency plans are in place
- Confirm date and time of transfer to home
- Confirm arrangements for transportation to home with accompanying escort, as needed

- Follow up to assure that plans were feasible and carried out
- Provide written materials regarding medications, supplies, and assistive devices as guides for caregivers, as needed
- Provide documentation to meet agency guidelines

3rd edition 2000

Background Readings:

Humphrey, C. J. & Milone-Nuzzo, P. (1996). *Orientation to home care nursing*. Gaithersberg, MD: Aspen.

Kelly, K. & McClelland, E. (1989). Discharge planning: Home care considerations. In I. Martinson & A. Widmer (Eds.), *Home care nursing*. Philadelphia: Saunders.

Lin, Y. (2006). Psychiatric home care nursing. In W. K. Mohr (Ed.), *Psychiatric-mental health nursing* (6th ed., pp. 339–352). Philadelphia: Lippincott Williams & Wilkins.

McClelland, E. & Tarbox, M. (1998). Discharge planning: Home care considerations. In I. Martinson, A. Widmer, & C. Portillo (Eds.), *Home care nursing* (2nd ed.). Philadelphia: Saunders.

Environmental Management: Safety 6486

Definition: Monitoring and manipulation of the physical environment to promote safety

Activities:

- Identify the safety needs of patient, based on level of physical and cognitive function and past history of behavior
- Identify safety hazards in the environment (i.e., physical, biological, and chemical)
- Remove hazards from the environment, when possible
- Modify the environment to minimize hazards and risk
- Provide adaptive devices (e.g., step stools and handrails) to increase the safety of the environment
- Use protective devices (e.g., restraints, side rails, locked doors, fences, and gates) to physically limit mobility or access to harmful situations
- Notify agencies authorized to protect the environment (e.g., health department, environmental services, Environmental Protection Agency [EPA], and police)
- Provide patient with emergency phone numbers (e.g., police, local health department, and poison control center)
- Monitor the environment for changes in safety status
- Assist patient in relocating to safer environment (e.g., referral for housing assistance)
- Initiate and/or conduct screening programs for environmental hazards (e.g., lead and radon)
- Educate high-risk individuals and groups about environmental hazards
- Collaborate with other agencies to improve environmental safety (e.g., health department, police, and EPA)

1st edition 1992; revised 1996, 2000

Background Readings:

Clark, M. J. (1992). Environmental influences on community health. In M. J. Clark (Ed.), *Nursing in the community* (pp. 342–365). Norwalk, CT: Appleton & Lange.

Kanak, M. F. (1992). Interventions related to safety. In G. M. Bulechek & J. C. McCloskey (Eds.), Symposium on nursing interventions. *Nursing Clinics of North America, 27*(2), 371–396.

Kozier, B. & Erb, G. (1991). *Fundamentals of nursing: Concepts and procedures* (4th ed.). Menlo Park, CA: Addison-Wesley.

Lancaster, J. (1992). Environmental health and safety. In M. Stanhope & J. Lancaster (Eds.), *Community health nursing* (3rd ed., pp. 293–309). St. Louis: Mosby.

Mulroy, E. A. (2004). A user-friendly approach to program evaluation and effective community interventions for families at risk of homelessness. *Social Work, 49*(4), 573–586.

U.S. Department of Health and Human Services. (1991). *Healthy people 2000: National health promotion and disease prevention objectives*. Washington, DC: U.S. Government Printing Office.

Environmental Management: Violence Prevention 6487

Definition: Monitoring and manipulation of the physical environment to decrease the potential for violent behavior directed toward self, others, or environment

Activities:

- Remove potential weapons from environment (e.g., sharps and ropelike objects such as guitar strings)
- Search environment routinely to maintain it as hazard-free
- Search patient and belongings for weapons/potential weapons during inpatient admission procedure, as appropriate
- Monitor the safety of items being brought to the environment by visitors
- Instruct visitors and other caregivers about relevant patient safety issues
- Limit patient use of potential weapons (e.g., sharps and ropelike objects)
- Monitor patient during use of potential weapons (e.g., razor)
- Place patient with potential for self-harm with a roommate to decrease isolation and opportunity to act on self-harm thoughts, as appropriate

E

- Assign single room to patient with potential for violence toward others
- Place patient in bedroom located near nursing station
- Limit access to windows, unless locked and shatterproof, as appropriate
- Lock utility and storage rooms
- Provide paper dishes and plastic utensils at meals
- Place patient in least restrictive environment that allows for necessary level of observation
- Provide ongoing surveillance of all patient access areas to maintain patient safety and therapeutically intervene, as needed
- Remove other individuals from the vicinity of a violent or potentially violent patient
- Maintain a designated safe area (e.g., seclusion room) for patient to be placed when violent
- Apply mitts, splints, helmets, or restraints to limit mobility and ability to initiate self-harm, as appropriate
- Provide plastic, rather than metal, clothes hangers, as appropriate

1st edition 1992; revised 2013

Background Readings:

Bracken, M. I., Messing, J. T., Campbell, J.C., La Flair, L. N. & Kub, J. (2010). Intimate partner violence and abuse among female nurses and nursing personnel: Prevalence and risk factors. *Issues in Mental Health Nursing, 31*(2), 137–148.

Campbell, J.C., Webster, D.W., Glass, N. (2009). The danger assessment: Validation of a lethality risk assessment instrument for intimate partner femicide. *Journal of Interpersonal Violence, 24*(4), 653–674.

Constantino, R. E. & Privitera, M. R. (2010). Prevention terminology: Primary, secondary, tertiary and an evolution of terms. In M. R. Privitera (Ed.), *Workplace violence in mental and general healthcare settings* (pp. 15–22). Sudbury, MA: Jones and Bartlett.

Cutcliffe, J. R. & Barker, P. (2004). The Nurses' Global Assessment of Suicide Risk (NGASR): Developing a tool for clinical practice. *Journal of Psychiatric and Mental Health Nursing, 11*(4), 393–400.

Delaney, K. R., Esparza, D., Hinderliter, D., Lamb, K., & Mohr, W. K. (2006). Violence and abuse within the community. In W. K. Mohr (Ed.), *Psychiatric-mental health nursing* (6th ed., pp. 353–376). Philadelphia: Lippincott Williams & Wilkins.

Larsson, P., Nilsson, S., Runeson, B., & Gustafsson, B. (2007). Psychiatric nursing care of suicidal patients described by the sympathy-acceptance-understanding-competence model for confirming nursing. *Archives of Psychiatric Nursing, 21*(4), 222–232.

Moracco, K. & Cole, T. (2009). Preventing intimate partner violence: Screening is not enough. *JAMA: Journal of the American Medical Association, 302*(5), 568–570.

Ramsay, J., Carter, Y., Davidson, L., Dunne, D., Eldridge, S., Hegarty, K., et al. (2009). Advocacy interventions to reduce or eliminate violence and promote the physical and psychosocial well-being of women who experience intimate partner abuse. *Cochrane Database of Systematic Reviews* 2009, Issue 3. Art. No.: CD005043. doi: 10.1002/14651858.CD005043.pub2.

Schmidt, H. & Ivanoff, A. (2007). Behavioral prescriptions for treating self-injurious and suicidal behaviors. In O. J. Thienhaus & M. Piasecki (Eds.), *Correctional psychiatry: Practice guidelines and strategies* (pp. 7/1–7/23). Kingston, NJ: Civic Research Institute.

Environmental Management: Worker Safety 6489

Definition: Monitoring and manipulation of the worksite environment to promote safety and health of workers

Activities:

- Maintain confidential health records on employees
- Determine employee's fitness for work
- Identify worksite environmental hazards and stressors (i.e., physical, biological, chemical, and ergonomic)
- Identify applicable Occupation Safety and Health Administration (OSHA) standards and worksite compliance with standards
- Inform workers of their rights and responsibilities under OSHA (i.e., OSHA poster, copies of Act, and copies of standards)
- Inform workers of hazardous substances to which they may be exposed
- Use labels or signs to warn workers of potential worksite hazards
- Maintain records of occupational injuries and illnesses on forms acceptable to OSHA and participate in OSHA inspections
- Keep log of occupational injuries and illnesses for workers
- Identify risk factors for occupational injuries and illnesses through reviewing records for patterns of injuries and illnesses
- Initiate modification of the environment to eliminate or minimize hazards (e.g., training programs to prevent back injuries)
- Initiate worksite screening programs for early detection of work-related and nonoccupational illnesses and injuries (e.g., blood pressure, hearing and vision, and pulmonary function tests)
- Initiate worksite health promotion programs based on health risk assessments (e.g., smoking cessation, stress management, and immunizations)
- Identify and treat acute conditions at worksite
- Develop emergency protocols and train selected employees on emergency care
- Coordinate follow-up care for work-related injuries and illnesses

2nd edition 1996

Background Readings:

American Association of Occupational Health Nurses. (1988). *Standards for occupational health nursing practice*. Atlanta: Author.

Centers for Disease Control. (1986). Leading work-related diseases and injuries—United States. *MMWR-Morbidity & Mortality Weekly Report, 35*(8), 113–116.

Clemen-Stone, S., Eigsti, D. G., & McGuire, S. L. (1991). Occupational health nursing. In S. Clemen-Stone, D. G. Eigsti, & S. L. McGuire (Eds.), *Comprehensive family and community health nursing* (3rd ed., pp. 616–657). St. Louis: Mosby.

Department of Health and Human Services. (1991). *Healthy people 2000: National health promotion and disease prevention objectives* (DHHS Publication No. PHS 91-50213). Washington, DC: U.S. Government Printing Office.

Department of Labor Occupational Safety and Health Administration. (1994). *All about OSHA*. Washington, DC: U.S. Government Printing Office.

Environmental Risk Protection   8880

Definition: Preventing and detecting disease and injury in populations at risk from environmental hazards

Activities:

- Assess environment for potential and actual risk
- Analyze the level of risk associated with the environment (e.g., living habits, work, atmosphere, water, housing, food, waste, radiation, and violence)
- Inform populations at risk about the environmental hazards
- Monitor incidents of illness and injury related to environmental hazards
- Maintain knowledge associated with specific environmental standards (e.g., Environmental Protection Agency (EPA) and Occupation Safety and Health Administration (OSHA) regulations)
- Notify agencies authorized to protect the environment of known hazards
- Collaborate with other agencies to improve environmental safety
- Advocate for safer environmental designs, protection systems, and use of protective devices
- Support programs to disclose environmental hazards
- Screen populations at risk for evidence of exposure to environmental hazards
- Participate in data collection related to incidence and prevalence of exposure to environmental hazards

3rd edition 2000

Background Readings:

Humphrey, C. J. & Milone-Nuzzo, P. (1996). *Orientation to home care nursing.* Gaithersberg, MD: Aspen.

Klainberg, M., Holzemer, S., Leonard, M., & Arnold, J. (1998). *Community health nursing: An alliance for health.* New York: McGraw-Hill.

Kuss, T., Proulx-Girouard, L., Lovitt, S., Katz, C.B., & Kennelly, P. (1997). A public health nursing model. *Public Health Nursing, 14*(2), 81–91.

Nester, R. M. (1996). Occupational safety and health administration: Building partnerships. *AAOHN Journal, 44*(10), 493–499.

Stanhope, M. & Lancaster, J. (Eds.). (1996). *Community health nursing: Promoting health of aggregates, families and individuals* (4th ed.). St. Louis: Mosby.

Stevens, P. E. & Hall, J. M. (1993). Environmental health. In J. M. Swanson & M. Albrecht (Eds.), *Community health nursing: Promoting the health of aggregates.* Philadelphia: Saunders.

E

Examination Assistance   7680

Definition: Providing assistance to the patient and another health care provider during a procedure or exam

Activities:

- Ensure consent is completed, as appropriate
- Explain the rationale for the procedure
- Provide sensory preparation information, as appropriate
- Use developmentally appropriate language when explaining procedures to children
- Ensure availability of emergency equipment and medications before procedure
- Assemble appropriate equipment
- Keep threatening equipment out of view, as appropriate
- Provide a private environment
- Include parent/significant other, as appropriate
- Position and drape patient, as appropriate
- Restrain patient, as appropriate
- Explain need for restraints, as appropriate
- Prepare procedure site, as appropriate
- Maintain universal precautions
- Maintain strict aseptic technique, as appropriate
- Explain each step of the procedure to patient
- Monitor patient status during procedure
- Provide patient with emotional support, as indicated
- Provide distraction during procedure, as appropriate
- Assist patient to maintain positioning during procedure
- Reinforce expected behavior during examination of a child
- Facilitate use of equipment, as appropriate
- Note amount and appearance of fluids removed, as appropriate
- Collect, label, and arrange for transport of specimens, as appropriate
- Provide site care and dressing, as appropriate
- Ensure that follow-up tests (e.g., x-ray examinations) are done
- Instruct patient on postprocedure care
- Monitor patient after procedure, as appropriate

2nd edition 1996

Background Readings:

Manion, J. (1990). Preparing children for hospitalization, procedures or surgery. In M. J. Craft & J. A. Denehy (Eds.), *Nursing interventions for infants and children* (pp. 74–92). Philadelphia: Saunders.

Millar, S., Sampson, L. K., & Soukup, S. M. (1985). *AACN procedure manual for critical care.* Philadelphia: Saunders.

Exercise Promotion 0200

Definition: Facilitation of regular physical activity to maintain or advance to a higher level of fitness and health

Activities:
- Appraise individual's health beliefs about physical exercise
- Explore prior exercise experiences
- Determine individual's motivation to begin/continue exercise program
- Explore barriers to exercise
- Encourage verbalization of feelings about exercise or need for exercise
- Encourage individual to begin or continue exercise
- Assist in identifying a positive role model for maintaining the exercise program
- Assist individual to develop an appropriate exercise program to meet needs
- Assist individual to set short-term and long-term goals for the exercise program
- Assist individual to schedule regular periods for the exercise program into weekly routine
- Perform exercise activities with individual, as appropriate
- Include family/caregivers in planning and maintaining the exercise program
- Inform individual about health benefits and physiological effects of exercise
- Instruct individual about appropriate type of exercise for level of health, in collaboration with physician and/or exercise physiologist
- Instruct individual about desired frequency, duration, and intensity of the exercise program
- Monitor individual's adherence to exercise program/activity
- Assist individual to prepare and maintain a progress graph/chart to motivate adherence with the exercise program
- Instruct individual about conditions warranting cessation of or alteration in the exercise program
- Instruct individual on proper warm-up and cool-down exercises
- Instruct individual in techniques to avoid injury while exercising
- Instruct individual in proper breathing techniques to maximize oxygen uptake during physical exercise
- Provide reinforcement schedule to enhance individual's motivation (e.g., increased endurance estimation; weekly weigh-in)
- Monitor individual's response to exercise program
- Provide positive feedback for individual's efforts

1st edition 1992; revised 2000, 2004

Background Readings:

Allan, J. D. & Tyler, D. O. (1999). Exercise promotion. In G. M. Bulechek & J. C. McCloskey (Eds.), *Nursing interventions: Effective nursing treatments* (3rd ed., pp. 130–148). Philadelphia: Saunders.

Bennett, C. (2001). Exercise promotion. In M. Craft-Rosenberg & J. Denehy (Eds.), *Nursing interventions for infants, children, and families* (pp. 555–572). Thousand Oaks, CA: Sage.

Glick, O. J. (1992). Interventions related to activity and movement. In G. M. Bulechek & J. C. McCloskey (Eds.), Symposium on nursing interventions. *Nursing Clinics of North America, 27*(2), 541–568.

NIH Consensus Development Panel of Physical Activity and Cardiovascular Health. (1996). Physical activity and cardiovascular health. *Journal of the American Medical Association, 276*(3), 241–246.

Rippe, J., Ward, A., Porcari, M. S., Freedson, P., O'Hanley, S., & Wilkie, S. (1989). The cardiovascular benefits of walking. *Practical Cardiology, 15*(1), 66–72.

Topp, R. (1991). Development of an exercise program for older adults: Pre-exercise testing, exercise prescription and program maintenance. *Nurse Practitioner, 16*(10), 16–28.

Exercise Promotion: Strength Training 0201

Definition: Facilitating regular resistive muscle training to maintain or increase muscle strength

Activities:
- Conduct preexercise health screening to identify risks for exercise using standardized physical activity readiness scales and/or complete history and physical exam
- Obtain medical clearance for initiating a strength-training program, as appropriate
- Assist patient to express own beliefs, values, and goals for muscle fitness and health
- Provide information about muscle function, exercise physiology, and consequences of disuse
- Determine muscle fitness levels using exercise field or laboratory tests (e.g., maximum lift, number of list per unit of time)
- Provide information about types of muscle resistance that can be used (e.g., free weights, weight machines, rubberized stretch bands, weighted objects, aquatic)
- Assist to set realistic short-term and long-term goals and to take ownership of the exercise plan
- Assist to develop ways to minimize effects of procedural, emotional, attitudinal, financial, or comfort barriers to resistance muscle training
- Assist to obtain resources needed to engage in progressive muscle training
- Assist to develop a home/work environment that facilitates engaging in the exercise plan
- Instruct to wear clothing that prevents overheating or cooling
- Assist to develop a strength training program consistent with muscle fitness level, musculoskeletal constraints, functional health goals, exercise equipment resources, personal preference, and social support
- Specify level of resistance, number of repetitions, number of sets, and frequency of "training" sessions according to fitness level and presence/absence of exercise risk factors
- Instruct to rest briefly after each set, as needed
- Specify type and duration of warm-up/cooldown activity (e.g., stretches, walking, calisthenics)
- Demonstrate proper body alignment (posture) and lift form for exercising each major muscle group
- Use reciprocal movements to avoid injury in selected exercises
- Assist to talk through/perform the prescribed movement patterns without weights until correct form is learned

- Modify movements and methods of applying resistance for chair-bound or bed-bound patients
- Instruct to recognize sign/symptoms of exercise tolerance/intolerance during and after exercise sessions (e.g., light-headedness; SOB; more than usual muscle, skeletal, or joint pain; weakness; extreme fatigue; angina; profuse sweating; palpitations)
- Instruct to conduct exercise sessions for specific muscle groups every other day to facilitate muscle adaptation to training
- Instruct to perform three training sessions with each muscle group each week until training goals are achieved and then place on a maintenance program
- Instruct to avoid strength training exercise during temperature extremes
- Assist to determine rate of progressively increasing muscle work (i.e., amount of resistance and number of repetitions and sets)
- Provide illustrated, take-home, written instructions for general guidelines and movement form for each muscle group
- Assist to develop a record-keeping system that includes amount of resistance, and number of repetitions and sets to monitor progress in muscle fitness
- Reevaluate muscle fitness levels monthly
- Establish a follow-up schedule to maintain motivation, assist in problem solving, and monitor progress

- Assist to alter programs or develop other strategies to prevent boredom and dropout
- Collaborate with family and other health professionals (e.g., activity therapist, exercise physiologist, occupational therapist, recreational therapist, physical therapist) in planning, teaching, and monitoring a muscle training program

3rd edition 2000

Background Readings:

Hyatt, G. (1996). Strength training for the aging adult. In J. Clark (Ed.), *Exercise programming for older adults* (pp. 27–36). New York: Haworth Press.

Mobily, K. & Mobily, P. (1996). Progressive resistive training. In M. Titler (Ed.), *Gerontological nursing interventions research center, research development and dissemination core.* Iowa City: The University of Iowa.

Robbins, G., Fowers, D., & Burgess, S. (1997). *A wellness way of life.* Madison, WI: Brown-Benchmark.

Roberts, S. (1997). Principles of prescribing exercise. In S. Roberts, R. Robergs, & F. Hanson (Eds.), *Clinical exercise testing and prescription: Theory and application* (pp. 235–261). Boca Raton, FL: CRC Press.

Sharpe, F. & McConnell, C. (1992). Exercise beliefs and behaviors among older employees: A health promotion trial. *The Gerontologist, 32*(4), 444–449.

Southard, D. & Lombard, D. (1997). Principles of health behavior change. In S. Roberts, F. Robergs, & F. Hanson (Eds.), *Clinical exercise testing and prescription: Theory and application.* Boca Raton, NY: CRC Press.

E

Exercise Promotion: Stretching   0202

Definition: Facilitation of systematic slow-stretch-hold muscle exercises to induce relaxation, to prepare muscles/joints for more vigorous exercise, or to increase or maintain body flexibility

Activities:
- Obtain medical clearance for instituting a stretching exercise plan, as needed
- Assist patient to explore own beliefs, motivation, and level of neuromusculoskeletal fitness
- Assist to develop realistic short-term and long-term goal(s), based on current fitness level and lifestyle
- Provide information about aging-related changes in neuro-musculoskeletal structure and the effects of disuse
- Provide information about options for sequence, specific stretching activities, place, and time
- Assist to develop a schedule for exercise consistent with age, physical status, goals, motivation, and lifestyle
- Assist to develop an exercise plan that incorporates an orderly sequence of stretching movements, increments in the duration of the hold phase of the movement, and increments in number of repetitions for each slow-stretch-hold movement, consistent with level of musculoskeletal fitness or presence of pathology
- Instruct to begin exercise routine in muscle/joint groups that are least stiff or sore and gradually move to more restricted muscle/joint groups
- Instruct to slowly extend muscle/joint to point of full stretch (or reasonable discomfort) and hold for specified time and slowly release the stretched muscles
- Instruct to avoid quick, forceful, or bouncing movement to prevent overstimulation of the myotatic reflex or excessive muscle soreness

- Instruct in ways to monitor own adherence to schedule and progress toward goal(s) (e.g., increments in joint ROM, awareness of releasing muscle tension, increasing duration of "hold" phase and number of repetitions without pain and fatigue, and increases in tolerance to vigorous exercise)
- Provide illustrated, take-home, written instructions for each movement component
- Coach return demonstrations of exercises, as needed
- Monitor adherence to technique and schedule at specified follow-up time and place
- Monitor exercise tolerance (e.g., presence of such symptoms as breathlessness, rapid pulse, pallor, lightheadedness, and joint/muscle pain or swelling) during exercise
- Reevaluate exercise plan if symptoms of low exercise tolerance persist after cessation of exercise
- Collaborate with family members in planning, teaching, and monitoring an exercise plan

2nd edition 1996

Background Readings:

Allan, J. D. & Tyler, D. O. (1999). Exercise promotion. In G. M. Bulechek & J. C. McCloskey (Eds.), *Nursing interventions: Effective nursing treatments* (3rd ed., pp. 130–148). Philadelphia: Saunders.

Burke, E. J. & Humphreys, J. H. L. (1992). *Fit to exercise* (pp. 90–96). London: Pelham Books.

Maas, M. (1991). Impaired physical mobility. In M. Maas, K. Buckwalter, & M. Hardy (Eds.), *Nursing diagnoses and interventions for the elderly* (pp. 274–277). Redwood City, CA: Addison-Wesley.

Piscopo, J. (1985). *Fitness and aging* (pp. 169–189). New York: John Wiley & Sons.

Pollock, M. L. & Wilmore, J. H. (1990). *Exercise in health and disease: Evaluation and prescription for prevention and rehabilitation* (2nd ed.). Philadelphia: Saunders.

Sharkey, B. J. (1990). *Physiology of fitness* (3rd ed., pp. 66, 78, 331–335). Champaign, IL: Human Kinetics Books.

Sorenson, A. J. & Poh, A. E. (1989). Physical fitness. In P. Swinford & J. Webster (Eds.), *Promoting wellness: A nurse's handbook* (pp. 108–109, 122–125). Rockville, MD: Aspen.

E

Exercise Therapy: Ambulation   0221

Definition: Promotion and assistance with walking to maintain or restore autonomic and voluntary body functions during treatment and recovery from illness or injury

Activities:
- Dress patient in nonrestrictive clothing
- Assist patient to use footwear that facilitates walking and prevents injury
- Provide low-height bed, as appropriate
- Place bed-positioning switch within easy reach
- Encourage to sit in bed, on side of bed ("dangle"), or in chair, as tolerated
- Assist patient to sit on side of bed to facilitate postural adjustments
- Consult physical therapist about ambulation plan, as needed
- Instruct in availability of assistive devices, if appropriate
- Instruct patient how to position self throughout the transfer process
- Use a gait belt to assist with transfer and ambulation, as needed
- Assist patient to transfer, as needed
- Provide cueing card(s) at head of bed to facilitate learning to transfer
- Apply/provide assistive device (cane, walker, or wheelchair) for ambulation, if the patient is unsteady
- Assist patient with initial ambulation and as needed
- Instruct patient/caregiver about safe transfer and ambulation techniques
- Monitor patient's use of crutches or other walking aids
- Assist patient to stand and ambulate specified distance and with specified number of staff
- Assist patient to establish realistic increments in distance for ambulation
- Encourage independent ambulation within safe limits
- Encourage patient to be "up ad lib," if appropriate

1st edition 1992; revised 2000

Background Readings:
Alora, J. (1981). Exercise and skeletal health. *Journal of the American Geriatric Society, 29*(3), 104–107.

Donohue, K., Miller, C., & Craig, B. (1988). Chronic alterations in mobility. In P. H. Mitchell (Ed.), *AANN's neuroscience nursing: Phenomena and practice* (pp. 319–343). Norwalk, CT: Appleton & Lange.

Glick, O. J. (1992). Interventions related to activity and movement. In G. M. Bulechek & J. C. McCloskey (Eds.), Symposium on nursing interventions. *Nursing Clinics of North America, 27*(2), 541–568.

Lubkin, I. (1990). *Chronic illness: Impact and interventions* (2nd ed.). Boston: Jones & Bartlett.

McFarland, G. K. & McFarlane, E. A. (1997). *Nursing diagnosis and intervention* (3rd ed.). St. Louis: Mosby.

Moorhouse, M., Geissler, A., & Doenges, M. (1987). *Critical care plans, guidelines for patient care.* Philadelphia: F. A. Davis.

Smith, E. L. & Gillian, C. (1983). Physical activity prescription for the older adult. *The Physician & Sports Medicine, 11*(8), 91–182.

Snyder, M. (1992). Exercise. In M. Snyder (Ed.), *Independent nursing interventions* (2nd ed., pp. 67–77). Albany: Delmar.

Exercise Therapy: Balance   0222

Definition: Use of specific activities, postures, and movements to maintain, enhance, or restore balance

Activities:
- Determine patient's ability to participate in activities requiring balance
- Collaborate with physical, occupational, and recreational therapists in developing and executing exercise program, as appropriate
- Evaluate sensory functions (e.g., vision, hearing, and proprioception)
- Provide opportunity to discuss factors that influence fear of falling
- Provide safe environment for practice of exercises
- Instruct patient on the importance of exercise therapy in maintaining and improving balance
- Encourage low-intensity exercise programs with opportunities to share feelings
- Instruct patient on balance exercises, such as standing on one leg, bending forward, stretching and resistance, as appropriate
- Assist with ankle strengthening and walking programs
- Provide information on alternative therapies such as yoga and Tai Chi
- Adjust environment to facilitate concentration
- Provide assistive devices (e.g., cane, walker, pillows, or pads) to support patient in performing exercise
- Assist patient to formulate realistic, measurable goals
- Reinforce or provide instruction about how to position self and perform movements to maintain or improve balance during exercises or activities of daily living
- Assist patient to participate in stretching exercises while lying, sitting, or standing

- Assist patient to move to sitting position, stabilize trunk with arms placed at side on bed/chair, and rock trunk over supporting arms
- Assist to stand (or sit) and rock body from side to side to stimulate balance mechanisms
- Encourage patient to maintain wide base of support, if needed
- Assist patient to practice standing with eyes closed for short periods at regular intervals to stimulate proprioception
- Monitor patient's response to balance exercises
- Conduct a home assessment to identify existing environmental and behavioral hazards, if applicable
- Provide resources for balance, exercise, or fall-education programs
- Refer to physical and/or occupational therapy for vestibular habituation training exercises

1st edition 1992; revised 2008

Background Readings:

Baum, E. E., Jarjoura, D., Polen, A. E., Faur, D., & Rutecki, G. (2004). Effectiveness of a group exercise program in a long-term care facility: A randomized pilot trial. *Journal of American Medical Directors Association*, 4(2), 74–80.

Choi, J. H., Moon, J. S., & Song, R. (2005). Effects of sun-style tai chi exercise on physical fitness and fall prevention in fall-prone older adults. *Journal of Advanced Nursing*, 51(2), 150–157.

Deiner, D. & Mitchell, M. (2005). Impact of a multifactorial fall prevention program upon falls of older frail adults attending an adult health day care center. *Topics in Geriatric Rehabilitation*, 21(3), 247–257.

Hansson, E. E., Mansson, N., & Hakansson, A. (2005). Balance performance and self-perceived handicap among dizzy patients in primary health care. *Scandinavian Journal of Primary Health Care*, 23(4), 215–220.

Gentleman, B. & Malozemoff, W. (2001). Falls and feelings: Description of a psychological group nursing intervention. *Journal of Gerontological Nursing*, 27(10), 35–39.

Liu-Ambrose, T., Khan, K. M., Eng, J. J., Lord, S. R., & McKay, H. A. (2004). Balance confidence improves with resistance or agility training. Increase is not correlated with objective changes in fall risk and physical abilities. *Gerontology*, 50(6), 373–382.

Norre, M. & Beckers, A. (1989). Vestibular habituation training for positional vertigo in elderly patients. *Archives of Gerontology and Geriatrics*, 8 (2), 117.

Oken, B., Zajdel, D., Kishiyama, S., Flegal, K., Dehen, C., Haas, M., et al. (2006). Randomized, controlled, six-month trial of yoga in healthy seniors: Effects on cognition and quality of life. *Alternative Therapy Health Medicine*, 12(1), 40–47.

Schoenfelder, D. & Rubinstein, L. (2004). An exercise program to improve fall-related outcomes in elderly nursing home residents. *Applied Nursing Research*, 17(1), 21–31.

Exercise Therapy: Joint Mobility   0224

Definition: Use of active or passive body movement to maintain or restore joint flexibility

Activities:
- Determine limitations of joint movement and effect on function
- Collaborate with physical therapy in developing and executing an exercise program
- Determine patient motivation level for maintaining or restoring joint movement
- Explain to patient/family the purpose and plan for joint exercises
- Monitor location and nature of discomfort or pain during movement/activity
- Initiate pain control measures before beginning joint exercise
- Dress patient in nonrestrictive clothing
- Protect patient from trauma during exercise
- Assist patient to optimal body position for passive/active joint movement
- Encourage active range-of-motion (ROM) exercises, according to regular, planned schedule
- Perform passive (PROM) or assisted (AROM) exercises, as indicated
- Instruct patient/family how to systematically perform PROM, AROM, or active ROM exercises
- Provide written discharge instructions for exercise
- Assist patient to develop a schedule for active ROM exercises
- Encourage patient to visualize body motion before beginning movement
- Assist with regular rhythmic joint motion within limits of pain, endurance, and joint mobility
- Encourage patient to sit in bed, on side of bed ("dangle"), or in chair, as tolerated
- Encourage ambulation, if appropriate
- Determine progress toward goal achievement
- Provide positive reinforcement for performing joint exercises

1st edition 1992; revised 2000

Background Readings:

Glick, O. J. (1992). Interventions related to activity and movement. In G. M. Bulechek & J. C. McCloskey (Eds.), Symposium on nursing interventions. *Nursing Clinics of North America*, 27(2), 541–568.

Hickey, J. (1992). *The clinical practice of neurological and neurosurgical nursing* (3rd ed.). Philadelphia: Lippincott.

Hogue, C. (1985). Mobility. In E. G. Schneider (Ed.), *The teaching nursing home*. New York: Raven Press.

Lewis, C. B. (1989). *Improving mobility in older persons*. Rockville, MD: Aspen.

Lubkin, I. (1990). *Chronic illness: Impact and interventions* (2nd ed.). Boston: Jones & Bartlett.

McFarland, G. K. & McFarlane, E. A. (1997). *Nursing diagnosis and intervention* (3rd ed.). St. Louis: Mosby.

Moorhouse, M., Geissler, A., & Doenges, M. (1987). *Critical care plans, guidelines for patient care*. Philadelphia: F. A. Davis.

Pender, N. J. (1987). *Health promotion nursing practice* (2nd ed.). Norwalk, CT: Appleton & Lange.

Snyder, M. (1992). Exercise. In M. Snyder (Ed.), *Independent nursing interventions* (2nd ed., pp. 67–77). Albany: Delmar.

Sullivan, P. & Markos, P. (1993). *Clinical procedures in therapeutic exercise*. Norwalk, CT: Appleton & Lange.

Vogt, G., Miller, M., & Esluer, M. (1985). *Mosby's manual of neurological care*. St. Louis: Mosby.

Exercise Therapy: Muscle Control

0226

Definition: Use of specific activity or exercise protocols to enhance or restore controlled body movement

Activities:

- Determine patient's readiness to engage in activity or exercise protocol
- Collaborate with physical, occupational, and recreational therapists in developing and executing exercise program, as appropriate
- Consult physical therapy to determine optimal position for patient during exercise and number of repetitions for each movement pattern
- Evaluate sensory functions (e.g., vision, hearing, and proprioception)
- Explain rationale for type of exercise and protocol to patient/family
- Provide patient privacy for exercising, if desired
- Adjust lighting, room temperature, and noise level to enhance patient's ability to concentrate on the exercise activity
- Sequence daily care activities to enhance effects of specific exercise therapy
- Initiate pain control measures before beginning exercise/activity
- Dress patient in nonrestrictive clothing
- Assist to maintain trunk and/or proximal joint stability during motor activity
- Apply splints to achieve stability of proximal joints involved with fine motor skills, as prescribed
- Reevaluate need for assistive devices at regular intervals in collaboration with physical therapist, occupational therapist, or respiratory therapist
- Assist patient to sitting/standing position for exercise protocol, as appropriate
- Reinforce instructions provided to patient about the proper way to perform exercises to minimize injury and maximize effectiveness
- Determine accuracy of body image
- Reorient patient to body awareness
- Reorient patient to movement functions of the body
- Coach patient to visually scan affected side of body when performing activities of daily living (ADLs) or exercises, if indicated
- Provide step-by-step cueing for each motor activity during exercise or ADLs
- Instruct patient to "recite" each movement as it is being performed
- Use visual aids to facilitate learning how to perform ADLs or exercise movements, as appropriate
- Provide restful environment for patient after periods of exercise
- Assist patient to develop exercise protocol for strength, endurance, and flexibility
- Assist patient to formulate realistic, measurable goals
- Use motor activities that require attention to and use of both sides of the body
- Incorporate ADLs into exercise protocol, if appropriate
- Encourage patient to practice exercises independently, as indicated
- Assist patient with/encourage patient to use warm-up and cool-down activities before and after exercise protocol
- Use tactile (and/or tapping) stimuli to minimize muscle spasm
- Assist patient to prepare and maintain a progress graph/chart to motivate adherence with exercise protocol
- Monitor patient's emotional, cardiovascular, and functional responses to exercise protocol
- Monitor patient's self-exercise for correct performance
- Evaluate patient's progress toward enhancement/restoration of body movement and function
- Provide positive reinforcement for patient's efforts in exercise and physical activity
- Collaborate with home caregivers regarding exercise protocol and ADLs
- Assist patient/caregiver to make prescribed revisions in home exercise plan, as indicated

1st edition 1992; revised 2000

Background Readings:

Donohue, K., Miller, C., & Craig, B. (1988). Chronic alterations in mobility. In P. H. Mitchell (Ed.), *AANN's neuroscience nursing: Phenomena and practice* (pp. 319–343). Norwalk, CT: Appleton & Lange.

Glick, O. J. (1992). Interventions related to activity and movement. In G. M. Bulechek & J. C. McCloskey (Eds.), Symposium on nursing interventions. *Nursing Clinics of North America, 27*(2), 541–568.

Hickey, J. (1992). *The clinical practice of neurological and neurosurgical nursing* (3rd ed.). Philadelphia: Lippincott.

Hogue, C. (1985). Mobility. In E. G. Schneider (Ed.), *The teaching nursing home*. New York: Raven Press.

Lewis, C. B. (1989). *Improving mobility in older persons*. Rockville, MD: Aspen.

Lubkin, I. (1990). *Chronic illness: Impact and intervention* (2nd ed.). Boston: Jones & Bartlett.

McFarland, G. K. & McFarlane, E. A. (1997). *Nursing diagnosis and intervention* (3rd ed.). St. Louis: Mosby.

Moorhouse, M., Geissler, A., & Doenges, M. (1987). *Critical care plans, guidelines for patient care*. Philadelphia: F. A. Davis.

Pender, N. J. (1987). *Health promotion nursing practice* (2nd ed.). Norwalk, CT: Appleton & Lange.

Sullivan, P. & Markos, P. (1993). *Clinical procedures in therapeutic exercise*. Norwalk, CT: Appleton & Lange.

Vogt, G., Miller, M., & Esluer, M. (1985). *Mosby's manual of neurological care*. St. Louis: Mosby.

Eye Care   1650

Definition: Prevention or minimization of threats to eye or visual integrity

Activities:

- Monitor for redness, exudate, or ulceration
- Instruct patient not to touch eye
- Monitor corneal reflex
- Remove contact lenses, as appropriate
- Apply eye shield, as appropriate
- Patch the eyes, as needed
- Alternate eye patch for diplopia
- Apply lubricating eyedrops, as appropriate
- Apply lubricating ointment, as appropriate
- Tape eyelids shut, as appropriate
- Apply moisture chamber, as appropriate

1st edition 1992; revised 2000

Background Readings:

Ackerman, L. L. (1992). Interventions related to neurological care. In G. M. Bulechek & J. C. McCloskey (Eds.), Symposium on nursing interventions. *Nursing Clinics of North America, 27*(2), 325–346.

American Association of Critical Care Nurses. (2006). Core curriculum for critical care nursing (6th ed.) [J. G. Alspach, Ed.]. Philadelphia: Saunders.

Craven, R. F. & Hirnle, C. J. (2003). Self-care hygiene. In *Fundamentals of nursing: Human health and function* (4th ed., pp. 703–752). Philadelphia: Lippincott Williams & Wilkins.

Hickey, J. V. (1992). *The clinical practice of neurological and neurosurgical nursing* (3rd ed.). Philadelphia: Lippincott.

Wincek, J. & Turrnam, M. S. (1989). Exposure keratitis in comatose children. *Journal of Neuroscience Nursing, 21*(4), 241–244.

E

Fall Prevention 6490

Definition: Instituting special precautions with patient at risk for injury from falling

Activities:

- Identify cognitive or physical deficits of the patient that may increase potential of falling in a particular environment
- Identify behaviors and factors that affect risk of falls
- Review history of falls with patient and family
- Identify characteristics of environment that may increase potential for falls (e.g., slippery floors and open stairways)
- Monitor gait, balance, and fatigue level with ambulation
- Ask patient for perception of balance, as appropriate
- Share with patient observations about gait and movement
- Suggest changes in gait to patient
- Coach patient to adapt to suggested gait modifications
- Assist unsteady individual with ambulation
- Provide assistive devices (e.g., cane and walker) to steady gait
- Encourage patient to use cane or walker, as appropriate
- Instruct patient about use of cane or walker, as appropriate
- Maintain assistive devices in good working order
- Lock wheels of wheelchair, bed, or gurney during transfer of patient
- Place articles within easy reach of the patient
- Instruct patient to call for assistance with movement, as appropriate
- Teach patient how to fall as to minimize injury
- Post signs to remind patient to call for help when getting out of bed, as appropriate
- Monitor ability to transfer from bed to chair and vice versa
- Use proper technique to transfer patient to and from wheelchair, bed, toilet, and so on
- Provide elevated toilet seat for easy transfer
- Provide chairs of proper height, with backrests and armrests for easy transfer
- Provide bed mattress with firm edges for easy transfer
- Use side rails of appropriate length and height to prevent falls from bed, as needed
- Place a mechanical bed in lowest position
- Provide a sleeping surface close to the floor, as needed
- Provide seating on bean bag chair to limit mobility, as appropriate
- Place a foam wedge in seat of chair to prevent patient from arising, as appropriate
- Use partially-filled water mattress on bed to limit mobility, as appropriate
- Provide the dependent patient with a means of summoning help (e.g., bell or call light) when caregiver is not present
- Answer call light immediately
- Assist with toileting at frequent, scheduled intervals
- Use a bed alarm to alert caretaker that individual is getting out of bed, as appropriate
- Mark doorway thresholds and edges of steps, as needed
- Remove low-lying furniture (e.g., footstools and tables) that present a tripping hazard
- Avoid clutter on floor surface
- Provide adequate lighting for increased visibility
- Provide nightlight at bedside
- Provide visible handrails and grab bars
- Place gates in open doorways leading to stairways
- Provide nonslip, nontrip floor surfaces
- Provide a nonslip surface in bathtub or shower
- Provide sturdy, nonslip step stools to facilitate easy reaches

- Provide storage areas that are within easy reach
- Provide heavy furniture that will not tip if used for support
- Orient patient to physical "setup" of room
- Avoid unnecessary rearrangement of physical environment
- Ensure that patient wears shoes that fit properly, fasten securely, and have nonskid soles
- Instruct patient to wear prescription glasses, as appropriate, when out of bed
- Educate family members about risk factors that contribute to falls and how they can decrease these risks
- Suggest home adaptations to increase safety
- Instruct family on importance of handrails for stairs, bathrooms, and walkways
- Assist family in identifying hazards in the home and modifying them
- Suggest safe footwear
- Instruct patient to avoid ice and other slippery outdoor surfaces
- Develop ways for patient to participate safely in leisure activities
- Institute a routine physical exercise program that includes walking
- Post signs to alert staff that patient is at high risk for falls
- Collaborate with other health care team members to minimize side effects of medications that contribute to falling (e.g., orthostatic hypotension and unsteady gait)
- Provide close supervision and/or a restraining device (e.g., infant seat with seat belt) when placing infants/young children on elevated surfaces (e.g., table and highchair)
- Remove objects that provide young child with climbing access to elevated surfaces
- Maintain crib side rails in elevated position when caregiver is not present, as appropriate
- Provide a "bubble top" on hospital cribs of pediatric patients who may climb over elevated side rails, as appropriate
- Fasten the latches securely on access panel of incubator when leaving bedside of infant in incubator, as appropriate

1st edition 1992; revised 2000, 2004

Background Readings:

Foley, G. (1999). The multidisciplinary team: Partners in patient safety. *Cancer Practice, 7*(3), 108.

Kanak, M. F. (1992). Interventions related to safety. In G. M. Bulechek & J. C. McCloskey (Eds.), Symposium on nursing interventions. *Nursing Clinics of North America, 27*(2), 371–396.

Maciorowski, L. F., Monro, B. H., Dietrick-Gallagher, M., McNew, C. D., Sheppard-Hinkel, E., Wanich, C., et al. (1989). A review of the patient fall literature. *Journal of Nursing Quality Assurance, 3*(1), 18–27.

Stolley, J. M., Lewis, A., Moore, L., & Harvey, P. (2001). Risk for injury: Falls. In M. Maas, K. Buckwalter, M. Hardy, T. Tripp-Reimer, M. Titler, & J. Specht (Eds.), *Nursing care of older adults: Diagnoses, outcomes, and interventions* (pp. 23–33). St. Louis: Mosby.

Sullivan, R. P. (1999). Recognize factors to prevent patient falls. *Nursing Management, 30*(5), 37–40.

Tack, K. A., Ulrich, B., & Kehr, C. (1987). Patient falls: Profiles for prevention. *Journal of Neuroscience Nursing, 19*(2), 83–89.

Tideiksaar, R. (1997). *Falling in old age: Prevention and management.* New York: Springer.

F

Family Integrity Promotion   7100

Definition: Promotion of family cohesion and unity

Activities:
- Be a listener for the family members
- Establish trusting relationship with family members
- Determine family understanding of condition
- Determine family feelings regarding their situation
- Assist family to resolve unrealistic feelings of guilt or responsibility, as warranted
- Determine typical family relationships for each family
- Monitor current family relationships
- Identify typical family coping mechanisms
- Identify conflicting priorities among family members
- Assist family with conflict resolution
- Counsel family members on additional effective coping skills for their own use
- Respect privacy of individual family members
- Provide for family privacy
- Tell family members it is safe and acceptable to use typical expressions of affection when in a hospital setting
- Facilitate a tone of togetherness within/among the family
- Provide family members with information about the patient's condition regularly, according to patient preference
- Collaborate with family in problem solving and decision-making
- Encourage family to maintain positive relationships
- Facilitate open communication among family members
- Provide for care of patient by family members, as appropriate
- Facilitate family visitation
- Refer family to support group of other families dealing with similar problems
- Refer for family therapy, as indicated

1st edition 1992; revised 2008

Background Readings:

Keefe, M. R., Barbaos, G. A., Froese-Fretz, A., Kotzer, A. M., & Lobo, M. (2005). An intervention program for families with irritable infants. *MCH American Journal of Maternal Child Nursing, 30*(4), 230–236.

McBride, K. L., White, C. L., Sourial, R., & Mayo, N. (2004). Post discharge nursing interventions for stroke survivors and their families. *Journal of Advanced Nursing, 47*(2), 192–200.

Mu, P. F., Kuo, H. C., & Chang, K. P. (2005). Boundary ambiguity, coping patterns and depression in mothers caring for children with epilepsy in Taiwan. *International Journal of Nursing Studies, 42*(3), 273–282.

F

Family Integrity Promotion: Childbearing Family   7104

Definition: Facilitation of the growth of individuals or families who are adding an infant to the family unit

Activities:
- Establish trusting relationship with parent(s)
- Listen to families concerns, feelings, and questions
- Respect and support family's cultural value system
- Identify family interaction patterns
- Assist family in identifying strengths and weaknesses
- Identify normal family coping mechanisms
- Assist family in developing adaptive coping mechanisms to deal with the transition to parenthood
- Monitor parent's adaptation to parenthood
- Prepare parent(s) for expected role changes involved in becoming a parent
- Educate parent(s) about potential role conflict and role overload
- Promote self-efficacy in carrying out parental role
- Prepare parent(s) for responsibilities of parenthood
- Encourage parents to articulate their values, beliefs, and expectations regarding parenthood
- Assist parents in having realistic role expectations about parenthood
- Assist parents in dealing with suggestions, criticisms, and concerns about parental role expectations and performance from others (e.g., parents, grandparents, coworkers, friends)
- Education parents about the effects of sleep deprivation on family functioning
- Reinforce positive parenting behaviors
- Assist parents in gaining skills needed to perform tasks appropriate to family developmental stage
- Assist parents in balancing work, parental, and marital roles
- Assist mother in making plans for returning to work, as appropriate
- Provide parent(s) an opportunity to express their feelings about parenthood
- Identify effect of newborn on family dynamics and equilibrium
- Encourage parents to spend time together as a couple to maintain marital satisfaction
- Encourage parents to discuss household maintenance role responsibilities
- Encourage verbalization of feelings, perceptions, and concerns about the birth experience
- Explain causes and manifestations of postpartum depression
- Encourage parent(s) to maintain individual hobbies or outside interests
- Encourage family to attend sibling preparation classes, as appropriate
- Provide information about sibling preparation, as appropriate
- Give family information on sibling rivalry, as appropriate
- Discuss reaction of sibling(s) to newborn, as appropriate
- Assist family in identifying support systems
- Encourage family to use support systems, as appropriate
- Assist family in developing new support networks, as appropriate
- Offer to be an advocate for the family

1st edition 1992; revised 2008

Background Readings:

Cowan, C. P. & Cowan, P. A. (1995). Interventions to ease the transition to parenthood: Why they are needed and what they can do. *Family Relations, 44*(4), 412–423.

Newman, B. M. (2000). The challenges of parenting infants and young children. In P. C. McKenry & S. J Price (Eds.), *Families & change: Coping with stressful events and transitions* (2nd ed., pp. 43–70). Thousand Oaks, CA: Sage.

Swartz, M. K. & Knafl, K. (2006). Enhancement of family support systems. In M. Craft-Rosenberg & M. J. Krajicek (Eds.), *Nursing excellence for children & families* (pp. 77–95). New York: Springer.

Family Involvement Promotion   7110

Definition: Facilitating participation of family members in the emotional and physical care of the patient

Activities:

- Establish a personal relationship with the patient and family members who will be involved in care
- Identify family members' capabilities for involvement in care of the patient
- Create a culture of flexibility for the family
- Determine physical, emotional, and educational resources of primary caregiver
- Identify patient's self-care deficits
- Identify family members' preferences for involvement with patient
- Identify family members' expectations for the patient
- Anticipate and identify family needs
- Encourage the family members and the patient to assist in the development of a plan of care, including expected outcomes and implementation of the plan of care
- Encourage the family members and patient to be assertive in interactions with health care professionals
- Monitor family structure and roles
- Monitor involvement in patient's care by family members
- Encourage care by family members during hospitalization or care in a long-term care facility
- Provide crucial information to family members about the patient in accordance with patient preference
- Facilitate understanding of the medical aspects of the patient's condition for family members
- Provide the support needed for the family to make informed decisions
- Identify family members' perception of the situation, precipitating events, patient's feelings, and patients' behaviors
- Identify other situational stressors for family members
- Identify individual family members' physical symptoms related to stress (e.g., tearfulness, nausea, vomiting, distractibility)
- Determine level of patient dependence on family members, as appropriate for age or illness
- Encourage focus on any positive aspects of the patient's situation
- Identify and respect coping mechanisms used by family members
- Identify with family members the patient's coping difficulties
- Identify with family members the patient's strengths and abilities with family
- Inform family members of factors that may improve patient's condition
- Encourage family members to keep or maintain family relationships, as appropriate
- Discuss options for type of home care, such as group living, residential care, or respite care, as appropriate
- Facilitate management of the medical aspects of illness by family members

1st edition 1992; revised 2000, 2004, 2008

Background Readings:

Gosline, M. B. (2003). Client participation to enhance socialization for frail elders. *Geriatric Nursing, 24*(5), 286–289.

Powaski, K. M. (2006). Nursing interventions in pediatric palliative care. *Child and Adolescent Psychiatric Clinics of North America, 15*(3), 717–37.

Schumacher, K. L., Koresawa, S., West, C., Hawkins, C., Johnson, C., Wais, E., et al. (2002). Putting cancer pain management regimens into practice at home. *Journal of Pain Symptom Management, 23*(5), 369–382.

Family Mobilization   7120

Definition: Utilization of family strengths to influence patient's health in a positive direction

Activities:

- Be a listener for family members
- Establish trusting relationships with family members
- View family members as potential experts in the care of the patient
- Identify strengths and resources within the family, in family members, and in their support system and community
- Determine the readiness and ability of family members to learn
- Provide information frequently to the family to assist them in identifying the patient's limitations, progress, and implications for care
- Foster mutual decision-making with family members, related to the patient's care plan
- Teach home caregivers about the patient's therapy, as appropriate
- Explain to family members the need for continuing of professional health care, as appropriate
- Collaborate with family members in planning and implementing patient therapies and life-style changes
- Support family activities in promoting patient health or management of condition, when appropriate
- Assist family members to identify health services and community resources that can be used to enhance the health status of the patient
- Monitor the current family situation
- Refer family members to support groups, as appropriate
- Determine expected patient outcome achievement systematically

1st edition 1992; revised 2004, 2008

Background Readings:

Deatrick, J. A. (2006). Family partnerships in nursing care. In M. Craft-Rosenberg & M. Krajicek (Eds.), *Nursing excellence for children & families.* New York: Springer.

Gerdner, L. A., Buckwalter, K. C., & Reed, D. (2002). Impact of a psychoeducational intervention of caregiver response to behavioral problems. *Nursing Research, 51*(6), 363–374.

Sylvain, H. & Talbot, L. R. (2002). Synergy towards health: A nursing intervention model for women living with fibromyalgia, and their spouses. *Journal of Advanced Nursing, 38*(3), 264–273.

Family Planning: Contraception
6784

Definition: Assisting patient in determining and providing method of pregnancy prevention

Activities:
- Appraise patient's knowledge and understanding of contraceptive choices
- Instruct patient on physiology of human reproduction, including both female and male reproductive systems, as needed
- Conduct relevant physical exam if indicated by patient history
- Determine ability and motivation for using a method
- Determine level of commitment to consistently use method
- Discuss religious, cultural, developmental, socioeconomical, and individual considerations pertaining to contraceptive choice
- Discuss methods of contraception (e.g., medication-free, barrier, hormonal, intrauterine device, and sterilization) including effectiveness, side effects, contraindications, and signs and symptoms that warrant reporting to a health care professional
- Assist adolescents to obtain contraceptive information in a confidential manner
- Assist female patient to determine ovulation through basal body temperature, changes in vaginal secretions, and other physiological indicators
- Provide contraception to patient, if indicated
- Discuss emergency contraception, as needed
- Provide emergency contraception (e.g., morning after pill, copper intrauterine device), as appropriate
- Instruct on safe sex activities, as indicated
- Refer patient to other health care professional or community resources (e.g., social worker and home health care professional), as needed
- Determine financial resources for contraception and refer for community resources, as appropriate

1st edition 1992; revised 2013

Background Readings:

Cheng, L., Gulmezoglu, A. M., Piaggio, G., Ezcurra, E. E., & Van Look, P. (2008). Interventions for emergency contraception. *Cochrane Database of Systematic Reviews,* Issue 2. Art. No.: CD001324. doi: 10.1002/14651858.CD001324.pub3.

Lopez, L. M., Tolley, E. E., Grimes, D. A., & Chen-Mok, M. (2009). Theory-based interventions for contraception. *Cochrane Database of Systematic Reviews,* Issue 1. Art. No.: CD007249. doi: 10.1002/14651858.CD007249.pub2.

Oringanje, C., Meremikwu, M. M., Eko, H., Esu, E., Meremikwu, A., Ehiri, J. E. (2009). Interventions for preventing unintended pregnancies among adolescents. *Cochrane Database of Systematic Reviews,* Issue 4. Art. No.: CD005215. doi: 10.1002/14651858.CD005215.pub2.

U.S. Department of Health and Human Services. (2000). *Healthy People 2010: Understanding and improving health* (2nd ed.). Washington, DC: Government Printing Office.

Ward, S. L. & Hisley, S. M. (2009). *Maternal-child nursing care: Optimizing outcomes for mothers, children, & families.* Philadelphia: F. A. Davis.

Family Planning: Infertility
6786

Definition: Management, education, and support of the patient and significant other undergoing evaluation and treatment for infertility

Activities:
- Explain female reproductive cycle to patient, as needed
- Assist female patient to determine ovulation through basal body temperature, changes in vaginal secretions, and other physiological indicators
- Prepare patient physically and psychologically for gynecological examination
- Explain purpose of procedure and sensations the patient might experience during the procedure
- Determine patient's understanding of test results and recommended therapy
- Support patient through infertility history and evaluation, acknowledging stress often experienced in obtaining detailed history and during lengthy evaluation and treatment process
- Assist with expressions of grief and disappointment and feelings of failure
- Encourage expressions of feelings about sexuality, self-image, and self-esteem
- Determine extent to which patient (and significant other) are engaging in magical thinking
- Assist individuals to redefine concepts of success and failure, as needed
- Refer patient to support group for infertile couples, as appropriate
- Assist with problem solving to help couple evaluate alternatives to biologic parenthood
- Determine effect of infertility on couple's relationship

1st edition 1992; revised 1996

Background Readings:

Bernstein, J., Brill, M., Levin, S., & Seibel, M. (1992). Coping with infertility: A new nursing perspective. *NAACOG's Clinical Issues in Perinatal & Women's Health Nursing, 3*(2), 335–342.

Bobak, I. M., Jensen, M., & Lowdermilk, D. L. (1993). *Maternity & gynecologic care: The nurse and the family* (5th ed.). St. Louis: Mosby.

Hahn, S. J. (2001). Reproductive technology management. In M. Craft-Rosenberg & J. Denehy (Eds.), *Nursing interventions for infants, children, and families* (pp. 19–32). Thousand Oaks, CA: Sage.

James, C. A. (1992). The nursing role in assisted reproductive technologies. *NAACOG's Clinical Issues in Perinatal & Women's Health Nursing, 3*(2), 328–334.

Olshansky, E. F. (1992). Redefining the concepts of success and failure in infertility treatment. *NAACOG's Clinical Issues in Perinatal & Women's Health Nursing, 3*(2), 343–346.

Pillitteri, A. (2007). *Maternal and child health nursing: Care of the childbearing and childrearing family* (5th ed.). Philadelphia: Lippincott Williams & Wilkins.

F

F

Family Planning: Unplanned Pregnancy 6788

Definition: Facilitation of decision-making regarding pregnancy outcome

Activities:
- Determine whether patient has made a choice about outcome of pregnancy
- Encourage patient and significant other to explore options regarding outcomes of pregnancy, including termination, keeping the infant, or relinquishing the infant for adoption
- Discuss alternatives to abortion with patient and significant other
- Discuss factors related to unplanned pregnancy (e.g., multiple partners, drug and/or alcohol use, and likelihood of sexually transmitted disease)
- Assist patient in identifying support system
- Encourage patient to involve support system during decision-making process
- Support patient and significant other in decision about pregnancy outcome
- Clarify misinformation about contraceptive use
- Refer to community agencies that have services that will support patient in acting on decision regarding pregnancy outcome, as

well as other health concerns (e.g., sexually transmitted diseases and substance abuse)

1st edition 1992; revised 1996

Background Readings:
Bobak, I. M., Jensen, M., & Lowdermilk, D. L. (1993). *Maternity & gynecologic care: The nurse and the family* (5th ed.). St. Louis: Mosby.
O'Campo, P., Faden, R. R., Gielen, A. C., Kass, N., & Anderson, J. (1993). Contraceptive practices among single women with an unplanned pregnancy: Partner influences. *Family Planning Perspectives, 25*(5), 215–219.
Pillitteri, A. (2007). Reproductive life planning. In *Maternal and child health nursing: Care of the childbearing and childrearing family* (5th ed.). Philadelphia: Lippincott Williams & Wilkins.
Sulak, P. J. & Haney, A. F. (1993). Unwanted pregnancies: Understanding contraceptive use and benefits in adolescents and older women. *American Journal of Obstetrics & Gynecology, 168*(6), 2042–2048.

Family Presence Facilitation 7170

Definition: Facilitation of the family's presence in support of an individual undergoing resuscitation and/or invasive procedures

Activities:
- Introduce yourself to the staff treating the patient and family
- Determine suitability of the physical location for family presence
- Obtain consensus from the staff for the family's presence and the timing of the family's presence
- Apprise the treatment team of the family's emotional reaction to patient's condition, as appropriate
- Obtain information concerning the patient's status, response to treatment, identified needs
- Introduce yourself and other members of the support team to the family and patient
- Communicate information concerning the patient's current status in a timely manner
- Assure family that best care possible is being given to patient
- Use the patient's name when speaking to the family
- Determine the patient's and the family's emotional, physical, psychosocial, and spiritual support needs and initiate measures to meet those needs, as necessary
- Determine the psychological burden of prognosis for family
- Foster realistic hope, as appropriate
- Advocate for family, as appropriate
- Prepare the family, assuring they have been informed about what to expect, what they will see, hear, and/or smell
- Inform family of behavior expectations and limits
- Provide a dedicated staff person to assure that family members are never left unattended at the bedside
- Accompany the family to and from the treatment or resuscitation area, announce their presence to the treatment staff each time the family enters the treatment area
- Provide information and explanations of the interventions, medical/nursing jargon, and expectations of the patient's response to treatment

- Escort the family from the bedside if requested by the staff providing direct care
- Provide the opportunity for the family to ask questions and to see, touch, and speak to the patient prior to transfers
- Assist the patient or family members in making telephone calls, as needed
- Offer and provide comfort measures and support, including appropriate referrals, as needed
- Participate in the evaluation of staff's and own emotional needs
- Assist in identifying need for critical incident stress debriefing, individual defusing of events, etc., as appropriate
- Participate, initiate, and/or coordinate family bereavement follow-up at established intervals, as appropriate

4th edition 2004

Background Readings:
American Heart Association. (2000). Guidelines for cardiopulmonary resuscitation and emergency cardiovascular care. Part 2: Ethical aspects of CPR and ECC. *Circulation, 102*(Suppl. 8), I12–I21.
Eichhorn, D. J., Meyers, T. A., Guzzetta, C. E., Clark, A. P., Klein, J. D., & Calvin, A. O. (2001). During invasive procedures and resuscitation: Hearing the voice of the patient. *American Journal of Nursing, 101*(5), 48–55.
Emergency Nurses Association. (1998). Emergency Nurses Association position statement: Family presence at the bedside during invasive procedures and/or resuscitation. *Journal of Emergency Nursing, 21*(2), 26A.
Emergency Nurses Association. (2000). *Presenting the option for family presence* (2nd ed.). Des Plaines, IL: Author.
Hampe, S. O. (1975). Needs of a grieving spouse in a hospital setting. *Nursing Research, 24*(2), 113–120.

McPhee, A. T. (1983). Let the family in. *Nursing, 13*(1), 120.

Meyers, T. A., Eichborn, D. J., & Guzzetta, C. E. (1998). Do families want to be present during CPR? A retrospective survey. *Journal of Emergency Nursing, 24*(5), 405.

Meyers, T. A., Eichborn, D. J., Guzzetta, C. E., Clark, A. P., Klein, J. D., Taliaferro, E., et al. (2000). Family presence during invasive procedures and resuscitation. *American Journal of Nursing, 100*(2), 32–42.

Family Process Maintenance   7130

Definition: Minimization of family process disruption effects

Activities:

- Determine typical family processes
- Determine disruption in typical family processes
- Identify effects of role changes on family process
- Encourage continued contact with family members, as appropriate
- Keep opportunities for visiting flexible to meet needs of family members and patient
- Discuss strategies for normalizing family life with family members
- Assist family members to implement normalizing strategies for their situation
- Discuss existing social support mechanisms for the family
- Assist family members to use existing support mechanisms
- Minimize family routine disruption by facilitating family routines and rituals, such as private meals together or family discussions for communication and decision-making
- Provide mechanisms for family members staying with patient to communicate with other family members (e.g., telephones, e-mail messages, and pictures, tape recordings, photographs, and videotapes)
- Provide opportunities for ongoing parental care of hospitalized children, when the patient is a child
- Provide opportunities for adult family members to maintain ongoing commitments to their jobs, if possible, or to use the Family Medical Leave Act in the United States
- Assist family members to facilitate home visits by patient, when appropriate
- Identify home care needs and how these might be incorporated into family lifestyle
- Design schedules of home care activities that minimize disruption of family routine
- Teach family time management/organization skills when performing home care, as needed

1st edition 1992; revised 2008

Background Readings:

Broome, M. E. & Huth, M. M. (2001). Preparation for hospitalization, surgery and procedures. In M. Craft-Rosenberg & J. Denehy (Eds.), *Nursing interventions for infants, children, and families* (pp. 281–298). Thousand Oaks, CA: Sage.

Daugherty, J., Saarmann, L., Riegel, B., Sornborger, K., & Moser, D. (2002). Can we talk? Developing a social support nursing interventions for couples. *Clinical Nurse Specialist, 16*(4), 211–218.

Drageset, J. (2004). The importance of activities of daily living and social contact for loneliness: A survey among residents in nursing homes. *Scandinavian Journal of Caring Sciences, 18*(1), 65–71.

Finfgeld-Connett, D. (2005). Clarification of social support. *Journal of Nursing Scholarship, 37*(1), 4–9.

Titler, M. G., Cohen, M. Z., & Craft, M. J. (1991). Impact of critical hospitalization: Perceptions of patients, spouses, children, and nurses. *Heart & Lung, 20*(2), 174–181.

Family Support   7140

Definition: Promotion of family values, interests, and goals

Activities:

- Assure family that best care possible is being given to patient
- Appraise family's emotional reaction to patient's condition
- Determine the psychological burden of prognosis for family
- Foster realistic hope
- Listen to family concerns, feelings, and questions
- Facilitate communication of concerns/feelings between patient and family or between family members
- Promote trusting relationship with family
- Accept the family's values in a nonjudgmental manner
- Answer all questions of family members or assist them to get answers
- Orient family to the health care setting, such as hospital unit or clinic
- Provide assistance in meeting basic needs for family, such as shelter, food, and clothing
- Identify nature of spiritual support for family
- Identify congruence between patient, family, and health professional expectations
- Reduce discrepancies in patient, family, and health professional expectations through use of communication skills
- Assist family members in identifying and resolving a conflict in values
- Respect and support adaptive coping mechanisms used by family
- Provide feedback for family regarding their coping
- Counsel family members on additional effective coping skills for their own use
- Provide spiritual resources for family, as appropriate
- Provide family with information about patient's progress frequently, according to patient preference
- Teach the medical and nursing plans of care to family
- Provide necessary knowledge of options to family that will assist them to make decisions about patient care

- Include family members with patient in decision making about care, when appropriate
- Encourage family decision making in planning long-term patient care affecting family structure and finances
- Acknowledge understanding of family decision about postdischarge care
- Assist family to acquire necessary knowledge, skills, and equipment to sustain their decision about patient care
- Advocate for family, as appropriate
- Foster family assertiveness in information seeking, as appropriate
- Provide opportunities for visitation by extended family members, as appropriate
- Introduce family to other families undergoing similar experiences, as appropriate
- Give care to patient in lieu of family to relieve them and/or when family is unable to give care
- Arrange for ongoing respite care, when indicated and desired
- Provide opportunities for peer group support
- Refer for family therapy, as appropriate
- Tell family members how to reach the nurse
- Assist family members through the death and grief processes, as appropriate

1st edition 1992; revised 1996

Background Readings:

Craft, M. J. (1987). Health care preferences of rural teens. *Journal of Pediatric Nursing, 2*(1), 3–13.

Craft, M. J. & Craft, J. (1989). Perceived changes in siblings of hospitalized children: A comparison of parent and sibling report. *Children's Health Care, 18*(1), 42–49.

Craft, M. J. & Willadsen, J. A. (1992). Interventions related to family. In G. M. Bulechek & J. C. McCloskey (Eds.), Symposium on nursing interventions. *Nursing Clinics of North America, 27*(2), 517–540.

Gilliss, C., Highley, B., Roberts, B., & Martinson, I. (1989). *Toward a science of family nursing.* Menlo Park, CA: Addison-Wesley.

Goldenberg, I. & Goldenberg, H. (1985). *Family therapy: An overview* (2nd ed.). Monterey, CA: Brooks/Cole.

Leske, J. S. (1992). Needs of adult family members after critical illnesses: Prescriptions for interventions. *Critical Care Nursing Clinics of North America, 4*(4), 587–596.

Peirce, A. G., Wright, F., & Fulmer, T. T. (1992). Needs of family during critical illness of elderly patients. *Critical Care Nursing Clinics of North America, 4*(4), 597–606.

Titler, M. G. & Walsh, S. M. (1992). Visiting critically ill adults: Strategies for practice. *Critical Care Nursing Clinics of North America, 4*(4), 623–633.

Family Therapy 7150

Definition: Assisting family members to move their family toward a more productive way of living

Activities:

- Use family-history taking to encourage family discussion
- Determine family communication patterns
- Identify how family solves problems
- Determine how family makes decisions
- Determine if abuse is occurring in the family
- Identify family strengths/resources
- Identify usual roles within the family system
- Identify specific disturbances related to role expectations
- Determine if any family members are dealing with substance abuse
- Determine family alliances
- Identify areas of dissatisfaction and/or conflict
- Determine recent or impending events that have threatened the family
- Help family members communicate more effectively
- Facilitate family discussion
- Help members prioritize and select the most immediate family issue to address
- Help family members clarify what they need and expect from each other
- Facilitate strategies to reduce stress
- Provide education and information
- Help family enhance existing positive coping strategies
- Share therapy plan with family
- Ask family members to participate in homework assignments of experiential activities, such as eating some of their meals together
- Provide challenges within family discussion to encourage new behavior
- Discuss hierarchical relationship of subsystem members
- Assist family members to change how they relate to other family members
- Facilitate restructuring family subsystems, as appropriate
- Help family set goals toward a more competent way of handling dysfunctional behavior
- Monitor family boundaries
- Monitor for adverse therapeutic responses
- Plan termination and evaluation strategies

1st edition 1992; revised 2008

Background Readings:

Craft, M. J. & Willadsen, J. A. (1992). Interventions related to family. In G. M. Bulechek & J. C. McCloskey (Eds.), Symposium on nursing interventions. *Nursing Clinics of North America, 27*(2), 517–540.

Friedman, M. M., Bowden, V. R., & Jones, E. G. (2003). *Family nursing: Research, theory, and practice* (5th ed.). Upper Saddle River, NJ: Prentice Hall.

Goldenberg, I. & Goldenberg, H. (2004). *Family therapy: An overview* (6th ed.). Pacific Grove, CA: Thomson Learning.

Johnson, G., Kent, G., & Leather, J. (2005). Strengthening the parent-child relationship: A review of family interventions and their use in medical settings. *Child: Care Health & Development, 31*(1), 25–32.

Kelly, M. & Newstead, L. (2004). Family intervention in routine practice: It is possible! *Journal of Psychiatric & Mental Health Nursing, 11*(1), 64–72.

Minuchen, S. & Fishmen, H. C. (1981). *Family therapy techniques.* Cambridge: Harvard University Press.

Rojano, R. (2004). The practice of community family therapy. *Family Practice, 43*(1), 59–77.

Walsh, F. (2003). Family resilience: A framework for clinical practice. *Family Process, 42*(1), 1–18.

Feeding   1050

Definition: Providing nutritional intake for patient who is unable to feed self

Activities:
- Identify prescribed diet
- Set food tray and table attractively
- Create a pleasant environment during mealtime (e.g., put bed-pans, urinals, and suctioning equipment out of sight)
- Provide for adequate pain relief before meals, as appropriate
- Provide for oral hygiene before meals
- Identify presence of swallowing reflex, if necessary
- Sit down while feeding to convey pleasure and relaxation
- Offer opportunity to smell foods to stimulate appetite
- Ask patient preference for order of eating
- Fix foods as patient prefers
- Maintain in an upright position, with head and neck flexed slightly forward during feeding
- Place food in the unaffected side of the mouth, as appropriate
- Place food in the person's vision if he or she has a visual-field defect
- Choose different-colored dishes to help distinguish item, if perceptual deficit
- Follow feedings with water, if needed
- Protect with a bib, as appropriate
- Ask the patient to indicate when finished, as appropriate
- Record intake, if appropriate
- Avoid disguising drugs in food
- Avoid presenting drink or bite up to mouth while still chewing

- Provide a drinking straw, as needed or desired
- Provide finger foods, as appropriate
- Provide foods at most appetizing temperature
- Avoid distracting patient during swallowing
- Feed unhurriedly/slowly
- Maintain attention to patient during feeding
- Postpone feeding, if patient is fatigued
- Check mouth for residue at end of meal
- Wash face and hands after meal
- Encourage parents/family to feed patient

1st edition 1992; revised 2008

Background Readings:

Evans-Stoner, N. J. (1999). Feeding. In G. M. Bulechek & J. C. McCloskey (Eds.), *Nursing interventions: Effective nursing treatments* (3rd ed., pp. 31–46). Philadelphia: Saunders.

Harkreader, H. C. (2004). *Fundamentals of nursing: Caring and clinical judgment.* Philadelphia: Saunders.

Pelletier, C. A. (2004). What do certified nurse assistants actually know about dysphagia and feeding nursing home residents? *American Journal of Speech-Language Pathology, 13*(2), 99–113.

Styker, R. (1977). *Rehabilitative aspects of acute and chronic nursing care.* Philadelphia: Saunders.

Fertility Preservation   7160

Definition: Providing information, counseling, and treatment that facilitate reproductive health and the ability to conceive

Activities:
- Discuss factors related to infertility (e.g., maternal age >35 and sexually transmitted diseases)
- Encourage conception before age 35, as appropriate
- Teach patient how to prevent sexually transmitted diseases
- Inform patient of signs and symptoms of sexually transmitted diseases and importance of early, aggressive treatment
- Perform pelvic examination, as appropriate
- Obtain cervical cultures, as appropriate
- Prescribe treatment, as indicated, for sexually transmitted disease or vaginal infection
- Advise patient to seek evaluation and treatment for sexually transmitted disease if partner exhibits any symptoms, even if patient experiences no symptoms
- Advise patient to have partner treated for sexually transmitted disease, if culture is positive
- Report positive sexually transmitted disease cultures, as required by law
- Discuss effects of different contraceptive methods on future fertility
- Counsel patient about contraceptive use
- Advise patient to avoid use of intrauterine devices
- Inform patients about occupational and environmental hazards to fertility (e.g., radiation, chemicals, stress, infections, other environmental factors, and shift rotation)

- Inform patient about more conservative options that are likely to preserve fertility when gynecological or abdominal surgery is indicated
- Refer patient for thorough physical examination for health problems affecting fertility (e.g., amenorrhea, diabetes, endometriosis, and thyroid disease)
- Encourage early, aggressive treatment for endometriosis
- Review lifestyle habits that may alter fertility (e.g., smoking, substance use, alcohol consumption, nutrition, exercise, and sexual behavior)
- Refer to wellness or lifestyle modification program, as appropriate
- Inform patient about the effects of alcohol, tobacco, drugs, and other factors on sperm production and male sexual function
- Refer patient with history indicative of possible fertility disorder for early diagnosis and treatment
- Assist patient in receiving occupational support for fertility treatment
- Inform patient to consider the potential or lack of potential reversibility of different methods of sterilization
- Advise patient considering sterilization to consider procedure irreversible

2nd edition 1996

Background Readings:

Keating, C. E. (1992). The role of the expanded function nurse in fertility preservation. *NAACOG's Clinical Issues in Perinatal and Women's Health Nursing, 3*(2), 293–300.

Keleher, K. C. (1991). Occupational health: How work environments can affect reproductive capacity and outcome. *Nurse Practitioner, 16*(9), 23–30, 33–34, 37.

Pillitteri, A. (2007). The infertile couple. In *Maternal and child health nursing: Care of the childbearing and childrearing family* (5th ed., pp. 113–154). Philadelphia: Lippincott Williams & Wilkins.

Wilson, B. (1991). The effect of drugs on male sexual function and fertility. *Nurse Practitioner, 16*(9), 12–17, 21–22.

Fever Treatment 3740

Definition: Management of symptoms and related conditions associated with an increase in body temperature mediated by endogenous pyrogens

Activities:

- Monitor temperature and other vital signs
- Monitor skin color and temperature
- Monitor intake and output, being aware of changes in insensible fluid loss
- Administer medications or IV fluids (e.g., antipyretics, antibacterial agents, and antishivering agents)
- Do not administer aspirin to children
- Cover the patient with blanket or light clothing, depending on phase of fever (i.e., provide warm blanket for chill phase; provide light clothing or bed linens for fever and flush phases)
- Encourage fluid consumption
- Facilitate rest, applying activity restrictions if needed
- Administer oxygen, as appropriate
- Administer a tepid sponge bath with caution (i.e., administer for patients with very high temperature, do not administer during chill phase, and avoid chilling patient)
- Increase air circulation
- Monitor for fever-related complications and signs and symptoms of fever-causing condition (e.g., seizure, decreased level of consciousness, abnormal electrolyte status, acid-base imbalance, cardiac arrhythmia, and abnormal cellular changes)
- Ensure other signs of infection are monitored in elderly persons, as they may display only a low-grade fever or no fever during infection
- Ensure safety measures are in place should patient become restless or delirious
- Moisturize dry lips and nasal mucosa

1st edition 1992; revised 2013

Background Readings:

Craven, R. F. & Hirnle, C. J. (2009). The body's defense against infection. In *Fundamentals of nursing: Human health and function* (6th ed., pp. 1033–1070). Philadelphia: Lippincott Williams & Wilkins.

Smith, S. F., Duell, D. J., & Martin, B. C. (2008). *Clinical nursing skills: Basic to advanced skills* (7th ed.). Upper Saddle River, NJ: Pearson Prentice Hall.

Financial Resource Assistance 7380

Definition: Assisting an individual/family to secure and manage finances to meet health care needs

Activities:

- Determine patient's current use of health care system and the financial impact of this use
- Assist patient to identify financial needs, including analysis of assets and liabilities
- Determine patient's cognitive ability to read, fill out forms, balance checkbook, and manage money
- Determine patient's daily living expenses
- Prioritize patient's daily living needs and assist patient to develop a plan to meet those needs
- Devise a plan of care to encourage patient/family to access appropriate levels of care in the most cost-effective manner
- Inform patient of services available through state and federal programs
- Determine if patient is eligible for waiver programs
- Refer patient who may be eligible for state or federally funded programs to appropriate individuals
- Inform patient of available resources and assist in accessing resources (e.g., medication assistance program, county relief program)
- Assist patient to develop a budget and/or make referral to appropriate financial resource person (e.g., financial planner, estate planner, consumer counselor), as needed
- Assist patient to fill out applications for available resources, as needed
- Assist patient in long-term care placement planning, as needed
- Assist patient to assure money is in secure place (i.e., bank), as needed
- Assist patient in obtaining a burial fund, as appropriate
- Encourage family to be involved in financial management, as appropriate
- Represent economic needs of patients at multidisciplinary conferences, as needed
- Collaborate with community agencies to provide needed services to patient

3rd edition 2000

Background Readings:

Antonello, S. J. (1996). *Social skills development: Practical strategies for adolescents and adults with developmental disabilities.* Boston: Allyn & Bacon.

Bush, G. W. (1990). Calculating the cost of long-term living: A four-step process. *Journal of Head Trauma Rehabilitation, 5*(1), 47–56.

Horner, M., Rawlins, P., & Giles, K. (1987). How parents of children with chronic conditions perceive their own needs. *Maternal Child Nursing, 12*(1), 40–43.

Klug, R. M. (1991). Understanding private insurance for funding pediatric home care. *Pediatric Nursing, 17*(2), 197–198.

McDowell, I. & Newell, C. (1996). *Measuring health: A guide to rating scales and questionnaires* (2nd ed.). New York: Oxford University Press.

Olen, D. R. (1984). *Teaching life skills to children: A practical guide for parents and teachers.* New York: Paulist Press.

Peterson, D. A. (1983). *Facilitating education for older learners.* San Francisco: Jossey Bass.

Pfeffer, R. I., Kurosaki, T. T., Harrah, C. H. Jr., Chance, J. M., & Filos, S. (1992). Measurement of functional activities in older adults in the community. *Journal of Gerontology, 37*(3), 323–329.

Schmall, V. L. (1995). Family caregiver education and training: Enhancing self-efficacy. *Journal of Case Management, 4*(4), 156–162.

Social Security Administration, Office of Disability. (1998). *Disability evaluation under social security.* (SSA Publication No. 64-039). Baltimore, MD: Author.

Fire-Setting Precautions   6500

Definition: Prevention of fire-setting behaviors

Activities:
- Search patient for incendiary materials (e.g., matches/lighters) on admission and each time that patient returns to care environment (e.g., from a pass or a recreational activity)
- Search patient environment on routine basis to remove fire-setting materials
- Determine appropriate behavioral expectations and consequences, given the patient's level of cognitive functioning and capacity for self-control
- Communicate rules, behavioral expectations, and consequences to patient
- Communicate risk to other care providers
- Provide ongoing surveillance in an environment that is free of fire-setting materials
- Provide close supervision, if patient is allowed to smoke
- Obtain verbal contract from patient to refrain from fire-setting activity
- Encourage the expression of feelings in an appropriate manner
- Assist patient, as appropriate, with impulse control training
- Increase surveillance and security (e.g., area restriction or seclusion), if risk of fire-setting behavior increases

2nd edition 1996

Background Readings:

Schultz, J. M. & Dark, S. L. (1990). *Manual of psychiatric nursing care plans* (3rd ed.). Philadelphia: Lippincott.

Swaffer, T., Haggett, M., & Oxley, T. (2001). Mentally disordered fire setters: A structured intervention programme. *Clinical Psychology and Psychotherapy, 8*(6), 468–475.

Taylor, J. L., Thorne, I., Robertson, A., & Avery, G. (2002). Evaluation of a group intervention for convicted arsonists with mild borderline intellectual disabilities. *Criminal Behaviour and Mental Health, 12*(4), 282–293.

First Aid   6240

Definition: Providing immediate care for minor burns, injuries, poisoning, bites, and stings

Activities:
- Instruct others to call for help, if needed
- Employ precautionary measures to reduce risk of infection while giving care
- Monitor vital signs, as appropriate
- Note characteristics of the wound or burn including drainage, color, size, and odor
- Institute appropriate care of wound or burn
- Institute measures (e.g., pressure, pressure dressing, positioning) to reduce or minimize bleeding
- Use rest, ice, compression, and elevation (RICE) for extremity bone, joint, and muscle injuries
- Splint affected extremity
- Cleanse skin exposed to poison ivy, oak, or sumac (i.e., use water and soap or liberal amount of rubbing alcohol) and stinging nettle (i.e., use water and soap)
- Flush tissue exposed to chemicals (except lye or white phosphorous) with water
- Remove embedded stinger and venom sac from insect sting or tentacles from marine animal sting by scraping a hard object over site (e.g., fingernail, credit card, and comb)
- Remove tick from the skin using tweezers or specialized tick-removal tool
- Administer medication (e.g., prophylactic antibiotic, vaccination, antihistamine, antiinflammatory, and analgesic), as appropriate
- Relieve itching (i.e., administer medication, apply calamine lotion or baking soda paste, and instruct patient to bathe in colloidal oatmeal)
- Report animal bites to appropriate authority (e.g., police or animal control)
- Provide instructions for necessary follow-up care

- Instruct patient on care of injury
- Coordinate medical transport, as needed

1st edition 1992; revised 2013

Background Readings:
American Academy of Orthopaedic Surgeons. (2005). *First aid, CPR, and AED* (4th ed.) [A. Thygerson, A. & B. Gulli, (Eds.)]. Sudbury, MA: Jones and Bartlett.

Boy Scouts of America. (2009). *The Boy Scout handbook* (12th ed.) Irving, TX: Author.

Pfeiffer, R. P., Thygerson, A., & Palmieri, N. F. (2009). *Sports first aid and injury prevention* [B. Gulli & E. W. Ossman, Medical Eds.]. Sudbury, MA: Jones and Bartlett.

Fiscal Resource Management 8550

Definition: Procuring and directing the use of financial resources to assure the development and continuation of programs and services

Activities:
- Develop a business plan
- Develop a cost-benefit analysis of programs and services
- Maintain a budget appropriate to the services provided
- Identify sources of financing services
- Generate grant applications
- Identify marketing efforts to enhance programs
- Identify "in-kind" (contributed) resources that support programs and services
- Analyze economic viability of program based on trends
- Implement relevant policies and procedures to secure reimbursement
- Maximize potential reimbursement (e.g., program certification, qualified providers)
- Use appropriate accounting methods to assure accurate and designated use of funds
- Use appropriate methods to address fiduciary responsibility
- Evaluate outcomes and cost effectiveness of the program
- Make appropriate changes in financial management in response to evaluation

3rd edition 2000

Background Readings:
Branowiki, P. A. & Shermont, H. (1997). Maximizing resources: A microanalysis assessment tool. *Nursing Management, 28*(5), 65–70.
Grimaldi, P. L. (1996). Financial management: Unsettling times for public health care providers. *Nursing Management, 27*(9), 14, 16–17.
Klainberg, M., Holzemer, S., Leonard, M., & Arnold, J. (1998). *Community health nursing: An alliance for health.* New York: McGraw-Hill.
Stanhope, M. & Lancaster, J. (1996). *Community health nursing: Promoting health of aggregates, families, and individuals* (4th ed.). St. Louis: Mosby.
Storfjell, J. L., & Jessup, S. (1996). Bringing the gap between finances and clinical operations with activity based cost management. *Journal of Nursing Administration, 26*(12), 12–17.

Flatulence Reduction 0470

Definition: Prevention of flatus formation and facilitation of passage of excessive gas

Activities:
- Teach patient how flatus is produced and methods for alleviation
- Teach patient to avoid situations that cause excessive air swallowing, such as chewing gum, drinking carbonated beverages, eating rapidly, sucking through straws, chewing with mouth open, or talking with mouth full
- Teach patient to avoid foods that cause flatulence, such as beans, cabbage, radishes, onions, cauliflower, and cucumbers
- Discuss use of dairy products
- Monitor for bloated feeling, abdominal distension, cramping pains, and excessive passage of gas from the mouth or anus
- Monitor bowel sounds
- Monitor vital signs
- Provide for adequate exercise (e.g., ambulate)
- Insert lubricated nasogastric tube or rectal tube into the rectum, as appropriate; tape in place; and insert distal end of tube into a receptacle
- Administer a laxative, suppository, or enema, as appropriate
- Monitor side effects of medication administration
- Limit oral intake, if lower gastrointestinal system is inactive
- Position on left side with knees flexed, as appropriate
- Offer antiflatulence medications, as appropriate

1st edition 1992; revised 1996

Background Readings:
Craven, R. F. & Hirnle, C. J. (2000). *Fundamentals of nursing: Human health and function* (3rd ed., pp. 1086, 1098, 1102). Philadelphia: Lippincott.
Evans-Smith, P. (2005). *Taylor's clinical nursing skills* (pp. 513–515). Philadelphia: Lippincott Williams & Wilkins.
Levy, D. J. & Rosenthal, W. S. (1985). Gastrointestinal gas. *Hospital Medicine, 21*(4), 13, 17–19, 22–25.
Ribakove, B. M. (1982). Gas . . . flatus. *Health, 14*(12), 48–49.
Vaughn, J. B. & Nemcek, M. A. (1986). Postoperative flatulence: Causes and remedies. *Today's OR Nurse, 8*(10), 19–23.

Fluid/Electrolyte Management 2080

Definition: Regulation and prevention of complications from altered fluid and/or electrolyte levels

Activities:
- Monitor for abnormal serum electrolyte levels, as available
- Monitor for changes in pulmonary or cardiac status indicating fluid overload or dehydration
- Monitor for signs and symptoms of worsening overhydration or dehydration (e.g., moist crackles in lung sounds, polyuria or oliguria, behavior changes, seizures, frothy or thick viscous saliva, edematous or sunken eyes, rapid shallow breathing)
- Obtain laboratory specimens for monitoring of altered fluid or electrolyte levels (e.g., hematocrit, BUN, protein, sodium, and potassium levels), as appropriate
- Weigh daily and monitor trends
- Give fluids, as appropriate
- Promote oral intake (e.g., provide oral fluids that are the patient's preference, place in easy reach, provide a straw, and provide fresh water), as appropriate
- Administer prescribed nasogastric replacement based on output, as appropriate
- Irrigate nasogastric tubes with normal saline, per agency policy and as indicated
- Provide free water with tube feedings, per agency policy and as indicated
- Administer fiber as prescribed for the tube-fed patient to reduce fluid and electrolyte loss through diarrhea
- Minimize the number of ice chips consumed or amount of oral intake by patients with gastric tubes connected to suction
- Minimize intake of foods and drinks with diuretic or laxative effects (e.g., tea, coffee, prunes, herbal supplements)
- Maintain an appropriate intravenous infusion, blood transfusion, or enteral flow rate, especially if not regulated by a pump
- Ensure that intravenous solution containing electrolytes is administered at a constant flow rate, as appropriate
- Monitor laboratory results relevant to fluid balance (e.g., hematocrit, BUN, albumin, total protein, serum osmolality, and urine specific gravity levels)
- Monitor laboratory results relevant to fluid retention (e.g., increased specific gravity, increased BUN, decreased hematocrit, and increased urine osmolality levels)
- Monitor hemodynamic status, including CVP, MAP, PAP, and PCWP levels, if available
- Keep an accurate record of intake and output
- Monitor for signs and symptoms of fluid retention
- Restrict free water intake in the presence of dilutional hyponatremia with serum Na level below 130 mEq per liter
- Institute fluid restriction, as appropriate
- Monitor vital signs, as appropriate
- Correct preoperative dehydration, as appropriate
- Monitor patient's response to prescribed electrolyte therapy
- Monitor for manifestations of electrolyte imbalance
- Provide prescribed diet appropriate for specific fluid or electrolyte imbalance (e.g., low-sodium, fluid-restricted, renal, and no added salt)
- Administer prescribed supplemental electrolytes, as appropriate
- Administer prescribed electrolyte binding or excreting resins, as appropriate
- Monitor for side effects (e.g., nausea, vomiting, diarrhea) of prescribed supplemental electrolytes
- Watch patient's buccal membranes, sclera, and skin for indications of altered fluid and electrolyte balance (e.g., dryness, cyanosis, and jaundice)
- Consult physician if signs and symptoms of fluid and/or electrolyte imbalance persist or worsen
- Institute measures to control excessive electrolyte loss (e.g., by resting the gut, changing type of diuretic, or administering antipyretics), as appropriate
- Institute measures to rest the bowel (i.e., restrict food or fluid intake and decrease intake of milk products), if appropriate
- Follow quick-acting glucose with long-acting carbohydrates and proteins for management of acute hypoglycemia, as appropriate
- Prepare patient for dialysis (e.g., by assisting with catheter placement for dialysis), as appropriate
- Monitor for fluid loss (e.g., bleeding, vomiting, diarrhea, perspiration, and tachypnea)
- Promote a positive body image and self-esteem if concerns are expressed as a result of excessive fluid retention, if appropriate
- Assist patients with impaired mental or physical conditions (e.g., dysphagia, cognitive impairment, mentally challenged, reduction in physical strength or coordination) to achieve adequate fluid balance
- Assist patients with undesirable sequelae from prescribed therapeutic regimen (e.g., patient with fear of urinary frequency or incontinence from diuretic limits own fluid intake) to achieve adequate fluid balance
- Instruct patient and family about rationale for fluid restrictions, hydration measures, or supplemental electrolyte administration, as indicated

1st edition 1992; revised 2013

Background Readings:
Allsopp, K. (2010). Caring for patients with kidney failure. *Emergency Nurse, 18*(10), 12–16.
Harvey, S. & Jordan, S. (2010). Diuretic therapy: Implications for nursing practice. *Nursing Standard, 24*(43), 40–50.
Murch, P. (2005). Optimizing the fluid management of ventilated patients with suspected hypovolemia. *Nursing in Critical Care, 10*(6), 279–288.
Ostendorf, W. R. (2011). Fluid, electrolyte and acid-base balances. In P. A. Potter, A. G. Perry, P. Stockert, & A. Hall (Eds.), *Basic nursing* (7th ed., pp. 466–521). St. Louis: Mosby.
Scales, K. & Pilsworth, J. (2008). The importance of fluid balance in clinical practice. *Nursing Standard, 22*(47), 50–58.
Tang, V.C.Y. & Lee, E.W.Y. (2010). Fluid balance chart: Do we understand it? *Clinical Risk, 16*(1), 10–13.
Welch, K. (2010). Fluid balance. *Learning Disability Practice, 13*(6), 33–38.
Young, E., Sherrard-Jacob, A., Knapp, K., Craddock, T. S., Kemper, C., Falvo, R., et al. (2009). Perioperative fluid management. *AORN Journal, 89*(1), 167–182.

F

Fluid Management 4120

Definition: Promotion of fluid balance and prevention of complications resulting from abnormal or undesired fluid levels

Activities:

- Weigh daily and monitor trends
- Count or weigh diapers, as appropriate
- Maintain accurate intake and output record
- Insert urinary catheter, if appropriate
- Monitor hydration status (e.g., moist mucous membranes, adequacy of pulses, and orthostatic blood pressure), as appropriate
- Monitor laboratory results relevant to fluid retention (e.g., increased specific gravity, increased BUN, decreased hematocrit, and increased urine osmolality levels)
- Monitor hemodynamic status, including CVP, MAP, PAP, and PCWP, if available
- Monitor vital signs, as appropriate
- Monitor for indications of fluid overload/retention (e.g., crackles, elevated CVP or pulmonary capillary wedge pressure, edema, neck vein distention, and ascites), as appropriate
- Monitor patient's weight change before and after dialysis, if appropriate
- Assess location and extent of edema, if present
- Monitor food/fluid ingested and calculate daily caloric intake, as appropriate
- Administer IV therapy, as prescribed
- Monitor nutrition status
- Give fluids, as appropriate
- Administer prescribed diuretics, as appropriate
- Administer IV fluids at room temperature
- Promote oral intake (e.g., provide a drinking straw, offer fluids between meals, change ice water routinely, make freezer pops using child's favorite juice, cut gelatin into fun squares, use small medicine cups), as appropriate
- Instruct patient on nothing by mouth (NPO) status, as appropriate
- Administer prescribed nasogastric replacement based on output, as appropriate
- Distribute the fluid intake over 24 hours, as appropriate
- Encourage significant other to assist patient with feedings, as appropriate
- Offer snacks (e.g., frequent drinks and fresh fruits/fruit juice), as appropriate
- Restrict free water intake in the presence of dilutional hyponatremia with serum Na level below 130 mEq per liter
- Monitor patient's response to prescribed electrolyte therapy
- Consult physician if signs and symptoms of fluid volume excess persist or worsen
- Arrange availability of blood products for transfusion, if necessary
- Prepare for administration of blood products (e.g., check blood with patient identification and prepare infusion setup), as appropriate
- Administer blood products (e.g., platelets and fresh frozen plasma), as appropriate

1st edition 1992; revised 2000

Background Readings:

American Association of Critical Care Nurses. (2006). *Core curriculum for critical care nursing* (6th ed.) [J. G. Alspach, Ed.]. Philadelphia: Saunders.

Baer, C. L. (1993). Fluid and electrolyte balance. In M. R. Kinney, D. R. Packa, & S. B. Dunbar (Eds.), *AACN's clinical reference for critical-care nursing* (pp. 173–208). St. Louis: Mosby.

Cullen, L. M. (1992). Interventions related to fluid and electrolyte balance. In G. M. Bulechek & J. C. McCloskey (Eds.), Symposium on nursing interventions. *Nursing Clinics of North America, 27*(2), 569–598.

Horne, M. & Swearingen, P. (1997). *Pocket guide to fluids and electrolytes* (3rd ed.). St. Louis: Mosby.

Kokko, J. & Tannen, R. (1990). *Fluids and electrolytes* (2nd ed.). Philadelphia: Saunders.

Wong, D. L. (1995). *Whaley and Wong's nursing care of infants and children* (5th ed.). St. Louis: Mosby.

Fluid Monitoring 4130

Definition: Collection and analysis of patient data to regulate fluid balance

Activities:

- Determine history of amount and type of fluid intake and elimination habits
- Determine possible risk factors for fluid imbalance (e.g., albumin loss state, burns, malnutrition, sepsis, nephrotic syndrome, hyperthermia, diuretic therapy, renal pathologies, cardiac failure, diaphoresis, liver dysfunction, strenuous exercise, heat exposure, infection, postoperative state, polyuria, vomiting, and diarrhea)
- Determine if patient is experiencing thirst or symptoms of fluid changes (e.g., dizziness, change of mentation, lightheadedness, apprehension, irritability, nausea, twitching)
- Examine capillary refill by holding the patient's hand at the same level as their heart and pressing on the pad of their middle finger for five seconds, releasing pressure and counting time until color returns (i.e., should be less than 2 seconds)
- Examine skin turgor by grasping tissue over a bony area such as the hand or shin, pinching the skin gently, holding it for a second and releasing (i.e., skin will fall back quickly if patient is well hydrated)
- Monitor weight
- Monitor intake and output
- Monitor serum and urine electrolyte values, as appropriate
- Monitor serum albumin and total protein levels
- Monitor serum and urine osmolality levels
- Monitor BP, heart rate, and respiratory status
- Monitor orthostatic blood pressure and change in cardiac rhythm, as appropriate
- Monitor invasive hemodynamic parameters, as appropriate
- Keep an accurate record of intake and output (e.g., oral intake, enteral intake, IV intake, antibiotics, fluids given with

medications, nasogastric (NG) tubes, drains, vomit, rectal tubes, colostomy drainage, and urine)
- Insure that all intake and output on all patients with intravenous therapy, subcutaneous infusions, enteral feedings, NG tubes, urinary catheters, vomiting, diarrhea, wound drains, chest drains, and medical conditions that affect fluid balance (e.g., heart failure, renal failure, malnutrition, burns, sepsis)
- Record incontinence episodes in patients requiring accurate intake and output
- Correct mechanical problems (e.g., kinked or blocked catheter) in patients experiencing sudden cessation of urine output
- Monitor mucous membranes, skin turgor, and thirst
- Monitor color, quantity, and specific gravity of urine
- Monitor for distended neck veins, crackles in the lungs, peripheral edema, and weight gain
- Monitor for signs and symptoms of ascites
- Note presence or absence of vertigo on rising
- Administer fluids, as appropriate
- Assure that all IV and enteral intake devices are operating at the correct rates, especially if not regulated by a pump
- Restrict and allocate fluid intake, as appropriate
- Consult physician for urine output less than 0.5ml/kg/hr or adult fluid intake less than 2000 in 24 hours, as appropriate
- Administer pharmacological agents to increase urinary output, as appropriate
- Administer dialysis, as appropriate, noting patient response

- Maintain accurate fluid container reference charts to assure standardization of container measurements
- Audit intake and output graphs periodically to ensure good practice patterns

1st edition 1992; revised 2013

Background Readings:

Allsopp, K. (2010). Caring for patients with kidney failure. *Emergency Nurse,* 18(10), 12–16.

Harvey, S. & Jordan, S. (2010). Diuretic therapy: Implications for nursing practice. *Nursing Standard, 24*(43), 40–50.

Murch, P. (2005). Optimizing the fluid management of ventilated patients with suspected hypovolemia. *Nursing in Critical Care, 10*(6), 279–288.

Ostendorf, W. R. (2011). Fluid, electrolyte and acid-base balances. In P. A. Potter, A. G. Perry, P. Stockert, & A. Hall (Eds.), *Basic nursing* (7th ed., pp. 466–521). St. Louis: Mosby.

Scales, K. & Pilsworth, J. (2008). The importance of fluid balance in clinical practice. *Nursing Standard, 22*(47), 50–58.

Tang, V. C. Y. & Lee, E. W. Y. (2010). Fluid balance chart: Do we understand it? *Clinical Risk, 16*(1), 10–13.

Welch, K. (2010). Fluid balance. *Learning Disability Practice, 13*(6), 33–38.

Young, E., Sherrard-Jacob, A., Knapp, K., Craddock, T. S., Kemper, C., Falvo, R., et al. (2009). Perioperative fluid management. *AORN Journal, 89*(1), 167–182.

F

Fluid Resuscitation   4140

Definition: Administering prescribed intravenous fluids rapidly

Activities:
- Obtain and maintain a large-bore IV
- Collaborate with physicians to ensure administration of both crystalloids (e.g., normal saline and lactated Ringer's) and colloids (e.g., Hesban, and Plasmanate), as appropriate
- Administer IV fluids, as prescribed
- Obtain blood specimens for cross-matching, as appropriate
- Administer blood products, as prescribed
- Monitor hemodynamic response
- Monitor oxygen status
- Monitor for fluid overload
- Monitor output of various body fluids (e.g., urine, nasogastric drainage, and chest tube)

- Monitor BUN, creatinine, total protein, and albumin levels
- Monitor for pulmonary edema and third spacing

1st edition 1992; revised 2008

Background Readings:

Urden, L. D., Stacy, K. M., & Lough, M. E. (2006). *Thelan's critical care nursing: Diagnosis and management* (5th ed.). St. Louis: Mosby.

Thompson, J. M., McFarland, G. K., Hirsch, J. E., & Tucker, S. M. (2002). *Mosby's clinical nursing* (5th ed.). St. Louis: Mosby.

Foot Care   1660

Definition:: Cleansing and inspecting the feet for the purposes of relaxation, cleanliness, and healthy skin

Activities:
- Inspect skin for irritation, cracking, lesions, corns, calluses, deformities, or edema
- Inspect patient's shoes for proper fit
- Administer foot soaks, as needed
- Dry carefully between toes
- Apply lotion

- Clean nails
- Apply moisture-absorbing powder, as indicated
- Discuss with patient his/her usual foot care routine
- Instruct patient/family on the importance of foot care
- Offer positive feedback about self-care foot activities
- Monitor patient's gait and weight distribution on feet
- Monitor cleanliness and general condition of shoes and stockings

- Instruct patient to inspect inside of shoes for rough areas
- Monitor hydration level of feet
- Monitor for arterial insufficiency in lower legs
- Monitor legs and feet for edema
- Instruct patient to monitor temperature of feet using the back of the hand
- Instruct patient in the importance of inspection, especially when sensation is diminished
- Cut normal thickness toenails when soft, using a toenail clipper and using the curve of the toe as a guide
- Refer to podiatrist for trimming of thickened nails, as appropriate
- Inspect nails for thickness, discoloration
- Teach patient how to prepare and trim nails

1st edition 1992; revised 2004

Background Readings:

Christensen, M. H., Funnell, M. M., Ehrlich, M. R., Fellows, E. P., & Floyd, J. C. (1991). How to care for the diabetic foot. *American Journal of Nursing, 91*(3), 50–57.

Craven, R. F. & Hirnle, C. J. (2003). Self-care hygiene. In *Fundamentals of nursing: Human health and function* (4th ed., pp. 703–752). Philadelphia: Lippincott Williams & Wilkins.

Evanski, P. M. (1991). Easing the pain of common foot problems. *Patient Care, 25*(2), 38–44, 47–50, 52–54.

Harley, J. R. (1993). Preventing diabetic foot disease. *Nurse Practitioner, 18*(10), 37–44.

Maier, T. (1991). The foot and foot wear. *Nursing Clinics of North America, 26*(1), 223–231.

Smith, S. & Duell, D. (1992). *Clinical nursing skills* (3rd ed.). Los Altos, CA: National Nursing Review.

Forensic Data Collection   7940

Definition: Collection and recording of pertinent patient data for a forensic report

Activities:

- Establish rapport with the patient or significant other, as appropriate
- Establish collaborative working relationship with all additional examiners
- Complete all parts of the examination, including normals
- Record omissions in examinations, including rationale for omission
- Provide facts only (e.g., what was examined, what was normal [pertinent negatives], what was abnormal) as seen at the time of examination
- Describe physical injuries by size, color, type of injury, location (add depth and trajectory, if indicated)
- Measure in inches and increments of inches, including the greatest perpendicular dimensions of irregular wounds
- Describe wounds simply and with basic colors as much as possible (e.g., red, blue, purple, maroon)
- Determine wound location in two dimensions (length and midline standpoint) with body divided into anterior midline and posterior midline, describing in terms of how far right or left of midline
- Measure consistently from center of the lesion being described
- Record all contusions immediately as marks will fade and be lost as evidence
- Record directionality in abrasions using piling up of skin cells on the side opposite of the force
- Differentiate lacerations from incised wounds and stab wounds
- Note the order of wounds and why each is known to be first, second, etc., if possible
- Avoid long lists of probable injurious instruments (implies uncertainty and incompetence with examination)
- Determine wound trajectory
- Describe gunshot wounds completely (e.g., sooting, stippling, abrasion ring, or absence of sooting, etc.)
- Describe gunshot wounds as the face of a clock and identify in the report where 12:00 is on the body
- Describe any surrounding bruising or discolorations to gunshot wounds, including any muzzle imprints
- Use body diagrams and photographs to supplement written report
- Adhere to rules about information that must be added to each body diagram (e.g., case number, victim name, examination

date and time, time finished, names and identification numbers of those present during examination)

- Draw in all identifying features (e.g., scars, tattoos, nail polish, body piercings, skin lesions)
- Draw scars in their orientation on the body
- Take injury photos similar to crime scene photography (e.g., victim as part of crime scene, case number in every photograph) assuring case number does not cover or shadow injuries
- Obtain initial photographs as overall entire body photographs before the injuries are cleaned
- Obtain next set of photos as mid-range and closer up with identifiers or landmarks (e.g., nipple in a chest wound)
- Obtain final photos as close-up photos (injury fills nearly entire frame with small identifying number) before and after cleaning
- Ensure that two photographs are obtained in pointer shots (one with and one without pointer) assuring nothing covered in photo with pointer
- Ensure that photographs of injuries are taken perpendicular to the skin surface to prevent distortion
- Ensure that photographs include a measuring scale for perspective
- Ensure that color scales are added to photographs of colored injuries to avoid color distortion
- Wash injured areas and blot dry before photographing to avoid wetness glare and ensure jury use
- Describe clothing (e.g., brand, size), jewelry, and personal property
- Record where items found (e.g., yellow metal watch on the left wrist)
- Record pertinent information related to items (e.g., gunshot wound with soot on the shirt)
- Ensure all items are photographed
- Diagram all medical interventions (e.g., EKG pads, endotracheal tubes, IVs, Foleys)
- Collect and package all specimens in clearly labeled paper bags
- Record date, time, type, and collection method for all specimens
- Use correct chain-of-evidence protocol for all specimens
- Record additional information or events that unfold later as an Addendum Report
- Describe all responses to additional information or events that unfold later (e.g., sexual assault examination completed

24 hours later after evidence presented indicating a sexual assault occurred)
- Plan daily follow-up visits with victims, if possible, to document developing injury patterns
- Prepare reports as customary for state legal evidence requirements (e.g., complete date; military time; black ink; no correction fluid; numbered pages, including all diagrams and worksheets; all pages initialed, no blanks)
- Follow hospital or medical examiner protocol for saving original reports; if self-employed, save own originals
- Provide log sheet where all contact about case is recorded in file with case
- Generate a report entitled Amended Report for any report that needs to be rewritten or corrected due to an error, including date and time of new report, why generated, and description of error in original report, and include correction
- Obtain information from additional examiners (e.g., medical examiner, emergency room physician, emergency room nurse) when unable to obtain information per self (e.g., wound trajectory, wound depth)

- Document information, informant and title, date and time of data collection, when obtaining information from additional examiners
- Provide for appropriate counseling and follow-up care for victims and family, as indicated

5th edition 2008

Background Readings:

Burgess, A. W., Brown, K., Bell, K., Ledray, L. E., & Poarch, J. C. (2005). Sexual abuse of older adults: Assessing for signs of a serious crime and reporting it. *American Journal of Nursing, 105*(10), 66–71.
Calianno, C. & Martin-Boyan, A. (2006). When is it appropriate to photograph a patient's wound? *Advances in Skin & Wound Care, 19*(6), 304–307.
Cohen, S. S. (2003). *Trauma nursing secrets.* Philadelphia, PA: Hanley & Belfus Medical.
Hoyt, C. A. (2006). Integrating forensic science into nursing processes in the ICU. *Critical Care Nursing Quarterly, 29*(3), 259–270.
Lynch, V. A. (2006). *Forensic nursing.* St. Louis: Mosby.

Forgiveness Facilitation   5280

Definition: Assisting an individual's willingness to replace feelings of anger and resentment toward another, self, or higher power, with beneficence, empathy, and humility

Activities:
- Identify patient's beliefs that may hinder/help in "letting go" of an issue
- Acknowledge when anger and resentment are justifiable
- Identify source of anger and resentment, when possible
- Listen empathetically without moralizing or offering platitudes
- Explore forgiveness as a process
- Help the patient explore feelings of anger, bitterness, and resentment
- Use presence, touch, and empathy, as appropriate, to facilitate the process
- Explore possibilities of making amends and reconciliation with self, others, and/or higher power
- Assist the patient to examine the health and healing dimension of forgiveness
- Assist patient to overcome blocks to healing by using spiritual practices (e.g., prayers of praise, guidance, and discernment; healing, touch, visualization of healing, and thanksgiving), as appropriate
- Teach the art of emotional release and relaxation
- Assist client to seek out arbitrator (objective party) to facilitate process of individual or group concern

- Invite use of faith tradition rituals, as appropriate (e.g., anointing, confession, reconciliation)
- Communicate God's/higher power's or inner self's forgiveness through prayer, scripture, other readings, as appropriate
- Communicate acceptance for the individual's level of progress

3rd edition 1996; revised 2008

Background Readings:

Brush, B. L., McGee, E. M., Cavanaugh, B., & Woodward, M. (2001). Forgiveness: A concept analysis. *Journal of Holistic Nursing, 19*(1), 27–41.
Burkhardt, M. A. & Nagai-Jacobson, M. G. (2002). *Spirituality: Living our connectedness.* Albany, NY: Delmar.
Enright, R. D. (2001). *Forgiveness is a choice.* Washington, DC: American Psychological Association.
Enright, R. D. & Fitzgibbons, R. P. (2000). *Helping clients to forgive.* Washington, DC: American Psychological Association.
Festa, L. M. & Tuck, I. (2000). A review of forgiveness literature and with implications for nursing practice. *Holistic Nursing Practice, 14*(4), 77–86.
Worthington, E. L. Jr. (1998). An empathy-humility-commitment model of forgiveness applied within family dyads. *Journal of Family Therapy, 20*(1), 59–76.

Gastrointestinal Intubation 1080

Definition: Insertion of a tube into the gastrointestinal tract

Activities:
- Select type and size of nasogastric tube to insert, considering use and rationale for insertion
- Explain to the patient and family the rationale for using a gastrointestinal tube
- Insert the tube according to agency protocol
- Provide the patient with a glass of water or ice chips to swallow during insertion, as appropriate
- Position patient on right side to facilitate movement of the tube into the duodenum, as appropriate
- Administer medication to increase peristalsis, as appropriate
- Determine correct placement of the tube by observing for signs and symptoms of tracheal entry, checking color and/or pH level of aspirate, inspecting oral cavity, and/or noting placement on x-ray film, if appropriate

1st edition 1992; revised 1996

Background Readings:

Boyes, R. J. & Kruse, J. A. (1992). Nasogastric and nasoenteric intubation. *Critical Care Clinics, 8*(4), 865–878.

Evans-Smith, P. (2005). *Taylor's clinical nursing skills* (pp. 440–444). Philadelphia: Lippincott Williams & Wilkins.

Metheny, N. (1988). Measures to test placement of nasogastric and nasointestinal feeding tubes: A review. *Nursing Research, 37*(6), 324–329.

Metheny, N. (1993). Minimizing respiratory complications of nasoenteric tube feedings: State of the science. *Heart & Lung, 22*(3), 213–223.

Rakel, B. A., Titler, M., Gsoode, C., Barry-Walker, J., Budreau, G., & Buckwalter, K. C. (1994). Nasogastric and nasointestinal feeding tube placement: An integrated review of research. *AACN Clinical Issues in Critical Care Nursing, 5*(2), 194–206.

Thelan, L. A. & Urden, L. D. (1993). *Critical care nursing: Diagnosis and management* (2nd ed.). St. Louis: Mosby.

Thompson, J. M., McFarland, G. K., Hirsch, J. E., & Tucker, S. M. (1998). *Mosby's clinical nursing* (4th ed.). St. Louis: Mosby.

Genetic Counseling 5242

Definition: Use of an interactive helping process focusing on assisting an individual, family, or group, manifesting or at risk for developing or transmitting a birth defect or genetic condition, to cope

Activities:
- Provide privacy and ensure confidentiality
- Establish a therapeutic relationship based on trust and respect
- Determine the patient's purpose, goals, and agenda for the genetic counseling session
- Determine knowledge base, myths, perceptions, and misperceptions related to a birth defect or genetic condition
- Determine presence and quality of family support, other support systems, and previous coping skills
- Provide estimates of patient's risk based upon phenotype (patient characteristics), family history (pedigree analysis), calculated risk information, or genotype (genetic testing results)
- Provide estimates of occurrence or recurrence risk for patient and at-risk family members
- Provide information on the natural history of the disease or condition, treatment and/or management strategies, and prevention strategies, if known
- Provide information about the risks, benefits, and limitations of treatment/management options, as well as options for dealing with recurrence risk in a nondirective manner
- Provide decision-making support as patients consider their options
- Prioritize areas of risk reduction in collaboration with the individual, family, or group
- Monitor response when patient learns about own genetic risk factors
- Allow expression of feelings
- Support patient's coping process
- Institute crisis support skills, as needed
- Provide referral to genetic health care specialists, as necessary
- Provide referral to community resources, including genetic support groups, as needed
- Provide patient a written summary of genetic counseling session, as indicated

1st edition 1992; revised 2000

Background Readings:

Braithwaite, D., Emery, J., Walter, F., Prevost, T., & Sutton, S. (2004). Psychological impact of genetic counseling for familial cancer: Review and meta-analysis. *Journal of the National Cancer Institute, 96*(2), 122–133.

Cohen, F. L. (2005). *Clinical genetics in nursing practice* (3rd ed.). New York: Springer.

Pieterse, A. H., van Dulmen, S., van Dijk, S., Bensing, J. M., & Ausems, M. G. E. M. (2006). Risk communication in completed series of breast cancer genetic counseling visits. *Genetics in Medicine, 8*(11), 688–696.

Scanlon, C. & Fibison, W. (1995). *Managing genetic information: Implications for nursing practice.* Washington, DC: American Nurses Association.

Skirton, H., Patch, C., & Williams, J. (2005). *Applied genetics in healthcare.* Oxford: Taylor & Francis.

Williams, J. K. (2001). Genetic counseling. In M. Craft-Rosenberg & J. Denehy (Eds.), *Nursing interventions for infants, children, and families* (pp. 201–220). Thousand Oaks, CA: Sage.

Grief Work Facilitation   5290

Definition: Assistance with the resolution of a significant loss

Activities:
- Identify the loss
- Assist the patient to identify the nature of the attachment to the lost object or person
- Assist the patient to identify the initial reaction to the loss
- Encourage expression of feelings about the loss
- Listen to expressions of grief
- Encourage discussion of previous loss experiences
- Encourage the patient to verbalize memories of the loss, both past and current
- Make empathetic statements about grief
- Encourage identification of greatest fears concerning the loss
- Instruct in phases of the grieving process, as appropriate
- Support progression through personal grieving stages
- Include significant others in discussions and decisions, as appropriate
- Assist to identify personal coping strategies
- Encourage patient to implement cultural, religious, and social customs associated with the loss
- Communicate acceptance of discussing loss
- Answer children's questions associated with the loss
- Use clear words, such as *dead* or *died*, rather than euphemisms
- Encourage children to discuss feelings
- Encourage expression of feelings in ways comfortable to the child, such as writing, drawing, or playing
- Assist the child to clarify misconceptions
- Identify sources of community support
- Support efforts to resolve previous conflict, as appropriate
- Reinforce progress made in the grieving process
- Assist in identifying modifications needed in lifestyle

1st edition 1992; revised 2004

Background Readings:
Craven, R. F. & Hirnle, C. J. (2000). Loss and grieving. In *Fundamentals of nursing: Human health and function* (3rd ed., pp. 1299–1324). Philadelphia: Lippincott.
Collison, C. & Miller, S. (1987). Using images of the future in grief work. *Image: Journal of Nursing Scholarship, 19*(1), 9–11.
Egan, K. A. & Arnold, K. L. (2003). Grief and bereavement care. *American Journal of Nursing, 103*(9), 42–52.
Gifford, B. J. & Cleary, B. B. (1990). Supporting the bereaved. *American Journal of Nursing, 90*(2), 48–53.
Hampe, S. D. (1975). Needs of a grieving spouse in a hospital setting. *Nursing Research, 24*(2), 113–119.
Whiting, G. & Buckwalter, K. (1991). Dysfunctional grieving. In M. Maas, K. Buckwalter, & M. Hardy (Eds.), *Nursing diagnoses and interventions for the elderly* (pp. 505–518). Redwood City, CA: Addison-Wesley.

Grief Work Facilitation: Perinatal Death   5294

Definition: Assistance with the resolution of a perinatal loss

Activities:
- Encourage participation in decisions about discontinuing life support
- Assist in keeping infant alive until parents arrive
- Baptize the infant, as appropriate
- Encourage parents in holding infant while it dies, as appropriate
- Determine how and when the fetal or infant death was diagnosed
- Discuss plans that have been made (e.g., burial, funeral, and infant name)
- Discuss decisions that will need to be made about funeral arrangements, autopsy, genetic counseling, and family participation
- Describe mementos that will be obtained, including footprints, handprints, pictures, caps, gowns, blankets, diapers, and blood pressure cuffs, as appropriate
- Discuss available support groups, as appropriate
- Discuss differences between male and female patterns of grieving, as appropriate
- Obtain infant footprints, handprints, length, and weight, as needed
- Prepare infant for viewing by bathing and dressing, including parents in activities, as appropriate
- Encourage family members to view and hold infant for as long as desired
- Discuss appearance of infant based on gestational age and length of demise
- Focus on normal features of infant, while sensitively discussing anomalies
- Encourage family time alone with infant, as desired
- Provide referrals to chaplain, social service, grief counselor, and genetic counselor, as appropriate
- Create keepsakes and present to family before discharge, as appropriate
- Discuss characteristics of normal and abnormal grieving, including triggers that precipitate feelings of sadness
- Notify laboratory or funeral home, as appropriate, for disposition of body
- Transfer infant to morgue or prepare body to be transported by family to funeral home

2nd edition 1996

Background Readings:
Davis, D. L., Stewart, M., & Harmon, R. J. (1988). Perinatal loss: Providing emotional support for bereaved parents. *Birth, 15*(4), 242–246.
Gilbert, E. S. & Harmon, J. S. (1998). *Manual of high risk pregnancy and delivery* (2nd ed.). St. Louis: Mosby.
Klingbeil, C. G. (1986). Extended nursing care after a perinatal loss: Theoretical implications. *Neonatal Network, 5*(3), 21–28.

Page-Lieberman, J. & Hughes, C. B. (1990). How fathers perceive perinatal death. *MCN, American Journal of Maternal Child Nursing, 15*(5), 320–323.

Primeau, M. R. & Recht, C. K. (1994). Professional bereavement photographs: One aspect of a perinatal bereavement program. *Journal of Obstetric, Gynecologic, and Neonatal Nursing, 23*(1), 22–25.

Wilkins, J. E. (2001). Grief work facilitation: Perinatal loss. In M. Craft-Rosenberg & J. Denehy (Eds.), *Nursing interventions for infants, children, and families* (pp. 241–256). Thousand Oaks, CA: Sage.

York, C. R. & Stichler, J. F. (1985). Cultural grief expressions following infant death. *Dimensions of Critical Care Nursing, 4*(2), 120–127.

Guided Imagery   6000

Definition: Purposeful use of imagination to achieve a particular state, outcome, or action or to direct attention away from undesirable sensations

Activities:

- Screen for severe emotional problems, history of psychiatric illness, or hallucinations
- Screen for current decreased energy level, inability to concentrate, or other symptoms that may interfere with cognitive ability to create focus on mental images
- Describe the rationale for and the benefits, limitations, and types of guided imagery techniques available
- Elicit information on past coping experiences to determine whether guided imagery might be helpful
- Discuss ability to create vivid mental images and to experience them as if they were real
- Determine capability for doing non-nurse guided imagery (e.g., alone or with tape)
- Encourage the individual to choose from a variety of guided imagery techniques (e.g., nurse-guided, taped)
- Suggest that the individual assume a comfortable position, with unrestricted clothing and eyes closed
- Provide comfortable environment without interruptions, as possible (e.g., using headphones)
- Discuss an image the patient has experienced that is pleasurable and relaxing, such as lying on a beach, watching a new snowfall, floating on a raft, or watching the sun set
- Individualize the images chosen, considering religious or spiritual beliefs, artistic interest, or other individual preferences
- Described the scene using as many of the five senses as possible
- Make suggestions to induce relaxation (e.g., peaceful images, pleasant sensations, or rhythmic breathing), as appropriate
- Use modulated voice when guiding the imagery experience
- Have the patient travel mentally to the scene and assist in describing the setting in detail
- Use permissive directions and suggestions when leading the imagery, such as "perhaps," "if you wish," or "you might like"
- Have the patient slowly experience the scene; how does it look? smell? sound? feel? taste?
- Use words or phrases that convey pleasurable images, such as floating, melting, releasing, and so on
- Develop cleansing or clearing portion of imagery (e.g., all pain appears as red dust and washes downstream in a creek as you enter)
- Assist the patient to develop a method of ending the imagery technique, such as counting slowly while breathing deeply, and slow movements and thoughts of being relaxed, refreshed, and alert
- Encourage patient to express thoughts and feelings regarding the experience
- Prepare patient for unexpected (but often therapeutic) experiences, such as crying
- Instruct patient to practice the imagery, if possible
- Tape-record the imaged experience, if useful
- Plan with patient an appropriate time to do guided imagery
- Use the imagery techniques preventively
- Plan follow-up to assess effects of imagery and any resultant changes in sensation and perception
- Use guided imagery as an adjuvant strategy to pain medications or in conjunction with other measures, as appropriate
- Evaluate and document response to guided imagery

1st edition 1992; revised 2008

Background Readings:

Dossey, B. (1995). Using imagery to help heal your patient. *American Journal of Nursing, 95*(6), 41–46.

Eller, L. S. (1999). Guided imagery interventions for symptom management. In J. Fitzpatrick (Ed.), *Annual review of nursing research* (Vol. 17, pp. 57–84). New York: Springer.

Herr, K. A. & Mobily, P. R. (1999). Pain management. In G. M. Bulechek & J. C. McCloskey (Eds.), *Nursing interventions: Effective nursing treatments* (3rd ed., pp. 149–171). Philadelphia: Saunders.

Kwekkeboom, K., Kneip, J., & Pearson, L. (2003). A pilot study to predict success with guided imagery for cancer pain. *Pain Management Nursing, 4*(3), 112–123.

McCaffery, M. & Pasero, C. (1999). Practical nondrug approaches to pain. In M. McCaffery & C. Pasero (Eds.), *Pain: Clinical manual* (2nd ed., pp. 399–427). St. Louis: Mosby.

Post-White, J. (1998). Imagery. In M. Snyder & R. Lindquist (Eds.), *Complementary/alternative therapies in nursing* (3rd ed., pp. 103–122). New York: Springer.

Van Kuiken, D. (2004). A meta-analysis of the effect of guided imagery practice on outcomes. *Journal of Holistic Nursing, 22*(2), 164–179.

Guilt Work Facilitation   **5300**

Definition: Helping another to cope with painful feelings of actual or perceived responsibility

Activities:

- Guide patient/family in identifying painful feelings of guilt
- Help patient/family identify and examine the situations in which these feelings are experienced or generated
- Assist patient/family members to identify their behaviors in the guilt situation
- Help patient/family understand that guilt is a common reaction to trauma, abuse, grief, catastrophic illness, or accidents
- Use reality testing to help the patient/family identify possible irrational beliefs
- Help patient/family to identify destructive displacement of feelings onto other individuals sharing responsibility in the situation
- Facilitate discussion of the impact of the situation on family relationships
- Facilitate genetic counseling, as appropriate
- Refer patient/family to the appropriate trauma, abuse, grief, illness, caregiver, or survivor group for education and support
- Facilitate spiritual support, as appropriate
- Teach patient to use thought stopping technique and thought substitution in conjunction with deliberate muscle relaxation when persistent thoughts of guilt enter the mind
- Guide the patient through steps of self-forgiveness when one's guilt is valid
- Assist the patient/family to identify options for prevention, restitution, atonement, and resolution when appropriate

1st edition 1992; revised 2008

Background Readings:

Antai-Otong, D. (2003). Crisis intervention and management: The role of adaptation. In D. Antai-Otong (Ed.), *Psychiatric nursing: Biological and behavioral concepts* (pp. 841–862). Clifton Park, NY: Thomson Delmar Learning.

Kemp, C. (2004). Grief and loss. In K. M. Fortinash & P. A. Holloday Worret (Eds.), *Psychiatric mental health nursing* (3rd ed., pp. 573–588). St. Louis: Mosby.

Stuart, G. (2005). Self concept responses and dissociative disorders. In G. W. Stuart & M. T. Laraia (Eds.), *Principles and practice of psychiatric nursing* (8th ed., pp. 303–329). St. Louis: Mosby.

Sundeen, S. (2005). Psychiatric rehabilitation and recovery. In G. W. Stuart & M. T. Laraia (Eds.), *Principles and practice of psychiatric nursing* (8th ed., pp. 239–257). St. Louis: Mosby.

Veenema, T. G. & Shroeder-Bruce, K. (2002). The aftermath of violence: Children, disaster, and posttraumatic stress disorder. *Journal of Pediatric Health Care, 16*(5), 235–244.

G

Hair and Scalp Care

1670

Definition: Promotion of healthy, clean, and attractive hair and scalp

Activities:

- Monitor condition of hair and scalp, including abnormalities (e.g., dry, coarse, or brittle hair, pest infestation, dandruff, and nutritional deficiencies)
- Provide treatment for abnormalities or notify appropriate health care provider
- Prepare supplies for cleansing hair (e.g., basin, shampoo board, waterproof pad, towel, shampoo, and conditioner)
- Assist patient into comfortable position
- Use hydrogen peroxide or alcohol to dissolve matted blood, if present, prior to cleansing hair
- Place commercially-prepared, disposable cleansing cap on patient's head and massage head to work solution through hair and scalp, being sure to use cap according to manufacturer's instructions
- Wash and condition hair, massaging shampoo and conditioner into scalp and hair
- Avoid chilling during cleansing (i.e., adjust room temperature and provide warmed towels)
- Dry hair with hair dryer on a low setting to avoid burning scalp
- Brush or comb hair, using wide-toothed comb or pick, as needed
- Apply small amount of oil to dry or flaking areas of scalp
- Style hair
- Monitor patient response to hair loss, providing support if indicated (i.e., assist in selecting a hat, wig, or scarf; refer to community agency; and discuss hair transplants and drugs to stimulate hair growth)
- Arrange for barber or hairdresser to cut hair
- Prepare supplies for shaving (e.g., shaving cream, towel, and safety or electric razor)
- Shave body hair, if desired, using an electric razor for patients at risk for excessive bleeding
- Perform hair removal procedures using scissors, hair clippers, or chemical depilatory agents prior to surgical procedure, being sure to refer to institutional policies and physician's order
- Instruct patient or parent on hair care (e.g., cleansing infant scalp and hair and preventing pest infestation)
- Provide referral, as appropriate

1st edition 1992; revised 2008, 2013

Background Readings:

Craven, R. F., & Hirnle, C. J. (2009). *Fundamentals of nursing: Human health and function* (6th ed.). Philadelphia: Lippincott Williams & Wilkins.

Smith, S. F., Duell, D. J., & Martin, B. C. (2008). *Clinical nursing skills: Basic to advanced skills* (7th ed.). Upper Saddle River, NJ: Pearson Prentice Hall.

Titler, M. G., Pettit, D., Bulechek, G. M., McCloskey, J. C., Craft, M. J., Cohen, M. Z., et al. (1991). Classification of nursing interventions for care of the integument. *Nursing Diagnosis, 2*(2), 45–56.

Hallucination Management

6510

Definition: Promoting the safety, comfort, and reality orientation of a patient experiencing hallucinations

Activities:

- Establish a trusting, interpersonal relationship with the patient
- Monitor and regulate the level of activity and stimulation in the environment
- Maintain a safe environment
- Provide appropriate level of surveillance/supervision to monitor patient
- Record patient behaviors that indicate hallucinations
- Maintain a consistent routine
- Assign consistent caregivers on a daily basis
- Promote clear and open communication
- Provide patient with opportunities to discuss hallucinations
- Encourage patient to express feelings appropriately
- Refocus patient to topic if patient's communication is inappropriate to circumstances
- Monitor hallucinations for presence of content that is violent or self-harmful
- Encourage patient to develop control/responsibility over own behavior, if ability allows
- Encourage patient to discuss feelings and impulses rather than acting on them
- Encourage patient to validate hallucinations with trusted others (e.g., reality testing)
- Point out, if asked, that you are not experiencing the same stimuli
- Avoid arguing with patient about the validity of the hallucinations
- Focus discussion upon the underlying feelings rather than the content of the hallucinations (e.g., "It appears as if you are feeling frightened")
- Provide antipsychotic and antianxiety medications on a routine and PRN basis
- Provide medication teaching to patient and significant others
- Monitor patient for medication side effects and desired therapeutic effects
- Provide for safety and comfort of patient and others when patient is unable to control behavior (e.g., limit setting, area restriction, physical restraint, and seclusion)

- Discontinue or decrease medications (after consulting with prescribing caregiver) that may be causing hallucinations
- Provide illness teaching to patient/significant others if hallucinations are illness based (e.g., delirium, schizophrenia, and depression)
- Educate family and significant others about ways to deal with patient who is experiencing hallucinations
- Monitor self-care ability
- Assist with self-care, as needed
- Monitor physical status of patient (e.g., body weight, hydration, and soles of feet in patient who paces)
- Provide for adequate rest and nutrition
- Involve patient in reality-based activities that may distract from the hallucinations (e.g., listening to music)

1st edition 1992; revised 1996

Background Readings:

Bostrum, A. C., & Boyd, M. A. (2005). Schizophrenia. In M. A. Boyd (Ed.), *Psychiatric nursing: Contemporary practice* (3rd ed., pp. 265–310). Philadelphia: Lippincott Williams & Wilkins.

Eklund, E. S. (1991). Perception/cognition, altered. In G. K. McFarland & M. D. Thomas (Eds.), *Psychiatric mental health nursing: Application to the nursing process* (pp. 332–357). Philadelphia: Lippincott.

Moller, M. D. (1989). *Understanding and communicating with a person who is hallucinating.* [Videotape]. Omaha, NE: NurSeminars.

Norris, J. (1987). Schizophrenia and schizophreniform disorders. In J. Norris, M. Kunes-Cornell, S. Stockard, P. M. Ehrhart, & G. R. Newton (Eds.), *Mental health-psychiatric nursing: A continuum of care* (pp. 785–811). New York: John Wiley & Sons.

Varcarolis, E. M. (2000). *Psychiatric nursing clinical guide* (pp. 230–232). Philadelphia: Saunders.

H

Healing Touch 1390

Definition: Providing a noninvasive, biofield therapy using touch and compassionate intentionality to influence the energy system of a person, affecting their physical, emotional, mental, and spiritual health and healing

Activities:
- Create a comfortable, private environment without distractions
- Determine willingness to have body touched
- Identify mutual goals for the session
- Advise the patient to ask questions whenever they arise
- Place patient in a comfortable and safe position that facilitates relaxation (e.g., chair, recliner, or massage table may be used if the body can be safely supported)
- Remove constricting items (e.g., eyeglasses, shoes, and belt)
- Keep the patient comfortably clothed
- Drape only to provide temperature comfort
- Center self by focusing awareness on inner self
- Ground self by attuning to Earth's energy
- Attune to the patient's energy field
- Set intention to work for the patient's highest good
- Conduct an assessment of the patient's energy field (aura) and energy centers to determine whether clearing, balancing, or energizing techniques are to be used
- Determine the specific healing touch approach to promote healing (e.g., unruffling or smoothing the energy field, full body connection, Etheric Vitality, magnetic unruffled, magnetic pain drain, spiral meditation, pyramid technique)
- Use hands to clear, balance, and energize the patient's field
- Continue until the energy fields and energy centers feel balanced, smooth, connected, symmetrical, and flowing
- Repeat an energy assessment to identify what changes have occurred
- Instruct the patient to gently move their body and stretch before they get up
- Touch the patient's body to help them ground or connect with the Earth's energy if they experience dizziness when they get up
- Offer client a glass of water to replenish the water lost with the energy movement
- Provide feedback to the patient regarding the energetic work in terms they understand
- Ask the patient to describe what they experienced or noted during and after the session
- Record the characteristics of the energy work
- Record the physical, mental, and emotional responses to the session

6th edition 2013

Background Readings:

Hover-Kramer, D. (2004). *Healing touch: A guidebook for practitioners.* Albany NY: Delmar: Thomson.

Hutchison, P. (1999). Healing touch. An energetic approach. *American Journal of Nursing, 99*(4), 43–48.

Umbreit, A. (2006). Healing touch. In M. Snyder & R. Lindquist (Eds.), *Complementary/alternative therapies in nursing* (5th ed.). New York: Springer.

Wardell, D. W., & Weymouth, K. K. (2004). Review of studies of healing touch. *Journal of Nursing Scholarship, 36*(2), 147–154.

Health Care Information Exchange 7960

Definition: Providing patient care information to other health professionals

Activities:

- Identify referring nurse and location
- Identify essential demographic data
- Describe pertinent past health history
- Identify current nursing and medical diagnoses
- Identify resolved nursing and medical diagnoses, as appropriate
- Describe plan of care, including diet, medications, and exercise
- Describe nursing interventions being implemented
- Identify equipment and supplies necessary for care
- Summarize progress of patient toward goals
- Identify anticipated date of discharge or transfer
- Identify planned return appointment for follow-up care
- Describe role of family in continuing care
- Identify capabilities of patient and family in implementing care after discharge
- Identify other agencies providing care
- Request information from health professionals in other agencies
- Coordinate care with other health professionals
- Discuss patient's strengths and resources
- Share concerns of patient or family with other health care providers
- Share information from other health professionals with patient and family, as appropriate

Background Readings:

Craven, R. F., & Hirnle, C. J. (2003). Communication of the nursing process: Documenting and reporting. In *Fundamentals of nursing: Human health and function* (4th ed., pp. 229–251). Philadelphia: Lippincott Williams & Wilkins.

Jenkins, C. A., Schullz, M. Hanson, J. Bruera. E. (2000). Demographic, symptom and medication profiles of cancer patients seen by a palliative care consult team in a tertiary referral hospital. *Journal of Pain & Symptom Management, 19*(3), 174–184.

Job, T. (1999). A system for determining the priority of referrals within a multidisciplinary community mental health team. *British Journal of Occupation Therapy, 62*(11), 486–490.

Kozier, B., Erb, G., Berman, A., & Snyder, S. (2004). Documenting and reporting. In *Fundamentals of nursing: Concepts, processes, and practice.* (7th ed., pp. 328–349). Upper Saddle River, NJ: Prentice Hall.

Kron, T., & Gray, A. (1987). *The management of patient care. Putting leadership skills to work* (6th ed.). Philadelphia: Saunders.

Smith, F. A. (2000). The function of consumer health information centers in hospitals. *Medical Library Association News, 327,* 23.

Summerton, H. (1998). Discharge planning: Establishing an effective coordination team. *British Journal of Nursing 7*(20), 1263–1267.

2nd edition 1996; revised 2004

Health Education 5510

Definition: Developing and providing instruction and learning experiences to facilitate voluntary adaptation of behavior conducive to health in individuals, families, groups, or communities

Activities:

- Target high-risk groups and age ranges that would benefit most from health education
- Target needs identified in Healthy People 2010: National Health Promotion and Disease Prevention Objectives, or other local, state, and national needs
- Identify internal or external factors that may enhance or reduce motivation for healthy behavior
- Determine personal context and social-cultural history of individual, family, or community health behavior
- Determine current health knowledge and lifestyle behaviors of individual, family, or target group
- Assist individuals, families, and communities in clarifying health beliefs and values
- Identify characteristics of target population that affect selection of learning strategies
- Prioritize identified learner needs based on client preference, skills of nurse, resources available, and likelihood of successful goal attainment
- Formulate objectives for health education program
- Identify resources (e.g., personnel, space, equipment, money, etc.) needed to conduct program
- Consider accessibility, consumer preference, and cost in program planning
- Strategically place attractive advertising to capture attention of target audience
- Avoid use of fear or scare techniques as strategy to motivate people to change health or lifestyle behaviors
- Emphasize immediate or short-term positive health benefits to be received by positive lifestyle behaviors rather than long-term benefits or negative effects of noncompliance
- Incorporate strategies to enhance the self-esteem of target audience
- Develop educational materials written at a readability level appropriate to target audience
- Teach strategies that can be used to resist unhealthy behavior or risk taking rather than give advice to avoid or change behavior
- Keep presentation focused and short, and begin and end on main point
- Use group presentations to provide support and lessen threat to learners experiencing similar problems or concerns, as appropriate
- Use peer leaders, teachers, and support groups in implementing programs to groups less likely to listen to health professionals or adults (i.e., adolescents), as appropriate
- Use lectures to convey the maximum amount of information, when appropriate
- Use group discussions and role-playing to influence health beliefs, attitudes, and values

- Use demonstrations/return demonstrations, learner participation, and manipulation of materials when teaching psychomotor skills
- Use computer-assisted instruction, television, interactive video, and other technologies to convey information
- Use teleconferencing, telecommunications, and computer technologies for distance learning
- Involve individuals, families, and groups in planning and implementing plans for lifestyle or health behavior modification
- Determine family, peer, and community support for behavior conducive to health
- Utilize social and family support systems to enhance effectiveness of lifestyle or health behavior modification
- Emphasize importance of healthy patterns of eating, sleeping, exercising, etc. to individuals, families, and groups who model these values and behaviors to others, particularly children
- Use variety of strategies and intervention points in educational program
- Plan long-term follow-up to reinforce health behavior or lifestyle adaptations
- Design and implement strategies to measure client outcomes at regular intervals during and after completion of program
- Design and implement strategies to measure program and cost effectiveness of education, using this data to improve the effectiveness of subsequent programs

- Influence development of policy that guarantees health education as an employee benefit
- Encourage policy where insurance companies give consideration for premium reductions or benefits for healthful lifestyle practices

2nd edition 1996; revised 2000

Background Readings:

APHA Technical Report. (1987). Criteria for the development of health promotion and education programs. *American Journal of Public Health*, 77(1), 89–92.

Bastable, S. B. (2003). *Nurse as educator: Principles of teaching and learning for nursing practice*. Sudbury, MA: Jones and Bartlett.

Craven, R. F., & Hirnle, C. J. (2003). Health and wellness. In *Fundamentals of nursing: Human health and function* (4th ed., pp. 255–266). Philadelphia: Lippincott Williams & Wilkins.

Kozier, B., Erb, G., Berman, A., & Snyder, S. (2004). Health promotion. In *Fundamentals of nursing: Concepts, processes, and practice*. (7th ed., pp. 118–139). Upper Saddle River, NJ: Prentice Hall.

Pender, N. J., Murdaugh, C. L., & Parsons, M. A. (2002). *Health promotion in nursing practice* (4th ed.). Upper Saddle River, NJ: Prentice Hall.

U.S. Department of Health and Human Services. (2000). *Healthy people 2010: Understanding and improving health* (2nd ed.). Washington, DC: U.S. Government Printing Office.

H

Health Literacy Enhancement   5515

Definition: Assisting individuals with limited ability to obtain, process, and understand information related to health and illness

Activities:
- Create a health care environment where a patient with impaired literacy can seek help without feeling ashamed or stigmatized
- Use appropriate and clear communication
- Use plain language
- Simplify language whenever possible
- Use a slow speaking pace
- Avoid medical jargon and use of acronyms
- Communicate with consideration for culture-suitability, age-suitability, and gender-suitability
- Determine patient's experience with the health care system, including health promotion, health protection, disease prevention, health care and maintenance, and health care system navigation
- Determine health literacy status at initiation of contact with the patient through informal and/or formal assessments
- Determine patient's learning style
- Observe for impaired health literacy cues (e.g., failing to complete written forms, missing appointments, not taking medications appropriately, inability to identify medications or describe reasons for taking them, deferring to family members for information about health condition, asking multiple questions about topics already covered in handouts and brochures, avoiding reading things in front of health care providers)
- Obtain interpreter services as needed
- Provide essential written and oral information to a patient in his/her first language

- Determine what the patient already knows about his/her health condition or risks and relate new information to what is already known
- Provide one-to-one teaching or counseling whenever feasible
- Provide understandable written materials (i.e., use short sentences and common words with fewer syllables, highlight key points, use an active voice, use large print, have a user-friendly layout and design, group similar content into segments, emphasize behaviors and action that should be taken, use pictures or diagrams to clarify and decrease the reading burden)
- Use strategies to enhance understanding (i.e., start with the most important information first, focus on key messages and repeat, limit the amount of information presented at any one time, use examples to illustrate important points, relate to the individual's experience, use a storytelling style)
- Use multiple communication tools (e.g., audiotapes, videotapes, digital video devices, computers, pictograms, models, diagrams).
- Evaluate patient understanding by having patient repeat back in own words or demonstrate skill.
- Encourage the individual to ask questions and seek clarification (e.g., What is my main problem? What do I need to do? Why is it important for me to do this?)
- Assist the individual in anticipating their experiences in the health care system (e.g., being asked questions, seeing different health professionals, needing to let providers know when information is not understood, getting the results from laboratory tests, making and keeping appointments)

- Encourage use of effective measures for coping with impaired health literacy (e.g., being persistent when asking for help, bringing a written list of questions or concerns to each health care encounter, depending on oral explanations or demonstrations of tasks, seeking the assistance of family or friends in getting health information)

5th edition 2008

Background Readings:

Baker, D. W. (2006). The meaning and measure of health literacy. *Journal of General Internal Medicine, 21*(8), 878–883.

DeWalt, D. A., Berkman, N. D., Sheridan, S., Lohr, K. N., & Pignone, M. P. (2004). Literacy and health outcomes: A systematic review of the literature. *Journal of General Internal Medicine, 19*(12), 1228–1239.

Doak, C. C, Doak, L. G., & Root, J. H. (1996). *Teaching patients with low literacy skills* (2nd ed.). Philadelphia: Lippincott.

Dubrow, J. (2004). *Adequate literacy and health literacy: Prerequisites for informed health care decision making.* Washington, DC: AARP Public Policy Institute.

Institute of Medicine. (2004). *Health literacy: A prescription to end confusion.* Washington, DC: National Academies Press.

Osborne, H. (2005). *Health literacy from A to Z. Practical ways to communicate your health message.* Sudbury, MA: Jones and Bartlett.

Schwartzberg, J. G., VanGeest, J. B., & Wang, C. (Eds.). (2005). *Understanding health literacy: Implications for medicine and public health.* Chicago: American Medical Association Press.

Speros, C. (2005). Health literacy: Concept analysis. *Journal of Advanced Nursing, 50*(6), 633–640

Weiss, B. D., Mays, M. Z., Martz, W., Castro, K. M., DeWalt, D. A., Pignone, M. P., et al. (2005). Quick assessment of literacy in primary care: The newest vital sign. *Annals of Family Medicine, 3*(6), 514-522.

H

Health Policy Monitoring   7970

Definition: Surveillance and influence of government and organization regulations, rules, and standards that affect nursing systems and practices to ensure quality care of patients

Activities:

- Review proposed policies and standards in organizational, professional, and governmental literature, and in the popular media
- Assess implications and requirements of proposed policies and standards for quality patient care
- Compare requirements of policies and standards with current practices
- Assess negative and positive effects of health policies and standards on nursing practice, patient, and cost outcomes
- Identify and resolve discrepancies between health policies and standards and current nursing practice
- Acquaint policy makers with implications of current and proposed policies and standards for patient welfare
- Lobby policy makers to make changes in health policies and standards to benefit patients
- Testify in organizational, professional, and public forums to influence the formulation of health policies and standards that benefit patients
- Assist consumers of health care to be informed of current and proposed changes in health policies and standards and the implications for health outcomes

2nd edition 1996

Background Readings:

Dean-Barr, S. L. (1994). Standards and guidelines: How do they assure quality? In J. McCloskey & H. K. Grace (Eds.), *Current issues in nursing* (4th ed.). St. Louis: Mosby.

Donahue, M. (1985). Advocacy. In G. M. Bulechek & J. C. McCloskey (Eds.), *Nursing interventions: Treatments for nursing diagnoses* (pp. 338–351). Philadelphia: Saunders.

Maas, M., & Mulford, C. (1989). Structural adaptation of organizations: Issues and strategies for nurse executives. In *Series on Nursing Administration* (Vol. 2) (pp. 3–40). St. Louis: Mosby.

Mason, D. J., Leavitt, J. K., & Chaffee, M. W. (2007). *Policy and politics in nursing and health care.* Philadelphia: Saunders.

Specht, J. (1992). Implications of the ethics and economics of health care rationing for nursing administration. In M. Johnson (Ed.), *Economic myths and realities: Doing more with no more. Series on Nursing Administration* (Vol. 4) (pp. 19–36). St. Louis: Mosby.

Warner, D. M., Holloway, D. C., & Grazier, K. L. (1984). *Decision making and control for health administration.* Ann Arbor, MI: Health Administration Press.

Health Screening   6520

Definition: Detecting health risks or problems by means of history, examination, and other procedures

Activities:
- Determine target population for health screening
- Advertise health-screening services to increase public awareness
- Provide easy access to screening services (e.g., time and place)
- Schedule appointments to enhance efficiency and individualized care
- Use valid, reliable health screening instruments
- Instruct on rationale and purpose of health screenings and self-monitoring
- Obtain informed consent for health-screening procedures, as appropriate
- Provide for privacy and confidentiality
- Provide for comfort during screening procedures
- Obtain health history, as appropriate, including description of health habits, risk factors, and medications
- Obtain family health history, as appropriate
- Perform physical assessment, as appropriate
- Measure blood pressure, height, weight, percent body fat, cholesterol and blood sugar levels, and urinalysis, as appropriate
- Perform (or refer for) Pap smear, mammography, prostate check, EKG, testicular examination, and vision check, as appropriate
- Obtain specimens for analysis
- Complete appropriate Department of Health or other records for monitoring abnormal results, such as high blood pressure
- Provide appropriate self-monitoring information during screening
- Provide results of health screenings to patient
- Inform patient of limitations and margin of error of specific screening tests
- Counsel patient who has abnormal findings about treatment alternatives or need for further evaluation
- Refer patient to other health care providers, as necessary
- Provide follow-up contact for patient with abnormal findings

1st edition 1992; revised 1996

Background Readings:
Ahlbom, A., & Norell, S. (1990). *Introduction to modern epidemiology* (2nd ed.). Chestnut Hill, MA: Epidemiology Resources.
Ferren-Carter, K. (1991). The health fair as an effective health promotion strategy. *AAOHN Journal, 39*(11), 513–516.
Goeppinger, J., & Labuhn, K. T. (1992). Self-health care through risk appraisal and reduction. In M. Stanhope & J. Lancaster (Eds.), *Community health nursing* (3rd ed., pp. 578–591). St. Louis: Mosby.
Hornsey, J. (1991). Screening by program. *Occupational Health, 43*(5), 150–151.
Kozier, B., Erb, G., Berman, A., & Snyder, S. (2004). Health assessment. In *Fundamentals of nursing: Concepts, processes, and practice.* (7th ed., pp. 523–625). Upper Saddle River, NJ: Prentice Hall.
Leatherman, J., & Davidhizar, R. (1992). Health screening on a college campus by nursing students. *Journal of Community Health Nursing, 9*(1), 43–51.
May, A., (1992). Implementing an annual screening program. *Health Visitor, 65*(7), 240–241.
Smeltzer, S. C., & Bare, B. G. (2004). Health assessment. In *Brunner & Suddarth's textbook of medical surgical nursing* (Vol. 1) (10th ed., pp. 59–79). Philadelphia: Lippincott Williams & Wilkins.
Smith, R. A., Cokkinides, V., von Eschenbach, A. C., Levin, B., Cohen, C., Runowicz, C. D., et al. (2002). American Cancer Society guidelines for the early detection of cancer. *CA: A Cancer Journal for Clinicians, 52*(1), 8–22.
Summer, J. (1991). Screening the elderly. *Nursing Times, 87*(3), 60–82.

H

Health System Guidance   7400

Definition: Facilitating a patient's location and use of appropriate health services

Activities:
- Explain the immediate health care system, how it works, and what the patient/family can expect
- Assist patient or family to coordinate health care and communication
- Assist patient or family to choose appropriate health care professionals
- Instruct patient on what type of services to expect from each type of health care provider (e.g., nurse specialists, registered dietitians, registered nurses, licensed practical nurses, physical therapists, cardiologists, internists, optometrists, and psychologists)
- Inform the patient about different types of health care facilities (e.g., general hospital, specialty hospital, teaching hospital, walk-in clinic, and outpatient surgical clinic), as appropriate
- Inform the patient of accreditation and state health department requirements for judging the quality of a facility
- Inform patient of appropriate community resources and contact persons
- Advise use of second opinion
- Inform patient of right to change health care provider
- Inform the patient the meaning of signing a consent form
- Provide patient with copy of Patient's Bill of Rights
- Inform patient how to access emergency services by telephone and vehicle, as appropriate
- Encourage patient to go to the emergency room, if appropriate
- Identify and facilitate communication among health care providers and patient/family, as appropriate
- Inform patient/family how to challenge a decision made by a health care provider, as needed
- Encourage consultation with other health care professionals, as appropriate
- Request services from other health professionals for patient, as appropriate

- Coordinate referrals to relevant health care providers, as appropriate
- Review and reinforce information given by other health care professionals
- Provide information on how to obtain equipment
- Coordinate/schedule time needed by each service to deliver care, as appropriate
- Inform patient of the cost, time, alternatives, and risks involved in a specific test or procedure
- Give written instructions for purpose and location of post-hospitalization/outpatient activities, as appropriate
- Give written instructions for purpose and location of health care activities, as appropriate
- Discuss outcome of visit with other health care providers, as appropriate
- Identify and facilitate transportation needs for obtainment of health care services
- Provide follow-up contact with patient, as appropriate
- Monitor adequacy of current health care follow-up
- Provide report to posthospital caregivers, as appropriate
- Encourage the patient/family to ask questions about services and charges
- Comply with regulations for third-party reimbursement
- Assist individual to complete forms for assistance, such as housing and financial aid, as needed
- Notify patient of scheduled appointments, as appropriate

1st edition 1992; revised 2000, 2004

Background Readings:

Arnold, E., & Boggs, K. (1989). *Interpersonal relationships: Professional communication skills for nurses.* Philadelphia: Saunders.

Craven, R. F., & Hirnle, C. J. (2003). Case management. In *Fundamentals of nursing: Human health and function* (4th ed., pp. 379–390). Philadelphia: Lippincott Williams & Wilkins.

Dunne, P. J. (1998). The emerging health care delivery system. *American Association of Respiratory Care Times, 22*(1), 24–28.

Matthews, P. (2000). Planning for successful outcomes in the new millennium. *Topics in Health Information Management, 20*(3), 55–64.

Viscardis, L. (1998). The family-centered approach to providing services: A parent perspective. *Physical & Occupation Therapy in Pediatrics, 18*(1), 41–53.

Zarbock, S. G. (1999). Sharing in all dimensions: Providing nourishment at home. *Home Care Provider 4*(3), 106–107.

Heat/Cold Application 1380

Definition: Stimulation of the skin and underlying tissues with heat or cold for the purpose of decreasing pain, muscle spasms, or inflammation

Activities:

- Explain the use of heat or cold, the reason for the treatment, and how it will affect the patient's symptoms
- Screen for contraindications to cold or heat, such as decreased or absent sensation, decreased circulation, and decreased ability to communicate
- Select a method of stimulation that is convenient and readily available (e.g., waterproof plastic bags with melting ice; frozen gel packs; chemical ice envelope; ice immersion; cloth or towel in freezer for cold; hot water bottle; electric heating pad; hot, moist compresses; immersion in tub or whirlpool; paraffin wax; sitz bath; radiant bulb; or plastic wrap for heat)
- Determine availability and safe working condition of all equipment used for heat or cold application
- Determine condition of skin and identify any alterations requiring a change in procedure or contraindications to stimulation
- Select stimulation site, considering alternate sites when direct application is not possible (e.g., adjacent to, distal to, between affected areas and the brain, and contralateral)
- Wrap the heat or cold application device with a protective cloth, if appropriate
- Use a moist cloth next to the skin to increase the sensation of cold or heat, when appropriate
- Use ice after an ankle sprain to reduce edema, followed by rest, compression, and elevation
- Instruct how to avoid tissue damage associated with heat or cold
- Check the temperature of the application, especially when using heat
- Determine duration of application based on individual verbal, behavioral, and biological responses
- Time all applications carefully
- Apply cold or heat directly on or near the affected site, if possible
- Avoid using heat or cold on tissue that has been exposed to radiation therapy
- Inspect the site carefully for signs of skin irritation or tissue damage throughout the first 5 minutes and then frequently during the treatment
- Finish with a cold treatment to encourage vasoconstriction when alternating heat and cold applications for an injured athlete
- Evaluate general condition, safety, and comfort throughout the treatment
- Position to allow movement from the temperature source, if needed
- Instruct not to adjust temperature settings independently without prior instruction
- Change sites of cold or heat application or switch form of stimulation if relief is not achieved
- Instruct that cold application may be painful briefly, with numbness about 5 minutes after the initial stimulation
- Instruct on indications for, frequency of, and procedure for application
- Instruct to avoid injury to the skin after stimulation
- Evaluate and document response to heat and cold application

1st edition 1992, revised 2013

Background Readings:

Berman, A., Snyder, S., Kozier, B., & Erb, G. (2008). Skin integrity and wound care. In *Kozier & Erb's Fundamentals of nursing: Concepts, processes, and practice.* (8th ed., pp. 902–938). Upper Saddle River, NJ: Prentice Hall.

Smeltzer, S. C., Bare, B. G., Hinkle, J. L., & Cheever, K. H. (2010). Pain management. In *Brunner & Suddarth's textbook of medical surgical nursing* (Vol. 1) (12th ed., pp. 230–262). Philadelphia: Lippincott Williams & Wilkins.

Thompson, C., Kelsberg, G., & St. Anna, L. (2003). Heat or ice for acute ankle sprain. *Journal of Family Practice, 52*(8), 642–643.

White, L. (2005). *Foundations of nursing* (2nd ed., p. 471). Clifton Park, NY: Thomson Delmar Learning.

Hemodialysis Therapy   2100

Definition: Management of extracorporeal passage of the patient's blood through a dialyzer

Activities:

- Draw blood sample and review blood chemistries (e.g., blood urea nitrogen; serum creatinine; serum Na, K, and PO_4 levels) pretreatment
- Record baseline vital signs: weight, temperature, pulse, respirations, and blood pressure
- Explain hemodialysis procedure and its purpose
- Check equipment and solutions, according to protocol
- Use sterile technique to initiate hemodialysis and for needle insertions and catheter connections
- Use gloves, eyeshield, and clothing to prevent direct contact with blood
- Initiate hemodialysis, according to protocol
- Anchor connections and tubing securely
- Check system monitors (e.g., flow rate, pressure, temperature, pH level, conductivity, clots, air detector, negative pressure for ultrafiltration, and blood sensor) to ensure patient safety
- Monitor blood pressure, pulse, respirations, temperature, and patient response during dialysis
- Administer heparin, according to protocol
- Monitor clotting times and adjust heparin administration appropriately
- Adjust filtration pressures to remove an appropriate amount of fluid
- Institute appropriate protocol if patient becomes hypotensive
- Discontinue hemodialysis according to protocol
- Compare postdialysis vitals and blood chemistries to predialysis values
- Avoid taking blood pressure or doing intravenous punctures in arm with fistula
- Provide catheter or fistula care, according to protocol
- Work collaboratively with patient to adjust diet regulations, fluid limitations, and medications to regulate fluid and electrolyte shifts between treatments
- Teach patient to self-monitor signs and symptoms that indicate need for medical treatment (e.g., fever, bleeding, clotted fistula, thrombophlebitis, and irregular pulse)
- Work collaboratively with patient to relieve discomfort from side effects of the disease and treatment (e.g., cramping, fatigue, headaches, itching, anemia, bone demineralization, body image changes, and role disruption)
- Work collaboratively with patient to adjust length of dialysis, diet regulations, and pain and diversion needs to achieve optimal benefit of the treatment

1st edition; revised 1996, 2004

Background Readings:

Fearing, M. O., & Hart, L. K. (1992). Dialysis therapy. In G. M. Bulechek & J. C. McCloskey (Eds.), *Nursing interventions: Essential nursing treatments* (2nd ed., pp. 587–601). Philadelphia: Saunders.

Smeltzer, S. C., & Bare, B. G. (2004). Management of patients with upper or lower urinary tract dysfunction. In *Brunner & Suddarth's textbook of medical surgical nursing* (Vol. 2) (10th ed., pp. 1271–1308). Philadelphia: Lippincott Williams & Wilkins.

Thompson, J. M., McFarland, G. K., Hirsch, J. E., & Tucker, S. M. (1998). *Mosby's clinical nursing* (4th ed.). St. Louis: Mosby.

H

Hemodynamic Regulation   4150

Definition: Optimization of heart rate, preload, afterload, and contractility

Activities:

- Perform a comprehensive appraisal of hemodynamic status (i.e., check blood pressure, heart rate, pulses, jugular venous pressure, central venous pressure, right and left atrial and ventricular pressures, and pulmonary artery pressure), as appropriate
- Use multiple parameters to determine patient's clinical status (i.e., proportional pulse pressure is considered the definitive parameter)
- Monitor and document proportional pulse pressure (i.e., systolic blood pressure minus diastolic blood divided by systolic blood pressure, resulting in a proportion or percentage)
- Provide frequent physical examination in at-risk populations (e.g., heart failure patients)
- Alleviate patient anxieties by providing accurate information and correcting any misconceptions
- Instruct patient and family on hemodynamic monitoring (e.g., medications, therapies, purposes of equipment)
- Explain the aims of care and how progress will be measured
- Recognize presence of early warning signs and symptoms of compromised hemodynamic system (e.g., dyspnea, decreased ability to exercise, orthopnea, profound fatigue, dizziness, lightheadedness, edema, palpitations, paroxysmal nocturnal dyspnea, sudden weight gain)
- Determine volume status (i.e., Is patient hypervolemic, hypovolemic, or in a balanced fluid level?)
- Monitor for signs and symptoms of volume status problems (e.g., neck vein distension, elevated pressure in the right internal jugular vein, positive abdominal jugular neck vein reflex, edema, ascites, crackles, dyspnea, orthopnea, paroxysmal nocturnal dyspnea)
- Determine perfusion status (i.e., Is patient cold, lukewarm, or warm?)
- Monitor for signs and symptoms of perfusion status problems (e.g., symptomatic hypotension; cool extremities, including arms and legs; mental obtundation or constant sleepiness; elevation in serum levels of creatinine and BUN; hyponatremia; narrow pulse pressure; and proportional pulse pressure of 25% or less)
- Auscultate lung sounds for crackles or other adventitious sounds
- Recognize that adventitious lung sounds are not the sole indicator of hemodynamic issues

- Auscultate heart sounds
- Monitor and document blood pressure, heart rate, rhythm, and pulses
- Monitor pacemaker functioning, if appropriate
- Monitor systemic and pulmonary vascular resistance, as appropriate
- Monitor cardiac output and cardiac index and left-ventricular stroke work index, as appropriate
- Administer positive inotropic and contractility medications
- Administer antiarrhythmic medications, as appropriate
- Monitor effects of medications
- Monitor peripheral pulses, capillary refill, and temperature and color of extremities
- Elevate the head of the bed, as appropriate
- Elevate foot of bed, as appropriate
- Monitor for peripheral edema; jugular vein distension; S_3 and S_4 heart sounds; dyspnea; gains in weight; and organ distension, especially in the lungs or liver
- Monitor pulmonary capillary and artery wedge pressure and central venous and right-atrial pressure, as appropriate
- Monitor electrolyte levels
- Maintain fluid balance by administering IV fluids or diuretics, as appropriate
- Administer vasodilator and vasoconstrictor medication, as appropriate
- Monitor intake and output, urine output, and patient weight, as appropriate
- Evaluate effects of fluid therapy
- Insert urinary catheter, if appropriate
- Minimize environmental stressors
- Collaborate with physician, as indicated

1st edition 1992: revised 2013

Background Readings:

Albert, N., Trochelman, K., Li, J., & Lin, S. (2010). Signs and symptoms of heart failure: Are you asking the right questions. *American Journal of Critical Care, 19*(5), 443–453.

American Association of Critical Care Nurses. (2006). *Core curriculum for critical care nursing* (6th ed.) [J. G. Alspach, Ed.]. Philadelphia: Saunders.

Blissitt, P. (2006). Hemodynamic monitoring in the care of the critically ill neuroscience patient. *AACN Advanced Critical Care, 17*(3), 327–340.

Whitlock, A., & MacInnes, J. (2010). Acute heart failure: Patient assessment and management. *British Journal of Cardiac Nursing, 5*(11),516–525.

Hemofiltration Therapy   2110

Definition: Cleansing of acutely ill patient's blood via a hemofilter controlled by the patient's hydrostatic pressure

Activities:

- Determine baseline vital signs and weight
- Draw blood sample and review blood chemistries (e.g., BUN; serum creatinine; serum Na, Ca, K, and PO_4 levels) before therapy
- Determine and record patient's hemodynamic function
- Explain procedure to patient and significant others, as appropriate
- Obtain written consent
- Adjust technology to account for patient's multiple system pathologies (e.g., place patient on rotating-airflow bed)
- Use sterile technique to flush and prime the arterial tubing, venous tubing, and hemofilter with heparinized saline, and to connect to other tubing as required
- Remove all air bubbles from hemofiltration system
- Administer heparin loading dose per protocol or physician's order
- Use mask, glove, and apron to prevent contact with blood
- Use sterile technique to initiate venous and arterial access per protocol
- Anchor connections and tubing securely
- Apply restraints, as appropriate
- Monitor ultrafiltration rate, adjusting rate per protocol or physician's order
- Monitor hemofiltration system for leaks at connections, clotting of filter or tubing
- Monitor patient's multiple system parameters per protocol
- Monitor and care for access sites and lines according to protocol
- Monitor for signs and symptoms of infection
- Instruct patient/family about precautions posttreatment

3rd edition 2000

Background Readings:

Gutch, C., Stoner, M., & Corea, A. (1993). *Review of hemodialysis for nurses and dialysis personnel* (5th ed.). St. Louis: Mosby.

Holloway, N. (1988). *Nursing the critically ill adult* (3rd ed.). Menlo Park, CA: Addison-Wesley.

Kinney, M., Packa, D., & Dunbar, S. (1998). *AACN's reference for critical-care nursing* (4th ed.). St. Louis: Mosby.

Smeltzer, S. C., & Bare, B. G. (2004). Management of patients with upper or lower urinary tract dysfunction. In *Brunner & Suddarth's textbook of medical surgical nursing* (Vol. 2) (10th ed., pp. 1271–1308). Philadelphia: Lippincott Williams & Wilkins.

High-Risk Pregnancy Care   6800

Definition: Identification and management of a high-risk pregnancy to promote healthy outcomes for mother and baby

Activities:

- Determine the presence of medical factors that are related to poor pregnancy outcome (e.g., diabetes, hypertension, lupus erythmatosus, herpes, hepatitis, HIV, and epilepsy)
- Review obstetrical history for pregnancy-related risk factors (e.g., prematurity, postmaturity, preeclampsia, multifetal pregnancy, intrauterine growth retardation, abruption, previa, Rh sensitization, premature rupture of membranes, and family history of genetic disorder)
- Recognize demographic and social factors related to poor pregnancy outcome (e.g., maternal age, race, poverty, late or no prenatal care, physical abuse, and substance abuse)
- Determine client knowledge of identified risk factors
- Encourage expression of feelings and fears about lifestyle changes, fetal well-being, financial changes, family functioning, and personal safety
- Provide educational materials that address the risk factor and usual surveillance tests and procedures
- Instruct client in self-care techniques to increase the chance of a healthy outcome (e.g., hydration, diet, activity modifications, importance of regular prenatal check-ups, normalization of blood sugars, and sexual precautions, including abstinence)
- Instruct about alternate methods of sexual gratification and intimacy
- Refer as appropriate for specific programs (e.g., smoking cessation, substance abuse treatment, diabetes education, preterm birth prevention education, abuse shelter, and sexually transmitted disease clinic)
- Instruct client on use of prescribed medication (e.g., insulin, tocolytics, antihypertensives, antibiotics, anticoagulants, and anticonvulsants)
- Instruct client on self-monitoring skills, as appropriate (e.g., vital signs, blood glucose testing, uterine activity monitoring, and continuous subcutaneous medication delivery)
- Write guidelines for signs and symptoms that require immediate medical attention (e.g., bright red vaginal bleeding, change in amniotic fluid, decreased fetal movement, four or more contractions/hour before 37 weeks of gestation, headache, visual disturbances, epigastric pain, and rapid weight gain with facial edema)
- Discuss fetal risks associated with preterm birth at various gestational ages
- Tour the neonatal intensive care unit if preterm birth is anticipated (e.g., multifetal pregnancy)
- Teach fetal movement counts
- Conduct tests to evaluate fetal status and placental function, such as nonstress, oxytocin challenge, biophysical profiles, and ultrasound tests
- Obtain cervical cultures, as appropriate
- Assist with fetal diagnostic procedures (e.g., amniocentesis, chorionic villus sampling, percutaneous umbilical blood sampling, and Doppler blood flow studies)
- Assist with fetal therapy procedures (e.g., fetal transfusions, fetal surgery, selective reduction, and termination procedure)
- Interpret medical explanations for test and procedure results
- Administer $Rh_o(D)$ immune globulin (e.g., RhoGAM or Gamulin Rh), as appropriate, to prevent Rh sensitization after invasive procedures
- Establish plan for clinic follow-up
- Provide anticipatory guidance for likely interventions during birth process (e.g., Electronic Fetal Monitoring: Intrapartum, Labor Suppression, Labor Induction, Medication Administration, Cesarean Section Care)
- Encourage early enrollment in prenatal classes or provide childbirth education materials for patients on bed rest
- Provide anticipatory guidance for common experiences that high-risk mothers have during the postpartum period (e.g., exhaustion, depression, chronic stress, disenchantment with childbearing, loss of income, partner discord, and sexual dysfunction)
- Refer to high-risk mother support group, as needed
- Refer to home care agencies (e.g., specialized perinatal nursing services, perinatal case management, and public health nursing)
- Monitor physical and psychosocial status closely throughout pregnancy
- Report deviations from normal in maternal and/or fetal status immediately to physician or nurse midwife
- Document patient education, lab results, fetal testing results, and client responses

2nd edition 1996

Background Readings:

Association of Women's Health, Obstetric, and Neonatal Nurses. (1993). *Didactic content and clinical skills verification for professional nurse providers of basic, high-risk and critical-care intrapartum nursing.* Washington, DC: Author.

Field, P. A., & Marck, P. (1994). *Uncertain motherhood: Negotiating the risks of the childbearing years.* Thousand Oaks, CA: Sage.

Gilbert, E. S., & Harmon, J. S. (1998). *Manual of high risk pregnancy and delivery* (2nd ed.). St. Louis: Mosby.

Mattson, S, & J. E. Smith (Eds.). (1993). *Core curriculum for maternal-newborn nursing.* Philadelphia: Saunders.

Pillitteri, A. (2007). High-risk pregnancy: A women with a preexisting or newly acquired illness. In *Maternal and child health nursing: Care of the childbearing and childrearing family* (5th ed., pp. 344–397). Philadelphia: Lippincott Williams & Wilkins.

Pillitteri, A. (2007). High-risk pregnancy: A woman who develops a complication of pregnancy. In *Maternal and child health nursing: Care of the childbearing and childrearing family* (5th ed., pp. 398–442). Philadelphia: Lippincott Williams & Wilkins.

Pillitteri, A. (2007). High-risk pregnancy: A women with special needs. In *Maternal and child health nursing: Care of the childbearing and childrearing family* (5th ed., pp. 461–483). Philadelphia: Lippincott Williams & Wilkins.

H

Home Maintenance Assistance 7180

Definition: Helping the patient/family to maintain the home as a clean, safe, and pleasant place to live

Activities:
- Determine patient's home maintenance requirements
- Involve patient/family in deciding home maintenance requirements
- Suggest necessary structural alterations to make home accessible
- Provide information on how to make home environment safe and clean
- Assist family members to develop realistic expectations of themselves in performance of their roles
- Advise the alleviation of all offensive odors
- Suggest services for pest control, as needed
- Facilitate cleaning of dirty laundry
- Suggest services for home repair, as needed
- Discuss cost of needed maintenance and available resources
- Offer solutions to financial difficulties
- Order homemaker services, as appropriate
- Help family use social support network
- Provide information on respite care, as needed
- Coordinate use of community resources

1st edition 1992; revised 2004

Background Readings:
Craven, R. F., & Hirnle, C. J. (2003). Case management. In *Fundamentals of nursing: Human health and function* (4th ed., pp. 379–390). Philadelphia: Lippincott Williams & Wilkins.
Dickerson, A. E. (1993). Age differences in functional performance. *American Journal of Occupational Therapy, 47*(8), 686–692.
Scott, E. (2001). The potential benefits of infection control measures in the home. *American Journal of Infection Control, 29*(4), 247-249.

Hope Inspiration 5310

Definition: Enhancing the belief in one's capacity to initiate and sustain actions

Activities:
- Assist patient/family to identify areas of hope in life
- Inform the patient about whether the current situation is a temporary state
- Demonstrate hope by recognizing the patient's intrinsic worth and viewing the patient's illness as only one facet of the individual
- Expand the patient's repertoire of coping mechanisms
- Teach reality recognition by surveying the situation and making contingency plans
- Assist the patient to devise and revise goals related to the hope object
- Help the patient expand spiritual self
- Avoid masking the truth
- Facilitate the patient's incorporating a personal loss into his/her body image
- Facilitate the patient's/family's reliving and savoring past achievements and experiences
- Emphasize sustaining relationships, such as mentioning the names of loved ones to the unresponsive patient
- Employ guided life review and/or reminiscence, as appropriate
- Involve the patient actively in own care
- Develop a plan of care that involves degree of goal attainment, moving from simple to more complex goals
- Encourage therapeutic relationships with significant others
- Teach family about the positive aspects of hope (e.g., develop meaningful conversational themes that reflect love and need for the patient)
- Provide patient/family opportunity to be involved with support groups
- Create an environment that facilitates patient practicing religion, as appropriate

1st edition 1992; revised 2008

Background Readings:
Brown, P. (1989). The concept of hope: Implications for care of the critically ill. *Critical Care Nurse, 9*(5), 97–105.
Forbes, S. B. (1994). Hope: An essential human need in the elderly. *Journal Gerontological Nursing, 20*(6), 5–10.
Herth, K. (1990). Fostering hope in terminally-ill people. *Journal of Advanced Nursing, 15*(11), 1250–1259.
Miller, J. F. (2000). Inspiring hope. In J. F. Miller (Ed.), *Coping with chronic illness: Overcoming powerlessness* (3rd ed., pp. 523–546). Philadelphia: F. A. Davis.
Pilkington, F. B. (1999). The many facets of hope. In R. R. Parse (Ed.), *Hope: An international human becoming perspective* (pp. 9–44). Sudbury, MA: Jones and Bartlett.
Poncar, P. J. (1994). Inspiring hope in the oncology patient. *Journal of Psychosocial Nursing, 32*(1), 33–38.
Snyder, C. R., Sympson, S. C., Ybasco, F. C., Borders, T. F., Babyak, M. A., & Higgins, R. L. (1996). Development and validation of the State Hope Scale. *Journal of Personality and Social Psychology, 70*(2), 321–335.

Hormone Replacement Therapy 2280

Definition: Facilitation of safe and effective use of hormone replacement therapy

Activities:
- Determine reason for choosing hormone replacement therapy
- Review alternatives to hormone replacement therapy
- Monitor patient for therapeutic effect
- Monitor for adverse effects
- Review information regarding beneficial and adverse effects of the different hormonal components (e.g., estrogen, progesterone, androgen)
- Review information regarding interaction effects of adjunct therapies (e.g., calcium and vitamin D supplementation, exercise, thiazide use)
- Review information regarding the different methods of administration (e.g., oral continuous combined, oral sequential, dermal, vaginal)
- Facilitate the decision to continue/discontinue
- Facilitate changes in hormone replacement therapy with primary care provider, as appropriate
- Recommend patients make short-term annual decisions about continuation
- Adjust medications or medication dose, as appropriate

4th edition 2004

Background Readings:

Blackwood, M., Creasman, W., & Speroff, L. (2001). Postmenopausal hormone therapy: Informed patients, shared decisions. *Women's Health in Primary Care*, (Suppl. 1), 28–34.

Pillitteri, A. (2007). Reproductive and sexual health. In *Maternal and child health nursing: Care of the childbearing and childrearing family* (5th ed., pp. 90–92). Philadelphia: Lippincott Williams & Wilkins.

Smeltzer, S. C., & Bare, B. G. (2004). Assessment and management of female physiologic processes. In *Brunner & Suddarth's textbook of medical surgical nursing* (Vol. 2) (10th ed., pp. 1368–1409). Philadelphia: Lippincott Williams & Wilkins.

Speroff, L., Glass, R., Kase, N. (1999). *Clinical gynecologic endocrinology and infertility* (6th ed., pp. 725–779). Philadelphia: Lippincott Williams & Wilkins.

Wingo, P., McTiernan, A. (2000). The risks and benefits of hormone replacement therapy: Weighing the evidence. In M. Goldman & M. Hatch (Eds.), *Women and health* (pp. 1169–1187). San Diego, CA: Academic Press.

H

Humor 5320

Definition: Facilitating the patient to perceive, appreciate, and express what is funny, amusing, or ludicrous in order to establish relationships, relieve tension, release anger, facilitate learning, or cope with painful feelings

Activities:
- Determine the types of humor appreciated by the patient
- Determine the patient's typical response to humor (e.g., laughter or smiles)
- Determine the time of day that patient is most receptive
- Avoid content areas about which patient is sensitive
- Discuss advantages of laughter with patient
- Select humorous materials that create moderate arousal for the individual
- Make available a selection of humorous games, cartoons, jokes, videos, tapes, books, and so on
- Point out humorous incongruity in a situation
- Encourage visualization with humor (e.g., picture a forbidding authority figure dressed only in underwear)
- Encourage silliness and playfulness
- Remove environmental barriers that prevent or diminish the spontaneous occurrence of humor
- Monitor patient response and discontinue humor strategy if ineffective
- Avoid use with patient who is cognitively impaired
- Demonstrate an appreciative attitude about humor
- Respond positively to humor attempts made by patient

1st edition 1992; revised 2008

Background Readings:

Buxman, K. (1991). Make room for laughter. *American Journal of Nursing*, 91(12), 46–51.

Kolkmeier, L. G. (1988). Play and laughter: Moving toward harmony. In B. M. Dosseyk, L. Keegan, C. E. Guzetta, & L. G. Kolkmeier (Eds.), *Holistic nursing: A handbook for practice* (pp. 289–304). Rockville, MD: Aspen.

Smith, K. (2006). Humor. In M. Snyder & R. Lindquist (Eds.), *Complimentary/alternative therapies in nursing*, (5th ed., pp. 93–106). New York: Springer.

Sullivan, J. L., & Deane, D. M. (1988). Humor and health. *Journal of Gerontological Nursing*, 14(1), 20–24.

H

Hyperglycemia Management 2120

Definition: Preventing and treating above-normal blood glucose levels

Activities:
- Monitor blood glucose levels, as indicated
- Monitor for signs and symptoms of hyperglycemia: polyuria, polydipsia, polyphagia, weakness, lethargy, malaise, blurring of vision, or headache
- Monitor urine ketones, as indicated
- Monitor ABG, electrolyte, and betahydroxybutyrate levels, as available
- Monitor orthostatic blood pressure and pulse, as indicated
- Administer insulin, as prescribed
- Encourage oral fluid intake
- Monitor fluid status (including input and output), as appropriate
- Maintain IV access, as appropriate
- Administer IV fluids, as needed
- Administer potassium, as prescribed
- Consult physician if signs and symptoms of hyperglycemia persist or worsen
- Assist with ambulation if orthostatic hypotension is present
- Provide oral hygiene, if necessary
- Identify possible cause of hyperglycemia
- Anticipate situations in which insulin requirements will increase (e.g., intercurrent illness)
- Restrict exercise when blood glucose levels are greater than 250 mg/dl, especially if urine ketones are present
- Instruct patient and significant others on prevention, recognition, and management of hyperglycemia
- Encourage self-monitoring of blood glucose levels
- Assist patient to interpret blood glucose levels
- Review blood glucose records with patient and/or family
- Instruct on urine ketone testing, as appropriate
- Instruct on indications for, and significance of, urine ketone testing, if appropriate
- Instruct patient to report moderate or large urine ketone levels to the health professional
- Instruct patient and significant others on diabetes management during illness, including use of insulin and/or oral agents, monitoring fluid intake, carbohydrate replacement, and when to seek health professional assistance, as appropriate
- Provide assistance in adjusting regimen to prevent and treat hyperglycemia (e.g., increasing insulin or oral agent), as indicated
- Facilitate adherence to diet and exercise regimen
- Test blood glucose levels of family members

1st edition 1992; revised 2004

Background Readings:

Guthrie, D. W. (Ed.). (1988). *Diabetes education: Core curriculum for health professionals.* Chicago: American Association of Diabetes Educators.

Smeltzer, S. C., & Bare, B. G. (2004). Assessment and management of patients with diabetes mellitus. *Brunner & Suddarth's textbook of medical surgical nursing* (Vol. 2) (10th ed., pp. 1150–1203). Philadelphia: Lippincott Williams & Wilkins.

Thompson, J. M., McFarland, G. K., Hirsch, J. E., & Tucker, S. M. (1998). *Mosby's clinical nursing* (4th ed.). St. Louis: Mosby.

Hyperthermia Treatment 3786

Definition: Management of symptoms and related conditions associated with an increase in body temperature resulting from thermoregulation dysfunction

Activities:
- Ensure patent airway
- Monitor vital signs
- Administer oxygen, as needed
- Discontinue presumed causative medication (e.g., selective serotonin reuptake inhibitors (SSRI), monoamine oxidase inhibitors (MAOI), or tricyclic antidepressant) for patient experiencing neuroleptic malignant syndrome
- Discontinue physical activity
- Remove patient from heat source, moving to cooler environment
- Loosen or remove clothing
- Apply external cooling methods (e.g., cold packs to neck, chest, abdomen, scalp, armpits, and groin and cooling blanket), as appropriate
- Place patient in cooled water as tolerated to avoid shivering
- Wet the body surface and fan the patient
- Avoid alcohol sponge bath
- Provide oral rehydrating solution (e.g., sports drink) or other cold fluid
- Do not offer flood or liquid by mouth for patient with neurological impairment
- Do not administer salt tablets
- Establish IV access
- Administer IV fluids, using cooled solutions, as appropriate
- Apply internal cooling methods (e.g., iced gastric, bladder, peritoneal, or thoracic lavage), as appropriate
- Administer antishivering medication, as needed
- Do not administer aspirin or other antipyretic
- Insert nasogastric tube, as appropriate
- Insert urinary catheter
- Discontinue cooling activities when core body temperature reaches 39°C
- Monitor for abnormalities in mental status (e.g., confusion, bizarre behavior, anxiety, loss of coordination, agitation, seizure, and coma)
- Monitor core body temperature using appropriate device (e.g., rectal or esophageal probe)

- Obtain laboratory values for serum electrolytes, urinalysis, cardiac enzymes, liver enzymes, and complete blood count, monitoring results
- Monitor urine output
- Monitor arterial blood gases
- Monitor for hypoglycemia
- Monitor electrocardiography results
- Monitor for complications (e.g., renal impairment, acid-base imbalance, coagulopathy, pulmonary edema, cerebral edema, and multiple organ dysfunction syndrome)
- Provide or arrange for transportation to hospital for further treatment
- Instruct patient on risk factors for heat-related illness (e.g., high environmental temperature, high humidity, dehydration, physical exertion, obesity, extremes of age, certain drugs, and heart disease)
- Instruct patient on measures to prevent heat-related illness (e.g., prevent sun over exposure; ensure adequate intake of nutritious foods and fluids before, during, and after physical activity; seek settings where air conditioning is available; and wear lightweight, light-colored, and loose-fitting clothing)

- Instruct patient on early signs and symptoms of heat-related illness and when to seek assistance from health care professional

6th edition 2013

Background Readings:
Badjatia, N. (2009). Hyperthermia and fever control in brain injury. *Critical Care Medicine*, 37(7), S250–S257.
Laskowski-Jones, L. (2010). Care of patients with common environmental emergencies. In D. D. Ignatavicius & M. L. Workman (Eds.), *Medical-surgical nursing: Patient-centered collaborative care* (6th ed., 141–168). St. Louis: Saunders.
McDermott, B. P., Casa, D. J., Ganio, M. S., Lopez, R. M., Yeargin, S. W., Armstrong, L. E., et al. (2009). Acute whole-body cooling for exercise-induced hyperthermia: A systematic review. *Journal of Athletic Training*, 44(1), 84–93.
Smeltzer, S. C., Bare, B. G., Hinkle, J. L., & Cheever, K. H. (2008). Emergency nursing. In *Brunner & Suddarth's textbook of medical surgical nursing* (11th ed., pp. 2516–2557). Philadelphia: Lippincott Williams & Wilkins.

H

Hypervolemia Management   4170

Definition: Reduction in extracellular and/or intracellular fluid volume and prevention of complications in a patient who is fluid overloaded

Activities:
- Weigh daily at consistent times (e.g., after voiding, before breakfast) and monitor trends
- Monitor hemodynamic status, including HR, BP, MAP, CVP, PAP, PCWP, CO, and CI, if available
- Monitor respiratory pattern for symptoms of pulmonary edema (e.g., anxiety, air hunger, orthopnea, dyspnea, tachypnea, cough, frothy sputum production, and shortness of breath)
- Monitor for adventitious lung sounds
- Monitor for adventitious heart sounds
- Monitor for jugular venous distention
- Monitor for peripheral edema
- Monitor for laboratory evidence of hemoconcentration (e.g., sodium, BUN, hematocrit, urine specific gravity), if available
- Monitor for laboratory evidence of the potential for increased plasma oncotic pressure (e.g., increased protein and albumin), if available
- Monitor for laboratory evidence of the underlying cause for hypervolemia (e.g., B-type natriuretic peptide for heart failure; BUN, Cr, and GFR for renal failure), if available
- Monitor intake and output
- Administer prescribed medications to reduce preload (e.g., furosemide, spironolactone, morphine, and nitroglycerin)
- Monitor for evidence of reduced preload (e.g., increased urine output; improvement in adventitious lung sounds; decreased BP, MAP, CVP, PCWP, CO, CI)
- Monitor for evidence of excessive medication effect (e.g., dehydration, hypotension, tachycardia, hypokalemia)
- Instruct patient on the use of medications to reduce preload
- Administer intravenous infusions (e.g., fluids, blood products) slowly to prevent a rapid increase in preload

- Restrict free water intake in patients with dilutional hyponatremia
- Avoid the use of hypotonic IV fluids
- Elevate head of bed to improve ventilation, as appropriate
- Facilitate endotracheal intubation and initiation of mechanical ventilation for patients with severe pulmonary edema, as appropriate
- Maintain prescribed mechanical ventilator settings (e.g., FiO_2, mode, volume or pressure settings, PEEP), as appropriate
- Use closed-system suction for patient with pulmonary edema on mechanical ventilation with PEEP, as appropriate
- Prepare patient for dialysis (e.g., assist with dialysis catheter insertion), as appropriate
- Maintain dialysis vascular access device
- Determine patient's weight change before and after each dialysis session
- Monitor patient's hemodynamic response during and after each dialysis session
- Determine volume of infused dialysate and returned effluent after each peritoneal dialysis exchange
- Monitor returned peritoneal effluent for indications of complications (e.g., infection, excessive bleeding, and clots)
- Reposition the patient with dependent edema frequently, as appropriate
- Monitor skin integrity in immobile patients with dependent edema
- Promote skin integrity (e.g., prevent shearing, avoid excessive moisture, and provide adequate nutrition) in immobile patients with dependent edema, as appropriate
- Instruct the patient and family on use of intake and output record, as appropriate

- Instruct patient and family on the planned interventions to treat hypervolemia
- Restrict dietary intake of sodium, as indicated
- Promote a positive body image and self-esteem if concerns are expressed as a result of excessive fluid retention

1st edition; revised 2013

Background Readings:

Heitz, U., Horne, M. M., & Spahn, D. L. (2005). *Pocket guide to fluids, electrolytes, and acid-base balance* (5th ed.). St. Louis: Mosby.

Leeper, B. (2006). Cardiovascular system. In M. Chulay & S. M. Burns (Eds.), *AACN essentials of critical care nursing* (pp. 215-246). New York: McGraw-Hill.

Miller, L. R. (2006). Hemodynamic monitoring. In M. Chulay & S. M. Burns (Eds.). *AACN essentials of critical care nursing* (pp. 65-110). New York: McGraw-Hill.

Salvador, D. R. K., Punzalan, F. E., & Ramos, G. C. (2005). Continuous infusion versus bolus injection of loop diuretics in congestive heart failure. *Cochrane Database of Systematic Reviews, 3*, CD003178.

Schroeder, K. (2012). Acute renal failure. In E. T. Bope & R. D. Kellerman (Eds.), *Conn's current therapy 2012* (pp. 873-877). Philadelphia: Elsevier Saunders.

Stark, J. (2006). The renal system. In American Association of Critical Care Nurses, *Core curriculum for critical care nursing* (6th ed. pp. 525–610) [J. G. Alspach, Ed.]. Philadelphia: Saunders.

Winkel, E., Kao, W. (2012). Heart failure. In E. T. Bope & R. D. Kellerman (Eds.), *Conn's current therapy 2012* (pp. 432-436). Philadelphia: Elsevier Saunders.

H

Hypnosis 5920

Definition: Assisting a patient to achieve a state of attentive, focused concentration with suspension of some peripheral awareness to create changes in sensation, thoughts, or behavior

Activities:

- Obtain history of the problem to be treated by hypnosis
- Determine goals for hypnosis with patient
- Determine patient's receptivity to using hypnosis
- Correct myths and misconceptions of hypnosis
- Ensure the patient has accepted the treatment
- Evaluate the suitability of the patient by assessing their hypnotic suggestibility
- Determine patient's history with trance states, such as daydreaming and "highway hypnosis"
- Confirm the presence of a trusting relationship
- Prepare a quiet comfortable environment
- Take precautions to prevent interruptions
- Instruct patient on purpose for the intervention
- Instruct patient that he/she will induce the trance state and retain control
- Sit comfortably, half-facing the patient, when appropriate
- Discuss with patient hypnotic suggestions to be used before induction
- Select an induction technique (e.g., Chevreul pendulum illusion, relaxation, imaging walking down a staircase, eye closure, arm levitation, simple muscle relaxation, visualization exercises, attention to breathing, repetition of key words/phrases, and others)
- Use patient's language as much as possible
- Give a small number of suggestions in an assertive manner
- Combine suggestions with naturally occurring events
- Convey permissive attitude to aid in trance induction
- Use a rhythmical, soothing, monotone voice during patient induction
- Pace statements with patient's respirations
- Encourage patient to take deep breaths to intensify the state of relaxation and decrease tension
- Assist patient to escape to a pleasant place, using guided imagery
- Assist the patient to identify appropriate deepening techniques (e.g., movement of a hand to the face, imagery escalation technique, fractionation, and others)
- Avoid guessing what the patient is thinking
- Assist patient to use all senses during the process
- Determine whether to use directive or nondirective imagery with the patient, as appropriate
- Facilitate quick induction through a specific cue (verbal or visual) with experience
- Instruct patient that the level of trance is not important to successful hypnosis
- Facilitate patient's coming out of the trance by counting to a prearranged number, as appropriate
- Assist patient to come out of the trance at own pace, as appropriate
- Provide positive feedback to patient after each episode
- Encourage patient to use self-induction independent of the nurse to manage problem under treatment
- Identify situations, such as painful procedures, where patient requires additional staff support for effective induction

1st edition 1992; revised 2008

Background Readings:

Fontaine, K. L. (2005). Hypnotherapy and guided imagery. In K. L. Fountaine (Ed.), *Complementary & alternative therapies for nursing practice.* (2nd ed., pp. 301–338). Upper Saddle River, NJ: Prentice Hall.

Freeman, L. (2004). Hypnosis. In L. Freeman (Ed.), *Mosby's complementary & alternative medicine: A research-based approach* (2nd ed., pp. 237–274). St. Louis: Mosby.

Lynn, S. J., & Kirsch, I. (2006). *Essentials of clinical hypnosis: An evidence-based approach.* Washington, DC: American Psychological Association.

Rankin-Box, D. (2001). Hypnosis. In D. Rankin-Box (Ed.), *The nurse's handbook of complementary therapies* (2nd ed., pp. 208–214). Edinburgh: Bailliere Tindall.

Zahourek R. P. (1985). *Clinical hypnosis and therapeutic suggestion in nursing.* Orlando. FL: Grune & Stratton.

Hypoglycemia Management   2130

Definition: Preventing and treating low blood glucose levels

Activities:

- Identify patient at risk for hypoglycemia
- Determine recognition of hypoglycemia signs and symptoms
- Monitor blood glucose levels, as indicated
- Monitor for signs and symptoms of hypoglycemia, (e.g., shakiness, tremor, sweating, nervousness, anxiety, irritability, impatience, tachycardia, palpitations, chills, clamminess, light-headedness, pallor, hunger, nausea, headache, tiredness, drowsiness, weakness, warmth, dizziness, faintness, blurred vision, nightmares, crying out in sleep, paresthesia, difficulty concentrating, difficulty speaking, incoordination, behavior change, confusion, coma, seizure)
- Provide simple carbohydrate, as indicated
- Provide complex carbohydrate and protein, as indicated
- Administer glucagon, as indicated
- Contact emergency medical services, as necessary
- Administer intravenous glucose, as indicated
- Maintain IV access, as appropriate
- Maintain patent airway, as necessary
- Protect from injury, as necessary
- Review events prior to hypoglycemia to determine probable cause
- Provide feedback regarding appropriateness of self-management of hypoglycemia
- Instruct patient and significant others on signs and symptoms, risk factors, and treatment of hypoglycemia
- Instruct patient to have simple carbohydrate available at all times
- Instruct patient to obtain and carry/wear appropriate emergency identification
- Instruct significant others on the use and administration of glucagon, as appropriate
- Instruct on interaction of diet, insulin/oral agents, and exercise
- Provide assistance in making self-care decisions to prevent hypoglycemia, (e.g., reducing insulin/oral agents and/or increasing food intake for exercise)
- Encourage self-monitoring of blood glucose levels
- Encourage ongoing telephone contact with diabetes care team for consultation regarding adjustments in treatment regimen
- Collaborate with patient and diabetes care team to make changes in insulin regimen, (e.g., multiple daily injections), as indicated
- Modify blood glucose goals to prevent hypoglycemia in the absence of hypoglycemia symptoms
- Inform patient of increased risk of hypoglycemia with intensive therapy and normalization of blood glucose levels
- Instruct patient regarding probable changes in hypoglycemia symptoms with intensive therapy and normalization of blood glucose levels

1st edition 1992; revised 2000

Background Readings:

American Diabetes Association. (1994). *Medical management of insulin-dependent (Type I) diabete*s (2nd ed.) [J. V. Santiago, Ed.]. Alexandria, VA: Author.

American Diabetes Association. (1995). *Intensive diabetes management.* Alexandria, VA: Author.

Ahern, J. & Tamborlane, W. V. (1997). Steps to reduce the risks of severe hypoglycemia. *Diabetes Spectrum, 10*(1), 39–41.

Cryer, P. E., Fisher J. N., & Shamoon, H. (1994). Hypoglycemia. *Diabetes Care, 17*(7), 734–755.

Levandoski, L. A. (1993). Hypoglycemia. In V. Peragallo-Dittko (Ed.), *A core curriculum for diabetes education* (pp. 351–372). Chicago: American Association of Diabetes Educators and AADE Education and Research Foundation.

Smeltzer, S. C., & Bare, B. G. (2004). Assessment and management of patients with diabetes mellitus. In *Brunner & Suddarth's textbook of medical surgical nursing* (Vol. 2) (10th ed., pp. 1150–1203). Philadelphia: Lippincott Williams & Wilkins.

H

Hypothermia Induction Therapy   3790

Definition: Attaining and maintaining core body temperature below 35° C and monitoring for side effects and/or prevention of complications

Activities:

- Monitor vital signs, as appropriate
- Monitor patient's temperature, using a continuous core temperature monitoring device, as appropriate
- Place patient on a cardiac monitor
- Institute active external cooling measures (e.g., ice packs, water cooling blanket, circulating water cooling pads), as appropriate
- Institute active internal cooling measures (e.g., intravascular cooling catheters), as appropriate
- Monitor skin color and temperature
- Monitor for shivering
- Use facial or hand warming or insulative wraps to diminish shivering response, as appropriate
- Give appropriate medication to prevent or control shivering
- Monitor for and treat arrhythmias, as appropriate
- Monitor for electrolyte imbalance
- Monitor for acid-base imbalance
- Monitor intake and output
- Monitor respiratory status

- Monitor coagulation studies, including prothrombin time, activated partial thromboplastin time, and platelet counts, as indicated
- Monitor the patient closely for signs and symptoms of persistent bleeding
- Monitor white blood cell count, as appropriate
- Monitor hemodynamic status (e.g., PCWP, CO, SVR), using invasive hemodynamic monitoring, as appropriate
- Promote adequate fluid and nutritional intake

5th edition 2008

Background Readings:

Holtzclaw, B. J. (2004). Shivering in acutely ill vulnerable populations. *AACN Clinical Issues*, 15(2), 267-279.

McIlvoy, L. H. (2005). The effect of hypothermia and hyperthermia on acute brain injury. *AACN Clinical Issues*, 16(4), 488–500.

Wright, J. E. (2005). Therapeutic hypothermia in traumatic brain injury. *Critical Care Nursing Quarterly*, 28(2), 150–161.

Zeitzer, M. B. (2005). Inducing hypothermia to decrease neurologic deficit: Literature review. *Journal of Advanced Nursing*, 52(2), 189–199.

Hypothermia Treatment   3800

H

Definition: Heat loss prevention, rewarming, and surveillance of a patient whose core body temperature is abnormally low as a result of noninduced circumstances

Activities:

- Monitor patient's temperature, using most appropriate measuring device and route
- Remove patient from cold environment
- Remove patient's cold, wet clothing
- Place patient in supine position, minimizing orthostatic changes
- Minimize stimulation of the patient (i.e., handle gently and avoid excessive movement) to avoid precipitating ventricular fibrillation
- Encourage patient with uncomplicated hypothermia to consume warm, high-carbohydrate liquids without alcohol or caffeine
- Share body heat, using minimal clothing to facilitate heat transfer between victim and rescuer
- Apply passive rewarming (e.g., blanket, head covering, and warm clothing)
- Apply active external rewarming (e.g., heating pad placed on truncal area prior to extremities, hot water bottles, forced air warmer, warmed blanket, radiant light, warmed packs, and convective air heaters)
- Avoid active external rewarming for the severely hypothermic patient
- Apply active internal rewarming or "core rewarming" (e.g., warmed IV fluids, warmed humid oxygen, cardiopulmonary bypass, hemodialysis, continuous arteriovenous rewarming, and warm lavage of body cavities)
- Monitor for complications associated with extracorporeal rewarming (e.g., acute respiratory distress syndrome, acute renal failure, and pneumonia)
- Initiate CPR for patients without spontaneous circulation and being aware that defibrillation attempts may be ineffective until core temperature is above 30 °C

- Administer medications using caution (e.g., be aware of unpredictable metabolism, monitor for increased action or toxicity, and consider withholding IV medications until core temperature is above 30 °C)
- Monitor for symptoms associated with mild hypothermia (e.g., tachypnea, dysarthria, shivering, hypertension, and diuresis), moderate hypothermia (e.g., atrial arrhythmias, hypotension, apathy, coagulopathy, and decreased reflexes), and severe hypothermia (e.g., oliguria, absent neurological reflexes, pulmonary edema, and acid-base abnormalities)
- Monitor for rewarming shock
- Monitor skin color and temperature
- Identify medical, environmental, and other factors that may precipitate hypothermia (e.g., cold water immersion, illness, traumatic injury, shock states, immobilization, weather, extremes of age, medications, alcohol intoxication, malnutrition, hypothyroidism, diabetes, and malnutrition)

1st edition 1992; revised 2013

Background Readings:

Ireland, S., Murdoch, K., Ormrod, P., Saliba, E., Endacott, R., Fitzgerald, M., et al. (2006). Nursing and medical staff knowledge regarding the monitoring and management of accidental or exposure hypothermia in adult major trauma patients. *International Journal of Nursing Practice*, 12(6), 308–318.

Laskowski-Jones, L. (2010). Care of patients with common environmental emergencies. In D. D. Ignatavicius & M. L. Workman (Eds.), *Medical-surgical nursing: Patient-centered collaborative care* (6th ed., pp. 141–168). St. Louis: Saunders.

Smith, S. F., Duell, D. J., & Martin, B. C. (2008). *Clinical nursing skills: Basic to advanced skills* (7th ed.). Upper Saddle River, NJ: Pearson Prentice Hall.

Hypovolemia Management   4180

Definition: Expansion of intravascular fluid volume in a patient who is volume depleted

Activities:

- Weigh daily at consistent times (e.g., after voiding, before breakfast) and monitor trends
- Monitor hemodynamic status, including HR, BP, MAP, CVP, PAP, PCWP, CO, and CI, if available
- Monitor for evidence of dehydration (e.g., poor skin turgor, delayed capillary refill, weak/thready pulse, severe thirst, dry mucous membranes, and decreased urine output)
- Monitor for orthostatic hypotension and dizziness upon standing
- Monitor for sources of fluid loss (e.g., bleeding, vomiting, diarrhea, excessive perspiration, and tachypnea)
- Monitor intake and output
- Monitor vascular access device insertion site for infiltration, phlebitis, and infection, as appropriate
- Monitor for laboratory evidence of blood loss (e.g., hemoglobin, hematocrit, fecal occult blood test), if available
- Monitor for laboratory evidence of hemoconcentration (e.g., sodium, BUN, urine specific gravity), if available
- Monitor for laboratory and clinical evidence of impending acute kidney injury (e.g., increased BUN, increased creatinine, decreased GFR, myoglobinemia, and decreased urine output)
- Encourage oral fluid intake (i.e., distribute fluids over 24 hours and give fluids with meals), unless contraindicated
- Offer a beverage of choice every 1 to 2 hours while awake, unless contraindicated
- Maintain patent IV access
- Calculate fluid needs based on body surface area and size of burn, as appropriate
- Administer prescribed isotonic IV solutions (e.g., normal saline or lactated Ringer's solution) for extracellular rehydration at an appropriate flow rate, as appropriate
- Administer prescribed hypotonic IV solutions (e.g., 5% dextrose in water or 0.45% sodium chloride) for intracellular rehydration at an appropriate flow rate, as appropriate
- Administer prescribed isotonic IV fluid bolus at an appropriate flow rate to maintain hemodynamic integrity
- Administer prescribed colloid suspensions (e.g., Hespan, albumin, or Plasmanate) for replacement of intravascular volume, as appropriate
- Administer prescribed blood products to increase plasma oncotic pressure and replace blood volume, as appropriate
- Monitor for evidence of blood transfusion reaction, as appropriate
- Institute autotransfusion of blood loss, if appropriate
- Monitor for evidence of hypervolemia and pulmonary edema during IV rehydration
- Administer IV fluids at room temperature
- Use an IV pump to maintain a steady intravenous infusion flow rate
- Monitor skin integrity in immobile patients with dry skin
- Promote skin integrity (e.g., prevent shearing, avoid excessive moisture, and provide adequate nutrition) in immobile patients with dry skin, as appropriate
- Assist patient with ambulation in case of postural hypotension
- Instruct the patient to avoid rapid position changes, especially from supine to sitting or standing
- Implement modified Trendelenburg positioning (e.g., legs elevated above heart level with rest of body supine) when hypotensive to optimize cerebral perfusion while minimizing myocardial oxygen demand
- Monitor oral cavity for dry and/or cracked mucous membranes
- Provide oral fluids (or moistened mouth swabs) frequently to maintain oral mucous membrane integrity, unless contraindicated
- Facilitate oral cleaning (e.g., toothbrush with toothpaste, non-alcohol based mouthwash) twice daily
- Position for peripheral perfusion
- Administer prescribed vasodilators with caution (e.g., nitroglycerin, nitroprusside, and calcium channel blockers) when rewarming a postoperative patient, as appropriate
- Administer prescribed atrial natriuretic peptide (ANP) to prevent acute kidney injury, as appropriate
- Instruct the patient and/or family on the use of intake and output record, as appropriate
- Instruct the patient and/or family on measures instituted to treat the hypovolemia

1st edition 1992; revised 2013

Background Readings:

Heitz, U., Horne, M. M., & Spahn, D. L. (2005). *Pocket guide to fluids, electrolytes, and acid-base balance* (5th ed.). St. Louis: Mosby.

Leeper, B. (2006). Cardiovascular system. In M. Chulay & S. M. Burns (Eds.), *AACN essentials of critical care nursing* (pp. 215-246). New York: McGraw-Hill.

Mentes, J. C. (2008). Managing oral hydration. In E. Capezuti, D. Zwicker, M. Mezey, and T. Fulmer (Eds.), *Evidence-based geriatric nursing protocols for best practice* (3rd ed., pp. 391-402). New York: Springer.

Miller, L. R. (2006). Hemodynamic monitoring. In M. Chulay & S. M. Burns (Eds.). *AACN essentials of critical care nursing* (pp. 65-110). New York: McGraw-Hill.

Nigwekar, S. U., Navaneethan, S. D., Parikh, C. R., & Hix, J. K. (2009). Atrial natriuretic peptide for preventing and treating acute kidney injury. *Cochrane Database of Systematic Reviews, 4,* CD006028.

Smeltzer, S. C., & Bare, B. G. (2004). Fluid and electrolytes: Balance and distribution. In *Brunner & Suddarth's textbook of medical surgical nursing* (Vol. 1) (10th ed., pp. 256–259). Philadelphia: Lippincott Williams & Wilkins.

Stark, J. (2006). The renal system. In American Association of Critical Care Nurses, *Core curriculum for critical care nursing* (6th ed., pp. 525–610). [J. G. Alspach, Ed.]. Philadelphia: Saunders.

H

Immunization/Vaccination Management 6530

Definition: Monitoring immunization status, facilitating access to immunizations, and providing immunizations to prevent communicable disease

Activities:
- Teach parent(s) recommended immunizations necessary for children, their route of medication administration, reasons and benefits of use, adverse reactions, and side effects schedule (e.g., hepatitis B, diphtheria, tetanus, pertussis, H. influenza, polio, measles, mumps, rubella, and varicella)
- Inform individuals of immunization protective against illness but not presently required by law (e.g., influenza, pneumococcal, and hepatitis B vaccinations)
- Teach individual/families about vaccinations available in the event of special incidence and/or exposure (e.g., cholera, influenza, plague, rabies, Rocky Mountain spotted fever, smallpox, typhoid fever, typhus, yellow fever, and tuberculosis)
- Provide vaccine information statements prepared by Centers for Disease Control and Prevention
- Provide and update diary for recording date and type of immunizations
- Identify proper administration techniques, including simultaneous administration
- Identify latest recommendations regarding use of immunizations
- Follow the five rights of medication administration
- Note patient's medical history and history of allergies
- Administer injections to infant in the anterolateral thigh, as appropriate
- Document vaccination information, per agency protocol (e.g., manufacturer, lot number, expiration date, etc.)
- Inform families which immunizations are required by law for entering preschool, kindergarten, junior high, high school, and college
- Audit school immunization records for completeness on a yearly basis
- Notify individual/family when immunizations are not up-to-date
- Follow the American Academy of Pediatrics, American Academy of Family Physicians, and U.S. Public Health Service guidelines for immunization administration
- Inform travelers of vaccinations appropriate for travel to foreign countries
- Identify true contraindications for administering immunizations (anaphylactic reaction to previous vaccine and moderate or severe illness with or without fever)
- Recognize that a delay in series administration does not indicate restarting the schedule

- Secure informed consent to administer vaccine
- Help family with financial planning to pay for immunizations (e.g., insurance coverage and health department clinics)
- Identify providers who participate in the federal "Vaccine for Children" program, which provides free vaccines
- Inform parent(s) of comfort measures helpful after medication administration to child
- Observe patient for a specified period of time after medication administration
- Schedule immunizations at appropriate time intervals
- Determine immunization status at every health care visit (including emergency room and hospital admission) and provide immunizations as needed
- Advocate for programs and policies that provide free or affordable immunizations to all populations
- Support national registry to track immunization status

1st edition 1992; revised 2000, 2004

Background Readings:

Centers for Disease Control. (1997). Recommended childhood immunization schedule: United States 1997. *Mortality and Morbidity Weekly Report,* *46*(2), 35–40.

Centers for Disease Control. (2002). Recommended adult immunization schedule: United States 2002-2003. *Mortality and Morbidity Weekly Report,* *51*(40), 904–908.

Kozier, B., Erb, G., Berman, A., & Snyder, S. (2004). Asepsis. In *Fundamentals of nursing: Concepts, processes, and practice.* (7th ed., pp. 628–668). Upper Saddle River, NJ: Prentice Hall.

Lambert, J. (1995). Every child by two: A program of the American Nurses Foundation. *American Nurse, 27*(8), 12

Lerner-Durjava, L. (1998). Needle-free injections. *Nursing, 28*(7), 52–53

Scarbrough, M. L. & Landis, S. E. (1997). A pilot study for the development of a hospital-based immunization program. *Clinical Nurse Specialist,* *11*(2), 70–75.

Scudder, L. (1995). Child immunization initiative: Politics and health policy in action. *Nursing Policy Forum, 1*(3), 20–29.

West, A. R. & Kopp, M. (1999). *Making a difference: Immunizing infants and children.* Washington, DC: American Nurse Foundation.

Impulse Control Training 4370

Definition: Assisting the patient to mediate impulsive behavior through application of problem-solving strategies to social and interpersonal situations

Activities:
- Select a problem-solving strategy that is appropriate to the patient's developmental level and cognitive functioning
- Use a behavior modification plan, as appropriate, to reinforce the problem-solving strategy that is being taught

- Assist patient to identify the problem or situation that requires thoughtful action
- Teach patient to cue himself or herself to "stop and think" before acting impulsively
- Assist patient to identify courses of possible action and their costs/benefits

I

- Assist patient to choose the most beneficial course of action
- Assist patient to evaluate the outcome of the chosen course of action
- Provide positive reinforcement (e.g., praise and rewards) for successful outcomes
- Encourage patient to self-reward for successful outcomes
- Assist patient to evaluate how unsuccessful outcomes could have been avoided by different behavioral choices
- Provide opportunities for patient to practice problem solving (role-playing) within the therapeutic environment
- Provide models who demonstrate the steps of the problem-solving strategy in the context of situations that are meaningful to the patient
- Encourage patient to practice problem solving in social and interpersonal situations outside the therapeutic environment, followed by evaluation of outcome

2nd edition 1996

Background Readings:

Alexander, D. I. (1991). Impulse control, altered. In G. K. McFarland, & M. D. Thomas (Eds.), *Psychiatric mental health nursing: Application of the nursing process* (pp. 282–285). Philadelphia: Lippincott.
Limandri, B. J., & Boyd, M. A. (2005). Personality and impulse control disorders. In M. A. Boyd (Ed.), *Psychiatric nursing: Contemporary practice* (3rd ed., pp. 420–470). Philadelphia: Lippincott Williams & Wilkins.
Kendall, P. C. (1977). On the efficacious use of verbal self-instructional procedures with children. *Cognitive Therapy and Research, 1*(4), 331–334.
Kendall, P. C. & Braswell, L. (1985). *Cognitive-behavioral therapy for impulsive children.* New York: The Guilford Press.
Kendall, P. C., & Finch, A. J. (1979). Developing nonimpulsive behavior in children. Cognitive-behavioral strategies for self control. In P. C. Kendall, & S. D. Hollon (Eds.), *Cognitive behavioral interventions: Theory, research, & procedures* (pp. 37–78). New York: Academic Press.
Meichenbaum, D., & Goodman, J. (1971). Training impulsive children to talk to themselves: A means of developing self-control. *Journal of Abnormal Psychology, 77*(2), 115–126.

Incident Reporting   7980

Definition: Written and verbal reporting of any event in the process of patient care that is inconsistent with desired patient outcomes or routine operations of the health care facility

Activities:
- Identify events (e.g., patient falls, blood transfusion reactions, and equipment malfunction) that require reporting, as defined in agency policy
- Notify physician to evaluate patient, as appropriate
- Notify nursing supervisor, as appropriate
- Document in patient record that physician was notified
- Complete incident report form(s) to include factual information, patient hospital number, medical diagnosis, and date of admission
- Document factual information about the event in the patient record
- Document nursing assessments and interventions after the event
- Identify and report medical device failures leading to patient injury, as appropriate
- Maintain confidentiality of incident report, according to agency policy
- Initiate Medical Device Reporting System for deaths or serious injury resulting from medical devices
- Discuss event with involved staff to determine what, if any, corrective action is necessary

2nd edition 1996

Background Readings:

Benson-Flynn, J. (2001). Incident reporting: Clarifying occurrences, incidents, and sentinel events. *Home Healthcare Nurse, 19*(11), 701–706.
Feutz-Harper, S. (1989). Documentation principles and pitfalls. *Journal of Nursing Administration, 19*(12), 7–9.
Kozier, B., Erb, G., Berman, A., & Snyder, S. (2004). Legal aspects of nursing. In *Fundamentals of nursing: Concepts, processes, and practice.* (7th ed., pp. 46–67). Upper Saddle River, NJ: Prentice Hall.
Peters, G. (1991). Details are not incidental. *Geriatric Nursing, 12*(2), 90–93.

Incision Site Care   3440

Definition: Cleansing, monitoring, and promotion of healing in a wound that is closed with sutures, clips, or staples

Activities:
- Explain the procedure to the patient, using sensory preparation
- Inspect the incision site for redness, swelling, or signs of dehiscence or evisceration
- Note characteristics of any drainage
- Monitor the healing process in the incision site
- Cleanse the area around the incision with an appropriate cleansing solution
- Swab from the clean area toward the less clean area
- Monitor incision for signs and symptoms of infection
- Use sterile, cotton-tipped applicators for efficient cleansing of tight-fitting wire sutures, deep and narrow wounds, or wounds with pockets
- Cleanse the area around any drain site or drainage tube last
- Maintain the position of any drainage tube
- Apply closure strips, as appropriate
- Apply antiseptic ointment, as ordered
- Remove sutures, staples, or clips, as indicated
- Change the dressing at appropriate intervals
- Apply an appropriate dressing to protect the incision

- Facilitate the patient's viewing of the incision
- Instruct the patient on how to care for the incision during bathing or showering
- Teach the patient how to minimize stress on the incision site
- Teach the patient and/or the family how to care for the incision, including signs and symptoms of infection

1st edition 1992; revised 2000

Background Readings:

Kozier, B., Erb, G., Berman, A., & Snyder, S. (2004). Perioperative nursing. In *Fundamentals of nursing: Concepts, processes, and practice.* (7th ed., pp. 896–937). Upper Saddle River, NJ: Prentice Hall.

Perry, A. G., & Potter, P. A. (1998). *Clinical nursing skills and techniques* (4th ed.). St. Louis: Mosby.

Infant Care   6820

Definition: Provision of developmentally-appropriate, family-centered care to the child under 1 year of age

Activities:

- Encourage consistent assignment of professional caregivers
- Monitor infant's height and weight
- Monitor intake and output
- Incorporate parent preferences for bathing, when possible
- Change diapers
- Feed infant foods that are developmentally appropriate
- Provide opportunities for nonnutritive sucking
- Keep side rails of crib up when not caring for infant
- Remove small items from crib (e.g., syringe covers and alcohol wipes)
- Monitor safety of infant's environment
- Provide developmentally-appropriate safe toys and activities for infant
- Provide information to parent about child development and child rearing
- Provide visual, auditory, tactile, and kinetic stimulation during play
- Structure play and care around infant's temperament
- Talk to infant while giving care
- Encourage parent to participate in care activities (e.g., bathing, feeding, medication administration, or dressing changes)
- Instruct parent to perform special care for infant
- Reinforce parent skill in performing special care for infant
- Inform parent about infant's status
- Involve parent in the decision-making process, providing support throughout process
- Explain rationale for treatments and procedures to parent
- Give parent the option of being present for procedure or returning upon its completion
- Apply restraints when indicated and monitor throughout use
- Comfort infant through rocking, holding, cuddling, swaddling
- Monitor infant for signs of pain, including kicking, legs drawn up, steady crying, and difficulty consoling
- Use pain management strategies (e.g., distraction, parent's involvement, positioning, swaddling, or environmental manipulation)
- Explain to parent that regression is normal during times of stress, such as illness or hospitalization
- Encourage family to visit and stay overnight in hospital
- Provide emotional and spiritual support to parent (e.g., be available to listen, assist with maintaining or creating coping strategies or referral)
- Maintain infant's daily routine during hospitalization, when possible
- Provide quiet, uninterrupted environment during nap time and nighttime

1st edition 1992; revised 2013

Background Readings:

Algren, C. L. (2007). Family-centered care of the child during illness and hospitalization. In M. J. Hockenberry & D. Wilson (Eds.), *Wong's nursing care of infants and children* (8th ed., pp. 1046–1082). St. Louis: Mosby.

Hopia, H., Tomlinson, P. S., Paavilainen, E., & Astedt-Kurki, P. (2005). Child in hospital: Family experiences and expectations of how nurses can promote family health. *Journal of Clinical Nursing, 14*(2), 212–222.

Pillitteri, A. (2007). The family with an infant. In *Maternal and child health nursing: Care of the childbearing and childrearing family* (5th ed., pp. 824–859). Philadelphia: Lippincott Williams & Wilkins.

Ward, S. L., & Hisley, S. M. (2009). Caring for the child in the hospital and in the community. In *Maternal-child nursing care: Optimizing outcomes for mothers, children, & families* (pp. 664–700). Philadelphia: F. A. Davis.

Ward, S. L., & Hisley, S. M. (2009). Caring for the family across care settings. In *Maternal-child nursing care: Optimizing outcomes for mothers, children, & families* (pp. 701–714). Philadelphia: F. A. Davis.

Infant Care: Newborn   6824

Definition: Provision of care to the infant during the transition from birth to extrauterine life and subsequent period of stabilization

Activities:

- Clear secretions from oral and nasal passages
- Perform Apgar evaluation at 1 and 5 minutes after birth
- Weigh and measure newborn
- Monitor newborn's temperature
- Maintain adequate body temperature of newborn (i.e., dry infant immediately after birth, wrap newborn in blanket if not to be placed in warmer, apply stockinette cap and instruct parent to keep head covered, and place newborn in isolette or under warmer as needed)
- Monitor respiratory rate and breathing pattern
- Respond to signs of respiratory distress (e.g., tachypnea, nasal flaring, grunting, retractions, rhonchi, and rales)
- Monitor newborn's heart rate
- Monitor newborn's color
- Place newborn skin-to-skin with parent, as appropriate
- Measure head circumference
- Determine gestational age
- Compare newborn's weight with estimated gestational age
- Put newborn to the breast immediately after birth
- Monitor newborn's first feeding
- Monitor newborn's suck reflex during feeding
- Burp newborn with the head elevated
- Monitor newborn's weight
- Monitor intake and output
- Record newborn's first voiding and bowel movement
- Assist parent in giving newborn initial bath after temperature has stabilized
- Regularly hold or touch newborn in isolette
- Provide prophylactic eye care
- Compare maternal and newborn blood groups and types
- Swaddle newborn to promote sleep and provide a sense of security
- Position newborn on back or side after feeding
- Elevate head of mattress of bassinet or isolette to promote respiratory function
- Use blanket roll at newborn's back to position on side, placing dependent arm forward to decrease likelihood of rolling into prone position
- Reinforce or provide information about newborn's nutritional needs
- Determine condition of newborn's cord prior to transfusion using umbilical vein
- Cleanse umbilical cord with prescribed preparation
- Keep umbilical cord dry and exposed to air by diapering newborn below cord
- Monitor umbilical cord for redness and drainage
- Cleanse and apply petroleum jelly dressing to circumcision
- Apply diapers loosely after circumcision
- Apply restraints when indicated and appropriate monitoring throughout use
- Monitor newborn's response to circumcision
- Monitor for hypoglycemia and anomalies if mother has diabetes
- Monitor for signs of hyperbilirubinemia, if appropriate
- Instruct parent to recognize symptoms of hyperbilirubinemia
- Protect newborn from sources of infection in hospital environment
- Determine newborn's readiness state before providing care
- Make eye contact and talk to newborn while giving care
- Provide a quiet, soothing environment
- Respond to newborn's cues for care to facilitate the development of trust
- Promote and facilitate family bonding and attachment with newborn
- Provide information and facilitate the screening of newborn for metabolic disorder(s)
- Instruct parent to recognize signs of breathing difficulty
- Instruct parent to place newborn on back when sleeping

6th edition 2013

Background Readings:

Pillitteri, A. (2007). Nursing care of a newborn and family. In *Maternal and child health nursing: Care of the childbearing and childrearing family* (5th ed., pp. 679–721). Philadelphia: Lippincott Williams & Wilkins.

Ward, S. L., & Hisley, S. M. (2009). Caring for the normal newborn. In *Maternal-child nursing care: Optimizing outcomes for mothers, children, & families* (pp. 563–602). Philadelphia: F. A. Davis.

Wheeler, B., & Wilson, D. (2007). Health promotion of the newborn and family. In M. J. Hockenberry & D. Wilson (Eds.), *Wong's nursing care of infants and children* (8th ed., pp. 257–309). St. Louis: Mosby.

Wong, D. L., Hockenberry, M. J., Wilson, D., Perry, S. E., & Lowdermilk, D. L. (2006). Nursing care of the newborn. In *Maternal child nursing care* (3rd ed., pp. 727–767). St. Louis: Mosby.

Wong, D. L., Hockenberry, M. J., Wilson, D., Perry, S. E., & Lowdermilk, D. L. (2006). Physiologic adaptations of the newborn. In *Maternal child nursing care* (3rd ed., pp. 691–726). St. Louis: Mosby.

I

I

Infant Care: Preterm 6826

Definition: Aligning caretaking practices with the preterm infant's individual developmental and physiological needs to support growth and development

Activities:

- Create a therapeutic and supportive relationship with parent
- Provide space for parent on unit and at infant's bedside
- Provide parent with accurate, factual information regarding the infant's condition, treatment, and needs
- Inform parent about developmental considerations in preterm infants
- Facilitate parent-infant bonding/attachment
- Instruct parent to recognize infant cues and states
- Demonstrate how to elicit infant's visual or auditory attention
- Assist parent in planning care responsive to infant cues and states
- Point out infant's self-regulatory activities (e.g., hand to mouth, sucking, use of visual or auditory stimulus)
- Provide "time out" when infant exhibits signs of stress (e.g., finger splaying, poor color, fluctuation of heart and respiratory rates)
- Instruct parent how to console infant using behavioral quieting techniques (e.g., placing hand on infant, positioning, and swaddling)
- Create individualized development plan and update regularly (e.g., Neonatal Individualized Development Care and Assessment Program [NIDCAP])
- Avoid over-stimulation by stimulating one sense at a time (i.e., avoid talking while handling and looking at while feeding)
- Provide boundaries that maintain flexion of extremities while still allowing room for extension (e.g., nesting, swaddling, bunting, hammock, hat, and clothing)
- Provide supports to maintain positioning and prevent deformities (e.g., back rolls, nesting, bunting, and head donuts)
- Reposition infant frequently
- Provide midline orientation of arms to facilitate hand-to-mouth activities
- Provide water mattress and sheepskin as appropriate
- Use smallest diaper to prevent hip abduction
- Monitor stimuli (e.g., light, noise, handling, and procedures) in infant's environment and reduce when possible
- Decrease environmental ambient light
- Shield eyes of infant when using lights with high foot-candles wattage
- Alter environmental lighting to provide diurnal rhythmicity
- Decrease environmental noise (i.e., turn down and respond quickly to monitor alarms and telephones and move conversation away from bedside)
- Position incubator away from sources of noise (e.g., sinks, doors, telephone, high activity, radio, and traffic pattern)
- Time infant care and feeding around sleep and wake cycle
- Gather and prepare necessary equipment away from bedside
- Cluster care to promote longest possible sleep interval and energy conservation
- Position infant for sleeping in prone upright position on parent's bared chest, if appropriate
- Provide comfortable chair in quiet area for feeding
- Use slow, gentle movements when handling, feeding, and caring for infant
- Position and support throughout feeding maintaining flexion and midline position (e.g., shoulder and truncal support, foot bracing, hand holding, use of bunting, or swaddling)
- Feed in upright position to promote tongue extension and swallowing
- Promote parent participation in feeding
- Support breastfeeding
- Monitor intake and output
- Use a pacifier during gavage feeding and between feedings for nonnutritive sucking to promote physiologic stability and nutritional status
- Facilitate state transition and calming during painful, stressful-but-necessary procedures
- Establish consistent and predictable routines to promote regular sleep and wake cycles
- Provide stimulation using recorded instrumental music, mobiles, massage, rocking, and touch
- Monitor and manage oxygenation needs
- Cover eyes and genitalia with opaque shield for child receiving phototherapy
- Remove eye mask during feedings and regularly to monitor for discharge or corneal irritation
- Monitor hematocrit and administer blood transfusions when necessary
- Inform parent about prevention measures for SIDS (Sudden Infant Death Syndrome)

6th edition 2013

Background Readings:

Becker, P. T., Grunwald, P. C., Moorman, J., & Stuhr, S. (1991). Outcomes of developmentally supportive nursing care for very low birth weight infants. *Nursing Research, 40*(3), 150–155.

Brown, G. (2009). NICU noise and the preterm infant. *Neonatal Network, 28*(3), 165–173.

Johnston, A. M., Bullock, C. E., Graham, J. E., Reilly, M. C., Rocha, C., Hoopes, R. D., et al. (2006). Implementation and case study results of potentially better practices for family-centered care: The family-centered care map. *Pediatrics, 118*(Suppl. 2), S108–S114.

Pinelli, J., & Symington, A. J. (2005). Non-nutritive sucking for promoting physiologic stability and nutrition in preterm infants. *Cochrane Database of Systematic Reviews,* Issue 4. Art. No.: CD001071. DOI: 10.1002/14651858. CD001071.pub2.

Symington, A. J, & Pinelli, J. (2006). Developmental care for promoting development and preventing morbidity in preterm infants. *Cochrane Database of Systematic Reviews,* Issue 2. Art. No.: CD001814. DOI: 10.1002/14651858.CD001814.pub2.

Wallin, L., & Eriksson, M. (2009). Newborn individual developmental care and assessment program (NIDCAP): A systematic review of the literature. *Worldviews on Evidence-Based Nursing, 6*(2), 54–69.

Ward, S. L., & Hisley, S. M. (2009). Caring for the newborn at risk. In *Maternal-child nursing care: Optimizing outcomes for mothers, children, & families.* (pp. 603–637). Philadelphia: F. A. Davis.

Infection Control   6540

Definition: Minimizing the acquisition and transmission of infectious agents

Activities:
- Allocate the appropriate square feet per patient, as indicated by Centers for Disease Control and Prevention (CDC) guidelines
- Clean the environment appropriately after each patient use
- Change patient care equipment, per agency protocol
- Isolate persons exposed to communicable disease
- Place on designated isolation precautions, as appropriate
- Maintain isolation techniques, as appropriate
- Limit the number of visitors, as appropriate
- Teach improved hand washing to health care personnel
- Instruct patient on appropriate hand washing techniques
- Instruct visitors to wash hands on entering and leaving the patient's room
- Use antimicrobial soap for hand washing, as appropriate
- Wash hands before and after each patient care activity
- Institute universal precautions
- Wear gloves as mandated by universal precaution policy
- Wear scrub clothes or gown when handling infectious material
- Wear sterile gloves, as appropriate
- Scrub the patient's skin with an antibacterial agent, as appropriate
- Shave and prep the area, as indicated in preparation for invasive procedures and/or surgery
- Maintain an optimal aseptic environment during bedside insertion of central lines
- Maintain an aseptic environment while changing TPN tubing and bottles
- Maintain a closed system while doing invasive hemodynamic monitoring
- Change peripheral IV and central line sites and dressings according to current CDC guidelines
- Ensure aseptic handling of all IV lines
- Ensure appropriate wound care technique
- Use intermittent catheterization to reduce the incidence of bladder infection
- Teach patient to obtain midstream urine specimens at first sign of return of symptoms, as appropriate
- Encourage deep breathing and coughing, as appropriate
- Promote appropriate nutritional intake
- Encourage fluid intake, as appropriate
- Encourage rest
- Administer antibiotic therapy, as appropriate
- Administer an immunizing agent, as appropriate
- Instruct patient to take antibiotics, as prescribed
- Teach patient and family about signs and symptoms of infection and when to report them to the health care provider
- Teach patient and family members how to avoid infections
- Promote safe food preservation and preparation

1st edition 1992; revised 2000

Background Readings:

Degroot-Kosolcharoen, J., & Jones, J. M. (1989). Permeability of latex and vinyl gloves to water and blood. *American Journal of Infection Control*, *17*(4), 196–201.

Ehrenkranz, J. J., Eckert, D. G., & Phillips, P. M. (1989). Sporadic bacteremia complicating central venous catheter use in a community hospital. *American Journal of Infection Control*, *17*(2), 69–76.

Kozier, B., Erb, G., Berman, A., & Snyder, S. (2004). Asepsis. In *Fundamentals of nursing: Concepts, processes, and practice*. (7th ed., pp. 628–668). Upper Saddle River, NJ: Prentice Hall.

Larsen, E., Mayur, K., & Laughon, B. A. (1989). Influence of two hand washing frequencies on reduction in colonizing flora with three hand washing products used by health care personnel. *American Journal of Infection Control*, *17*(2), 83–88.

Pottinger, J., Burns, S., & Manske, C. (1989). Bacterial carriage by artificial versus natural nails. *American Journal of Infection Control*, *17*(6), 340–344.

Pugliese, G., & Lampinen, T. (1989). Prevention of human immunodeficiency virus infection: Our responsibilities as health care professionals. *American Journal of Infection Control*, *17*(1), 1–22.

Thompson, J. M., McFarland, G. K., Hirsch, J. E., & Tucker, S. M. (1998). Mosby's clinical nursing (4th ed.). St. Louis: Mosby.

Turner, J. & Lovvorn, M. (1992). Communicable diseases and infection control practices in community health nursing. In M. Stanhope & J. Lancaster (Eds.), *Community health nursing* (3rd ed., pp. 312–331). St. Louis: Mosby.

Infection Control: Intraoperative   6545

Definition: Preventing nosocomial infection in the operating room

Activities:
- Damp dust flat surfaces and lights in operating room
- Monitor and maintain room temperature between 20° and 24° C
- Monitor and maintain relative humidity between 20% and 60%
- Monitor and maintain laminar airflow
- Limit and control traffic
- Verify that prophylactic antibiotics have been administered, as appropriate
- Use universal precautions
- Ensure that operating personnel are wearing appropriate attire
- Use designated isolation precautions, as appropriate
- Monitor isolation techniques, as appropriate
- Verify integrity of sterile packaging
- Verify sterilization indicators
- Open sterile supplies and instruments using aseptic technique
- Scrub, gown, and glove, as per agency policy
- Assist with gowning and gloving of team members
- Assist with draping the patient, ensuring protection of eyes, and minimizing pressure to body parts
- Separate sterile from nonsterile supplies
- Monitor sterile field for break-in sterility and correct breaks, as indicated

- Maintain integrity of catheters and intravascular lines
- Inspect skin and tissue around surgical site
- Apply drip towels to prevent pooling of antimicrobial prep solution
- Apply antimicrobial solution to surgical site, as per agency policy
- Remove drip towels
- Obtain cultures, as needed
- Contain contamination when it occurs
- Administer antibiotic therapy, as appropriate
- Maintain a neat and orderly room to limit contamination
- Apply and secure surgical dressings
- Remove drapes and supplies to limit contamination
- Clean and sterilize instruments, as appropriate
- Coordinate cleaning and preparation of the operating room for the next patient

2nd edition 1996; revised 2013

Background Readings:

Association of periOperative Registered Nurses. (2010). *Perioperative standards and recommended practices.* Denver: Author.

Berenguer, C. M., Ochsner, M. G., Jr., Lord, S. A., & Senkowski, C. K. (2010). Improving surgical site infections: Using National Surgical Quality Improvement Program data to institute surgical care improvement project protocols in improving surgical outcomes. *Journal of the American College Surgeons, 210*(5), 737–741.

Facility Guidelines Institute. (2010). *Guidelines for design and construction of health care facilities.* Chicago: Author.

Kozier, B., Erb, G., Berman, A., & Snyder, S. (2004). Asepsis. In *Fundamentals of nursing: Concepts, processes, and practice* (7th ed., pp. 628–668). Upper Saddle River, NJ: Prentice Hall.

Stulberg, J. J., Delaney, C. P., Neuhauser, D. V., Aron, D. C., Fu, P., & Koroukian, S. M. (2010). Adherence to surgical care improvement project measures and the association with postoperative infections. *JAMA: Journal of the American Medical Association, 303*(24), 2479–2485.

Infection Protection 6550

> *Definition:* Prevention and early detection of infection in a patient at risk

Activities:

- Monitor for systemic and localized signs and symptoms of infection
- Monitor vulnerability to infection
- Review histories of international and global travel
- Monitor absolute granulocyte count, WBC, and differential results
- Follow neutropenic precautions, as appropriate
- Limit the number of visitors, as appropriate
- Avoid close contact between pet animals and immunocompromised hosts
- Screen all visitors for communicable disease
- Maintain asepsis for patient at risk
- Maintain isolation techniques, as appropriate
- Provide appropriate skin care to edematous areas
- Inspect skin and mucous membranes for redness, extreme warmth, or drainage
- Inspect condition of any surgical incision or wound
- Obtain cultures, as needed
- Promote sufficient nutritional intake
- Encourage fluid intake, as appropriate
- Encourage rest
- Monitor for change in energy level or malaise
- Encourage increased mobility and exercise, as appropriate
- Encourage deep breathing and coughing, as appropriate
- Administer an immunizing agent, as appropriate
- Instruct patient to take antibiotics as prescribed
- Maintain judicial use of antibiotics
- Do not attempt antibiotic treatment for viral infections
- Teach the patient and patient's family the differences between viral and bacterial infections
- Teach the patient and family about signs and symptoms of infection and when to report them to the health care provider
- Teach patient and family members how to avoid infections
- Eliminate fresh fruits, vegetables, and pepper in the diet of patients with neutropenia
- Remove fresh flowers and plants from patient areas, as appropriate
- Provide private room, as needed
- Ensure water safety by instituting hyperchlorination and hyperheating, as appropriate
- Report suspected infections to infection control personnel
- Report positive cultures to infection control personnel

1st edition 1992, revised 2013

Background Readings:

Cookson, B., Mathai, E., Allegranzi, B., Pessoa-Silva, C. L., Bagheri Nejad, S., Schneider, A., et al. (2009). Comparison of national and subnational guidelines for hand hygiene. *Journal of Hospital Infection, 72*(3), 202–210.

Gammon, J., Morgan-Samuel, H., & Gould, D. (2008). A review of the evidence for suboptimal compliance of healthcare practitioners to standard/universal infection control precautions. *Journal of Clinical Nursing, 17*(2), 157–167.

Gardam, M. A., Lemieux, C., Reason, P., van Dijk, M., & Goel, V. (2009). Healthcare-associated infections as patient safety indicators. *Healthcare-Papers, 9*(3), 8–24.

Gould, I. M. (2009). Controversies in infection: Infection control or antibiotic stewardship to control healthcare-acquired infection? *Journal of Hospital Infection, 73*(4), 386–391.

Kozier, B., Erb, G., Berman, A., & Snyder, S. (2004). Asepsis. In *Fundamentals of nursing: Concepts, processes, and practice.* (7th ed., pp. 628–668). Upper Saddle River, NJ: Prentice Hall.

Loveless, T. J. (2008). Infection protection. *Evidence-based nursing care guidelines medical-surgical interventions* (pp. 472–477). St. Louis: Mosby.

Insurance Authorization   7410

Definition: Assisting the patient and provider to secure payment for health services or equipment from a third party

Activities:

- Explain reasons for obtaining preapproval for health services or equipment
- Explain consent for release of information
- Obtain signature of patient or responsible adult on release of information form
- Obtain information and signature of patient or responsible adult on assignment of benefits form, as needed
- Provide information to third-party payer about the necessity of the health service or equipment
- Obtain or write a prescription for equipment, as appropriate
- Submit prescription for equipment to the third-party payer
- Record evidence of preapproval (e.g., validation number) on the patient's chart, as necessary
- Inform patient or responsible adult of the status of the preapproval request
- Discuss financial responsibilities of client (e.g., out-of-pocket expenses), as appropriate
- Notify appropriate health professional if approval refused by the third-party payer
- Negotiate alternative modalities of care, as appropriate, if approval is refused (e.g., outpatient status or change in care/acuity level)
- Provide preapproval information to other departments, as necessary
- Document care provided, as required
- Assist with the completion of claim forms, as needed
- Facilitate communication with third-party payers, as needed
- Collaborate with other health professionals about continued need for health services, as appropriate
- Document continued need for health services, as required
- Provide necessary information (e.g., name, Social Security number, and provider) to third-party payer for billing, as needed
- Assist client to access needed health services or equipment

2nd edition 1996

Background Readings:

Grossman, J. (1987). The psychiatric, alcohol and drug algorithm: A decision model for the nurse reviewer. *Quality Review Bulletin, 13*(9), 302–308.

Kozier, B., Erb, G., Berman, A., & Snyder, S. (2004). Health care delivery systems. In *Fundamentals of nursing: Concepts, processes, and practice.* (7th ed., pp. 88–105). Upper Saddle River, NJ: Prentice Hall.

LeNoble, E. (1991). Pre-admission possible. *The Canadian Nurse, 14*(2), 18–20.

Pechansky, R., & Macnee, C.L. (1993). Ensuring excellence: Reconceptualizing quality assurance, risk management, and utilization review. *Quality Review Bulletin, 19*(6), 182–189.

Stone, C. L., & Krebs, K. (1990). The use of utilization review nurses to decrease reimbursement denials. *Home Healthcare Nurse, 8*(3), 13–17.

I

Intracranial Pressure (ICP) Monitoring   2590

Definition: Measurement and interpretation of patient data to regulate intracranial pressure

Activities:

- Assist with ICP monitoring device insertion
- Provide information to patient and family/significant others
- Calibrate the transducer
- Level external transducer to consistent anatomical reference point
- Prime flush system, as appropriate
- Set monitor alarms
- Record ICP pressure readings
- Monitor quality and characteristics of ICP waveform
- Monitor cerebral perfusion pressure
- Monitor neurological status
- Monitor patient's ICP and neurological response to care activities and environmental stimuli
- Monitor amount, rate, and characteristics of cerebrospinal fluid (CSF) drainage
- Maintain position of CSF collection chamber, as ordered
- Monitor intake and output
- Prevent device dislodgment
- Maintain sterility of monitoring system
- Monitor pressure tubing for air bubbles, debris, or clotted blood
- Change transducer, flush system, and drainage bag, as indicated
- Change and/or reinforce insertion site dressing, as necessary
- Monitor insertion site for infection or leakage of fluid
- Obtain CSF drainage samples, as appropriate
- Monitor temperature and WBC count
- Check patient for nuchal rigidity
- Administer antibiotics
- Position the patient with head and neck in a neutral position, avoiding extreme hip flexion
- Adjust head of bed to optimize cerebral perfusion
- Monitor effect of environmental stimuli on ICP
- Space nursing care to minimize ICP elevation
- Alter suctioning procedure to minimize increase in ICP with catheter introduction (e.g., give lidocaine and limit number of suction passes)
- Monitor CO_2 levels and maintain within specified parameters
- Maintain systemic arterial pressure within specified range
- Administer pharmacological agents to maintain ICP within specified range
- Notify physician for elevated ICP that does not respond to treatment protocols

1st edition 1992; revised 2008

Background Readings:

American Association of Neuroscience Nurses. (1997). *Clinical guidelines series: Intracranial pressure monitoring.* Glenview, IL: Author.

Arbour, R. (2004). Intracranial hypertension: Monitoring and nursing assessment. *Critical Care Nurse, 24*(5), 19–32.

Barker, E. (2002). Intracranial pressure and monitoring. In E. Barker (Ed.), *Neuroscience nursing: A spectrum of care* (2nd ed., pp. 379–408). St. Louis: Mosby.

Hickey, J. V. (2003). Intracranial hypertension: Theory and management of increased intracranial pressure. In J. V. Hickey (Ed.), *The clinical practice of*

neurological and neurosurgical nursing (5th ed., pp. 285–318). Philadelphia: Lippincott Williams & Wilkins.

Kirkness, C. & March, K. (2004). Intracranial pressure management. In M. K. Bader & L. R. Littlejohns (Eds.), *AANN core curriculum for neuroscience nursing* (pp. 249–267). Philadelphia: Saunders.

Mitchell, P. H. (2001). Decreased behavioral arousal. In C. Stewart-Amidei & J. A. Kunkel (Eds.), *AANN's neuroscience nursing: Human responses to neurologic dysfunction* (2nd ed., pp. 93–118). Philadelphia: Saunders.

Intrapartal Care 6830

Definition: Monitoring and management of stages one and two of the birth process

Activities:

- Determine whether patient is in labor
- Determine whether membranes are ruptured
- Admit to birthing area
- Determine patient's childbirth preparation and goals
- Encourage family participation in the birth process, consistent with patient goals
- Prepare patient for labor per protocol, practitioner request, and patient preference
- Drape patient to ensure privacy during examination
- Perform Leopold maneuver to determine fetal position
- Perform vaginal exams, as appropriate
- Monitor maternal vital signs between contractions, per protocol or as needed
- Auscultate the fetal heart every 30 to 60 minutes in early labor, every 15 to 30 minutes during active labor, and every 5 to 10 minutes in second stage, depending on risk status
- Auscultate fetal heart rate between contractions to establish baseline
- Monitor fetal heart rate during and after contractions to detect decelerations or accelerations
- Apply electronic fetal monitor, per protocol or as appropriate, to obtain additional information
- Report abnormal fetal heart rate changes to primary practitioner
- Palpate contractions to determine frequency, duration, intensity, and resting tone
- Encourage ambulation during early labor
- Monitor pain level during labor
- Explore positions that improve maternal comfort and maintain placental perfusion
- Teach breathing, relaxation, and visualization techniques
- Provide alternative methods of pain relief consistent with patient's goals (e.g., simple massage, effleurage, aromatherapy, hypnosis, and transcutaneous electrical nerve stimulation [TENS])
- Provide ice chips, wet washcloth, or hard candy
- Encourage patient to empty bladder every 2 hours
- Assist labor coach or family in providing comfort and support during labor
- Administer analgesics to promote comfort and relaxation during labor
- Observe effects of medication on mother and fetus
- Advise patients of options for anesthesia that would require referral to another practitioner
- Assist with regional analgesia/anesthesia, as appropriate
- Perform or assist with amniotomy, as appropriate

- Auscultate fetal heart rate before and after amniotomy
- Reevaluate position of fetus and cord after amniotomy
- Document characteristics of fluid, fetal heart rate, and contraction pattern after spontaneous or artificial rupture of membranes
- Cleanse perineum and change absorbent pads regularly
- Monitor progress of labor, including vaginal discharge, cervical dilation, effacement, position, and fetal descent
- Keep patient and labor coach informed of progress
- Explain purpose of required labor interventions
- Obtain informed consent before invasive procedures
- Monitor family coping during labor
- Perform vaginal exam to determine complete cervical dilation, fetal position, and station
- Teach pushing techniques for second stage labor, based on the woman's birth preparation and preference
- Coach during second stage labor
- Monitor pushing progress, fetal descent, fetal heart rate, and maternal vital signs, per protocol
- Encourage spontaneous bearing-down efforts during the second stage
- Evaluate pushing efforts and length of time in second stage
- Recommend pushing changes to enhance fetal descent
- Massage perineum to stretch and relax tissue
- Apply warm compresses, as appropriate
- Assist coach to continue supportive activities
- Prepare delivery supplies
- Document events of labor
- Notify primary practitioner at the appropriate time to scrub for attending delivery

1st edition 1992; revised 1996

Background Readings:

Martin, E. J. (1990). *Intrapartum management modules.* Baltimore: Williams & Wilkins.

May, K. A., & Mahlmeister, L. R. (1994). *Maternal and neonatal nursing: Family-centered care* (3rd ed.). Philadelphia: Lippincott.

Nurses Association of the American College of Obstetricians and Gynecologists. (1990). *Fetal heart rate auscultation: OGN nursing practice resource.* Washington, DC: Author.

Pillitteri, A. (2007). Caring for a woman during vaginal birth. In *Maternal and child health nursing: Care of the childbearing and childrearing family* (5th ed., pp. 487–541). Philadelphia: Lippincott Williams & Wilkins.

Varney, H. (1987). *Nurse-midwifery* (2nd ed.). St. Louis: Mosby.

Intrapartal Care: High-Risk Delivery   **6834**

Definition: Assisting with vaginal delivery of multiple or malpositioned fetuses

Activities:
- Inform patient and support person of extra procedures and personnel to anticipate during birth process
- Communicate changes in maternal or fetal status to primary practitioner, as appropriate
- Prepare appropriate equipment, including electronic fetal monitor, ultrasound, anesthesia machine, neonatal resuscitation supplies, forceps (e.g., Piper), and extra infant warmers
- Notify extra assistants to attend birth (e.g., neonatologist, neonatal intensive care nurses, and anesthesiologist)
- Provide assistance for gowning and gloving obstetrical team
- Continue electronic monitoring
- Coach during second stage pushing
- Alert primary practitioner to abnormalities in maternal vital signs or fetal heart tracing(s)
- Encourage support person to assist with comfort measures
- Use universal precautions
- Perform perineal scrub
- Perform or assist with manual rotation of fetal head from occiput posterior to anterior position, as appropriate
- Record time of delivery of first twin or of breech to the level of the umbilicus
- Assist with amniotomy of additional amniotic membranes, as needed
- Continue to monitor heart rate(s) of second or third fetus
- Perform ultrasound to locate fetal position, as appropriate
- Follow fetal head with hand to promote flexion during breech delivery, as directed by primary practitioner
- Support body as primary practitioner delivers aftercoming head
- Assist with application of forceps or vacuum extractor, as needed
- Assist with administration of maternal anesthesic, as needed (e.g., intubation)
- Record time of birth(s)
- Assist with neonatal resuscitation, as needed
- Document procedures (e.g., anesthesia, forceps, vacuum extraction, suprapubic pressure, McRobert maneuver, and neonatal resuscitation) used to facilitate birth
- Explain newborn characteristics related to high-risk birth (e.g., bruising and forceps marks)
- Observe closely for postpartum hemorrhage
- Assist mother to recover from anesthesic, as appropriate
- Encourage parental interaction with newborn(s) soon after delivery

2nd edition 1996

Background Readings:
Eganhouse, D. J. (1992). Fetal monitoring of twins. *Journal of Obstetric, Gynecologic, and Neonatal Nursing, 21*(1), 16–22.

Gilbert, E. S., & Harmon, J. S. (1993). *Manual of high-risk pregnancy and delivery.* St. Louis: Mosby.

Mattson, S., & Smith, J. E. (Eds.). (1993). *Core curriculum for maternal-newborn nursing.* Philadelphia: Saunders.

Pillitteri, A. (2007). The woman who develops a complication during labor and birth. In *Maternal and child health nursing: Care of the childbearing and childrearing family* (5th ed., pp. 588–618). Philadelphia: Lippincott Williams & Wilkins.

Intravenous (IV) Insertion   **4190**

Definition: Insertion of a cannulated needle into a peripheral vein for the purpose of administering fluids, blood, or medications

Activities:
- Verify order for IV therapy
- Instruct patient about procedure
- Maintain strict aseptic technique
- Identify whether patient is allergic to any medications, iodine, or tape
- Identify whether patient has a clotting problem or is taking any medications that would affect clotting
- Provide emotional support, as appropriate
- Place the patient in a supine position
- Ask parents to hold and comfort a child, as appropriate
- Assure patient comfort in positioning
- Ask patient to hold still while performing venipuncture
- Remove all clothing from the targeted extremity
- Select an appropriate vein for venipuncture, considering the patient's preference, past experience with IVs, and non-dominant hand
- Consider assessment factors when examining veins for cannula insertion (e.g., patient age, purpose of catheter, cannula gauge, cannula material, cannula proximity to joints, condition of extremity, condition of patient, skill of practitioner)
- Start IVs in the opposite arm for patients with arteriovenous fistulas or shunts, or conditions contraindicating cannulation (e.g., lymphedema, mastectomy, lymphectomy, radiation therapy)
- Choose an appropriate type of needle, based on purpose and length of expected use
- Choose an 18-gauge needle, if possible, for blood administration in adults
- Apply heat compresses, if needed, for increased blood flow for vein visualization (e.g., warm dry towels)
- Apply topical analgesia, as indicated, per agency protocol
- Adhere to time requirements for topical analgesia effectiveness (i.e., some topical analgesic medications require 2 hours to take effect)

- Apply a tourniquet 3 to 4 inches above the anticipated puncture site, as appropriate
- Apply enough tourniquet pressure to impede venous circulation but not arterial flow
- Instruct patient to hold the extremity lower than the heart to allow for maximum blood flow to the selected site
- Massage patient's arm from proximal to distal end, as appropriate
- Lightly tap the puncture area after applying the tourniquet, as appropriate
- Request patient to open and close hand several times, as appropriate
- Cleanse area with an appropriate solution, based on agency protocol
- Administer 1% or 2% lidocaine at the insertion site, based on agency protocol
- Insert needle according to manufacturer's instructions, using only needles with sharps injury prevention features
- Determine correct placement by observing for blood in flash chamber or in tubing
- Remove tourniquet as soon as possible
- Tape needle securely in place
- Connect needle to IV tubing or flush and connect to saline lock, as appropriate and per agency protocol
- Apply a small transparent dressing over IV insertion site
- Label IV site dressing with date, gauge, and initials, per agency protocol

- Apply arm board, being careful not to compromise circulation, as appropriate
- Maintain universal precautions

1st edition 1992; revised 2013

Background Readings:

Berman, A., Snyder, S., Kozier, B., & Erb, G. (2008). Fluid, electrolyte, and acid-base balance. In *Kozier & Erb's fundamentals of nursing: Concepts, processes, and practice.* (8th ed., pp. 1423–1483). Upper Saddle River, NJ: Prentice Hall.

Emergency Nurses Association. (2011). *Position statement: Percutaneous sharps/needlestick injuries.* Des Plaines, IL: Author.

Fink, R. M., Hjort, E., Wenger, B., Cook, P. F., Cunningham, M., Orf, A., et al. (2009). The impact of dry versus moist heat on peripheral IV catheter insertion in a hematology-oncology outpatient population. *Oncology Nursing Forum, 36*(4), E198–E204.

Ingram, P., & Lavery, I. (2007). Peripheral intravenous cannulation: Safe insertion and removal technique. *Nursing Standard, 22*(1), 44–48.

Kuensting, L. L., DeBoer, S., Holleran, R., Shultz, B. L., Steinmann, R. A., & Venella, J. (2009). Difficult venous access in children: Taking control. *Journal of Emergency Nursing, 35*(5), 419–424.

Valdovinos, N. C., Reddin, C., Bernard, C., Shafer, B., & Tanabe, P. (2009). The use of topical anesthesia during intravenous catheter insertion in adults: A comparison of pain scores using LMX-4 versus placebo. *Journal of Emergency Nursing, 35*(4), 299–230.

Intravenous (IV) Therapy   4200

Definition: Administration and monitoring of intravenous fluids and medications

Activities:

- Verify order for IV therapy
- Instruct patient about procedure
- Maintain strict aseptic technique
- Examine the solution for type, amount, expiration date, character of the solution, and lack of damage to container
- Perform the five rights prior to starting infusion or administering medications (right drug, dose, patient, route, and frequency)
- Select and prepare an IV infusion pump, as indicated
- Spike container with appropriate tubing
- Administer IV fluids at room temperature, unless otherwise ordered
- Identify whether patient is taking medication that is incompatible with medication ordered
- Administer IV medications, as prescribed, and monitor for results
- Monitor intravenous flow rate and intravenous site during infusion
- Monitor for fluid overload and physical reactions
- Monitor for IV patency before administration of IV medication
- Replace IV cannula, apparatus, and infusate every 48 to 72 hours, according to agency protocol
- Maintain occlusive dressing
- Perform IV site checks according to agency protocol
- Perform IV site care according to agency protocol
- Monitor vital signs

- Monitor amount of intravenous potassium to not exceed 200 mEq per 24 hours, for adults as appropriate
- Flush intravenous lines between administration of incompatible solutions
- Record intake and output as appropriate
- Monitor for signs and symptoms associated with infusion phlebitis and local infection
- Document prescribed therapy, per agency protocol
- Maintain universal precautions

1st edition 1992; revised 2004

Background Readings:

Craven, R. F. & Hirnle, C. J. (2003).Intravenous therapy. In *Fundamentals of nursing: Human health and function* (3rd ed., pp. 575–609). Philadelphia: Lippincott Williams & Wilkins.

Hadaway, L. C. (2000). Managing IV therapy "high-alert" drugs keep nurse managers ever watchful. *Nursing Management, 31*(10), 38–40.

Intravenous Nurses Society. (1998). Revised intravenous nursing standards of practice. *Journal of Intravenous Nursing, 21*(1S), S1–S95.

Kozier, B., Erb, G., Berman, A., & Snyder, S. (2004). Fluid, electrolyte, and acid-base balance. In *Fundamentals of nursing: Concepts, processes, and practice.* (7th ed., pp. 1351–1409). Upper Saddle River, NJ: Prentice Hall.

Perry, A. G. & Potter, P. A. (2002). Clinical nursing skills and techniques (5th ed., 559–616). St. Louis: Mosby.

Invasive Hemodynamic Monitoring 4210

Definition: Measurement and interpretation of invasive hemodynamic parameters to determine cardiovascular function and regulate therapy as appropriate

Activities:
- Assist with insertion and removal of invasive hemodynamic lines
- Assist with Allen test for evaluation of collateral ulnar circulation before radial artery cannulation, if appropriate
- Assist with chest x-ray examination after insertion of pulmonary artery catheter
- Monitor heart rate and rhythm
- Zero and calibrate equipment every 4 to 12 hours, as appropriate, with transducer at the level of the right atrium
- Monitor blood pressure (systolic, diastolic, and mean), central venous/right atrial pressure, pulmonary artery pressure (systolic, diastolic, and mean), and pulmonary capillary/artery wedge pressure
- Monitor hemodynamic waveforms for changes in cardiovascular function
- Compare hemodynamic parameters with other clinical signs and symptoms
- Use closed-system cardiac output setup
- Obtain cardiac output by administering cardiac output injectate within 4 seconds and average three injections that are within less than 1 L of each other
- Monitor pulmonary artery and systemic arterial waveforms; if dampening occurs, check tubing for kinks or air bubbles, check connections, aspirate clot from tip of catheter, gently flush system, or assist with repositioning of catheter
- Document pulmonary artery and systemic arterial waveforms
- Monitor peripheral perfusion distal to catheter insertion site every 4 hours or as appropriate
- Monitor for dyspnea, fatigue, tachypnea, and orthopnea
- Monitor for forward progression of pulmonary catheter resulting in spontaneous wedge, and notify physician if it occurs
- Refrain from inflating balloon more frequently than every 1 to 2 hours, or as appropriate
- Monitor for balloon rupture (e.g., assess for resistance when inflating balloon and allow balloon to passively deflate after obtaining pulmonary capillary/artery wedge pressure)
- Prevent air emboli (e.g., remove air bubbles from tubing; if balloon rupture is suspected, refrain from attempts to reinflate balloon and clamp balloon port)
- Maintain sterility of ports
- Maintain closed-pressure system to ports, as appropriate
- Perform sterile dressing changes and site care, as appropriate
- Inspect insertion site for signs of bleeding or infection
- Change IV solution and tubing every 24 to 72 hours, based on protocol
- Monitor laboratory results to detect possible catheter-induced infection
- Administer fluid and/or volume expanders to maintain hemodynamic parameters within specified range
- Administer pharmacological agents to maintain hemodynamic parameters within specified range
- Instruct patient and family on therapeutic use of hemodynamic monitoring catheters
- Instruct patient on activity restriction while catheters remain in place

1st edition 1992; revised 2000, 2004

Background Readings:

American Association of Critical Care Nurses. (2006). *Core curriculum for critical care nursing* (6th ed.) [J. G. Alspach, Ed.]. Philadelphia: Saunders.

Barcelona, M., Patague, L., Bunoy, M. Gloriani, M., Justice, B., & Robinson, L. (1985). Cardiac output determination by the thermodilution method: Comparison of ice temperature injectate versus room temperature injectate contained in prefilled syringes or closed injectate delivery system. *Heart & Lung, 14*(3), 232–235.

Cullen, L. M. (1992). Interventions related to circulatory care. In G. M. Bulechek & J. C. McCloskey (Eds.), Symposium on nursing interventions. *Nursing Clinics of North America, 27*(2), 445–476.

Daily, E., & Mersch, J. (1987). Thermodilution cardiac output using room and ice temperature injectate: Comparison with the Fick method. *Heart & Lung, 16*(3), 294–300.

Groom, L., Frisch, S., & Elliot, M. (1990). Reproducibility and accuracy of pulmonary artery pressure measurement in supine and lateral positions. *Heart & Lung, 19*(2), 147–151.

Lipp-Ziff, E., & Kawanishi, D. (1991). A technique for improving accuracy of the pulmonary artery diastolic pressure as an estimate of left ventricular end-diastolic pressure. *Heart & Lung, 20*(2), 107–115.

Smeltzer, S. C., & Bare, B. G. (2004). Assessment of cardiovascular function. In *Brunner & Suddarth's textbook of medical surgical nursing* (Vol. 1) (10th ed., pp. 646–681). Philadelphia: Lippincott Williams & Wilkins.

Titler, M. G. (1992). Interventions related to surveillance. In G. M. Bulechek & J. C. McCloskey (Eds.), Symposium on nursing interventions. *Nursing Clinics of North America, 27*(2), 495–516.

I

Journaling 4740

Definition: Promotion of writing as a means to provide opportunities to reflect upon and analyze past events, experiences, thoughts, and feelings

Activities:

- Discuss experiences with similar interventions and receptiveness to intervention
- Establish purpose and goals
- Explain various approaches to journaling and decide on a journaling technique (e.g., free flowing, topical, or intensive journaling)
- Determine a time frame to complete task
- Encourage writing without interruption at least 3 times a week for 20 minutes
- Ensure the environment is optimal for task completion (e.g., client is in a comfortable position, room is well lit, client has glasses)
- Minimize emotional, visual, audio, olfactory, and visceral distractions
- Maintain privacy and assure confidentiality
- Allow the person to select media and method (e.g., pen, pencil, marker, journal, computer, tape recorder, etc.)
- Gather all necessary supplies
- Instruct the person to date journal entries for future reference and reflection
- Encourage writing in the order that things occur without topic restrictions
- Encourage the describing and telling of events in terms of stories, images, and associated thoughts and feelings
- Describe experiences in terms of the five senses, as applicable
- Promote expressing deepest thoughts and feelings
- Instruct to pay no attention to punctuation, spelling, sentence structure, and/or grammar
- Determine ability to continue with intervention independently in the future
- Review journal entries at defined intervals
- Monitor achievement of the established goals

5th edition 2008

Background Readings:

Butcher, H. K. (2004). Written expression and the potential to enhance knowing participation in change. *Visions: The Journal of Rogerian Nursing Science, 12*(1), 37–50.

DeSalvo, L. (2000). *Writing as a way of healing: How telling our stories transforms our lives.* Boston: Beacon Press.

Lepore, S. J., & Smyth, J. M. (2002*). The writing cure: How expressive writing promotes health and emotional well-being.* Washington, DC: American Psychological Association.

Pennebaker, J. W. (1997). *Opening up: The healing power of expressing emotions.* New York: Guilford.

Pennebaker, J. W. (1997). Writing about emotional experiences as a therapeutic process. *Psychological Science, 8*(3), 162–166.

Rew. L. (2005). Self-reflection: Consulting the truth within. In B. M. Dossey, L. Keegan, & C. E. Guzzetta (Eds.), *Holistic nursing: A handbook for practice* (4th ed., pp. 429–447). Sudbury, MA: Jones and Bartlett.

Stone, M. (1998). Journaling with clients. *The Journal of Individual Psychology, 54*(4), 535–545.

Synder, M. (2006). Journaling. In M. Snyder and R. Lindquist (Eds.), *Complementary/alternative therapies in nursing* (5th ed., pp. 165–173). New York: Springer.

J

Kangaroo Care 6840

Definition: Facilitation of skin-to-skin contact between parent or other caregiver and physiologically-stable preterm infant

Activities:

- Explain advantages and implications of providing skin-to-skin contact with infant
- Monitor parent factors influencing involvement in care (e.g., willingness, health, availability, and presence of support system)
- Ensure that infant's physiological status meets guidelines for participation in care
- Prepare a quiet, private, and warm environment
- Provide parent with a reclining or rocking chair
- Instruct parent to wear comfortable, open-front clothing
- Instruct parent how to transfer infant from incubator, warmer bed, or bassinet while managing equipment and tubing
- Position diaper-clad infant in prone, upright position on parent's bare chest
- Turn infant head to one side in a slightly extended position to facilitate eye contact with parent and keep airway open
- Avoid forward flexion and hyperextension of infant head
- Infant's hips and arms should be flexed
- Secure infant and parent position (i.e., tie binding cloth around infant-parent dyad, wrap parent's clothing around infant, and place blanket over dyad)
- Instruct parent how to move infant in and out of binding cloth
- Encourage parent to focus on infant, rather than high techno-logical setting and equipment
- Encourage parent to gently stroke infant in prone upright position
- Encourage parent to gently rock infant in prone upright position
- Encourage auditory stimulation of infant
- Support parent in nurturing and providing hands-on care for infant
- Instruct parent to hold infant with full, encompassing hands
- Encourage parent to identify infant's behavioral cues
- Point out infant physiological state changes to parent
- Encourage parent to sit, stand, walk, and engage in other activities of interest while providing skin-to-skin contact
- Encourage postpartum mothers to ambulate every 90 minutes while providing skin-to-skin contact, to prevent thrombolytic disease
- Instruct parent to decrease activity when infant shows signs of overstimulation, distress, or avoidance
- Encourage parent to let the infant sleep during care
- Encourage breastfeeding during care, as appropriate
- Encourage parent to provide care at least 60 minutes, if possible, to avoid frequent and potentially-stressful changes
- Instruct parent to gradually increase time of each skin-to-skin contact, with length eventually becoming as continuous as possible
- Monitor parent's emotional reaction to and concerns regarding kangaroo care
- Monitor infant's physiological status (e.g., color, temperature, heart rate, and apnea)
- Instruct parent how to monitor infant's physiological status
- Support parent to continue skin-to-skin contact at home
- Discontinue care if infant becomes physiologically compromised or agitated

2nd edition 1996; revised 2013

Background Readings:

Askin, D. F., & Wilson, D. (2007). The high risk newborn and family. In M. J. Hockenberry & D. Wilson (Eds.), *Wong's nursing care of infants and children* (8th ed., pp. 344–421). St. Louis: Mosby.

Breitbach, K. M. (2001). Kangaroo care. In M. Craft-Rosenberg & J. Denehy (Eds.), *Nursing interventions for infants, children, and families* (pp. 151–162). Thousand Oaks, CA: Sage.

Johnston, C. C., Filion, F., Campbell-Yeo, M., Goulet, C., Bell, L. McNaughton, K., et al. (2008). Kangaroo mother care diminishes pain from heel lance in very preterm neonates: A crossover trial. *BMC Pediatrics, 8*(13). 10.1186/1472-2431.

Renfrew, M. J., Craig, D., Dyson, L., McCormick, F., Rice, S., King, S.E., et al. (2009). Breastfeeding promotion for infants in neonatal units: A systematic review and economic analysis. *Health Technology Assessment, 13*(40), 1–146.

Smith, K. M. (2007). Sleep and kangaroo care: Clinical practice in the newborn intensive care unit where the baby sleeps. *Journal of Perinatology and Neonatal Nursing, 21*(2), 151–157.

Suman, R. P., Udani, R., & Nanavati, R. (2008). Kangaroo mother care for low birth weight infants: A randomized controlled trial. *Indian Pediatrics, 45*(1), 17–23.

World Health Organization Department of Reproductive Health and Research. (2003). *Kangaroo mother care: A practical guide.* Geneva, Switzerland: Author.

K

Labor Induction 6850

Definition: Initiation or augmentation of labor by mechanical or pharmacological methods

Activities:

- Determine medical and/or obstetrical indication for induction
- Review obstetrical history for pertinent information that may influence induction, such as gestational age and length of prior labor and contraindications such as complete placenta previa, classical uterine incision, and pelvic structural deformities
- Monitor maternal and fetal vital signs before induction
- Perform or assist with application of mechanical or pharmaco-logical agents (e.g., laminaria and prostaglandin gel) at the appropriate intervals, as needed, to enhance cervical readiness
- Monitor for side effects of procedures used to ready cervix
- Reevaluate cervical status and verify presentation before initiating further induction measures
- Perform or assist with amniotomy, if cervical dilatation is adequate and vertex is well engaged
- Determine fetal heart rate by auscultation or electronic fetal monitoring postamniotomy and per protocol
- Encourage ambulation if no contraindications are present for both mother and fetus
- Observe for onset or change in uterine activity
- Initiate IV medication (e.g., oxytocin) to stimulate uterine activity, as needed, after physician consultation
- Monitor labor progress closely, being alert to signs of abnormal labor progress
- Avoid uterine hyperstimulation by infusing oxytocin to achieve adequate contraction frequency, duration, and relaxation
- Observe for signs of uteroplacental insufficiency (e.g., late decelerations) during the process of induction
- Reduce or increase uterine stimulant (e.g., oxytocin), as needed or per protocol, until birth is imminent

2nd edition 1996

Background Readings:

Day, M. L., & Snell, B. J. (1993). Use of prostaglandins for induction of labor. *Journal of Nurse-Midwifery, 38*(2), 42S–48S.

Gilbert, E. S., & Harmon, J. S. (1998). *Manual of high risk pregnancy & delivery* (2nd ed.). St. Louis: Mosby.

Nurses Association of the American College of Obstetricians and Gynecologists. (1988). OGN nursing practice resource. *The nurse's role in the induction/augmentation of labor.* Washington, DC: Author.

Nurses Association of the American College of Obstetricians and Gynecologists. (2004). *Core curriculum for maternal-newborn nursing* (3rd ed.) [S. Mattson, & J. E. Smith, Eds.]. Philadelphia: Saunders.

Pillitteri, A. (2007). The woman who develops a complication during labor and birth. In *Maternal and child health nursing: Care of the childbearing and childrearing family* (5th ed., pp. 588–618). Philadelphia: Lippincott Williams & Wilkins.

Pozaic, S. (1992). Induction and augmentation of labor. In L. K. Mandeville & N. H. Troiano (Eds.), *High-risk intrapartum nursing* (pp. 101–144, 287–288). Philadelphia: Lippincott.

Labor Suppression 6860

Definition: Controlling uterine contractions prior to 37 weeks of gestation to prevent preterm birth

Activities:

- Review history for risk factors commonly related to preterm labor (e.g., multifetal pregnancy, uterine anomalies, prior history of preterm birth, early cervical change, and uterine irritability)
- Determine fetal age, based on last menstrual period, early sonogram, fundal height measurements, date of quickening, and date of audible fetal heart tones
- Interview about onset and duration of preterm labor symptoms
- Ask about activities preceding onset of preterm labor symptoms
- Determine status of amniotic membranes
- Perform cervical exam for dilation, effacement, softening, and position
- Palpate fetal position, station, and presentation
- Obtain urine and cervical cultures
- Document uterine activity, using palpation, as well as electronic fetal monitoring
- Obtain baseline maternal weight
- Position mother laterally to optimize placental perfusion
- Discuss bed rest and activity limits during acute phase of labor suppression
- Initiate oral or intravenous hydration
- Note contraindications to use of tocolytics (e.g., chorioamnionitis, preeclampsia, hemorrhage, fetal demise, or severe intrauterine growth retardation)
- Initiate subcutaneous or IV tocolytics, per physician order or protocol, if hydration does not reduce uterine activity
- Monitor maternal vital signs, fetal heart rate, and uterine activity every 15 minutes during initiation of IV tocolysis
- Monitor for side effects of tocolytic therapy, including loss of deep tendon reflexes, if magnesium sulfate is administered
- Educate the patient and family about normal tocolytic side effects (e.g., tremors, headache, palpitations, anxiety, nausea, vomiting, flushing, and warmth)
- Provide interventions to reduce discomforts of normal side effects (e.g., relaxation therapy, anxiety reduction, and therapeutic touch)
- Educate patient and family about abnormal tocolytic side effects (e.g., chest pain, shortness of breath, tachycardia, or recurrent contractions) to report to physician
- Obtain baseline EKG, as appropriate
- Monitor intake and output
- Auscultate lungs
- Begin oral or subcutaneous tocolysis, per physician order, after achieving adequate uterine quiescence

- Determine patient and family knowledge of fetal development and preterm birth, as well as motivation to prolong pregnancy
- Involve patient and family in plan for home care
- Begin discharge teaching for home care, including medication regimens, activity restrictions, diet and hydration, sexual abstinence, and ways to avoid constipation
- Teach contraction palpation techniques
- Provide written patient education material for family
- Provide referrals to assist family with child care, home maintenance, and diversional activities, as appropriate
- Discuss signs of recurrent preterm labor and reinforce the need to reseek care immediately, if symptoms return and continue for 1 hour
- Provide written discharge instructions, including explicit directions for reseeking medical care

2nd edition 1996

Background Readings:

Eganhouse, D. J. (1994). Development of a nursing program for preterm birth prevention. *Journal of Obstetric, Gynecologic, and Neonatal Nursing,* 23(9), 756–766.

Gilbert, E. S., & Harmon, J. S. (1998). *Manual of high-risk pregnancy & delivery* (2nd ed.). St. Louis: Mosby.

Nance, N. (1990). Module 8: Caring for the woman at risk for preterm labor or with premature rupture of membranes. In E. J. Martin (Ed.), *Intrapartum management modules* (pp. 259–284). Baltimore: Williams & Wilkins.

Pillitteri, A. (2007). High-risk pregnancy: A woman who develops a complication of pregnancy. In *Maternal and child health nursing: Care of the childbearing and childrearing family* (5th ed., pp. 398–442). Philadelphia: Lippincott Williams & Wilkins.

Wheeler, D. G. (1994). Preterm birth prevention. *Journal of Nurse-Midwifery,* 39(2), 665–805.

Laboratory Data Interpretation   7690

Definition: Critical analysis of patient laboratory data in order to assist with clinical decision-making

Activities:
- Be familiar with accepted abbreviations for particular institution
- Use the reference ranges from the laboratory that is performing the particular test(s)
- Recognize physiological factors that can affect laboratory values, including gender, age, pregnancy, diet (especially hydration), time of day, activity level, and stress
- Recognize the effect of drugs on laboratory values, including prescription drugs, as well as over-the-counter medications
- Note time and site of specimen collection, as applicable
- Use peak drug levels when testing for toxicity
- Recognize that trough drug levels are useful for demonstrating satisfactory therapeutic level
- Consider influences of pharmacokinetics (e.g., half-life, peak, protein binding, and excretion) when evaluating toxic and therapeutic levels of drugs
- Consider that multiple test abnormalities are more likely to be significant than single test abnormalities
- Compare test results with other related laboratory and/or diagnostic tests
- Compare results with previous values obtained when the patient was not ill (if available) to determine baseline values
- Monitor sequential test results for trends or gross changes
- Consult appropriate references/texts for clinical implication of unfamiliar tests
- Recognize that incorrect test results most often result from clerical errors
- Perform confirmation of grossly abnormal test results with close attention to patient and specimen identification, condition of specimen, and prompt delivery to the laboratory
- Report results of lab tests to patient, as appropriate
- Send split samples to the laboratory for verification of results, if appropriate
- Report sudden changes in laboratory values to physician immediately
- Report critical values (as determined by institution) to physician immediately
- Analyze whether results obtained are consistent with patient behavior and clinical status

2nd edition 1996

Background Readings:

Call-Schmidt, T. (2001). Interpreting lab results: A primer. *MEDSURG Nursing,* 10(4), 179–184.

Corbett, J. V. (2000). *Laboratory tests and diagnostic procedures with nursing diagnoses* (5th ed.). Upper Saddle River, NJ: Prentice Hall.

Kee, J. F. (2001). *Handbook of laboratory and diagnostic tests with nursing implications* (4th ed.). Upper Saddle River, NJ: Prentice Hall.

Pagana, K. D. & Pagana, T. J. (2001). *Mosby's diagnostic and laboratory test reference* (5th ed.). St. Louis: Mosby.

Perry, A. C., & Potter, P. A. (2002). *Clinical nursing skills & techniques* (5th ed., pp. 1148–1149). St. Louis: Mosby.

Titler, M. G. (1992). Interventions related to surveillance. In G. M. Bulechek & J. C. McCloskey (Eds.), Symposium on nursing interventions. *Nursing Clinics of North America,* 27(2), 495–516.

Lactation Counseling   5244

Definition: Assisting in the establishment and maintenance of successful breastfeeding

Activities:

- Provide information about psychological and physiological benefits of breastfeeding
- Determine mother's desire and motivation to breastfeed as well as perception of breast-feeding
- Correct misconceptions, misinformation, and inaccuracies about breastfeeding
- Encourage mother's significant other, family, or friends to provide support (i.e., offer praise, encouragement, and reassurance, perform household tasks, and ensure that mother is receiving adequate rest and nutrition)
- Provide educational material, as needed
- Encourage attendance to breastfeeding classes and support groups
- Provide mother the opportunity to breastfeed after birth, when possible
- Instruct on infant's feeding cues (e.g., rooting, sucking, and quiet alertness)
- Assist in ensuring proper infant attachment to breast (i.e., monitor proper infant alignment, areolar grasp and compression, and audible swallowing)
- Instruct on various feeding positions (e.g., cross-cradle, football hold, and side-lying)
- Instruct mother on signs of milk transfer (e.g., milk leakage, audible swallowing, and "let down" sensations)
- Discuss ways to facilitate milk transfer (e.g., relaxation techniques, breast massage, and a quiet environment)
- Inform about the difference between nutritive and nonnutritive sucking
- Monitor infant's ability to suck
- Demonstrate suck training, if necessary (i.e., use a clean finger to stimulate suck reflex and latch on)
- Instruct mother to allow infant to finish first breast before offering second breast
- Instruct on how to break suction of nursing infant, if necessary
- Instruct mother on nipple care
- Monitor for nipple pain and impaired skin integrity of nipples
- Discuss techniques to avoid or minimize engorgement and associated discomfort (e.g., frequent feedings, breast massage, warm compresses, milk expression, ice packs applied after feeding or pumping, and antiinflammatory medications)
- Instruct on signs, symptoms, and management strategies for plugged ducts, mastitis, and candidiasis infection
- Discuss needs for adequate rest, hydration, and well-balanced diet
- Assist in determining need for supplemental feedings, pacifiers, and nipple shields
- Encourage mother to wear a well-fitting, supportive bra
- Instruct on record keeping of nursing and pumping sessions, if indicated
- Instruct about infant stool and urination patterns
- Discuss frequency of normal feeding patterns, including cluster feedings and growth spurts
- Encourage continued lactation upon return to work or school
- Discuss options for milk expression, including nonelectrical pumping (e.g., hand and manual) and electrical pumping (e.g., single and double; hospital-grade pump for mother of preterm infant)
- Instruct on appropriate handling of expressed milk (e.g., collection, storage, thawing, preparation, fortification, and warming)
- Instruct patient to contact lactation consultant to assist in determining status of milk supply (i.e., whether insufficiency is perceived or actual)
- Discuss strategies aimed at optimizing milk supply (e.g., breast massage, frequent milk expression, complete emptying of breasts, kangaroo care, and medications)
- Provide instruction and support in accordance with healthcare institution's policy on lactation for the mother of preterm infant (i.e., instruct on frequency of pumping, when to expect milk supply to increase, normal feeding patterns based on gestational age, and weaning from pump when infant is able to nurse well)
- Instruct on signs and symptoms warranting reporting to a healthcare practitioner or lactation consultant
- Provide discharge instructions and arrange for follow-up care tailored to patient's specific needs (e.g., mother of healthy term infant, multiples, preterm infant, or ill infant)
- Refer to a lactation consultant
- Assist with relactation, if needed
- Discuss options for weaning
- Instruct mother to consult her healthcare practitioner before taking any medications while breastfeeding, including over-the-counter medications and oral contraceptives
- Discuss methods of contraception
- Encourage employers to provide opportunities for lactating mothers to express and store breast milk during the workday

2nd edition 1996; revised 2013

Background Readings:

Dyson, L., McCormick, F. M., & Renfrew, M. J. (2005). Interventions for promoting the initiation of breastfeeding. *Cochrane Database of Systematic Reviews*, Issue 2. Art. No.: CD001688. doi: 10.1002/14651858. CD001688.pub2.

Hill, P. D. (2001). Lactation counseling. In M. Craft-Rosenberg & J. Denehy (Eds.), *Nursing interventions for infants, children, and families* (pp. 61–76). Thousand Oaks, CA: Sage.

Kramer, M. S., & Kakuma, R. (2002). The optimal duration of exclusive breastfeeding: A systematic review. Geneva, Switzerland: World Health Organization.

Lang, S. (2002). *Breastfeeding special care babies.* (2nd ed.). New York: Bailliere Tindall.

Riordan, J. (2005). *Breastfeeding and human lactation* (3rd ed.). Sudbury, MA: Jones and Bartlett.

Ward, S. L., & Hisley, S. M. (2009). Caring for the postpartal woman and her family. In *Maternal-child nursing care: Optimizing outcomes for mothers, children, & families.* (pp. 469–509). Philadelphia: F. A. Davis.

Walker, M. (2006). *Breastfeeding management for the clinician: Using the evidence.* Sudbury, MA: Jones and Bartlett.

Lactation Suppression 6870

Definition: Facilitating the cessation of milk production while minimizing painful engorgement

Activities:
- Discuss options for milk expression (e.g., hand, manual, and electrical pumping)
- Instruct patient to express enough milk via hand, manual, or electrical pumping to reduce breast pressure but not enough to empty breast
- Assist patient in securing a good quality breast pump for use
- Assist patient in determining schedule (e.g., frequency and duration) for milk expression based on individual factors (e.g., length of time since giving birth, frequency of emptying breasts, and amount of milk currently being produced)
- Monitor breast engorgement and associated discomfort or pain
- Instruct patient on measures to reduce discomfort or pain (i.e., ice packs or cold cabbage leaves applied to breasts and analgesics)
- Administer lactation suppression drug, if appropriate
- Encourage patient to wear supportive, well-fitting bra continuously until lactation is suppressed
- Provide anticipatory guidance on physiological changes (i.e., uterine cramping and presence of scant milk post-lactation suppression)
- Discuss feelings, concerns, or issues patient may have pertaining to lactation cessation

1st edition 1992; revised 2013

Background Readings:

Moore, D. B., & Catlin, A. (2003). Pediatric ethics, issues, & commentary. Lactation suppression: Forgotten aspect of care for the mother of a dying child. *Pediatric Nursing, 29*(5), 383–384.

Oladapo, O. T., & Fawole, B. (2009). Treatments for suppression of lactation. *Cochrane Database of Systematic Reviews*, Issue 1. Art. No.: CD005937. doi:10.1002/14651858.CD005937.pub2.

Pillitteri, A. (2007). Nutritional needs of a newborn. In *Maternal and child health nursing: Care of the childbearing and childrearing family* (5th ed., pp. 722–746). Philadelphia: Lippincott Williams & Wilkins.

Riordan, J. (2005). *Breastfeeding and human lactation* (3rd ed.). Sudbury, MA: Jones and Bartlett.

Walker, M. (2006). *Breastfeeding management for the clinician: Using the evidence.* Sudbury, MA: Jones & Bartlett.

L

Laser Precautions 6560

Definition: Limiting the risk of laser-related injury to the patient

Activities:
- Provide appropriate laser, fiber(s), filters, lenses, and attachments
- Provide appropriate eye protection
- Verify that instruments and supplies are laser-safe
- Verify that ointments and solutions are nonflammable
- Provide a rectal pack, as appropriate
- Cover windows, as appropriate
- Set up and connect plume evacuator, as appropriate
- Provide high-filtration masks, as appropriate
- Place laser use sign on entrances to room
- Check fire-extinguishing supplies/equipment
- Set up laser, as per protocol
- Inspect electrical cords
- Inspect laser fibers for breaks
- Activate area entryway control system, as appropriate
- Test fire laser
- Instruct patient about importance of not moving during laser use, as appropriate
- Instruct patient about importance of eye wear, as appropriate
- Immobilize patient's body part, as appropriate
- Protect tissue around laser site with moistened towels or sponges
- Remove other pedals from the area
- Adjust laser settings, as per physician or agency protocol
- Monitor patient for potential injury
- Monitor environment for possible fire
- Monitor environment for flammable substance or breaks in precautions
- Return laser key to designated secure location
- Sterilize laser lenses, as appropriate
- Record information, as per protocol

2nd edition 1996

Background Readings:

Association of Operating Room Nurses. (1993). *Standards and recommended practices.* Denver, CO: Author.

Ball, K. (1995). *Lasers: The perioperative challenge* (2nd ed.). St. Louis: Mosby.

Fairchild, S. (1993). *Perioperative nursing: Principles and practice* (3rd ed.). Sudbury, MA: Jones and Bartlett.

Kneedler, J., & Dodge, G. (1994). *Perioperative patient care: The nursing perspective.* Sudbury, MA: Jones and Bartlett.

Smeltzer, S. C., & Bare, B. G. (2004). Intraoperative nursing management. In *Brunner & Suddarth's textbook of medical surgical nursing* (Vol. 1) (10th ed., pp. 417–435). Philadelphia: Lippincott Williams & Wilkins.

Latex Precautions

6570

Definition: Reducing the risk of a systemic reaction to latex

Activities:
- Question patient or appropriate other about history of neural tube defect (e.g., spina bifida) or congenital urological condition (e.g., exstrophy of the bladder)
- Question patient or appropriate other about history of systemic reactions to natural rubber latex (e.g., facial or scleral edema, tearing eyes, urticaria, rhinitis, and wheezing)
- Question patient or appropriate other about allergies to foods such as bananas, kiwi, avocado, mango, and chestnuts
- Refer patient to allergist for allergy testing, as appropriate
- Record allergy or risk in patient's medical record
- Place allergy band on patient
- Post sign indicating latex precautions
- Survey environment and remove latex products
- Monitor latex-free environment
- Monitor patient for signs and symptoms of a systemic reaction
- Report information to physician, pharmacist, and other care providers, as indicated
- Administer medications, as appropriate
- Instruct patient and family about risk factors for developing a latex allergy
- Instruct patient and family about signs and symptoms of a reaction
- Instruct patient and family about latex content in household products and substitution with nonlatex products, as appropriate
- Instruct patient to wear a medical alert tag
- Instruct patient and family about emergency treatment (e.g., epinephrine), as appropriate
- Instruct visitors about latex-free environment (e.g., latex balloons)

2nd edition 1996; revised 2004

Background Readings:

Floyd, P. T. (2000). Latex allergy update. *Journal of Peri Anesthesia Nursing*, *15*(1), 26–30.

Kelly, K. J., & Walsh-Kelly, C. M. (1998). Latex allergy: A patient and health-care system emergency. *Annals of Emergency Medicine*, *32*(6), 723–729.

Kim, K. T., Graves, P. B., Safadi, G. S., Alhadeff, G., Metcalfe, J. (1998). Implementation recommendations for making health care facilities latex safe. *AORN*, *67*(3), 615–632.

Miller, K. K. & Weed, P. (1998). The latex allergy trigger admission tool: An algorithm to identify which patient would benefit from latex safe precautions. *Journal of Emergency Nursing*, *24*(2), 145–152.

Smeltzer, S. C., & Bare, B. G. (2004). Assessment and management of patients with allergic disorders. In *Brunner & Suddarth's textbook of medical surgical nursing* (Vol. 2) (10th ed., pp. 1580–1604). Philadelphia: Lippincott Williams & Wilkins.

Tarlo, S. M. (1998). Latex allergy: A problem for both healthcare professionals and patients. *Ostomy/Wound Management*, *44*(8), 80–88.

Learning Facilitation

5520

Definition: Promoting the ability to process and comprehend information

Activities:
- Begin the instruction only after the patient demonstrates readiness to learn
- Set mutual, realistic learning goals with the patient
- Identify learning objectives clearly and in measurable terms
- Adjust the instruction to the patient's level of knowledge and understanding
- Tailor the content to the patient's cognitive, psychomotor, and affective abilities
- Provide information appropriate to developmental level
- Provide an environment conducive to learning
- Arrange the information in a logical sequence
- Arrange the information from simple to complex, known to unknown, or concrete to abstract, as appropriate
- Differentiate "critical" content from "desirable" content
- Adapt the information to comply with the patient's lifestyle and routines
- Relate the information to the patient's personal desires and needs
- Provide information that is consistent with the patient's values and beliefs
- Provide information that is compatible with the patient's locus of control
- Ensure that the material is current and up-to-date
- Provide educational materials to illustrate important and complex information
- Use multiple teaching modalities, as appropriate
- Use familiar language
- Explain unfamiliar terminology
- Relate new content to previous knowledge, as appropriate
- Present the information in a stimulating manner
- Incorporate animation in multimedia presentations when possible and appropriate
- Provide instructional pamphlets, videos, and online resources, when appropriate
- Introduce the patient to persons who have undergone similar experiences, as appropriate
- Encourage the patient's active participation
- Encourage the patient to share valid experiences throughout the learning experience
- Use self-paced instruction, when possible
- Avoid setting time limits
- Encourage free expression of different opinions and ideas
- Provide adequate time for mastery of content, as appropriate
- Keep teaching sessions short, as appropriate
- Simplify instructions, as appropriate
- Repeat important information
- Provide verbal prompts and reminders, as appropriate

- Provide memory aids, as appropriate
- Avoid demands for abstract thinking, if patient can think only in concrete terms
- Ensure that consistent information is being provided by various members of the health care team
- Use demonstration and return demonstration, as appropriate
- Provide opportunities for practice, as appropriate
- Provide frequent feedback about learning progress
- Correct information misinterpretations, as appropriate
- Reinforce behavior, as appropriate
- Provide time for the patient to ask questions and discuss concerns
- Answer questions in a clear, concise manner
- Refer the patient to appropriate online resources, including support groups

1st edition 1992; revised 2013

Background Readings:

Bastable, S. B. (2003). *Nurse as educator: Principles of teaching and learning for nursing practice*. Sudbury, MA: Jones and Bartlett.

Berman, A., Snyder, S., Kozier, B., & Erb, G. (2008). Teaching. In *Kozier & Erb's fundamentals of nursing: Concepts, process, and practice* (8th ed., pp. 487–511). Upper Saddle River, NJ: Prentice Hall.

Chang, M. (2007). Patient education: Addressing cultural diversity ad health literacy issues. *Urologic Nursing, 27*(5), 411–417.

Craven, R. F., & Hirnle, C. J. (2009). Client education. In *Fundamentals of nursing: Human health and function* (6th ed., pp. 344–363). Philadelphia: Lippincott Williams & Wilkins.

Fry, H. (2009). *A handbook for teaching and learning in higher education: Enhancing academic practice* (3rd ed.). New York: Routledge.

Stern, C. (2005). Knowledge retention from preoperative patient information. *International Journal of Evidence-Based Healthcare, 3*(3), 45–63.

Learning Readiness Enhancement   5540

Definition: Improving the ability and willingness to receive information

Activities:
- Provide a nonthreatening environment
- Establish rapport
- Establish teacher credibility, as appropriate
- Maximize the patient's hemodynamic status to facilitate brain oxygenation (e.g., positioning and medication adjustments), as appropriate
- Fulfill the patient's basic physiological needs (e.g., hunger, thirst, warmth, and oxygen)
- Decrease the patient's level of fatigue, as appropriate
- Control the patient's pain, as appropriate
- Avoid the use of medications that may alter the patient's perception (e.g., narcotics and hypnotics), as appropriate
- Monitor the patient's level of orientation/confusion
- Increase the patient's orientation to reality, as appropriate
- Maximize sensory input by use of eyeglasses, hearing aids, and so on, as appropriate
- Minimize the degree of sensory overload/underload, as appropriate
- Satisfy the patient's safety needs (e.g., security, control, and familiarity), as appropriate
- Monitor the patient's emotional state
- Assist the patient to deal with intense emotions (e.g., anxiety, grief, and anger), as appropriate
- Encourage verbalization of feelings, perceptions, and concerns
- Provide time for the patient to ask questions and discuss concerns
- Address the patient's specific concerns, as appropriate
- Establish a learning environment as early in contact with patient as possible
- Facilitate the patient's acceptance of the situation, as appropriate
- Assist the patient to develop confidence in ability, as appropriate
- Enlist participation of family/significant others, as appropriate
- Explain how the information will help the patient meet goals, as appropriate
- Explain how the patient's past unpleasant experiences with health care differs from the current situation, as appropriate
- Assist the patient to realize the severity of the illness, as appropriate
- Assist the patient to realize that treatment options exist, as appropriate
- Assist the patient to realize susceptibility to complications, as appropriate
- Assist the patient to realize the ability to prevent illness or condition, as appropriate
- Assist the patient to realize ability to control the progression of the illness, as appropriate
- Assist the patient to realize that current situation differs from past stressful situation, as appropriate
- Assist the patient to see alternative actions that are less risky to lifestyle, as appropriate
- Provide a trigger or cue (e.g., motivating comments/rationale and new information) toward appropriate action, as appropriate

1st edition 1992; revised 2004

Background Readings:

Bastable, S. B. (2003). *Nurse as educator: Principles of teaching and learning for nursing practice*. Sudbury, MA: Jones and Bartlett.

Craven, R. F., & Hirnle, C. J. (2003). Client education. In *Fundamentals of nursing: Human health and function* (4th ed., pp. 361–378). Philadelphia: Lippincott Williams & Wilkins.

Kozier, B., Erb, G., Berman, A., & Snyder, S. (2004). Teaching. In *Fundamentals of nursing: Concepts, processes, and practice*. (7th ed., pp. 445–468). Upper Saddle River, NJ: Prentice Hall.

Rakel, B. A. (1992). Interventions related to patient teaching. In G. M. Bulechek & J. C. McCloskey (Eds.), Symposium on nursing interventions. *Nursing Clinics of North America, 27*(2), 397–424.

Redman, B. K. (1993). Assessment of motivation to learn & the need for patient education. In B. K. Redman (Ed.), *The process of patient education* (7th ed., pp. 16-43). St. Louis: Mosby.

L

Leech Therapy

3460

Definition: Application of medicinal leeches to help drain replanted or transplanted tissue engorged with venous blood

Activities:

- Use leeches only if patient has an intact arterial blood supply, to prevent infection from the endosymbiotic bacterium present in the gut of the leech
- Instruct patient that the leech's salivary glands secrete a local anesthetic that helps mask the sensation of the bite
- Instruct patient that a local anesthetic will not be needed in replanted tissue because the nerves are newly reanastomosed
- Instruct patient that leeches secrete hirudin, an anticoagulant, so site will ooze up to 50 ml of blood for 24 to 48 hours after removal
- Reassure the patient that leech therapy is an accepted medical treatment
- Use universal precautions
- Use each leech for only one patient to prevent transfer of infection from another patient
- Cleanse the flap or digit with sterile water and dry it with a sterile cloth
- Instruct the patient to not touch leech or remove the leeches manually once applied
- Surround the site with towels and/or gauze to prevent the leech from migrating
- Enhance the leech's interest in attaching by placing a drop of 5% dextrose and water on the site
- Gently apply leech to site, using forceps
- Ensure that both the anterior and posterior ends of the leech attach to the affected area
- Continuously monitor leech until it is fully distended (10 to 15 minutes after attachment) and drops off patient
- Remove leeches that do not drop off by gently stroking with an alcohol pad
- Refrigerate unused leeches in a container filled with salt solution (spring or distilled water) and covered with netting
- Handle leeches carefully after feeding to prevent regurgitation of gut contents
- Place leeches in a small container of alcohol for incineration
- Cleanse the treated area every 1 to 2 hours with a half-and-half solution of hydrogen peroxide and sterile water to prevent bloody drainage from hardening and constricting blood flow
- Administer antibiotics as appropriate to prevent iatrogenic *A. hydrophilia* infection
- Monitor hemoglobin and hematocrit at least once a day, as appropriate
- Document the patient's response to treatment

2nd edition 1996; revised 2004

Background Readings:

Kocent, L. S., & Spinner, S. S. (1992). Leech therapy: New procedures for an old treatment. *Pediatric Nursing, 18*(5), 481–483, 542.

Peel, K. (1993). Making sense of leeches. *Nursing Times, 89*(27), 34–35.

Shinnkman, R. (2000). Worms and squirms: Maggots, leeches making a comeback in modern medicine. *Modern Healthcare, 30*(43), 54.

Voge, C. & Lehnherr, S. M. (1999). Getting attached to leeches. *Nursing 99, 29*(11), 46–47.

Life Skills Enhancement

5326

Definition: Developing an individual's ability to independently and effectively deal with the demands and challenges of everyday life

Activities:

- Establish rapport by using empathy, warmth, spontaneity, organization, patience, and persistence
- Determine the life skill learning needs of the patient, family, group, or community
- Appraise the patient's educational level
- Determine level of knowledge of the life skill
- Appraise the patient's current level of skill and understanding of the content
- Appraise the patient's learning style
- Mutually agree upon goals for the life skills program
- Determine number of sessions and length of time of the program
- Enhance motivation by setting achievable incremental goals
- Appraise the patient's cognitive, psychomotor, and affective abilities and disabilities
- Determine the patient's ability to learn specific information (i.e., consider the patient's developmental level, physiological status, orientation, pain, fatigue, unfulfilled basic needs, emotional state, and adaptation to illness)
- Determine the patient's motivation to learn specific information (i.e., consider the patient's health beliefs, past noncompliance, bad experiences with health care or learning, and conflicting goals)
- Select appropriate teaching methods and strategies
- Select appropriate educational materials
- Tailor the content to the patient's cognitive, psychomotor, and affective abilities and disabilities
- Break more complex skills into their stepwise components to enable incremental progress
- Adjust instruction to facilitate learning, as appropriate
- Provide an environment conducive to learning
- Use role-playing of appropriate behaviors with scenarios that simulate real life interpersonal interactions
- Provide positive feedback contingent on improvements in the patient's improved learning skill
- Use assignments to practice and enhance the performance of new skills in real life situations
- Instruct on strategies designed to enhance communication skills, if needed
- Provide assertiveness training, if needed

- Use strategies to enhance the patient's self awareness
- Provide appropriate social skills training, if needed
- Assist the patient to solve problems in a constructive manner
- Instruct patient how to manage conflict, if needed
- Instruct patient in setting priorities and decision making
- Assist patient in values clarification
- Provide instruction on time management, if needed
- Provide instruction on diet, nutrition, and food preparation, if needed
- Instruct patient in the use of stress management techniques, as appropriate
- Instruct patient on how to manage their illness symptoms, if appropriate
- Instruct patient on medication management, if appropriate
- Instruct the patient on workplace fundamentals (e.g., improving job performance, leaning about specific workplace and performance expectations, making friends and appropriate socializing)
- Identify and arrange for participation in leisure activities
- Provide assistance in managing finances and creating a budget, if indicated
- Include the family or significant others, as appropriate

6th edition 2013

Background Readings:

Bartels, S. J., Forester, B., Mueser, K. T., Miles. K. M., Dums, A. R., Pratt, S. I., et al. (2004). Enhanced skills training and health care management for older persons with severe mental illness. *Community Mental Health Journal*, 40(1), 75–90.

Bellack, A. S., Mueser, K. T., Gingerich, S., & Agresta, J. (2004). *Social skills training for schizophrenia: A step-by-step guide* (2nd ed.). New York: Guilford Press.

Grawe, R. W., Hagen, R., Espeland, B., & Mueser, K. T. (2007). The better life program: Effects of group skills training for persons with severe mental illness and substance abuse disorders. *Journal of Mental Health*, 15(5), 625–634.

Liberman, R. P. (2007). Dissemination and adoption of social skills training: Social validation of an evidence-based treatment for the mentally disabled. *Journal of Mental Health*, 15(5), 595–623.

Liberman, R. P., Glynn, S. M., Blair, K. E., Ross, D., & Marder, S. R. (2002). In vivo amplified skills training: Promoting generalization of independent living skills for clients with schizophrenia. *Psychiatry*, 65(2), 137–155.

World Health Organization. (1999). *Partners in life skills education: Conclusions from a United Nations inter-agency meeting.* Geneva, Switzerland: Author.

Limit Setting   4380   **L**

Definition: Establishing the parameters of desirable and acceptable patient behavior

Activities:

- Use a consistent, matter-of-fact, nonjudgmental approach
- State, limit, or identify (with patient input, when appropriate) undesirable patient behavior
- Communicate the limit in positive terms (e.g., "keep your clothes on", rather than "that behavior is inappropriate")
- Discuss concerns with patient about behavior
- Establish consequences (with patient input, when appropriate) for occurrence or nonoccurrence of desired behaviors
- Discuss with patient, when appropriate, what is desirable behavior in a given situation or setting
- Establish reasonable expectations for patient behavior, based on the situation and the patient
- Avoid arguing or bargaining about the consequences and established behavioral expectations with the patient
- Communicate the established consequences and behavioral expectations to the patient in a language that is easily understood and nonpunitive
- Communicate the established consequences and behavioral expectations with the treatment team for consistency and continuity in care
- Assist patient, when necessary and appropriate, to show the desired behaviors
- Monitor patient for occurrence or nonoccurrence of the desired behaviors
- Initiate the established consequences for the occurrence or nonoccurrence of the desired behaviors
- Modify consequences and behavioral expectations, as needed, to accommodate reasonable changes in the patient's situation
- Decrease limit setting, as patient behavior approximates the desired behaviors

1st edition 1992; revised 2008

Background Readings

Deering, C. (2006). Therapeutic relationships and communication. In W. Mohr (Ed.), *Psychiatric mental health nursing* (6th ed., pp. 55–78). Philadelphia: Lippincott Williams & Wilkins.

Lowe, T., Wellman, N., & Taylor, R. (2003). Limit-setting and decision-making in the management of aggression. *Journal of Advanced Nursing*, 41(2), 154–161.

Rickelman, B. L. (2006). The client who displays angry, aggressive, or violent behavior. In W. Mohr (Ed.), *Psychiatric mental health nursing* (6th ed., pp. 659–686). Philadelphia: Lippincott Williams & Wilkins.

Videbeck, S. L. (2006). *Psychiatric mental health nursing* (3rd ed.). Philadelphia: Lippincott Williams & Wilkins.

Listening Visits   5328

Definition: Empathic listening to genuinely understand an individual's situation and work collaboratively over a number of home visits to identify and generate solutions to reduce depressive symptoms

Activities:

- Screen for depression to establish baseline
- Establish the purpose and proposed number of visits
- Establish an agreeable place and time for the visits
- Display interest in the patient
- Maintain patient confidentiality and privacy
- Use personal strengths to establish relationship with patient
- Use open-ended questions to encourage expression of thoughts, feelings, and concerns
- Use silence to encourage the expression of thoughts, feelings, and concerns
- Avoid barriers to active listening (i.e., minimizing feelings, offering easy solutions, interrupting, talking about self, and premature closure)
- Focus completely on the interaction by suppressing prejudice, bias, assumptions, preoccupying personal concerns, and other distractions
- Use nonverbal behavior to facilitate communication (i.e., be aware of physical stance conveying nonverbal messages)
- Listen for the unexpressed message and feeling, as well as content, of the conversation
- Explore patient's behavior, feelings, and cognition about a situation
- Assist patient to name feelings and emotion associated with situation
- Clarify the message through the use of questions and feedback
- Identify the predominant themes
- Assist patient to generate a comprehensive list of current problems
- Assist patient to identify most important problem
- Assist patient to generate a list of solutions
- Assist patient to evaluate the disadvantages and advantages of the list generated
- Encourage patient to select desired solutions
- Assist patient to develop a plan to carry out the solution
- Explore progress toward resolution of the problem at subsequent visit
- Evaluate depression symptoms at appropriate intervals
- Refer patient to other health care providers, as necessary

6th edition 2013

Background Readings:

Cooper, P. J., Murray, L., Wilson, A., & Romaniuk, H. (2003). Controlled trial of the short- and long-term effect of psychological treatment of post-partum depression. I. Impact on maternal mood. *British Journal of Psychiatry, 182*(5), 412–419.

Holden, J. M., Sagovsky, R., & Cox, J. L. (1989). Counseling in a general practice setting: Controlled study of health visitor intervention in treatment of postnatal depression. *British Medical Journal, 298*(6668), 223–226.

Morrell, C. J., Slade, P., Warner, R., Paley, G., Dixon, S., Walters, S. J., et al. (2009). Clinical effectiveness of health visitor training in psychologically informed approaches for depression in postnatal women: Pragmatic cluster randomised trial in primary care, *British Medical Journal, 338*, a3045 [online].

Segre, L. S. (2011). Postpartum depression. In M. C. Rosenberg & S. R. Pehler (Eds.), *Encyclopedia of family health* (pp. 833–835). Thousand Oaks, CA: Sage.

Wickberg, B., & Hwang, C. P. (1996). Counseling of postnatal depression: A controlled study on a population based Swedish sample. *Journal of Affective Disorders, 39*(3), 209–216.

Lower Extremity Monitoring   3480

Definition: Collection, analysis, and use of patient data to categorize risk and prevent injury to the lower extremities

Activities:

- Inspect skin for evidence of poor hygiene
- Inspect lower extremities for presence of edema
- Inspect toenails for changes (e.g., thickening, fungal infection, ingrownness, and evidence of improper trimming)
- Inspect skin for color, temperature, hydration, hair growth, texture, cracking, or fissuring
- Inspect between the toes for maceration, cracking, or fissuring
- Inquire about changes in feet and current or past history of foot ulcers or amputation
- Determine mobility status (i.e., walks without assistance, walks with assistance of an assistive device, or does not walk-uses a wheelchair)
- Inspect foot for deformities including cocked-up toes, prominent metatarsal heads, and high or low arch or Charcot changes
- Monitor muscle strength in ankle and foot
- Inspect foot for evidence of pressure (i.e., the presence of localized redness, increased temperatures, blisters, corns, or callus formation)
- Inquire about the presence of parasthesias (e.g., numbness, tingling, or burning)
- Palpate thickness of fat pads over metatarsal heads
- Palpate dorsalis pedis and posterior tibial pulses
- Determine ankle pressure index, as indicated
- Inquire about the presence of intermittent claudication, rest pain, or night pain
- Determine capillary refill time
- Monitor level of protective sensation using Semmes-Weinstein nylon monofilament
- Determine vibration perception threshold
- Determine proprioceptive responses
- Elicit deep tendon reflexes (i.e., ankle and knee), as indicated
- Monitor gait and weight distribution on feet (e.g., observe walking and determine wear pattern on shoes)
- Monitor condition of shoes and socks (i.e., clean and in good repair)
- Monitor appropriateness of shoes (i.e., low-heeled with a shoe shape that matches foot shape; adequate depth of toe box; soles

made of material that will absorb shock; adjustable fit by lace or straps; uppers made of breathable, soft, and flexible materials; changes made for gait and limb length disorders; and potential for modification, if necessary)
- Monitor appropriateness of socks (i.e., absorbent material and nonconstricting)
- Monitor joint mobility (e.g., ankle dorsiflexion and subtalar joint motion)
- Perform ongoing surveillance of the lower extremities to determine need for referral, at least four times per year
- Use level of risk for injury as a guide for determining appropriate referrals
- Identify specialty foot care services required (e.g., orthotics or prescription footwear, callus trimming, toenail trimming, mobility evaluation and exercises, foot deformity evaluation and management, treatment of skin or nail deformities/infection, correction of abnormal gait or weight-bearing, and/or evaluation and management of impaired arterial circulation)
- Consult with physician regarding recommendation for further evaluation and therapy (e.g., x-ray), as needed
- Provide patient/family/significant others with information about recommended specialty foot care services
- Identify patient/family/significant others' preference for referral health professional or agency, as appropriate
- Determine patient's financial resources for payment for specialty foot care services
- Provide assistance in obtaining necessary financial resources (e.g., contact social services), as appropriate
- Contact health professional/agency as appropriate to arrange for specialty foot care services (i.e., schedule an appointment)
- Complete written referral, as appropriate

4th edition 2004

Background Readings:

American Diabetes Association. (1998). Preventive foot care in people with diabetes. *Diabetes, 21*(12), 2178–2179.

Collier, J. H. & Brodbeck, C. A. (1993). Assessing the diabetic foot: Plantar callus and pressure sensation. *The Diabetes Educatior, 19*(6), 503–508.

Craven, R. F., & Hirnle, C. J. (2003). Health assessment of human function. In *Fundamentals of nursing: Human health and function* (4th ed., pp. 393–442). Philadelphia: Lippincott Williams & Wilkins.

Culleton, J. L. (1999). Preventing diabetic foot complications. *Postgraduate Medicine, 106*(1), 78–84.

Halpin-Landry, J. E., & Goldsmith, S. (1999). Feet first, diabetic care. *American Journal of Nursing, 99*(2), 26–33.

Jacobs, A. M., & Appleman, K. K. (1999). Foot-ulcer prevention in the elderly patient. *Clinics in Geriatric Medicine, 15*(2), 351–369.

Mayfield, J. A., Reiber, G. E., Sanders, L. J., Janise, D., & Pogach, L. M., (1998). Preventive foot care in people with diabetes. *Diabetes Care, 21*(12), 2161–2177.

McNeely, M. J., Boyko, E. J., Ahroni, J. H., Stensel, V. L., Reiber, G. E., Smith, D. G., et al. (1995). The independent contributions of diabetic neuropathy and vasculopathy in foot ulceration. *Diabetes Care, 18*(2), 216–219.

Smeltzer, S. C., & Bare, B. G. (2004). Assessment and management of patients with diabetes mellitus. In *Brunner & Suddarth's textbook of medical surgical nursing* (Vol. 2) (10th ed., pp. 1149–1203). Philadelphia: Lippincott Williams & Wilkins.

Spollett, G. R. (1998). Preventing amputations in the diabetic population. *Nursing Clinics of North America, 33*(4), 629–641.

L

Malignant Hyperthermia Precautions 3840

Definition: Prevention or reduction of hypermetabolic response to pharmacological agents used during surgery

Activities:

- Ask patient about personal or family history of malignant hyperthermia, unexpected deaths from anesthetic, muscle disorder, or unexplained postoperative fever
- Refer patient with family history of malignant hyperthermia for further testing to determine risk (e.g., muscle contracture test, molecular genetic test)
- Notify surgical team of patient history or risk status
- Maintain emergency equipment for malignant hyperthermia, per protocol
- Review malignant hyperthermia emergency care with staff, per protocol
- Monitor vital signs, including core body temperature
- Provide anesthesia machine free of precipitating anesthetic agents for patient at risk for malignant hyperthermia or discontinue use of anesthesia machine for patient experiencing malignant hyperthermia
- Place cooling water mattress under patient at risk for malignant hyperthermia at start of procedure
- Use nontriggering anesthetic agents for patient at risk for or experiencing malignant hyperthermia (e.g., opioids, benzodiazepines, local anesthetics, nitrous oxide, and barbiturates)
- Avoid or discontinue use of triggering agents (e.g., succinylcholine used alone or in conjunction with volatile inhalation agents, such as halothane, enflurane, isoflurane, sevoflurane, or desflurane)
- Monitor for signs of malignant hyperthermia (e.g., hypercarbia, hyperthermia, tachycardia, tachypnea, metabolic acidosis, arrhythmias, cyanosis, mottled skin, muscle rigidity, profuse sweating, and unstable blood pressure)
- Discontinue procedure, if possible
- Provide emergency management supplies
- Obtain blood and urine samples
- Monitor for abnormalities in laboratory values (e.g., increased end-tidal carbon dioxide level with decreased oxygen saturation, increased serum calcium, increased potassium, unexplained metabolic acidosis, hematuria, and myoglobinuria)
- Monitor electrocardiography results
- Intubate or assist with intubation if endotracheal tube is not already in place
- Hyperventilate with 100% oxygen using highest flow rate possible
- Prepare and administer medications (e.g., dantrolene sodium, sodium bicarbonate, insulin, antidysrhythmic agents other than calcium channel blockers, and osmotic or loop diuretics)

- Administer iced saline
- Apply cooling blanket or commercial cooling device over torso
- Rub or wrap extremities with cold, wet, or iced towels
- Lavage stomach, bladder, rectum, and open body cavities with sterile, iced, normal saline
- Insert nasogastric tube, rectal tube, and urinary catheter, as necessary
- Monitor urine output
- Administer sufficient IV fluids to maintain urine output
- Initiate second IV line
- Assist with arterial and central venous pressure line insertion
- Avoid use of drugs, including calcium chloride or gluconate, cardiac glycosides, adrenergics, atropine, and lactated Ringer solutions
- Decrease environmental stimuli
- Observe for signs of late complications (e.g., consumption coagulopathy, renal failure, hypothermia, pulmonary edema, hyperkalemia, neurological sequelae, muscle necrosis, and reoccurrence of symptoms after treatment of initial episode)
- Provide patient and family education (i.e., discuss needed precautions for future anesthetic administration, discuss methods for determining malignant hyperthermia risk)
- Refer patient and family to Malignant Hyperthermia Association of the United States
- Refer for genetic counseling
- Report incident to the North American Malignant Hyperthermia Registry and the Medic Alert Hotline

2nd edition 1996; revised 2013

Background Readings:

Chard, R. (2010). Care of intraoperative patients. In D. D. Ignatavicius & M. L. Workman (Eds.), *Medical-surgical nursing: Patient-centered collaborative care* (6th ed., pp. 264–284). St. Louis: Saunders.

Hernandez, J. F., Secrest, J. A., Hill, L., & McClarty, S. J. (2009). Scientific advances in the genetic understanding and diagnosis of malignant hyperthermia. *Journal of PeriAnesthesia Nursing, 24*(1), 19–34.

Hommertzheim, R., & Steinke, E. E. (2006). Malignant hyperthermia: The perioperative nurse's role. *AORN Journal, 83*(1), 149–164.

Kaplow, R. (2010). Care of postanesthesia patients. *Critical Care Nursing, 30*(1), 60-62.

Nagelhout, J. J., & Plaus, K. L. (2010). *Handbook of nurse anesthesia* (4th ed.). St. Louis: Saunders.

Massage 1480

Definition: Stimulation of the skin and underlying tissues with varying degrees of hand pressure to decrease pain, produce relaxation, and/or improve circulation

Activities:
- Screen for contraindications such as decreased platelets, decreased skin integrity, deep vein thrombosis, areas with open lesions, redness or inflammation, tumors, and hypersensitivity to touch
- Assess the client's willingness to have a massage
- Establish a period of time for massage that achieves the desired response
- Select the area or areas of the body to be massaged
- Wash hands with warm water
- Prepare a warm, comfortable, private environment, without distractions
- Place in a comfortable position that facilitates massage
- Drape to expose only area to be massaged, as needed
- Drape unexposed areas with blankets, sheets, or bath towels as needed
- Use lotion, oil, or dry powder to reduce friction (no lotion or oils on head or scalp), assessing for any sensitivity or contraindications
- Warm lotion or oil in palm of hands or by running bottle under warm water for several minutes
- Massage using continuous, even, long strokes; kneading; or vibration with palms, fingers, and thumbs
- Adapt massage area, technique, and pressure to patient's perception of comfort and purpose of massage
- Massage the hands or feet if other areas are inconvenient or if more comfortable for the patient
- Encourage patient to deep breathe and relax during massage
- Encourage patient to advise of any part of the massage that is uncomfortable
- Instruct patient at completion of massage to rest until ready and then to move slowly
- Use massage alone or in conjunction with other measures, as appropriate
- Evaluate and document response to massage

1st edition 1992; revised 2008

Background Readings:
Altman, G. B. (2004). *Delmar's fundamental and advanced nursing skills* (2nd ed.). Clifton Park, NY: Delmar Learning.
Coe, A. B., & Anthony, M. L. (2005). Understanding bodywork for the patient with cancer. *Clinical Journal of Oncology Nursing 9*(6), 733–739.
Fontaine, K. L. (2005). Complementary and alternative therapies for nursing practice (2nd ed.). Upper Saddle River, NJ: Pearson Education.
Smith, M. C., Kemp, J., Hemphill, L. & Vojir, C. P. (2002). Outcomes of therapeutic massage for hospitalized cancer patients. *Journal of Nursing Scholarship, 34*(3), 257–267.
Smith, S. F., Duell, D. J., & Martin, B. C., (2004). *Clinical nursing skills: Basic to advanced skills* (6th ed.). Upper Saddle River, NJ: Prentice Hall.
Snyder, M., & Tseng, Y. (2002). Massage. In M. Snyder & R. Lindquist (Eds.), *Complementary/alternative therapies in nursing* (4th ed., pp. 223–233). New York: Springer.
Wang, H. L., & Keck, J. F. (2004). Foot and hand massage as an intervention for postoperative pain. *Pain Management Nursing, 5*(2), 59–65.

M

Mechanical Ventilation Management: Invasive 3300

Definition: Assisting the patient receiving artificial breathing support through a device inserted into the trachea

Activities:
- Monitor for conditions indicating a need for ventilation support (e.g., respiratory muscle fatigue, neurological dysfunction secondary to trauma, anesthesia, drug overdose, refractory respiratory acidosis)
- Monitor for impending respiratory failure
- Consult with other health care personnel in selection of a ventilator mode (initial mode usually volume control with breath rate, FiO_2 level and targeted tidal volume specified)
- Obtain baseline total body assessment of patient initially and with each change of caregiver
- Initiate setup and application of the ventilator
- Ensure that ventilator alarms are on
- Instruct the patient and family about the rationale and expected sensations associated with use of mechanical ventilators
- Routinely monitor ventilator settings, including temperature and humidification of inspired air
- Check all ventilator connections regularly
- Monitor for decrease in exhaled volume and increase in inspiratory pressure
- Administer muscle paralyzing agents, sedatives, and narcotic analgesics, as appropriate
- Monitor for activities that increase oxygen consumption (e.g., fever, shivering, seizures, pain, or basic nursing activities) that may supersede ventilator support settings and cause oxygen desaturation
- Monitor for factors that increase patient/ventilator work of breathing (e.g., morbid obesity, pregnancy, massive ascites, lowered head of bed, biting of ET, condensation in ventilator tubes, clogged filters)
- Monitor for symptoms that indicate increased work of breathing (e.g., increased heart or respiratory rate, increased blood pressure, diaphoresis, changes in mental status)
- Monitor the effectiveness of mechanical ventilation on patient's physiological and psychological status
- Initiate relaxation techniques, as appropriate
- Provide care to alleviate patient distress (e.g., positioning, tracheobronchial toileting, bronchodilator therapy, sedation and/or analgesia, frequent equipment checks)
- Provide patient with a means for communication (e.g., paper and pencil, alphabet board)

- Empty condensed water from water traps
- Ensure change of ventilator circuits every 24 hours
- Use aseptic technique in all suctioning procedures, as appropriate
- Monitor ventilator pressure readings, patient/ventilator synchronicity, and patient breath sounds
- Perform suctioning based on presence of adventitious breath sounds and/or increased inspiratory pressure
- Monitor pulmonary secretions for amount, color, and consistency and regularly document findings
- Stop NG feedings during suctioning and 30 to 60 minutes before chest physiotherapy
- Silence ventilator alarms during suctioning to decrease frequency of false alarms
- Monitor patient's progress on current ventilator settings and make appropriate changes as ordered
- Monitor for adverse effects of mechanical ventilation (e.g., tracheal deviation, infection, barotrauma, volutrauma, reduced cardiac output, gastric distension, subcutaneous emphysema)
- Monitor for mucosal damage to oral, nasal, tracheal, or laryngeal tissue from pressure from artificial airways, high cuff pressures, or unplanned extubations
- Use commercial tube holders rather than tape or strings to fixate artificial airways to prevent unplanned extubations
- Position to facilitate ventilation/perfusion matching ("good lung down"), as appropriate
- Collaborate with physician to use pressure support or PEEP to minimize alveolar hypoventilation, as appropriate
- Collaborate routinely with physician and respiratory therapist to coordinate care and assist patient to tolerate therapy
- Perform chest physiotherapy, as appropriate
- Promote adequate fluid and nutritional intake
- Promote routine assessments for weaning criteria (e.g., hemodynamic, cerebral, metabolic stability, resolution of condition prompting intubation, ability to maintain patent airway, ability to initiate respiratory effort)
- Provide routine oral care with soft moist swabs, antiseptic agent, and gentle suctioning

- Monitor effects of ventilator changes on oxygenation: ABG, SaO_2, SvO_2, end-tidal CO_2, Qsp/Qt, A-aDO_2, patient's subjective response
- Monitor degree of shunt, vital capacity, V_d/V_t, MVV, inspiratory force, and FEV_1 for readiness to wean from mechanical ventilation, based on agency protocol
- Document all changes to ventilator settings, with rationale for changes
- Document all patient responses to ventilator and ventilator changes (e.g., chest movement observation/auscultation, changes in x-ray, changes in ABGs)
- Monitor for postextubation complications (e.g., stridor, glottic swelling, laryngospasm, tracheal stenosis)
- Ensure emergency equipment at bedside at all times (e.g., manual resuscitation bag connected to oxygen, masks, suction equipment/supplies), including preparations for power failures

1st edition 1992; revised 2000, 2008

Background Readings:

American Association of Critical Care Nurses. (2006). *Core curriculum for critical care nursing* (6th ed.) [J. G. Alspach, Ed.]. Philadelphia: Saunders.

American Heart Association. (2005). Guidelines for cardiopulmonary resuscitation and emergency cardiovascular care. *Circulation, 112*(24), 1–211.

Fenstermacher, D. & Hong, D. (2004). Mechanical ventilation: What have we learned. *Critical Care Nursing Quarterly, 27*(3), 258–294.

Knipper, J. S., & Alpen, M. A. (1992). Ventilatory support. In G. M. Bulechek & J. C. McCloskey (Eds.), *Nursing interventions: Essential nursing treatments* (2nd ed., pp. 531–543). Philadelphia: Saunders.

Lynn-McHale, D. J., & Carlson, K. K. (2005). *AACN procedure manual for critical care* (5th ed.). Philadelphia: Saunders.

Manno, M. S. (2005). Managing mechanical ventilation. *Nursing 2005, 35*(12), 36–42.

Smeltzer, S. C., & Bare, B. G. (2004). *Brunner & Suddarth's textbook of medical-surgical nursing* (Vol. 1) (10th ed.). Philadelphia: Lippincott Williams and Wilkins.

Urden, L. D., Stacy, K. M., & Lough, M. E. (2006). *Thelan's critical care nursing: Diagnosis and management* (5th ed.). St. Louis: Mosby.

M

Mechanical Ventilation Management: Noninvasive   3302

Definition: Assisting a patient receiving artificial breathing support that does not necessitate a device inserted into the trachea

Activities:

- Monitor for conditions indicating appropriateness of noninvasive ventilation support (e.g., acute exacerbations of COPD, asthma, noncardiogenic and cardiogenic pulmonary edema, acute respiratory failure due to community acquired pneumonia, obesity hypoventilation syndrome, obstructive sleep apnea)
- Monitor for contraindications to noninvasive ventilation support (e.g., hemodynamic instability, cardiovascular or respiratory arrest, unstable angina, acute myocardial infarction, refractory hypoxemia, severe respiratory acidosis, decreased level of consciousness, problems with securing/placing noninvasive equipment, facial trauma, inability to cooperate, morbidly obese, thick secretions, or bleeding)
- Consult with other health care personnel in selection of a noninvasive ventilator type (e.g., pressure limited [bilevel positive airway pressure], volume-cycled flow-limited, or CPAP)

- Consult with other health care personnel and patient in selection of noninvasive device (e.g., nasal or face mask, nasal plugs, nasal pillow, helmet, oral mouthpiece)
- Obtain baseline total body assessment of patient initially and with each change of caregiver
- Instruct the patient and family about the rationale and expected sensations associated with use of noninvasive mechanical ventilators and devices
- Place patient in semi-Fowler position
- Apply noninvasive device assuring adequate fit and avoidance of large air leaks (take particular care with edentulous or bearded patients)
- Apply facial protection as needed to avoid pressure damage to skin
- Initiate setup and application of the ventilator
- Observe patient continuously in first hour after application to assess tolerance

- Ensure that ventilator alarms are on
- Routinely monitor ventilator settings, including temperature and humidification of inspired air
- Check all ventilator connections regularly
- Monitor for decrease in exhaled volume and increase in inspiratory pressure
- Monitor for activities that increase oxygen consumption (e.g., fever, shivering, seizures, pain, or basic nursing activities) that may supersede ventilator support settings and cause oxygen desaturation
- Monitor for symptoms that indicate increased work of breathing (e.g., increased heart or respiratory rate, increased blood pressure, diaphoresis, changes in mental status)
- Monitor the effectiveness of mechanical ventilation on patient's physiological and psychological status
- Initiate relaxation techniques, as appropriate
- Ensure periods of rest daily (e.g., 15 to 30 minutes every 4 to 6 hours)
- Provide care to alleviate patient distress (e.g., positioning; treat side effects such as rhinitis, dry throat, or epistaxis; give sedation and/or analgesia; frequent equipment checks; cleansing or change of noninvasive device)
- Provide patient with a means for communication (e.g., paper and pencil, alphabet board)
- Empty condensed water from water traps
- Ensure change of ventilator circuits every 24 hours
- Use aseptic technique, as appropriate
- Monitor patient and ventilator synchronicity and patient breath sounds
- Monitor patient's progress on current ventilator settings and make appropriate changes as ordered
- Monitor for adverse effects (e.g., eye irritation, skin breakdown, occluded airway from jaw displacement with mask, dyspnea, anxiety, claustrophobia, gastric distension)
- Monitor for mucosal damage to oral, nasal, tracheal, or laryngeal tissue
- Monitor pulmonary secretions for amount, color, and consistency, and regularly document findings
- Collaborate routinely with physician and respiratory therapist to coordinate care and assist patient to tolerate therapy
- Perform chest physiotherapy, as appropriate
- Promote adequate fluid and nutritional intake

- Promote routine assessments for weaning criteria (e.g., resolution of condition prompting ventilation, ability to maintain adequate respiratory effort)
- Provide routine oral care with soft moist swabs, antiseptic agent, and gentle suctioning
- Document all changes to ventilator settings, with rationale for changes
- Document all patient responses to ventilator and ventilator changes (e.g., chest movement observation/auscultation, changes in x-ray, changes in ABGs)
- Ensure emergency equipment at bedside at all times (e.g., manual resuscitation bag connected to oxygen, masks, suction equipment/supplies), including preparations for power failures

5th edition 2008

Background Readings:

American Association of Critical Care Nurses. (2006). *Core curriculum for critical care nursing* (6th ed.) [J. G. Alspach, Ed.]. Philadelphia: Saunders.

American Heart Association. (2005). Guidelines for cardiopulmonary resuscitation and emergency cardiovascular care. *Circulation, 112*(24), 1–211.

Fenstermacher, D., & Hong, D. (2004). Mechanical ventilation: What have we learned. *Critical Care Nursing Quarterly, 27*(3), 258–294.

Knipper, J. S., & Alpen, M. A. (1992). Ventilatory support. In G. M. Bulechek and J. C. McCloskey (Eds.), *Nursing interventions: Essential nursing treatments* (2nd ed., pp. 531–543). Philadelphia: Saunders.

Lynn-McHale, D. J. & Carlson, K. K. (2005). *AACN procedure manual for critical care* (5th ed.). Philadelphia: Saunders.

Manno, M. S. (2005). Managing mechanical ventilation. *Nursing 2005, 35*(12), 36–42.

Smeltzer, S. C., & Bare, B. G. (2004). *Brunner & Suddarth's textbook of medical-surgical nursing* (10th ed.). Philadelphia: Lippincott Williams and Wilkins.

Stoltzfus, S. (2006). The role of noninvasive mechanical ventilation. *Dimensions of Critical Care Nursing, 25*(2), 66–70.

Urden, L. D., Stacy, K. M., & Lough, M. E. (2006). *Thelan's critical care nursing: Diagnosis and management* (5th ed.). St. Louis: Mosby.

M

Mechanical Ventilation Management: Pneumonia Prevention   3304

Definition: Care of a patient at risk for developing ventilator-associated pneumonia

Activities:
- Wash hands before and after patient care activity, particularly after emptying fluids from ventilator circuitry
- Wear gloves and protective equipment and clothing for oral care and change gloves to prevent cross-contamination during oral care
- Monitor oral cavity, lips, tongue, buccal mucosa, and condition of teeth
- Monitor oral cavity for dental plaque, inflammation, bleeding, candidiasis, purulent matter, calculus, and staining
- Brush teeth and tongue with toothpaste or an antiseptic oral rinse using circular motion with a soft toothbrush or suction toothbrush

- Rinse toothbrush after each use and change at regular intervals
- Brush gingiva gently if patient is edentulous
- Assist with the application of a debriding agent or mouth wash to gingiva, teeth, and tongue with swab, according to agency protocol
- Use water rinses instead of a debriding agent with patients who have mucositis or altered oral mucosa
- Assist with swabbing perpendicular to gum line while applying gentle pressure to help facilitate the removal of debris and mucus
- Consider providone-iodine oral antiseptic in patients with severe head injury
- Consult dentistry, if needed

- Apply oral moisturizer to oral mucosa and lips, as needed
- Facilitate use of yankauer or soft suction for oral care, as needed
- Facilitate subglottic suctioning prior to repositioning patient supine (bed, chair, road trip), repositioning endotracheal tube (ET), and deflating the ET cuff
- Suction the trachea, then oral cavity, and then nasal pharynx to remove secretions above the ET cuff to decrease the risk of aspiration
- Rinse yankauer and inline deep suction lines after each use and change every day
- Consider use of continuous subglottic suctioning and drainage with specifically designed ET in patients who have mechanical ventilation longer than 72 hours
- Keep head of bed elevated to 30-45 degrees unless contraindicated (i.e., hemodynamic instability), particularly during enteral tube feedings
- Turn patient frequently (at least every 2 hours)
- Facilitate daily interruptions of sedation, in consultation with the physician team
- Consider using a cuffed ET with in-line or subglottic suctioning
- Maintain an endotracheal cuff pressure of at least 20 cm
- Monitor the depth of the ET
- Consider use of oral intubation over nasal intubation
- Keep ET tapes clean and dry
- Monitor the effectiveness of mechanical ventilation on patient's physiological and psychosocial status
- Check all ventilator connections regularly
- Monitor daily for evidence of readiness for extubation
- Monitor patient for signs and symptoms of respiratory infection (e.g., restlessness, coughing, fever, increased heart rate, change in secretions, leukocytosis, infiltrates in chest x-ray)
- Monitor and document oxygen saturation

- Avoid histamine receptor blocking agents and proton pump inhibitors unless patient is at high risk for developing a stress ulcer
- Instruct patient and family about oral care routine

6th edition 2013

Background Readings:

Cason, C. L., Tyner, T. Saunders, S., & Broome, L. (2007). Nurses' implementation of guidelines for ventilator-associated pneumonia from the Centers for Disease Control and Prevention. *American Journal of Critical Care*, 16(1), 28–36.

Centers for Disease Control and Prevention. (2003). *Guidelines for preventing health-care-associated pneumonia.* Atlanta, GA: Author.

Chan, E. Y., Ruest, A., Meade, M., & Cook, D. J. (2007). Oral decontamination for prevention of pneumonia in mechanically ventilated adults: Systematic review and meta-analysis. *British Medical Journal*, 334(7599), 889.

Efraiti, S., Deutsch, I., Antonelli, M., Hockey, P., Rozenblum, R., & Gurman, G. M. (2010). Ventilator-associated pneumonia: Current status and future recommendations. *Journal of Clinical Monitoring and Computing*, 24(2), 161–168.

Munro, C. L., Grap, M. J., Jablonski, R., & Boyle, A. (2006). Oral health measurement in nursing research: State of the science. *Biological Research for Nursing*, 8(1), 35–42.

Muscadere, J., Dodek, P., Keenan, S. Fowler, R., Cook, D., & Heyland, D. (2008). Comprehensive evidence-based clinical practice guidelines for ventilator-associated pneumonia: Prevention. *Journal of Critical Care*, 23(1), 126–137.

Pineda, L. A., Saliba, R. G., & El Solh, A. A. (2006). Effect of oral decontamination with chlorhexidine on the incidence of nosocomial pneumonia: A meta-analysis. *Critical Care*, 10(1), R35.

Tolentino-Delosreyes, A. F., Ruppert, S. D., & Shiao, P. K. (2007). Evidence-based practice: Use of the ventilator bundle to prevent ventilator-associated pneumonia. *American Journal of Critical Care*, 16(1), 20–27.

M

Mechanical Ventilatory Weaning   3310

Definition: Assisting the patient to breathe without the aid of a mechanical ventilator

Activities:

- Determine patient readiness for weaning (e.g., hemodynamically stable, condition requiring ventilation resolved, current condition optimal for weaning)
- Monitor predictors of ability to tolerate weaning based on agency protocol (e.g., degree of shunt, vital capacity, Vd/Vt, MVV, inspiratory force, FEV_1, negative inspiratory pressure)
- Monitor to assure patient is free of significant infection prior to weaning
- Monitor for optimal fluid and electrolyte status
- Collaborate with other health team members to optimize patient's nutritional status, assuring that 50% of the diet's non-protein caloric source is fat rather than carbohydrate
- Position patient for best use of ventilatory muscles and to optimize diaphragmatic descent
- Suction the airway, as needed
- Administer chest physiotherapy, as appropriate
- Consult with other health care personnel in selecting a method for weaning
- Initiate weaning with trial periods (e.g., 30 to 120 minutes of ventilator-assisted spontaneous breathing)
- Alternate periods of weaning trials with sufficient periods of rest and sleep

- Avoid delaying return of patient with fatigued respiratory muscles to mechanical ventilation
- Set a schedule to coordinate other patient care activities with weaning trials
- Promote the best use of the patient's energy by initiating weaning trials after the patient is well rested
- Monitor for signs of respiratory muscle fatigue (e.g., abrupt rise in $PaCO_2$, rapid, shallow ventilation, paradoxical abdominal wall motion), hypoxemia, and tissue hypoxia while weaning is in process
- Administer medications that promote airway patency and gas exchange
- Set discrete, attainable goals with the patient for weaning
- Use relaxation techniques, as appropriate
- Coach the patient during difficult weaning trials
- Assist the patient to distinguish spontaneous breaths from mechanically delivered breaths
- Minimize excessive work of breathing that is nontherapeutic by eliminating extra dead space, adding pressure support, administering bronchodilators, and maintaining airway patency, as appropriate
- Avoid pharmacological sedation during weaning trials, as appropriate
- Provide some means of patient control during weaning

- Stay with the patient and provide support during initial weaning attempts
- Instruct patient about ventilator setting changes that increase the work of breathing, as appropriate
- Provide the patient with positive reinforcement and frequent progress reports
- Consider using alternate methods of weaning as determined by patient's response to the current method
- Instruct the patient and family about what to expect during various stages of weaning
- Prepare discharge arrangements through multidisciplinary involvement with patient and family

1st edition 1992; revised 1996, 2008

Background Readings:

American Association of Critical Care Nurses. (2006). *Core curriculum for critical care nursing* (6th ed.) [J. G. Alspach, Ed.]. Philadelphia: Saunders.

A Collective Task Force Facilitated by the American College of Chest Physicians, the American Association of Respiratory Care and the American College of Critical Care Medicine. (2002). Evidenced-based guidelines for weaning and discontinuing ventilatory support. *Respiratory Care, 47*(1), 69–90.

Evidence-based Practice Center McMaster University. (2000). *Criteria for weaning from mechanical ventilation. Summary, Evidence report/Technology Assessment: Number 23* (Publication No. 00-E028). Rockville, MD: Agency for Healthcare Research and Quality.

Fenstermacher, D., & Hong, D. (2004). Mechanical ventilation: What have we learned. *Critical Care Nursing Quarterly, 27*(3), 258–294.

Lynn-McHale, D. J., & Carlson, K. K. (2005). *AACN procedure manual for critical care* (5th ed.). Philadelphia: Saunders.

Manno, M. S. (2005). Managing mechanical ventilation. *Nursing 2005, 35*(12), 36–42.

Phelan, B. A., Cooper, D. A., & Sangkachand, P. (2002). Prolonged mechanical ventilation and tracheotomy in the elderly. *AACN Clinical Issue, 13*(1), 84–93.

Smeltzer, S. C., & Bare, B. G. (2004). *Brunner & Suddarth's textbook of medical-surgical nursing* (10th ed.). Philadelphia: Lippincott Williams and Wilkins.

Urden, L. D., Stacy, K. M., & Lough, M. E. (2006). *Thelan's critical care nursing: Diagnosis and management* (5th ed.). St. Louis: Mosby.

Medication Administration 2300

Definition: Preparing, giving, and evaluating the effectiveness of prescription and nonprescription drugs

M

Activities:
- Maintain agency policies and procedures for accurate and safe administration of medications
- Maintain an environment that maximizes safe and efficient administration of medications
- Avoid interruptions when preparing, verifying, or administering medications
- Follow the five rights of medication administration
- Verify the prescription or medication order before administering the drug
- Prescribe or recommend medications, as appropriate, according to prescriptive authority
- Monitor for possible medication allergies, interactions, and contraindications, including over-the-counter medications and herbal remedies
- Note patient's allergies before delivery of each medication and hold medications, as appropriate
- Notify the patient of medication type, reason for administration, expected actions, and adverse effects prior to administering, as appropriate
- Ensure that hypnotics, narcotics, and antibiotics are either discontinued or reordered on their renewal date
- Note expiration date on medication container
- Prepare medications using appropriate equipment and techniques for the drug administration modality
- Verify changes in medication form prior to administering (e.g., crushed enteric tablets, oral liquids in intravenous syringe, unusual packaging)
- Use bar code assisted medication administration when possible
- Avoid administration of medications not properly labeled
- Dispose of unused or expired drugs, according to agency guidelines
- Monitor vital signs and laboratory values before medication administration, as appropriate
- Assist patient in taking medication
- Give medication using appropriate technique and route

- Use orders, agency policies, and procedures to guide appropriate method of medication administration
- Instruct patient and family about expected actions and adverse effects of the medication
- Validate and document patient and family understanding of expected actions and adverse effects of the medication
- Monitor patient to determine need for PRN medications, as appropriate
- Monitor patient for the therapeutic effect of all medications
- Monitor patient for adverse effects, toxicity, and interactions of the administered medications
- Sign out narcotics and other restricted drugs, according to agency protocol
- Document medication administration and patient responsiveness (i.e., include medication generic name, dose, time, route, reason for administration, and effect achieved), according to agency protocol

1st edition 1992; revised 2013

Background Readings:

Biron, A. D., Lavoie-Tremblay, M., & Loiselle, C. G. (2009). Characteristics of work interruptions during medication administration. *Journal of Nursing Scholarship, 41*(4), 330–336.

Elliott, M., & Liu, Y. (2010). The nine rights of medication administration: An overview. *British Journal of Nursing (BJN), 19*(5), 300–305.

Helmons, P. J., Wargel, L. N., & Daniels, C. E. (2009). Effect of bar-code-assisted medication administration on medication administration errors and accuracy in multiple patient care areas. *American Journal of Health-System Pharmacy, 66*(13), 1202–1210.

Hewitt, P. (2010). Nurses' perceptions of the causes of medication errors: An integrative literature review. *MEDSURG Nursing, 19*(3), 159–156.

Kozier, B., Erb, G., Berman, A., & Snyder, S. (2004). Medications. In *Fundamentals of nursing: Concepts, processes, and practice.* (7th ed., pp. 829–901). Upper Saddle River, NJ: Prentice Hall.

Medication Administration: Ear 2308

Definition: Preparing and instilling otic medications

Activities:

- Follow the five rights of medication administration
- Note patient's medical history and history of allergies
- Determine patient's knowledge of medication and understanding of method of administration
- Position patient in a side-lying position with ear to be treated facing up, or have patient sit in chair
- Straighten ear canal by pulling auricle down and back (child) or upward and outward (adult)
- Instill medication holding dropper 1 cm above ear canal
- Instruct patient to remain in side-lying position 5 to 10 minutes
- Apply gentle pressure or massage to tragus of ear with finger
- Teach and monitor self-administration technique, as appropriate
- Document medication administration and patient responsiveness according to agency protocol

3rd edition 2000; revised 2004

Background Readings:

Craven, R. F., & Hirnle, C. J. (2003). Medication administration. In *Fundamentals of nursing: Human health and function* (4th ed., pp. 513–574). Philadelphia: Lippincott Williams & Wilkins.

Kozier, B., Erb, G., Berman, A., & Snyder, S. (2004). Medications. In *Fundamentals of nursing: Concepts, processes, and practice.* (7th ed., pp. 785–854). Upper Saddle River, NJ: Prentice Hall.

Naegle, M. A. (1999). Medication management. In G. M. Bulechek & J. C. McCloskey (Eds.), *Nursing interventions: Effective nursing treatments* (3rd ed., pp. 234–242). Philadelphia: Saunders.

Perry, A. G. & Potter, P. A. (2002). *Clinical nursing skills and techniques* (5th ed., pp. 436–452, 475–479). St. Louis: Mosby.

Rice, J. (2002). *Medications and mathematics for the nurse* (9th ed.). Albany, NY: Delmar.

Medication Administration: Enteral 2301

Definition: Delivering medications through a tube inserted into the gastrointestinal system

M

Activities:

- Follow the five rights of medication administration
- Note patient's medical history and history of allergies
- Determine patient's knowledge of medication and understanding of method of administration (e.g., nasogastric tube, orogastric tube, gastrostomy tube)
- Determine any contraindications to patient receiving oral medication via tube (e.g., bowel inflammation, reduced peristalsis, recent gastrointestinal surgery, attached to gastric suction)
- Prepare medication (e.g., crush or mix with fluids, as appropriate)
- Inform patient of expected actions and possible adverse effects of medications
- Check placement of the tube by aspirating gastrointestinal contents, checking the pH level of the aspirate, or obtaining x-ray film, as appropriate
- Schedule medication to be in accord with formula feeding
- Place patient into high Fowler position, if not contraindicated
- Aspirate stomach contents, return aspirate by flushing with 30 ml of air or appropriate amount for age, and flush tube with 30 ml of water, as appropriate
- Remove plunger from syringe and pour medication into syringe
- Administer medication by allowing medication to flow freely from barrel of syringe, using plunger only as needed to facilitate flow
- Flush tube with 30 ml of warm water, or appropriate amount for age, after medication administration
- Monitor patient for therapeutic effects, adverse effect, drug toxicity, and drug interactions
- Document medication administration and patient responsiveness according to agency protocol

1st edition 1992; revised 1996, 2004

Background Readings:

Bozzetti, F., Braga, M., Gianotti, L., Gavazzi, C., & Mariani, L. (2001). Postoperative enteral versus perenteral nutrition in malnourished patients with gastrointestinal cancer: A randomised multicentre trial. *Lancet*, 358(9292), 1487–1492.

Craven, R. F., & Hirnle, C. J. (2003). Medication administration. In *Fundamentals of nursing: Human health and function* (4th ed., pp. 513–574). Philadelphia: Lippincott Williams & Wilkins.

Keidan, I., & Gallagher, T. J. (2000). Electrocardiogram-guided placement of enteral feeding tubes. *Critical Care Medicine*, 28(7), 2631–2633.

Kozier, B., Erb, G., Berman, A., & Snyder, S. (2004). Medications. In *Fundamentals of nursing: Concepts, processes, and practice.* (7th ed., pp. 785–854). Upper Saddle River, NJ: Prentice Hall.

Miller, D., & Miller, H. (2000). To crush or not to crush: What to consider before giving medications to a patient with a tube or who has trouble swallowing. *Nursing 2000*, 30(2), 50–52.

Naegle, M. A. (1999). Medication management. In G. M. Bulechek & J. C. McCloskey (Eds.), *Nursing interventions: Effective nursing treatments* (3rd ed., pp. 234–242). Philadelphia: Saunders.

Perry, A. G., & Potter, P. A. (2002). Clinical nursing skills & techniques (5th ed., pp. 436–452, 461–465, 756–762). St. Louis: Mosby.

Rumalla, A., & Baron, T. H. (2000). Results of direct percutaneous endoscopic jejunostomy, an alternative method for providing jejunal feeding. *Mayo Clinic Proceedings*, 75(8), 807–810.

Spalding, H. K., Sullivan, K. J., Soremi, O., Gonzalez, F., & Goodwin, S. R. (2000). Bedside placement of transpyloric feeding tubes in the pediatric intensive care unit using gastric insufflation. *Critical Care Medicine*, 28(6), 2041–2044.

Trujillo, E. B., Robinson, M. K., & Jacobs, D. O. (2001). Feeding critically ill patients: Current concepts. *Critical Care Nurse*, 21(4), 60–69.

Medication Administration: Eye 2310

Definition: Preparing and instilling ophthalmic medications

Activities:
- Follow the five rights of medication administration
- Note patient's medical history and history of allergies
- Determine patient's knowledge of medication and understanding of method of administration
- Position patient supine or sitting in a chair with neck slightly hyperextended; ask patient to look at ceiling
- Instill medication onto the conjunctival sac using aseptic technique
- Apply gentle pressure to nasolacrimal duct if medication has systemic effects
- Instruct patient to close eye gently to help distribute medication
- Monitor for local, systemic, and adverse effects of medication
- Teach and monitor self-administration technique, as appropriate
- Document medication administration and patient responsiveness according to agency protocol

3rd edition 2000

Background Readings:
Craven, R. F., & Hirnle, C. J. (2003). Medication administration. In *Fundamentals of nursing: Human health and function* (4th ed., pp. 513–574). Philadelphia: Lippincott Williams & Wilkins.

Kozier, B., Erb, G., Berman, A., & Snyder, S. (2004). Medications. In *Fundamentals of nursing: Concepts, processes, and practice*. (7th ed., pp. 785–854). Upper Saddle River, NJ: Prentice Hall.

Naegle, M. A. (1999). Medication management. In G. M. Bulechek & J. C. McCloskey (Eds.), *Nursing interventions: Effective nursing treatments* (3rd ed., pp. 234–242). Philadelphia: Saunders.

Perry, A. G., & Potter, P. A. (2002). *Clinical nursing skills & techniques* (5th ed., pp. 436–452, 470–475). St. Louis: Mosby.

Rice, J. (2002). *Medications and mathematics for the nurse* (9th ed.). Albany, NY: Delmar.

Medication Administration: Inhalation 2311

Definition: Preparing and administering inhaled medications

M

Activities:
- Follow the five rights of medication administration
- Note patient's medical history and history of allergies
- Determine patient's knowledge of medication and understanding of method of administration
- Determine patient's ability to manipulate and administer medication
- Assist patient to use inhaler as prescribed
- Instruct patient on use of aerochamber (spacer) with the inhaler, as appropriate
- Shake inhaler
- Remove inhaler cap and hold inhaler upside down
- Assist patient to position inhaler in mouth or nose
- Instruct patient to tilt head back slightly and exhale completely
- Instruct patient to press down on inhaler to release medication while inhaling slowly
- Have patient take slow, deep breaths, with a brief end-inspiratory pause, and passive exhalation while using a nebulizer
- Have patient hold breath for 10 seconds, as appropriate
- Have patient exhale slowly through nose or pursed lips
- Instruct patient to repeat inhalations as ordered, waiting at least 1 minute between inhalations
- Instruct patient to wait between inhalations if two metered-dose inhalers are prescribed, per agency protocol
- Instruct patient in removing medication canister and cleaning inhaler in warm water
- Monitor patient's respirations and auscultate lungs, as appropriate
- Monitor for effects of medication and instruct patient and caregivers on desired effects and possible side effects of medication
- Teach and monitor self-administration technique, as appropriate
- Document medication administration and patient responsiveness, according to agency protocol

3rd edition 2000; revised 2004

Background Readings:
Craven, R. F., & Hirnle, C. J. (2003). Medication administration. In *Fundamentals of nursing: Human health and function* (4th ed., pp. 513–574). Philadelphia: Lippincott Williams & Wilkins.

Kozier, B., Erb, G., Berman, A., & Snyder, S. (2004). Medications. In *Fundamentals of nursing: Concepts, processes, and practice*. (7th ed., pp. 785–854). Upper Saddle River, NJ: Prentice Hall.

Naegle, M. A. (1999). Medication management. In G. M. Bulechek & J. C. McCloskey (Eds.), *Nursing interventions: Effective nursing treatments* (3rd ed., pp. 234–242). Philadelphia: Saunders.

Perry, A. G., & Potter, P. A. (2002). Clinical nursing skills & techniques (5th ed., pp. 436–452, 485–493). St. Louis: Mosby.

Rice, J. (2002). *Medications and mathematics for the nurse* (9th ed.). Albany, NY: Delmar.

Smeltzer, S. C., & Bare, B. G. (2004). Management of patients with chronic obstructive pulmonary disease. In *Brunner & Suddarth's textbook of medical surgical nursing* (Vol. 1) (10th ed., pp. 568–598). Philadelphia: Lippincott Williams & Wilkins.

Medication Administration: Interpleural 2302

Definition: Administration of medication through a catheter for diffusion within the pleural cavity

Activities:
- Follow agency policies and protocols for management and monitoring of interpleural catheters
- Follow the five rights of medication administration
- Note patient's medical history and history of allergies
- Determine patient's comfort level
- Instruct patient about the purpose, benefits, and rationale for use of the interpleural catheter and medication
- Monitor patient vital signs
- Maintain aseptic technique
- Affirm correct catheter placement with chest x-ray examination, as appropriate
- Monitor patient's pain before and after catheter insertion, as appropriate
- Aspirate interpleural catheter fluid before all injections of medication
- Check for no blood return before medication administration
- Observe aspirate for color and amount of return
- Withhold medication if more than 2 cc of fluid returns when checking interpleural catheter
- Prepare all medications aseptically
- Administer medication for pain relief through interpleural catheter intermittently or by continuous drip
- Position patient to avoid pressure on interpleural catheter
- Use monitoring modalities to interpret physiologic responses and initiate nursing interventions to ensure optimal patient care
- Monitor for shortness of breath or unequal or abnormal breath sounds
- Note any leakage that may occur from interpleural catheter
- Observe for pain relief, side effects, or adverse reactions from medication administered
- Connect catheter to medication administration pump, as appropriate
- Document medication administration in accordance with established agency policies
- Provide for the patient's total care needs while receiving analgesia, as needed
- Anticipate potential complications of the analgesia technique in relation to the device and medication(s) being used
- Recognize emergency situations and institute treatment in compliance with established agency policies, procedures, and guidelines
- Encourage early ambulation with the use of the interpleural catheter, as appropriate
- Change dressing, as appropriate
- Observe for signs and symptoms of infection at interpleural catheter insertion site
- Remove interpleural catheter as ordered and per agency policy

1st edition 1992; revised 2013

Background Readings:

Arkansas State Board of Nursing. (2010). Position statement 98-1: Administration of analgesia by specialized catheter (epidural, intrathecal, intrapleural). *ASBN Update, 14*(5), 24–25.

Pasero, C., Eksterowicz, N., Primeau, M., & Cowley, C. (2007). Registered nurse management and monitoring of analgesia by catheter techniques: Position statement. *Pain Management Nursing, 8*(2), 48–54.

Pasero, C., Eksterowicz, N., Primeau, M., & Cowley, C. (2008). The registered nurse's role in the management of analgesia by catheter techniques. *Journal of PeriAnesthesia Nursing, 23*(1), 53–56.

Shrestha, B. R., Tabadar, S., Maharjan, S., & Amatya, S. R. (2003). Interpleural catheter technique for perioperative pain management. *Kathmandu University Medical Journal, 1*(1), 46–47.

Weinberg, L., Scurrah, N., Parker, F., Story, D., & McNicol, L. (2010). Interpleural analgesia for attenuation of postoperative pain after hepatic resection. *Anaesthesia, 65*(7), 721–728.

Medication Administration: Intradermal 2312

Definition: Preparing and giving medications via the intradermal route

Activities:
- Follow the five rights of medication administration
- Note patient's medical history and history of allergies
- Determine patient's understanding of purpose of injection and skin testing
- Select correct needle and syringe based on type of injection
- Note expiration dates of drug
- Prepare dose correctly from ampule or vial
- Select appropriate injection site and inspect skin for bruises, inflammation, edema, lesions, or discoloration
- Use aseptic technique
- Insert needle at a 5- to 15-degree angle
- Inject medication slowly while watching for small bleb on skin surface
- Monitor patient for allergic reaction
- Mark injection site and read site at the appropriate interval after the injection (e.g., 48 to 72 hours)
- Monitor for expected effects of specific allergen or medication
- Document area of injection and appearance of skin at injection site
- Document appearance of injection site after the appropriate interval

3rd edition 2000

Background Readings:

Craven, R. F., & Hirnle, C. J. (2003). Medication administration. In *Fundamentals of nursing: Human health and function* (4th ed., pp. 513–574). Philadelphia: Lippincott Williams & Wilkins.

Kozier, B., Erb, G., Berman, A., & Snyder, S. (2004). Medications. In *Fundamentals of nursing: Concepts, processes, and practice*. (7th ed., pp. 785–854). Upper Saddle River, NJ: Prentice Hall.

Naegle, M. A. (1999). Medication management. In G. M. Bulechek & J. C. McCloskey (Eds.), *Nursing interventions: Effective nursing treatments* (3rd ed., pp. 234–242). Philadelphia: Saunders.

Perry, A. G., & Potter, P. A. (2002). *Clinical nursing skills & techniques* (5th ed., pp. 436–452, 519–522). St. Louis: Mosby.

Rice, J. (2002). *Medications and mathematics for the nurse* (9th ed.). Albany, NY: Delmar.

Medication Administration: Intramuscular (IM)   2313

Definition: Preparing and giving medications via the intramuscular route

Activities:
- Follow the five rights of medication administration
- Note patient's medical history and history of allergies
- Consider indications and contraindications for intramuscular injection
- Determine patient's knowledge of medication and understanding of method of administration
- Select correct needle and syringe based on patient and medication information
- Note expiration dates of drugs
- Prepare dose correctly from ampule, vial, or prefilled syringe
- Select appropriate injection site; palpate site for edema, masses, or tenderness; avoid areas of scarring, bruising, abrasion, or infection
- Position nondominant hand at proper anatomic landmark, spread skin tightly
- Administer injection using aseptic technique and proper protocol
- Inject needle quickly at a 90-degree angle
- Aspirate prior to injection; if no blood is aspirated, inject medication slowly, wait 10 seconds after injecting medication, then smoothly withdraw needle and release skin
- Apply gentle pressure at injection site; avoid massaging site
- Monitor patient for acute pain at injection site
- Monitor patient for sensory or motor alteration at or distal to injection site
- Monitor for expected and unexpected medication effects
- Discard mixed medications that are not properly labeled
- Document medication administration and patient responsiveness, according to agency protocol

3rd edition 2000; revised 2004

Background Readings:

Craven, R. F., & Hirnle, C. J. (2003). Medication administration. In *Fundamentals of nursing: Human health and function* (4th ed., pp. 513–574). Philadelphia: Lippincott Williams & Wilkins.

Kozier, B., Erb, G., Berman, A., & Snyder, S. (2004). Medications. In *Fundamentals of nursing: Concepts, processes, and practice.* (7th ed., pp. 785–854). Upper Saddle River, NJ: Prentice Hall.

Naegle, M. A. (1999). Medication management. In G. M. Bulechek & J. C. McCloskey (Eds.), *Nursing interventions: Effective nursing treatments* (3rd ed., pp. 234–242). Philadelphia: Saunders.

Perry, A. G., & Potter, P. A. (2002). *Clinical nursing skills & techniques* (5th ed., pp. 436–452, 528–534). St. Louis: Mosby.

M

Medication Administration: Intraosseous   2303

Definition: Insertion of a needle through the bone cortex into the medullary cavity for the purpose of short-term, emergency administration of fluid, blood, or medication

Activities:
- Follow the five rights of medication administration
- Note patient's medical history and history of allergies
- Determine patient's comfort level
- Determine patient's knowledge of medication and understanding of method of administration
- Immobilize the extremity
- Select an appropriate site for insertion by assessing landmarks to ensure proper needle placement away from the epiphyseal growth plate
- Assist with insertion of intraosseous lines
- Prepare the site with solution using aseptic technique
- Administer 1% lidocaine at insertion point, as appropriate
- Choose an appropriate size needle with a stylet (bone marrow biopsy/aspiration needle or 13- to 20-gauge rigid needle with stylet)
- Insert needle with stylet at 60- to 90-degree angle directed inferiorly
- Remove inner stylet, as necessary
- Aspirate for bone marrow content to confirm needle placement, according to agency protocol
- Flush needle with solution, according to agency protocol
- Secure needle in place with tape and apply appropriate dressing, according to agency protocol
- Connect tubing to needle and allow fluids to run by gravity or under pressure, as required by flow rate
- Anchor IV lines to extremity
- Identify compatibility of medications and fluids in infusion
- Determine flow rate, and adjust accordingly
- Monitor for signs and symptoms of extravasation of fluids or medications, infection, or fat embolism
- Document site, needle type and size, type of fluid and medication, flow rate, and patient response, as per agency protocol
- Report patient response to therapy, according to agency protocol
- Establish IV access and discontinue intraosseous line after patient condition stabilizes

2nd edition 1996; revised 2004

Background Readings:

Calkins, M. D., Fitzgerald, G., Bentley, T. B., & Burris, D. (2000). Intraosseous infusion devices: A comparison for potential use in special operations. *The Journal of Trauma: Injury, Infection, and Critical Care, 48*(6), 1068–1074.

Dubick, M. A. & Holcomb, J. B. (2000). A review of intraosseous vascular access: Current status and military application. *Military Medicine, 165*(7), 552–559.

Hurren, J. S. (2000). Can blood taken from intraosseous cannulations be used for blood analysis? *Burns, 26*(8), 727–730.

Miccolo, M. (1990). Intraosseous infusion. *Critical Care Nurse, 10*(10), 35–47.

Naegle, M. A. (1999). Medication management. In G. M. Bulechek & J. C. McCloskey (Eds.), *Nursing interventions: Effective nursing treatments* (3rd ed., pp. 234–242). Philadelphia: Saunders.

Medication Administration: Intraspinal 2319

Definition: Administration and monitoring of medication via an established epidural or intrathecal route

Activities:

- Follow the five rights of medication administration
- Note patient's medical history and history of allergies
- Determine patient's comfort level
- Determine patient's knowledge of medication and understanding of method of administration
- Monitor patient's vital signs
- Monitor neurological status
- Maintain aseptic technique
- Monitor patient's mobility, and motor and sensory functions, as appropriate
- Aspirate cerebral spinal fluid before injection of medication and evaluate for blood or cloudy returns prior to administering an intrathecal bolus injection
- Aspirate epidural catheter gently with an empty syringe, checking for a return of air only, prior to administering an epidural bolus injection
- Aseptically prepare preservative-free medication through filter needle
- Observe aspirate for amount and color of return
- Inject medication slowly per physician order, according to agency protocol
- Monitor epidural or intrathecal catheter insertion site for signs of infection
- Monitor dressing on epidural or intrathecal catheter insertion site for presence of clear drainage
- Notify physician if epidural or intrathecal dressing is wet
- Affirm catheter is secured to patient's skin
- Tape all tubing connections as appropriate
- Mark tubing as either intrathecal or epidural, as appropriate
- Check infusion pump for proper calibration and operation, per agency protocol
- Monitor IV set up, flow rate, and solution at regular intervals
- Monitor for central nervous system infection (e.g., fever, change in level of consciousness, nausea, and vomiting)
- Document medication administration and patient response, according to agency protocol

4th edition 2004

Background Readings:

Alpen, M. A. & Morse, C. (2001). Managing the pain of traumatic injury. *Critical Care Nursing Clinics of North America, 13*(2), 243–257.

Craven, R. F., & Hirnle, C. J. (2003). Pain perception and management. In *Fundamentals of nursing: Human health and function* (4th ed., pp. 1167–1198). Philadelphia: Lippincott Williams & Wilkins.

Francois, B., Vacher, P., Roustan, J., Salle, J. Y., Vidal, J., Moreau, J. J., et al. (2001). Intrathecal Baclofen after traumatic brain injury: Early treatment using a new technique to prevent spasticity. *The Journal of Trauma Injury, Infection, and Critical Care, 50*(1), 158–161.

Lehne, R. A. (2001). *Pharmacology for nursing care* (4th ed., p. 236). Philadelphia: Saunders.

Naegle, M. A. (1999). Medication management. In G. M. Bulechek & J. C. McCloskey (Eds.), *Nursing interventions: Effective nursing treatments* (3rd ed., pp. 234–242). Philadelphia: Saunders.

National Institutes of Health (2001). Living with cancer chemotherapy. http://www.cc.nih.gov/ccc/patient_education/CaTxeng/intrathec.pdf.

Smith S. F. & Duell, D. J. (1996). *Clinical nursing skills: Basic to advanced skills* (4th ed., pp. 426–427). Stamford, CT: Appleton & Lange.

Medication Administration: Intravenous (IV) 2314

Definition: Preparing and giving medications via the intravenous route

Activities:

- Follow the five rights of medication administration
- Note patient's medical history and history of allergies
- Determine patient's knowledge of medication and understanding of method of administration
- Check for IV drug incompatibilities
- Note expiration date of drugs and solutions
- Set up proper equipment for medication administration
- Prepare the appropriate concentration of IV medication from ampule or vial
- Verify placement and patency of IV catheter within vein
- Maintain sterility of patent IV system
- Administer IV medication at the appropriate rate
- Mix solution gently if adding medication to IV fluid container
- Select injection port of IV tubing closest to patient, occlude IV line above port, and aspirate prior to injecting intravenous bolus into an existing line
- Flush intravenous lock with appropriate solution before and after medication administration, as per agency protocol
- Complete medication additive label and apply to IV fluid container, as appropriate
- Maintain IV access, as appropriate
- Monitor patient to determine response to medication
- Monitor IV set up, flow rate, and solution at regular intervals, per agency protocol
- Monitor for infiltration and phlebitis at infusion site
- Document medication administration and patient responsiveness, according to agency protocol

3rd edition 2000; revised 2004

Background Readings:

Craven, R. F., & Hirnle, C. J. (2003). Intravenous therapy. In *Fundamentals of nursing: Human health and function* (4th ed., pp. 575–610). Philadelphia: Lippincott Williams & Wilkins.

Kozier, B., Erb, G., Berman, A., & Snyder, S. (2004). Fluid, electrolytes, and acid-base balance. In *Fundamentals of nursing: Concepts, processes, and practice.* (7th ed., pp. 1351–1409). Upper Saddle River, NJ: Prentice Hall.

Naegle, M. A. (1999). Medication management. In G. M. Bulechek & J. C. McCloskey (Eds.), *Nursing interventions: Effective nursing treatments* (3rd ed., pp. 234–242). Philadelphia: Saunders.

Perry, A. G., & Potter, P. A. (2002). *Clinical nursing skills & techniques* (5th ed., pp. 436–452, 534–551). St. Louis: Mosby.

Rice, J. (2002). *Medications and mathematics for the nurse* (9th ed.). Albany, NY: Delmar.

M

Medication Administration: Nasal 2320

Definition: Preparing and giving medications via nasal passages

Activities:

- Follow the five rights of medication administration
- Note patient's medical history and history of allergies
- Determine patient's knowledge of medication and understanding of method of administration
- Instruct patient to blow nose gently prior to administration of nasal medication, unless contraindicated
- Assist patient to supine position and position head appropriately, depending on which sinuses are to be medicated when administering nose drops
- Instruct patient to breathe through mouth during administration when administering nose drops
- Hold dropper 1 cm above nares and instill prescribed number of drops
- Instruct patient to remain supine for 5 minutes after administering nose drops
- Instruct patient to remain upright and to not tilt head backward when administering nasal spray
- Insert nozzle into nostril and squeeze bottle quickly and firmly when administering nasal spray
- Instruct patient not to blow nose for several minutes after administration
- Monitor patient to determine response to medication
- Document medication administration and patient response, according to agency protocol

4th edition 2004

Background Readings:

Craven, R. F., & Hirnle, C. J. (2003). Medication administration. In *Fundamentals of nursing: Human health and function* (4th ed., pp. 513–574). Philadelphia: Lippincott Williams & Wilkins.

Kozier, B., Erb, G., Berman, A., & Snyder, S. (2004). Medications. In *Fundamentals of nursing: Concepts, processes, and practice.* (7th ed., pp. 785–854). Upper Saddle River, NJ: Prentice Hall.

Naegle, M. A. (1999). Medication management. In G. M. Bulechek & J. C. McCloskey (Eds.), *Nursing interventions: Effective nursing treatments* (3rd ed., pp. 234–242). Philadelphia: Saunders.

Perry, A. G., & Potter, P. A. (2002). *Clinical nursing skills & techniques* (5th ed., pp. 436–452, 482–485). St. Louis: Mosby.

Medication Administration: Oral 2304

M

Definition: Preparing and giving medications by mouth

Activities:

- Follow the five rights of medication administration
- Note patient's medical history and history of allergies
- Determine patient's knowledge of medication and understanding of method of administration
- Determine any contraindications to patient receiving oral medication (e.g., difficulty swallowing, nausea/vomiting, bowel inflammation, reduced peristalsis, recent gastrointestinal surgery, attached to gastric suction, NPO, decreased level of consciousness)
- Check for possible drug interactions and contraindications
- Ensure that hypnotics, narcotics, and antibiotics are either discontinued or reordered on their renewal date
- Note the expiration date on the medication container
- Give medications on an empty stomach or with food, as appropriate
- Mix offensive-tasting medications with food or fluids, as appropriate
- Mix medication with flavored syrup from the pharmacy, as appropriate
- Crush medication and mix with small amount of soft food (e.g., applesauce), as appropriate
- Inform patient of expected actions and possible adverse effects of medications
- Instruct patient of proper administration of sublingual medication
- Place sublingual medications under the patient's tongue and instruct not to swallow the pill
- Have client place buccal medication in mouth against mucous membranes of the cheek until it dissolves
- Instruct the patient not to eat or drink until the sublingual or buccal medication is completely dissolved
- Assist patient with ingestion of medications, as appropriate
- Monitor patient for possible aspiration, as appropriate
- Perform mouth checks after delivery of medications, as appropriate
- Instruct the patient or family member on how to administer the medication
- Monitor patient for therapeutic effects, adverse effects, drug toxicity, and drug interactions
- Document medications administered and patient responsiveness, according to agency protocol

1st edition 1992; revised 2000, 2004

Background Readings:

Craven, R. F., & Hirnle, C. J. (2003). Medication administration. In *Fundamentals of nursing: Human health and function* (4th ed., pp. 513–574). Philadelphia: Lippincott Williams & Wilkins.

Kozier, B., Erb, G., Berman, A., & Snyder, S. (2004). Medications. In *Fundamentals of nursing: Concepts, processes, and practice.* (7th ed., pp. 785–854). Upper Saddle River, NJ: Prentice Hall.

Naegle, M. A. (1999). Medication management. In G. M. Bulechek & J. C. McCloskey (Eds.), *Nursing interventions: Effective nursing treatments* (3rd ed., pp. 234–242). Philadelphia: Saunders.

Perry, A. G., & Potter, P. A. (2002). *Clinical nursing skills & techniques* (5th ed., pp. 436–452, 455–461). St. Louis: Mosby.

Rice, J. (2002). *Medications and mathematics for the nurse* (9th ed.). Albany, NY: Delmar.

Medication Administration: Rectal 2315

Definition: Preparing and inserting rectal suppositories

Activities:
- Follow the five rights of medication administration
- Note patient's medical history and history of allergies
- Determine patient's knowledge of medication and understanding of method of administration
- Review medical record for history of rectal surgery or bleeding
- Determine for any presenting signs and symptoms of gastrointestinal alterations (e.g., constipation or diarrhea)
- Determine patient's ability to retain suppository
- Assist patient to left side-lying Sim position with upper leg flexed upward
- Lubricate gloved index finger of dominant hand and rounded end of suppository
- Instruct patient to take slow deep breaths through mouth and to relax anal sphincter
- Insert suppository gently through anus, past internal anal sphincter, and against rectal wall
- Instruct patient to remain flat or on side for 5 minutes
- Monitor for effects of medication
- Teach and monitor self-administration technique as appropriate
- Document medication administration and patient responsiveness according to agency protocol

3rd edition 2000; revised 2004

Background Readings:

Craven, R. F., & Hirnle, C. J. (2003). Medication administration. In *Fundamentals of nursing: Human health and function* (4th ed., pp. 513–574). Philadelphia: Lippincott Williams & Wilkins.

Kozier, B., Erb, G., Berman, A., & Snyder, S. (2004). Medications. In *Fundamentals of nursing: Concepts, processes, and practice*. (7th ed., pp. 785–854). Upper Saddle River, NJ: Prentice Hall.

Naegle, M. A. (1999). Medication management. In G. M. Bulechek & J. C. McCloskey (Eds.), *Nursing interventions: Effective nursing treatments* (3rd ed., pp. 234–242). Philadelphia: Saunders.

Perry, A. G., & Potter, P. A. (2002). *Clinical nursing skills & techniques* (5th ed., pp. 436–452, 498–501). St. Louis: Mosby.

Rice, J. (2002). *Medications and mathematics for the nurse* (9th ed.). Albany, NY: Delmar.

Medication Administration: Skin 2316

Definition: Preparing and applying medications to the skin

Activities:
- Follow the five rights of medication administration
- Note patient's medical history and history of allergies
- Determine patient's knowledge of medication and understanding of method of administration
- Determine patient's skin condition over area that medication will be applied
- Remove previous dose of medication and cleanse skin
- Measure the correct amount of topically applied systemic medications, using standardized measurement devices
- Apply topical agent as prescribed
- Apply transdermal patches and topical medications to non-hairy areas of the skin, as appropriate
- Spread the medication evenly over the skin, as appropriate
- Rotate application sites of topical systemic medications
- Monitor for local, systemic, and adverse effects of the medication
- Teach and monitor self-administration techniques, as appropriate
- Document medication administration and patient responsiveness, according to agency protocol

3rd edition 2000

Background Readings:

Craven, R. F., & Hirnle, C. J. (2003). Medication administration. In *Fundamentals of nursing: Human health and function* (4th ed., pp. 513–574). Philadelphia: Lippincott Williams & Wilkins.

Kozier, B., Erb, G., Berman, A., & Snyder, S. (2004). Medications. In *Fundamentals of nursing: Concepts, processes, and practice*. (7th ed., pp. 785–854). Upper Saddle River, NJ: Prentice Hall.

Naegle, M. A. (1999). Medication management. In G. M. Bulechek & J. C. McCloskey (Eds.), *Nursing interventions: Effective nursing treatments* (3rd ed., pp. 234–242). Philadelphia: Saunders.

Perry, A. G., & Potter, P. A. (2002). *Clinical nursing skills & techniques* (5th ed., pp. 436–452, 465–469). St. Louis: Mosby.

Medication Administration: Subcutaneous 2317

Definition: Preparing and giving medications via the subcutaneous route

Activities:
- Follow the five rights of medication administration
- Note patient's medical history and history of allergies
- Determine patient's knowledge of medication and understanding of method of administration
- Consider indications and contraindications for subcutaneous injection
- Note expiration dates of drugs
- Select correct needle and syringe based on patient and medication information
- Prepare dose correctly from ampule or vial
- Select appropriate injection site
- Rotate insulin injection sites systematically within one anatomic region
- Palpate injection site for edema, masses, or tenderness; avoid areas of scarring, bruising, abrasion, or infection
- Use abdominal sites when administering heparin subcutaneously
- Administer injection using aseptic technique
- Inject needle quickly at a 45- to 90-degree angle depending on size of patient
- Apply gentle pressure to site; avoid massaging site
- Monitor for expected and unexpected medication effects
- Educate patient, family member, and or significant other regarding injection technique
- Document medication administration and patient responsiveness, according to agency protocol

3rd edition 2000; revised 2004

Background Readings:

Craven, R. F., & Hirnle, C. J. (2003). Medication administration. In *Fundamentals of nursing: Human health and function* (4th ed., pp. 513–574). Philadelphia: Lippincott Williams & Wilkins.

Kozier, B., Erb, G., Berman, A., & Snyder, S. (2004). Medications. In *Fundamentals of nursing: Concepts, processes, and practice.* (7th ed., pp. 785–854). Upper Saddle River, NJ: Prentice Hall.

Naegle, M. A. (1999). Medication management. In G. M. Bulechek & J. C. McCloskey (Eds.), *Nursing interventions: Effective nursing treatments* (3rd ed., pp. 234–242). Philadelphia: Saunders.

Perry, A. G., & Potter, P. A. (2002). *Clinical nursing skills & techniques* (5th ed., pp. 436–452, 523–528). St. Louis: Mosby.

Rice, J. (2002). *Medications and mathematics for the nurse* (9th ed.). Albany, NY: Delmar.

M

Medication Administration: Vaginal 2318

Definition: Preparing and inserting vaginal medications

Activities:
- Follow the five rights of medication administration
- Note patient's medical history and history of allergies
- Determine patient's knowledge of medication and understanding of method of administration
- Have client void prior to administration
- Apply water-soluble lubricant to rounded end of suppository; lubricate gloved index finger of dominant hand
- Insert rounded end of suppository along posterior wall of vaginal canal 3 to 4 inches or insert applicator approximately 2 to 3 inches
- Instruct patient to remain on her back for at least 10 minutes
- Maintain good perineal hygiene
- Monitor for effects of medication
- Teach and monitor self-administration technique, as appropriate
- Document medication administration and patient responsiveness, according to agency protocol

3rd edition 2000; revised 2004

Background Readings:

Craven, R. F., & Hirnle, C. J. (2003). Medication administration. In *Fundamentals of nursing: Human health and function* (4th ed., pp. 513–574). Philadelphia: Lippincott Williams & Wilkins.

Kozier, B., Erb, G., Berman, A., & Snyder, S. (2004). Medications. In *Fundamentals of nursing: Concepts, processes, and practice.* (7th ed., pp. 785–854). Upper Saddle River, NJ: Prentice Hall.

Naegle, M. A. (1999). Medication management. In G. M. Bulechek & J. C. McCloskey (Eds.), *Nursing interventions: Effective nursing treatments* (3rd ed., pp. 234–242). Philadelphia: Saunders.

Perry, A. G., & Potter, P. A. (2002). *Clinical nursing skills & techniques* (5th ed., pp. 436–452, 494–498). St. Louis: Mosby.

Medication Administration: Ventricular Reservoir 2307

Definition: Administration and monitoring of medication through an indwelling catheter into the lateral ventricle of the brain

Activities:
- Follow the five rights of medication administration
- Note patient's medical history and history of allergies
- Determine patient's comfort level
- Determine patient's knowledge of medication and understanding of method of administration
- Monitor neurological status
- Monitor vital signs
- Maintain aseptic technique
- Shave hair over reservoir, as per agency protocol
- Fill reservoir with cerebral spinal fluid by applying pressure gently with index finger
- Collect cerebral spinal fluid specimen, as appropriate, per order or agency protocol
- Aspirate cerebral spinal fluid before injection of medication and evaluate for blood or cloudy returns
- Inject medication slowly, per physician order and according to agency protocol
- Apply pressure with index finger to reservoir to ensure mixing of medication with cerebral spinal fluid
- Apply dressing to site, as appropriate
- Monitor for central nervous system infection (e.g., fever, change in level of consciousness, nausea, and vomiting)
- Document medication administration and patient response, according to agency protocol

2nd edition 1996; revised 2000, 2004

Background Readings:
Access device guidelines: Catheters module; cancer chemotherapy guidelines. (1998). Pittsburgh, PA: Oncology Nursing Society.

Almadrones, L., Campana, P., & Dantis, E. C. (1995). Arterial, peritoneal, and intraventricular access devices. *Seminars in Oncology Nursing, 11*(3), 194–202.

Craig, C. (2000). Current treatment approaches for neoplastic meningitis: Nursing management of patients receiving Depocyt. *Oncology Nursing Forum, 27*(8), 1225–1230.

Cummings, R. (1992). Understanding external ventricular drainage. *Journal of Neuroscience Nursing, 24*(2), 84–87.

Naegle, M. A. (1999). Medication management. In G. M. Bulechek & J. C. McCloskey (Eds.), *Nursing interventions: Effective nursing treatments* (3rd ed., pp. 234–242). Philadelphia: Saunders.

M

Medication Management 2380

Definition: Facilitation of safe and effective use of prescription and over-the-counter drugs

Activities:
- Determine what drugs are needed, and administer according to prescriptive authority and/or protocol
- Discuss financial concerns related to medication regimen
- Determine patient's ability to self-medicate, as appropriate
- Monitor effectiveness of the medication administration modality
- Monitor patient for the therapeutic effect of the medication
- Monitor for signs and symptoms of drug toxicity
- Monitor for adverse effects of the drug
- Monitor serum blood levels (e.g., electrolytes, prothrombin, medications), as appropriate
- Monitor for nontherapeutic drug interactions
- Review periodically with the patient and/or family the types and amounts of medications taken
- Discard old, discontinued, or contraindicated medications, as appropriate
- Facilitate changes in medication with physician, as appropriate
- Monitor for response to changes in medication regimen, as appropriate
- Determine the patient's knowledge about medication
- Monitor adherence with medication regimen
- Determine factors that may preclude the patient from taking drugs as prescribed
- Develop strategies with the patient to enhance compliance with prescribed medication regimen
- Consult with other health care professionals to minimize the number and frequency of drugs needed for a therapeutic effect
- Teach patient and/or family members the method of drug administration, as appropriate
- Teach patient and/or family members the expected action and side effects of the medication
- Provide patient and family members with written and visual information to enhance self-administration of medications, as appropriate
- Develop strategies to manage side effects of drugs
- Obtain physician order for patient self-medication, as appropriate
- Establish a protocol for the storage, restocking, and monitoring of medications left at the bedside for self-medication purposes
- Investigate possible financial resources for acquisition of prescribed drugs, as appropriate
- Determine impact of medication use on patient's lifestyle
- Provide alternatives for timing and modality of self-administered medications to minimize lifestyle effects
- Assist the patient and family members in making necessary lifestyle adjustments associated with certain medications, as appropriate
- Instruct patient when to seek medical attention
- Identify types and amounts of over-the-counter drugs used
- Provide information about the use of over-the-counter drugs and how they may influence the existing condition
- Determine whether the patient is using culturally-based home health remedies and the possible effects on use of over-the-counter and prescribed medications
- Review with the patient strategies for managing medication regimen
- Provide patient with a list of resources to contact for further information about the medication regimen

- Contact patient and family postdischarge, as appropriate, to answer questions and discuss concerns associated with the medication regimen
- Encourage the patient to have screening tests to determine medication effects

1st edition 1992; revised 1996, 2000, 2004

Background Readings:

Abrams, A. C., Pennington, S. S., & Lammon, C. B. (2007). *Clinical drug therapy: Rationales for nursing practice* (8th ed.). Philadelphia: Lippincott Williams & Wilkins.

Craven, R. F., & Hirnle, C. J. (2003). Medication administration. In *Fundamentals of nursing: Human health and function* (4th ed., pp. 513–574). Philadelphia: Lippincott Williams & Wilkins.

Le Sage, J. (1991). Polypharmacy in geriatric patients. *Nursing Clinics of North America, 26*(2), 273–290.

Malseed, R. T. (1990). *Pharmacology drug therapy and nursing considerations* (3rd ed.). Philadelphia: Lippincott.

Mathewson, M. J. (1986). *Pharmacotherapeutics: A nursing approach.* Philadelphia: F. A. Davis.

Weitzel, E. A. (1992). Medication management. In G. M. Bulechek & J. C. McCloskey (Eds.), *Nursing Interventions: Essential nursing treatments* (2nd ed., pp. 213–220). Philadelphia: Saunders.

Medication Prescribing 2390

Definition: Prescribing medication for a health problem

Activities:

- Evaluate signs and symptoms of current health problem
- Determine past health history and medication use
- Identify known allergies
- Determine patient's/family's ability to administer medication
- Identify medications that are indicated for current problems
- Prescribe medications according to prescriptive authority and/or protocol
- Write prescription, using name of medication and including dose and directions for administration
- Spell out problematic abbreviations that are easily misunderstood (e.g., micrograms, milligrams, units)
- Verify that decimal points used in dosages are clearly seen by using leading zeros (e.g., 0.2 vs. .2)
- Avoid the use of trailing zeros (e.g., 2 vs. 2.0)
- Utilize electronic prescribing methods, as available
- Utilize standardized abbreviations, acronyms, and symbols
- Verify that all medication orders are written accurately, completely, and with the necessary discrimination for their intended use
- Follow recommendations for starting doses of medication (e.g., milligrams per kilogram body weight, body surface area, or lowest effective dose)
- Consult with physician or pharmacist, as appropriate
- Consult *Physician's Desk Reference* and other references, as necessary
- Consult with representatives from drug companies, as appropriate
- Teach patient and/or family members the method of drug administration, as appropriate
- Teach patient and/or family members the expected action and side effects of the medication
- Provide alternatives for timing and modality of self-administered medications to minimize lifestyle effects
- Instruct patient and family about how to fill prescription, as necessary
- Instruct patient/family when to seek additional assistance
- Monitor for the therapeutic and adverse effects of the medication, as appropriate
- Maintain knowledge of medications used in practice, including indications for use, precautions, adverse effects, toxic effects, and dosing information, as required by prescriptive authority rules and regulations

2nd edition 1996; revised 2004

Background Readings:

Anonymous. (2001). ARNP prescriptive authority rules approved at joint meeting. *Washington Nurse, 31*(2), 24.

Anonymous. (2001). Issue: Nurses impact 2001: Recognizing nursing's independent license: Prescriptive authority for APNs. *Michigan Nurse, 74*(Suppl. 3), 13–14.

Freeman, G. (Ed.). (2002). Medication errors related to poor communications. *Healthcare Risk Management, 24*(1), 9–10.

Talley, S. & Richens, S. (2001). Prescribing practices of advanced practice psychiatric nurses: Part 1—demographic, educational, and practice characteristics. *Archives of Psychiatric Nursing, 15*(5), 205–213.

Woodbridge, H. B. (1998). Basics of prescription writing. In R. E. Rakel, *Essentials of family practice* (2nd ed., pp. 166–171). Philadelphia: Saunders.

Medication Reconciliation 2395

Definition: Comparison of the patient's home medications with the admission, transfer, and/or discharge orders to ensure accuracy and patient safety

Activities:
- Use a standardized tool to elicit all medication information, including prescribed medications, over-the-counter medications, and dietary and herbal supplements
- Obtain a complete medication history by examining medication vials or list, verifying with patient and family, and/or communicating with physicians and pharmacy, as needed
- Document drug name, dosage, frequency, and route on medication list
- Determine when medications were last taken
- Compare medication list to indications and medical history to ensure list is accurate and complete
- Reconcile medications at all transition points including admission, transfer, and discharge
- Reconcile medications with changes in patient condition or with medication changes
- Communicate discrepancies to ordering practitioners, as needed
- Instruct patient and family to maintain an updated medication list and reconcile with physician at each appointment or hospital admission
- Instruct patient and family to obtain all medications though one pharmacy to decrease risk of error
- Instruct patient and family to take an active role in medication management

5th edition 2008

Background Readings:
Gleason, K., Groszek, J., Sullivan, C., Barnard, C., & Noskin, G. (2004). Reconciliation of discrepancies in medication histories and admission orders of newly hospitalized patients. *American Journal of Health System Pharmacy, 61*(16), 1689–1695.
Manno, M., & Hayes, D. (2006). How medication reconciliation saves lives. *Nursing, 36*(3), 63–64.
Sullivan, C., Gleason, K., Rooney, D., Groszek, J., & Barnard, C. (2005). Medication reconciliation in the acute care setting. *Journal of Nursing Care Quality, 20*(2), 95–98.
Thompson, C. (2005). JCAHO views medication reconciliation as adverse-event prevention. *American Journal of Health System Pharmacy, 62*(15), 1528–1530.
Young, D. (2005). IMO panel reviews lessons for medication safety. *American Journal of Health System Pharmacy, 62*(13), 1340–1341.

M

Meditation Facilitation 5960

Definition: Facilitating a person to alter his/her level of awareness by focusing specifically on an image or thought

Activities:
- Prepare a quiet environment
- Instruct patient to sit quietly in a comfortable position
- Instruct patient to close eyes if desirable
- Instruct patient to relax all muscles and remain relaxed
- Assist patient to select a mental device for repetition during procedure (e.g., repeating a word such as "one")
- Instruct patient to say the mental device silently to self while breathing out through the nose
- Continue with the breathing exercise, focusing on the mental device chosen (e.g., "one") as long as needed or desired
- When finished, instruct patient to sit quietly for several minutes with eyes open
- Inform patient to ignore distracting thoughts by returning to the mental device being used
- Inform patient to perform the procedure once or twice daily, but not within 2 hours after meals

Background Readings:
Craven, R. F., & Hirnle, C. J. (2003). Health and wellness. In *Fundamentals of nursing: Human health and function* (4th ed., pp. 255–266). Philadelphia: Lippincott Williams & Wilkins.
Graves, P., & Lancaster, J. (1992). Stress management and crisis intervention. In M. Stanhope, & J. Lancaster (Eds.), *Community health nursing* (3rd ed., pp. 612–631). St. Louis: Mosby.
Kozier, B., Erb, G., Berman, A., & Snyder, S. (2004). Complementary and alternative healing modalities. In *Fundamentals of nursing: Concepts, processes, and practice.* (7th ed., pp. 223–243). Upper Saddle River, NJ: Prentice Hall.
McCaffery, M., & Beebe, A. (1989). *Pain: Clinical manual for nursing practice* (pp. 194, 202–203). St. Louis: Mosby.

1st edition 1992; revised 2000

Memory Training 4760

Definition: Facilitation of memory

Activities:

- Discuss with patient/family any practical memory problems experienced
- Stimulate memory by repeating patient's last expressed thought, as appropriate
- Reminisce about past experiences with patient, as appropriate
- Implement appropriate memory techniques, such as visual imagery, mnemonic devices, memory games, memory cues, association techniques, making lists, using computers, using name tags, or rehearsing information
- Assist in associate-learning tasks, such as practice learning and recalling verbal and pictorial information presented, as appropriate
- Provide for orientation training, such as patient rehearsing personal information and dates, as appropriate
- Provide opportunity for concentration, such as a game matching pairs of cards, as appropriate
- Provide opportunity to use memory for recent events, such as questioning patient about a recent outing, as appropriate
- Guide new learning, such as locating geographical features on a map, as appropriate
- Provide for picture recognition memory, as appropriate
- Structure the teaching methods according to patient's organization of information
- Refer to occupational therapy, as appropriate
- Encourage patient to participate in group memory training programs, as appropriate
- Monitor patient's behavior during therapy
- Identify and correct the patient errors in orientation
- Monitor changes in memory with training

1st edition 1992; revised 2004

Background Readings:

Craven, R. F., & Hirnle, C. J. (2003). Cognitive process. In *Fundamentals of nursing: Human health and function* (4th ed., pp. 1219–1252). Philadelphia: Lippincott Williams & Wilkins.

Drofman, D. R., & Ager, C. L. (1989). Memory and memory training: Some treatment implications for use with the well elderly. *Physical and Occupational Therapy in Geriatrics, 7*(3), 21–41.

Godfrey, H. P., & Knight, R. G. (1988). Memory training and behavioral rehabilitation of a severely head-injured adult. *Archives of Physical and Medical Rehabilitation, 69*(6), 458–460.

Schmidt, I. W., Dijkstra, H. T., Berg, I. J., Deelman, B. G. (1999). Memory training for remembering names in older adults. *Clinical Gerontologist, 20*(2), 57–73.

Schmidt, I. W., Berg, I. J., Deelman, B. G. (2000). Memory training for remembering texts in older adults. *Clinical Gerontologist, 21*(4), 67–90.

M

Milieu Therapy 4390

Definition: Use of people, resources, and events in the patient's immediate environment to promote optimal psychosocial functioning

Activities:

- Determine factors in environment that contribute to patient's behavior
- Consider needs of others in addition to needs of particular individual
- Make resources necessary for self-care available
- Enhance the normality of the environment through use of clocks, calendars, railings, furniture, and so on
- Facilitate open communication between patient, nurses, and other staff
- Include patient in decisions about own care
- Write behavioral expectations and agreements for the patient's and others' reference, when appropriate
- Provide one-on-one nursing care, as appropriate
- Support formal and informal group activities to promote sharing, cooperation, compromise, and leadership
- Examine own attitudes toward issues of patients' rights, self-determination, social control, and deviancy
- Ensure staff presence and supervision
- Minimize restrictions that diminish privacy or self-control (autonomy)
- Encourage use of personal property
- Minimize, as much as possible, the use of locked doors, medications, and strict regulations of activity or property
- Provide a telephone in a private space
- Provide attractively furnished areas for private conversations with other patients, family, and friends
- Provide books, magazines, and arts and crafts materials in accordance with patient's recreational, cultural, and educational background and needs
- Monitor individual behavior that may be disruptive or detrimental to overall well-being of others
- Limit the number of unmedicated psychotic patients at any time through controlled admissions and varying lengths of medication-free trials, as appropriate

1st edition 1992; revised 1996

Background Readings:

Boyd, M. A. (2005). Psychiatric-mental health nursing interventions. In M. A. Boyd (Ed.), *Psychiatric nursing: Contemporary practice* (3rd ed., pp. 218–232). Philadelphia: Lippincott Williams & Wilkins.

Love, C. C., & Buckwalter, K. (1991). Reactive depression. In M. Maas, K. Buckwalter, & M. Hardy (Eds.), *Nursing diagnoses and interventions for the elderly* (pp. 419–432). Redwood City, CA: Addison-Wesley.

Wilson, H. S., & Kneisl, C. R. (1992). *Psychiatric nursing* (4th ed.). Redwood City, CA: Addison-Wesley.

Mood Management

Definition: Providing for safety, stabilization, recovery, and maintenance of a patient who is experiencing dysfunctionally depressed or elevated mood

Activities:

- Evaluate mood (e.g., signs, symptoms, personal history) initially, and on a regular basis, as treatment progresses
- Administer self-report questionnaires (e.g., Beck Depression Inventory, functional status scales), as appropriate
- Determine whether patient presents safety risk to self or others
- Consider hospitalization of the mood-disordered patient who poses a safety risk, is unable to meet his or her self-care needs, and/or lacks social support
- Initiate necessary precautions to safeguard the patient or others at risk for physical harm (e.g., suicide, self-harm, elopement, violence)
- Provide or refer a patient for substance abuse treatment, if substance abuse is a factor contributing to the mood disorder
- Adjust or discontinue medications that may be contributing to mood disorders (e.g., per appropriately licensed advanced practice nurses)
- Refer patient for evaluation and/or treatment of any underlying medical illness that may be contributing to a dysfunctional mood (e.g., thyroid disorders, etc.)
- Monitor self-care ability (e.g., grooming, hygiene, food/fluid intake, elimination)
- Assist with self-care, as needed
- Monitor physical status of patient (e.g., body weight and hydration)
- Monitor and regulate level of activity and stimulation in environment in accord with patient's needs
- Assist patient to maintain a normal cycle of sleep/wakefulness (e.g., scheduled rest times, relaxation techniques, sedating medications, limit caffeine)
- Assist patient to assume increasing responsibility for self-care as he or she is able to do so
- Provide opportunity for physical activity (e.g., walking, riding the exercise bike)
- Monitor cognitive functioning (e.g., concentration, attention, memory, ability to process information, and decision-making ability)
- Use simple, concrete, here-and-now language during interactions with the cognitively compromised patient
- Use memory aides and visual cues to assist the cognitively compromised patient
- Limit decision-making opportunities for the cognitively compromised patient
- Teach patient decision-making skills, as needed
- Encourage patient to engage in increasingly more complex decision making as he or she is able
- Encourage patient to take an active role in treatment and rehabilitation, as appropriate
- Provide or refer for psychotherapy (e.g., cognitive behavioral, interpersonal, marital, family, group), when appropriate
- Interact with the patient at regular intervals to convey caring and/or to provide an opportunity for patient to talk about feelings
- Assist patient to consciously monitor mood (e.g., 1 to 10 rating scale, journaling)
- Assist patient to identify thoughts and feelings underlying the dysfunctional mood
- Limit amount of time that patient is allowed to express negative feelings and/or accounts of past failures
- Assist patient to ventilate feelings in an appropriate manner (e.g., punching bag, art therapy, and vigorous physical activity)
- Assist patient to identify precipitants of dysfunctional mood (e.g., chemical imbalances, situational stressors, grief/loss, and physical problems)

- Assist patient to identify aspects of precipitants that can/cannot be changed
- Assist in identification of available resources and personal strengths/abilities that can be used in modifying the precipitants of dysfunctional mood
- Teach new coping and problem-solving skills
- Encourage the patient, as he/she can tolerate, to engage in social interactions and activities with others
- Provide social skills and/or assertiveness training, as needed
- Provide the patient with feedback regarding the appropriateness of his or her social behaviors
- Utilize limit setting and behavioral management strategies to assist the manic patient to refrain from intrusive and disruptive behavior
- Utilize restrictive interventions (e.g., area restriction, seclusion, physical restraint, chemical restraint) to manage unsafe or inappropriate behavior that is not responsive to less restrictive behavior management interventions
- Manage and treat hallucinations and/or delusions that may accompany the mood disorder
- Prescribe, adjust, and discontinue medications used to treat the dysfunctional mood (e.g., per appropriately licensed advanced practice nurse)
- Administer mood-stabilizing medications (e.g., antidepressants, lithium, anticonvulsants, antipsychotics, anxiolytics, hormones, and vitamins)
- Monitor patient for medication side effects and impact on mood
- Treat and/or manage medication side effects or adverse drug reactions from medications used to treat mood disorders
- Draw and monitor serum blood levels of medications (e.g., tricyclic antidepressants, lithium, anticonvulsants), as appropriate
- Monitor and promote the patient's medication compliance
- Assist physician with the provision of electroconvulsive therapy (ECT) treatments, when they are indicated
- Monitor the physiological and mental status of the patient immediately after ECT
- Assist with the provision of "phototherapy" to elevate mood
- Provide procedural teaching to patient and significant others of patient who is receiving ECT or phototherapy
- Monitor patient's mood for response to ECT or phototherapy
- Provide medication teaching to patient/significant others
- Provide illness teaching to patient/significant others, if dysfunctional mood is illness based (e.g., depression, mania, and premenstrual syndrome)
- Provide guidance about development and maintenance of support systems (e.g., family, friends, spiritual resources, support groups, and counseling)
- Assist patient to anticipate and cope with life changes (e.g., new job, leave of absence from work, new peer group)
- Provide outpatient follow-up at appropriate intervals, as needed

2nd edition 1996; revised 2000

Background Readings:

Chitty, C. K. (1996). Clients with mood disorders. In H. S. Wilson & C. R. Kneisel (Eds.), *Psychiatric nursing* (pp. 323–359). Redwood City, CA: Addison-Wesley.

Fortinash, K. M., & Holoday-Worret, P. A. (1995). Mood disorders. In K. M. Fortinash & P. A. Holoday-Worret (Eds.), *Psychiatric nursing care plans* (pp. 48–73). St. Louis: Mosby.

Hagerty, B. (1996). Mood disorders: Depression and mania. In K. M. Fortinash & P. A. Holoday-Worret (Eds.), *Psychiatric mental health nursing* (pp. 251–283). St. Louis: Mosby.

McFarland, G. K., Wasli, E., & Gerety, E. K. (1997). Mood disorders. In G. K. McFarland, E. Wasli, & E. K. Gerety (Eds.), *Nursing diagnoses and process in psychiatric mental health nursing* (pp. 243–262). Philadelphia: Lippincott.

Schultz, J. M., & Videbeck, S. D. (1998). *Lippincott's manual of psychiatric nursing care plans*. Philadelphia: Lippincott Williams & Wilkins.

Stuart, G. (1998). Emotional responses and mood disorders. In G. W. Stuart & S. J. Sundeen (Eds.), *Principles and practice of psychiatric nursing* (6th ed., pp. 413–451). St. Louis: Mosby.

Tommasini, N. R. (1995). The client with a mood disorder (depression). In D. Antai-Otong & G. Kongable (Eds.), *Psychiatric nursing: Biological and behavioral concepts* (pp. 157–189). Philadelphia: Saunders.

Wood, S. J. (2005). Mood disorders. In M. A. Boyd (Ed.), *Psychiatric nursing: Contemporary practice* (3rd ed., pp. 333–373). Philadelphia: Lippincott Williams & Wilkins.

Multidisciplinary Care Conference

8020

Definition: Planning and evaluating patient care with health professionals from other disciplines

Activities:

- Summarize health status data pertinent to patient care planning
- Identify current nursing diagnoses
- Describe nursing interventions being implemented
- Describe patient and family response to nursing interventions
- Seek input about effectiveness of nursing interventions
- Discuss progress toward goals
- Revise patient care plan, as necessary
- Solicit input for patient care planning
- Establish mutually agreeable goals
- Review discharge plans
- Discuss referrals, as appropriate
- Recommend changes in treatment plan, as necessary
- Provide data to facilitate evaluation of patient care plan
- Clarify responsibilities related to implementation of patient care plan

2nd edition 1996

Background Readings:

Kozier, B., Erb, G., Berman, A., & Snyder, S. (2004). Health care delivery systems. In *Fundamentals of nursing: Concepts, processes, and practice*. (7th ed., pp. 88–105). Upper Saddle River, NJ: Prentice Hall.

Kozier, B., Erb, G., Berman, A., & Snyder, S. (2004). Planning. In *Fundamentals of nursing: Concepts, processes, and practice*. (7th ed., pp. 292–314). Upper Saddle River, NJ: Prentice Hall.

Mariano, C. (1989). The case for interdisciplinary collaboration. *Nursing Outlook*, 37(6), 285–288.

Richardson, A. T. (1986). Nurses interfacing with other members of the team. In D. A. England (Ed.), *Collaboration in Nursing* (pp. 163–185). Rockville, MD: Aspen.

M

Music Therapy

4400

Definition: Using music to help achieve a specific change in behavior, feeling, or physiology

Activities:

- Define the specific change in behavior and/or physiology that is desired (e.g., relaxation, stimulation, concentration, pain reduction)
- Determine the individual's interest in music
- Identify the individual's musical preferences
- Inform the individual as to the purpose of the music experience
- Choose particular music selections representative of the individual's preferences
- Assist the individual in assuming a comfortable position
- Limit extraneous stimuli (e.g., lights, sounds, visitors, telephone calls) during the listening experience
- Make music tapes/compact discs and equipment available to the individual
- Ensure that tapes/compact discs and equipment are in good working order
- Provide headphones, as indicated
- Ensure that the volume is adequate but not too high
- Avoid turning music on and leaving it on for long periods
- Facilitate the individual's active participation (e.g., playing an instrument or singing) if this is desired and feasible within the setting
- Avoid stimulating music after an acute head injury

1st edition 1992; revised 2000, 2004

Background Readings:

Chlan, L. (1998). Music therapy. In M. Snyder & R. Lindquist (Eds.), *Complementary/alternative therapies in nursing* (3rd ed., pp. 243–257). New York: Springer.

Craven, R. F., & Hirnle, C. J. (2003). Cognitive processes. In *Fundamentals of nursing: Human health and function* (4th ed., pp. 1219–1252). Philadelphia: Lippincott Williams & Wilkins.

Gerdner, L. A. & Buckwalter, K. C. (1999). Music therapy. In G. M. Bulechek & J. C. McCloskey (Eds.), *Nursing interventions: Effective nursing treatments* (3rd ed, pp. 451–468). Philadelphia: Saunders.

Kozier, B., Erb, G., Berman, A., & Snyder, S. (2004). Complementary and alternative healing modalities. In *Fundamentals of nursing: Concepts, processes, and practice* (7th ed., pp. 223–243). Upper Saddle River, NJ: Prentice Hall.

Tanabe, P., Thomas, R., Paice, J., Spiller, M., & Marcantonio, R. (2001). The effect of standard care, ibuprofen, and music on pain relief and patient satisfaction in adults with musculoskeletal trauma. *Journal of Emergency Nursing*, 27(2), 124–131.

White, J. M. (2001). Music as intervention: A notable endeavor to improve patient outcomes. *Nursing Clinics of North America*, 36(1), 83–92.

Mutual Goal Setting   **4410**

Definition: Collaborating with patient to identify and prioritize care goals, then developing a plan for achieving those goals

Activities:
- Encourage the identification of specific life values
- Assist patient and significant other to develop realistic expectations of themselves in performance of their roles
- Determine patient's recognition of own problem
- Encourage the patient to identify own strengths and abilities
- Assist the patient in identifying realistic, attainable goals
- Construct and use goal attainment scaling, as appropriate
- Identify with patient the goals of care
- State goals in positive terms
- Assist the patient in breaking down complex goals into small, manageable steps
- Recognize the patient's value and belief system when establishing goals
- Encourage the patient to state goals clearly, avoiding the use of alternatives
- Avoid imposing personal values on patient during goal setting
- Explain to the patient that only one behavior should be modified at a time
- Assist the patient in prioritizing (weighting) identified goals
- Clarify with the patient the roles of the health care provider and the patient, respectively
- Explore with the patient ways to best achieve the goals
- Assist the patient in examining available resources to meet the goals
- Assist the patient in developing a plan to meet the goals
- Assist the patient in setting realistic time limits
- Assist the patient in prioritizing activities used for goal achievement
- Appraise the patient's current level of functioning with regard to each goal
- Facilitate the patient in identification of individualized expected outcomes for each goal
- Assist the patient in identifying a specific measurement indicator (e.g., behavior, social event) for each goal
- Prepare behavioral outcomes for use in goal attainment scaling
- Help the patient focus on expected, rather than desired, outcomes
- Encourage the acceptance of partial goal satisfaction
- Develop a scale of upper and lower levels related to expected outcomes for each goal
- Identify scale levels that are defined by behavioral or social events for each goal
- Assist the patient in specifying the period of time in which each indicator will be measured
- Explore with the patient methods of measuring progress toward goals
- Coordinate with the patient periodic review dates for assessment of progress toward goals
- Review the scale (as developed with the patient) during review dates for assessment of progress
- Calculate a goal attainment score
- Reevaluate goals and plan as appropriate

1st edition 1992; revised 2000

Background Readings:

Boyd, M. A. (2005). Psychiatric-mental health nursing interventions. In M. A. Boyd (Ed.), *Psychiatric nursing: Contemporary practice* (3rd ed., pp. 218–232). Philadelphia: Lippincott Williams & Wilkins.

Hefferin, E. A. (1979). Health goal setting: Patient-nurse collaboration at Veterans Administration facilities. *Military Medicine, 144*(12), 814–822.

Horsley, J. A., Crane, J., Haller, K. B., & Reynolds, M. A. (1982). *Mutual goal setting in patient care. CURN Project.* New York: Grune & Stratton.

Simons, M. R. (1992). Interventions related to compliance. In G. M. Bulechek & J. C. McCloskey (Eds.), Symposium on nursing interventions. *Nursing Clinics of North America, 27*(2) 477–494.

Stanley, B. (1984). Evaluation of treatment goals: The use of goal attainment scaling. *Journal of Advanced Nursing, 9*(4), 351–356.

Webster, J. (2002). Client-centered goal planning. *Nursing Times, 98*(6), 36–37.

M

Nail Care   1680

Definition: Promotion of clean, neat, attractive nails and prevention of skin lesions related to improper care of nails

Activities:

- Monitor or assist with cleaning of nails, according to individual's self-care ability
- Monitor or assist with trimming of nails, according to individual's self-care ability
- Soak nails in warm water, clean under nails with orange stick, and push back cuticles with a cuticle stick
- Moisturize area around nails to prevent dryness
- Monitor nails for any changes
- Remove nail polish before taking patient to surgery, as appropriate
- Assist patient to apply nail polish, as desired

1st edition 1992; revised 2004

Background Readings:

Perry, A. G., & Potter, P. A. (2002). *Clinical nursing skills & techniques* (5th ed., pp. 145–150). St. Louis: Mosby.

Titler, M. G., Pettit, D., Bulechek, G. M., McCloskey, J. C., Craft, M. J., Cohen, M. Z., et al. (1991). Classification of nursing interventions for care of the integument. *Nursing Diagnosis, 2*(2), 45–56.

Nasal Irrigation   3316

Definition: Enhancing nasal mucosa functioning using saline lavage

Activities:

- Consider contraindications prior to procedure (e.g., patients with facial trauma not fully healed and patients with neurologic or musculoskeletal problems that increase aspiration risk)
- Prepare irrigating solution, using premade packets or household ingredients
- Mix 1 teaspoon salt and ½ teaspoon baking soda with 1 pint lukewarm, potable water, adjusting salinity and temperature of solution according to institutional guidelines or patient preference, if necessary
- Use salt that does not contain iodine, anticaking agents, or preservatives to avoid irritation to the nasal mucosa (i.e., use kosher, canning, or pickling salt)
- Draw up solution using low positive pressure device (e.g., bulb syringe or spray bottle) or gravity-based pressure device (e.g., neti-pot or other commercial nasal saline rinse product)
- Position patient over sink or basin with head tilted downward and rotated so that one nostril is above the other
- Gently insert applicator tip or spout into uppermost nostril until a comfortable seal is formed while avoiding pressing tip or spout into the septum
- Instill approximately half of prepared solution into nostril
- Instruct patient to breathe normally through mouth
- Monitor evacuation of fluid return from lower nostril (e.g., amount, color, consistency)
- Repeat procedure in other nostril
- Adjust head position as needed to avoid the draining of solution into back of throat or ears
- Encourage patient to blow nose gently
- Irrigate nasal passages 1 to 3 times per day or as prescribed
- Cleanse irrigating device after each use
- Prepare fresh solution daily
- Discontinue if patient experiences pain, nosebleeds, or other problems
- Instruct patient on techniques for self-irrigation
- Administer nasal medication, if necessary
- Provide referral to health care provider

6th edition 2013

Background Readings:

Azar, A. E. & Muller, B. A. (2006). A practical evidence-based approach to rhinosinusitis. *The Journal of Respiratory Disease, 27*(9), 372–379.

Harvey, R., Hannan, S. A., Badia, L., & Scadding, G. (2007). Nasal saline irrigations for the symptoms of chronic rhinosinusitis. *Cochrane Database of Systematic Reviews,* Issue 3. Art. No.: CD006394. DOI: 10.1002/14651858. CD006394.pub2.

Kassel, J. C., King, D., & Spurling, G. K. P. (2010). Saline nasal irrigation for acute upper respiratory tract infections. *Cochrane Database of Systematic Reviews,* Issue 3. Art. No.: CD006821. DOI: 10.1002/14651858.CD006821. pub2.

Moyad, M. A. (2009). Conventional and alternative medical advice for cold and flu prevention: What should be recommended and what should be avoided? *Urologic Nursing, 29*(6), 455–458.

Rabago, D. & Zgierska, A. (2009). Saline nasal irrigation for upper respiratory conditions. *American Family Physician, 80*(10), 1117–1119, 1121–1122.

Steele, R. W. (2005). Chronic sinusitis in children. *Clinical Pediatrics, 44*(6), 465–471.

N

Nausea Management 1450

Definition: Prevention and alleviation of nausea

Activities:
- Encourage patient to monitor own nausea experience
- Encourage patient to learn strategies for managing own nausea
- Perform complete assessment of nausea, including frequency, duration, severity, and precipitating factors, using such tools as Self-Care Journal, Visual Analog Scales, Duke Descriptive Scales, and Rhodes Index of Nausea and Vomiting (INV) Form 2
- Observe for nonverbal cues of discomfort, especially for infants, children, and those unable to communicate effectively, such as individuals with Alzheimer's disease
- Evaluate past experiences with nausea (e.g., pregnancy and car sickness)
- Obtain a complete pretreatment history
- Obtain dietary history containing the person's likes, dislikes, and cultural food preferences
- Evaluate the impact of nausea experience on quality of life (e.g., appetite, activity, job performance, role responsibility, and sleep)
- Identify factors (e.g., medication and procedures) that may cause or contribute to nausea
- Ensure that effective antiemetic drugs are given to prevent nausea when possible (except for nausea related to pregnancy)
- Control environmental factors that may evoke nausea (e.g., aversive smells, sound, and unpleasant visual stimulation)
- Reduce or eliminate personal factors that precipitate or increase the nausea (anxiety, fear, fatigue, and lack of knowledge)
- Identify strategies that have been successful in relieving nausea
- Demonstrate acceptance of nausea and collaborate with the patient when selecting a nausea control strategy
- Consider the cultural influence on nausea response while implementing intervention
- Encourage patient not to tolerate nausea but to be assertive with health providers in obtaining pharmacological and nonpharmacological relief
- Teach the use of nonpharmacological techniques (e.g., biofeedback, hypnosis, relaxation, guided imagery, music therapy, distraction, acupressure) to manage nausea
- Encourage the use of nonpharmacological techniques before, during, and after chemotherapy, before nausea occurs or increases, and along with other nausea control measures
- Inform other health care professionals and family members of any nonpharmacological strategies being used by the nauseated person
- Promote adequate rest and sleep to facilitate nausea relief
- Use frequent oral hygiene to promote comfort, unless it stimulates nausea
- Encourage eating small amounts of food that are appealing to the nauseated person
- Instruct in high-carbohydrate and low low-fat food, as appropriate
- Give cold, clear liquid, odorless and colorless food, as appropriate
- Monitor recorded intake for nutritional content and calories
- Weigh regularly
- Provide information about the nausea, such as causes of the nausea and how long it will last
- Assist to seek and provide emotional support
- Monitor effects of nausea management throughout

3rd edition 2000

Background Readings:

Fessele, K. S. (1996). Managing the multiple causes of nausea and vomiting in the patient with cancer. *Oncology Nursing Forum, 23*(9), 1409–1417.

Grant, M. (1987). Nausea, vomiting, and anorexia. *Seminars in Oncology Nursing, 3*(4), 227–286.

Hogan, C. M. (1990). Advances in the management of nausea and vomiting. *Nursing Clinics of North America, 25*(2), 475–497.

Hablonski, R. S. (1993). Nausea: The forgotten symptom. *Holistic Nursing Practice, 7*(2), 64–72.

Larson, P., Halliburton, P., & Di Julio, J. (1993). Nausea, vomiting, and retching. In V. Carrier-Kohlman, A. M. Lindsey, & C. M. West (Eds.), *Pathophysiological phenomena in nursing human responses to illness* (pp. 255–274). Philadelphia: Saunders.

Rhodes, V.A. (1990). Nausea, vomiting, and retching. *Nursing Clinics of North America, 25*(4), 885–900.

Timby, B. K., & Smith, N. E. (2007). Caring for clients with disorders of the upper gastrointestinal tract. In *Introductory medical-surgical nursing* (9th ed., pp. 821–846). Philadelphia: Lippincott Williams & Wilkins.

N

Neurologic Monitoring 2620

Definition: Collection and analysis of patient data to prevent or minimize neurologic complications

Activities:
- Monitor pupillary size, shape, symmetry, and reactivity
- Monitor level of consciousness
- Monitor level of orientation
- Monitor trend of Glasgow Coma Scale
- Monitor recent memory, attention span, past memory, mood, affect, and behaviors
- Monitor vital signs: temperature, blood pressure, pulse, and respirations
- Monitor respiratory status: ABG levels, pulse oximetry, depth, pattern, rate, and effort
- Monitor invasive hemodynamic parameters, as appropriate
- Monitor ICP and CPP
- Monitor corneal reflex
- Monitor cough and gag reflex
- Monitor muscle tone, motor movement, gait, and proprioception
- Monitor for pronator drift
- Monitor grip strength

- Monitor for tremor
- Monitor facial symmetry
- Monitor tongue protrusion
- Monitor for tracking response
- Monitor EOMs and gaze characteristics
- Monitor for visual disturbance: diplopia, nystagmus, visual-field cuts, blurred vision, and visual acuity
- Note complaint of headache
- Monitor speech characteristics: fluency, presence of aphasias, or word-finding difficulty
- Monitor response to stimuli: verbal, tactile, and noxious
- Monitor sharp/dull or hot/cold discrimination
- Monitor for paresthesia: numbness and tingling
- Monitor sense of smell
- Monitor sweating patterns
- Monitor Babinski response
- Monitor for Cushing response
- Monitor craniotomy/laminectomy dressing for drainage
- Monitor response to medications
- Consult with coworkers to confirm data, as appropriate
- Identify emerging patterns in data
- Increase frequency of neurological monitoring, as appropriate
- Avoid activities that increase intracranial pressure
- Space required nursing activities that increase intracranial pressure
- Notify physician of change in patient condition
- Institute emergency protocols, as needed

1st edition 1992; revised 1996

Background Readings:

Ackerman, L. L. (1992). Interventions related to neurological care. In G. M. Bulechek & J. C. McCloskey (Eds.), Symposium on nursing interventions. *Nursing Clinics of North America, 27*(2), 325–346.

American Association of Critical Care Nurses. (2006). *Core curriculum for critical care nursing* (6th ed.) [J. G. Alspach, Ed.]. Philadelphia: Saunders.

Ammons, A. M. (1990). Cerebral injuries and intracranial hemorrhages as a result of trauma. *Nursing Clinics of North America, 25*(1), 23–34.

Crimlisk, J. T., & Grande, M. M. (2004). Neurologic assessment skills for the acute medical surgical nurse. *Orthopaedic Nursing, 23*(1), 3–11.

Crosby, L., & Parsons, L. C. (1989). Clinical neurologic assessment tool: Development and testing of an instrument to index neurologic status. *Heart & Lung, 18*(2), 121–125.

Lehman, C. A., Hayes, J. M., LaCroix, M., Owen, S. V., & Nauta, H. J. (2002). Developing and implementation of a problem-focused neurological assessment system. *Journal of Neuroscience Nursing, 35*(4), 185–192.

Mitchell, P. H., & Ackerman, L. L. (1992). Secondary brain injury reduction. In G. M. Bulechek & J. C. McCloskey (Eds.), *Nursing interventions: Essential nursing treatments* (2nd ed., pp. 558–573). Philadelphia: Saunders.

Timby, B. K., & Smith, N. E. (2007). Introduction to the nervous system. In *Introductory medical-surgical nursing* (9th ed., pp. 653–665). Philadelphia: Lippincott Williams & Wilkins.

Titler, M. G. (1992). Interventions related to surveillance. In G. M. Bulechek & J. C. McCloskey (Eds.), Symposium on nursing interventions. *Nursing Clinics of North America, 27*(2), 495–516.

Nonnutritive Sucking   6900   **N**

Definition: Provision of sucking opportunities for the infant

Activities:

- Select a smooth pacifier or pacifier substitute that meets standards to prevent airway obstruction
- Use a pacifier that has been cleaned or sterilized daily, is used with only one patient, and has had no contact with contaminated areas
- Place largest soft pacifier the infant can tolerate on top of the infant's tongue
- Position infant to allow tongue to drop to floor of mouth
- Position thumb and index finger under infant's mandible to support sucking reflex, if needed
- Move infant's tongue rhythmically with the pacifier if needed to encourage sucking
- Rub infant's cheek gently to stimulate the suck reflex
- Provide pacifier to encourage sucking during tube feeding and for 5 minutes following the tube feeding
- Provide pacifier to encourage sucking at least every 4 hours for infants receiving long-term hyperalimentation
- Use pacifier after feedings if infant demonstrates continual need to suck
- Rock and hold infant while infant sucks on pacifier, when possible
- Play soft, appropriate music
- Position infant to prevent loss of pacifier
- Inform parent(s) on importance of meeting infant sucking needs
- Encourage breastfeeding mother to allow nonnutritive sucking at breast after feeding complete
- Inform parents of alternatives to nipple sucking (e.g., thumb, parent's finger, pacifier)
- Instruct parent(s) on the use of nonnutritive sucking

1st edition 1992; revised 2000

Background Readings:

Hill, A. S., Kurkowski, T. B., & Garcia, J. (2000). Oral support measures used in feeding the preterm infant. *Nursing Research, 49*(1), 2–9.

Pickler, R. H. (2001). Nonnutritive sucking. In M. Craft-Rosenberg & J. Denehy (Eds.), *Nursing interventions for infants, children, and families* (pp. 139–150). Thousand Oaks, CA: Sage.

Standley, J. M. (2000). The effect of contingent music to increase nonnutritive sucking of premature infants. *Pediatric Nursing, 26*(5), 493–499.

Normalization Promotion 7200

Definition: Assisting parents and other family members of children with chronic illnesses or disabilities in providing normal life experiences for their children and families

Activities:

- Promote development of membership of child into family system without letting child become central focus of family
- Assist family to view affected child as a child first, rather than a chronically ill or disabled individual
- Provide opportunities for child to have normal childhood experiences
- Encourage interaction with normal peers
- Deemphasize uniqueness of child's condition
- Encourage parents to make child appear as normal as possible
- Assist family in avoiding potentially embarrassing situations with child
- Assist family in making changes in home environment that decrease reminders of child's special needs
- Determine accessibility of activity and child's ability to participate in activity
- Identify adaptations needed to accommodate child's limitations so child can participate in normal activities
- Communicate information about child's condition to those who need this information to provide safe supervision or appropriate educational opportunities for child
- Assist family in altering prescribed therapeutic regime to fit normal schedule, when appropriate
- Assist family in advocating for child in school system to ensure access to appropriate education programs
- Encourage child to participate in school and community activities appropriate for developmental and ability level
- Encourage parents to have same parenting expectations and techniques for affected child as with other children in family, as appropriate
- Encourage parents to spend time with all children in family

- Involve siblings in care and activities of child, as appropriate
- Determine need for respite care for parents or other care providers
- Identify resources for respite care in community
- Encourage parents to take time to care for their personal needs
- Provide information to family about child's condition, treatment, and associated support groups for families
- Encourage parents to balance involvement in special programs for child's special needs and normal family and community activities
- Encourage family to maintain usual social network and support system
- Encourage family to maintain usual family habits, rituals, and routines

2nd edition 1996

Background Readings:

Bossert, E., Holaday, B., Harkins, A., & Turner-Henson, A. (1990). Strategies of normalization used by parents of chronically ill school age children. *Journal of Child and Adolescent Psychiatric and Mental Health Nursing, 3*(2), 57–61.

Knafl, K. A., & Deatrick, J. A. (1986). How families manage chronic conditions: An analysis of the concept of normalization. *Research in Nursing & Health, 9*(3), 215–222.

Knafl, K. A., Deatrick, J. A., & Kirby, A. (2001). Normalization promotion. In M. Craft-Rosenberg & J. Denehy (Eds.), *Nursing interventions for infants, children, and families* (pp. 373–388). Thousand Oaks, CA: Sage.

Wong, D. L. (1997). *Whaley & Wong's essentials of pediatric nursing* (5th ed., p. 527). St. Louis: Mosby.

Nutrition Management 1100

Definition: Providing and promoting a balanced intake of nutrients

Activities:

- Determine patient's nutritional status and ability to meet nutritional needs
- Identify patient's food allergies or intolerances
- Determine patient's food preferences
- Instruct patient about nutritional needs (i.e., discuss dietary guidelines and food pyramids)
- Assist patient in determining guidelines or food pyramids (e.g., Vegetarian Food Pyramid, Food Guide Pyramid, and Food Pyramid for Seniors Over 70) most suited in meeting nutritional needs and preferences
- Determine number of calories and type of nutrients needed to meet nutrition requirements
- Provide food selection while offering guidance towards healthier choices, if necessary
- Adjust diet, as necessary (i.e., provide high protein foods; suggest using herbs and spices as an alternative to salt provide

sugar substitute; increase or decrease calories; increase or decrease vitamins, minerals, or supplements)
- Provide optimal environment for meal consumption (e.g., clean, well-ventilated, relaxed, and free from strong odors)
- Perform or assist patient with oral care prior to eating
- Ensure patient uses well-fitting dentures, if appropriate
- Administer medications prior to eating (e.g., pain relief, antiemetics), if needed
- Encourage patient to sit in upright position in chair, if possible
- Ensure food is served in attractive manner and at temperature most suited for optimal consumption
- Encourage family to bring patient's favorite foods while in hospital or care facility, as appropriate
- Assist patient with opening packages, cutting food, and eating, if needed
- Instruct patient on necessary diet modifications, as necessary (e.g., NPO, clear liquid, full liquid, soft, or diet as tolerated)

- Instruct patient on diet requirements for disease state (i.e, for patients with renal disease, restrict sodium, potassium, protein, and fluids)
- Instruct patient on specific dietary needs based on development or age (e.g., increased calcium, protein, fluid, and calories for lactating women; increased fiber intake to prevent constipation among older adults)
- Offer nutrient-dense snacks
- Ensure that diet includes foods high in fiber content to prevent constipation
- Monitor calorie and dietary intake
- Monitor trends in weight loss and gain
- Instruct patient to monitor calorie and dietary intake (e.g., food diary)
- Encourage safe food preparation and preservation techniques
- Assist patient in accessing community nutritional programs (e.g., Women, Infants, and Children, food stamps, and home-delivered meals)
- Provide referral, if necessary

1st edition 1992; revised 2013

Background Readings:

Craven, R. F., & Hirnle, C. J. (2009). Nutrition. In *Fundamentals of nursing: Human health and function* (6th ed., pp. 947–988). Philadelphia: Lippincott Williams & Wilkins.

Ignatavicius, D. D. (2010). Care of patients with malnutrition and obesity. In D. D. Ignatavicius & M. L. Workman (Eds.), *Medical-surgical nursing: Patient-centered collaborative care* (6th ed., pp. 1386–1410). St. Louis: Saunders.

Kaiser, L., Allen, L. H., & American Dietetic Association. (2008). Position of the American Dietetic Association: Nutrition and lifestyle for a healthy pregnancy outcome. *Journal of the American Dietetic Association, 108*(3), 553–561.

U.S. Department of Agriculture (USDA) and U.S. Department of Health and Human Services (HHS). (2010). *Dietary guidelines for Americans, 2010* (7th ed.). Washington, DC: Government Printing Office.

Nutrition Therapy   1120

Definition: Administration of food and fluids to support metabolic processes of a patient who is malnourished or at high risk for becoming malnourished

Activities:
- Complete a nutritional assessment, as appropriate
- Monitor food/fluid ingested and calculate daily caloric intake, as appropriate
- Monitor appropriateness of diet orders to meet daily nutritional needs, as appropriate
- Determine, in collaboration with the dietitian, the number of calories and type of nutrients needed to meet nutrition requirements, as appropriate
- Determine food preferences with consideration of cultural and religious preferences
- Select nutritional supplements, as appropriate
- Encourage patient to select semisoft food if lack of saliva hinders swallowing
- Encourage intake of high-calcium foods, as appropriate
- Encourage intake of foods and fluids high in potassium, as appropriate
- Ensure that diet includes foods high in fiber content to prevent constipation
- Provide patient with high-protein, high-calorie, nutritious finger foods and drinks that can be readily consumed, as appropriate
- Assist patient to select soft, bland, and nonacidic foods, as appropriate
- Determine need for enteral tube feedings
- Administer enteral feedings, as appropriate
- Discontinue use of tube feedings, as oral intake is tolerated
- Administer hyperalimentation fluids, as appropriate
- Ensure availability of progressive therapeutic diet
- Provide needed nourishment within limits of prescribed diet
- Encourage bringing home-cooked food to the institution, as appropriate
- Suggest trial elimination of foods containing lactose, as appropriate
- Offer herbs and spices as an alternative to salt
- Structure the environment to create a pleasant and relaxing atmosphere
- Present food in an attractive, pleasing manner, giving consideration to color, texture, and variety
- Provide oral care before meals, as needed
- Assist patient to a sitting position before eating or feeding
- Monitor lab values, as appropriate
- Instruct patient and family about prescribed diet
- Refer for diet teaching and planning, as needed
- Give patient and family written examples of prescribed diet

1st edition 1992; revised 2004

Background Readings:

American Society for Parenteral and Enteral Nutrition, Board of Directors. (2001). Standards of practice for nutrition support nurses. *Nutrition Support Nurses Standards, 16*(1), 56–62.

Bowers, S. (1999). Nutrition support for malnourished, acutely ill adults. *MEDSURG Nursing, 8*(3), 145–146.

Cluskey, M. & Kim, Y. K. (2001). Use and perceived effectiveness of strategies for enhancing food and nutrient intakes among elderly persons in long-term care. *Journal of the American Dietetic Association, 101*(1), 111–114.

Creamer, K. M., Schotik Chan, D., Sutton, C., DeLeon, C., Moreno, C., Shoupe, B. A. (2001). A comprehensive pediatric inpatient nutrition support package: A multi-disciplinary approach. *Nutrition in Clinical Practice, 16*(4), 246–257.

Dudek, S. G. (2007). *Nutrition essentials for nursing practice* (5th rev. ed.). Philadelphia: Lippincott Williams & Wilkins.

N

Nutritional Counseling

5246

Definition: Use of an interactive helping process focusing on the need for diet modification

Activities:

- Establish a therapeutic relationship based on trust and respect
- Establish the length of the counseling relationship
- Determine patient's food intake and eating habits
- Facilitate identification of eating behaviors to be changed
- Establish realistic short-term and long-term goals for change in the nutritional status
- Use accepted nutritional standards to assist client in evaluating adequacy of dietary intake
- Provide information, as necessary, about the health need for diet modification: weight loss, weight gain, sodium restriction, cholesterol reduction, fluid restriction, and so on
- Post attractive food guide material in the patient's room (i.e., The Food Guide Pyramid)
- Help patient to consider factors of age, stage of growth and development, past eating experiences, injury, disease, culture, and finances in planning ways to meet nutritional requirements
- Discuss patient's knowledge of the basic four food groups, as well as perceptions of the needed diet modification
- Discuss nutritional requirements and patient's perceptions of prescribed/recommended diet
- Discuss patient's food likes and dislikes
- Assist patient to record what is usually eaten in a 24-hour period
- Review with patient measurements of fluid intake and output, hemoglobin values, blood pressure readings, or weight gains and losses, as appropriate
- Discuss food buying habits and budget constraints
- Discuss the meaning of food to patient
- Determine attitudes and beliefs of significant others about food, eating, and the patient's needed nutritional change
- Evaluate progress of dietary modification goals at regular intervals
- Assist patient in stating feelings and concerns about achievement of goals
- Praise efforts to achieve goals
- Provide referral/consultation with other members of the health care team, as appropriate

1st edition 1992; revised 1996

Background Readings:

Busse, G. (1985). Nutritional counseling. In G. M. Bulechek & J. C. McCloskey (Eds.), *Nursing interventions: Treatments for nursing diagnoses* (pp. 113–126). Philadelphia: Saunders.

Dudek, S. G. (2007). *Nutrition essentials for nursing practice* (5th rev. ed.). Philadelphia: Lippincott Williams & Wilkins.

Gabello, W. J. (1993). Dietary counseling. *Patient Care, 27*(5), 168–174, 177, 181–184.

Nutritional Monitoring

1160

Definition: Collection and analysis of patient data pertaining to nutrient intake

Activities:

- Weigh patient
- Monitor growth and development
- Obtain anthropometric measurements of body composition (e.g., body mass index, waist measurement, and skinfold measures)
- Monitor trends in weight loss and gain (i.e., in pediatric patients, plot height and weight on standardized growth chart)
- Identify recent changes in body weight
- Determine appropriate amount of weight gain during antepartum period
- Monitor skin turgor and mobility
- Identify abnormalities in skin (e.g., excessive bruising, poor wound healing, and bleeding)
- Identify abnormalities in hair (e.g., dry, thin, coarse, and breaks easily)
- Monitor for nausea and vomiting
- Identify abnormalities in bowel elimination (e.g., diarrhea, blood, mucus, and irregular or painful elimination)
- Monitor caloric and dietary intake
- Identify recent changes in appetite and activity
- Monitor type and amount of usual exercise
- Discuss role of social and emotional aspects of food consumption
- Determine meal patterns (e.g., food likes and dislikes, overconsumption of fast food, missed meals, hurried eating, parent-child interaction during feeding, and frequency and length of infant feedings)
- Monitor for pale, reddened, and dry conjunctival tissue
- Identify abnormalities in nails (e.g., spoon-shaped, cracked, split, broken, brittle, and ridged)
- Perform swallowing evaluation (e.g., motor function of facial, oral, and tongue muscles; swallowing reflex; and gag reflex)
- Identify abnormalities in oral cavity (e.g., inflammation; spongy, receding, or bleeding gums; dry, cracked lips; sores; scarlet, raw tongue; and hyperemic and hypertrophic papillae)
- Monitor mental state (e.g., confusion, depression, and anxiety)
- Identify abnormalities in musculoskeletal system (e.g., muscle wasting, painful joints, bone fractures, and poor posture)
- Conduct laboratory testing, monitoring results (e.g., cholesterol, serum albumin, transferrin, prealbumin, 24-hour urinary nitrogen, blood urea nitrogen, creatinine, hemoglobin, hematocrit, cellular immunity, total lymphocyte count, and electrolyte levels)
- Determine energy recommendation (e.g., Recommended Dietary Allowance) based on patient factors (e.g., age, weight, height, gender, and physical activity level)

- Determine factors affecting nutritional intake (e.g., knowledge, availability, and accessibility of quality food products in all food categories; religious and cultural influences; gender; ability to prepare food; social isolation; hospitalization; inadequate chewing; impaired swallowing; periodontal disease; poor-fitting dentures; decreased taste sensitivity; use of drugs or medications; and disease or postsurgical states)
- Review other sources of data pertaining to nutritional status (e.g., patient food diary and written logs)
- Initiate treatment or provide referral, as appropriate

1st edition 1992; revised 2013

Background Readings:

Craven, R. F., & Hirnle, C. J. (2009). Nutrition. In *Fundamentals of nursing: Human health and function* (6th ed., pp. 947–988). Philadelphia: Lippincott Williams & Wilkins.

Dudek, S. G. (2007). *Nutrition essentials for nursing practice* (5th rev. ed.). Philadelphia: Lippincott Williams & Wilkins.

Roman-Vinas, B., Serra-Majem, L., Ribas-Barba, L., Ngo, J., Garcia-Alvarez, A., Wijnhoven, T., et al. (2009). Overview of methods used to evaluate the adequacy of nutrient intakes for individuals and populations. *British Journal of Nutrition, 101*(Suppl. 2), S6–S11.

Smith, S. F., Duell, D. J., & Martin, B. C. (2008). *Clinical nursing skills: Basic to advanced skills* (7th ed., pp. 208–248). Upper Saddle River, NJ: Pearson Prentice Hall.

N

Oral Health Maintenance 1710

Definition: Maintenance and promotion of oral hygiene and dental health for the patient at risk for developing oral or dental lesions

Activities:

- Establish a mouth care routine
- Apply lubricant to moisten lips and oral mucosa, as needed
- Monitor teeth for color, shine, and presence of debris
- Identify the risk for development of stomatitis secondary to drug therapy
- Encourage and assist patient to rinse mouth
- Monitor for therapeutic effects of topical anesthetics, oral protective pastes, and topical or systemic analgesics, as appropriate
- Instruct and assist patient to perform oral hygiene after eating and as often as needed
- Monitor for signs and symptoms of glossitis and stomatitis
- Consult physician or dentist about readjustment of wires/appliances and alternative methods of oral care if irritation of oral mucous membranes occurs from these devices
- Consult physician if oral dryness, irritation, and discomfort persist
- Facilitate toothbrushing and flossing at regular intervals
- Recommend the use of a soft-bristle toothbrush
- Instruct person to brush teeth, gums, and tongue
- Recommend a healthy diet and adequate water intake
- Arrange for dental checkups, as needed
- Assist with denture care, as needed
- Encourage denture wearers to brush gums and tongue and rinse the oral cavity daily
- Discourage smoking and tobacco chewing
- Instruct patient to chew sugarless gum to increase saliva and cleanse teeth

1st edition 1992; revised 2004

Background Readings:

Locker, D. (1992). Smoking and oral health in older adults. *Canadian Journal of Public Health*, 83(6), 429–432.

Payton, L. (2000). The winning smile. *Arkansas Nursing News*, 16(3), 27–30.

Perry, A. G., & Potter, P. A. (2002). *Clinical nursing skills & techniques* (5th ed., pp. 117–118, 132–140). St. Louis: Mosby.

Stiefel, K. A., Damron, S., Sowers, N. J., & Velez, L. (2000). Improving oral hygiene for the seriously ill patient: Implementing research-based practice. *MEDSURG Nursing*, 9(1), 40–46.

Titler, M. G., Pettit, D., Bulechek, G. M., McCloskey, J. C., Craft, M. J., Cohen, M. Z., et al. (1991). Classification of nursing interventions for care of the integument. *Nursing Diagnosis*, 2(2), 45–56.

Walton, J. C., Miller, J., & Tordecilla, L. (2001). Elder oral assessment and care. *MEDSURG Nursing*, 10(1), 37–44.

Oral Health Promotion 1720

Definition: Promotion of oral hygiene and dental care for a patient with normal oral and dental health

Activities:

- Monitor condition of patient's mouth (e.g., lips, tongue, mucous membranes, teeth, gums, and dental appliances and their fit)
- Provide oral health screening and risk assessment
- Determine patient's usual dental hygiene routine, identifying areas to be addressed, if necessary
- Instruct patient or patient's family on frequency and quality of proper oral health care (e.g., flossing, brushing, rinsing, adequate nutrition, use of fluoride-containing water, supplement, or other preventive product, and other considerations based on patient's developmental level and self-care ability)
- Assist patient in brushing teeth, gums, and tongue; rinsing; and flossing, as needed
- Assist patient wearing dentures in oral care, as needed (i.e., remove, cleanse, and reinsert dentures; brush gums, remaining teeth, and tongue; and massage gums with brush or fingers)
- Provide oral care for unconscious patient, using appropriate precautions (i.e., turn patient's head to side or place in side-lying position when possible, insert bite block or padded tongue blade, avoid putting fingers in mouth, use small amounts of liquid, and use bulb syringe or other suction device)
- Cleanse infant's mouth using dry gauze or washcloth
- Apply lubricant to moisten lips and oral mucosa, as needed
- Assist patient or patient's family in identifying and obtaining oral care products most suited to meet needs (e.g., toothbrush with easy-to-grasp handle, powered toothbrush, dental floss holder, immersion cleanser for dentures, and athletic mouthguard)
- Discuss role of sugar in development of caries (i.e., encourage patient to limit natural sugar intake; suggest use of artificial sweeteners in diet, particularly xylitol; and instruct parent on appropriate use of bottles and sippy cups and their contents)
- Discourage smoking and tobacco chewing (i.e., instruct patient on effects of tobacco use, implement tobacco-use prevention measures, and provide tobacco-cessation assistance)
- Discuss importance of regular dental checkups, including timing of child's first visit to dental health professional
- Provide community-level services (i.e., assist patient in meeting needs for transportation and translational services, use health fairs and cultural events as opportunities for education, and develop public service announcements)
- Provide referral, as needed

1st edition 1992; revised 2013

Background Readings:

Brickhouse, T. H. (2010). Family oral health education. *General Dentistry*, 58(3), 212–219.

Clarke, W., Periam, C., & Zoitopoulos, L. (2009). Oral health promotion for linguistically and culturally diverse populations: Understanding the local non-English-speaking population. *Health Education Journal*, 68(2), 119–129.

Craven, R. F., & Hirnle, C. J. (2009). Self-care and hygiene. In *Fundamentals of nursing: Human health and function* (6th ed., pp. 703–755). Philadelphia: Lippincott Williams & Wilkins.

Harris, N. O., Garcia-Godoy, F., & Nathe, C. N. (Eds.). (2009). *Primary preventive dentistry* (7th ed.). Upper Saddle River, NJ: Pearson.

Petersen, P. E., & Kwan, S. (2010). The 7th Global Conference on Health Promotion: Towards integration of oral health (Nairobi, Kenya 2009). *Community Dental Health*, 27(2), 129–36.

Smith, S. F., Duell, D. J., & Martin, B. C. (2008). Personal hygiene. In *Clinical nursing skills: Basic to advanced skills* (7th ed., pp. 208–248). Upper Saddle River, NJ: Pearson Prentice Hall.

Yevlahova, D., & Satur, J. (2009). Models for individual oral health promotion and their effectiveness: A systematic review. *Australian Dental Journal*, 54(3), 190–197.

Oral Health Restoration   1730

Definition: Promotion of healing for a patient who has an oral mucosa or dental lesion

Activities:

- Monitor condition of patient's mouth (e.g., lips, tongue, mucous membranes, teeth, gums, and dental appliances and their fit), including character of abnormalities (e.g., size, color, and location of internal or external lesions or inflammation, and other signs of infection)
- Monitor changes in taste, swallowing, quality of voice, and comfort
- Obtain order from health care provider to perform oral hygiene, if applicable
- Determine necessary frequency for oral care, encouraging patient or patient's family to adhere to schedule or assisting with oral care, as needed
- Instruct patient to use soft-bristled toothbrush or disposable mouth sponge
- Instruct patient on appropriate selection of floss use and type (i.e., avoid use if at risk for bleeding; use waxed floss to prevent tissue trauma)
- Administer mouth rinse to patient (e.g., anesthetic, effervescent, saline, coating, antifungal, or antibacterial solution)
- Administer medication (e.g., analgesics, anesthetics, antimicrobials, and antiinflammatory agents), if needed
- Remove dentures, encouraging patient to use only for meals
- Apply lubricant to moisten lips and oral mucosa, as needed
- Discourage smoking and tobacco chewing
- Discourage alcohol consumption
- Instruct patient or patient's family on frequency and quality of proper oral health care (e.g., flossing, brushing, rinsing, adequate nutrition, use of fluoride-containing water, supplement, or other preventive product, and other considerations based on patient's developmental level and self-care ability)
- Instruct patient to avoid oral hygiene products containing glycerin, alcohol, or other drying agents
- Instruct patient to keep toothbrushes and other cleaning equipment clean

- Discuss importance of adequate nutritional intake (i.e., address malnutrition caused by deficiencies in folate, zinc, iron, and complex B vitamins; encourage consumption of high-protein, high vitamin C-containing foods)
- Encourage avoidance of spicy, salty, acidic, dry, rough, or hard foods
- Instruct patient to avoid foods causing allergic response (e.g., coffee, cheese, nuts, citrus fruits, gluten, and potatoes), if applicable
- Encourage patient to increase water intake
- Instruct patient to avoid hot foods and liquids, preventing burns and further irritation
- Instruct patient on signs and symptoms of stomatitis, including when to report to health care provider
- Provide referral

1st edition 1992; revised 2013

Background Readings:

Dietzen, K. K. (2010). Care of patients with oral cavity problems. In D. D. Ignatavicius & M. L. Workman (Eds.) *Medical-surgical nursing: Patient-centered collaborative care* (6th ed., pp. 1231–1242). St. Louis: Saunders.

Harris, D. J., Eilers, J., Harriman, A., Cashavelly, B. J., Maxwell, C. (2008). Putting evidence into practice: Evidence-based interventions for the management of oral mucositis. *Clinical Journal of Oncology Nursing*, 12(1), 141–152.

Potting, C., Mistiaen, P., Poot, E., Blijlevens, N., Donnelly, P., & van Achterberg, T. (2008). A review of quality assessment of the methodology used in guidelines and systematic reviews on oral mucositis. *Journal of Clinical Nursing*, 18(1), 3–12.

Scardina, G. A., Pisano, T., & Messina, P. (2010). Oral mucositis: Review of literature. *New York State Dental Journal*, 76(1), 34–38.

Sciubba, J. J. (2007). Oral mucosal diseases in the office setting part I: Aphthous stomatitis and herpes simplex infections. *General Dentistry*, 55(4), 347–355.

Order Transcription 8060

Definition: Transferring information from order sheets to the nursing patient care planning and documentation system

Activities:
- Ensure that order sheet is stamped with patient identification
- Ensure that order sheet is in correct patient chart
- Ensure that orders are written or cosigned by a licensed health care provider with clinical privileges
- Repeat verbal order back to the physician to ensure accuracy
- Avoid taking verbal orders by or through other providers
- Ensure that verbal orders are documented per agency policy before noting
- Clarify confusing or illegible orders
- Evaluate appropriateness of orders and ensure that all needed information is provided
- Consult with a pharmacist whenever you have doubts about an unfamiliar drug or dose that is prescribed
- Document any disagreement with a physician's order after discussion of the order with the physician and a supervisor
- Sign name, title, date, and time to each order noted
- Transfer order to appropriate Kardex, worksheet, medication form, lab slip, or care plan
- Schedule appointments, as appropriate
- Note start and stop dates on medications, per agency policy
- Note patient allergies when transcribing medication orders
- Inform team members to initiate treatment

2nd edition 1996

Background Readings:

Carson, W. (1994). What you should know about physician verbal orders. *American Nurse, 26*(3), 30–31.

Davis, N. M., (1994). Clarifying questionable orders. *American Journal of Nursing, 94*(4), 16.

Festa, J. (1983). *The law and liability: A guide for nurses.* New York: John Wiley & Sons.

Kozier, B., Erb, G., Berman, A., & Snyder, S. (2004). Documenting and reporting. In *Fundamentals of nursing: Concepts, processes, and practice.* (7th ed., pp. 328–351). Upper Saddle River, NJ: Prentice Hall.

Organ Procurement 6260

Definition: Guiding families through the donation process to ensure timely retrieval of vital organs and tissue for transplant

Activities:
- Review institutional policy and procedures for organ donation
- Review potential donor medical history for contraindications to donation
- Anticipate organ suitability for donation, depending on criteria of death
- Determine whether patient has an organ donation card
- Provide emotional support for families when donation is desired but contraindicated
- Alert organ procurement team of potential donor
- Participate in obtaining specimens to verify donor suitability
- Prepare to articulate current criteria for brain death in terms that family members can understand
- Obtain consent for organ donation from family, as appropriate
- Collaborate with the family to complete separate consent forms that specifically name the organs and tissues authorized for removal
- Allow family time for grieving
- Provide emotional support for family
- Answer commonly asked questions about financial responsibility for procurement, criteria for transplant, and length of procedure
- Take actions to preserve viability of organ (e.g., intravenous fluids and ventilation)
- Participate in organ procurement procedures, as appropriate
- Provide postmortem care
- Offer family postmortem viewing of body, when possible
- Participate in postprocedure conference

2nd edition 1996

Background Readings:

Adams, E. F., Just, G., De Young, S., & Temmler, L. (1993). Organ donation: Comparison of nurses' participation in two states. *American Journal of Critical Care, 2*(4), 310–316.

Chabalewski, F., & Norris, M. K. G. (1994). The gift of life: Talking to families about organ and tissue donation. *American Journal of Nursing, 94*(6), 28–33.

Goodell, A.S. (1993). Anencephalic tissue transplantation. *The Canadian Nurse, 89*(5), 36–38.

Grover, L.E.K. (1993). The potential role of accident and emergency departments in cadaveric organ donation. *Accident and Emergency Nursing, 1*(1), 8–13.

Kawamoto, K. L. (1992). Organ procurement in the operating room: Implications for perioperative nurses. *AORN Journal, 55*(6), 1541–1546.

Smith, K. A. (1992). Demystifying organ procurement: Initiating the protocols, understanding the sequence of events. *AORN Journal, 55*(6), 1530–1540.

Ostomy Care   0480

Definition: Maintenance of elimination through a stoma and care of surrounding tissue

Activities:
- Instruct patient/significant other in the use of ostomy equipment/care
- Have patient/significant other demonstrate use of equipment
- Assist patient in obtaining needed equipment
- Apply appropriately fitting ostomy appliance, as needed
- Monitor for incision/stoma healing
- Monitor for postoperative complications such as intestinal obstruction, paralytic ileus, anastomotic leaks, or mucocutaneous separation, as appropriate
- Monitor stoma/surrounding tissue healing and adaptation to ostomy equipment
- Change/empty ostomy bag, as appropriate
- Irrigate ostomy, as appropriate
- Assist patient in providing self-care
- Encourage patient/significant other to express feelings and concerns about changes in body image
- Explore patient's care of ostomy
- Explain to the patient what the ostomy care will mean to his/her day-to-day routine
- Assist patient to plan time for care routine
- Instruct patient how to monitor for complications (e.g., mechanical breakdown, chemical breakdown, rash, leaks, dehydration, infection)
- Instruct patient on mechanisms to reduce odor
- Monitor elimination patterns
- Assist patient to identify factors that affect elimination pattern
- Instruct patient/significant other in appropriate diet and expected changes in elimination function
- Provide support and assistance while patient develops skill in caring for stoma/surrounding tissue
- Teach patient to chew thoroughly, avoid foods that caused digestive upset in the past, add new foods one at a time, and drink plenty of fluids
- Instruct in Kegel exercises if patient has ileoanal reservoir
- Instruct patient to intubate and drain Indiana pouch whenever it feels full (every 4 to 6 hours)
- Discuss concerns about sexual functioning, as appropriate
- Encourage visitation by persons from support group who have same condition
- Express confidence that patient can resume normal life with ostomy
- Encourage participation in ostomy support groups after discharge

1st edition 1992; revised 2000, 2004

Background Readings:
Bradley, M. & Pupiales, M. (1997). Essential elements of ostomy care. *American Journal of Nursing, 97*(7), 38–46.
Craven, R. F. & Hirnle, C. J. (2000). *Fundamentals of nursing: Human health and function* (3rd ed., pp. 1109–1112). Philadelphia: Lippincott Williams & Wilkins.
Innes, B. S. (1986). Meeting bowel elimination needs. In K. C. Sorenson & J. Luckmann (Eds.), *Basic nursing* (pp. 827–851). Philadelphia: Saunders.
O'Shea, H. S. (2001). Teaching the adult ostomy patient. *Journal of Wound Ostomy and Continence Nurses Society, 28*(1), 47–54.

O

Oxygen Therapy   3320

Definition: Administration of oxygen and monitoring of its effectiveness

Activities:
- Clear oral, nasal, and tracheal secretions, as appropriate
- Restrict smoking
- Maintain airway patency
- Set up oxygen equipment and administer through a heated, humidified system
- Administer supplemental oxygen as ordered
- Monitor the oxygen liter flow
- Monitor position of oxygen delivery device
- Instruct patient about importance of leaving oxygen delivery device on
- Periodically check oxygen delivery device to ensure that the prescribed concentration is being delivered
- Monitor the effectiveness of oxygen therapy (e.g., pulse oximetry, ABGs), as appropriate
- Assure replacement of oxygen mask/cannula whenever the device is removed
- Monitor patient's ability to tolerate removal of oxygen while eating
- Change oxygen delivery device from mask to nasal prongs during meals, as tolerated
- Observe for signs of oxygen-induced hypoventilation
- Monitor for signs of oxygen toxicity and absorption atelectasis
- Monitor oxygen equipment to ensure that it is not interfering with the patient's attempts to breathe
- Monitor patient's anxiety related to need for oxygen therapy
- Monitor for skin breakdown from friction of oxygen device
- Provide for oxygen when patient is transported
- Instruct patient to obtain a supplementary oxygen prescription before air travel or trips to high altitude, as appropriate
- Consult with other health care personnel regarding use of supplemental oxygen during activity and/or sleep
- Instruct patient and family about use of oxygen at home
- Arrange for use of oxygen devices that facilitate mobility and teach patient accordingly
- Convert to alternate oxygen delivery device to promote comfort, as appropriate

1st edition 1992; revised 2000

Background Readings:

American Association of Critical Care Nurses. (2006). *Core curriculum for critical care nursing* (6th ed.) [J. G. Alspach, Ed.]. Philadelphia: Saunders.

Gottlie, B. J. (1988). Breathing and gas exchange. In M. Kinney, D. Packa, & S. Dunbar (Eds.), *AACN's clinical reference for critical-care nursing* (2nd ed., pp. 160–192). St. Louis: Mosby.

Lewis, S. M. & Collies, I. C. (1996). *Medical-surgical nursing: Assessment and management of clinical problems* (4th ed.). St. Louis: Mosby.

Nelson, D. M. (1992). Interventions related to respiratory care. In G. M. Bulechek & J. C. McCloskey (Eds.), Symposium on nursing interventions. *Nursing Clinics of North America, 27*(2), 301–323.

Suddarth, D. (1991). *The Lippincott manual of nursing practice* (5th ed., pp. 210–226). Philadelphia: Lippincott.

Thelan, L. A., & Urden, L. D. (1998). *Critical care nursing: Diagnosis and management* (3rd ed.). St. Louis: Mosby.

U.S. Department of Health and Human Services. (1994). *Unstable angina: Diagnosis and management*. Rockville, MD: Agency for Health Care Policy and Research.

O

Pacemaker Management: Permanent   4091

Definition: Care of the patient receiving permanent support of cardiac pumping though the insertion and use of a pacemaker

Activities:
- Provide information to patient and family related to pacemaker implantation (e.g., indications, functions, universal programming codes, potential complications)
- Provide concrete objective information related to the effects of pacemaker therapy to reduce patient uncertainty, fear, and anxiety about treatment-related symptoms
- Document pertinent data in patient permanent record for initial insertion of pacemaker (e.g., manufacturer, model number, serial number, implant date, mode of operation, programmed parameters, upper and lower rate limits for rate-responsive devices, type of lead fixation, unipolar or bipolar lead system, capability for pacing and/or shock delivery, delivery system for shocks)
- Assure confirmation of pacemaker placement post-implantation in initial insertion with baseline chest x-ray
- Monitor for signs of improved cardiac output at specified intervals after initiation of pacing (e.g., improved urine output, warm and dry skin, freedom from chest pain, stable vital signs, absence of JVD and crackles, improved level of consciousness), per facility protocol
- Palpate peripheral pulses at specified intervals per facility protocol to ensure adequate perfusion with paced beats
- Monitor for potential complications associated with pacemaker insertion (e.g., pneumothorax, hemothorax, myocardial perforation, cardiac tamponade, hematoma, PVCs, infections, hiccups, muscle twitches)
- Monitor for failure to pace and determine cause (e.g., lead dislodgement, fracture, or migration), as appropriate
- Monitor for failure to capture and determine cause (e.g., lead dislodgement or malposition, pacing at voltage below capture threshold, faulty connections, lead fracture, ventricular perforation), as appropriate
- Monitor for failure to sense and determine cause (e.g., sensitivity set too high, malposition of catheter lead, lead fracture, lead insulation break), as appropriate
- Obtain chest x-ray immediately in the event of suspected lead fracture, patch crinkling, lead dislodgement, or lead migration
- Monitor for symptoms of arrhythmias, ischemia, or heart failure (e.g., dizziness, syncope, palpitations, chest pain, shortness of breath), particularly with each outpatient contact
- Monitor for pacemaker problems that have occurred between scheduled checkup visits
- Monitor for arm swelling or increased warmth on side ipsilateral to implanted endovascular leads
- Monitor for redness or swelling at the device site
- Perform a comprehensive appraisal of peripheral circulation (i.e., check peripheral pulses, edema, capillary refill, skin temperature, and diaphoresis) in any initial assessment of pacemaker patients and before initiating corrective actions
- Determine type and mode of pacemaker, including universal pacemaker code information for the five positions, before initiating corrective actions
- Gather additional data, if possible, from patient's permanent record (e.g., date of implantation, frequency of use, programming changes and parameters) before initiating corrective actions
- Ensure ongoing monitoring of bedside EKG by qualified individuals
- Note frequency and duration of dysrhythmias

- Monitor hemodynamic response to dysrhythmias
- Facilitate acquisition of a 12-lead EKG, as appropriate
- Monitor sensorium and cognitive abilities
- Monitor blood pressure at specified intervals and with changes in patient condition
- Monitor heart rate and rhythm at specified intervals and with changes in patient condition
- Monitor drug and electrolyte levels for patients receiving concurrent antiarrhythmic medications
- Monitor for metabolic conditions with adverse effects on pacemakers (acid-base disturbances, myocardial ischemia, hyperkalemia, severe hyperglycemia [greater than 600 mg/dl], renal failure, hypothyroidism)
- Instruct patient related to the potential hazards for electromagnetic interference from outside sources (i.e., keep at least 6 inches away from sources of interference, do not leave cell phones in the "on" mode in a shirt pocket over the pacemaker)
- Instruct patient related to sources of highest electromagnetic interference (e.g., arc welding equipment, electronic muscle stimulators, radio transmitters, concert speakers, large motor-generator systems, electric drills, hand-held metal detectors, magnetic resonance imaging, radiation treatments)
- Instruct patient to check manufacturer warnings when in doubt about household appliances
- Instruct patient related to potential hazards from environmental interactions (e.g., inappropriate pacing or rhythm sensing, shortened generator life, cardiac arrhythmias, cardiac arrest)
- Instruct patient related to the potential hazards from metabolic disruptions (e.g., potential to increase pacer or capture thresholds)
- Instruct patient on the need for regular checkups with primary cardiologist
- Instruct patient to consult primary cardiologist for all changes in medications
- Instruct patient with new pacemaker to refrain from operating motor vehicles until permitted per primary cardiologist (usually 3 months minimally)
- Instruct patient in the need for regular monitoring of pacemaker sensing and capture thresholds
- Instruct patient in the need for regular interrogation of pacemaker by cardiologist for evidence of electromagnetic interference
- Instruct patient in the need to obtain chest x-ray minimally annually for continued pacemaker placement confirmation
- Instruct patient of the signs and symptoms of dysfunctional pacemaker (e.g., bradycardia <30 beats per minute, dizziness, weakness, fatigue, chest discomfort, angina, shortness of breath, orthopnea, pedal edema, paroxysmal nocturnal dyspnea, dyspnea on exertion, hypotension, near-syncope, frank syncope, cardiac arrest)
- Instruct patient to carry manufacturer identification card at all times
- Instruct patient to wear a medical alert bracelet or necklace that identifies patient as a pacemaker patient
- Instruct patient on the special considerations at government security gates or the airport (e.g., always inform security guard of implantable pacemaker, walk through security gates, DO NOT allow hand-held metal detectors near the device site, always walk

P

quickly through metal detection devices or ask to be searched by hand, do not lean on or stand near detection devices for long periods)
- Instruct patient that hand-held metal detectors contain magnets that can reset the pacemaker and cause malfunction
- Instruct patient's family that no harm comes to a person touching a patient who is receiving a pacemaker discharge

5th edition 2008

Background Readings:

American Association of Critical Care Nurses. (2006). *Core curriculum for critical care nursing* (6th ed.) [J. G. Alspach, Ed.]. Philadelphia: Saunders.

Geiter, H. B. (2004). Getting back to basics with permanent pacemakers, part 1. *Nursing 2004, 34*(10), 32cc1–32cc4.

Geiter, H. B. (2004). Getting back to basics with permanent pacemakers, part 2. *Nursing 2004, 34*(11), 32cc1–32cc2.

Hogle, W. P. (2001). Pacing the standard of nursing practice in radiation oncology. *Clinical Journal of Oncology Nursing, 5*(6), 253–256, 267–268.

Mattingly, E. (2004). Arrhythmia management devices and electromagnetic interference. *AANA Journal, 72*(2), 129–136.

Smeltzer, S. C., & Bare, B. G. (2004). *Brunner & Suddarth's textbook of medical-surgical nursing* (10th ed.). Philadelphia: Lippincott Williams and Wilkins.

Yeo, T. P., & Berg, N. C. (2005). Counseling patients with implanted cardiac devices. *The Nurse Practitioner, 29*(12), 58–65.

Pacemaker Management: Temporary 4092

Definition: Temporary support of cardiac pumping though the insertion and use of a temporary pacemaker

Activities:
- Determine indications for temporary pacing and duration of intended pacing support
- Determine intended mechanics of pacing (e.g., internal or external, unipolar or bipolar, transthoracic, epicardial, or central venous catheter) including appropriateness of type of pulse generator selected
- Perform a comprehensive appraisal of peripheral circulation (i.e., check peripheral pulses, edema, capillary refill), skin temperature and diaphoresis
- Ensure ongoing monitoring of bedside EKG by qualified individuals
- Note frequency and duration of dysrhythmias
- Monitor hemodynamic response to dysrhythmias
- Facilitate acquisition of a 12-lead EKG, as appropriate
- Monitor sensorium and cognitive abilities
- Monitor blood pressure at specified intervals and with changes in patient condition
- Monitor heart rate and rhythm at specified intervals and with changes in patient condition
- Instruct patient related to the chosen pacemaker (e.g., purpose, indications, mechanics, duration)
- Ensure externally paced patients are aware of possibility of discomfort and availability of sedation for comfort and/or relaxation
- Obtain informed consent for insertion of the selected temporary pacemaker
- Prepare skin on chest and back by washing with soap and water and trim body hair with scissors, not razor, as necessary
- Prepare the chosen pacemaker for use, per facility protocol (i.e., ensure battery is fresh, identify atrial and ventricular wire sets, identify positive and negative leads for each pair of wires, identification labels as indicated/preferred)
- Assist with insertion or placement of selected device, as appropriate
- Apply external transcutaneous pacemaker electrodes to clean, dry skin on the left anterior chest and to the posterior chest, as appropriate
- Provide sedation and analgesia for patients with external transcutaneous pacemaker, as indicated
- Set rate according to patient need, as directed by physician (general guidelines 90 to 110 beats per minute surgical patients, 70 to 90 beats per minute medical patients, 80 beats per minute cardiac arrest patients)
- Set the milliamperage (mA) according to patient (general adult guidelines: nonurgent 10 mA, emergent 15 to 20 mA) and increase mA until capture is present
- Monitor patient response to mA setting at regular intervals in anticipation of fluctuations resulting from endothelial sheath formation around electrode tips
- Set the sensitivity (general adult guidelines: 2 to 5 millivolt, if failure to sense occurs, turn millivolt DOWN; if sensing beats not actually present, turn millivolt UP)
- Initiate pacing by slowly increasing mA level delivered until consistent capture (capture threshold) occurs (general guidelines of mA output at 1.5 to 3 times higher than threshold, and minimally 15 to 20 mA in emergent conditions)
- Obtain chest x-ray examination after insertion of invasive temporary pacemaker
- Monitor for presence of paced rhythm or resolution of initiating dysrhythmia
- Monitor for signs of improved cardiac output at specified intervals after initiation of pacing (e.g., improved urine output, warm and dry skin, freedom from chest pain, stable vital signs, absence of JVD and crackles, improved level of consciousness) per facility protocol
- Palpate peripheral pulses at specified intervals per facility protocol to ensure adequate perfusion with paced beats
- Inspect skin frequently to prevent potential burns for patients with external transcutaneous pacemaker
- Monitor for potential complications associated with pacemaker insertion (e.g., pneumothorax, hemothorax, myocardial perforation, cardiac tamponade, hematoma, PVCs, infections, hiccups, muscle twitches)
- Observe for changes in cardiac or hemodynamic status that indicate a need for modifications in pacemaker status
- Monitor for failure to pace and determine cause (e.g., battery failure, lead dislodgement, wire fracture, disconnected wire or cable), as appropriate
- Monitor for failure to capture and determine cause (e.g., lead dislodgement or malposition, battery failure, pacing at voltage below capture threshold, faulty connections, lead fracture, ventricular perforation), as appropriate
- Monitor for failure to sense and determine cause (e.g., sensitivity set too high, battery failure, malposition of catheter lead, lead fracture, pulse generator failure, lead insulation break), as appropriate

- Monitor for conditions that potentially influence capture and sensing (e.g., fluid status changes, pericardial effusion, electrolyte or metabolic abnormalities, certain medications, tissue inflammation, tissue fibrosis, tissue necrosis)
- Perform capture and sensitivity threshold testing every 24 to 48 hours with newly inserted pacers to determine best generator settings (contraindicated in patients paced 90% or more of the time)
- Perform threshold testing separately for atrial and ventricular chambers
- Provide appropriate incisional care for pacemakers with insertion sites (e.g., dressing change, antimicrobial and sterile occlusive dressing), per facility protocol
- Ensure that all equipment is grounded, in good working order, and carefully located (e.g., in a location where it will not be dropped on the floor)
- Ensure that wires are of a length to deter inadvertent dislodging of electrodes
- Wear gloves when adjusting electrodes
- Insulate electrode wires when not in use (e.g., cover unused thoracic wires with the fingertip of a disposable glove)
- Instruct patient and family member(s) regarding symptoms to report (e.g., dizziness, fainting, prolonged weakness, nausea, palpitations, chest pain, difficulty breathing, discomfort at insertion or external electrode site, electrical shocks)
- Teach patient and family member(s) precautions and restrictions required while temporary pacemaker is in place (e.g., limitation of movement, avoid handling the pacemaker)

4th edition 2004; revised 2008

Background Readings:

American Association of Critical Care Nurses. (2006). *Core curriculum for critical care nursing* (6th ed.) [J. G. Alspach, Ed.]. Philadelphia: Saunders.

Lynn-McHale, D. J. & Carlson, K. K. (2005). *AACN procedure manual for critical care* (5th ed.). Philadelphia: Saunders.

Overbay, D. & Criddle, L. (2004). Mastering temporary invasive cardiac pacing. *Critical Care Nurse, 24*(3), 25–32.

Smeltzer, S. C., & Bare, B. G. (2004). *Brunner & Suddarth's textbook of medical-surgical nursing* (10th ed.). Philadelphia: Lippincott Williams and Wilkins.

Yeo, T. P., & Berg, N. C. (2005). Counseling patients with implanted cardiac devices. *The Nurse Practitioner, 29*(12), 58–65.

Pain Management   1400

Definition: Alleviation of pain or a reduction in pain to a level of comfort that is acceptable to the patient

Activities:

- 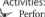 Perform a comprehensive assessment of pain to include location, characteristics, onset/duration, frequency, quality, intensity or severity of pain, and precipitating factors
- Observe for nonverbal cues of discomfort, especially in those unable to communicate effectively
- Assure patient attentive analgesic care
- Use therapeutic communication strategies to acknowledge the pain experience and convey acceptance of the patient's response to pain
- Explore patient's knowledge and beliefs about pain
- Consider cultural influences on pain response
- Determine the impact of the pain experience on quality of life (e.g., sleep, appetite, activity, cognition, mood, relationships, performance of job, and role responsibilities)
- Explore with patient the factors that improve/worsen pain
- Evaluate past experiences with pain to include individual or family history of chronic pain or resulting disability, as appropriate
- Evaluate, with the patient and the health care team, the effectiveness of past pain control measures that have been used
- Assist patient and family to seek and provide support
- Utilize a developmentally appropriate assessment method that allows for monitoring of change in pain and that will assist in identifying actual and potential precipitating factors (e.g., flow chart, daily diary)
- Determine the needed frequency of making an assessment of patient comfort and implement monitoring plan
- Provide information about the pain, such as causes of the pain, how long it will last, and anticipated discomforts from procedures
- Control environmental factors that may influence the patient's response to discomfort (e.g., room temperature, lighting, noise)
- Reduce or eliminate factors that precipitate or increase the pain experience (e.g., fear, fatigue, monotony, and lack of knowledge)
- Consider the patient's willingness to participate, ability to participate, preference, support of significant others for method, and contraindications when selecting a pain relief strategy
- Select and implement a variety of measures (e.g., pharmacological, nonpharmacological, interpersonal) to facilitate pain relief, as appropriate
- Teach principles of pain management
- Consider type and source of pain when selecting pain relief strategy
- Encourage patient to monitor own pain and to intervene appropriately
- Teach the use of nonpharmacological techniques (e.g., biofeedback, TENS, hypnosis, relaxation, guided imagery, music therapy, distraction, play therapy, activity therapy, acupressure, hot/cold application, and massage) before, after, and, if possible, during painful activities; before pain occurs or increases; and along with other pain relief measures
- Explore patient's current use of pharmacological methods of pain relief
- Teach about pharmacological methods of pain relief
- Encourage patient to use adequate pain medication
- Collaborate with the patient, significant other, and other health professionals to select and implement nonpharmacological pain relief measures, as appropriate
- Provide the person optimal pain relief with prescribed analgesics
- Implement the use of patient-controlled analgesia (PCA), if appropriate

- Use pain control measures before pain becomes severe
- Medicate prior to an activity to increase participation, but evaluate the hazard of sedation
- Assure pretreatment analgesia and/or nonpharmacologic strategies prior to painful procedures
- Verify level of discomfort with patient, note changes in the medical record, inform other health professionals working with the patient
- Evaluate the effectiveness of the pain control measures used through ongoing assessment of the pain experience
- Institute and modify pain control measures on the basis of the patient's response
- Promote adequate rest/sleep to facilitate pain relief
- Encourage patient to discuss his/her pain experience, as appropriate
- Notify physician if measures are unsuccessful or if current complaint is a significant change from patient's past experience of pain
- Inform other health care professionals/family members of nonpharmacologic strategies being used by the patient to encourage preventive approaches to pain management
- Utilize a multidisciplinary approach to pain management, when appropriate
- Consider referrals for patient, family, and significant others to support groups, and other resources, as appropriate
- Provide accurate information to promote family's knowledge of and response to the pain experience

- Incorporate the family in the pain relief modality, if possible
- Monitor patient satisfaction with pain management at specified intervals

1st edition 1992; revised 1996, 2004

Background Readings:

Herr, K. A., & Mobily, P. R. (1992). Interventions related to pain. In G. M. Bulechek & J. C. McCloskey (Eds.), Symposium on nursing interventions. *Nursing Clinics of North America, 27*(2), 347–370.

McCaffery, M., & Pasero, C. (1999). *Pain: Clinical manual for nursing practice* (2nd ed.). St. Louis: Mosby.

McGuire, L. (1994). The nurse's role in pain relief. *MEDSURG Nursing, 3*(2), 94–107.

Mobily, P. R. & Herr, K. A. (2000). Pain. In M. Maas, K. Buckwalter, M. Hardy, T. Tripp-Reimer, M. Titler, & J. Specht (Eds.), *Nursing diagnosis, interventions, and outcomes for elders* (2nd ed., pp. 455-475). Thousand Oaks, CA: Sage.

Perry, A. G., & Potter, P. A. (2000). *Clinical nursing skills and techniques* (pp. 84–101). St. Louis: Mosby.

Rhiner, M., & Kedziera, P. (1999). Managing breakthrough pain: A new approach. *American Journal of Nursing*, (Suppl.), 3–12.

Titler, M. G., & Rakel, B. A. (2001). Nonpharmacologic treatment of pain. *Critical Care Nursing Clinics of North America, 13*(2), 221–232.

Victor, K. (2001). Properly assessing pain in the elderly. *RN, 64*(5), 45–49.

Parent Education: Adolescent   5562

Definition: Assisting parents to understand and help their adolescent children

Activities:
- Ask parents to describe the characteristics of their adolescent child
- Discuss parent-child relationship during earlier, school-aged years
- Understand the relationship between the parent's behavior and child's age-appropriate goals
- Identify personal factors that impact on the success of the educational program (e.g., cultural values, presence of any negative experiences with social service providers, language barriers, time commitment, scheduling issues, travel, and general lack of interest)
- Identify the presence of family stressors (e.g., parental depression, drug addiction, alcoholism, low literacy, limited education, domestic violence, marital conflict, blending of families after divorce, and excessive punishment of children)
- Discuss disciplining of parents themselves when they were adolescents
- Instruct parent on normal physiological, emotional, and cognitive characteristics of adolescents
- Identify developmental tasks or goals of the adolescent period of life
- Identify defense mechanisms used most commonly by adolescents, such as denial and intellectualization
- Address the effects of adolescent cognitive development on information processing
- Address the effects of adolescent cognitive development on decision making

- Have parents describe methods of discipline used before adolescent years and their feelings of success with these measures
- Provide online resources, books, and literature designed to teach parents about teen parenting
- Describe the importance of power and control issues for both parents and adolescents during adolescent years
- Instruct parents about essential communication skills that will increase their ability to empathize with their adolescent and assist their adolescent to problem solve
- Instruct parents about methods of communicating their love to adolescents
- Explore parallels between school-aged dependency on parents and adolescent dependency on peer group
- Reinforce normalcy of adolescent vacillation between desire for independence and regression to dependence
- Discuss effects of adolescent separation from parents on spousal relationships
- Share strategies for managing adolescent's perception of parental rejection
- Facilitate expression of parental feelings
- Assist parents to identify reasons for their responses to adolescents
- Identify avenues to assist adolescent to manage anger
- Instruct parents how to use conflict for mutual understanding and family growth
- Role play strategies for managing family conflict
- Discuss with parents issues over which they will accept compromise and issues over which they cannot compromise

- Discuss necessity and legitimacy of limit setting for adolescents
- Address strategies for limit setting for adolescents
- Instruct parents to use reality and consequences to manage adolescent behavior
- Refer parents to support group or parenting classes, as appropriate

1st edition 1992; revised 2013

Background Readings:

American Academy of Child and Adolescent Psychiatry. (1999). *Your adolescent: Emotional, behavioral, and cognitive development from early adolescence through the teen years* [D. Pruitt, Ed.]. New York: Harper Collins.

Cline, F., & Fay, J. (2006). *Parenting teens with love and logic: Preparing adolescents for responsible adulthood* (updated ed.). Colorado Springs, CO: Piñon Press.

Dinkmeyer, D., McKay, G. D., & McKay, J. L. (2007). *Parenting teenagers: Systematic training for effective parenting of teens.* Bowling Green, KY: STEP.

Pillitteri, A. (2007). The family with an adolescent. In *Maternal and child health nursing: Care of the childbearing and childrearing family* (5th ed., pp. 941–974). Philadelphia: Lippincott Williams & Wilkins.

Parent Education: Childrearing Family   5566

Definition: Assisting parents to understand and promote the physical, psychological, and social growth and development of their toddler, preschool, or school-aged child

Activities:

- Ask parent to describe the behaviors of the child
- Understand the relationship between the parent's behavior and child's age-appropriate goals
- Design an education program that builds on the family's strengths
- Involve parents in the design and content of the education program
- Identify personal factors that impact on the success of the education program (e.g., cultural values, presence of any negative experiences with social service providers, language barriers, time commitment, scheduling issues, travel, and general lack of interest)
- Identify the presence of family stressors (e.g., parental depression, drug addiction, alcoholism, low literacy, limited education, domestic violence, marital conflict, blending of families after divorce, and excessive punishment of children)
- Identify appropriate developmental tasks or goals for the child
- Identify defense mechanisms used most by age group
- Facilitate parents' discussion of methods of discipline available, selection, and results obtained
- Instruct parent on normal physiological, emotional, and behavioral characteristics of child
- Provide online resources, books, and literature designed to teach parents about parenting
- Provide parents with readings and other materials that will be helpful in performing parenting role
- Instruct parents on the importance of a balanced diet, three meals a day, and nutritious snacks
- Review nutritional requirements for specific age groups
- Review dental hygiene facts with parents
- Review grooming facts with parents
- Review safety issues with parents (e.g., children meeting strangers, water safety, bicycle safety)
- Discuss avenues parents can use to assist children in managing anger
- Discuss approaches parents can use to assist children to express feelings positively
- Help parents identify evaluation criteria for day care and school settings
- Inform parents of community resources
- Identify and instruct parents on how to use a variety of strategies in managing child's behavior
- Encourage parents to try different childrearing strategies, as appropriate
- Encourage parents to observe other parents interacting with children
- Role play childrearing techniques and communication skills
- Refer parents to support group or parenting classes, as appropriate

1st edition 1992; revised 2013

Background Readings:

American Academy of Child and Adolescent Psychiatry. (1998). *Your child: Emotional, behavioral, and cognitive development from birth to preadolescent* [D. Pruitt, Ed.]. New York: Harper Collins.

Hockenberry, M., & Tashiro, J. (2005). *Wong's essentials of pediatric nursing* (7th ed.). St. Louis: Mosby.

Licence, K. (2004). Promoting and protecting the health of children and young people. *Child: Care, Health, and Development, 30*(6), 623–635.

Riesch, S. K., Anderson, L. S., Krueger, H. A. (2006). Parent–child communication processes: Preventing children's health-risk behavior. *Journal for Specialists in Pediatric Nursing, 11*(1), 41–56.

Schor, E. (1999). *Caring for your school age child: Ages 5 to 12.* New York: Bantam.

Shelov, S., & Altman T. R. (2009). *Caring for your baby and young child: Birth to age 5* (5th ed.). New York: Bantam.

Shonkoff, J. P., & Phillips. D. A. (Eds.). (2000). *From neurons to neighborhoods: The science of early childhood development.* Washington, DC: National Academy Press.

P

Parent Education: Infant   5568

Definition: Instruction on nurturing and physical care needed during the first year of life

Activities:

- Determine parent(s)' knowledge and readiness and ability to learn about infant care
- Monitor learning needs of the family
- Provide anticipatory guidance about developmental changes during the first year of life
- Assist parent(s) in articulating ways to integrate infant into family system
- Teach parent(s) skills to care for newborn
- Instruct parent(s) on formula preparation and selection
- Give parent(s) information about pacifiers
- Give information about adding solid foods to diet during the first year
- Instruct parent(s) on appropriate fluoride supplementation
- Give information about developing dentition and oral hygiene during the first year
- Discuss alternatives to a bedtime bottle to prevent nursing bottle caries
- Provide anticipatory guidance about changing elimination patterns during the first year
- Instruct parent(s) on how to treat and prevent diaper rash
- Provide anticipatory guidance about changing sleep patterns during the first year
- Demonstrate ways in which parent(s) can stimulate infant's development
- Encourage parent(s) to hold, cuddle, massage, and touch infant
- Encourage parent(s) to talk and read to infant
- Encourage parent(s) to provide pleasurable auditory and visual stimulation
- Encourage parent(s) to play with infant
- Give examples of safe toys or available things in home that can be used as toys
- Encourage parent(s) to attend parenting classes
- Provide parent(s) with written materials appropriate to identified knowledge needs
- Reinforce parent(s)' ability to apply teaching to child care skills
- Provide parent(s) with support when learning infant caretaking skills
- Assist parent(s) in interpreting infant cues, nonverbal cues, crying, and vocalizations
- Provide anticipatory guidance about changing sleep patterns during the first year

- Provide information on newborn behavioral characteristics
- Demonstrate reflexes to parent(s) and explain their significance to infant care
- Discuss infant's capabilities for interaction
- Assist parent(s) to identify behavioral characteristics of infant
- Demonstrate infant's abilities and strengths to parent(s)
- Explain and demonstrate infant states
- Demonstrate quieting techniques
- Monitor parent skill in recognizing the infant's physiological needs
- Reinforce caregiver role behaviors
- Reinforce skills parent does well in caring for infant to promote confidence
- Provide parent(s) with information about making home environment safe for infant
- Provide information about safety needs of infant while in a motor vehicle
- Instruct parent(s) on how to reach health professionals
- Place follow-up telephone call 1-2 weeks after encounter
- Provide information about community resources

3rd edition 2000

Background Readings:

American Academy of Pediatrics & American College of Obstetricians and Gynecologists. (1992). Postpartum and follow-up care. In *Guidelines for perinatal care* (3rd ed., pp. 91–116). Evanston, IL: Author.

Barnes, L. P. (1994). Infant care: Teaching the basics. *Maternal Child Nursing, 19*(2), 117.

Betz, C. L., Hunsberger, M. M., & Wright, S. (1994). Families with neonates. In *Nursing care of children* (pp. 107–142). Philadelphia: Saunders.

Denehy, J. A. (1990). Anticipatory guidance. In M. J. Craft & J. A. Denehy (Eds.), *Nursing interventions for infants and children* (pp. 53–68). Philadelphia: Saunders.

Denehy, J. A. (1992). Interventions related to parent-infant attachment. In G.M. Bulechek & J.C. McCloskey (Eds.), Symposium on nursing interventions. *Nursing Clinics of North America, 27*(2), 425–444.

Mott, S. R., James, S. R. & Sperhc, A. M. (1990). *Nursing care of children and families* (2nd ed.). Redwood City, CA: Addison-Wesley.

Pillitteri, A. (2007). The family with an infant. In *Maternal and child health nursing: Care of the childbearing and childrearing family* (5th ed., pp. 824–859). Philadelphia: Lippincott Williams & Wilkins.

Parenting Promotion   8300

Definition: Providing parenting information, support, and coordination of comprehensive services to high-risk families

Activities:

- Identify and enroll high-risk families in follow-up program
- Encourage mothers to receive early and regular prenatal care
- Visit mothers in the hospital before discharge to begin establishing trusting relationship and schedule follow-up visit
- Make home visits as indicated by level of risk
- Assist parents to have realistic expectations appropriate to developmental and ability level of child
- Assist parents with role transition and expectations of parenthood

- Refer to home male visitors to work with fathers, as appropriate
- Provide anticipatory guidance needed at different developmental levels
- Provide pamphlets, books, and other materials to develop parenting skills
- Discuss age-appropriate behavior management strategies
- Assist parents to identify unique temperament of infant
- Teach parents to respond to behavior cues exhibited by their infant
- Model and encourage parental interaction with children

- Refer to parent support groups, as appropriate
- Assist parents in developing, maintaining, and using social support systems
- Listen to parents' problems and concerns nonjudgmentally
- Provide positive feedback and structured successes at parenting skills to foster self-esteem
- Assist parents to develop social skills
- Teach and model coping skills
- Enhance problem-solving skills through role modeling, practice, and reinforcement
- Provide toys through toy lending library
- Monitor child health status, well-child checks, and immunization status
- Monitor parental health status and health maintenance activities
- Arrange transportation to well-child visits or other services, as necessary
- Refer to community resources, as appropriate
- Coordinate community agencies working with family
- Provide linkage to job training or employment, as needed
- Inform parents where to receive family planning services
- Monitor consistent and correct use of contraceptives, as appropriate
- Assist in arranging day care, as needed
- Refer for respite care, as appropriate
- Refer to domestic violence center, as needed

- Refer for substance abuse treatment, as needed
- Collect and record data as indicated for follow-up and program evaluation

3rd edition 2000

Background Readings:

Clarke, B. A. & Strauss, S. S. (1992). Nursing role supplementation for adolescent parents: Prescriptive nursing practice. *Journal of Pediatric Nursing, 7*(5), 312–318.

Denehy, J. A. (2001). Parenting promotion. In M. Craft-Rosenberg & J. Denehy (Eds.), *Nursing interventions for infants, children, and families* (pp. 99–118). Thousand Oaks, CA: Sage.

Fuddy, L., & Thompson, R. A. (2001). Healthy start: A statewide system of family support for the prevention of child abuse and neglect. In G. B. Melton, R. A. Thompson, & M. A. Small (Eds.), *Toward a child-centered, neighborhood-based child protection system: A report of the consortium on children, families, and the law* (pp. 214–232). Westport, CT: Praeger.

Hardy, J. B. & Streett, R. (1989). Family support and parenting education in the home: An effective extension of clinic-based preventive health care services for poor children. *Journal of Pediatrics, 115*(6), 927–931.

Olds, D. L., & Kitzman, H. (1993). Review of research on home visiting for pregnant women and parents of young children. *The Future of Children 3*(3), 53–92.

Pass Facilitation   7440

Definition: Arranging a leave for a patient from a health care facility

Activities:

- Obtain physician order for pass, as appropriate
- Establish objectives for the pass
- Provide information about restrictions and length of time for pass
- Provide information needed for emergency use on pass
- Determine who is responsible for patient, as appropriate
- Discuss pass with responsible person describing nursing care/self-care, as needed
- Prepare medication to be taken on pass, and instruct responsible person
- Provide assistive devices/equipment, as appropriate
- Offer suggestions for appropriate pass activities, as needed
- Help pack personal belongings for pass, as needed
- Provide time for patient, family, and friends to ask questions and express concerns
- Obtain signature of patient or responsible person on "sign-out" form

- Instruct appropriate person that information will be needed about medication, food, and alcohol intake while on pass
- Evaluate whether objectives for pass were met on return

2nd edition 1996

Background Readings:

March, C. S. (1992). *The complete care plan manual for long-term care.* Chicago: American Hospital.

Nurse's Reference Library. (1987). *Patient teaching: Learning needs, discharge preparation, tips and checklists.* Springhouse, PA: Springhouse.

Rakel, B. A. (1992). Interventions related to patient teaching. In G. M. Bulechek & J. C. McCloskey (Eds.), Symposium on nursing interventions. *Nursing Clinics of North America, 27*(2), 397–423.

P

Patient Contracting   4420

Definition: Negotiating an agreement with an individual that reinforces a specific behavior change

Activities:

- Determine the individual's mental and cognitive ability to enter into a contract
- Encourage the individual to identify own strengths and abilities
- Assist the individual in identifying the health practices he/she wishes to change

- Identify with individual the goals of care
- Encourage the individual to identify own goals, not those he/she believes the health care provider expects
- Avoid focusing on diagnosis or disease process alone when assisting the individual in identifying goals
- Assist the individual in identifying realistic, attainable goals

- Assist the individual in identifying appropriate short-term and long-term goals
- Encourage the individual to write down his/her own goals, if possible
- State goals as easily observed behaviors
- State goals in positive terms
- Assist the individual in breaking down complex goals into small, manageable steps
- Clarify with the individual roles of the health care provider and the individual, respectively
- Explore with the individual ways to best achieve the goals
- Assist the individual in examining available resources to meet the goals
- Assist the individual in developing a plan to meet the goals
- Assist the individual in identifying present circumstances in the environment, which may interfere with the achievement of goals
- Assist the individual in identifying methods of overcoming environmental circumstances that may interfere with goal achievement
- Explore with the individual methods for evaluating accomplishment of the goals
- Foster an open, accepting environment for the creation of the contract
- Facilitate involvement of significant others in the contracting process, if desired by the individual
- Facilitate the making of a written contract, including all agreed-upon elements
- Assist the individual in setting time or frequency requirements for performance of behaviors/actions
- Assist the individual in setting realistic time limits
- Together with the individual, identify a target date for termination of the contract
- Coordinate with the individual opportunities for review of the contract and goals
- Facilitate renegotiation of contract terms, if necessary
- Assist the individual in discussing his/her feelings about the contract
- Observe individual for signs of incongruence that may indicate lack of commitment to fulfilling the contract

- Identify with the individual consequences or sanctions for not fulfilling the contract, if desired
- Have the contract signed by all involved parties
- Provide the individual with a copy of the signed and dated contract
- Encourage the individual to identify appropriate, meaningful reinforcers/rewards
- Encourage the individual to choose a reinforcer/reward that is significant enough to sustain the behavior
- Specify with the individual timing of delivery of reinforcers/rewards
- Identify additional rewards with the individual if original goals are exceeded, if desired
- Instruct the individual on various methods of observing and recording behaviors
- Assist the individual in developing some form of flowchart to assist in tracking the progress toward goals
- Assist the individual in identifying even small successes
- Explore with the individual reasons for success, or lack of it

1st edition 1992; revised 2004

Background Readings:
McConnell, E. S. (2000). Health contract calendars: A tool for health professionals with older adults. *The Gerontologist, 40*(2), 235–239.
Newell, M. (1997). Patient contracting for improved outcomes. *The Journal of Care Management, 3*(4), 76–87.
Sherman, J. M., Baumstein, S., & Hendeles, L. (2001). Intervention strategies for children poorly adherent with asthma medications; one center's experience. *Clinical Pediatrics, 40*(5), 253–258.
Simons, M. R. (1999). Patient contracting. In G. M. Bulechek & J. C. McCloskey (Eds.), *Nursing interventions: Effective nursing treatments* (3rd ed., pp. 385–397). Philadelphia: Saunders.
Snyder, M. (1992). Contracting. In M. Snyder, *Independent nursing interventions* (2nd ed., pp. 145–154). Albany, NY: Delmar.

Patient-Controlled Analgesia (PCA) Assistance 2400

Definition: Facilitating patient control of analgesic administration and regulation

Activities:
- Collaborate with physicians, patient, and family members in selecting the type of narcotic to be used
- Recommend administration of aspirin and nonsteroidal antiinflammatory drugs in conjunction with narcotics, as appropriate
- Recommend discontinuation of opioid administration by other routes
- Avoid use of meperidine hydrochloride (Demerol)
- Ensure that patient is not allergic to analgesic to be administered
- Instruct patient and family to monitor pain intensity, quality, and duration
- Instruct patient and family to monitor respiratory rate and blood pressure
- Establish nasogastric, venous, subcutaneous, or spinal access, as appropriate
- Validate that the patient can use a PCA device (i.e., is able to communicate, comprehend explanations, and follow directions)
- Collaborate with patient and family to select appropriate type of patient-controlled infusion device
- Instruct patient and family members how to use the PCA device

- Assist patient and family to calculate appropriate concentration of drug to fluid, considering the amount of fluid delivered per hour via the PCA device
- Assist patient or family member to administer an appropriate bolus loading dose of analgesic
- Instruct the patient and family to set an appropriate basal infusion rate on the PCA device
- Assist the patient and family to set the appropriate lockout interval on the PCA device
- Assist the patient and family in setting appropriate demand doses on the PCA device
- Consult with patient, family members, and physician to adjust lockout interval, basal rate, and demand dosage, according to patient responsiveness
- Instruct patient how to titrate doses up or down, depending on respiratory rate, pain intensity, and pain quality
- Instruct patient and family members on the action and side effects of pain-relieving agents
- Document patient's pain, amount and frequency of drug dosing, and response to pain treatment in a pain flow chart

- Monitor closely for respiratory depression in at-risk patients (e.g., older than 70 years; history of sleep apnea; concurrent use of PCA with a central nervous system depressant; obesity; upper abdominal or thoracic surgery and PCA bolus of greater than 1mg; history of renal, hepatic, pulmonary, or cardiac impairment)
- Recommend a bowel regimen to avoid constipation
- Consult with clinical pain experts for a patient who is having difficulty achieving pain control

1st edition 1992; revised 2013

Background Readings:

Berman, A., Snyder, S., Kozier, B., & Erb, G. (2008). Pain management. In *Kozier & Erb's fundamentals of nursing: Concepts, processes, and practice.* (8th ed., pp. 1187–1230). Upper Saddle River, NJ: Prentice Hall.

Chumbley, G., & Mountford, L. (2010). Patient-controlled analgesia infusion pumps for adults. *Nursing Standard, 25*(8), 35–40.

Craft, J. (2010). Patient-controlled analgesia: Is it worth the painful prescribing process? *Baylor University Medical Center Proceedings, 23*(4), 434–438.

Franson, H. (2010). Postoperative patient-controlled analgesia in the pediatric population: A literature review. *AANA Journal, 78*(5), 374–378.

Patient Identification   6574

Definition: Positive verification of a patient's identity

Activities:
- Explain to the patient the importance of proper identification throughout the health encounter
- Ask the patient their first and last name, and date of birth
- Verify that the information provided by the patient is the same as the information in the identification device (e.g., wristbands, bed tag, fingerprint recognition software, palm vein scanner) and medical record
- Select the most appropriate location(s) for placing the identification device(s)
- Ensure that identification device(s) are put in appropriate locations
- Have on hand a number of replacement bands and an easy process for a new bracelet to be stamped and applied should a wristband be removed
- Standardize the format of the wristbands across the health care institution
- Compare the information provided by the patient with the information in the identification device before every administration of care (e.g., administering medications, performing invasive procedures, conducting diagnostic tests, transferring patient)
- Use at least two patient identifiers when laboratory samples are obtained or medications or blood products are administered
- Conduct verification of patient at multiple points in time when procedure is complex and involves several stages
- Use identification by family member or good friend when patient cannot provide information
- Institute a "stop-the-line" policy if a misidentification error is suspected (i.e., do not carry out the intended action until positive identification is made)
- Educate the patient about the risks related to an incorrect identification
- Compare the information provided by a family member with the information in the identification device to confirm a patient's death
- Ensure a best practice for patient identification by instituting a clearly written, easy to understand agency policy

6th edition, 2013

Background Readings:

AORN (2006). Best practices for preventing wrong site, wrong person, and wrong procedure errors in perioperative settings. *AORN Journal 84* (Suppl. 1), S13–S29.

Beyea, S. C. (2003). Patient identification: A crucial aspect on patient safety. *AORN Journal, 78*(3), 478, 481.

Bittle, M. J., Charache, P., & Wassilchalk, D. M. (2007). Registration-associated patient misidentification in an academic medical centre: Causes and corrections. *Joint Commission Journal on Quality and Patient Safety, 33*(1), 25–33.

Clarke, J. R., Johnson, J., & Finley, E. (2007). Getting surgery right. *Annals of Surgery, 246*(3), 395–403.

Edwards, P. (2008). Ensuring correct site surgery. *Journal of Perioperative Practice, 18*(4), 168–171.

Gray, J. E., Suresh, G., Ursprung, R., Edwards, W. H., Nickerson, J., Shiono, P. H., et al. (2006). Patient misidentification in the neonatal intensive care unit: Quantification of risk. *Pediatrics, 117*(1), e43–e47.

Hain, P. D., Joers, B., Rush, M., Slayton, J. Throop, P., Hoagg, S., et al. (2010). An intervention to decrease patient identification band errors in a children's hospital. *Quality Safety Health Care, 19*(3), 244–247.

High Tech Patient ID, Information technologists design system to recognize palm vein patterns (2007, October). *Science Daily* <http://www.science-daily.com/videos/2007/1009-high_tech_patient_id.htm>.

Patient Rights Protection   7460

Definition: Protection of health care rights of a patient, especially a minor, incapacitated, or incompetent patient unable to make decisions

Activities:
- Provide patient with "Patient's Bill of Rights"
- Provide environment conducive for private conversations between patient, family, and health care professionals
- Protect patient's privacy during activities of hygiene, elimination, and grooming
- Determine whether patient's wishes about health care are known in the form of advance directives (e.g., living will, durable power of attorney for health care)
- Honor patient's right to receive appropriate pain management for acute, chronic, and terminal conditions

- Determine who is legally empowered to give consent for treatment or research
- Work with physician and hospital administration to honor patient and family wishes
- Refrain from forcing the treatment
- Note religious preference
- Know the legal status of living wills in the state
- Honor a patient's wishes expressed in a living will or durable power of attorney for health care, as appropriate
- Honor written "Do Not Resuscitate" orders
- Assist the dying person with unfinished business
- Note on medical record any observable facts bearing on the testator's mental competency to make a will
- Intervene in situations involving unsafe or inadequate care
- Be aware of mandatory reporting requirements in the state
- Limit viewing of the patient's record to immediate health care providers
- Maintain confidentiality of patient health information

1st edition 1992; revised 2004

Background Readings:

American Hospital Association. (2001). *Ethical conduct for health care institutions.* Chicago, IL: Author.

American Hospital Association. (2003). *The patient care partnership* <http://www.aha.org/aha/issues/Communicating-With-Patients/pt-care-partnership.html/>.

Perry, A. G. & Potter, P. A. (2002). *Clinical nursing skills and techniques* (5th ed., pp. 4–6). St. Louis: Mosby.

Ryan, B. (2004). Advance directives: Your role. *RN, 67*(5), 59–62.

Timby, B. K., & Smith, N. E. (2007). Legal and ethical issues. In *Introductory medical-surgical nursing* (9th ed., pp. 34–47). Philadelphia: Lippincott Williams & Wilkins.

Weiler, K. & Moorhead, S. (1999). Patient rights protection. In G. M. Bulechek & J. C. McCloskey (Eds.), *Nursing interventions: Effective nursing treatments* (3rd ed., pp. 624–636). Philadelphia: Saunders.

Peer Review 7700

Definition: Systematic evaluation of a peer's performance compared with professional standards of practice

Activities:
- Develop and use policies to guide function of the peer review committee and review process, as necessary
- Participate in establishment of protocols and standards for professional practice
- Participate in committee meetings, as appropriate
- Coordinate evaluation process, as necessary
- Observe peer during performance of service, as required for evaluation
- Identify performance requiring support of peers
- Perform evaluations of selected peers (including self, when required)
- Provide input in areas of strength and development needs, as indicated
- Review credentials of selected peer, as necessary
- Recommend promotion or clinical advancement, as appropriate
- Provide supervision and counseling, as appropriate
- Provide opportunity for feedback
- Develop shared responsibility for change or improvement, as necessary
- Coordinate appropriate continuing education and training, as necessary
- Participate in grievance proceedings, as needed

2nd edition 1996

Background Readings:

American Nurses Association. (1988). *Peer review guidelines.* Kansas City, MO: Author.

Mann, L., Barton, C., Presti, M., & Hirsch J. (1990). Peer review in performance appraisal. *Nursing Administrative Quarterly, 14*(4), 9–14.

Quigley, P., Hixon, A., & Janzen, S. (1991). Promoting autonomy and professional practice: A program of clinical privileging. *Journal of Nursing Quality Assurance, 5*(3), 27–32.

Supples, J. (1993). Self-regulation in the nursing profession: Response to substandard practice. *Nursing Outlook, 41*(1), 20–24.

Titlebaum, H., Hart, C., & Romano-Egan, J. (1992). Interagency psychiatric consultation liaison nursing peer review and peer board: Quality assurance and employment. *Archives of Psychiatric Nursing, 7*(2), 125–131.

Pelvic Muscle Exercise 0560

Definition: Strengthening and training the levator ani and urogenital muscles through voluntary, repetitive contraction to decrease stress, urge, or mixed types of urinary incontinence

Activities:
- Determine ability to recognize urge to void
- Instruct individual to tighten, then relax, the ring of muscle around urethra and anus, as if trying to prevent urination or bowel movement
- Instruct individual to avoid contracting the abdomen, thighs, and buttocks; holding breath; or straining down during the exercise
- Assure that the individual can differentiate between the desired drawing up-and-in muscle contraction and the undesired bearing down effort
- Instruct female individual to identify the levator ani and urogenital muscles by placing a finger in the vagina and squeezing
- Instruct individual to perform muscle tightening exercises, working up to 300 contractions each day, holding the contractions for

10 seconds each and resting at least 10 seconds between each contraction, per agency protocol
- Inform individual that it takes 6 to 12 weeks for exercises to be effective
- Provide positive feedback for doing exercises as prescribed
- Teach individual to monitor response to exercise by attempting to stop urine flow no more often than once a week
- Incorporate biofeedback or electrical stimulation for selected individuals when assistance is indicated to identify correct muscles to contract and/or to elicit desired strength of muscle contraction
- Provide written instructions describing the intervention and the recommended number of repetitions
- Discuss daily record of continence with individual to provide reinforcement

2nd edition 1996; revised 2000, 2004

Background Readings:

DeLancey, J. O. (1994). Structural support of the urethra as it relates to stress urinary incontinence: The hammock hypothesis. *American Journal of Obstetrics & Gynecology, 170*(6), 1713–1720.

Dougherty, M., Bishop, K., Mooney, R., Gimotty, P., & Williams, B. (1993). Graded pelvic muscle exercise: Effect on stress urinary incontinence. *Journal of Reproductive Medicine, 39*(9), 684–691.

Johnson, V. Y. (2001). How the principles of exercise physiology influence pelvic floor muscle training. *Journal of Wound, Ostomy, and Continence Nursing, 28*(3), 150–155.

Palmer, M. H. (2001). A long-term study of patient outcomes with pelvic muscle re-education for urinary incontinence. *Journal of Wound, Ostomy, and Continence Nursing, 28*(4), 199–205.

Sampselle, C. (1993). The urine stream interruption test: Using a stopwatch to assess pelvic muscle strength. *Nurse Practitioner, 18*(1), 14–20.

Perineal Care   1750

Definition: Maintenance of perineal skin integrity and relief of perineal discomfort

Activities:
- Assist with hygiene
- Keep the perineum dry
- Provide cushion for chair, as appropriate
- Inspect condition of incision, or tear(s) (e.g., episiotomy, laceration, circumcision)
- Apply cold pack, as appropriate
- Apply a heat cradle or heat lamp, as appropriate
- Instruct patient on rationale and use of sitz baths
- Provide and assist with sitz baths, as necessary
- Clean the perineum thoroughly at regular intervals
- Maintain patient in comfortable position
- Apply absorbent pads to absorb drainage, as appropriate
- Apply protective barrier (e.g., zinc oxide, petrolatum), as appropriate
- Apply prescribed medication (e.g., antibacterial, antifungal), as appropriate
- Document characteristics of drainage, as appropriate
- Provide scrotal support, as appropriate
- Provide pain medications, as appropriate
- Instruct patient or significant other, as appropriate, regarding inspection of perineum for pathology (e.g., infection, skin breakdown, rash, abnormal discharge)

1st edition 1992; revised 2013

Background Readings:

Albers, L. L., & Borders, N. (2007). Minimizing genital tract trauma and related pain following spontaneous vaginal birth. *Journal of Midwifery & Womens Health, 52*(3), 246–253.

Driver, D. S. (2007). Perineal dermatitis in critical care patients. *Critical Care Nurse, 27*(4), 42–47.

Gray, M., Ratliff, C., & Donovan, A. (2002). Protecting perineal skin integrity. Incontinent patients present unique challenges to successful skin care management. *Nursing Management, 33*(12), 61–63.

Leventhal, L. C., de Oliveira, S. M., Nobre, M. R., & da Silva, F. M. (2011). Perineal analgesia with an ice pack after spontaneous vaginal birth: A randomized controlled trial. *Journal of Midwifery & Womens Health, 56*(2), 141–146.

Nix, D., & Ermer-Seltun J. (2004). A review of perineal skin care protocols and skin barrier product use. *Ostomy Wound Management, 50*(12), 59–67.

Potter, P. A., & Perry, A. G. (2009). *Fundamentals of nursing* (7th ed.). St. Louis: Mosby.

Ward, S. L., & Hisley, S. M. (2009). *Maternal-child nursing care: Optimizing outcomes for mothers, children and families* (1st ed., pp. 472–473, 487, 576, 843). Philadelphia: F. A. Davis.

P

Peripheral Sensation Management   2660

Definition: Prevention or minimization of injury or discomfort in the patient with altered sensation

Activities:
- Monitor sharp or dull and hot or cold discrimination
- Monitor for paresthesia (e.g., numbness, tingling, hyperesthesia, hypoesthesia, and level of pain), as appropriate
- Encourage patient to use the unaffected body part to determine temperature of food, liquids, bathwater, and so on
- Encourage patient to use the unaffected body part to identify location and texture of objects
- Instruct patient or family to monitor position of body parts while bathing, sitting, lying, or changing position
- Instruct patient or family to examine skin daily for alteration in skin integrity

- Monitor fit of bracing devices, prosthesis, shoes, and clothing
- Instruct patient or family to use thermometer to test water temperature
- Encourage use of thermal insulated mitts when handling cooking utensils
- Encourage use of gloves or other protective clothing over affected body part when body part is in contact with objects that, because of their thermal, textural, or other inherent characteristics, may be potentially hazardous
- Avoid or carefully monitor use of heat or cold, such as heating pads, hot water bottles, and ice packs
- Encourage patient to wear well-fitting, low-heeled, soft shoes
- Place cradle over affected body parts to keep bed clothes off affected areas
- Check shoes, pockets, and clothing for wrinkles or foreign objects
- Instruct patient to use timed intervals, rather than presence of discomfort, as a signal to alter position
- Use pressure-relieving devices, as appropriate
- Protect body parts from extreme temperature changes
- Immobilize the head, neck, and back, as appropriate
- Monitor ability to void or defecate
- Establish a means of voiding, as appropriate
- Establish a means of bowel evacuation, as appropriate
- Administer analgesics, corticosteroids, anticonvulsants, tricyclic antidepressants, or local anesthesias, as necessary
- Monitor for thrombophlebitis and venous thromboembolism
- Discuss or identify causes of abnormal sensations or sensation changes
- Instruct patient to visually monitor position of body parts, if proprioception is impaired

1st edition 1992; revised 2013

Background Readings:

Bader M. E., & Littlejohns, L. R. (Eds.). (2004). AANN *Core curriculum for neuroscience nursing* (4th ed.). New York: WB Saunders.

Barker, E. (2007). *Neuroscience nursing: A spectrum of care* (3rd ed.). St. Louis: Mosby Elsevier.

Gore, M., Brandenburg, N. A., Dukes, E., Hoffman, D. L., Tai, K., & Stacey, B. (2005). Pain severity in diabetic peripheral neuropathy is associated with patient functioning, symptoms levels of anxiety and depression, and sleep. *Journal of Pain and Symptom Management, 30*(4), 374–385.

Hickey, J. V. (2009). *The clinical practice of neurological and neurosurgical nursing* (6th ed.). Philadelphia: Lippincott Williams & Wilkins.

Paice, J. A. (2009). Clinical challenges: Chemotherapy-induced peripheral neuopathy. *Seminars in Oncolocy Nursing, 25*(2), S8–S19.

Pugh, S., Mathiesen, C., Meighan, M., Summer, D., & Zrelak, P. (2008). *Guide to the care of the hospitalized patient with ischemic stroke.* (2nd ed., pp. 5–38). Glenview, IL: American Association of Neuroscience Nurses.

Ratliff, C., Tomaselli, N., Goldberg, M., Bonham, P., Crawford, P., Flemister, B., et al. (2010). *Guideline for prevention and management of pressure ulcers.* Mt. Laurel, NJ: Wound, Ostomy, and Continence Nurses Society.

Smith, C. M., & Cotter, V. (2008). Age-related changes in health. In E. Capezuti, D. Zwicker, M. Mezey, & T. Fulmer, (Eds.), *Evidence-based geriatric nursing protocols for best practice* (3rd ed., pp. 431–458). New York: Springer.

Peripherally Inserted Central Catheter (PICC) Care   4220

Definition: Insertion and maintenance of a peripherally inserted catheter for access into the central circulation

Activities:

- Identify the intended use of the catheter to determine the type needed (i.e., vesicants or potentially irritating drugs should be run through a centrally inserted line, not a peripheral line)
- Explain the purpose of the catheter, benefits, and risks associated with its use to patient/family
- Obtain consent for the insertion procedure
- Select an appropriate size and type of catheter to meet patient needs
- Select most accessible and least used antecubital vein available (usually the basilic or cephalic vein of the dominant arm)
- Assure patient is appropriate candidate for insertion (i.e., veins must be visible or palpable; skin site should not have evidence of infection or bruising; patient should not have underlying sepsis, abnormal bleeding, history of noncompliance with previous line, or absence of proper consent)
- Determine desired placement of the catheter tip (e.g., superior vena cava or brachiocephalic and axillary or subclavian veins)
- Instruct patient that the dominant arm is used when placement is in the superior vena cava to increase blood flow and prevent edema
- Position patient supine for insertion with arm at a 90-degree angle to body
- Measure the circumference of the upper arm
- Measure the distance for catheter insertion
- Prep the site for insertion, according to agency protocol
- Instruct patient to turn head toward arm to be cannulated and drop chin to chest during insertion
- Insert the catheter using sterile technique and according to manufacturer's instructions and agency protocol
- Connect extension tubing and aspirate for blood return
- Flush with prepared heparin and saline, as appropriate and per agency protocol
- Secure the catheter and apply a sterile transparent dressing, per agency protocol
- Date and time the dressing
- Verify catheter tip placement by x-ray examination, as appropriate and per agency protocol
- Avoid use of affected arm for blood pressure measurement and phlebotomy
- Monitor for immediate complications, such as bleeding, nerve or tendon damage, cardiac decompression, respiratory distress, or catheter embolism
- Monitor for signs of phlebitis (e.g., pain, redness, warm skin, edema)
- Use sterile technique to change the insertion-site dressing, according to agency protocol
- Instruct patient/family on dressing change technique, as appropriate
- Flush the line after each use with an appropriate solution, per agency protocol
- Declot line according to agency protocol, as appropriate
- Instruct patient and family about heparinization and medication administration techniques, as appropriate
- Remove catheter according to manufacturer's instructions and per agency protocol

- Document reason for removal and condition of catheter tip
- Instruct the patient to report signs of infection (e.g., fever, chills, drainage from insertion site)
- Obtain a skin culture and blood culture (sample from the line and other arm) if purulent drainage is noted
- Culture catheter tip, as appropriate
- Maintain universal precautions

1st edition 1992; revised 2004, 2013

Background Readings:

Camara, D. (2001). Minimizing risks associated with peripherally inserted central catheters in the NICU. The *American Journal of Maternal/Child Nursing, 26*(1), 17.

Infusion Nursing Society. (2011). *Infusion nursing standards of practice.* Norwood, MA: Author.

Mitchell, M. D., Anderson, B. J., Williams, K., & Umscheid, C. A. (2009). Heparin flushing and other interventions to maintain patency of central venous catheters: A systematic review. *Journal of Advanced Nursing, 65*(10), 2007–2021.

Moureau, N. (2006). Vascular safety: It's all about PICCs. *Nursing Management, 37*(5), 22–27, 50–51.

Schmid, M. W. (2000). Risks & complications of peripherally and centrally inserted intravenous catheters. *Perioperative Critical Care, 12*(2), 165–174.

Visscher, M., deCastro, M. V., Combs., L., Perkins, L., Winer, J., Schwegman, N., et al. (2009). Effect of chlorhexidine gluconate on the skin integrity at PICC line sites. *Journal of Perinatology, 29*(12), 802–807.

Yap, Y., Karapetis, C., Lerose, S., Iyer, S., & Koczwara, B. (2006). Reducing the risk of peripherally inserted central catheter line complications in the oncology setting. *European Journal of Cancer Care, 15*(4), 342–347.

Peritoneal Dialysis Therapy   2150

Definition: Administration and monitoring of dialysis solution into and out of the peritoneal cavity

Activities:

- Explain the selected peritoneal dialysis procedure and purpose
- Warm the dialysis fluid before instillation
- Assess patency of catheter, noting difficulty in inflow/outflow
- Maintain record of inflow/outflow volumes and individual/cumulative fluid balance
- Have patient empty bladder before peritoneal catheter insertion
- Avoid excess mechanical stress on peritoneal dialysis catheters (e.g., coughing, dressing change, infusing large volumes)
- Monitor blood pressure, pulse, respirations, temperature, and patient response during dialysis
- Ensure aseptic handling of peritoneal catheter and connections
- Draw laboratory samples and review blood chemistries (e.g., blood urea nitrogen, serum creatinine, and serum Na, K, and PO_4 levels)
- Obtain cell count cultures of peritoneal effluent, if indicated
- Record baseline vital signs: weight, temperature, pulse, respirations, and blood pressure
- Measure and record abdominal girth
- Measure and record daily weight
- Anchor connections and tubing securely
- Check equipment and solutions, according to protocol
- Administer dialysis exchanges (inflow, dwell, and outflow), according to protocol
- Monitor for signs of infection (e.g., peritonitis and exit site inflammation/drainage)
- Monitor for signs of respiratory distress
- Monitor for bowel perforation or fluid leaks
- Work collaboratively with patient to adjust length of dialysis, diet regulations, and pain and diversion needs to achieve optimal benefit of the treatment
- Teach patient to monitor for signs and symptoms that indicate need for medical treatment (e.g., fever, bleeding, respiratory distress, irregular pulse, cloudy outflow, and abdominal pain)
- Teach procedure to patient requiring home dialysis

1st edition 1992; revised 1996, 2004

Background Readings:

Fearing, M. O., & Hart, L. K. (1992). Dialysis therapy. In G. M. Bulechek & J. C. McCloskey (Eds.), *Nursing interventions: Essential nursing treatments* (2nd ed., pp. 587–601). Philadelphia: Saunders.

Smeltzer, S. C., & Bare, B. G. (2004). Management of patients with upper or lower urinary tract dysfunction. In *Brunner & Suddarth's textbook of medical surgical nursing* (Vol. 2) (10th ed., pp. 1271–1308). Philadelphia: Lippincott Williams & Wilkins.

P

Pessary Management   0630

Definition: Placement and monitoring of a vaginal device for treating stress urinary incontinence, uterine retroversion, genital prolapse, or incompetent cervix

Activities:

- Review patient history for contraindications for pessary therapy (e.g., pelvic infections, lacerations, or space occupying lesions; noncompliance; or endometriosis)
- Determine estrogen requirements, as appropriate
- Discuss maintenance regimen with patient prior to fitting pessary (e.g., fit is trial and error, frequent follow-up visits are required, cleaning procedures)
- Discuss sexual activity needs prior to selecting pessary
- Review manufacturer's directions regarding specific type of pessary
- Select type of pessary, as appropriate
- Instruct to empty bladder and rectum
- Perform speculum exam to visualize status of vaginal mucosa
- Perform pelvic examination
- Insert pessary following manufacturer's instructions

- Ask patient to change positions (e.g., stand, squat, walk, and bear down slightly)
- Perform second exam in upright position to verify fit
- Instruct on method for pessary removal, as appropriate
- Instruct on contraindications for intercourse or douching, based upon pessary type
- Instruct to report discomfort; dysuria; changes in color, consistency, or frequency of vaginal discharge
- Prescribe medication to reduce irritation, as appropriate
- Determine ability to perform self-care of pessary
- Schedule appointment to recheck pessary fit at 24 hours and 72 hours, and then as appropriate
- Recommend yearly Pap exams, as appropriate
- Determine therapeutic response to pessary use
- Observe for presence of vaginal discharge or odor
- Palpate placement of pessary
- Remove pessary, as appropriate
- Inspect vagina for excoriation, laceration, or ulceration
- Clean and inspect pessary, per manufacturer's directions
- Replace or refit pessary, as appropriate
- Schedule ongoing practitioner follow up at intervals of 1 to 3 months
- Perform dilute vinegar or hydrogen peroxide douches, as needed
- Apply topical estrogen to reduce inflammation, as needed

3rd edition 2000

Background Readings:

Deger, R. B., Menzin, A. W., & Mikuta, J. J. (1993). The vaginal pessary: Past and present. *Postgraduate Obstetrics & Gynecology, 13*(18), 1–8.

Miller, D. S. (1992). Contemporary use of the pessary. In W. Droegemueller & J. J. Sciarra (Eds.), *Gynecology & Obstetrics* (Vol. 1, ch. 39). Philadelphia: Lippincott.

Smeltzer, S. C., & Bare, B. G. (2004). Management of patients with female reproductive disorders. In *Brunner & Suddarth's textbook of medical surgical nursing* (Vol. 2) (10th ed., pp. 1410–1444). Philadelphia: Lippincott Williams & Wilkins.

Sulak, P. J., Kuehl, T. J. & Schull, B. L. (1993). Vaginal pessaries and their use in pelvic relaxation. *The Journal of Reproductive Medicine, 38*(12), 919–923.

Wood, N. J. (1992). The use of vaginal pessaries for uterine prolapse. *Nurse Practitioner, 17*(7), 31–38.

Zeitlin, M. P. & Lebherz, T. B. (1992). Pessaries in the geriatric patient. *Journal of American Geriatrics Society, 40*(6), 635–639.

Phlebotomy: Arterial Blood Sample   4232

Definition: Obtaining a blood sample from an uncannulated artery to assess oxygen and carbon dioxide levels and acid-base balance

Activities:

- Maintain universal precautions
- Palpate brachial or radial artery for pulse
- Perform Allen test before radial artery puncture
- Cleanse area with an appropriate solution
- Withdraw a small amount of heparin into syringe to coat the syringe barrel and needle lumen
- Eject all air bubbles from syringe
- Stabilize artery by pulling skin taut
- Insert needle directly over pulse at 45- to 60-degree angle
- Obtain 3- to 5-cc specimen of blood
- Withdraw needle when sample is obtained
- Apply pressure over site for 5 to 15 minutes
- Cap syringe and place in ice immediately
- Label specimen, according to agency protocol
- Arrange for immediate transport of specimen to lab
- Apply pressure bandage over site, as appropriate
- Record temperature, oxygen percent, delivery method, site of puncture, and circulatory assessment after puncture
- Interpret results and adjust treatment, as appropriate

2nd edition 1996; revised 2004

Background Readings:

Evans-Smith, P. (2005). Oxygenation. In *Taylor's clinical nursing skills* (pp. 543–628). Philadelphia: Lippincott Williams & Wilkins.

Garza, D., & Becan-McBride, K. (1984). *Phlebotomy handbook* (pp. 105–107). Norwalk, CT: Appleton-Century-Crofts.

Kozier, B., Erb, G., Berman, A., & Snyder, S. (2004). Fluid, electrolyte, and acid-base balance. In *Fundamentals of nursing: Concepts, processes, and practice* (7th ed., pp. 1351–1410). Upper Saddle River, NJ: Prentice Hall.

Miller, K. (1985). Arterial puncture. In S. Millar, L. Sampson, & S. Soukup (Eds.), *AACN procedure manual for critical care* (pp. 54–61). Philadelphia: Saunders.

Phlebotomy: Blood Unit Acquisition   4234

Definition: Procuring blood and blood products from donors

Activities:

- Maintain standard precautions
- Adhere to agency protocol for donor screening and acceptance (e.g., drug abuse and HIV status)
- Obtain demographic information from donor
- Obtain written consent from donor authorizing collection and use of blood
- Ensure that donor has eaten 4 to 6 hours before donating blood
- Determine hemoglobin and hematocrit levels
- Measure weight and vital signs before donation
- Ensure availability of emergency equipment
- Ensure that skin at site of venipuncture is free of lesions
- Maintain strict aseptic technique
- Assemble equipment

- Place donor in semirecumbent position during donation process
- Cleanse skin with an iodine preparation prior to venipuncture, according to agency protocol
- Perform venipuncture
- Connect blood-collecting tubing and bag
- Ensure that blood collected in bag mixes with anticoagulant
- Instruct individual to elevate arm and apply firm pressure for 2 to 3 minutes after completion of blood or blood product donation process
- Place pressure bandage or dressing over venipuncture site, as appropriate
- Instruct individual to remain recumbent for another 1 to 2 minutes, or longer if faintness or weakness is experienced
- Encourage donor to remain seated for 10 to 15 minutes after donation
- Instruct individual to eat food and drink fluids immediately after donation
- Label and store blood, according to agency protocol
- Stay with donor during and immediately after collection of blood
- Instruct individual to leave the pressure bandage on for several hours after donation

- Instruct individual to avoid heavy lifting for several hours after donation
- Instruct individual to avoid smoking for 1 hour and alcoholic beverages for 3 hours after donation
- Instruct individual to increase fluid intake for 2 days after donation
- Instruct individual to eat well-balanced meals for 2 weeks after donation

2nd edition 1996; revised 2004

Background Readings:

Beekmann, S. E., Vaughn, T. E., McCoy, K. D., Ferguson, K. J., Torner, J. C., Woolson, R. F., et al. (2001). Hospital blood borne pathogens programs: Program characteristics and blood and body fluid exposure rates. *Infection Control and Hospital Epidemiology, 22*(2), 73–82.

Ernst, D. J. & Ernst, C. (2001). *Phlebotomy for nurses and nursing personnel.* Ramsey, IN: HealthStar Press.

Garza, D. & Becan-McBride, K. (1999). Phlebotomy handbook: Blood collection essentials (5th ed., pp. 227–252). Stamford, CT: Appleton & Lange.

Perry, A. G. & Potter, P. A. (2002). *Clinical nursing skills and techniques* (5th ed., pp. 1188–1196). St. Louis: Mosby.

Phlebotomy: Cannulated Vessel   4235

Definition: Aspirating a blood sample through an indwelling vascular catheter for laboratory tests

Activities:
- Assemble equipment, wash hands, and don gloves
- Stop any intravenous infusion that could contaminate the blood sample
- Remove cap or tubing to access port, cleanse port with alcohol and allow to dry
- Follow manufacturer's instructions to obtain a sample from an indwelling catheter
- Apply tourniquet central to peripheral intravenous site, only if necessary
- Connect needleless adapter and vacutainer, or syringe, to vascular access port, open pathway to patient by adjusting stopcocks or opening clamps
- Gently aspirate blood into appropriate specimen tube or syringe; discard the first amount determined by catheter used, laboratory tests ordered, and agency policy; collect blood needed for laboratory tests
- Remove tourniquet, if applicable
- Flush port and catheter with appropriate solution, monitoring closely to prevent introducing air bubbles or clots into the line
- Place clean cap on access port and resume any interrupted infusions
- Fill specimen tubes from vacutainer syringe in appropriate order (e.g., heparinized tube last)

- Label and package specimens according to agency policy, send to appropriate laboratory
- Place all sharps and contaminated items in appropriate receptacle

4th edition 2004

Background Readings:

Darovic, G. & Vanriper, S. (1995). Arterial pressure monitoring. In G. Darovic (Ed.), *Hemodynamic monitoring: Invasive and noninvasive clinical applications* (2nd ed., pp. 205–207). Philadelphia: Saunders.

Evans-Smith, P. (2005). Fluid, electrolyte, and acid-base balance. In *Taylor's clinical nursing skills* (pp. 629–672). Philadelphia: Lippincott Williams & Wilkins.

Laxson, C. & Titler, M. (1994). Drawing coagulation studies from arterial lines: An integrative literature review. *American Journal of Critical Care, 3*(1), 16–24.

Mohler, M. Sato, Y., Bobick, K. & Wise, L. (1988). The reliability of blood sampling from peripheral intravenous infusion lines: Complete blood cell counts, electrolyte panels, and survey panels. *Journal of Intravenous Nursing, 21*(4), 209–214.

Kennedy, C., Angermuller, S., King, R., Noviello, S., Walker, J., Warden, J., et al. (1996). A comparison of hemolysis rates using intravenous catheters versus venipuncture tubes for obtaining blood samples. *Journal of Emergency Nursing, 22*(6), 566–569.

P

Phlebotomy: Venous Blood Sample 4238

Definition: Removal of a sample of venous blood from an uncannulated vein

Activities:
- Review physician's order for sample to be drawn
- Verify correct patient identification
- Minimize anxiety for the patient by explaining the procedure and rationale, as appropriate
- Provide a private environment
- Select vein, considering amount of blood needed, mental status, comfort, age, availability and condition of blood vessels, and presence of arteriovenous fistulas or shunts
- Select appropriate size and type of needle
- Select appropriate blood specimen tube
- Promote vessel dilation through the use of a tourniquet, gravity, application of heat, milking the vein, or fist clenching and relaxation
- Cleanse area with an appropriate solution
- Cleanse site with circular motion, starting at the point of anticipated venipuncture and moving in an outward circle
- Maintain strict aseptic technique
- Maintain universal precautions
- Ask patient to hold still while performing venipuncture
- Insert needle at a 20- to 30-degree angle in the direction of venous blood return
- Observe for blood return in the needle
- Withdraw sample of blood
- Remove needle from the vein and immediately apply pressure to the site with dry gauze
- Apply dressing, as appropriate
- Label specimen(s) with patient name, date and time of collection, and other information, as appropriate
- Send labeled specimen to appropriate laboratory
- Place all sharps (needles) in sharps container

2nd edition 1996

Background Readings:

Brown, B. (1984). *Hematology: Principles and procedures* (4th ed., pp. 1–8). Philadelphia: Lea & Febiger.

Cudworth, K. L. (1985). When you have to draw blood from a femoral vein. *RN, 48*(3), 47–49.

Evans-Smith, P. (2005). Fluid, electrolyte, and acid-base balance. In *Taylor's clinical nursing skills* (pp. 629–672). Philadelphia: Lippincott Williams & Wilkins.

Wahid, S. R. (1993). New technique for starting IV lines (Wahid's maneuver) (Letter to the editor). *Journal for Emergency Nursing, 19*(3), 186–187.

Phototherapy: Mood/Sleep Regulation 6926

Definition: Administration of doses of bright light in order to elevate mood and/or normalize the body's internal clock

Activities:
- Obtain a physician's order for phototherapy (i.e., frequency, distance, intensity, and duration of phototherapy), as appropriate
- Instruct the patient/significant other about the treatment (i.e., indications for use, treatment procedure)
- Assist the patient to obtain the appropriate light source for the treatment
- Assist patient to set up the light source, as prescribed, in preparation for the treatment
- Support the patient's use of the treatment
- Supervise the patient, as needed, during the treatment
- Monitor for side effects of the treatment (e.g., headache, eyestrain, nausea, insomnia, hyperactivity)
- Terminate the treatment if patient develops side effects
- Notify the treating physician of side effects
- Modify the treatment, as ordered, to decrease/eliminate side effects
- Document the treatment and patient's response

4th edition 2004

Background Readings:

Elmore, S. K. (1991). Seasonal affective disorder, Part II: Phototherapy, an expanded role of the psychosocial nurse. *Archives of Psychiatric Nursing 5*(6), 365–372.

Frisch, N. C. (2001). Complimentary and somatic therapies (2001). In N. C. Frisch & L. E. Frisch (Eds.), *Psychiatric mental health nursing* (2nd ed., pp. 743–757). Albany, NY: Delmar.

Hagerty, B. (2000). Mood disorders: Depression and mania. In K. M. Fortinash & P. A. Holoday-Worret (Eds.), *Psychiatric mental health nursing* (pp. 258–262). St. Louis: Mosby.

Stuart, G. (1998). Somatic therapies. In G. W. Sturart & M. T. Laraia (Eds.), *Principles and practice of psychiatric nursing* (6th ed., pp. 604–617). St. Louis: Mosby.

Terman, M. & Terman, J. S. (1999). Bright light therapy: Side effects and benefits across the symptoms spectrum. *Journal of Clinical Psychiatry, 60*(11), 799–808.

Townsend, M. (2000). *Psychiatric/mental health concepts of care* (3rd ed.). Philadelphia: F. A. Davis.

University of Iowa Hospitals & Clinics Department of Nursing. (2001). Light therapy. In *Behavioral Health Service (BHS) – Psychiatric. Section II (16).* Iowa City, IA: Author.

P

Phototherapy: Neonate   6924

Definition: Use of light therapy to reduce bilirubin levels in newborn infants

Activities:
- Review maternal and infant history for risk factors for hyper-bilirubinemia (e.g., Rh or ABO incompatibility, polycythemia, sepsis, prematurity, malpresentation)
- Observe for signs of jaundice
- Order serum bilirubin levels, as appropriate, per protocol or primary practitioner request
- Report lab values to primary practitioner
- Place infant in isolette
- Instruct family on phototherapy procedures and care
- Apply patches to cover both eyes, avoiding excessive pressure
- Remove eye patches every 4 hours or when lights are off for parental contact and feeding
- Monitor eyes for edema, drainage, and color
- Place phototherapy lights above infant at appropriate height
- Check intensity of lights daily
- Monitor vital signs per protocol or as needed
- Change infant position every 4 hours or per protocol
- Monitor serum bilirubin levels per protocol or practitioner request
- Evaluate neurological status every 4 hours or per protocol
- Observe for signs of dehydration (e.g., depressed fontanels, poor skin turgor, loss of weight)
- Weigh daily
- Encourage eight feedings per day
- Encourage family to participate in light therapy
- Instruct family on home phototherapy, as appropriate

2nd edition 1996; revised 2000

Background Readings:
Merenstien, G., & Gardner, S. (1993). *Handbook of neonatal intensive care.* St. Louis: Mosby.
Pillitteri, A. (2007). Nursing care of the high-risk newborn and family. In *Maternal and child health nursing: Care of the childbearing and childrearing family* (5th ed., pp. 747–795). Philadelphia: Lippincott Williams & Wilkins.

Physical Restraint   6580

Definition: Application, monitoring, and removal of mechanical restraining devices or manual restraints used to limit physical mobility of patient

Activities:
- Obtain a physician's order, if required by institutional policy, to use a physically restrictive intervention or to reduce use
- Provide patient with a private, yet adequately supervised, environment in situations where a patient's sense of dignity may be diminished by the use of physical restraints
- Provide sufficient staff to assist with safe application of physical restraining devices or manual restraints
- Designate one nursing staff member to direct staff and communicate with the patient during the application of physical restraints
- Use appropriate hold when manually restraining patient in emergency situations or during transport
- Identify for patient and significant others those behaviors that necessitated the intervention
- Explain procedure, purpose, and time period of the intervention to patient and significant others in understandable and nonpunitive terms
- Explain to patient and significant others the behaviors necessary for termination of the intervention
- Monitor the patient's response to procedure
- Avoid tying restraints to side rails of bed
- Secure restraints out of patient's reach
- Provide appropriate level of supervision/surveillance to monitor patient and to allow for therapeutic actions, as needed
- Provide for patient's psychological comfort, as needed
- Provide diversional activities, (e.g., television, read to patient, visitors, mobiles), when appropriate, to facilitate patient cooperation with the intervention
- Administer PRN medications for anxiety or agitation
- Monitor skin condition at restraint site(s)
- Monitor color, temperature, and sensation frequently in restrained extremities
- Provide for movement and exercise, according to patient's level of self-control, condition, and abilities
- Position patient to facilitate comfort and prevent aspiration and skin breakdown
- Provide for movement of extremities in patient with multiple restraints by rotating the removal/reapplication of one restraint at a time (as safety permits)
- Assist with periodic changes in body position
- Provide the dependent patient with a means of summoning help (e.g., bell or call light) when caregiver is not present
- Assist with needs related to nutrition, elimination, hydration, and personal hygiene
- Evaluate, at regular intervals, patient's need for continued restrictive intervention
- Involve patient in activities to improve strength, coordination, judgment, and orientation
- Involve patient, when appropriate, in making decisions to move to a more/less restrictive form of intervention
- Remove restraints gradually (i.e., one at a time if in four-point restraints), as self-control increases
- Monitor patient's response to removal of restraints
- Process with the patient and staff, on termination of the restrictive intervention, the circumstances that led to the use of the intervention, as well as any patient concerns about the intervention itself
- Provide the next appropriate level of restrictive action (e.g., area restriction or seclusion), as needed
- Implement alternatives to restraints, such as sitting in chair with table over lap, self-releasing waist belt, geri-chair without tray table, or close observation, as appropriate
- Teach family the risks and benefits of restraints and restraint reduction

P

- Document the rationale for use of restrictive intervention, patient's response to the intervention, patient's physical condition, nursing care provided throughout the intervention, and rationale for terminating the intervention

1st edition 1992; revised 1996

Background Readings:

Craig, C., Ray, F., & Hix, C. (1989). Seclusion and restraint: Decreasing the discomfort. *Journal of Psychosocial Nursing and Mental Health Services, 27*(7), 16–19.

Craven, R. F. & Hirnle, C. J. (2003). *Fundamentals of nursing: Human health and function* (4th ed.). Philadelphia: Lippincott Williams & Wilkins.

Evans, L. K., & Strumpf, N. E. (1989). Tying down the elderly: A review of the literature on physical restraint. *Journal of the American Geriatric Society, 37*(1), 65–74.

Harper-Jaques, S., & Reimer, M. (2005). Management of aggression and violence. In M. A. Boyd (Ed.), *Psychiatric nursing: Contemporary practice* (3rd ed., pp. 802–822). Philadelphia: Lippincott Williams & Wilkins.

Kanak, M. F. (1992). Interventions related to safety. In G. M. Bulechek & J. C. McCloskey (Eds.), Symposium on nursing interventions. *Nursing Clinics of North America, 27*(2), 371–396.

Munns, D., & Nolan, L. (1990). Potential for violence: Self-directed or directed at others. In M. Maas, K. C. Buckwalter, & M. Hardy (Eds.), *Nursing diagnoses and interventions for the elderly* (pp. 551–560). Redwood City, CA: Addison-Wesley.

Yorker, B. C. (1988). The nurse's use of restraint with a neurologically impaired patient. *Journal of Neuroscience Nursing, 20*(6), 390–392.

Physician Support 7710

Definition: Collaborating with physicians to provide quality patient care

Activities:

- Establish a professional working relationship with the medical staff
- Participate in orientation of medical staff
- Help physicians to learn routines of the patient care unit
- Participate in educational programs for the medical staff
- Encourage open, direct communication between physicians and nurses
- Coach residents and physicians through unfamiliar routines
- Alert physicians to changes in scheduled procedures
- Discuss patient care concerns or practice-related issues directly with physician(s) involved
- Assist patient to voice concerns to physician
- Report changes in patient status, as appropriate
- Report variation in physician practice within the quality assurance or risk management system, as appropriate
- Participate on multidisciplinary committees to address clinical issues
- Provide information to appropriate physician groups to encourage practice changes or innovations, as needed
- Follow up on physician requests for new equipment or supplies
- Process practice changes through the appropriate administrative channels once physician groups have been educated about the need for change
- Provide feedback to physicians about changes in practice, equipment, and staffing
- Include physicians in in-services for new equipment or practice changes
- Encourage physicians to participate in collaborative education programs
- Use multidisciplinary projects and committees as forums to educate physicians about related nursing issues
- Support collaborative research and quality assurance activities

2nd edition 1996

Background Readings:

Alpert, H. B., Goldman, L. D., Kilroy, C. M., & Pike, A. W. (1992). 7 Gryzmish: Toward an understanding of collaboration. *Nursing Clinics of North America, 27*(1), 47–59.

Baggs, J., & Schmitt, M. (1988). Collaboration between nurses and physicians. *Image: Journal of Nursing Scholarship, 20*(3), 145–149.

Burke, M., Boal, J., & Mitchell, R. (2004). A new look at the old. Communicating for better care: Improving nurse-physician communication. *American Journal of Nursing, 104*(12), 40–48.

Pike, A. W. (1991). Moral outrage and moral discourse in nurses-physician collaboration. *Journal of Professional Nursing, 7*(6), 351–363.

Pike, A., McHugh, M., Cannery, K. C., Miller, N. E., Reiley, P., & Seibert, C. P. (1993). A new architecture for quality assurance: Nurse-physician collaboration. *Journal of Nursing Quality, 7*(3), 1–8.

Pneumatic Tourniquet Precautions 6590

Definition: Applying a pneumatic tourniquet, while minimizing the potential for patient injury from use of the device

Activities:

- Verify correct functioning of pneumatic tourniquet by checking the regulator against a calibrated gauge
- Select a tourniquet cuff of appropriate width and length for extremity
- Verify the correct functioning of the cuff by inflating the cuff and checking for leaks in the cuff and tubing
- Instruct patient about purpose of tourniquet and sensations expected, as appropriate (e.g., tingling, numbness, and dull ache)
- Inspect skin at the site of tourniquet cuff
- Evaluate baseline peripheral pulses, sensation, and ability to move digits of involved extremity
- Wrap cotton roll around extremity under site of tourniquet cuff, ensuring that cotton is wrinkle free

- Apply and secure tourniquet cuff around the extremity, avoiding neurovascular sites and ensuring that skin is not pinched
- Protect the skin and cuff from prep and irrigation solutions, as appropriate
- Adjust the tourniquet pressure, as instructed by physician or by agency policy
- Exsanguinate extremity by elevating and wrapping with an elastic bandage before cuff inflation
- Inflate the cuff, as instructed by physician
- Monitor patient continuously during use and on deflation of tourniquet
- Verify tourniquet pressure and cuff inflation periodically during use
- Monitor tourniquet equipment and pressure continuously when used for an IV block
- Notify physician of tourniquet times at regular intervals, as per agency policy
- Deflate the tourniquet cuff, as instructed by physician or by agency policy
- Deflate the tourniquet cuff used for an IV block incrementally
- Remove the tourniquet cuff

- Inspect skin under the tourniquet cuff after removal of cuff
- Evaluate the strength of peripheral pulses, sensation, and ability to move digits after deflation or removal of the cuff
- Document tourniquet identification number, cuff site, pressure, inflation and deflation times, condition of skin under cuff, and peripheral circulatory and neurological evaluation, as per agency policy

2nd edition 1996

Background Readings:

Association of Operating Room Nurses. (1994). Recommended practices for use of the pneumatic tourniquet. In *AORN 1994 Standards and recommended practices*. Denver, CO: Author.

Evans-Smith, P. (2005). Oxygenation. In *Taylor's clinical nursing skills* (pp. 543–628). Philadelphia: Lippincott Williams & Wilkins.

Fairchild, S. (1993). *Perioperative nursing: Principles and practice*. Sudbury, MA: Jones and Bartlett.

Kneedler, J., & Dodge, G. (1994). *Perioperative patient care: The nursing perspective*. Sudbury, MA: Jones and Bartlett.

Positioning   0840

Definition: Deliberative placement of the patient or a body part to promote physiological and/or psychological well being

Activities:
- Place on an appropriate therapeutic mattress/bed
- Provide a firm mattress
- Explain to the patient that he/she is going to be turned, as appropriate
- Encourage the patient to get involved in positioning changes, as appropriate
- Monitor oxygenation status before and after position change
- Premedicate patient before turning, as appropriate
- Place in the designated therapeutic position
- Incorporate preferred sleeping position into the plan of care, if not contraindicated
- Position in proper body alignment
- Immobilize or support the affected body part, as appropriate
- Elevate the affected body part, as appropriate
- Position to alleviate dyspnea (e.g., semi-Fowler position), as appropriate
- Provide support to edematous areas (e.g., pillow under arms and scrotal support), as appropriate
- Position to facilitate ventilation/perfusion matching ("good lung down"), as appropriate
- Encourage active or passive range-of-motion exercises, as appropriate
- Provide appropriate support for the neck
- Avoid placing a patient in a position that increases pain
- Avoid placing the amputation stump in the flexion position
- Minimize friction and shearing forces when positioning and turning the patient
- Apply a footboard to the bed
- Turn using the log roll technique
- Position to promote urinary drainage, as appropriate
- Position to avoid placing tension on the wound, as appropriate

- Prop with a backrest, as appropriate
- Elevate affected limb 20 degrees or greater, above the level of the heart, to improve venous return, as appropriate
- Instruct the patient how to use good posture and good body mechanics while performing any activity
- Monitor traction devices for proper setup
- Maintain position and integrity of traction
- Elevate head of the bed, as appropriate
- Turn as indicated by skin condition
- Develop a written schedule for repositioning, as appropriate
- Turn the immobilized patient at least every 2 hours, according to a specific schedule, as appropriate
- Use appropriate devices to support limbs (e.g., hand roll and trochanter roll)
- Place frequently used objects within reach
- Place bed-positioning switch within easy reach
- Place the call light within reach

1st edition 1992; revised 2000

Background Readings:

Kozier, B., Erb, G., Berman, A., & Snyder, S. (2004). Activity and exercise. In *Fundamentals of nursing: Concepts, processes, and practice* (7th ed., pp. 1058–1112). Upper Saddle River, NJ: Prentice Hall.

Metzler, D. & Finesilver, C. (1999). Positioning. In G. M. Bulechek, & J. C. McCloskey (Eds.), *Nursing interventions: Effective nursing treatments* (3rd ed., pp. 113–129). Philadelphia: Saunders.

Titler, M. G., Pettit, D., Bulechek, G. M., McCloskey, J. C., Craft, M. J., Cohen, M. Z., et al. (1991). Classification of nursing interventions for care of the integument. *Nursing Diagnosis, 2*(2), 45–56.

P

Positioning: Intraoperative   0842

Definition: Moving the patient or body part to promote surgical exposure while reducing the risk of discomfort and complications

Activities:
- Determine patient's range of motion and stability of joints
- Check peripheral circulation and neurological status
- Check skin integrity
- Use assistive devices for immobilization
- Lock wheels of stretcher and operating room bed
- Use an adequate number of personnel to transfer patient
- Support the head and neck during transfer
- Coordinate transfer and positioning with stage of anesthesia or level of consciousness
- Protect IV lines, catheters, and breathing circuits
- Protect the eyes, as appropriate
- Use assistive devices to support extremities and head
- Immobilize or support any body part, as appropriate
- Maintain patient's proper body alignment
- Place on an appropriate therapeutic mattress or pad
- Place in the designated surgical position (e.g., supine, prone, lateral chest, or lithotomy)
- Elevate extremities, as appropriate
- Apply padding to bony prominences
- Apply padding or avoid pressure to superficial nerves
- Apply safety strap and arm restraint, as needed
- Adjust operating bed, as appropriate

- Monitor positioning and traction devices, as appropriate
- Monitor patient's position intraoperatively
- Record position and devices used

2nd edition 1996

Background Readings:
Fairchild, S. (1993). *Perioperative nursing: Principles and practice.* Sudbury, MA: Jones and Bartlett.

Gruendemann, B. (1987). *Positioning plus: A clinical handbook on patient positioning for perioperative nurses.* Chatsworth, CA: Devon Industries.

Kozier, B., Erb, G., Berman, A., & Snyder, S. (2004). Perioperative nursing. In *Fundamentals of nursing: Concepts, processes, and practice* (7th ed., pp. 896–937). Upper Saddle River, NJ: Prentice Hall.

Ricker, L. E. (1998). Positioning the patient for surgery. In M. H. Meeker & J. C. Rothrock (Eds.), *Alexander's care of the patient in surgery* (10th ed., pp. 103–113). St. Louis: Mosby.

U.S. Department of Health and Human Services. (1992). *Pressure ulcers in adults: Prediction and prevention.* Rockville, MD: Agency for Health Care Policy and Research.

Positioning: Neurologic   0844

Definition: Achievement of optimal, appropriate body alignment for the patient experiencing, or at risk for, spinal cord injury or vertebral irritability

Activities:
- Immobilize or support the affected body part, as appropriate
- Place in the designated therapeutic position
- Refrain from applying pressure to the affected body part
- Support the affected body part
- Provide appropriate support for the neck
- Use appropriate body mechanics when positioning patient
- Provide a firm mattress
- Place on airflow bed, if possible
- Provide the patient with an adapted call system (e.g., low pressure, voice control, sip-and-puff straw like switch, chin movement switch), depending on level of motor function
- Maintain proper body alignment
- Position with head and neck in alignment
- Use heel boots to maintain ankles in neutral position
- Avoid positioning patient on bone flap removal site
- Position the head of bed as low as possible (measured by pulmonary function) to increase the surface area of the body and decrease pressure on bony prominences
- Turn, using the log roll technique, every 2 hours or more frequently, as indicated
- Stabilize the spine during position changes by keeping the spine in anatomical alignment (e.g., zero rotation)
- Monitor brain tissue oxygen and intracranial pressure in critically ill patients during positioning changes, as appropriate

- Apply an orthosis collar
- Instruct on orthosis collar care, as needed
- Monitor self-care ability while in orthosis collar or bracing device
- Apply and maintain a splinting or bracing device
- Monitor skin integrity under bracing device or orthosis collar
- Instruct on bracing device care, as needed
- Place a hand roll under the fingers
- Instruct the patient how to use good posture and good body mechanics while performing any activity
- Instruct on pin site care, as needed
- Monitor traction pin insertion site
- Perform traction or orthosis device pin insertion site care
- Monitor traction device setup
- Brace traction weights while moving patient
- Monitor for skin breakdown over bony prominences (e.g., sacrum, ischial tuberosities, heels)
- Provide passive range of motion to affected limbs, as determined by rehabilitation staff
- Instruct family members on how to assist patient to turn in bed and how to provide range of motion, as appropriate
- Encourage patient to participate in position changes (i.e., remind staff when it is time to be turned), as feasible
- Instruct on ways (e.g., tilt, recline) to provide pressure relief to decrease potential for skin breakdown when using a wheelchair

- Monitor for orthostatic hypotension when transferring to a sitting position in wheelchair
- Use a slide board to assist transfer to a chair or wheelchair for those patients with fair balance

1st edition 1992, revised 2013

Background Readings:

Fries, J. M. (2005). Critical rehabilitation of the patient with spinal cord injury. *Critical Care Nursing Quarterly, 28*(2), 179–197.

Ledwith, M. B., Bloom, S., Maloney-Wilensky, E., Coyle, B., Polomano, R., & LeRoux, P. D. (2010). Effect of body position on cerebral oxygenation and physiologic parameters in patients with acute neurological conditions. *Journal of Neuroscience Nursing, 42*(5), 280–287.

National Spinal Cord Injury Statistical Center. (2006). *The 2006 NSCISC statistical annual report for the model spinal cord injury care systems.* Birmingham, AL: Author.

Smeltzer, S. C., & Bare, B. G. (2004). Management of patients with neurologic trauma. In *Brunner & Suddarth's textbook of medical surgical nursing* (Vol. 2) (10th ed., pp. 1910–1941). Philadelphia: Lippincott Williams & Wilkins.

Sprigle, S., Maurer, C., & Sorenblum, S. E. (2010). Load redistribution in variable position wheelchairs in people with spinal cord injury. *Journal of Spinal Cord Medicine, 33*(1), 58–64.

Positioning: Wheelchair   0846

Definition: Placement of a patient in a properly selected wheelchair to enhance comfort, promote skin integrity, and foster independence

Activities:

- Select the appropriate wheelchair for the patient (e.g., standard adult, semi reclining, fully reclining, amputee, extra wide, narrow)
- Select a wheelchair with seat low to floor for patient who will get around using foot propelling
- Select a cushion tailored to the patient's needs
- Use appropriate body mechanics when positioning patient
- Check patient's position in the wheelchair while patient sits on selected pad and wears proper footwear
- Position the pelvis in the middle and as far back on the seat as possible
- Check that the iliac crests are level and aligned from side to side
- Ensure that there is at least 2 to 3 inches of clearance on each side of the chair
- Ensure that wheelchair allows at least 2 to 3 inches of clearance from the back of knee to front of sling seat
- Check that footrests have at least 2 inches of clearance from the floor
- Maintain the angle of the hips at 100 degrees, the knees at 105 degrees, and the ankles at 90 degrees, with the heel resting flat on the footrests
- Measure the distance from the cushion to just under the elbow, add 1 inch, and adjust the armrests to this height
- Adjust the backrest to provide the amount of support required, usually 10 to 15 degrees from vertical
- Incline the seat 10 degrees toward the back
- Position legs so they are 20 degrees from vertical
- Monitor for patient's inability to maintain correct posture in wheelchair
- Monitor for effects of prolonged sitting (e.g., pressure ulcers, skin tears, bruises, contractures, discomfort, incontinence, social isolation, falls)
- Provide modifications or appliances to wheelchair to correct for patient problems or muscle weakness
- Provide padding and other enhancements (e.g., contoured padded backs, padded leg rest panels, arm troughs, padded trays) for patients with special needs
- Facilitate small shifts of body weight frequently
- Determine appropriate time frame for patient to remain in wheelchair, based on health status
- Instruct patient on how to transfer from bed to wheelchair, as appropriate
- Provide trapeze or slide board to assist with transfer, as appropriate
- Instruct patient on how to operate wheelchair, as appropriate
- Instruct patient on exercises to increase upper body strength, as appropriate

1st edition 1992, revised 2013

Background Readings:

Gavin-Dreschnack, D. (2004). Effects of wheelchair posture on patient safety. *Rehabilitation Nursing, 29*(6), 221–226.

Gavin-Dreschnack, D., Nelson, A., Fitzgerald, S., Harrow, J., Sanchez-Anguiano, A., Ahmed, S., et al. (2005). Wheelchair-related falls: Current evidence and directions of improved quality of care. *Journal of Nursing Care Quality, 20*(2), 119–127.

Kozier, B., Erb, G., Berman, A., & Snyder, S. (2004). Activity and exercise. In *Fundamentals of nursing: Concepts, processes, and practice* (7th ed., pp. 1058–1112). Upper Saddle River, NJ: Prentice Hall.

Mayall, J. K., & Desharnais, G. (1995). *Positioning in a wheelchair* (2nd ed.). Thorofare, NJ: Slack.

Nelson, A. L., Groer, S., Palacious, P., Mitchell, D., Sabharwal, S., Kirby, R. L., et al. (2010). Wheelchair-related falls in veterans with spinal cord injury residing in the community: A prospective cohort study. *Archives of Physical Medicine Rehabilitation, 91*(8), 1166–1173.

P

Postanesthesia Care 2870

Definition: Monitoring and management of the patient who has recently undergone general or regional anesthesia

Activities:

- Review patient's allergies, including allergy to latex
- Administer oxygen, as appropriate
- Monitor oxygenation
- Ventilate, as appropriate
- Monitor quality and number of respirations
- Encourage patient to deep breathe and cough
- Obtain a report from the operating room nurse and anesthetist/anesthesiologist
- Monitor and record vital signs, including pain assessment, every 15 minutes or more often, as appropriate
- Monitor temperature
- Administer warming measures (e.g., warm blankets, convection blanket), as needed
- Monitor urinary output
- Provide nonpharmacological and pharmacological pain relief measures, as needed
- Administer antiemetic, as ordered
- Administer narcotic antagonists, as appropriate, per agency protocol
- Contact physician, as appropriate
- Monitor intrathecal anesthetic level
- Monitor return of sensorium and motor function
- Monitor neurological status
- Monitor level of consciousness
- Provide warm blankets, as appropriate
- Interpret diagnostic tests, as appropriate
- Check patient's hospital record to determine baseline vital signs, as appropriate
- Compare current status with previous status to detect improvements and deterioration in patient's condition
- Provide verbal or tactile stimulation, as appropriate
- Administer IV medication to control shivering, as per agency protocol
- Monitor surgical site, as appropriate
- Restrain patient, as appropriate
- Adjust the bed, as appropriate
- Provide privacy, as appropriate
- Provide emotional support to the patient and family, as appropriate
- Determine patient's status for discharge
- Provide patient report to the postoperative nursing unit
- Discharge patient to next level of care

2nd edition 1996; revised 2004

Background Readings:

American Society of Post-Anesthesia Nurses. (2002). *The standards of perianesthesia nursing practice.* Cherry Hill, NJ: Author.

Brenner, A. R. (2000). Preventing postoperative complications: What's old, what's new, what's tried-and-true. *Nursing Management, 31*(12), 17–23.

Burdern N. (Ed.). (2000). *Ambulatory surgical nursing* (2nd ed.). Philadelphia: Saunders.

Litwack, K. (1999). *Core curriculum for perianesthesia nursing practice* (4th ed.). Philadelphia: Saunders.

Wilson, M. (2001). Giving postanesthesia care in the critical care unit. *Dimensions in Critical Care Nursing, 19*(2), 38–43.

P

Postmortem Care 1770

Definition: Provision of care to the deceased patient and family

Activities:

- Remove external objects from body (e.g., clothing, tubes, monitors), as needed
- Cleanse the body
- Place incontinent pad under buttocks and between legs
- Raise the head of the bed slightly to prevent pooling of fluids in head or face
- Place dentures in mouth, if possible
- Close the eyes
- Maintain proper body alignment
- Notify various departments and personnel, according to policy
- Label and secure personal belongings
- Notify clergy, if requested by family
- Avoid restricting number of visitors
- Arrange for photographs
- Facilitate and support the family's viewing of the body
- Respect the family's religious beliefs and rituals
- Provide privacy and support for family members
- Answer questions concerning organ donation
- Answer questions concerning autopsy
- Label the body, according to policy, after the family has left
- Transfer the body to the morgue
- Notify mortician
- Notify coroner, as appropriate

1st edition 1992; revised 2013

Background Readings:

Ackerman, M. J. (2009). State of postmortem genetic testing known as the cardiac channel molecular autopsy in the forensic evaluation of unexplained sudden cardiac death in the young. *Pacing & Clinical Electrophysiology, 32*(Suppl. 2), S86–S89.

De Lisle-Porter, M., & Podruchny, A. M. (2009). The dying neonate: Family-centered end-of-life care. *Neonatal Network, 28*(2), 75–83.

Kozier, B., Erb, G., Berman, A., & Snyder, S. (2004). Loss, grieving, and death. In *Fundamentals of nursing: Concepts, processes, and practice* (7th ed., pp. 1032–1056). Upper Saddle River, NJ: Prentice Hall.

Perry, A. G., & Potter, P. A. (2006). *Clinical nursing skills and techniques* (6th ed.). St. Louis: Mosby.

Smith, T., Basa, E., Ewert-Flanagan, P., & Tilley, C. (2009). Incorporating spirituality into end-of-life and postmortem care. *Oncology Nursing Forum, 36*(3), 18.

Postpartal Care   6930

Definition: Providing care to a woman during the 6-week time period beginning immediately after childbirth

Activities:
- Monitor vital signs
- Monitor lochia for color, amount, odor, and presence of clots
- Have patient empty bladder before postpartum check and frequently thereafter
- Monitor fundal location, height, and tone, being sure to support the lower uterine segment during palpation
- Gently massage fundus until firm, as needed
- Monitor perineum or surgical incision and surrounding tissue (i.e., monitor for redness, edema, ecchymosis, discharge, and approximation of wound edges)
- Encourage early and frequent ambulation, assisting patient when needed
- Encourage the postoperative patient to perform respiratory exercises, assisting patient when needed
- Monitor patient's pain
- Comfort the patient experiencing shaking chills (i.e., provide warm blankets and offer beverages)
- Administer analgesics, as needed
- Instruct patient on nonpharmacologic relief of pain (e.g., sitz baths, ambulation, massage, imagery, ice packs, witch hazel pads, and distraction)
- Instruct patient on perineal care to prevent infection and reduce discomfort
- Perform or assist with perineal care (i.e., apply ice pack, encourage patient to take sitz baths, and apply dry heat)
- Monitor breasts for temperature and color and nipple condition
- Instruct patient on breast changes
- Monitor bladder, including intake and output (e.g., emptying of bladder, palpability, color, odor)
- Facilitate return to normal urinary functioning (i.e., assist with sitz baths, promote hydration, pour warm water on perineum, and encourage ambulation)
- Monitor bowels (e.g., date and time of last bowel movement, bowel sounds, presence of flatus)
- Facilitate return to normal bowel functioning (i.e., administer stool softener or laxative, instruct patient to increase consumption of fluids and fiber, encourage ambulation)
- Provide measures to reduce likelihood of deep vein thrombosis development (e.g., leg exercises and compression boot application)
- Monitor legs for Homans' sign and arrange for further testing, if needed
- Monitor patient's emotional status
- Encourage mother to discuss her labor and delivery experience
- Offer reassurance to patient on her ability to care for self and infant
- Provide information about mood changes (e.g., postpartum "blues," depression, and psychosis), including symptoms warranting further evaluation and treatment
- Monitor for symptoms of postpartum depression or psychosis
- Provide anticipatory guidance on physiological and psychological changes and their management
- Discuss activity and rest needs
- Discuss sexuality and contraceptive choices
- Monitor parent-infant attachment behaviors
- Facilitate optimal parent-infant attachment
- Instruct patient on nutritional needs, including the importance of a balanced diet and supplements, if indicated
- Instruct patient on infant's nutritional needs
- Provide adequate education and support on chosen feeding method
- Refer patient to lactation consultant, if indicated
- Instruct patient on danger signs that warrant immediate reporting (e.g., fever, depression)
- Administer Rh immune globulin and Rubella vaccine, if indicated
- Assist parent in scheduling newborn examination and postpartal examination
- Refer to appropriate resources for community support or follow-up care

1st edition 1992; revised 2013

Background Readings:
Brockington, I. (2004). Postpartum psychiatric disorders. *The Lancet, 363*(9405), 303–310.
Morten, A., Kohl, M., O'Mahoney, P., & Pelosi, K. (1991). Certified nurse-midwifery care of the postpartum client: A descriptive study. *Journal of Nurse-Midwifery, 36*(5), 276–288.
Ward, S. L., & Hisley, S. M. (2009). Caring for the postpartal woman and her family. In *Maternal-child nursing care: Optimizing outcomes for mothers, children, & families* (pp. 469–509). Philadelphia: F. A. Davis.

P

Preceptor: Employee   7722

Definition: Assisting and supporting a new or transferred employee through a planned orientation to a specific clinical area

Activities:
- Introduce new person to staff members
- Describe clinical focus of the unit/agency
- Communicate goals of the unit/agency
- Display an accepting attitude to individual assigned to the unit/agency
- Discuss the objectives of the orientation period
- Provide orientation checklist, as appropriate
- Tailor orientation to needs of new employee
- Discuss clinical ladder and/or other types of care providers and their specific responsibilities
- Review skills needed to fulfill clinical role
- Review fire and disaster plans, as appropriate
- Review code blue procedures, as appropriate
- Discuss use of policy and procedure manuals, as appropriate
- Instruct in use of clinical forms and other records, as appropriate

- Provide information and standards for universal precautions, as appropriate
- Discuss unit protocols, as appropriate
- Share work responsibilities during orientation, as appropriate
- Assist with locating needed supplies
- Orient to computer system, as appropriate
- Assist with new procedures, as appropriate
- Answer questions and discuss concerns, as appropriate
- Identify clinical specialists available for consultation, as appropriate
- Provide feedback on performance at specific intervals
- Include in unit social functions, as appropriate

2nd edition 1996

Background Readings:

Bastable, S. B. (2003). *Nurse as educator. Principles of teaching and learning for nursing practice*. Sudbury, MA: Jones and Bartlett.

Biancuzzo, M. (1994). Staff nurse preceptors: A program they "own." *Clinical Nurse Specialist, 8*(2), 97–102.

Davis, M.S., Savin, K.J., & Dunn, M. (1993). Teaching strategies used by expert nurse practitioner preceptors: A qualitative study. *Journal of the American Academy of Nurse Practitioners, 5*(1), 27–33.

Morrow, K.L. (1984). *Preceptorships in nursing staff development*. Rockville, MD: Aspen.

Preceptor: Student 7726

Definition: Assisting and supporting learning experiences for a student

Activities:
- Ensure patient's acceptance of students as caregivers
- Introduce students to staff members and patients
- Describe clinical focus of the unit/agency
- Communicate goals of the unit/agency
- Display an accepting attitude to student assigned to the unit/agency
- Recognize the importance of your behavior as a role model
- Discuss the objectives of the experience/program, as appropriate
- Encourage open communication between the staff and students
- Make recommendations for patient assignments or potential learning experiences available for students, considering course objectives, as appropriate
- Assist students to use policy and procedure manuals, as appropriate
- Orient students to the unit/agency
- Ensure that students know and understand fire and disaster policies and code blue procedures
- Assist students to locate needed supplies, as appropriate
- Provide information and standards for universal precautions
- Discuss care plan for assigned patient(s), as appropriate
- Guide students in the application of the nursing process, as appropriate
- Include students in care planning conferences, as appropriate
- Discuss any problems with students with the clinical instructor as soon as possible, as appropriate
- Provide observational experiences for activities beyond student's skill level
- Provide feedback to clinical instructor about student performance, as appropriate
- Provide constructive feedback to the student, when appropriate
- Assist student with new procedures, as appropriate
- Discuss issues in nursing practice with students based on specific patient situations, as appropriate
- Cosign charting with students, as appropriate
- Involve students in research activities, as appropriate
- Support student leadership experiences, as appropriate
- Serve as role model for developing collaborative relationships with other health care providers
- Inform clinical instructor of any changes in policy, as appropriate
- Orient to computer system, as appropriate

2nd edition 1996

Background Readings:

Bastable, S. B. (2003). *Nurse as educator: Principles of teaching and learning for nursing practice*. Sudbury, MA: Jones and Bartlett.

Reilly, D. (1992). *Clinical teaching in nursing education*. New York: National League for Nursing Press.

Shamian, J., & Inhaber, R. (1985). The concept and practice of preceptorships in nursing: A review of pertinent literature. *International Journal of Nursing Studies, 22*(2), 79–88.

Stuart-Siddal, S., & Haberlin, J. (Eds.). (1983). *Preceptorships in nursing education*. Rockville, MD: Aspen.

Preconception Counseling 5247

Definition: Screening and providing information and support to individuals of childbearing age before pregnancy to promote health and reduce risks

Activities:
- Establish a therapeutic, trusting relationship
- Obtain client history
- Develop a preconception, pregnancy-oriented health risk profile, based on history, prescription drug use, ethnic background, occupational and household exposures, diet, specific genetic disorders, and habits (e.g., smoking and alcohol and drug intake)
- Explore readiness for pregnancy with both partners
- Inquire about physical abuse

- Obtain a thorough sexual history, including frequency and timing of intercourse, use of spermicidal lubricants, and post-coital habits, such as douching
- Refer women with chronic medical conditions for a prepregnancy management plan
- Provide information related to risk factors
- Refer for genetic counseling for genetic risk factors
- Refer for prenatal diagnostic tests as needed for genetic, medical, or obstetrical risk factors
- Screen for or evaluate hemoglobin or hematocrit levels, Rh status, urine dipstick, toxoplasmosis, sexually transmitted diseases, rubella, and hepatitis
- Counsel about avoiding pregnancy until appropriate treatment has been given (e.g., rubella vaccine, Rho(D) immune globulin, immune serum globulin, or antibiotics)
- Screen individuals at risk or in populations at risk for tuberculosis, sexually transmitted disease, hemoglobinopathies, Tay-Sachs, and genetic defects
- Support decision making about advisability of pregnancy, based on identified risk factors
- Evaluate the need for a screening mammogram, based on the woman's age and desire for prolonged breastfeeding
- Encourage dental exam during preconception to minimize exposure to x-ray examinations and anesthetics
- Instruct about the relationships among early fetal development and personal habits, medication use, teratogens, and self-care requisites (e.g., prenatal vitamins and folic acid)
- Educate about ways to avoid teratogens (e.g., handling cat litter, smoking cessation, and alcohol substitutes)
- Refer to a teratogens information service to locate specific information about environmental agents
- Discuss specific ways to prepare for pregnancy, including the social, financial, and psychological demands of childbearing and childrearing
- Identify real or perceived barriers to family planning services and prenatal care and ways of overcoming barriers
- Discuss available methods of reproductive assistance and technology, as appropriate
- Encourage contraception until prepared for pregnancy
- Discuss timing of cessation of contraception to maximize accurate pregnancy dating

- Discuss methods of identifying fertility, signs of pregnancy, and ways to confirm pregnancy
- Discuss the need for early registration and compliance with prenatal care, including specific high-risk programs that may be appropriate
- Encourage attendance at early pregnancy and parenting classes
- Encourage women to learn details of health insurance coverage, including waiting periods and available provider options
- Recommend self-care needed during the preconception period
- Provide education and referrals to appropriate community resources
- Provide a copy of the written plan of care for the patients
- Provide or recommend follow-up care, as needed

2nd edition 1996; revised 2000

Background Readings:

American College of Obstetricians and Gynecologists. (1990). *ACOG guide to planning for pregnancy, birth, and beyond*. Washington, DC: Author.

Barron, M. L., Ganong, L. H., & Brown, M. (1987). An examination of preconception health teaching by nurse practitioners. *Journal of Advanced Nursing, 12*(5), 605–610.

Bushy, A. (1992). Preconception health promotion: Another approach to improve pregnancy outcomes. *Public Health Nursing, 9*(1), 10–14.

Cefalo, R. C., & Moos, M. K. (1988). *Preconceptional health promotion: A practical guide*. Rockville, MD: Aspen.

Chez, R. (1993). Preconception care. *Resident and Staff Physician, 89*(1), 49–51.

Department of Health and Human Services. (1990). *Healthy people 2000: National health promotion and disease prevention objectives*. Washington, DC: Author.

Institute of Medicine. (1985). *Preventing low birth weight* (pp. 119–174). Washington: National Academy Press.

Littleton, L. Y. & Enbretson, J. C. (2002). *Maternal, neonatal, & women's health nursing* (pp. 384–388). Albany, NY: Delmar.

Summers, L., & Price, R. A. (1993). Preconception care: An opportunity to maximize health in pregnancy. *Journal of Nurse-Midwifery, 38*(4), 188–198.

P

Pregnancy Termination Care   6950

Definition: Management of the physical and psychological needs of the woman undergoing a spontaneous or elective abortion

Activities:
- Prepare patient physically and psychologically for abortion procedure
- Explain sensations patient might experience
- Instruct on signs to report (e.g., increased bleeding, increased cramping, and passage of clots or tissue)
- Provide analgesics or antiemetics, as appropriate
- Administer medication to terminate pregnancy, as appropriate (e.g., prostaglandin suppositories; intraamniotic prostaglandin, saline, or potassium; or intravenous oxytocin)
- Encourage significant other to support patient before, during, or after abortion, if desired
- Monitor patient for bleeding and cramping

- Initiate intravenous line, as appropriate
- Observe for signs of spontaneous abortion (e.g., cessation of cramping, increased pelvic pressure, and loss of amniotic fluid)
- Perform vaginal exam, as appropriate
- Assist delivery, as appropriate, depending on gestational age of fetus
- Weigh blood loss, as appropriate
- Monitor vital signs
- Observe for signs of shock
- Save all passed tissue
- Administer oxytocics after delivery, as appropriate
- Provide teaching for procedures (e.g., suction curettage, dilation and curettage, and uterine evacuation)

- Administer Rho(D) immune globulin for Rh-negative status
- Instruct patient about postabortion self-care and monitoring of side effects
- Provide anticipatory guidance about grief reaction to fetal death
- Complete delivery record and report of death, as appropriate
- Obtain specimens for genetic studies or autopsy, as appropriate

1st edition 1992; revised 1996

Background Readings:

Bobak, I. M., Jensen, M., & Lowdermilk, D. L. (1993). *Maternity & gynecologic care: The nurse and the family* (5th ed.). St. Louis: Mosby.

Gilbert, E. S., & Harmon, J. S. (1993). *Manual of high-risk pregnancy & delivery.* St. Louis: Mosby.

Mattson, S., & Smith, J. E. (Eds.). (1993). *Core curriculum for maternal-newborn nursing.* Philadelphia: Saunders.

Pillitteri, A. (2007). Reproductive life planning. In *Maternal and child health nursing: Care of the childbearing and childrearing family* (5th ed., pp. 102–132). Philadelphia: Lippincott Williams & Wilkins.

Premenstrual Syndrome (PMS) Management 1440

Definition: Alleviation/attenuation of physical and/or behavioral symptoms occurring during the luteal phase of the menstrual cycle

Activities:
- Instruct individual in the prospective identification of the major premenstrual symptoms (e.g., bloating, cramping, irritability), use of a prospective calendar check list or symptom log, and the recording of timing and severity of each symptom
- Review symptom log/check list
- Collaborate with individual to prioritize most problematic symptoms
- Discuss the complexity of management and need for stepwise approach to alleviate individual symptoms
- Collaborate with the individual to select and institute stepwise approach to eliminating symptoms
- Provide information about symptom specific self-care measures (e.g., exercise and calcium supplementation)
- Prescribe symptom specific medication, as appropriate to practice level
- Monitor changes in symptoms
- Encourage individual to participate in PMS support group, if available
- Refer to a specialist, as appropriate

4th edition 2004

Background Readings:

Mortola, J. (2000). Premenstrual syndrome. In M. Goldman & M. Hatch (Eds.), *Women and health education* (pp. 114–125). San Diego, CA: Academic Press.

Smeltzer, S. C., & Bare, B. G. (2004). Management of patients with female reproductive disorders. In *Brunner & Suddarth's textbook of medical surgical nursing* (Vol. 2) (10th ed., pp. 1410–1444). Philadelphia: Lippincott Williams & Wilkins.

Speroff, L., Glass, R., & Kase, N. (1999). *Clinical gynecologic endocrinology and infertility* (6th ed., pp. 557–587). Philadelphia: Lippincott Williams & Wilkins.

Ugarriza, D., Klingner, S., & O'Brien, S. (1998). Premenstrual syndrome: Diagnosis and intervention. *The Nurse Practitioner, 23*(9), 40–58.

Prenatal Care 6960

Definition: Provision of health care during the course of pregnancy

Activities:
- Identify individual needs, concerns, and preferences, foster involvement in decision making, and identify and address barriers to care
- Discuss importance of participating in prenatal care throughout entire pregnancy, while encouraging involvement of patient's partner or other family member
- Encourage prenatal class attendance
- Monitor weight gain
- Monitor for hypertensive disorder (e.g., blood pressure; edematous ankles, hands, and face; and proteinuria)
- Monitor fetal heart tones
- Measure fundal height and compare with gestational age
- Monitor fetal movement
- Instruct patient on quickening and importance of monitoring fetal activity
- Monitor fetal presentation
- Review with patient changes noted on fetal growth and status
- Instruct patient on danger signs that warrant immediate reporting
- Discuss nutritional needs and concerns (e.g., balanced diet, folic acid, food safety, and supplements)
- Instruct patient on effects of exposure to or ingestion of harmful substances (e.g., alcohol, illicit drugs, teratogens, medications, herbs, and tobacco)
- Discuss activity level with patient (e.g., appropriate exercise, activities to avoid, and importance of rest)
- Provide genetic counseling and testing, if indicated
- Instruct patient on routine laboratory testing to occur throughout pregnancy (e.g., urinalysis, hemoglobin level, ultrasound, gestational diabetes, and HIV)
- Instruct patient on nonroutine tests and treatments (e.g., nonstress test, biophysical profile, Rh-immune globulin, and stripping of membranes), if needed
- Review results of testing with patient
- Discuss oral health care

- Discuss sexuality
- Monitor psychosocial status of patient and patient's partner
- Monitor for risk factors affecting patient or fetal health status (e.g., mental health disorder and intimate partner violence)
- Offer support and counsel to the patient presenting with an unplanned or unwanted pregnancy
- Offer anticipatory guidance about physiological and psychological changes and discomforts (e.g., nausea, vomiting, musculoskeletal changes, fears, and breast tenderness)
- Assist patient in identifying strategies to cope with changes and relieve discomforts associated with pregnancy
- Discuss changing body image with patient
- Review safety precautions to be taken during pregnancy (e.g., seat belt use, avoidance of hot tubs and saunas, and travel restrictions)
- Provide accurate information pertaining to risks, benefits, contraindications, and side effects of immunizations, if needed
- Assist patient in preparing for labor and delivery (i.e., discuss pain management options, review labor signs and symptoms, discuss special circumstances requiring medical intervention, and encourage planned involvement of patient's partner or family)
- Offer anticipatory guidance on infant care and considerations (e.g., circumcision, feeding, and selection of pediatric health care provider)

- Discuss postpartal concerns and considerations (e.g., family planning and contraception, returning to work or school, and physiological and psychological changes)
- Provide referral to appropriate service, if needed (e.g., supplemental food program, drug dependency treatment, and mental health counseling)

1st edition 1992; revised 2013

Background Readings:

Hanson, L., VandeVusse, L., Roberts, J., & Forristal, A. (2009). A critical appraisal of guidelines for antenatal care: Components of care and priorities in prenatal education. *Journal of Midwifery & Women's Health, 54*(6), 458–468.

Novick, G. (2009). Women's experience of prenatal care: An integrative review. *Journal of Midwifery & Women's Health, 54*(3), 226–237.

Pillitteri, A. (2007). *Maternal and child health nursing: Care of the childbearing and childrearing family* (5th ed.). Philadelphia: Lippincott Williams & Wilkins.

United States Department of Health and Human Services Expert Panel on the Content of Prenatal Care. (1989). *Caring for our future: The content of prenatal care.* Washington, DC: United States Public Health Service.

Preoperative Coordination   2880

Definition: Facilitating preadmission diagnostic testing and preparation of the surgical patient

Activities:
- Review planned surgery
- Obtain client history, as appropriate
- Complete a physical assessment, as appropriate
- Review physician's orders
- Order or coordinate diagnostic testing, as appropriate
- Describe and explain preadmission treatments and diagnostic tests
- Interpret diagnostic test results, as appropriate
- Obtain blood specimens, as appropriate
- Obtain urine specimen, as needed
- Notify physician of abnormal diagnostic results
- Inform patient and significant other of the date and time of surgery, time of arrival, and admission procedure
- Inform the patient and significant other of the location of receiving unit, surgery, and the waiting area
- Determine the patient's expectations about the surgery
- Reinforce information provided by other health care providers, as appropriate
- Obtain consent for treatment, as appropriate

- Provide time for the patient and significant other to ask questions and voice concerns
- Obtain financial clearance from third-party payers, as necessary
- Discuss postoperative discharge plans
- Determine ability of caretakers
- Telephone the patient to verify planned surgery

2nd edition 1996; revised 2000

Background Readings:

Burden, N. (1993). *Ambulatory surgical nursing.* Philadelphia: Saunders.

Kozier, B., Erb, G., Berman, A., & Snyder, S. (2004). Perioperative nursing. In *Fundamentals of nursing: Concepts, processes, and practice* (7th ed., pp. 896–937). Upper Saddle River, NJ: Prentice Hall.

Muldowny, E. (1993). Establishing a preadmission clinic: A model for quality service. *AORN Journal, 58*(6), 1183–1191.

U.S. Department of Health and Human Services. (1993). *Cataract in adults: Management of functional impairment.* Rockville, MD: Agency for Health Care Policy and Research.

P

Preparatory Sensory Information   5580

Definition: Describing in concrete and objective terms the typical sensory experiences and events associated with an upcoming stressful health care procedure/treatment

Activities:
- Identify the sequence of events and describe the environment associated with the procedure/treatment
- Identify the typical sensations (e.g., what will be seen, felt, smelled, tasted, heard) the majority of patients describe as associated with each aspect of the procedure/treatment

- Describe sensations in concrete, objective terms using patients' descriptive words, while omitting evaluative adjectives that reflect degree of sensation or emotional response to a sensation
- Present sensations and procedural/treatment events in the sequence most likely to be experienced
- Link the sensations to their cause when it may not be self-evident

- Describe how long the sensations and procedural events may be expected to last, or when they may be expected to change
- Personalize the information by using personal pronouns
- Provide an opportunity for the patient to ask questions and clarify misunderstandings

1st edition 1992; revised 2000

Background Readings:

Christman, N. J., Kirchhoff, K. T., & Oakley, M.G. (1999). Preparatory sensory information. In G. M. Bulechek & J. C. McCloskey (Eds.), *Nursing interventions: Effective nursing treatments* (3rd ed, pp. 398–408). Philadelphia: Saunders.

CURN Project (1981). *Preoperative sensory preparation to promote recovery.* New York: Grune & Stratton.

Johnson, J. E., Fieler, V. K., Jones, L. S., Wlasowicz, G. S., & Mitchell, M. L. (1997). *Self-regulation theory: Applying theory to your practice.* Pittsburgh, PA: Oncology Nursing Press.

Johnson, J. E., Fieler, V. K., Wlasowicz, G. S., Mitchell, M. L., & Jones, L. S. (1997). The effects of nursing care guided by self-regulation theory on coping with radiation therapy. *Oncology Nursing Forum, 24*(6),1041–1050.

Kozier, B., Erb, G., Berman, A., & Snyder, S. (2004). Perioperative nursing. In *Fundamentals of nursing: Concepts, processes, and practice* (7th ed., pp. 896–937). Upper Saddle River, NJ: Prentice Hall.

Sime, A. M. (1992). Sensation information. In M. Snyder (Ed.), *Independent nursing interventions* (2nd ed., pp. 165–170). Albany, NY: Delmar.

Prescribing: Diagnostic Testing 8080

Definition: Ordering a diagnostic test to identify or monitor a health problem

Activities:

- Evaluate signs and symptoms of current health problem
- Consider the status of the existing chronic health condition
- Review past medical history, medications, allergies, and past diagnostic testing pertinent to the presenting condition
- Evaluate the diagnostic utility of the test in addressing the specific clinical question (i.e., understand sensitivity and specificity of the diagnostic test for the presenting condition)
- Consult with accepted evidence-based practice guidelines, specialists, and other health care professionals, as appropriate
- Provide the patient or family members with the rationale for the proposed testing, including how the information would benefit clinical decision making or continued monitoring
- Allow for discussion and questions of the testing
- Provide alternatives to diagnostic testing, as appropriate
- Consider the availability and cost of the diagnostic testing and include the patient and family in the discussion
- Instruct the patient and family on what to expect of the diagnostic test
- Have a system in place to ensure test results are received when expected
- Identify a method that ensures accurate communication of test date, time, and location to the patient or caregiver

- Instruct the patient and family on the test date, time, location, and how to expect test results to be reported
- Employ a system that provides for the timely return of diagnostic test results and assurance that missing or delayed reports are noted and pursued
- Monitor for adverse effects of the diagnostic test
- Maintain knowledge of diagnostic testing used in practice (e.g., sensitivity or specificity, rationale, alternatives, standards of care, evidence-based practice, side effects, monitoring, and state regulations or policy issues)

6th edition 2013

Background Readings:

Buppert, C. (2008). *Nurse practitioner's business practice and legal guide* (3rd ed.). Sudbury, MA: Jones and Bartlett.

Chase, S. (2004). *Clinical judgment and communication in nurse practitioner practice.* Philadelphia: F. A. Davis

Dains, J. E., Baumann, L. C. & Scheibel, P. (2007). *Advanced health assessment & clinical diagnosis in primary care* (3rd ed). St. Louis: Mosby.

Prescribing: Nonpharmacologic Treatment 8086

Definition: Ordering nonpharmacologic treatment for a health problem

Activities:

- Determine signs and symptoms of current health problem
- Review past medical history, medications, allergies, and past diagnostic testing pertinent to the presenting condition
- Review past and current therapeutic treatments tried for the health problem, including the reasons for stopping treatment
- Document the effects of other treatments on the health problem
- Identify nonpharmacologic treatments (e.g., exercise, diet, physical therapy, occupational therapy, heat and cold treatment) that are indicated for current health problems

- Consult with accepted evidence-based practice guidelines, specialists, and other health care professionals, as appropriate
- Consider the availability and cost of the recommended treatment and include the patient and family in the discussion
- Provide the patient and family members with the rationale for the proposed treatment, expected outcome, and duration of the treatment
- Allow for questions and discussion related to the diagnosis and treatment and provide alternatives to the treatment
- Refer to appropriate service provider

- Monitor for adverse effects of the treatment
- Ensure for follow up to assess response to treatment
- Maintain knowledge of treatments commonly used in practice, including rationale, alternatives, standards of care, evidence-based practice, side effects, monitoring, and state regulations or policy issues

6th edition 2013

Background Readings:
Buppert, C. (2008). *Nurse practitioner's business practice and legal guide* (3rd ed.). Sudbury, MA: Jones and Bartlett.

Chase, S. (2004). *Clinical judgment and communication in nurse practitioner practice.* Philadelphia: F. A. Davis.
Dains, J. E., Baumann, L. C., & Scheibel, P. (2007). *Advanced health assessment & clinical diagnosis in primary care* (3rd ed.) St. Louis: Mosby.
Dunphy, L.M., Winland-Brown, J.E., Porter, B. O., & Thomas, D. J. (2007). *Primary care: The art and science of advanced practice* (2nd ed.). Philadelphia: F. A. Davis.

Presence   5340

Definition: Being with another, both physically and psychologically, during times of need

Activities:
- Demonstrate accepting attitude
- Verbally communicate empathy or understanding of the patient's experience
- Be sensitive to the patient's traditions and beliefs
- Establish trust and a positive regard
- Listen to the patient's concerns
- Use silence, as appropriate
- Touch patient to express concern, as appropriate
- Be physically available as a helper
- Remain physically present without expecting interactional responses
- Provide distance for the patient and family, as needed
- Offer to remain with patient during initial interactions with others on the unit
- Help patient to realize that you are available, but do not reinforce dependent behaviors
- Stay with patient to promote safety and reduce fear
- Reassure and assist parents in their supportive role with their child
- Stay with the patient and provide assurance of safety and security during periods of anxiety
- Offer to contact other support persons (e.g., priest/rabbi), as appropriate

1st edition 1992; revised 1996, 2000

Background Readings:
Frisch, N. C., & Frisch, L. E. (2002). Tools of psychiatric mental health nursing: Communication, nursing process, and the nurse-client-relationship. In *Psychiatric mental health nursing* (2nd ed., pp. 97–113). Albany, NY: Delmar.
Gardner, D. L. (1992). Presence. In G. M. Bulechek & J. C. McCloskey (Eds.), *Nursing interventions: Essential nursing treatments* (2nd ed., pp. 97–125). Philadelphia: Saunders.
Osterman, P. & Schwartz-Barcott, D. (1996). Presence: Four ways of being there. *Nursing Forum, 31*(2), 23–30.
Pederson, C. (1993). Presence as a nursing intervention with hospitalized children. *Maternal Child Nursing Journal, 21*(3), 75–81.

Pressure Management   3500

Definition: Minimizing pressure to body parts

Activities:
- Dress patient in nonrestrictive clothing
- Bivalve and spread a cast to relieve pressure
- Pad rough cast edges and traction connections, as appropriate
- Place on an appropriate therapeutic mattress/bed
- Place on a polyurethane foam pad, as appropriate
- Refrain from applying pressure to the affected body part
- Administer back rub/neck rub, as appropriate
- Elevate injured extremity
- Turn the immobilized patient at least every 2 hours, according to a specific schedule
- Facilitate small shifts of body weight
- Monitor skin for areas of redness and breakdown
- Monitor patient's mobility and activity
- Use an established risk assessment tool to monitor patient's risk factors (e.g., Braden scale)
- Use appropriate devices to keep heels and bony prominences off the bed
- Make bed with toe pleats
- Apply heel protectors, as appropriate
- Monitor the patient's nutritional status
- Monitor for sources of pressure and friction

1st edition 1992; revised 1996

Background Readings:

Bergman-Evans, B., Cuddigan, J., & Bergstrom, N. (1994). Clinical practice guidelines: Prediction and prevention of pressure ulcers. *Journal of Gerontological Nursing, 20*(9), 19–26, 52.

Braden, B. J. & Bergstrom, N. (1992). Pressure reduction. In G. M. Bulechek and J. C. McCloskey (Eds.), *Nursing interventions: Essential nursing treatments* (2nd ed., pp. 94–108). Philadelphia: Saunders.

Smeltzer, S. C., & Bare, B. G. (2004). Principles and practices of rehabilitation. In *Brunner & Suddarth's textbook of medical surgical nursing* (Vol. 1) (10th ed., pp. 158–187). Philadelphia: Lippincott Williams & Wilkins.

Titler, M. G., Pettit, D., Bulechek, G. M., McCloskey, J. C., Craft, M. J., Cohen, M. Z., et al. (1991). Classification of nursing interventions for care of the integument. *Nursing Diagnosis, 2*(2), 45–56.

Pressure Ulcer Care   3520

Definition: Facilitation of healing in pressure ulcers

Activities:
- Describe characteristics of the ulcer at regular intervals, including size (length x width x depth), stage (I-IV), location, exudate, granulation or necrotic tissue, and epithelization
- Monitor color, temperature, edema, moisture, and appearance of surrounding skin
- Keep the ulcer moist to aid in healing
- Apply moist heat to ulcer to improve blood perfusion and oxygen supply to area
- Cleanse the skin around the ulcer with mild soap and water
- Debride ulcer, as needed
- Cleanse the ulcer with the appropriate nontoxic solution, working in a circular motion from the center
- Use a 19-gauge needle and 35-cc syringe to clean deep ulcers
- Note characteristics of any drainage
- Apply a permeable adhesive membrane to the ulcer, as appropriate
- Apply saline soaks, as appropriate
- Apply ointments, as appropriate
- Apply dressings, as appropriate
- Administer oral medications, as appropriate
- Monitor for signs and symptoms of infection in the wound
- Position every 1 to 2 hours to avoid prolonged pressure
- Utilize specialty beds and mattresses, as appropriate
- Use devices on the bed (e.g., sheepskin) that protect the individual
- Ensure adequate dietary intake
- Monitor nutritional status
- Verify adequate caloric and high-quality protein intake
- Instruct family member/caregiver about signs of skin breakdown, as appropriate
- Teach individual or family member(s) wound care procedures
- Initiate consultation services of the enterostomal therapy nurse, as needed

1st edition 1992; revised 2000, 2004

Background Readings:

Bergstrom, N., Bennett, M. A., Carlson, C. E., et al. (1994). *Treatments of pressure ulcers: Clinical practice guideline.* Rockville, MD: Agency for Health Care Policy and Research, Public Health Service, U.S. Department of Health and Human Services.

Frantz, R. A. & Gardner, S. (1999). Pressure ulcer care. In G. M. Bulechek & J. C. McCloskey (Eds.), *Nursing interventions: Effective nursing treatments* (3rd ed., pp. 211–223). Philadelphia: Saunders.

Frantz, R. A., Gardner, S., Specht, J. K., & McIntire, G. (2001). Integration of pressure ulcer treatment protocol into practice: Clinical outcomes and care environment attributes. *Outcomes Management for Nursing Practice, 5*(3), 112–120.

Hirshberg, J., Coleman, J., Marchant, B., & Rees, R. S. (2001). TGF-[beta]3 in the treatment of pressure ulcers: A preliminary report. *Advances in Skin & Wound Care, 14*(2), 91–95.

Perry, A. G. & Potter, P. A. (2002). *Clinical nursing skills and techniques* (5th ed., pp. 175–191). St. Louis: Mosby.

Spungen, A. M., Koehler, K. M., Modeste-Duncan, R., Rasul, M., Cytryn, A. S., & Bauman, W.A. (2001). 9 clinical cases of nonhealing pressure ulcers in patients with spinal cord injury treated with an anabolic agent: A therapeutic trial. *Advances in Skin & Wound Care, 14*(3), 139–144.

Whitney, J. D., Salvadalena, G., Higa, L., & Mich, M. (2001). Treatment of pressure ulcers with noncontact normothermic wound therapy: Healing and warming effects. *Journal of Wound, Ostomy, and Continence Nursing, 28*(5), 244–252.

Pressure Ulcer Prevention   3540

Definition: Prevention of pressure ulcers for an individual at high risk for developing them

Activities:
- Use an established risk assessment tool to monitor individual's risk factors (e.g., Braden scale)
- Utilize methods of measuring skin temperature to determine pressure ulcer risk, as per agency protocol
- Encourage individual not to smoke and to avoid alcohol use
- Document any previous incidences of pressure ulcer formation
- Document weight and shifts in weight
- Document skin status on admission and daily
- Monitor any reddened areas closely
- Remove excessive moisture on the skin resulting from perspiration, wound drainage, and fecal or urinary incontinence
- Apply protective barriers, such as creams or moisture-absorbing pads, to remove excess moisture, as appropriate
- Turn every 1 to 2 hours, as appropriate
- Turn with care (e.g., avoid shearing) to prevent injury to fragile skin
- Post a turning schedule at the bedside, as appropriate

- Inspect skin over bony prominences and other pressure points when repositioning at least daily
- Avoid massaging over bony prominences
- Position with pillows to elevate pressure points off the bed
- Keep bed linens clean, dry, and wrinkle free
- Make bed with toe pleats
- Utilize specialty beds and mattresses, as appropriate
- Use devices on the bed (e.g., sheepskin) that protect the individual
- Avoid "donut" type devices to sacral area
- Moisturize dry, unbroken skin
- Avoid hot water and use mild soap when bathing
- Monitor for sources of pressure and friction
- Apply elbow and heel protectors, as appropriate
- Facilitate small shifts of body weight frequently
- Provide trapeze to assist patient in shifting weight frequently
- Monitor individual's mobility and activity
- Ensure adequate dietary intake, especially protein, vitamins B and C, iron, and calories, using supplements, as appropriate

- Assist individual in maintaining a healthy weight
- Instruct family member/caregiver on signs of skin breakdown, as appropriate

1st edition 1992; revised 1996, 2000, 2004

Background Readings:

Bergquist, S. & Frantz, R. (2001). Braden scale: Validity in community-based older adults receiving home health care. *Applied Nursing Research, 14*(1), 36–43.

Braden, B. J. & Bergstrom, N. (1999). Pressure ulcer reduction. In G. M. Bulechek & J. C. McCloskey (Eds.), *Nursing interventions: Essential nursing treatments* (3rd ed., pp. 193–210). Philadelphia: Saunders.

Cox, K. R., Laird, M., & Brown, J. M. (1998). Predicting and preventing pressure ulcers in adults. *Nursing Management, 29*(7), 41–45.

Murray, M., & Blaylock, B. (1994). Maintaining effective pressure ulcer prevention programs. *MEDSURG Nursing, 3*(2), 85–92.

Perry, A. G. & Potter, P. A. (2002). *Clinical nursing skills and techniques* (5th ed., pp. 165–174). St. Louis: Mosby.

Product Evaluation   7760

Definition: Determining the effectiveness of new products or equipment

Activities:

- Identify need for a new product or a change in a current product
- Select product(s) for evaluation
- Define perspective of analysis (benefit to patient or provider)
- Identify product efficacy and safety issues
- Contact other agencies using the product for additional information
- Define the objective of the evaluation
- Write trial criteria to be used during the evaluation
- Target appropriate areas in which to try a new product
- Conduct staff education needed to implement trial
- Complete trial evaluation forms
- Solicit input from other health care providers, as needed (e.g., biomedical engineers, pharmacists, physicians, and other agencies)
- Obtain patient evaluation of product, as appropriate
- Determine costs for new product implementation, including training, additional supplies, and maintenance agreements
- Make recommendations to the appropriate committee or individual coordinating the evaluation
- Participate in ongoing monitoring of product effectiveness

Background Readings:

Bryan, B. M., & Reineke, L. A. (1989). Assessing patient care devices: An objective methodology. *Nursing Management, 20*(6), 57–60.

Larson, E. L., & Peters, D. A. (1986). Integrating cost analyses in quality assurance. *Journal of Nursing Quality Assurance, 1*(1), 1–7.

Lipetzky, P. W. (1990). Cost analysis and the clinical nurse specialist. *Nursing Management, 21*(8), 25–28.

Myers, S. (1990). Material management: Nurses' involvement. *Nursing Management, 21*(8), 30–32.

Pranger, J. K. (1990). Service-wise purchasing: A nursing contribution. *Nursing Management, 21*(9), 46–49.

Stahler-Wilson, J. E., & Worman, F. R. (1991). A products nurse specialist: The complete clinical shopper. *Nursing Management, 22*(11), 36–38.

Takiguchi, S. A., Myers, S. A., Slavish, S., & Stucke, J. (1992). Product evaluation: Air-fluidized beds in an operational setting. *Nursing Management, 23*(6), 42–48.

2nd edition 1996

Program Development   8700

Definition: Planning, implementing, and evaluating a coordinated set of activities designed to enhance wellness, or to prevent, reduce, or eliminate one or more health problems for a group or community

Activities:

- Assist the group or community in identifying significant health needs or problems
- Prioritize health needs of problems identified
- Convene a task force, including appropriate community members, to examine the priority need or problem

- Educate members of the planning group regarding the planning process, as appropriate
- Identify alternative approaches to address the need(s) or problem(s)
- Evaluate alternative approaches detailing cost, resource needs, feasibility, and required activities

- Select the most appropriate approach
- Develop goals and objectives to address the need(s) or problem(s)
- Describe methods, activities, and a time frame for implementation
- Identify resources for and constraints on implementing the program
- Plan for evaluation of the program
- Gain acceptance for the program by the target group, providers, and related groups
- Hire personnel to implement and manage the program
- Procure equipment and supplies
- Market the program to the intended participants and to supporting individuals or groups
- Facilitate adoption of the program by the group or community
- Monitor the progress of program implementation
- Evaluate the program for relevance, efficiency, and cost-effectiveness
- Modify and refine the program

3rd edition 2000

Background Readings:

Allender, J., & Spradley, B. (2004). *Community health nursing: Promoting and protecting the public's health* (6th ed.). Philadelphia: Lippincott Williams & Wilkins.

Dignan, M. & Carr, P. (1992). *Program planning for health education and promotion* (2nd. ed.) Philadelphia: Lea & Febiger.

Progressive Muscle Relaxation 1460

Definition: Facilitating the tensing and releasing of successive muscle groups while attending to the resulting differences in sensation

Activities:
- Choose a quiet, comfortable setting
- Subdue the lighting
- Take precautions to prevent interruptions
- Seat patient in a reclining chair, or otherwise make comfortable
- Instruct patient to wear comfortable, unrestricted clothing
- Screen for neck or back orthopedic injuries to which hyperextension of the upper spine would add discomfort and complications
- Screen for increased intracranial pressure, capillary fragility, bleeding tendencies, severe acute cardiac difficulties with hypertension, or other conditions in which tensing muscles might produce greater physiological injury, and modify the technique, as appropriate
- Instruct patient in jaw relaxation exercise
- Have the patient tense, for 5 to 10 seconds, each of 8 to 16 major muscle groups
- Tense the foot muscles for no longer than 5 seconds to avoid cramping
- Instruct patient to focus on the sensations in the muscles while they are tense
- Instruct patient to focus on the sensations in the muscles while they are relaxed
- Check periodically with the patient to ensure that the muscle group is relaxed
- Have the patient tense the muscle group again, if relaxation is not experienced
- Monitor for indicators of nonrelaxation, such as movement, uneasy breathing, talking, and coughing
- Instruct the patient to breathe deeply and to slowly let the breath and tension out
- Develop a personal relaxation "patter" that helps the patient to focus and feel comfortable
- Terminate the relaxation session gradually
- Allow time for the patient to express feelings concerning the intervention
- Encourage the patient to practice between regular sessions with the nurse

1st edition 1992; revised 1996

Background Readings:

Greene, J. A. (2006). The client with an anxiety disorder. In W. K. Mohr (Ed.), *Psychiatric-mental health nursing* (6th ed., pp. 445–470). Philadelphia: Lippincott Williams & Wilkins.

McCaffery, M. & Beebe, A. (1989). *Pain: Clinical manual for nursing practice.* St. Louis: Mosby.

Scandrett, S., & Uecker, S. (1992). Relaxation training. In G. M. Bulechek & J. C. McCloskey (Eds.), *Nursing interventions: Essential nursing treatments* (2nd ed., pp. 434–461). Philadelphia: Saunders.

Snyder, M. (1998). Progressive muscle relaxation. In M. Snyder & R. Lindquist (Eds.) *Complementary/alternative therapies in nursing* (3rd ed., pp. 1–13). New York: Springer.

Prompted Voiding 0640

Definition: Promotion of urinary continence through the use of timed verbal toileting reminders and positive social feedback for successful toileting

Activities:
- Determine ability to recognize urge to void
- Keep a continence specification record for 3 days to establish voiding pattern
- Use for patients not exhibiting signs and symptoms of overflow and/or reflex urinary incontinence
- Establish interval of initial prompted voiding schedule, based upon voiding pattern
- Establish beginning and ending time for the prompted voiding schedule if not for 24 hours
- Approach within 15 minutes of prescribed prompted voiding intervals

- Allow time (5 seconds) to self-initiate a request for toileting assistance
- Determine patient awareness of continence status by asking if wet or dry
- Determine accuracy of response by physically checking clothing or linens, as appropriate
- Give positive feedback for accuracy of continence status response and success of maintaining continence between scheduled toileting times
- Prompt (maximum of 3 times) to use toilet or substitute, regardless of continence status
- Offer assistance with toileting, regardless of continence status
- Provide privacy for toileting
- Give positive feedback by praising desired toileting behavior
- Refrain from commenting on incontinence or refusal to toilet
- Inform patient of the time of next toileting session
- Teach patient to consciously hold urine between toileting sessions, if not cognitively impaired
- Teach patient to self-initiate requests to toilet in response to urge to void
- Document outcomes of toileting session in clinical record
- Discuss continence record with staff to provide reinforcement and encourage compliance with prompted voiding schedule on a weekly basis and as needed

3rd edition 2000

Background Readings:

Colling, J., Ouslander, J., Hadley, B. J., Eisch, J., & Campbell, E. (1992). The effects of patterned urge response toileting (PURT) on urinary incontinence among nursing home residents. *Journal of the American Geriatrics Society, 40*(2), 135–141.

Kaltreider, D. L., Hu, T. W., Igou, J. F., Yu, L. C., & Craighead, W. E. (1990). Can reminders curb incontinence. *Geriatric Nursing, 11*(1), 17–19.

Kozier, B., Erb, G., Berman, A., & Snyder, S. (2004). Urinary elimination. In *Fundamentals of nursing: Concepts, processes, and practice* (7th ed., pp. 1255–1290). Upper Saddle River, NJ: Prentice Hall.

Lyons, S. S., & Specht, J. K. P. (1999). *Research-based protocol: Prompted voiding for persons with urinary incontinence.* Iowa City, IA: The University of Iowa Gerontological Nursing Interventions Research Center.

Palmer, M., Bennett, R., Marks, J., McCormick, K., & Engel, B. (1994). UI: A program that works. *Journal of Long Term Care Administration, 22*(2), 19–25.

Specht, J.P., & Maas, M.L. (2001). Urinary incontinence: Functional, iatrogenic, overflow, reflex, stress, total, and urge. In M. Maas, K. Buckwalter, M. Hardy, T. Tripp-Reimer, M. Titler, & J. Specht (Eds.), *Nursing care of older adults: Diagnoses, outcomes & interventions* (pp. 252–278). St. Louis: Mosby.

Pruritus Management   3550

Definition: Preventing and treating itching

Activities:
- Determine the cause of the pruritus (i.e., contact dermatitis, systemic disorder, and medications)
- Perform a physical examination to identify skin disruptions (i.e., lesions, blisters, ulcers, and abrasions)
- Apply dressings or splints to hand or elbow during sleep to limit uncontrollable scratching, as appropriate
- Apply medicated creams and lotions, as appropriate
- Administer antipruritics, as indicated
- Administer opiate antagonists, as indicated
- Apply antihistamine cream, as appropriate
- Apply cold to relieve irritation
- Instruct patient to avoid perfumed bath soaps and oils
- Instruct patient to run a humidifier in the home
- Instruct the patient not to wear tight-fitting clothing and wool or synthetic fabrics
- Instruct patient to keep fingernails trimmed short
- Instruct patient to minimize sweating by avoiding warm/hot environments
- Instruct patient to limit bathing to once or twice a week, as appropriate

- Instruct patient to bathe in lukewarm water and pat skin dry
- Instruct patient to use the palm of the hand to rub over a wide area of the skin or pinch the skin gently between thumb and index finger to relieve itching
- Instruct patient with casts not to insert objects in cast opening to scratch skin

3rd edition 2000

Background Readings:

Banov, C. H., Epstein, J. H. & Grayson, L. D. (1992). When an itch persists. *Patient Care, 26*(5), 75–88.

Dewitt, S. (1990). Nursing assessment of the skin and dermatologic lesions. *Nursing Clinics of North America, 25*(1), 235–245.

Hagermark, O. & Wahlgren, C. F. (1995). Treatment of itch. *Seminars in Dermatology, 14*(4), 320–325.

Kam, P. C., & Tan, K. H. (1996). Pruritus – itching for a cause and relief. *Anesthesia, 51*(12), 1133–1138.

Smeltzer, S. C., & Bare, B. G. (2004). Management of patients with dermatologic problems. In *Brunner & Suddarth's textbook of medical surgical nursing* (Vol. 2) (10th ed., pp. 1654–1702). Philadelphia: Lippincott Williams & Wilkins.

P

Quality Monitoring

Definition: Systematic collection and analysis of an organization's quality indicators for the purpose of improving patient care

Activities:

- Identify patient care problems or opportunities to improve care
- Participate in development of quality indicators
- Incorporate standards from appropriate professional groups
- Use preestablished criteria when collecting data
- Interview patients, families, and staff, as appropriate
- Review patient care record for documentation of care, as needed
- Conduct data analysis, as appropriate
- Compare results of data collected with preestablished norms
- Consult with nursing staff or other health professionals to develop action plans, as appropriate
- Recommend changes in practice, based on findings
- Report findings at staff meetings
- Review and revise standards, as appropriate
- Participate on quality improvement committees, as appropriate
- Provide orientation about quality improvement for new employees at the unit level
- Participate on intradisciplinary and interdisciplinary problem-solving teams

2nd edition 1996

Background Readings:

Berwick, D. M. (1989). Continuous improvement as an ideal in health care. *New England Journal of Medicine, 320*(1), 53–56.

Crisler, K. S., & Richard, A. A. (2001). Using case mix and adverse event for outcome-based quality monitoring. *Home Healthcare Nurse, 19*(10), 613–621.

Fralic, M. F., Kowalski, P. M., & Llewellyn, F. A. (1991). The staff nurse as quality monitor. *American Journal of Nursing, 91*(4), 40–42.

Karon, S. L., & Zimmerman, D. R. (1998). Nursing home quality indicators and quality improvement initiatives. *Topics in Health Information Management, 18*(4), 46–58.

Kerfoot, K. M., & Watson, C. A. (1985). Research-based quality assurance: The key to excellence in nursing. In J. M. McCloskey & H. K. Grace (Eds.), *Current issues in nursing* (pp. 539–547). Boston: Blackwell Scientific.

Q

Radiation Therapy Management 6600

Definition: Assisting the patient to understand and minimize the side effects of radiation treatments

Activities:
- Monitor pretreatment screening workups for patients at risk for earlier onset, longer duration, and more distressing side effects
- Promote activities to modify the identified risk factors
- Monitor for side effects and toxic effects of treatment
- Provide information to patient and family regarding radiation effect on malignant cells
- Utilize recommended radiation precautions in the management of patients with cardiac pacemakers
- Monitor for alterations in skin integrity and treat appropriately
- Avoid use of adhesive tapes and other skin-irritating substances
- Provide special skin care to tissue folds that are prone to infection (e.g., buttocks, perineum, and groin)
- Avoid application of deodorants and aftershave lotions to treated areas
- Discuss the need for skin care, such as maintenance of dye markings, avoidance of soap, and other ointments, and protection during sunbathing or heat application
- Assist patient in planning for hair loss, as appropriate, by teaching about available alternatives such as wigs, scarves, hats, and turbans
- Teach patient to gently wash and comb hair and to sleep on a silk pillowcase to prevent further hair loss, as appropriate
- Reassure patient that hair will grow back after treatment is terminated, as appropriate
- Monitor for indications of infection of oral mucous membranes
- Encourage good oral hygiene with use of dental cleansing devices, such as unwaxed, non-shredding floss, sonic toothbrushes, or water pics, as appropriate
- Initiate oral health restoration activities, such as use of artificial saliva, saliva stimulants, non-alcohol based mouth sprays, sugarless mints, and fluoride treatments, as appropriate
- Teach patient on self-assessment of oral cavity, including signs and symptoms to report for further evaluation (e.g., burning, pain, and tenderness)
- Teach patient need for frequent dental follow-up care as dental caries can form rapidly
- Monitor patient for anorexia, nausea, vomiting, changes in taste, esophagitis, and diarrhea, as appropriate
- Promote adequate fluid and nutritional intake
- Promote therapeutic diet to prevent complications
- Discuss potential aspects of sexual dysfunction, as appropriate
- Teach implications of therapy on sexual function, including the time frame for contraceptive use, as appropriate
- Administer medications as needed to control side effects (e.g., antiemetics for nausea and vomiting)
- Monitor fatigue level by soliciting the patient's description of fatigue
- Teach patient and family techniques of energy management, as appropriate
- Assist patient in managing fatigue by planning frequent rest periods, spacing of activities, and limiting daily demands, as appropriate
- Encourage rest immediately after treatments
- Assist patient in achieving adequate comfort levels through the use of pain management techniques that are effective and acceptable to the patient
- Force fluids to maintain renal and bladder hydration, as appropriate
- Monitor for indications of urinary tract infection
- Teach patient and family about the effects of therapy on bone marrow functioning, as appropriate
- Instruct patient and family on ways to prevent infection, such as avoiding crowds, using good hygiene, and handwashing techniques, as appropriate
- Monitor for signs and symptoms of systemic infection, anemia, and bleeding
- Institute neutropenic and bleeding precautions, as indicated
- Facilitate patient's discussion of feelings about radiation therapy equipment, as appropriate
- Facilitate expression of fears about prognosis or success of treatments
- Provide concrete objective information related to the effects of therapy to reduce patient uncertainty, fear, and anxiety about treatment-related symptoms
- Instruct long-term survivors and their families of the possibility of second malignancies and the importance of reporting increased susceptibility to infection, fatigue, or bleeding
- Initiate and maintain protection according to agency protocol for patient receiving internal radiation treatment (e.g., gold seed placement or radiopharmaceutical agents)
- Explain protection protocols to patient, family, and visitors
- Offer diversional activities while patient is in radiation protection
- Limit visitor time in room, as appropriate
- Limit staff time in the room if patient is isolated for radiation precautions
- Distance oneself from the radiation sources while giving care (e.g., stand at the head of the bed of patient with uterine implants), as appropriate
- Shield oneself using a lead apron/shield while assisting with procedures involving radiation

1st edition 1992; revised 2008

Background Readings:

Barsevick, A. M., Whitmer, K., Sweeney, C., & Nail, L. M. (2002). A pilot study examining energy conservation for cancer treatment-related fatigue. *Cancer Nursing, 25*(5), 333–341.

Brooks-Brunn, J. A. (2000). Esophageal cancer: An overview. *MEDSURG Nursing; 9*(5), 248–254.

Bruce, S. D. (2004). Radiation-induced xerostomia: How dry is your patient. *Clinical Journal of Oncology Nursing, 8*(1), 61–68.

Christman, N. J. & Cain, L. B. (2004). The effects of concrete objective information and relaxation on maintaining usual activity during radiation therapy. *Oncology Nursing Forum, 31*(2), E39–E45.

Colella, J. & Scrofine, S. (2004). High-dose brachytherapy for treating prostate cancer: Nursing considerations. *Urologic Nursing, 24*(1), 39–44, 52.

D'haese, S., Bate, T., Claes, S., Boone, A., Vanvoorden, V., & Efficace, F. (2005). Management of skin reactions during radiotherapy: A study of nursing practice. *European Journal of Cancer Care, 14*(1), 28–42.

Hogle, W. P. (2001). Pacing the standard of nursing practice in radiation oncology. *Clinical Journal of Oncology Nursing, 5*(6), 253–256, 267–268.

Itano, J. K. & Taoka, K. T. (Eds.). (2005). *Core curriculum for oncology nursing* (4th ed.). Philadelphia: Elsevier Saunders.

R

Magnan, M. A. & Mood, D. W. (2003). The effects of health state, hemoglobin, global symptom distress, mood disturbance, and treatment site on fatigue onset, duration, and distress in patients receiving radiation therapy. *Oncology Nursing Forum, 30*(2), E33–E39.

Nail, L.M. (2002). Fatigue in patients with cancer. *Oncology Nursing Forum, 29*(3), 537–546.

Smith, M., Casey, L., Johnson, D., Gwede, C., & Riggin, O. Z. (2001). Music as a therapeutic intervention for anxiety in patients receiving radiation therapy. *Oncology Nursing Forum, 28*(5), 855–862.

Yarbro, C. H., Frogge, M. H., & Goodman, M. (2005). *Cancer nursing: Principles and practice.* Sudbury, MA: Jones and Bartlett.

Rape-Trauma Treatment 6300

Definition: Provision of emotional and physical support immediately following a reported rape

Activities:

- Provide support person to stay with patient
- Explain legal proceedings available to patient
- Explain rape protocol and obtain consent to proceed through protocol
- Document whether patient has showered, douched, or bathed since incident
- Document mental state, physical state (clothing, dirt, and debris), history of incident, evidence of violence, and prior gynecological history
- Determine presence of cuts, bruises, bleeding, lacerations, or other signs of physical injury
- Implement rape protocol (e.g., label and save soiled clothing, vaginal secretions, and vaginal hair combings)
- Secure samples for legal evidence
- Implement crisis intervention counseling
- Offer medication to prevent pregnancy, as appropriate
- Offer prophylactic antibiotic medication against venereal disease
- Inform patient of HIV testing, as appropriate
- Give clear, written instructions about medication use, crisis support services, and legal support
- Refer patient to rape advocacy program
- Document according to agency policy

1st edition 1992; revised 2000

Background Readings:

Boyd, M. R. (2005). Caring for abused persons. In M. A. Boyd (Ed.), *Psychiatric nursing: Contemporary practice* (3rd ed., pp. 823–856). Philadelphia: Lippincott Williams & Wilkins.

Burgess, A. W., Fehder, W. P., & Hartman, C. R. (1995). Delayed reporting of the rape victim. *Journal of Psychosocial Nursing and Mental Health Services, 33*(9), 21–29.

Fishwick, N., Parker, B., & Campbell, J. C. (2005). Care of survivors of abuse and violence. In G. W. Stuart & M. T. Laraia (Eds.), *Principles and practice of psychiatric nursing* (8th ed.). St. Louis: Mosby.

Haddix-Hill, K. (1997). The violence of rape. *Critical Care Nursing Clinics of North America, 9*(2), 167–174.

Morrison, G. & Butcher, H. K. (1997). Rape trauma syndrome. In G. K. McFarland & E. A. McFarlane (Eds.), *Nursing diagnoses and interventions: Planning for patient care* (3rd. ed., pp. 764–786). St. Louis: Mosby.

R

Reality Orientation 4820

Definition: Promotion of patient's awareness of personal identity, time, and environment

Activities:

- Address patient by name when initiating interaction
- Approach patient slowly and from the front
- Use a calm and unhurried approach when interacting with the patient
- Use a consistent approach (e.g., kind firmness, active friendliness, passive friendliness, matter-of-fact, and no demands) that reflects the particular needs and capabilities of the patient
- Speak in a distinct manner with an appropriate pace, volume, and tone
- Ask questions one at a time
- Avoid frustrating the patient by demands that exceed capacity (e.g., repeated orientation questions that cannot be answered, abstract thinking when patient can think only in concrete terms, activities that cannot be performed, decision making beyond preference or capacity)
- Inform patient of person, place, and time as needed
- Present reality in manner that preserves the patient's dignity (e.g., provides an alternate explanation, avoids arguing, and avoids attempts to convince the patient)
- Repeat patient's last expressed thought, as appropriate
- Interrupt confabulation by changing the subject or responding to the feeling or theme, rather than the content of the verbalization
- Give one simple direction at a time
- Use gestures and objects to increase comprehension of verbal communications
- Engage patient in concrete "here and now" activities (e.g., ADLs) that focus on something outside self that is concrete and reality oriented
- Provide physical prompting and posturing (e.g., moving patient's hand through necessary motions to brush teeth), as necessary for task completion
- Encourage use of aids that increase sensory input (e.g., eyeglasses, hearing aids, and dentures)

- Recommend patient wear personal clothing, assist as needed
- Provide objects that symbolize gender identity (e.g., purse or cap), as appropriate
- Use picture cues to promote appropriate use of items
- Avoid unfamiliar situations when possible
- Prepare patient for upcoming changes in usual routine and environment before their occurrence
- Provide for adequate rest and sleep, including short-term daytime naps as needed
- Provide caregivers who are familiar to the patient
- Encourage family to participate in care based on abilities, needs, and preferences
- Provide a consistent physical environment and daily routine
- Provide access to familiar objects, when possible
- Label items in environment to promote recognition
- Modulate human and environmental sensory stimuli (e.g., visiting sessions, sights, sounds, lighting, smells, and tactile stimulation) based on patient's needs.
- Use environmental cues (e.g., signs, pictures, clocks, calendars, and color coding of environment) to stimulate memory, reorient, and promote appropriate behavior
- Remove stimuli, when possible, that create misperception in a particular patient (e.g., pictures on the wall and television)
- Provide access to current news events (e.g., television, newspapers, radio, and verbal reports), when appropriate
- Involve patient in a reality orientation group setting/class when appropriate and available
- Provide psychoeducation to family and significant others regarding promotion of reality orientation
- Monitor for changes in orientation, cognitive and behavioral functioning, and quality of life

1st edition 1992; revised 2008

Background Readings

Bates, J., Boote, J., & Beverley, C. (2004). Psychosocial interventions for people with a milder dementing illness: A systematic review. *Journal of Advanced Nursing, 45*(6), 644–658.

Cacchione, P. Z., Culp, K., Laing, J., & Tripp-Reimer, T. (2003). Clinical profile of acute confusion in the long-term care setting. *Clinical Nursing Research, 12*(2), 145–158.

Foreman, M. D., Mion, L. C., Trygstad, L., Fletcher, K. (2003). Delirium: Strategies for assessing and treating. In M. Mezey, T. Fulmer, I. Abraham, & D. A. Zwicker (Eds.), *Geriatric nursing protocols for best practice* (2nd ed.). New York: Springer.

Hewitt, J. (2002). Psycho-affective disorder in intensive care units: A review. *Journal of Clinical Nursing, 11*(5), 575–584.

Minardi, H. & Hayes, N. (2003). Nursing older adults with mental health problems: Therapeutic interventions—part 2. *Nursing Older People, 15*(7), 20–24.

Onder, G., Zanetti, O, Giacobini, E. Frisoni, G. B., Bartorelli, L, Carbone, G., et al. (2005). Reality orientation therapy combined with cholinesterase inhibitors in Alzheimer's disease: Randomised control trial. *The British Journal of Psychiatry, 187*(5), 450–455.

Thomas, H., Feyz, M., LeBlanc, J., Brosseau, J., Champoux, M-C, Christopher, A., et al. (2003). North star project: Reality orientation in an acute care setting for patients with traumatic brain injuries. *Journal of Head Trauma Rehabilitation, 18*(3), 292–302.

Videbeck, S. L. (2006). *Psychiatric mental health nursing* (3rd ed.). Philadelphia: Lippincott Williams & Wilkins.

Recreation Therapy   5360

Definition: Purposeful use of recreation to promote relaxation and enhancement of social skills

Activities:

- Assist patient/family to identify deficits in mobility
- Assist to explore the personal meaning of favorite recreational activities
- Monitor physical and mental capacities to participate in recreational activities
- Include patient in the planning of recreational activities
- Assist patient to choose recreational activities consistent with physical, psychological, and social capabilities
- Assist in obtaining resources required for the recreational activity
- Assist patient to identify meaningful recreational activities
- Describe benefits of stimulation for a variety of sensory modalities
- Provide safe recreational equipment
- Observe safety precautions
- Supervise recreational sessions, as appropriate
- Provide new recreational activities that are age and ability appropriate, such as brewing root beer, making taffy, or visiting a horse farm
- Provide recreational activities aimed at reducing anxiety (e.g., cards or puzzles)
- Assist in obtaining transportation to recreational activities
- Provide positive reinforcement for participation in activities
- Monitor emotional, physical, and social response to recreational activity

1st edition 1992; revised 1996

Background Readings:

Carlo, S. & Deichman, E. S. (1990). Enlarging the circles of interest. *Nursing Homes, 39*(1), 16–17.

Donaghy, P. (1991). Recreation in a nursing home: A nursing success. *Australian Nurses Journal, 21*(4), 14–16.

Frish, N. (2002). Group therapy. In N. C. Frisch & L. Frisch (Eds.), *Psychiatric mental health nursing* (2nd ed., pp. 711–725). Albany, NY: Delmar.

Hutchinson, S. A. (1990). The PALS program: Intergenerational remotivation. *Journal of Gerontological Nursing, 16*(12), 18–26, 40–42.

Lyall, J. (1993). Beyond bingo . . . activity is central to the well-being of elderly people in residential homes. *Nursing Times, 89*(36), 16–17.

R

Rectal Prolapse Management   0490

Definition: Prevention and/or manual reduction of rectal prolapse

Activities:
- Identify patients with history of rectal prolapse
- Encourage avoidance of straining at stool, lifting, and excessive standing
- Instruct patient to regulate bowel function through diet, exercise, and medication, as appropriate
- Assist patient to identify specific activities that have triggered rectal prolapse episodes in the past
- Monitor for bowel incontinence
- Monitor status of rectal prolapse
- Position patient on left side with knees raised toward chest, when rectum is prolapsed
- Place a water- or saline-soaked cloth over the protruding bowel to protect it from drying
- Encourage patient to remain in side-lying position to facilitate return of bowel into rectum naturally
- Manually reduce rectal prolapse with lubricated, gloved hand, gently applying pressure to prolapse until it returns to a normal position, as necessary
- Check rectal area 10 minutes after manual reduction to ensure that prolapse is in correct position
- Identify frequency of occurrence of rectal prolapse
- Notify physician of change in frequency of occurrence or inability to manually reduce prolapse, as appropriate
- Assist in preoperative workup, as appropriate, helping to explain the tests and reduce anxiety for the patient who will undergo surgical repair

2nd edition 1996

Background Readings:

Abrams, W. B. & Berkow, R. (1990). *The Merck manual of geriatrics*. Rahway, NJ: Merck, Sharp & Dohme Research Laboratories.

Gillies, D. A. (1985). Nursing care for aged patients with rectal prolapse. *Journal of Gerontological Nursing, 11*(2), 29–33.

Referral   8100

Definition: Arrangement for services by another care provider or agency

Activities:
- Perform ongoing monitoring to determine the need for referral
- Identify preference for referral agency
- Identify health care providers' recommendation for referral, as needed
- Identify care required
- Determine whether appropriate supportive care is available in the home or community
- Determine whether rehabilitation services are available for use in the home
- Evaluate strengths and weaknesses of family or significant others for responsibility of care
- Evaluate accessibility of environmental needs for the patient in the home or community
- Determine appropriate equipment for use after discharge, as necessary
- Determine patient's financial resources for payment to another provider
- Arrange for appropriate home care services, as needed
- Inform patient of appropriate internet sites for use after discharge
- Encourage an assessment visit by receiving agency or other care provider, as appropriate
- Contact appropriate agency or health care provider
- Minimize time between discharge and appointment with next provider
- Complete appropriate written referral
- Send written referral and patient's plan of care electronically, as appropriate
- Provide patient or family member with a copy of the referral information, as appropriate
- Arrange mode of transportation
- Discuss patient's plan of care with next health care provider

1st edition 1992; revised 2013

Background Readings:

Berta, W., Barnsley, J., Bloom, J., Cockerill, R., Davis, D., Jaakkimainen, L., et al. (2008). Enhancing continuity of information: Essential components of a referral document. *Canadian Family Physician, 54*(10), 1432–1433.

Cummings, E., Showell, C., Roehrer, E., Churchill, B., Turner, B., Yee, K.C., et al. (2010). *A structured evidence-based literature review on discharge, referral and admission*. University of Tasmania, Australia: eHealth Services Research Group.

Edwards, N., Davies, B., Ploeg, J., Virani, T., & Skelly, J. (2007). Implementing nursing best practice guidelines: Impact on patient referrals. *BMC Nursing, 6*(4).

Heimly, V. (2009). Electronic referrals in healthcare: A review. In K. Adlassnig, B. Blobel, J. Mantas, & I. Masic (Eds.), *Medical informatics in a united and healthy Europe: Proceedings of MIE 2009*. Amsterdam, Netherlands: IOS Press.

Kim, Y., Chen, A.H., Keith, E., Yee, H. F., Jr., & Kushel, M. B. (2009). Not perfect, but better: Primary care providers' experiences with electronic referrals in a safety net health system. *Journal of General Internal Medicine, 24*(5), 614–619.

Reiki 1520

Definition: Using a specific sequence of hand positions and symbols to channel the universal life force for recharging, realigning, and rebalancing the human energy field

Activities:

- Create a calm and comfortable environment
- Use aroma or gentle music to create a healing atmosphere
- Wash your hands
- Ask about the chief complaints, such as the presence of pain in certain areas or the presence of a particular illness
- Have the Reiki receiver sit comfortably or lay down on a massage table, fully clothed, in a supine position
- Limit any unnecessary distractions
- Relax your mind and take a few deep breaths to focus yourself
- Remember, the Reiki does the work, not the practitioner
- Begin by sending Reiki from about 3 feet away, if possible, as a gentle way of beginning the session
- Follow a specific series of hand placements: over eyes, over ears, one hand on forehead and one hand on top of head, hands under head, over the neck, upper chest, upper abdomen, lower abdomen, thighs (one at a time), knees (one at a time), lower legs, ankles, feet, bottoms of feet, have client roll over on to stomach, shoulders, waist area, lower back, backs of legs as front of legs
- Draw or visualize Reiki symbols (e.g., power, mental or emotional, distance) as guided by your intuition
- Allow your intuition to guide your movements by placing hands on (or a few inches over) the part of the body that most requires healing
- Stay in each area for 5 to 15 minutes, or until you feel the energy flow more slowly, or your intuition informs you it is time to move hand position
- Ask for specific permission during the session to work on sexual organs or parts of the body that would be considered inappropriate, if so guided
- Move one hand at a time so that you maintain contact as much as possible
- Note whether the patient has experienced a relaxation response and any related changes

6th edition 2013

Background Readings:

Lee, M. S., Pittler, M. H., & Ernst, E. (2008). Effects of Reiki in clinical practice: A systematic review of randomized clinical trials. *International Journal of Clinical Practice, 62*(6), 947–954.

Lubeck, W., Petter, F. A., & Rand, W. L. (2001). *The spirit of Reiki: The complete handbook of the Reiki system.* Twin Lakes, WI: Lotus Press.

Miles, P. & True, G. (2003). Reiki—review of a biofield therapy history, theory, practice, and research. *Alternative Therapies in Health and Medicine, 9*(2), 62–72.

Ring, M. E. (2009). Reiki and pattern manifestations. *Nursing Science Quarterly, 22*(3), 250–258.

Shore, A. G. (2004). Long-term effects of energetic healing on symptoms of psychological depression and self-perceived stress. *Alternative Therapies in Health and Medicine, 10*(3), 42–48.

Vitale, A. (2007). An integrative review of Reiki touch therapy research. *Holistic Nursing Practice, 21*(4), 167–179.

Wardell, D. W. & Engebretson, J. (2001). Biological correlates of Reiki touch healing. *Journal of Advanced Nursing, 33*(4), 439–445.

Relaxation Therapy 6040

R

Definition: Use of techniques to encourage and elicit relaxation for the purpose of decreasing undesirable signs and symptoms such as pain, muscle tension, or anxiety

Activities:

- Describe the rationale for relaxation and the benefits, limits, and types of relaxation available (e.g., music, meditation, rhythmic breathing, jaw relaxation, and progressive muscle relaxation)
- Screen for current decreased energy level, inability to concentrate, or other concurrent symptoms that may interfere with cognitive ability to focus on relaxation technique
- Determine whether any relaxation intervention in the past has been useful
- Consider the individual's willingness to participate, ability to participate, preference, past experiences, and contraindications, before selecting a specific relaxation strategy
- Provide detailed description of chosen relaxation intervention
- Create a quiet, nondisrupting environment with dim lights and comfortable temperature, when possible
- Suggest that the individual assume a comfortable position, with unrestricted clothing and eyes closed
- Individualize the content of the relaxation intervention (e.g., by asking for suggestions of changes)
- Elicit behaviors that are conditioned to produce relaxation, such as deep breathing, yawning, abdominal breathing, or peaceful imaging
- Invite the patient to relax and let the sensations happen
- Use soft tone of voice with a slow, rhythmical pace of words
- Demonstrate and practice the relaxation technique with the patient
- Encourage return demonstrations of techniques, if possible
- Anticipate the need for the use of relaxation
- Provide written information about preparing and engaging in relaxation techniques
- Encourage frequent repetition or practice of technique(s) selected
- Provide undisturbed time, because patient may fall asleep
- Encourage control of when the relaxation technique is performed
- Regularly evaluate individual's report of relaxation achieved, and periodically monitor muscle tension, heart rate, blood pressure, and skin temperature, as appropriate
- Develop a tape of the relaxation technique for the individual to use, as appropriate

- Use relaxation as an adjuvant strategy with pain medication or in conjunction with other measures, as appropriate
- Evaluate and document the response to relaxation therapy

1st edition 1992; revised 2008

Background Readings:

Benson, H. & Klipper, M. Z. (2000). *Screen for current decreased energy level, inability to concentrate, or other concurrent symptoms that may interfere with cognitive ability to focus on relaxation technique.* New York: Harper Collins.

Herr, K. A. & Mobily, P. R. (1999). Pain management. In G. M. Bulechek & J. C. McCloskey (Eds.), *Nursing interventions: Effective nursing treatments* (3rd ed., pp. 149–171). Philadelphia: W. B. Saunders.

Mandle, C. L., Jacobs, S. C., Arcari, P. M., & Domar, A. D. (1996). The efficacy of relaxation response interventions with adult patients: A review of the literature. *Journal of Cardiovascular Nursing, 10*(3), 4–26.

McCaffery, M. & Pasero, C. (1999). Practical nondrug approaches to pain. In M. McCaffery & C. Pasero (Eds.), *Pain: Clinical manual* (2nd ed., pp. 399–427). St. Louis: Mosby.

Snyder, M. (1998). Progressive muscle relaxation. In M. Snyder & R. Lindquist (Eds.), *Complementary/alternative therapies in nursing* (3rd ed., pp. 1–14). New York: Springer.

Religious Addiction Prevention   5422

Definition: Prevention of a self-imposed controlling religious lifestyle

Activities:
- Identify individuals at risk for an excessive dependence upon religion, religious leaders, and/or religious practice
- Examine religious practices in terms of balanced relationships and beliefs
- Explore and encourage behaviors that contribute to growth and faith development
- Explore with individuals the elements of religious addiction and freedom for religious formation
- Explain how shame-based people are vulnerable to religious and ritual addiction
- Examine gratitude and forgiveness as ways of defending one's self from forming religious or other addictive processes
- Offer to pray for healthy, life-giving relationships with self, God/Higher Power, and others, as appropriate
- Educate individuals about the process of faith development

- Educate individuals about the dangers of using religion to control other persons
- Promote the formation of self-help groups or support groups to explore religious balance
- Identify and share resources of groups and professional counseling services within the community

3rd edition 2000

Background Readings:

Booth, L. (1991). *When God becomes a drug: Breaking the chains of religious addiction and abuse.* Los Angeles: Jeremy P. Tarcher.

Linn, M., Linn, S. F., & Linn, D. (1994). *Healing spiritual abuse and religious addiction.* Mahwah, NJ: Paulist Press.

Religious Ritual Enhancement   5424

Definition: Facilitating participation in religious practices

Activities:
- Identify patient's concerns regarding religious expression (e.g., lighting candles, fasting, circumcision ceremonies, or food practices)
- Coordinate or provide healing services, communion, meditation, or prayer in place of residence or other setting
- Encourage the use of and participation in usual religious rituals or practices that are not detrimental to health
- Provide video or audio tapes from religious services, as available
- Treat individual with dignity and respect
- Provide opportunities for discussion of various belief systems and world views
- Coordinate or provide transportation to worship site
- Encourage ritual planning and participation, as appropriate
- Encourage ritual attendance, as appropriate
- Explore alternative for worship
- Encourage discussion about religious concerns

- Listen and develop a sense of timing for prayer or ritual
- Refer to religious advisor of the patient's choice
- Assist with modifications of the ritual to meet the needs of the disabled or ill

3rd edition 2000; revised 2004

Background Readings:

Beck, R. & Metrick, S. (1990). *The art of ritual.* Berkley, CA: Celestial Arts.

LeMone, P. (2001). Spiritual distress. In M. L. Maas, K. C. Buckwalter, M. D. Hardy, T. Tripp-Reimer, M. G. Titler, & J. P. Specht (Eds.), *Nursing care of older adults: Diagnoses, outcomes and interventions* (pp. 782–793). St. Louis: Mosby.

Ramshaw, E. (1987). *Ritual and pastoral care.* Philadelphia: Fortress Press.

Walton, D. (1995, October). Adapting faith rituals. *Church of the Brethren Messenger* (p. 14).

Relocation Stress Reduction 5350

Definition: Assisting the individual to prepare for and cope with movement from one environment to another

Activities:
- Explore if the individual has had any previous relocations
- Include the individual in relocation plans, as appropriate
- Explore what is most important in the individual's life (e.g., family, friends, personal belongings)
- Encourage individual and family to discuss concerns regarding relocation
- Explore with the individual previous coping strategies
- Encourage the use of coping strategies
- Appraise individual's need/desire for social support
- Evaluate available support systems (e.g., extended family, community involvement, religious affiliations)
- Assign a "buddy" to the individual to help acquaint them to the new environment
- Encourage individual and/or family to seek counseling, as appropriate
- Make arrangements for individual's personal items to be in place prior to relocating
- Monitor for physiologic and psychological signs and symptoms of relocation (e.g., anorexia, anxiety, depression, increased demands, and hopelessness)
- Provide diversional activities (e.g., involvement in hobbies, usual activities)
- Assist the individual to grieve and work through the losses of home, friends, and independence
- Evaluate the impact of disruption of lifestyle, loss of home, and adaptation to a new environment

4th edition 2004

Background Readings:

Castle, N. G. (2001). Relocation of the elderly. *Medical Care Research & Review, 58*(3), 291–333.

Jackson, B., Swanson, C., Hicks, L. E., Prokop, L., Laughlin, J. (2000). Bridge of continuity from hospital to nursing home. Part II: Reducing relocation stress syndrome and interdisciplinary guide. *Continuum 2000, 20*(1), 9–14.

Morse, D. L. (2000). Relocation stress syndrome is real. *American Journal of Nursing 100*(8), 24AAAA–24BBBB, 24DDDD.

Puskar, K. R. & Rohay, J. M. (1999). School relocation and stress in teens. *Journal of School Nursing, 15*(1), 16–21.

Reed, J. & Morgan, D. (1999). Discharging older people from hospital to care homes: Implications for nursing. *Journal of Advanced Nursing 29*(4), 819–825.

Reminiscence Therapy 4860

Definition: Using the recall of past events, feelings, and thoughts to facilitate pleasure, quality of life, or adaptation to present circumstances

Activities:
- Choose a comfortable setting
- Set aside adequate time
- Identify, with the patient, a theme for each session (e.g., work life)
- Select an appropriately small number of participants for group reminiscence therapy
- Utilize effective listening and attending skills
- Determine which method of reminiscence (e.g., taped autobiography, journal, structured life review, scrapbook, open discussion, and storytelling) is most effective
- Introduce props (e.g., music for auditory, photo albums for visual, perfume for olfactory), addressing all five senses to stimulate recall
- Encourage verbal expression of both positive and negative feelings of past events
- Observe body language, facial expression, and tone of voice to identify the importance of recollections to the patient
- Ask open-ended questions about past events
- Encourage writing of past events
- Maintain focus of sessions, more on process than on an end product
- Provide support, encouragement, and empathy for participant(s)
- Use culturally sensitive props, themes, and techniques
- Assist the person to address painful, angry, or other negative memories
- Use the patient's photo albums or scrapbooks to stimulate memories
- Assist the patient in creating or adding to a family tree, or to write his/her oral history
- Encourage the patient to write to relatives or old friends
- Use communication skills, such as focusing, reflecting, and restating, to develop the relationship
- Comment on the affective quality accompanying the memories in an empathetic manner
- Use direct questions to refocus back to life events, as necessary
- Inform family members about the benefits of reminiscence
- Gauge the length of the session by the patient's attention span
- Give immediate positive feedback to cognitively impaired patients
- Acknowledge previous coping skills
- Repeat sessions weekly or more often over prolonged period
- Gauge the number of sessions by the patient's response and willingness to continue

1st edition 1992; revised 1996, 2000, 2004

Background Readings:

Brady, E. M. (1999). Stories at the hour of our death. *Home Healthcare Nurse, 17*(3), 176–180.

Burnside, I. (1994). Reminiscence and life review: Therapeutic interventions for older people. *Nurse Practitioner, 19*(4), 55–61.

Burnside, I. & Haight, B. (1992). Reminiscence and life review: Analyzing each concept. *Journal of Advanced Nursing, 17*(7), 855–862.

Coleman, P. G. (1999). Creating a life story: The task of reconciliation. *The Gerontologist, 39*(2), 133–139.

R

Haight, B. K. (2001). Life reviews: Helping Alzheimer's patients reclaim a fading past. *Reflections on Nursing Leadership, 27*(1), 20–22.

Hamilton, D. (1992). Reminiscence therapy. In G. Bulechek & J. McCloskey (Eds.), *Nursing interventions: Treatments for nursing diagnoses* (pp. 292–303). Philadelphia: W. B. Saunders.

Harrand, A. G. & Bollstetter, J. J. (2000). Developing a community-based reminiscence group for the elderly. *Clinical Nurse Specialist, 14*(1), 17–22.

Johnson, R. A. (1999). Reminiscence therapy. In G.M. Bulechek & J.C. McCloskey (Eds.), *Nursing interventions: Effective nursing treatments* (3rd ed., pp. 371–384). Philadelphia: W. B. Saunders.

Puentes, W. J. (2000). Using social reminiscence to teach therapeutic communication skills. *Geriatric Nursing, 21*(6), 315–318.

Reproductive Technology Management　　　7886

Definition: Assisting a patient through the steps of complex infertility treatment

Activities:

- Provide education about various treatment modalities (e.g., intrauterine insemination, in vitro fertilization-embryo transfer (IVF-ET), gamete intrafallopian transfer (GIFT), zygote intrafallopian transfer (ZIFT), donor sperm, donor oocytes, gestational carrier, and surrogacy)
- Discuss ethical dilemmas before initiating a particular treatment modality
- Explore feelings about assisted reproductive technology (e.g., known vs. anonymous oocyte or sperm donors, cryopreserved embryos, selective reduction, and use of a host uterus)
- Refer for preconception counseling, as needed
- Teach ovulation prediction and detection techniques (e.g., basal temperature and urine testing)
- Teach administration of ovulatory stimulants
- Schedule tests, as needed, based on the menstrual cycle
- Coordinate activities of the multidisciplinary team for treatment process
- Assist out-of-town individuals in locating housing while participating in the program
- Provide education to gamete donors and their partners
- Collaborate with in vitro fertilization team in screening and selecting gamete donors
- Explore psychosocial issues involving gamete donation before administering medications for comfort
- Coordinate synchronization of donor and recipient hormonal cycles
- Draw specimens for endocrine determination
- Perform ultrasound exams to ascertain follicular growth
- Participate in team conferences to correlate test results for evaluating oocyte maturity
- Set up equipment for oocyte retrieval
- Assist with freezing and preservation of embryos, as indicated
- Assist with fertilization procedures
- Prepare patient for embryo transfer
- Provide anticipatory guidance about typical emotional reactions, including extremes of anguish and joy
- Discuss risks, including the likelihood of miscarriage, ectopic pregnancy, and ovarian hyperstimulation
- Teach ectopic pregnancy precautions
- Teach symptoms of ovarian hyperstimulation to report
- Perform pregnancy tests
- Provide support for grieving when implantation fails to occur
- Schedule follow-up medication, tests, and ultrasound exams
- Assist with hormonal and ultrasound monitoring of early pregnancy
- Refer for genetic counseling, as needed, related to maternal age at conception
- Refer to infertility support groups, as needed
- Follow up with patients who have stopped treatment because of pregnancy, adoption, or the decision to remain childfree
- Assist patients to focus on life areas of success unrelated to fertility status
- Educate in methods of securing workplace support for necessary absences during treatment
- Provide counseling about financial and insurance issues
- Participate in reporting data about treatment outcomes to national registry

2nd edition 1996

Background Readings:

Bobak, I. M. & Jensen, M. (1993). *Maternity & gynecologic care: The nurse and the family* (5th ed.). St. Louis: Mosby.

Dunnington, R. M. & Estok, P. J. (1991). Potential psychological attachments formed by donors involved in fertility technology: Another side to infertility. *Nurse Practitioner, 16*(11), 41–48.

Field, P. A. & Marck, P. (1994). *Uncertain motherhood: Negotiating the risks of the childbearing years.* Thousand Oaks, CA: Sage.

Hahn, S. J., Butkowski, C. R., & Capper, L. L. (1994). Ovarian hyperstimulation syndrome: Protocols for nursing care. *Journal of Gynecologic, Obstetric, and Neonatal Nursing, 23*(3), 217–226.

James, C. (1992). The nursing role in assisted reproductive technologies. *NAACOG's Clinical Issues in Perinatal and Women's Health Nursing, 3*(2), 328–334.

Jones, S. L. (1994). Genetic-based and assisted reproductive technology of the 21st century. *Journal of Obstetric, Gynecologic, and Neonatal Nursing, 23*(2), 160–165.

Olshansky, E. F. (1992). Redefining the concepts of success and failure. *NAACOG's Clinical Issues in Perinatal and Women's Health Nursing, 3*(2), 343–346.

Pillitteri, A. (2007). Reproductive life planning. In *Maternal and child health nursing: Care of the childbearing and childrearing family* (5th ed., pp. 102–132). Philadelphia: Lippincott Williams & Wilkins.

Pillitteri, A. (2007). The infertile couple. In *Maternal and child health nursing: Care of the childbearing and childrearing family* (5th ed., pp. 133–153). Philadelphia: Lippincott Williams & Wilkins.

R

Research Data Collection 8120

Definition: Collecting research data

Activities:
- Adhere to Institutional Review Board (IRB) procedures of data collection site
- Inform investigator of facility rules for conducting research, as needed
- Facilitate completion of consent form, as appropriate
- Explain purpose of research during data collection, as appropriate
- Inform patient of the obligations of being a part of the study (e.g., surveys, laboratory tests, medications)
- Implement study protocol as specified and agreed upon
- Monitor patient's response to research protocol
- Collect data agreed upon for use in the study
- Provide private space for conducting interviews and/or data collection as needed
- Assist patients to complete study questionnaires or other data collection tool, as requested
- Perform activities per routine while under study observation
- Discuss with investigator any patient or agency rewards for participation
- Obtain summary of study results for participating staff and interested study subjects
- Communicate regularly with researcher about progress of data collection, as appropriate
- Record data findings clearly on provided forms
- Monitor amount of participation in research studies requested of patients and staff

2nd edition 1996; revised 2000

Background Readings:

American Nurses Association. (1985). *Human rights guidelines for nurses in clinical and other research.* Kansas City, MO: Author.

Bliesmer, M. & Earle, P. (1993). Research considerations: Nursing home quality perceptions. *Journal of Gerontological Nursing, 19*(6), 27–34.

Burns, N. & Grove, S. K. (2005). *The practice of nursing research: Conduct, critique, & utilization* (5th ed.). Philadelphia: Saunders.

Resiliency Promotion 8340

Definition: Assisting individuals, families, and communities in development, use, and strengthening of protective factors to be used in coping with environmental and societal stressors

Activities:
- Facilitate family cohesion
- Encourage family support
- Encourage the development and adherence to family routines and traditions (e.g., birthdays, holidays)
- Assist youth in viewing family as a resource for advice and support
- Facilitate family communication
- Encourage family to eat meals together on a regular basis
- Link youth to interested adults in community
- Provide family/community models for conventional behavior
- Motivate youth to pursue academic achievement and goals
- Encourage family involvement with child's schoolwork and activities
- Assist family in providing atmosphere conducive to learning
- Encourage family/community to value achievement
- Encourage family/community to value health
- Encourage positive health-seeking behaviors
- Assist parents in determining age-appropriate expectations for their child
- Encourage family to establish rules and consequences for child/youth behavior
- Assist parents in establishing norms for parental monitoring of friends and activities
- Assist youth in acquiring assertiveness skills
- Assist youth in role playing decision-making skills
- Assist youth in developing friendship-making skills
- Encourage family and youth attendance at religious services and/or activities
- Encourage youth involvement in school activities and/or voluntary clubs
- Provide opportunities for youth involvement in community volunteer activities
- Assist youth in developing social and global awareness
- Promote quality, caring schools in community
- Arrange to keep schools/gyms/libraries open after hours for activities
- Inform and involve community in youth programs
- Facilitate development and use of neighborhood resources
- Assist youth/families/communities in developing optimism for the future

3rd edition 2000

Background Readings:

Benson, P. (1993). *The troubled journey: A portrait of 6th–12th grade youth.* Minneapolis, MN: Search Institute.

Castiglia, P. T. (1993). Gangs. *Journal of Pediatric Health Care, 7*(1), 39–41.

Jessor, R. (1991). Risk behavior in adolescence: A psychosocial framework for understanding and action. *Journal of Adolescent Health, 12*(8), 597–605.

Keltner, B., Keltner, N. L., & Farren, E. (1990). Family routines and conduct disorders in adolescent girls. *Western Journal of Nursing Research, 12*(2), 161-174.

McCubbin, M. & Van Riper, M. (1996). Factors influencing family functioning and the health of family members. In S. M. H. Hanson & S. T. Boyd, (Eds.), *Family health care nursing: Theory, practice, and research* (pp. 101–121). Philadelphia: F. A. Davis.

Raphel, S. & Bennett, C. F. (2005). Child psychiatric nursing. In G. W. Stuart & M. T. Laraia (Eds.), *Principles and practice of psychiatric nursing* (8th ed., pp. 728–752). St. Louis: Mosby.

R

Respiratory Monitoring 3350

Definition: Collection and analysis of patient data to ensure airway patency and adequate gas exchange

Activities:
- Monitor rate, rhythm, depth, and effort of respirations
- Note chest movement, watching for symmetry, use of accessory muscles, and supraclavicular and intercostal muscle retractions
- Monitor for noisy respirations, such as crowing or snoring
- Monitor breathing patterns (e.g., bradypnea, tachypnea, hyperventilation, Kussmaul respirations, Cheyne-Stokes respirations, apneustic, Biot respiration, ataxic patterns)
- Monitor oxygen saturation levels continuously in sedated patients (e.g., SaO_2, SvO_2, SpO_2), per agency policy and as indicated
- Provide for noninvasive continuous oxygen sensors (e.g., finger, nose, or forehead devices) with appropriate alarm systems in at-risk patients (e.g., morbidly obese, confirmed obstructive sleep apnea, history of respiratory problems requiring oxygen therapy, extremes of age), per agency policy and as indicated
- Palpate for equal lung expansion
- Percuss anterior and posterior thorax from apices to bases bilaterally
- Note location of trachea
- Monitor for diaphragmatic muscle fatigue, as indicated by paradoxical motion
- Auscultate breath sounds, noting areas of decreased or absent ventilation and presence of adventitious sounds
- Determine the need for suctioning by auscultating for crackles and rhonchi over major airways
- Auscultate lung sounds after treatments to note results
- Monitor PFT values, particularly vital capacity, maximal inspiratory force, forced expiratory volume in 1 second (FEV_1), and FEV_1/FVC, as available
- Monitor mechanical ventilator readings, noting increases in inspiratory pressures and decreases in tidal volume, as appropriate
- Monitor for increased restlessness, anxiety, and air hunger
- Note changes in SaO_2, SvO_2, end tidal CO_2, and changes in ABG values, as appropriate
- Monitor patient's ability to cough effectively
- Note onset, characteristics, and duration of cough
- Monitor patient's respiratory secretions
- Provide frequent intermittent monitoring of respiratory status in at-risk patients (e.g., opioid therapy, newborn, mechanical ventilation, facial or chest burns, neuromuscular disorders)
- Monitor for dyspnea and events that improve and worsen it
- Monitor for hoarseness and voice changes every hour in patients with facial burns
- Monitor for crepitus, as appropriate
- Monitor chest x-ray reports
- Open the airway, using the chin lift or jaw thrust technique, as appropriate
- Place the patient on side, as indicated, to prevent aspiration; log roll if cervical aspiration suspected
- Institute resuscitation efforts, as needed
- Institute respiratory therapy treatments (e.g., nebulizer), as needed

1st edition 1992; revised 2013

Background Readings:

Becker, D. E., & Casabianca, A. B. (2009). Respiratory monitoring: Physiological and technical considerations. *Anesthesia Progress, 56*(1), 14–22.

Bodin, D. A. (2003). Telemetry: Beyond the ICU. *Nursing Management, 34*(8), 46–47, 49–50.

Carbery, C. (2008). Basic concepts in mechanical ventilation. *Journal of Perioperative Practice, 18*(3), 106–114.

Fetzer, S. J. (2011). Vital signs. In P. A. Potter, A. G. Perry, P. Stockert, & A. Hall (Eds.), *Basic nursing* (7th ed., pp. 278–280). St. Louis: Mosby Elsevier.

Hutchinson, D., & Whyte, K. (2008). Neuromuscular disease and respiratory failure. *Practical Neurology, 8*(4), 229–237.

Maddox, R. R., Williams, C. K., Oglesby, H., Butler, B., & Colclasure, B. (2006). Clinical experience with patient-controlled analgesia using continuous respiratory monitoring and a smart infusion system. *American Journal of Health-System Pharmacy, 63*(2), 157–164.

Pratt, E. S. (2011). Oxygenation. In P. A. Potter, A. G. Perry, P. Stockert, & A. Hall (Eds.), *Basic nursing* (7th ed., pp. 800–813). St. Louis: Mosby Elsevier.

R

Respite Care 7260

Definition: Provision of short-term care to provide relief for family caregiver

Activities:
- Establish a therapeutic relationship with patient and family
- Monitor endurance of caregiver
- Inform patient and family of available state funding for respite care
- Arrange for residential respite care
- Coordinate volunteers for in-home services, as appropriate
- Coordinate community support services (i.e., meals, day care, summer camp)
- Arrange for substitute caregiver
- Monitor skill level of respite care provider
- Follow usual routine of care
- Provide care, such as exercises, ambulation, and hygiene, as appropriate
- Provide a program of suitable activities, as appropriate
- Obtain emergency telephone numbers
- Determine how to contact usual caregiver
- Provide emergency care, as necessary
- Maintain normal home environment
- Provide a report to usual caregiver on return

1st edition 1992; revised 2013

Background Readings:

Barnard-Brak, L. & Thomson, D. (2009). How is taking care of caregivers of children with disabilities related to academic achievement. *Child Youth Care Forum, 38*(2), 91–102.

Barrett, M., Wheatland, B., Haselby, P., Larson, A., Kristjanson, L., & Whyatt, D. (2009). Palliative respite services using nursing staff reduces hospitalization of patients and improves acceptance among carers. *International Journal of Palliative Nursing, 15*(8), 389–395.

Cowen, P. S. & Reed, D. A. (2002). Effects of respite care for children with developmental disabilities: Evaluation of an intervention for at risk families. *Public Health Nursing, 19*(4), 273–283.

Donath, C., Winkler, A., & Grassel, E. (2009). Short-term residential care for dementia patients: Predictors for utilization and expected quality from a family caregiver's point of view. *International Psychogeriatrics, 21*(4), 703–710.

Molzahn, A. E., Gallagher, E., & McNulty, V. (2009). Quality of life associated with adult day centers. *Journal of Gerontological Nursing, 35*(8), 37–46.

Perry, J. & Bontinen, K. (2001). Evaluation of a weekend respite program for persons with Alzheimer disease. *Canadian Journal of Nursing Research, 33*(1), 81–95.

Salin, S., Kaunonen, M., & Astedt-Kurki, P. (2009). Informal carers of older family members: How they manage and what support they receive from respite care. *Journal of Clinical Nursing, 18*(4), 492–501.

Resuscitation 6320

Definition: Administering emergency measures to sustain life

Activities:

- Evaluate unresponsiveness to determine appropriate action
- Call for help if no breathing or no normal breathing and no response
- Call a code according to agency standard
- Obtain the automated external defibrillator (AED)
- Attach the AED and implement specified actions
- Assure rapid defibrillation, as appropriate
- Perform cardiopulmonary resuscitation (CPR) that focuses on chest compressions in adults and compressions with breathing efforts for children, as appropriate
- Initiate 30 chest compressions at specified rate and depth, allowing for complete chest recoil between compressions, minimizing interruptions in compressions, and avoiding excessive ventilation
- Assure patient's airway is open
- Provide two rescue breaths after initial 30 chest compressions completed
- Minimize the interval between stopping chest compressions and delivering a shock, if indicated
- Tailor rescue actions to the most likely cause of arrest (e.g., cardiac or respiratory arrest)
- Monitor the quality of CPR provided
- Monitor patient response to resuscitation efforts
- Use either the head tilt or jaw thrust maneuver to maintain an airway
- Clear oral, nasal, and tracheal secretions when possible and without interfering with chest compressions, as appropriate
- Administer manual ventilation when possible and without interfering with chest compressions, as appropriate
- Call for physician assistance, as needed
- Connect the person to an electrocardiogram (ECG) monitor, if needed, when defibrillation is completed
- Initiate an IV line and administer IV fluids, as indicated
- Check that electronic equipment is working properly
- Provide standby equipment
- Provide appropriate medications
- Apply cardiac or apnea monitor
- Obtain ECG
- Interpret ECG and deliver cardioversion or defibrillation as needed
- Evaluate changes in chest pain
- Assist with insertion of endotracheal tube (ET), as indicated
- Assess lung sounds after intubation for proper ET position
- Assist with performing chest x-ray examination after intubation
- Assure organized post cardiac arrest care (e.g., safe transport to appropriate nursing care unit)
- Offer family members opportunities to be present during resuscitation when in the best interests of the patient
- Support family members who are present during resuscitation (e.g., ensure safe environment, provide explanations and commentary, allow appropriate communication with patient, continually assess needs, provide opportunities to reflect on resuscitation efforts after event)
- Provide opportunities for team members to be involved in team debriefings or reflect on resuscitation efforts after event
- Document sequence of events

1st edition 1992; revised 2013

Background Readings:

Boucher, M. (2010). Family-witnessed resuscitation. *Emergency Nurse, 18*(5), 10–14.

Carlson, K. (Ed.). (2009). *Advanced critical care nursing.* Philadelphia: Saunders.

Field, J. M., Hazinski, M. F., Sayre, M. R., Chameides, L., Schexnayder, S. M., Hemphill, R., et al. (2010). Part 1: Executive summary: 2010 American Heart Association guidelines for cardiopulmonary resuscitation and emergency cardiovascular care. *Circulation, 122*(18 Suppl. 3), S640–S656.

Hazinski, M. F. (Ed.). (2010). *Highlights of the 2010 American Heart Association guidelines for CPR and ECC.* Dallas, TX: American Heart Association.

Urden, L., Stacy, K. M., & Lough, M. E. (2010). *Critical care nursing: Diagnosis and management* (6th ed.). St. Louis: Mosby Elsevier.

Wiegand, D. J. (Ed.). (2011). *AACN procedure manual for critical care* (6th ed.). St. Louis: Elsevier Saunders.

R

Resuscitation: Fetus 6972

Definition: Administering emergency measures to improve placental perfusion or correct fetal acid-base status

Activities:

- Monitor fetal vital signs, using auscultation and palpation or electronic fetal monitor, as appropriate
- Observe for abnormal (e.g., nonreassuring) fetal heart rate signs, such as bradycardia, tachycardia, nonreactivity, variable decelerations, late decelerations, prolonged decelerations, decreased long-term and/or short-term variability, and sinusoidal pattern
- Include mother and support person in explanation of measures needed to enhance fetal oxygenation
- Use universal precautions
- Reposition mother to lateral or hands-and-knees position
- Reevaluate fetal heart rate
- Apply oxygen at 6 to 8 L, if positioning is ineffective in correcting abnormal or nonreassuring pattern of fetal heart rate
- Initiate intravenous line, as appropriate
- Give a bolus of IV fluid, per physician order or protocol
- Monitor maternal vital signs
- Perform a vaginal exam with fetal scalp stimulation
- Apprise midwife or physician about outcome of resuscitation measures
- Document strip interpretation, activities performed, fetal outcome, and maternal response
- Once the amniotic membranes are ruptured, apply internal monitors to obtain more information about the fetal heart rate response to uterine activity
- Reassure and calm mother and support person(s)
- Decrease uterine activity by stopping oxytocin infusion, as appropriate
- Administer tocolytic medication to reduce contractions, as appropriate
- Perform amnioinfusion for abnormal (e.g., nonreassuring) variable decelerations in fetal heart rate or meconium-stained amniotic fluid
- Turn to left-lateral position for pushing during second-stage labor to improve placental perfusion
- Coach to decrease pushing efforts for abnormal (e.g., nonreassuring) fetal heart signs to allow reestablishment of placental perfusion
- Consult with obstetrician to obtain fetal blood sample, as appropriate
- Anticipate requirements for mode of delivery and neonatal support, based on fetal responses to resuscitation techniques

2nd edition 1996

Background Readings:

Galvan, B., Van Mullen, C., & Broekhuizen, F. (1989). Using amnioinfusion for the relief of repetitive variable decelerations during labor. *Journal of Obstetric, Gynecologic, and Neonatal Nursing, 18*(93), 222–229.

Knorr, L. J. (1989). Relieving fetal distress with amnioinfusion. *American Journal of Maternal/Child Nursing, 14*(5), 346–350.

Murray, M. (1988). *Essentials of electronic fetal monitoring. Antepartal and intrapartal fetal monitoring.* Washington, DC: Nurses Association of the American College of Obstetricians & Gynecologists.

Pillitteri, A. (2007). Nursing care of high-risk newborn and family. *Maternal and child health nursing: Care of the childbearing and childrearing family* (5th ed., pp. 747–795). Philadelphia: Lippincott Williams & Wilkins.

Roberts, J. E. (1989). Managing fetal bradycardia during second stage of labor. *American Journal of Maternal/Child Nursing, 14*(6), 394–398.

Resuscitation: Neonate 6974

Definition: Administering emergency measures to support newborn adaptation to extrauterine life

Activities:

- Set up equipment for resuscitation before birth
- Test resuscitation bag, suction, and oxygen flow to ensure proper function
- Place newborn under the radiant warmer
- Insert laryngoscope to visualize the trachea to suction for meconium-stained fluid, as appropriate
- Intubate with an endotracheal tube (ET) to remove meconium from the lower airway, as appropriate
- Reintubate and suction until the return is clear of meconium
- Use mechanical suction to remove meconium from lower airway
- Dry with a prewarmed blanket to remove amniotic fluid, to reduce heat loss, and to provide stimulation
- Position the newborn on back, with neck slightly extended to open airway
- Place a rolled blanket under the shoulders to assist with correct positioning, as appropriate
- Suction secretions from nose and mouth with a bulb syringe
- Provide tactile stimulation by rubbing the soles of the feet or rubbing the infant's back
- Monitor respirations
- Monitor heart rate
- Initiate positive-pressure ventilation for apnea or gasping
- Use 100% oxygen at 5 to 8 L to fill resuscitation bag
- Adjust bag to fill correctly
- Obtain a tight seal with a mask that covers the chin, mouth, and nose
- Ventilate at a rate of 40 to 60 breaths per minute using 20 to 40- cm of water for initial breaths and 15 to 20- cm of water for subsequent pressures
- Auscultate to ensure adequate ventilation
- Check heart rate after 15 to 30 seconds of ventilation
- Give chest compression for heart rate of <60 beats per minute or if >80 beats per minute with no increase
- Compress sternum 0.5 to 0.75 inches using a 3:1 ratio for delivering 90 compressions and 30 breaths per minute
- Check heart rate after 30 seconds of compressions
- Continue compressions until heart rate is >80 beats per minute
- Continue ventilations until adequate spontaneous respirations begin and color becomes pink

- Insert ET for prolonged ventilation or poor response to bag and mask ventilation
- Auscultate bilateral breath sounds for confirmation of ET placement
- Observe for rise of chest without gastric distention to check placement
- Secure airway to face with tape
- Insert an orogastric catheter if ventilation is given for more than 2 minutes
- Prepare medications, as needed (e.g., narcotic antagonists, epinephrine, volume expanders, and sodium bicarbonate)
- Administer medications per order
- Document time, sequence, and neonatal responses to all steps of resuscitation
- Provide explanation to parents, as appropriate
- Assist with neonatal transfer or transport, as appropriate

2nd edition 1996

Background Readings:

American Heart Association & American Academy of Pediatrics. (1990). *Textbook of neonatal resuscitation*. Elk Grove Village, IL: Author.

Keenan, W. J., Raye, J. R., & Schell, B. (1993, April). *NRP instructor update*. Elk Grove Village, IL: American Heart Association & American Academy of Pediatrics.

Pillitteri, A. (2007). Nursing care of high-risk newborn and family. *Maternal and child health nursing: Care of the childbearing and childrearing family* (5th ed., pp. 747–795). Philadelphia: Lippincott Williams & Wilkins.

Risk Identification   6610

Definition: Analysis of potential risk factors, determination of health risks, and prioritization of risk reduction strategies for an individual or group

Activities:

- Review past health history and documents for evidence of existing or previous medical and nursing diagnoses and treatments
- Review data derived from routine risk assessment measures
- Determine availability and quality of resources (e.g., psychological, financial, education level, family and other social, and community)
- Identify agency resources to assist in decreasing risk factors
- Maintain accurate records and statistics
- Identify biological, environmental, and behavioral risks and their interrelationships
- Identify typical coping strategies
- Determine past and current level of functioning
- Determine status of basic living needs
- Determine community resources appropriate for basic living and health needs
- Determine compliance with medical and nursing treatments
- Instruct on risk factors and plan for risk reduction
- Use mutual goal setting, as appropriate
- Consider criteria useful in prioritizing areas for risk reduction (e.g., awareness and motivation level, effectiveness, cost, feasibility, preferences, equity, stigmatization, and severity of outcomes if risks remain unaddressed)
- Discuss and plan for risk reduction activities in collaboration with individual or group
- Implement risk reduction activities
- Initiate referrals to health care personnel and/or agencies, as appropriate
- Plan for long-term monitoring of health risks
- Plan for long-term follow up of risk reduction strategies and activities

1st edition 1992; revised 2013

Background Readings:

Doll, L. S., Bonzo, S. E., Mercy, J. A., Sleet, D. A. (Eds.). (2007). *Handbook of injury and violence prevention* [E. N. Haas, Managing Ed.]. New York: Springer.

Kutcher, S. & Chehil, S. (2007). *Suicide risk management: A manual for health professionals*. Oxford: Blackwell.

Stanhope, M. & Lancaster, J. (2008). *Public health nursing: Population-centered health care in the community* (7th ed.). St. Louis: Mosby Elsevier.

R

Risk Identification: Childbearing Family   6612

Definition: Identification of an individual or family likely to experience difficulties in parenting, and prioritization of strategies to prevent parenting problems

Activities:

- Determine age of mother
- Determine developmental stage of parent
- Determine parity of mother
- Determine economic status of family
- Determine educational status of mother
- Determine marital status of mother
- Determine residential status of mother (e.g., place of residence, homelessness, living with someone, immigration status)
- Determine literacy
- Determine outcomes of all prior pregnancies
- Determine whether previous children born to mother are still in her care

- Ascertain understanding of English or other language used in community
- Determine prior involvement with social services
- Determine prior history of abuse and violence
- Determine prior history of depression or other mental illness
- Determine health and immunization status of siblings
- Monitor behaviors that may indicate a problem with attachment
- Review prenatal and intrapartal records for documented signs of prenatal attachment
- Review prenatal history for factors that predispose patient to complications
- Review, update, and complete information as pregnancy develops and at intrapartum, postpartum, and neonatal admissions, as needed
- Note medications that mother received during prenatal period
- Review prenatal history for possible stressors affecting neonatal glucose stores (e.g., diabetes, pregnancy-induced hypertension, and cardiac or renal disorders)
- Review history for abnormal prenatal growth patterns, as detected by ultrasonography or fundal changes
- Review maternal history of chemical dependency, noting duration, type of drugs used (including alcohol), and time and strength of last dose before delivery
- Determine the patient's feelings about an unplanned pregnancy
- Determine whether unplanned pregnancy is approved of by the family
- Determine whether unplanned pregnancy is supported by the family
- Document psychosocial adaptation to pregnancy by the patient, the father, other children and adults in the household, family members, and others in close relationship to the pregnant woman
- Note presence of multiple gestation and consider challenges of raising multiples
- Note any medications (e.g., sedative, anesthetic, or analgesic) administered to mother during intrapartal period
- Note maternal morbidities that could delay attachment (e.g., prolonged labor, infection, sedating medications)
- Note fetal and neonatal morbidities (e.g., fetal distress, hypoxia, oligohydramnios or polyhydramnios, hyperglycemia or hypoglycemia) that could delay its ability to interact with caretakers
- Identify reason for separation from newborn after birth

- Monitor parent-infant interactions, noting behaviors thought to indicate attachment
- Note attachment behaviors to multiples (e.g., twins, triplets)
- Promote family attachment through patient education
- Implement activities that promote attachment
- Evaluate behavioral assessment of neonates during early pediatric visits for possible indications of parenting adjustment problems
- Promote a postpartum maternal follow-up visit at 2 to 6 weeks to a qualified health care professional
- Promote newborn follow-up care at 2 and 6 weeks by a qualified health care professional
- Prioritize areas for risk reduction, in collaboration with the individual or family
- Plan for risk reduction activities, in collaboration with the individual or family
- Promote newborn safety by requiring newborn discharge into an approved car seat
- Refer to the appropriate community agency for follow up, if risk of parenting problems or a lag in attachment has been identified

1st edition 1992; revised 2013

Background Readings:

Fouquier, K. F. (2011). The concept of motherhood among three generations of African American women. *Journal of Nursing Scholarship, 43*(2), 145–153.

Lutz, K. F., Anderson, L. S., Pridham, K. A., Riesch, S. K., & Becker, P. T. (2009). Furthering the understanding of parent-child relationships: A nursing scholarship review series. Part 1: Introduction. *Journal for Specialists in Pediatric Nursing, 14*(4), 256–261.

Lutz, K. F., Anderson, L. S., Riesch, S. K., Pridham, K. A., & Becker, P. T. (2009). Furthering the understanding of parent-child relationships: A nursing scholarship review series. Part 2: Grasping the early parenting experience–the insider view. *Journal for Specialists in Pediatric Nursing, 14*(4), 262–283.

Taubman-Ben-Ari, O., Findler, L., & Kuint, J. (2010). Personal growth in the wake of stress: The case of mothers of preterm twins. *Journal of Psychology, 144*(2), 185–204.

Underdown, A. & Barlow, J. (2011). Interventions to support early relationships: Mechanisms identified within infant massage programmes. *Community Practitioner, 84*(4), 21–26.

Ward, S. L. & Hisley, S. M. (2009). *Maternal-child nursing care: Optimizing outcomes for mothers, children, & families*. Philadelphia: F. A. Davis.

R

Risk Identification: Genetic   6614

Definition: Identification and analysis of potential genetic risk factors in an individual, family, or group

Activities:

- Ensure privacy and confidentiality
- Obtain or review a complete health history, including prenatal and obstetrical history, developmental history, and past and present health status related to the confirmed or suspected genetic condition
- Obtain or review environment (e.g., potential teratogen and carcinogen exposures) and lifestyle (e.g., tobacco, alcohol, street or prescription drug exposure) history
- Determine presence and quality of family support, other support systems, and previous coping skills
- Obtain or review a comprehensive family history and construct at least a three-generation pedigree

- Obtain documented diagnosis of affected family members
- Review options for diagnostic testing that may confirm or predict the presence of a genetic disorder, such as biochemical or radiographic studies, chromosome analysis, linkage analyses, or direct DNA testing
- Provide information about the diagnostic procedures
- Discuss advantages, risks, and financial costs of diagnostic options
- Discuss insurance and possible job discrimination issues, as relevant
- Discuss issues in testing other family members, as relevant
- Initiate genetic counseling intervention based upon risk identification, as appropriate

- Refer to genetic health care specialists for genetic counseling, as needed
- Provide patient a written summary of the risk identification counseling, as indicated

3rd edition 2000

Background Readings:

Andrews, L. B., Fullerton, J. E., Holtzman, N. A. & Motulsky, A. G. (1994). *Assessing Genetic Risks: Implications for health and social policy*. Washington, DC: National Academy Press.

Cohen, F. L. (2005). *Clinical genetics in nursing practice* (3rd ed.). New York: Springer.

Nelson, H. D., Huffman, L. H., Fu, R., & Harris, E. L. (2005). Genetic risk assessment and BRCA mutation testing for breast and ovarian cancer susceptibility: Systematic evidence review for the U.S. Preventive Services Task Force. *Annals of Internal Medicine, 143*(5), 362–379.

Pieterse, A. H., van Dulmen, S., van Dijk, S., Bensing, J. M., & Ausems, M. G. E. M. (2006). Risk communication in completed series of breast cancer genetic counseling visits. *Genetics in Medicine, 8*(11), 688–696.

Pillitteri, A. (2007). Genetic assessment and counseling. In *Maternal and child health nursing: Care of the childbearing and childrearing family* (5th ed., pp. 157–180). Philadelphia: Lippincott Williams & Wilkins.

Skirton, H., Patch, C., & Williams, J. (2005). *Applied genetics in healthcare*. London: Taylor and Francis.

Stacey, D., DeGrasse, C., & Johnston, L. (2002). Addressing the support needs of women at high risk for breast cancer: Evidence-based care by advanced practice nurses. *Oncology Nursing Forum, 29*(6), E77–E84.

Role Enhancement 5370

Definition: Assisting a patient, significant other, and/or family to improve relationships by clarifying and supplementing specific role behaviors

Activities:

- Assist patient to identify various roles in life cycle
- Assist patient to identify usual role in family
- Assist patient to identify role transition periods throughout the lifespan
- Assist patient to identify role insufficiency
- Assist patient to identify behaviors needed for role development
- Assist patient to identify specific role changes required due to illness or disability
- Assist adult children to accept elderly parent's dependency and the role changes involved, as appropriate
- Encourage patient to identify a realistic description of change in role
- Assist patient to identify positive strategies for managing role changes
- Facilitate discussion of role adaptations of family to compensate for ill member's role changes
- Assist patient to imagine how a particular situation might occur and how a role would evolve
- Facilitate role rehearsal by having patient anticipate others' reactions to enactment
- Facilitate discussion of how siblings' roles will change with newborn's arrival, as appropriate
- Provide rooming-in opportunities to help clarify parents' roles, as appropriate
- Facilitate discussion of role adaptations related to children's leaving home (empty nest syndrome), as appropriate
- Serve as role model for learning new behaviors, as appropriate
- Facilitate opportunity for patient to role play new behaviors
- Facilitate discussion of expectations between patient and significant other in reciprocal role
- Teach new behaviors needed by patient/parent to fulfill a role
- Facilitate reference group interactions as part of learning new roles

1st edition 1992; revised 2008

Background Readings:

Bunten, D. (2001). Normal changes with aging. In M. L. Maas, K. C. Buckwalter, M. D. Hardy, T. T. Reimer, M. G. Titler, & J. P. Specht (Eds.), *Nursing care of older adults: Diagnoses, outcomes, & interventions* (pp. 615–618). St. Louis: Mosby.

Ebersole, P., Hess, P., Touhy, T., & Jett, K. (2005). *Gerontological nursing & healthy aging* (2nd ed.). St. Louis: Mosby.

Larsen, P. D., Lewis, P. R., & Lubkin, I. M. (2006). Illness behavior and roles. In I. M. Lubkin & P. D. Larsen (Eds.), *Chronic illness: Impact and interventions* (pp. 23–44.). Sudbury, MA: Jones and Bartlett.

Mercer, R. T. (2004). Becoming a mother versus maternal role attainment. *Journal of Nursing Scholarship, 36*(3), 226–232.

Miller, J. F. (2000). *Coping with chronic illness: Overcoming powerlessness* (3rd ed.). Philadelphia: F. A. Davis.

Moorhead, S. A. (1985). Role supplementation. In G. M. Bulechek & J. C. McCloskey (Eds.), *Nursing interventions: Treatments for nursing diagnoses* (pp. 152–159). Philadelphia: W. B. Saunders.

R

Seclusion

6630

Definition: Solitary containment in a fully protective environment with close surveillance by nursing staff for purposes of safety or behavior management

Activities:

- Obtain a physician's order, if required by institutional policy, to use a physically restrictive intervention
- Designate one nursing staff member to communicate with the patient and to direct other staff
- Identify for patient and significant others those behaviors that necessitated the intervention
- Explain procedure, purpose, and time period of the intervention to patient and significant others in understandable and nonpunitive terms
- Explain to patient and significant others the behaviors necessary for termination of the intervention
- Contract with patient (as patient is able) to maintain control of behavior
- Instruct on self-control methods, as appropriate
- Assist in dressing in clothing that is safe and in removing jewelry and eyeglasses
- Remove all items from seclusion area that patient might use to harm self or others
- Assist with needs related to nutrition, elimination, hydration, and personal hygiene
- Provide food and fluids in nonbreakable containers
- Provide appropriate level of supervision and surveillance to monitor patient and to allow for therapeutic actions, as needed
- Inform patient of video surveillance, as appropriate
- Explain reasons for the video monitoring
- Give careful consideration to who is responsible for watching the video monitor for changes in patient status
- Reassure patient of safety within the seclusion area during monitoring
- Distinguish direct visual inspection from checks performed through video monitoring and document appropriately
- Acknowledge your presence to patient periodically
- Administer PRN medications for anxiety or agitation
- Provide for patient's psychological comfort, as needed
- Monitor seclusion area for temperature, cleanliness, and safety
- Reduce sensory stimuli around the seclusion area
- Arrange for routine cleaning of seclusion area

- Evaluate, at regular intervals, patient's need for continued restrictive intervention
- Involve patient, when appropriate, in making decisions to move to a more or less restrictive intervention
- Determine patient's need for continued seclusion
- Document rationale for restrictive intervention, patient's response to intervention, patient's physical condition, nursing care provided throughout intervention, and rationale for terminating the intervention
- Process with the patient and staff, on termination of the restrictive intervention, the circumstances that led to the use of the intervention, as well as any patient concerns about the intervention itself
- Provide the next appropriate level of restrictive intervention (e.g., physical restraint or area restriction), as needed

1st edition 1992; revised 2013

Background Readings:

Byatt, N. & Guck, R. (2008). Safety in the psychiatric emergency service. In R. L. Glick, J. S. Berlin, A. B. Fishkind, & S. L. Zeller (Eds.), *Emergency psychiatry: Principles and practice* (pp. 33–44). Philadelphia: Lippincott Williams & Wilkins.

Happell, B. & Koehan, S. (2010). Attitudes to the use of seclusions: Has contemporary mental health policy made a difference? *Journal of Clinical Nursing, 19*(21-22), 3208–3217.

Harper-Jaques, S. & Reimer, M. (2005). Management of aggression and violence. In M. A. Boyd (Ed.), *Psychiatric nursing: Contemporary practice* (3rd ed., pp. 802–822). Philadelphia: Lippincott Williams & Wilkins.

Hyde, S., Fulbrook, P., Fenton, K., & Kilshaw, M. (2009). A clinical improvement project to develop and implement a decision-making framework for the use of seclusion. *International Journal of Mental Health Nursing, 18*(6), 398–408.

Needham, H. & Sands, N. (2010). Post-seclusion debriefing: A core nursing intervention. *Perspectives in Psychiatric Care 46*(3), 221–232.

Olsen, D. P. (1998). Ethical considerations of video monitoring of psychiatric patients in seclusion and restraint. *Archives of Psychiatric Nursing, 12*(2), 90–94.

S

Security Enhancement

5380

Definition: Intensifying a patient's sense of physical and psychological safety

Activities:

- Provide a nonthreatening environment
- Demonstrate calmness
- Spend time with patient
- Offer to remain with patient in a new environment during initial interactions with others
- Stay with the patient and provide assurance of safety and security during periods of anxiety
- Present change gradually
- Discuss upcoming changes (e.g., an interward transfer) before event

- Avoid causing intense emotional situations
- Give pacifier to infant, as appropriate
- Hold a young child or infant, as appropriate
- Facilitate a parent's staying overnight with the hospitalized child
- Facilitate maintenance of patient's usual bedtime rituals
- Encourage family to provide personal items for patient's use or enjoyment
- Listen to patient's/family's fears
- Encourage exploration of the dark, as appropriate
- Leave light on at night, as needed

- Discuss specific situations or individuals that threaten the patient or family
- Explain all tests and procedures to patient/family
- Answer questions about health status in an honest manner
- Help the patient/family identify what factors increase sense of security
- Assist patient to identify usual coping responses
- Assist patient to use coping responses that have been successful in the past

1st edition 1992

Background Readings:

Pillitteri, A. (2007). Nursing care and the ill child and family. In *Maternal and child health nursing: Care of the childbearing and childrearing family* (5th ed., pp. 1067–1105). Philadelphia: Lippincott Williams & Wilkins.

Reynolds, E. A. & Ramenofsky, M. L. (1988). The emotional impact of trauma on toddlers. *MCN: American Journal of Maternal Child Nursing, 13*(2), 106–109.

Schepp, K. G. (1990). Factors influencing the coping effort of mothers of hospitalized children. *Nursing Research, 40*(1), 42–46.

Sedation Management 2260

Definition: Administration of sedatives, monitoring of the patient's response, and provision of necessary physiological support during a diagnostic or therapeutic procedure

Activities:

- Review patient's health history and results of diagnostic tests to determine if patient meets agency criteria for conscious sedation by a registered nurse
- Ask patient or family about any previous experiences with conscious sedation
- Check for drug allergies
- Determine last food and fluid intake
- Review other medications patient is taking and verify absence of contraindications for sedation
- Instruct the patient and/or family about effects of sedation
- Obtain informed written consent
- Evaluate the patient's level of consciousness and protective reflexes before administering sedation
- Obtain baseline vital signs, oxygen saturation, EKG, height, and weight
- Ensure emergency resuscitation equipment is readily available, specifically a source to deliver 100% oxygen, emergency medications, and a defibrillator
- Initiate an IV line
- Administer medication as per physician's order or protocol, titrating carefully, according to patient's response
- Monitor the patient's level of consciousness and vital signs, oxygen saturation, and EKG, as per agency protocol
- Monitor the patient for adverse effects of medication, including agitation, respiratory depression, hypotension, undue somnolence, hypoxemia, arrhythmias, apnea, or exacerbation of a preexisting condition
- Ensure availability of and administer antagonists, as appropriate, per physician's order or protocol
- Determine if the patient meets discharge or transfer criteria (i.e., Aldrete scale), as per agency protocol
- Document actions and patient response, as per agency policy
- Discharge or transfer patient, as per agency protocol
- Provide written discharge instructions, as per agency protocol

2nd edition 1996; revised 2000, 2004

Background Readings:

American Academy of Pediatrics. (1992). Guidelines for monitoring and management of pediatric patients during and after sedation for diagnostic and therapeutic procedures. *Pediatrics, 89*(6), 1110–1114.

Holzman, R. S., Cullen, D. J., Eichron, J. H., & Philip, J. J. (1994). Guidelines for sedation by nonanesthesiologists during diagnostic and therapeutic procedures. *Clinical Anesthesia 6*(4), 265–276.

Karch, A. M. (2007). *2007 Lippincott's nursing drug guide*. Philadelphia: Lippincott Williams & Wilkins.

Somerson, S. J., Husted, C. W., & Sicilia, M. R. (1995). Insights into conscious sedation. *American Journal of Nursing 95*(6), 25–32.

Somerson, S. J., Somerson, S. W., & Sicilia, M. R. (1999). Conscious sedation. In G. M. Bulechek & J. C. McCloskey (Eds.), *Nursing interventions: Effective nursing treatments* (3rd ed., pp. 297–310). Philadelphia: W. B. Saunders.

Watson, D. (1990). *Monitoring the patient receiving local anesthesia*. Denver, CO: Association of Operating Room Nurses.

S

Seizure Management 2680

Definition: Care of a patient during a seizure and the postictal state

Activities:

- Maintain airway
- Turn onto side
- Guide movements to prevent injury
- Monitor direction of head and eyes during seizure
- Loosen clothing
- Remain with patient during seizure
- Establish IV access, as appropriate
- Apply oxygen, as appropriate
- Monitor neurological status
- Monitor vital signs
- Reorient after seizure

- Record length of seizure
- Record seizure characteristics (e.g., body parts involved, motor activity, and seizure progression)
- Document information about seizure
- Administer medication, as appropriate
- Administer anticonvulsants, as appropriate
- Monitor antiepileptic drug levels, as appropriate
- Monitor postictal period duration and characteristics

1st edition 1992; revised 2013

Background Readings:

American Association of Neuroscience Nurses. (2009). *Care of the patient with seizures. AANN Clinical Practice Guidelines Series* (2nd ed.). Glenview, IL: Author.

Clore, E. (2010). Seizure precautions for pediatric bedside nurses. *Pediatric Nursing, 36*(4), 191–194.

Fitzsimmons, B. & Bohan, E. (2009). Common neurosurgical and neurological disorders. In P. G. Morton & D. K. Fontaine (Eds.), *Critical care nursing: A holistic approach* (9th ed., pp. 873–918). Philadelphia: Lippincott Williams & Wilkins.

Smeltzer, S., Bare, B., Hinkle, J., & Cheever, K. (2010). Management of patients with neurological dysfunction. In *Brunner & Suddarth's textbook of medical-surgical nursing* (12th ed., pp. 1881–1888). Philadelphia: Lippincott Williams & Wilkins.

Therapeutics and Technology Assessment Subcommittee and Quality Standards Subcommittee of the American Academy of Neurology and the American Epilepsy Society. (2004). Efficacy and tolerability of the new antiepileptic drugs I: Treatment of new onset epilepsy. *Neurology, 62*(8), 1252–1260.

Seizure Precautions 2690

Definition: Prevention or minimization of potential injuries sustained by a patient with a known seizure disorder

Activities:

- Provide low-height bed, as appropriate
- Escort patient during off-ward activities, as appropriate
- Monitor drug regimen
- Monitor compliance in taking antiepileptic medications
- Have patient or significant other keep record of medications taken and occurrence of seizure activity
- Instruct patient not to drive
- Instruct patient about medications and side effects
- Instruct family or significant other about seizure first aid
- Monitor antiepileptic drug levels, as appropriate
- Instruct patient to carry medication alert card
- Remove potentially harmful objects from the environment
- Keep suction at bedside
- Keep Ambu bag at bedside
- Keep oral or nasopharyngeal airway at bedside
- Use padded side rails
- Keep side rails up
- Instruct patient on potential precipitating factors
- Instruct patient to call if aura occurs

1st edition 1992; revised 2013

Background Readings:

American Association of Neuroscience Nurses. (2009). *Care of the patient with seizures. AANN Clinical Practice Guidelines Series* (2nd ed.). Glenview, IL: Author.

Clore, E. (2010). Seizure precautions for pediatric bedside nurses. *Pediatric Nursing, 36*(4), 191–194.

Fitzsimmons, B. & Bohan, E. (2009). Common neurosurgical and neurological disorders. In P. G. Morton & D. K. Fontaine (Eds.), *Critical care nursing: A holistic approach* (9th ed., pp. 873–918). Philadelphia: Lippincott Williams & Wilkins.

Smeltzer, S., Bare, B., Hinkle, J., & Cheever, K. (2010). Management of patients with neurological dysfunction. In *Brunner & Suddarth's textbook of medical-surgical nursing* (12th ed., pp. 1881–1888). Philadelphia: Lippincott Williams & Wilkins.

Therapeutics and Technology Assessment Subcommittee and Quality Standards Subcommittee of the American Academy of Neurology and the American Epilepsy Society. (2004). Efficacy and tolerability of the new antiepileptic drugs I: Treatment of new onset epilepsy. *Neurology, 62*(8), 1252–1260.

Self-Awareness Enhancement 5390

Definition: Assisting a patient to explore and understand his/her thoughts, feelings, motivations, and behaviors

Activities:

- Encourage patient to recognize and discuss thoughts and feelings
- Assist patient to realize that everyone is unique
- Assist patient to identify the values that contribute to self-concept
- Assist patient to identify usual feelings about self
- Share observation or thoughts about patient's behavior or response
- Facilitate patient's identification of usual response patterns to various situations
- Assist patient to identify life priorities
- Assist patient to identify the impact of illness on self-concept
- Verbalize patient's denial of reality, as appropriate
- Confront patient's ambivalent (angry or depressed) feelings
- Make observation about patient's current emotional state
- Assist patient to accept dependency on others, as appropriate
- Assist patient to change view of self as victim by defining own rights, as appropriate

- Assist patient to be aware of negative self-statements
- Assist patient to identify guilty feelings
- Help patient identify situations that precipitate anxiety
- Explore with patient the need to control
- Assist patient to identify positive attributes of self
- Assist patient/family to identify reasons for improvement
- Assist patient to identify abilities, learning styles
- Assist patient to reexamine negative perceptions of self
- Assist patient to identify source of motivation
- Assist patient to identify behaviors that are self-destructive

- Facilitate self-expression with peer group
- Assist patient to recognize contradictory statements

1st edition 1992; revised 2004

Background Readings:

Craven, R. F., & Hirnle, C. J. (2003). *Fundamentals of nursing: Human health and function* (4th ed.). Philadelphia: Lippincott Williams & Wilkins.

Stuart, G. W., & Laraia, M. T. (2005). *Principles and practice of psychiatric nursing* (8th ed.). St. Louis: Mosby.

Self-Care Assistance

1800

Definition: Assisting another to perform activities of daily living

Activities:
- Consider the culture of the patient when promoting self-care activities
- Consider age of patient when promoting self-care activities
- Monitor patient's ability for independent self-care
- Monitor patient's need for adaptive devices for personal hygiene, dressing, grooming, toileting, and eating
- Provide a therapeutic environment by ensuring a warm, relaxing, private, and personalized experience
- Provide desired personal articles (e.g., deodorant, toothbrush, and bath soap)
- Provide assistance until patient is fully able to assume self-care
- Assist patient in accepting dependency needs
- Use consistent repetition of health routines as a means of establishing them
- Encourage patient to perform normal activities of daily living to level of ability
- Encourage independence, but intervene when patient is unable to perform

- Teach parents/family to encourage independence, to intervene only when the patient is unable to perform
- Establish a routine for self-care activities

1st edition 1992; revised 2008

Background Readings:

Armer, J. M., Conn, V. S., Decker, S. A., & Tripp-Reimer, T. (2001). Self-care deficit. In M. Maas, K. Buckwalter, M. Hardy, T. Tripp-Reimer, M. Titler, & J. Specht (Eds.), *Nursing care of older adults: Diagnoses, outcomes & interventions* (pp. 366–384). St. Louis: Mosby.

Hall, G. R. & Buckwalter, K. C. (2001). *Evidence-based protocol: Bathing persons with dementia.* Iowa City, IA: The University of Iowa, College of Nursing, Gerontological Nursing Interventions Research Center.

Kozier, B., Erb, G., Berman, A., & Snyder, S. J. (2004). *Fundamentals of nursing, concepts, process, and practice* (7th ed.). Upper Saddle River, NJ: Prentice Hall.

Perry, A. G. & Potter, P. A., (2006). *Clinical nursing skills and techniques* (6th ed.). St. Louis: Mosby.

Self-Care Assistance: Bathing/Hygiene

1801

S

Definition: Assisting patient to perform personal hygiene

Activities:
- Consider the culture of the patient when promoting self-care activities
- Consider age of patient when promoting self-care activities
- Determine amount and type of assistance needed
- Place towels, soap, deodorant, shaving equipment, and other needed accessories at bedside or in bathroom
- Provide desired personal articles (e.g., deodorant, toothbrush, bath soap, shampoo, lotion, and aromatherapy products)
- Provide a therapeutic environment by ensuring a warm, relaxing, private, and personalized experience
- Facilitate patient brushing teeth, as appropriate
- Facilitate patient bathing self, as appropriate
- Monitor cleaning of nails, according to patient's self-care ability
- Monitor patient's skin integrity

- Maintain hygiene rituals
- Facilitate maintenance of patient's usual bedtime routines, pre-sleep cues/props, and familiar objects (e.g., for children, a favorite blanket/toy, rocking, pacifier, or story; for adults, a book to read or a pillow from home), as appropriate
- Encourage parent/family participation in usual bedtime rituals, as appropriate
- Provide assistance until patient is fully able to assume self-care

1st edition 1992; revised 2008

Background Readings:

Craven, R. F. & Hirnle, C. J. (2000). *Fundamentals of nursing: Human health and function* (3rd ed., pp. 696–701). Philadelphia: Lippincott Williams & Wilkins.

Hall, G. R. & Buckwalter, K. C. (2001). *Evidence-based protocol: Bathing persons with dementia.* Iowa City, IA: The University of Iowa, College of Nursing, Gerontological Nursing Interventions Research Center.

Kozier, B., Erb, G., Berman, A., & Snyder, S. J. (2004). *Fundamentals of nursing, concepts, process, and practice* (7th ed.). Upper Saddle River, NJ: Prentice Hall.

Perry, A. G. & Potter, P. A., (2006). *Clinical nursing skills and techniques* (6th ed.). St. Louis: Mosby.

Tracy, C. A. (1992). Hygiene assistance. In G. M. Bulechek & J. C. McCloskey (Eds.), *Nursing interventions: Essential nursing treatments* (2nd ed., pp. 24–33). Philadelphia: W. B. Saunders.

Self-Care Assistance: Dressing/Grooming   1802

Definition: Assisting patient with clothes and appearance

Activities:
- Consider the culture of the patient when promoting self-care activities
- Consider age of patient when promoting self-care activities
- Inform patient of available clothing for selection
- Provide patient's clothes in accessible area (e.g., at bedside)
- Provide personal clothing, as appropriate
- Be available for assistance in dressing, as necessary
- Facilitate patient combing hair, as appropriate
- Facilitate patient shaving self, as appropriate
- Maintain privacy while the patient is dressing
- Help with laces, buttons, and zippers, as needed
- Use extension equipment for pulling on clothing, if appropriate
- Offer to launder clothing, as necessary
- Place removed clothing in laundry
- Offer to hang up clothing or place in dresser
- Offer to rinse special garments, such as nylons
- Provide fingernail polish, if requested
- Provide makeup, if requested
- Reinforce efforts to dress self
- Facilitate assistance of a barber or beautician, as necessary

1st edition 1992; revised 2008

Background Readings:
Craven, R. F. & Hirnle, C. J. (2003). *Fundamentals of nursing: Human health and function* (4th ed.). Philadelphia: Lippincott Williams & Wilkins.
Kozier, B., Erb, G., Berman, A., & Snyder, S. J. (2004). *Fundamentals of nursing, concepts, process, and practice* (7th ed.). Upper Saddle River, NJ: Prentice Hall.
Perry, A. G. & Potter, P. A. (2006). *Clinical nursing skills and techniques* (6th ed.). St. Louis: Mosby.
Smith, S. F., Duell, D. J., & Martin, B. C. (2004). *Clinical nursing skills: Basic to advanced skills* (6th ed.). Upper Saddle River, NJ: Prentice Hall.

Self-Care Assistance: Feeding   1803

Definition: Assisting a person to eat

Activities:
- Monitor patient's ability to swallow
- Identify prescribed diet
- Set food tray and table attractively
- Create a pleasant environment during mealtime (e.g., put bedpans, urinals, and suctioning equipment out of sight)
- Ensure proper patient positioning to facilitate chewing and swallowing
- Provide physical assistance, as needed
- Provide for adequate pain relief before meals, as appropriate
- Provide for oral hygiene before meals
- Fix food on tray, as necessary, such as cutting meat or peeling an egg
- Open packaged foods
- Avoid placing food on a person's blind side
- Describe location of food on tray for person with vision impairment
- Place patient in comfortable eating position
- Protect with a bib, as appropriate
- Provide a drinking straw, as needed or desired
- Provide foods at most appetizing temperature
- Provide preferred foods and drinks, as appropriate
- Monitor patient's weight, as appropriate
- Monitor patient's hydration status, as appropriate
- Encourage patient to eat in dining room, if available
- Provide social interaction as appropriate
- Provide adaptive devices to facilitate patient's feeding self (e.g., long handles, handle with large circumference, or small strap on utensils), as needed
- Use a cup with a large handle, if necessary
- Use unbreakable and weighted dishes and glasses, as necessary
- Provide frequent cueing and close supervision, as appropriate

1st edition 1992; revised 2008

Background Readings:
Evans, N. J. (1992). Feeding. In G. M. Bulechek & J. C. McCloskey (Eds.), *Nursing interventions: Essential nursing treatments* (2nd ed., pp. 48–60). Philadelphia: W. B. Saunders.
Kozier, B., Erb, G., Berman, A., & Snyder, S. J. (2004). *Fundamentals of nursing, concepts, process, and practice* (7th ed.). Upper Saddle River, NJ: Prentice Hall.
Perry, A. G. & Potter, P. A. (2006). *Clinical nursing skills and techniques* (6th ed.). St. Louis: Mosby.
Smith, S. F., Duell, D. J., & Martin, B. C. (2004). *Clinical nursing skills: Basic to advanced skills* (6th ed.). Upper Saddle River, NJ: Prentice Hall.

Self-Care Assistance: IADL   1805

Definition: Assisting and instructing a person to perform instrumental activities of daily living (IADL) needed to function in the home or community

Activities:
- Determine individual's need for assistance with IADL (e.g., shopping, cooking, housekeeping, laundry, use of transportation, managing money, managing medications, use of communication, and use of time)
- Determine needs for safety-related changes in the home (e.g., wider door frames to allow for wheelchair access to bathroom, removal of scatter rugs)
- Determine needs for home enhancements to offset disabilities (e.g., large numbers on telephones, increased volume of telephone ringer, laundry and other facilities located on main floor, side rails in hallways, grab bars in bathrooms)
- Provide for methods of contacting support and assistance people (e.g., lifeline; list of telephone numbers for police, fire, poison control, and assistance people)
- Instruct individual on alternative methods of transportation (e.g., buses and bus schedules, taxis, city or county transportation for disabled people)
- Provide cognitive enhancing techniques (e.g., up-to-date calendars, clearly legible and understandable lists such as medication times, easy-to-see clocks)
- Obtain transportation enhancements to offset disabilities (e.g., hand controls on cars, wide rear-view mirror), as appropriate
- Obtain tools to assist in daily activities (e.g., ability to reach items in cupboards, in closets, on countertops, on stovetops, and in refrigerator, and ability to operate household equipment such as stoves and microwaves)
- Determine financial resources and personal preferences regarding modifications to home or car
- Instruct individual to wear clothing with short or tight-fitting sleeves when cooking
- Verify adequacy of lighting throughout house, especially in working areas (e.g., kitchen, bathroom), and at night (e.g., appropriately placed nightlights)
- Instruct individual not to smoke in bed or while reclining, or after taking mind-altering medication
- Verify presence of safety equipment in home (e.g., smoke detectors, carbon monoxide detectors, fire extinguishers, hot water heater set to 120° F)
- Determine whether individual's monthly income is sufficient to cover ongoing expenses
- Obtain visual safety devices or techniques (e.g., painting edges of steps bright yellow, rearrange furniture for safety when walking, reduce clutter throughout walkways of house, install nonskid surfaces in showers and bathtubs)
- Assist individual in establishing methods and routines for cooking, cleaning, and shopping
- Instruct individual and caregiver on what to do in the event the individual suffers from a fall or other injury (e.g., what to do, how to gain access to emergency services, how to prevent further injury)
- Determine if physical or cognitive ability is stable or declining and respond to changes in either, accordingly
- Consult with occupational and/or physical therapist to deal with physical disability
- Instruct assisting person in completing appropriate setting-up tasks so that individual can complete task (e.g., chop up vegetables so individual can cook with them, place clothing to wear for the day in an easy-to-reach place, unpack groceries on countertop for eventual storage)
- Provide appropriate container for used sharps, as appropriate
- Instruct individual on appropriate and safe storage for medications
- Instruct individual on appropriate use of monitoring equipment (e.g., glucose-monitoring device, lancets)
- Instruct individual on appropriate methods of dressing wounds and appropriate disposal of soiled dressings
- Verify that individual is able to open medication containers
- Refer to family and community services, as needed

4th edition 2004

Background Readings:
Eliopoulos, C. (1999). *Manual of gerontologic nursing* (2nd ed.). St. Louis: Mosby.
Lawton, H. P. & Brody, E. M. (1969). Assessment of older people: Self maintaining and instrumental activities of daily living. *Gerontologist*, 9(3), 179–186.
Lueckenotte, A. (2000). *Gerontologic nursing* (2nd ed.). St. Louis: Mosby.
Perry, A. G. & Potter, P. A. (2002). *Clinical nursing skills and techniques* (5th ed., pp. 1093–1113). St. Louis: Mosby.

S

Self-Care Assistance: Toileting   1804

Definition: Assisting another with elimination

Activities:
- Consider the culture of the patient when promoting self-care activities
- Consider age of patient when promoting self-care activities
- Remove essential clothing to allow for elimination
- Assist patient to toilet/commode/bedpan/fracture pan/urinal at specified intervals
- Consider patient's response to lack of privacy
- Provide privacy during elimination
- Facilitate toilet hygiene after completion of elimination
- Replace patient's clothing after elimination
- Flush toilet/cleanse elimination utensil (commode, bedpan)
- Institute a toileting schedule, as appropriate

- Instruct patient/appropriate others in toileting routine
- Institute bathroom rounds, as appropriate and needed
- Provide assistive devices (e.g., external catheter or urinal), as appropriate
- Monitor patient's skin integrity

1st edition 1992; revised 2008

Background Readings:

Kozier, B., Erb, G., Berman, A., & Snyder, S. J. (2004). *Fundamentals of nursing, concepts, process, and practice* (7th ed.). Upper Saddle River, NJ: Prentice Hall.

Perry, A. G. & Potter, P. A. (2006). *Clinical nursing skills and techniques* (6th ed.). St. Louis: Mosby.

Smith, S. F., Duell, D. J., & Martin, B. C. (2004). *Clinical nursing skills: Basic to advanced skills* (6th ed.). Upper Saddle River, NJ: Prentice Hall.

Self-Care Assistance: Transfer 1806

Definition: Assisting a patient with limitation of independent movement to learn to change body location

Activities:

- Review chart for activity orders
- Determine current ability of patient to transfer self (e.g., mobility level, limitations of movement, endurance, ability to stand and bear weight, medical or orthopedic instability, level of consciousness, ability to cooperate, ability to comprehend instructions)
- Select transfer technique that is appropriate for patient
- Instruct patient in all appropriate techniques, with the goal of reaching the highest level of independence
- Instruct individual on techniques for transfer from one area to another (e.g., bed to chair, wheelchair to vehicle)
- Instruct individual in use of ambulatory aids (e.g., crutches, wheelchairs, walkers, trapeze bars, cane)
- Identify methods to prevent injury during transfer
- Provide assistive devices (e.g., bars attached to walls, ropes attached to headboard or footboard for help in moving to center or edge of bed) to help individual transfer independently, as appropriate
- Make sure equipment works before using it
- Demonstrate technique, as appropriate
- Determine amount and type of assistance needed
- Assist patient in receiving all necessary care (e.g., personal hygiene, gathering belongings) before performing the transfer, as appropriate
- Provide privacy, avoid drafts, and preserve the patient's modesty
- Use proper body mechanics during movements
- Keep patient's body in proper alignment during movements
- Raise and move patient with a hydraulic lift, as necessary

- Move patient using a transfer board, as necessary
- Use a belt to assist a patient who can stand with assistance, as appropriate
- Assist patient to ambulate using your body as a human crutch, as appropriate
- Maintain traction devices during move, as appropriate
- Evaluate patient at end of transfer for proper body alignment, nonocclusion of tubes, wrinkled linens, unnecessarily exposed skin, adequate patient level of comfort, raised side rails, and call bell within reach
- Provide encouragement to patient as he/she learns to transfer independently
- Document progress, as appropriate

4th edition 2004, revised 2008

Background Readings:

Lewis, S. M., Hetkemper, M. M., & Dirksen, S. R. (2003). *Medical-surgical nursing; Assessment and management of clinical problems.* St. Louis: Mosby.

Perry, A. G. & Potter, P. A. (2004). *Fundamentals of nursing* (6th ed.). St. Louis: Mosby.

Perry, A. G. & Potter, P. A. (2006). *Clinical nursing skills and techniques* (6th ed.). St. Louis: Mosby.

Smeltzer, S. C. & Bare, B. G. (2004). *Brunner & Suddarth's textbook of medical-surgical nursing* (10th ed.). Philadelphia: Lippincott Williams and Wilkins.

S

Self-Efficacy Enhancement 5395

Definition: Strengthening an individual's confidence in his/her ability to perform a health behavior

Activities:

- Explore individual's perception of his/her capability to perform the desired behavior
- Explore individual's perception of benefits of executing the desired behavior
- Identify individual's perception of risks of not executing the desired behavior
- Identify barriers to changing behavior
- Provide information about the desired behavior

- Assist individual to commit to a plan of action for changing behavior
- Reinforce confidence in making behavior changes and taking action
- Provide an environment supportive to learning knowledge and skills needed to carry out the behavior
- Use teaching strategies that are culturally appropriate and age-appropriate (e.g., games, computer assisted instruction, or conversation maps)

- Model/demonstrate desired behavior
- Engage in role play to rehearse behavior
- Provide positive reinforcement and emotional support during the learning process and while implementing the behavior
- Provide opportunities for mastery experiences (e.g., successful implementation of the behavior)
- Use positive persuasive statements regarding the individual's ability to carry out the behavior
- Encourage interaction with other individuals who are successfully changing their behavior (e.g., support group or group education participation)
- Prepare individual for the physiologic and emotional states that may be experienced during initial attempts to carry out a new behavior

5th edition 2008

Background Readings:

Bandura, A. (1997). *Self-efficacy: The exercise of control*. New York: W. H. Freeman.

Fisher, K. (2006). School nurses' perceptions of self-efficacy in providing diabetes care. *Journal of School Nursing, 22*(4), 223–228.

Lau-Walker, M. (2006). A conceptual care model for individualized care approach in cardiac rehabilitation: Combining both illness representation and self-efficacy. *British Journal of Health Psychology, 11*(pt. 1), 103–117.

Litarowsky, J. A., Murphy, S. O., & Canham, D. L. (2004). Evaluation of an anaphylaxis training program for unlicensed assistive personnel. *Journal of School Nursing, 20*(3), 279–284.

Long, J. D. & Stevens, K. R. (2004). Using technology to promote self-efficacy for healthy eating in adolescents. *Journal of Nursing Scholarship, 36*(2), 34–129.

Pender, N. J., Murdaugh, C. L., & Parsons, M. A. (2002). *Health promotion in nursing practice* (4th ed.). Upper Saddle River, NJ: Prentice Hall.

Self-Esteem Enhancement   5400

Definition: Assisting a patient to increase his or her personal judgment of self-worth

Activities:

- Monitor patient's statements of self-worth
- Determine patient's locus of control
- Determine patient's confidence in own judgment
- Encourage patient to identify strengths
- Assist patient to find self-acceptance
- Encourage eye contact in communicating with others
- Reinforce the personal strengths that patient identifies
- Encourage patient to engage in self-talk and verbalize positive affirmations to self daily
- Provide experiences that increase patient's autonomy, as appropriate
- Assist patient to identify positive responses from others
- Refrain from negatively criticizing
- Assist the patient to cope with bullying or teasing
- Convey confidence in patient's ability to handle situation
- Assist in setting realistic goals to achieve higher self-esteem
- Assist patient to accept dependence on others, as appropriate
- Assist patient to reexamine negative perceptions of self
- Encourage increased responsibility for self, as appropriate
- Assist patient to identify the impact of peer group on feelings of self-worth
- Explore previous achievements of success
- Explore reasons for self-criticism or guilt
- Encourage the patient to evaluate own behavior
- Encourage patient to accept new challenges
- Reward or praise patient's progress toward reaching goals
- Facilitate an environment and activities that will increase self-esteem
- Assist patient to identify significance of culture, religion, race, gender, and age on self-esteem

- Instruct parents on the importance of their interest and support in their children's development of a positive self-concept
- Instruct parents to set clear expectations and to define limits with their children
- Instruct parents to recognize children's accomplishments
- Monitor frequency of self-negating verbalizations
- Monitor lack of follow-through in goal attainment
- Monitor levels of self-esteem over time, as appropriate
- Make positive statements about patient

1st edition 1992; revised 2013

Background Readings:

Bode, C., van der Heij, A., Taal, E., & van de Laar, M. A. (2010). Body-self unity and self-esteem in patients with rheumatic diseases. *Psychology, Health & Medicine, 15*(6), 672–684.

Bunten, D. (2001). Normal changes with aging. In M. L. Maas, K. C. Buckwalter, M. D. Hardy, T. Tripp-Reimer, M. G. Titler, & J. P. Specht (Eds.), *Nursing care of older adults: Diagnoses, outcomes, & interventions* (p. 519). St. Louis: Mosby.

Lai, H., Lu, C., Jwo, J., Lee, P., Chou, W., & Wen, W. (2009). The effects of a self-esteem program incorporated into health and physical education classes. *Journal of Nursing Research, 17*(4), 233–240.

Lim, J., Kim, M., Kim, S., Kim, E., Lee, J., & Ko, Y. (2010). The effects of a cognitive-behavioral therapy on career attitude maturity, decision making style, and self-esteem of nursing students in Korea. *Nurse Education Today, 30*(8), 731–736.

Weber, S., Puskar, K., & Ren, D. (2010). Relationships between depressive symptoms and perceived social support, self-esteem, & optimism in a sample of rural adolescents. *Issues in Mental Health Nursing, 31*(9), 584–588.

S

Self-Hypnosis Facilitation 5922

Definition: Teaching and monitoring the use of a self-initiated hypnotic state for therapeutic benefit

Activities:
- Determine whether the patient is an appropriate candidate for self-hypnosis
- Utilize self-hypnosis as an adjunct to other treatment modalities (e.g., individual hypnotherapy by a therapist, individual psychotherapy, group therapy, family therapy, etc.)
- Introduce the patient to the concept of self-hypnosis as a therapeutic modality
- Identify with the patient those problems/issues that are amenable to treatment with self-hypnosis
- Obtain history of the problem to be treated by self-hypnosis
- Determine goals for self-hypnosis with patient
- Determine patient's receptivity about using self-hypnosis
- Correct myths and misconceptions of self-hypnosis
- Ensure the patient has accepted the treatment
- Evaluate the suitability of the patient by assessing their hypnotic suggestibility
- Provide the patient with an individualized procedure for the process of self-hypnosis that reflects his/her specific needs and goals
- Assist the patient to identify appropriate induction techniques (e.g., Chevreul pendulum illusion, relaxation, imagining walking down a staircase, eye closure, arm levitation, simple muscle relaxation, visualization exercises, attention to breathing, repetition of key words/phrases, and others)
- Assist the patient to identify appropriate deepening techniques (e.g., movement of a hand to the face, imagery escalation technique, fractionation, and others)
- Encourage the patient to become proficient at self-hypnosis by practicing the technique
- Contract for a practice schedule with the patient, if needed
- Monitor the patient's response to self-hypnosis on an ongoing basis
- Solicit the patient's feedback regarding his/her comfort with the procedure and experience of self-hypnosis
- Assist the patient to process and interpret what occurs as a result of the self-hypnosis sessions
- Recommend modifications in the patient's practice of self-hypnosis (frequency, intensity, specific techniques) based on his/her response and level of comfort
- Assist the patient to evaluate progress made towards therapy goals

4th edition 2004; revised 2008

Background Readings:

Fontaine, K. L. (2005). Hypnotherapy and guided imagery. In K. L. Fontaine, *Complementary & alternative therapies for nursing practice* (2nd ed., pp. 301–338). Upper Saddle River, NJ: Prentice Hall.

Freeman, L. (2004). Hypnosis. In L. Freeman, *Mosby's complementary & alternative medicine: A research-based approach* (2nd ed., pp. 237–274). St. Louis: Mosby.

Fromm, E. & Kahn, S. (1990). *Self-hypnosis. The Chicago paradigm.* New York: The Guilford Press.

Lynn, S. J. & Kirsch, I. (2006). *Essentials of clinical hypnosis: An evidence-based approach.* Washington, DC: American Psychological Association.

Rankin-Box, D. (2001). Hypnosis. In D. Rankin-Box (Ed.), *The nurse's handbook of complementary therapies* (2nd ed., pp. 208–214). Edinburgh: Bailliere Tindall.

Sanders, S. (1991). *Clinical self-hypnosis.* New York: The Guilford Press.

Zahourek, R. P. (1985). *Clinical hypnosis and therapeutic suggestion in nursing.* Orlando. FL: Grune & Stratton.

Zarren, J. I. & Eimer, B. N. (2002). *Brief cognitive hypnosis. Facilitating the change of dysfunctional behavior.* New York: Springer.

Self-Modification Assistance 4470

Definition: Reinforcement of self-directed change initiated by the patient to achieve personally important goals

Activities:
- Encourage the patient to examine personal values and beliefs and satisfaction with them
- Appraise the patient's reasons for wanting to change
- Assist the patient in identifying a specific goal for change
- Assist the patient in identifying target behaviors that need to change to achieve the desired goal
- Assist the patient in identifying the target behaviors' effects on their social and environmental surroundings
- Appraise the patient's present knowledge and skill level in relationship to the desired change
- Assist the patient in identifying the stages of change: precontemplation, contemplation, preparation, action, maintenance, and termination
- Appraise the patient's social and physical environment for extent of support of desired behaviors
- Explore with the patient potential barriers to change behavior
- Identify with the patient the most effective strategies for behavior change
- Explain to the patient the importance of self-monitoring in attempting behavior change
- Assist the patient in identifying the frequency with which specific behaviors occur
- Assist the patient in developing a portable, easy-to-use coding sheet to aid in recording behaviors (may be a graph or chart)
- Instruct the patient to record the incidence of behaviors for at least 3 days, up to 2 to 3 weeks
- Encourage the patient to identify appropriate, meaningful reinforcers and rewards
- Encourage the patient to choose a reinforcer or reward that is significant enough to sustain the behavior
- Assist the patient in developing a list of valued extrinsic and intrinsic rewards

- Encourage the patient to begin with extrinsic rewards and progress to intrinsic rewards
- Instruct the patient that reward list may include manners in which the nurse, family, or friends can assist the patient in behavior change
- Assist the patient in formulating a systematic plan for behavior change
- Encourage the patient to identify steps that are manageable in size and able to be accomplished in a set amount of time
- Foster moving toward primary reliance on self-reinforcement instead of family or nurse for rewards
- Instruct the patient on how to move from continuous reinforcement to intermittent reinforcement
- Assist the patient in evaluating progress by comparing records of previous behavior with present behavior
- Encourage the patient to develop a visual measure of changes in behavior (e.g., a graph)
- Foster flexibility during the shaping plan, promoting complete mastery of one step before advancing to the next
- Encourage the patient to adjust the shaping plan to enhance behavior change, if needed (e.g., size of steps or reward)
- Assist the patient in identifying the circumstances or situations in which the behavior occurs (e.g., cues, triggers)
- Assist the patient in identifying even small successes
- Explain to the patient the function of cues and triggers in producing behavior
- Assist the patient in appraising the physical, social, and interpersonal settings for the existence of cues and triggers
- Encourage the patient to develop a "cue analysis sheet," which illustrates links between cues and behaviors
- Instruct the patient on the use of "cue expansion", increasing the number of cues that prompt a desired behavior
- Instruct the patient on the use of "cue restriction or limitation", decreasing the frequency of cues that elicit an undesirable behavior
- Assist the patient in identifying methods of controlling behavioral cues
- Assist the patient in identifying existent behaviors that are habitual or automatic (e.g., brushing teeth and tying shoes)
- Assist the patient in identifying existing paired stimuli and habitual behavior (e.g., eating a meal and brushing teeth afterward)
- Encourage the patient to pair a desired behavior with an existing stimulus or cue (e.g., exercising after work every day)
- Encourage the patient to continue pairing desired behavior with existing stimuli until it becomes automatic or habitual
- Explore with the patient the option of using a technological device in organizing coding sheets, change data, cue analysis, and visual measures of change (e.g., computer, smart phone)
- Explore with the patient the potential use of imagery, meditation, or progressive relaxation in attempting behavior change
- Explore with the patient the possibility of using role playing to clarify behaviors

1st edition 1992; revised 2013

Background Readings:

Antony, M. M. (2005). Cognitive behavior therapy. In M. Hersen & J. Rosqvist (Eds.), *Encyclopedia of behavior modification and cognitive behavior therapy* (pp. 186–195). Thousand Oaks, CA: Sage.

Franklin, P. D., Farzanfar, R., & Thompson, D. D. (2008). E-health strategies to support adherence. In S. A. Shumaker, J. K. Ockene, & K. A. Riekert (Eds.), *Handbook of health behavior change* (3rd ed., pp. 169–190). New York: Springer.

Karoly, P. (2005). Self-control. In M. Hersen & J. Rosqvist (Eds.), *Encyclopedia of behavior modification and cognitive behavior therapy* (pp. 504–508). Thousand Oaks, CA: Sage.

Karoly, P. (2005). Self-monitoring. In M. Hersen & J. Rosqvist (Eds.), *Encyclopedia of behavior modification and cognitive behavior therapy* (pp. 521–525). Thousand Oaks, CA: Sage.

Prochaska, J. O., Johnson, S., & Lee. P. (2008). The transtheoretical model of behavior change. In S. A. Shumaker, J. K. Ockene, & K. A. Riekert (Eds.), *Handbook of health behavior change* (3rd ed., pp. 59–84). New York: Springer.

Stuart, G. W. (2009). *Principles and practice of psychiatric nursing* (9th ed.). St. Louis: Mosby.

Watson, D. L. & Tharp, R. G. (2006). *Self-directing behavior: Self-modification for personal adjustment* (9th ed.). Belmont, CA: Wadsworth.

Self-Responsibility Facilitation 4480

Definition: Encouraging a patient to assume more responsibility for own behavior

Activities:
- Hold patient responsible for own behavior
- Discuss with patient the extent of responsibility for present health status
- Determine whether patient has adequate knowledge about health care condition
- Encourage verbalizations of feelings, perceptions, and fears about assuming responsibility
- Monitor level of responsibility that patient assumes
- Encourage independence, but assist patient when unable to perform
- Discuss consequences of not dealing with own responsibilities
- Encourage admission of wrongdoing, as appropriate
- Set limits on manipulative behaviors
- Refrain from arguing or bargaining about the established limits with the patient
- Encourage patient to take as much responsibility for own self-care, as possible
- Assist parents in identifying age-appropriate tasks for which a child could be responsible, as appropriate
- Encourage parents to clearly communicate expectations for responsible behavior in child, as appropriate
- Encourage parents to follow through on expectations for responsible behavior in child, as appropriate
- Assist patients to identify areas in which they could readily assume more responsibility
- Facilitate family support for new level of responsibility sought or attained by patient

- Assist with creating a timetable to guide increased responsibility in the future
- Provide positive feedback for accepting additional responsibility and/or behavior change

1st edition 1992; revised 1996

Background Readings:

Arnold, L. J. (1990). Codependency. Part I: Origins, characteristics. *AORN Journal, 51*(5), 1341–1348.

Arnold, L. J. (1990). Codependency. Part II: The hospital as a dysfunctional family. *AORN Journal, 51*(6), 1581–1584.

Arnold, L. J. (1990). Codependency. Part III: Strategies for healing. *AORN Journal, 52*(1), 85–89.

Barnsteiner, J. H. & Gillis-Donovan, J. (1990). Being related and separate: A standard for therapeutic relationships. *MCN: American Journal of Maternal Child Nursing, 15*(4), 223–228.

Hall, S. F. & Wray, L. M. (1989). Codependency: Nurses who give too much. *American Journal of Nursing, 89*(11), 1456–1460.

Johnson, P. A. & Gaines, S. K. (1988). Helping families to help themselves. *MCN: American Journal of Maternal Child Nursing, 13*(5), 336–339.

Stuart, G. W. & Laraia, M. T. (2005). *Principles and practice of psychiatric nursing* (8th ed.). St. Louis: Mosby.

Sexual Counseling   5248

Definition: Use of an interactive process focusing on the need to make adjustments in sexual practice or to enhance coping with a sexual event or disorder

Activities:

- Establish a therapeutic relationship, based on trust and respect
- Establish the length of the counseling relationship
- Provide privacy and ensure confidentiality
- Inform patient early in the relationship that sexuality is an important part of life and that illness, medications, and stress (or other problems and events patient is experiencing) often alter sexual functioning
- Encourage patient to verbalize fears and to ask questions about sexual functioning
- Preface questions about sexuality with a statement that tells the patient that many people experience sexual difficulties
- Begin with the least sensitive topics and proceed to the more sensitive
- Collect the client's sexual history, paying close attention to normal patterns of functioning and the terms used by the patient to describe sexual function
- Determine the duration of sexual dysfunction and potential causes
- Monitor for stress, anxiety, and depression as possible causes of sexual dysfunction
- Determine the knowledge level of the patient and understanding about sexuality in general
- Provide information about sexual functioning, as appropriate
- Discuss the effect of health and illness on sexuality
- Discuss the effect of medications and supplements on sexuality, as appropriate
- Discuss the effect of changes in sexuality on significant others
- Discuss necessary modifications in sexual activity, as appropriate
- Help patient to express grief and anger about alterations in body functioning or appearance, as appropriate
- Avoid displaying aversion to an altered body part
- Introduce patient to positive role models who have successfully conquered a similar problem, as appropriate
- Provide factual information about sexual myths and misinformation that patient may verbalize
- Discuss alternative forms of sexual expression that are acceptable to patient, as appropriate
- Instruct the patient on use of medication(s) and devices to enhance ability to perform sexually, as appropriate
- Determine amount of sexual guilt associated with the patient's perception of the causative factors of illness
- Avoid prematurely terminating discussion of guilt feelings, even when these seem unreasonable
- Include the significant other in the counseling as much as possible, as appropriate
- Use humor and encourage patient to use humor to relieve anxiety or embarrassment, being careful to use humor that is appropriate to the situation, tactful, and respectful of patient beliefs and cultural background
- Provide reassurance that current and new sexual practices are healthy, as appropriate
- Provide reassurance and permission to experiment with alternative forms of sexual expression, as appropriate
- Provide referral or consultation with other members of the health care team, as appropriate
- Refer the patient to a sex therapist, as appropriate

1st edition 1992; revised 2013

Background Readings:

Barton-Burke, M. & Gustason, C. J. (2007). Sexuality in women with cancer. *Nursing Clinics of North America, 42*(4), 531–554.

Brassil, D. F. & Keller, M. (2002). Female sexual dysfunction: Definitions, causes, and treatment. *Urologic Nursing, 22*(4), 237–284.

Clayton, A. & Ramamurthy, S. (2008). The impact of physical illness on sexual dysfunction. *Advances in Psychosomatic Medicine, 29*, 70–88.

Ginsberg, T. B., Pomerantz, S. C., & Kramer-Feeley, V. (2005). Sexuality in older adults: Behaviours and preferences. *Age and Aging, 34*(5), 475–480.

Jaarsma, T., Steinke, E. E., & Gianotten, W. L. (2010). Sexual problems in cardiac patients: How to assess, when to refer. *Journal of Cardiovascular Nursing, 25*(2), 159–164.

Lewis, L. J. (2004). Examining sexual health discourses in a racial/ethnic context. *Archives of Sexual Behavior, 33*(3), 223–234.

Schwarz, E. R., Kapur, V., Bionat, S., Rastogi, S., Gupta, R., & Rosanio, S. (2008). The prevalence and clinical relevance of sexual dysfunction in women and men with chronic heart failure. *International Journal of Impotence Research, 20*(1), 85–91.

Steinke, E. E. (2005). Intimacy needs and chronic illness. *Journal of Gerontological Nursing, 31*(5), 40–50.

Steinke, E. E. & Jaarsma, T. (2008). Impact of cardiovascular disease on sexuality. In D. Moser & B. Riegel (Eds.), *Cardiac nursing: A companion to Braunwald's heart disease* (pp. 241–253). St. Louis: Saunders Elsevier.

S

Shift Report   8140

Definition: Exchanging essential patient care information with other nursing staff at change of shift

Activities:
- Review pertinent demographic data, including name, age, and room number
- Identify chief complaint and reason for admission, as appropriate
- Summarize significant past health history, as necessary
- Identify key medical and nursing diagnoses, as appropriate
- Identify resolved medical and nursing diagnoses, as appropriate
- Present information succinctly, focusing on recent and significant data needed by nursing staff assuming responsibility for care
- Describe treatment regimen, including diet, fluid therapy, medications, and exercise
- Identify laboratory and diagnostic tests to be completed during the next 24 hours
- Review recent pertinent laboratory and diagnostic test results, as appropriate
- Describe health status data, including vital signs and signs and symptoms present during the shift
- Describe nursing interventions being implemented
- Describe patient and family response to nursing interventions
- Summarize progress toward goals
- Summarize discharge plans, as appropriate

2nd edition 1996

Background Readings:
Donaghue, A. M. & Reiley, P. J. (1981). Some do's and don'ts for giving reports. *Nursing, 11*(11), 117.
Kron, T. & Gray, A. (1987). *The management of patient care: Putting leadership skills to work* (6th ed.). Philadelphia: W. B. Saunders.
Lamond, D. (2000). The information content of the nurse change of shift report: A comparative study. *Journal of Advanced Nursing, 31*(4), 794–804.
Priest, C. S. & Holmberg, S. K. (2000). A new model for the mental health nursing change of shift report. *Journal of Psychosocial Nursing and Mental Health Service, 38*(8), 36–45.
Richard, J. A. (1988). Congruence between intershift reports and patients' actual conditions. *Image, 20*(1), 4–6.

Shock Management   4250

Definition: Facilitation of the delivery of oxygen and nutrients to systemic tissue with removal of cellular waste products in a patient with severely altered tissue perfusion

Activities:
- Monitor vital signs, orthostatic blood pressure, mental status, and urinary output
- Position the patient for optimal perfusion
- Institute and maintain airway patency, as appropriate
- Monitor pulse oximetry, as appropriate
- Administer oxygen and/or mechanical ventilation, as appropriate
- Monitor ECG, as appropriate
- Utilize arterial line monitoring to improve accuracy of blood pressure readings, as appropriate
- Draw arterial blood gases (ABGs) and monitor tissue oxygenation
- Monitor trends in hemodynamic parameters (e.g., CVP, MAP, pulmonary capillary/artery wedge pressure)
- Monitor determinants of tissue oxygen delivery (e.g., PaO_2, SaO_2, hemoglobin levels, CO), if available
- Monitor sublingual carbon dioxide levels and/or gastric tonometry, as appropriate
- Monitor for symptoms of respiratory failure (e.g., low PaO_2, elevated $PaCO_2$ levels, respiratory muscle fatigue)
- Monitor laboratory values (e.g., CBC with differential, coagulation profile, ABG, lactate level, cultures, and chemistry profile)
- Insert and maintain large bore IV access
- Administer IV fluid challenge while monitoring hemodynamic pressures and urinary output, as appropriate
- Administer crystalloid or colloid intravenous fluids, as appropriate
- Administer packed red blood cells, fresh frozen plasma, and/or platelets, as appropriate
- Monitor for hyperdynamic state of septic shock post fluid resuscitation (e.g., increased CO, decreased SVR, flushed skin, or increased temperature)
- Administer vasopressors, as appropriate
- Administer antiarrhythmic agents, as appropriate
- Initiate early administration of antimicrobial agents and closely monitor their effectiveness, as appropriate
- Administer antiinflammatory agents and/or bronchodilators, as appropriate
- Monitor serum glucose and treat abnormal levels, as appropriate
- Monitor fluid status, including daily weights, hourly urine output, I&O
- Monitor renal function (e.g., BUN, Cr levels, creatinine clearance)
- Administer diuretics, as appropriate
- Administer continuous renal replacement therapy or hemodialysis, as appropriate
- Insert nasogastric tube to suction and monitor secretions, as appropriate
- Administer thrombolytics, as appropriate
- Administer recombinant activated protein C, as appropriate
- Administer low dose vasopressin, as appropriate
- Administer corticosteroids, as appropriate
- Administer inotropes, as appropriate
- Administer venodilators, as appropriate

S

- Administer DVT and stress ulcer prophylaxis, as appropriate
- Offer emotional support to the patient and family, encouraging realistic expectations

1st edition 1992; revised 2004, 2008

Background Readings:

Ahrens, T. & Tuggle, D. (2004). Surviving severe sepsis: Early recognition and treatment. *Critical Care Nurse*, (Oct. Suppl.), 2–15.

Albright, T. N., Selzman, C. H., & Zimmerman, M. A. (2002). Vasopressin in the cardiac surgery intensive care unit. *American Journal of Critical Care*, *11*(4), 326–330.

American Heart Association. (2005). 2005 American Heart Association guidelines for cardiopulmonary resuscitation and emergency cardiovascular care. *Circulation, 112*(24 Suppl.), IV1–IV203.

Bridges, E. J. & Dukes, S. (2005). Cardiovascular aspects of septic shock-pathophysiology, monitoring, and treatment. *Critical Care Nurse, 25*(2), 14–42.

Dellinger, R. P., Carlet, J. M., Masur, H., Gerlach, H., Calandra, T., Cohen, J., et al. (2004). Surviving sepsis campaign guidelines for management of severe sepsis and septic shock. *Critical Care Medicine, 32*(3), 858–873.

Flynn, M. B. & McLeskey, S. (2005). Shock, systemic inflammatory response syndrome, and multiple organ dysfunction syndrome. In P. G. Morton, D. K. Fontaine, C. M. Hudak, & B. M. Gallo, *Critical care nursing*. Philadelphia: Lippincott Williams & Wilkins.

Porth, C. M. (2004). *Essentials of pathophysiology: Concepts of altered health states*. Philadelphia: Lippincott Williams & Wilkins.

Smeltzer, S. C. & Bare, B. G. (2003). *Brunner & Suddarth's textbook of medical-surgical nursing* (10th ed.). Philadelphia: Lippincott Williams & Wilkins.

Tazbir, J. (2004). Sepsis and the role of activated protein C. *Critical Care Nurse, 24*(6), 40–45.

Shock Management: Cardiac   4254

Definition: Promotion of adequate tissue perfusion for a patient with severely compromised pumping function of the heart

Activities:

- Monitor for signs and symptoms of decreased cardiac output
- Auscultate lung sounds for crackles or other adventitious sounds
- Note signs and symptoms of decreased cardiac output
- Monitor for inadequate coronary artery perfusion (ST changes on EKG, elevated cardiac enzymes, angina), as appropriate
- Monitor coagulation studies, including prothrombin time (PT), partial thromboplastin time (PTT), fibrinogen, fibrin degradation/split products, and platelet counts, as appropriate
- Monitor and evaluate indicators of tissue hypoxia (mixed venous oxygen saturation, central venous oxygen saturation, serum lactate levels, sublingual capnometry)
- Administer supplemental oxygen, as appropriate
- Maintain optimal preload by administering IV fluids or diuretics, as appropriate
- Prepare patient for cardiac revascularization (percutaneous coronary intervention or coronary artery bypass graft)
- Administer positive inotropic/contractility medications, as appropriate
- Promote afterload reduction (e.g., with vasodilators, angiotensin converting enzyme inhibitors, or intraaortic balloon pumping), as appropriate
- Promote optimal preload while minimizing afterload (e.g., administer nitrates while maintaining pulmonary artery occlusion pressure within prescribed range), as appropriate
- Promote adequate organ system perfusion (with fluid resuscitation and/or vasopressors to maintain mean arterial pressure ≥60 mm Hg, as appropriate

1st edition 1992; revised 2008

Background Readings:

Antman, E., Anbe, D., Armstrong, P., Bates, E., Green, L., Hand, M., et al. (2004). ACC/AHA guidelines for the management of patients with ST-elevation myocardial infarction – executive summary. *Circulation, 110*(5), 588–636.

Bridges, E. J. & Dukes, M. S. (2005). Cardiovascular aspects of septic shock: Pathophysiology, monitoring, and treatment. *Critical Care Nurse, 25*(2), 14–40.

Hollenberg, S. M., Ahrens, T. S., Annane, D., Astiz, M. E., Chalfin, D. B., Dasta, J. F., et al. (2004). Practice parameters for hemodynamic support of sepsis in adult patients: 2004 update. *Critical Care Medicine, 32*(9), 1928–1948.

Irwin, R. S. & Rippe, J. M. (Eds.). (2003). *Irwin and Rippe's intensive care medicine* (5th ed.). Philadelphia: Lippincott Williams & Wilkins.

McCance, K. L. & Huether, S. E. (2002). *Pathophysiology: The biologic basis for disease in adults and children* (4th ed.). St. Louis: Mosby.

S

Shock Management: Vasogenic   4256

Definition: Promotion of adequate tissue perfusion for a patient with severe loss of vascular tone

Activities:
- Monitor for physiologic changes related to loss of vascular tone (e.g., note decreased BP, bradycardia, tachypnea, reduced pulse pressure, anxiety, oliguria)
- Place patient in a supine position with legs elevated to increase preload, as appropriate
- Consider Trendelenburg position if head injury has been ruled out
- Administer high flow oxygen, as appropriate
- Administer epinephrine via SQ, IV, or ET routes for anaphylaxis, if appropriate
- Assist in early endotracheal intubation, as appropriate
- Monitor ECG
- Administer atropine for bradycardia, as appropriate
- Utilize transcutaneous pacing, as appropriate
- Monitor pneumatic antishock garment, as appropriate
- Maintain two large-bore intravascular access sites
- Administer isotonic crystalloids as bolus doses, keeping systolic pressure at 90 mmHg or more, as appropriate
- Administer antihistamine and/or corticosteroid, as appropriate
- Administer vasopressors
- Treat overdoses with appropriate reversal agent
- Insert NG tube and administer charcoal lavage, as appropriate
- Monitor body temperature
- Avoid hypothermia with warming blankets
- Treat hyperthermia with antipyretic drugs, a cooling mattress, or a sponge bath
- Prevent or control shivering with medication or by wrapping the extremities
- Monitor trends in hemodynamic parameters (e.g., CVP, MAP, PAWP, or PCWP wedge pressure)
- Administer antibiotics, as appropriate
- Administer antiinflammatory medications, as appropriate
- Avoid stimuli that will precipitate neurogenic reaction (e.g., skin stimulation, distended bladder, or constipation)
- Monitor coagulation studies, including prothrombin time (PT), partial thromboplastin time (PTT), fibrinogen, fibrin degradation/split products, and platelet counts, as appropriate

1st edition 1992; revised 2008

Background Readings:

Ahrens, T. & Tuggle, D. (2004). Surviving severe sepsis: Early recognition and treatment. *Critical Care Nurse*, (Oct. Suppl.), 2–15.

American Heart Association. (2005). 2005 American Heart Association guidelines for cardiopulmonary resuscitation and emergency cardiovascular care. *Circulation, 112*(24 Suppl.), IV1–IV203.

Bridges, E. J. & Dukes, S. (2005). Cardiovascular aspects of septic shock: pathophysiology, monitoring, and treatment. *Critical Care Nurse, 25*(2), 14–42.

Dellinger, R. P., Carlet, J. M., Masur, H., Gerlach, H., Calandra, T., Cohen, J., et al. (2004). Surviving sepsis campaign guidelines for management of severe sepsis and septic shock. *Critical Care Medicine, 32*(3), 858–873.

Flynn, M. B. & McLeskey, S. (2005). Shock, systemic inflammatory response syndrome, and multiple organ dysfunction syndrome. In P.G. Morton, D. K., Fontaine, C. M., Hudak, & B. M. Gallo (Eds.), *Critical care nursing*. Philadelphia: Lippincott Williams & Wilkins.

Hollenberg, S. M., Ahrens, T. S., Annane, D., Astiz, M. E., Chalfin, D. B., Dasta, J. F., et al. (2004). Practice parameters for hemodynamic support of sepsis in adult patients: 2004 update. *Critical Care Medicine, 32*(9), 1928–1948.

Smeltzer, S. C. & Bare, B. G. (2003). *Brunner & Suddarth's textbook of medical-surgical nursing* (10th ed.). Philadelphia: Lippincott Williams & Wilkins.

Shock Management: Volume   4258

Definition: Promotion of adequate tissue perfusion for a patient with severely compromised intravascular volume

Activities:
- Monitor for sudden loss of blood, severe dehydration, or persistent bleeding
- Check all secretions for frank or occult blood
- Prevent blood volume loss (e.g., apply pressure to site of bleeding)
- Monitor for fall in systolic blood pressure to less than 90 mmHg or a fall of 30 mmHg in hypertensive patients
- Monitor sublingual carbon dioxide levels
- Monitor for signs/symptoms of hypovolemic shock (e.g., increased thirst, increased HR, increased SVR, decreased urine output, decreased bowel sounds, decreased peripheral perfusion, altered mental status, or altered respirations)
- Position the patient for optimal perfusion
- Insert and maintain large-bore IV access
- Administer IV fluids such as isotonic crystalloids or colloids, as appropriate
- Administer warmed IV fluids and blood products, as indicated
- Administer oxygen and/or mechanical ventilation, as appropriate
- Draw arterial blood gases and monitor tissue oxygenation
- Monitor hemoglobin/hematocrit level
- Administer blood products (e.g., packed red blood cells, platelets, or fresh frozen plasma), as appropriate
- Monitor coagulation studies, including prothrombin time (PT), partial thromboplastin time (PTT), fibrinogen, fibrin degradation/split products, and platelet counts, as appropriate
- Monitor lab studies (e.g., serum lactate, acid-base balance, metabolic profiles, and electrolytes)

1st edition 1992; revised 2008

Background Readings:

American Heart Association. (2005). 2005 American Heart Association guidelines for cardiopulmonary resuscitation and emergency cardiovascular care. *Circulation, 112*(24 Suppl.), IV1–IV203.

S

Flynn, M. B. & McLeskey, S. (2005). Shock, systemic inflammatory response syndrome, and multiple organ dysfunction syndrome. In P.G. Morton, D. K. Fontaine, C. M. Hudak, & B. M. Gallo (Eds.), *Critical care nursing*. Philadelphia: Lippincott Williams & Wilkins.

Kuhlman, D. K. (Ed.). (2003). *Resuscitation: Fluid therapy. Congress Review: Cutting edge therapeutics*. 32nd Critical Care Congress 2003 in San Antonio, TX. Des Plaines, IL: Society of Critical Care Medicine.

Porth, C. M. (2004). *Essentials of pathophysiology: Concepts of altered health states*. Philadelphia: Lippincott Williams & Wilkins.

Smeltzer, S. C. & Bare, B. G. (2003). *Brunner & Suddarth's textbook of medical-surgical nursing* (10th ed.). Philadelphia: Lippincott Williams & Wilkins.

Shock Prevention | 4260

Definition: Detecting and treating a patient at risk for impending shock

Activities:

- Monitor for early compensatory shock responses (e.g., normal blood pressure, narrowed pulse pressure, mild orthostatic hypotension (15 to 25 mmHg), slight delayed capillary refill, pale/cool skin or flushed skin, slight tachypnea, nausea and vomiting, increased thirst, or weakness)
- Monitor for early signs of systemic inflammatory response syndrome (e.g., increased temperature, tachycardia, tachypnea, hypocarbia, leukocytosis, or leucopenia)
- Monitor for early signs of allergic reactions (e.g., rhinitis, wheezing, stridor, dyspnea, itching, hives and wheals, cutaneous angioedema, GI upset, abdominal pain, diarrhea, anxiety, and restlessness)
- Monitor for early signs of cardiac compromise (e.g., declining CO and urinary output, increasing SVR and PCWP, crackles in the lungs, S_3 and S_4 heart sounds, and tachycardia)
- Monitor possible sources of fluid loss (e.g., chest tube, wound, and nasogastric drainage; diarrhea; vomiting; and increasing abdominal and extremity girth, hematemesis, or hematochezia)
- Monitor circulatory status (e.g., blood pressure, skin color, skin temperature, heart sounds, heart rate and rhythm, presence and quality of peripheral pulses, and capillary refill)
- Monitor for signs of inadequate tissue oxygenation (e.g., apprehension, increased anxiety, changes in mental status, agitation, oliguria, and cool, mottled periphery)
- Monitor pulse oximetry
- Monitor temperature and respiratory status
- Monitor ECG
- Monitor daily weights, intake, and output
- Monitor laboratory values, especially Hgb and Hct levels, clotting profile, ABG, lactate level, electrolyte levels, cultures, and chemistry profile
- Monitor invasive hemodynamic parameters (e.g., CVP, MAP, and central/mixed venous oxygen saturation), as appropriate
- Monitor sublingual CO_2 or gastric tonometry, as appropriate
- Note bruising, petechiae, and condition of mucous membranes
- Note color, amount, and frequency of stools, vomitus, and nasogastric drainage
- Test urine for blood and protein, as appropriate
- Monitor for signs/symptoms of ascites and abdominal or back pain
- Place patient in supine, legs elevated position (volume, vasogenic) or supine, head and shoulders elevated (cardiogenic), as appropriate
- Institute and maintain airway patency, as appropriate
- Administer IV and/or oral fluids, as appropriate
- Insert and maintain large-bore IV access, as appropriate
- Administer IV fluid challenge while monitoring hemodynamic pressures and urinary output, as appropriate
- Administer antiarrhythmics, diuretics, and/or vasopressors, as appropriate
- Administer packed red blood cells, fresh frozen plasma and/or platelets, as appropriate
- Initiate early administration of antimicrobial agents and closely monitor their effectiveness, as appropriate
- Administer oxygen and/or mechanical ventilation, as appropriate
- Administer antiinflammatory agents and/or bronchodilators, as appropriate
- Monitor blood glucose and administer insulin therapy, as appropriate
- Administer, IV, intraosseous, or endotracheal epinephrine, as appropriate
- Teach patient to avoid known allergens and how to use an anaphylaxis kit, as appropriate
- Perform skin testing to determine agents causing anaphylaxis and/or allergic reactions, as appropriate
- Advise patients at risk for severe allergic reactions to undergo desensitization therapy
- Advise patients at risk to wear or carry medical alert information
- Instruct patient and/or family on precipitating factors of shock
- Instruct patient and family about signs/symptoms of impending shock
- Instruct patient and family about steps to take with onset of shock symptoms

1st edition 1992; revised 2008

Background Readings:

Ahrens, T. & Tuggle, D. (2004). Surviving severe sepsis: Early recognition and treatment. *Critical Care Nurse*, (Oct. Suppl.), 2–15.

American Heart Association. (2005). *2005 American Heart Association guidelines for cardiopulmonary resuscitation and emergency cardiovascular care. Circulation, 112*(24 Suppl.), IV1–IV203.

Flynn, M. B. & McLeskey, S. (2005). Shock, systemic inflammatory response syndrome, and multiple organ dysfunction syndrome. In P. G. Morton, D. K. Fontaine, C. M. Hudak, & B. M. Gallo (Eds.), *Critical care nursing*. Philadelphia: Lippincott Williams & Wilkins.

Porth, C. M. (2004). *Essentials of pathophysiology: Concepts of altered health states*. Philadelphia: Lippincott Williams & Wilkins.

Smeltzer, S. C. & Bare, B. G. (2003). *Brunner & Suddarth's textbook of medical-surgical nursing* (10th ed.). Philadelphia: Lippincott Williams & Wilkins.

S

Sibling Support   7280

Definition: Assisting a sibling to cope with a brother or sister's illness/chronic condition/disability

Activities:

- Explore what sibling knows about brother or sister
- Appraise stress in sibling related to condition of affected brother or sister
- Appraise sibling's coping with illness/disability of brother or sister
- Facilitate family members' awareness of sibling's feelings
- Provide information about common sibling responses and what other family members can do to help
- Perform sibling advocacy role (e.g., in case of life-threatening situations when anxiety is high and parents or other family members are unable to perform that role)
- Recognize that each sibling responds differently
- Encourage parents or other family members to provide honest information to sibling
- Encourage parents to arrange for care of young sibling in their own home, if possible
- Assist sibling to maintain and/or modify usual routines and activities of daily living, as necessary
- Promote communication between well sibling and affected brother or sister
- Value each child individually, avoiding comparisons
- Help child to see differences/similarities between self and sibling with special needs
- Encourage sibling to visit affected brother or sister
- Explain to visiting sibling what is being done in care of affected brother or sister
- Encourage well sibling to participate in care of the affected brother or sister, as appropriate
- Teach well sibling ways to interact with affected sister/brother
- Permit siblings to settle own difficulties
- Recognize and respect sibling who may not be emotionally ready to visit an affected brother or sister
- Respect well sibling's reluctance to be with or to include child with special needs in activities
- Encourage maintenance of parental or family interactional patterns
- Assist parents to be fair in terms of discipline, resources, and attention
- Assist sibling to clarify and explore concerns
- Use drawings, puppetry, and dramatic play to see how younger sibling perceives events
- Clarify sibling concern for contracting the illness of the affected child, and develop strategies for coping with concern
- Teach pathology of disease to sibling, according to developmental stage and learning style
- Use concrete substitutes for sibling who is unable to visit affected brother or sister (e.g., pictures and videos)
- Explain to young siblings that they are not the cause of illness
- Teach sibling strategies for meeting own emotional and developmental needs
- Praise siblings when they have been patient, have sacrificed, or have been particularly helpful
- Acknowledge the personal strengths siblings have and their abilities to cope with stress successfully
- Provide referral to peer sibling group, as appropriate
- Provide community resource referrals to sibling, as necessary
- Communicate situation to the school nurse to promote support for younger sibling, in accord with parental wishes

1st edition 1992; revised 2000

Background Readings:

Craft, M. J. & Craft, J. (1989). Perceived changes in siblings of hospitalized children: A comparison of parent and sibling report. *Children's' Health Care, 18*(1), 42–49.

Craft, M. J. & Denehy, J. A. (Eds.). (1990). *Nursing interventions for infants and children.* Philadelphia: W. B. Saunders.

Craft, M. J. & Willadsen, J. A. (1992). Interventions related to family. In G. M. Bulechek & J. C. McCloskey (Eds.), Symposium on nursing interventions. *Nursing Clinics of North America, 27*(2), 517–540.

Pillitteri, A. (2007). Nursing care of the family coping with a child's long-term or terminal illness. In *Maternal and child health nursing: Care of the childbearing and childrearing family* (5th ed., pp. 1764–1783). Philadelphia: Lippincott Williams & Wilkins.

Ross-Alaolmolki, K. (1990). Coping with family loss: The death of a sibling. In M. J. Craft & J. A. Denehy (Eds.), *Nursing interventions for infants and children* (pp. 213–277). Philadelphia: W. B. Saunders.

S

Skin Care: Donor Site   3582

Definition: Prevention of wound complications and promotion of healing at the donor site

Activities:

- Verify that a complete history and physical have been obtained prior to skin graft surgery
- Provide adequate pain control (e.g., medication, music therapy, distraction, massage)
- Incorporate moist wound healing techniques for skin autografts
- Cover donor site for skin autografts postoperatively with an alginate and a transparent, semiocclusive dressing, as per agency protocol
- Inspect the dressing daily, as per agency protocol
- Monitor for signs of infection (e.g., fever, pain) and other postoperative complications
- Keep skin donor site clean, dry, and free from pressure
- Instruct individual to keep healed skin donor site soft and pliable with cream (e.g., lanolin, olive oil)
- Instruct individual to avoid exposing skin donor site to extremes in temperature, external trauma, and sunlight

4th edition 2004

Background Readings:

Mendez-Eastman, S. K. (2001). Skin grafting: Preoperative, intraoperative, and postoperative care. *Plastic Surgical Nursing, 21*(1), 49–51.

Smeltzer, S. C. & Bare, B. G. (1996). *Brunner & Suddarth's textbook of medical-surgical nursing* (Vol. I and II) (8th ed., pp. 805, 1535–1536, 1567). Philadelphia: J. B. Lippincott.

Skin Care: Graft Site   3583

Definition: Prevention of wound complications and promotion of graft site healing

Activities:

- Verify that a complete history and physical have been obtained prior to skin graft surgery
- Apply dressings made of cotton or gauze to maintain adequate tension on the graft site, as per agency protocol
- Provide adequate pain control (e.g., medication, music therapy, distraction, massage)
- Elevate graft site until graft-host circulation develops (approximately 1 week), then allow the graft site to be in a dependent position for progressively longer periods of time, per agency protocol
- Utilize needle aspiration to evacuate fluids from beneath the graft in order to maintain close contact between the recipient bed and the graft during the postoperative revascularization period
- Avoid "rolling" the blebs of fluid to the edge of the graft during the postoperative revascularization period
- Avoid friction and shearing forces at new graft site
- Limit patient activity to bed rest until graft adheres
- Instruct the patient to keep the affected part immobilized as much as possible during healing
- Inspect the dressing daily, as per agency protocol
- Monitor color, warmth, capillary refill, and turgor of graft, if not dressed
- Monitor for signs of infection (e.g., fever, pain) and other postoperative complications
- Incorporate aggressive efforts to prevent development of pneumonia, pulmonary emboli, and pressure ulcers during period of immobility
- Provide emotional support, understanding, and consideration to patient and family members in times when graft does not take
- Support patient to appropriately ventilate anger, hostility, and frustration if graft does not take
- Instruct patient on methods to protect the graft area from mechanical and thermal assaults (e.g., exposure to sun, use of heating pads)
- Instruct patient to utilize compression stockings, pads, or straps to protect the graft site
- Instruct patients to regularly apply artificial lubrication to graft site, as necessary
- Instruct patient that protection of graft site may be necessary for years following the graft
- Instruct patient that smoking decreases blood supply to the graft-recipient bed interface and increases chances of graft failure, and thus should be avoided

4th edition 2004

Background Readings:

Donato, M. C., Novicki, D. C., & Blume, P. A. (2000). Skin grafting: Historic and practical approaches. *Clinics in Podiatric Medicine and Surgery, 17*(4), 561–598.

Lewis, S. M., Heitkemper, M. M., & Dirksen, S. R. (2000). *Medical-surgical nursing: Assessment and management of clinical problems* (5th ed., pp. 515–516, 543–544). St. Louis: Mosby.

Mendez-Eastman, S. K. (2001). Skin grafting: Preoperative, intraoperative, and postoperative care. *Plastic Surgical Nursing, 21*(1), 49–51.

Smeltzer, S. C. & Bare, B. G. (1996). *Brunner & Suddarth's textbook of medical-surgical nursing* (8th ed., pp. 1534–1536, 1567). Philadelphia: J. B. Lippincott.

Waymack, P., Duff, R. G., & Sabolinski, M. (2000). The effect of a tissue engineered bilayered living skin analog, over meshed split-thickness autografts on the healing of excised burn wounds. *Burns, 26*(7), 609–619.

White, L. & Duncan, G. (2002). *Medical-surgical nursing: An integrated approach* (2nd ed., p. 522). Albany, NY: Delmar.

Skin Care: Topical Treatments   3584

Definition: Application of topical substances or manipulation of devices to promote skin integrity and minimize skin breakdown

Activities:

- Avoid using rough-textured bed linens
- Clean with antibacterial soap, as appropriate
- Dress patient in nonrestrictive clothing
- Dust the skin with medicated powder, as appropriate
- Remove adhesive tape and debris
- Provide support to edematous areas (e.g., pillow under arms and scrotal support), as appropriate
- Apply lubricant to moisten lips and oral mucosa, as needed
- Administer back rub/neck rub, as appropriate
- Change condom catheter, as appropriate
- Apply diapers loosely, as appropriate
- Place on incontinence pads, as appropriate
- Massage around the affected area
- Apply appropriately fitting ostomy appliance, as needed
- Cover the hands with mittens, as appropriate
- Provide toilet hygiene, as needed
- Refrain from giving local heat applications
- Refrain from using an alkaline soap on the skin
- Soak in a colloidal bath, as appropriate
- Keep bed linen clean, dry, and wrinkle free
- Turn the immobilized patient at least every 2 hours, according to a specific schedule
- Use devices on the bed (e.g., sheepskin) that protect the patient
- Apply heel protectors, as appropriate
- Apply drying powders to deep skinfolds
- Initiate consultation services of the enterostomal therapy nurse, as needed

- Apply clear occlusive dressing (e.g., Tegaderm or Duoderm), as needed
- Apply topical antibiotic to the affected area, as appropriate
- Apply topical antiinflammatory agent to the affected area, as appropriate
- Apply emollients to the affected area
- Apply topical antifungal agent to the affected area, as appropriate
- Apply topical debriding agent to the affected area, as appropriate
- Paint or spray skin warts with liquid nitrogen, as appropriate
- Inspect skin daily for those at risk of breakdown
- Document degree of skin breakdown
- Add moisture to environment with a humidifier, as needed

1st edition 1992; revised 1996, 2000

Background Readings:

Frantz, R. A. & Gardner, S. (1994). Management of dry skin. *Journal of Gerontological Nursing, 20*(9), 15–18.

Hardy, M. A., (1992). Dry skin care. In G. M. Bulechek & J. C. McCloskey (Eds.), *Nursing interventions: Essential nursing treatments* (2nd ed., pp. 34–47). Philadelphia: W. B. Saunders.

Kemp, M. G. (1994). Protecting the skin from moisture and associated irritants. *Journal of Gerontological Nursing, 20*(9), 8–14.

Kozier, B., Erb, G., Berman, A., & Snyder, S. (2004). Skin integrity and wound care. In *Fundamentals of nursing: Concepts, processes, and practice* (7th ed., pp. 855–895). Upper Saddle River, NJ: Prentice Hall.

Titler, M. G., Pettit, D., Bulechek, G. M., McCloskey, J. C., Craft, M. J., Cohen, M. Z., et al. (1991). Classification of nursing interventions for care of the integument. *Nursing Diagnosis, 2*(2), 45–56.

Skin Surveillance   3590

Definition: Collection and analysis of patient data to maintain skin and mucous membrane integrity

Activities:

- Inspect skin and mucous membranes for redness, extreme warmth, edema, or drainage
- Observe extremities for color, warmth, swelling, pulses, texture, edema, and ulcerations
- Inspect condition of surgical incision, as appropriate
- Use an assessment tool to identify patients at risk for skin breakdown (e.g., Braden Scale)
- Monitor skin color and temperature
- Monitor skin and mucous membranes for areas of discoloration, bruising, and breakdown
- Monitor skin for rashes and abrasions
- Monitor skin for excessive dryness and moistness
- Monitor for sources of pressure and friction
- Monitor for infection, especially of edematous areas
- Inspect clothing for tightness
- Document skin or mucous membrane changes
- Institute measures to prevent further deterioration (e.g., overlay mattress, repositioning schedule)
- Instruct family member/caregiver about signs of skin breakdown, as appropriate

1st edition 1992; revised 2008

Background Readings:

McCance, K. L. & Huether, S. E. (2006). *Pathophysiology: The biologic basis for disease in adults and children* (5th ed.). St. Louis: Mosby.

Perry, A. G. & Potter, P. A. (2006). *Clinical nursing skills and techniques* (6th ed.). St. Louis: Mosby.

Potter, P. A. & Perry, A. G. (2005). *Fundamentals of nursing* (6th ed.). St. Louis: Mosby.

Taylor, C., Lillis, C., & LeMone, P. (2007). *Fundamentals of nursing: The art and science of nursing care.* Philadelphia: Lippincott Williams and Wilkins.

Titler, M. G., Pettit, D., Bulechek, G. M., McCloskey, J. C., Craft, M. J., Cohen, M. Z., et al (1991). Classification of nursing interventions for care of the integument. *Nursing Diagnosis, 2*(2), 45–56.

Urden, L. D., Stacy, K. M., & Lough, M. E. (2006). *Thelan's critical care nursing: Diagnosis and management* (5th ed.). St. Louis: Mosby.

S

Sleep Enhancement   1850

Definition: Facilitation of regular sleep/wake cycles

Activities:

- Determine patient's sleep/activity pattern
- Approximate patient's regular sleep/wake cycle in planning care
- Explain the importance of adequate sleep during pregnancy, illness, psychosocial stresses, etc.
- Determine the effects of the patient's medications on sleep pattern
- Monitor/record patient's sleep pattern and number of sleep hours
- Monitor patient's sleep pattern, and note physical (e.g., sleep apnea, obstructed airway, pain/discomfort, and urinary frequency) and/or psychological (e.g., fear or anxiety) circumstances that interrupt sleep

- Instruct patient to monitor sleep patterns
- Monitor participation in fatigue-producing activities during wakefulness to prevent overtiredness
- Adjust environment (e.g., light, noise, temperature, mattress, and bed) to promote sleep
- Encourage patient to establish a bedtime routine to facilitate transition from wakefulness to sleep
- Facilitate maintenance of patient's usual bedtime routines, presleep cues/props, and familiar objects (e.g., for children, a favorite blanket/toy, rocking, pacifier, or story; for adults, a book to read, etc.), as appropriate

- Assist to eliminate stressful situations before bedtime
- Monitor bedtime food and beverage intake for items that facilitate or interfere with sleep
- Instruct patient to avoid bedtime foods and beverages that interfere with sleep
- Assist patient to limit daytime sleep by providing activity that promotes wakefulness, as appropriate
- Instruct patient how to perform autogenic muscle relaxation or other nonpharmacological forms of sleep inducement
- Initiate/implement comfort measures of massage, positioning, and affective touch
- Promote an increase in number of hours of sleep, if needed
- Provide for naps during the day, if indicated, to meet sleep requirements
- Group care activities to minimize number of awakenings; allow for sleep cycles of at least 90 minutes
- Adjust medication administration schedule to support patient's sleep/wake cycle
- Instruct the patient and significant others about factors (e.g., physiological, psychological, lifestyle, frequent work shift changes, rapid time zone changes, excessively long work hours, and other environmental factors) that contribute to sleep pattern disturbances
- Identify what sleep medications patient is taking
- Encourage use of sleep medications that do not contain REM sleep suppressor(s)

- Regulate environmental stimuli to maintain normal day-night cycles
- Discuss with patient and family sleep-enhancing techniques
- Provide pamphlet with information about sleep-enhancement techniques

1st edition 1992; revised 2004

Background Readings:

Craven, R. F. & Hirnle, C. J. (2003). Sleep and rest. In *Fundamentals of nursing: Human health and function* (4th ed., pp. 1143–1163). Philadelphia: Lippincott Williams & Wilkins.
Glick, O. J. (1992). Interventions related to activity and movement. In G. M. Bulechek & J. C. McCloskey (Eds.), Symposium on nursing interventions. *Nursing Clinics of North America*, 27(2), 541–554.
Guyton, A. (1991). *Textbook of medical physiology* (8th ed.). Philadelphia: W. B. Saunders.
Institute of Medicine. (2006). *Sleep disorders and sleep deprivation*. Washington, DC: National Academies Press.
McFarland, G. K. & McFarlane, E. A. (1997). *Nursing diagnosis and intervention* (3rd ed.). St. Louis: Mosby.
Prinz, P. N., Vitiello, M. V., Raskind, M. A., & Thorpy, M. J. (1990). Geriatrics: Sleep disorders and aging. *New England Journal of Medicine*, 322(8), 520–526.

Smoking Cessation Assistance   4490

Definition: Helping another to stop smoking

Activities:
- Record current smoking status and smoking history
- Determine patient's readiness to learn about smoking cessation
- Monitor patient's readiness to attempt to quit smoking
- Give clear, consistent advice to quit smoking
- Help patient identify reasons to quit and barriers to quitting
- Instruct patient on the physical symptoms of nicotine withdrawal (e.g., headache, dizziness, nausea, irritability, and insomnia)
- Reassure patient that physical withdrawal symptoms from nicotine are temporary
- Inform patient about nicotine replacement products (e.g., patch, gum, nasal spray, inhaler) to help reduce physical withdrawal symptoms
- Assist patient to identify psychosocial aspects (e.g., positive and negative feelings associated with smoking) that influence smoking behavior
- Assist patient in developing a smoking cessation plan that addresses psychosocial aspects that influence smoking behavior
- Assist patient to recognize cues that prompt him/her to smoke (e.g., being around others who smoke, frequenting places where smoking is allowed)
- Assist patient to develop practical methods to resist cravings (e.g., spend time with nonsmoking friends, frequent places where smoking is not allowed, relaxation exercises)
- Help choose best method for giving up cigarettes, when patient is ready to quit
- Help motivated patients to set a quit date
- Provide encouragement to maintain a smoke-free lifestyle (e.g., make the quit day a celebration day; encourage self-rewards at

specific intervals of smoke-free living, such as at 1 week, 1 month, 6 months; encourage saving money used previously on smoking materials to buy a special reward)
- Encourage patient to join a smoking cessation support group that meets weekly
- Refer to group programs or individual therapists, as appropriate
- Assist patient with any self-help methods
- Help patient plan specific coping strategies and resolve problems that result from quitting
- Advise to avoid dieting while trying to give up smoking because it can undermine chances of quitting
- Advise to work out a plan to cope with others who smoke and to avoid being around them
- Inform patient that dry mouth, cough, scratchy throat, and feeling on edge are symptoms that may occur after quitting; the patch or gum may help with cravings
- Advise to keep a list of "slips" or near slips, what causes them, and what patient learned from them
- Advise to avoid smokeless tobacco, dipping, and chewing as these can lead to addiction and/or health problems including oral cancer, gum problems, loss of teeth, and heart problems
- Manage nicotine replacement therapy
- Contact national and local resource organizations for resource materials
- Follow patient for 2 years after quitting if possible, to provide encouragement
- Arrange to maintain frequent telephone contact with patient (e.g., to acknowledge that withdrawal is difficult, to reinforce the importance of remaining abstinent, to offer congratulations on progress)

- Help patient deal with any lapses (e.g., reassure patient that he or she is not a "failure," reassure that much can be learned from this temporary regression; and assist patient in identifying reasons for the relapse)
- Support patient who begins smoking again by helping to identify what has been learned
- Encourage the relapsed patient to try again
- Promote policies that establish and enforce smoke-free environment
- Serve as a nonsmoking role model

1st edition 1992; revised 2000, 2004

Background Readings:

Lenaghan, N. A. (2000). The nurse's role in smoking cessation. *MEDSURG Nursing, 9*(6), 298–312.

O'Connell, K. A. (1990). Smoking cessation: Research on relapse crises. In J. J. Fitzpatrick, R. L. Taunton, & J. Z. Benoliel (Eds.), *Annual review of nursing research* (Vol. 8) (pp. 83–100). New York: Springer.
O'Connell, K. A. & Koerin, C. A. (1999). Smoking cessation assistance. In G. M. Bulechek & J. C. McCloskey (Eds.), *Nursing interventions: Effective nursing treatments* (3rd ed., pp. 438–450). Philadelphia: W. B. Saunders.
U.S. Department of Health and Human Services. (1997). *Smoking cessation: Clinical practice guideline No. 18.* Rockville, MD: Agency for Health Care Policy & Research.
Wewers, M. E. & Ahijeoych, K. L. (1996). Smoking cessation interventions in chronic illness. In J. J. Fitzpatrick & J. Norbeck. (Eds.), *Annual review of nursing research* (Vol. 14) (pp. 75–93). New York: Springer.

Social Marketing   8750

Definition: Use of marketing principles to influence the health beliefs, attitudes, and behaviors to benefit a target population

Activities:
- Maintain focus on the target audience through all activities
- Cultivate partnerships with the target audience and appropriate professionals
- Identify the overall goal to be achieved in collaboration with the target audience
- Identify the key formal, social, and governmental groups involved
- Conduct a needs assessment of the environment, identifying target audience desires
- Conduct organization or group assessment
- Identify appropriate quantitative and qualitative research to provide information, support, and indicators of success
- Design a plan of action based on mutually agreed-upon goals
- Nurture the voluntary basis of the planned social change
- Identify the product (behavior change), the price (consumer's actions), and the place (how the product reaches the consumer)
- Consider the financial resources necessary and available
- Identify specific activities for each goal, including naming of appropriate participants
- Implement the plan in collaboration with the target population
- Control the plan through monitoring of assigned tasks
- Provide appropriate reports on a timely basis
- Evaluate the plan for achievement of goals with consideration of sustainability and affordability
- Modify the plan as needed

5th edition 2008

Background Readings:

Brown, K. M., Bryant, C., Forthofer, M., Perrin, K., Quinn, G., Wolper, M., et al. (2000). Florida cares for women: Social marketing campaign a case study. *American Journal of Health Behavior, 24*(1), 44–52.
Grier, S. & Bryant, C. (2005). Social marketing in public health. *Annual Review of Public Health, 26,* 319–339.
Kotler, P. & Roberto, E. (1989). *Social marketing: Strategies for changing public behavior.* New York: The Free Press.
Pirani, S. & Reizes, R. (2005). The turning point social marketing national excellent collaborative: Integrating social marketing into routine public health practice. *Journal of Public Health Management Practice, 11*(2), 131–138
Smith, W. (2002). Social marketing: An evolving definition. *American Journal of Health Behavior, 24*(1), 11–17.
Szydlowski, S., Chattopadhyay, S., & Babela, R. (2005). Social marketing as a tool to improve behavioral health services for underserved populations in transition. *The Health Care Manager, 24*(1), 12–20.

S

Socialization Enhancement   5100

Definition: Facilitation of another person's ability to interact with others

Activities:
- Encourage enhanced involvement in already established relationships
- Encourage patience in developing relationships
- Promote relationships with persons who have common interests and goals
- Encourage social and community activities
- Promote sharing of common problems with others
- Encourage honesty in presenting oneself to others
- Promote involvement in totally new interests
- Encourage respect for the rights of others
- Facilitate the use of sensory deficit aids such as eyeglasses and hearing aids
- Encourage participation in group and/or individual reminiscence activities
- Facilitate patient participation in storytelling groups

- Refer patient to interpersonal skills group or program in which understanding of transactions can be increased, as appropriate
- Allow testing of interpersonal limits
- Give feedback about improvement in care of personal appearance or other activities
- Help patient increase awareness of strengths and limitations in communicating with others
- Use role playing to practice improved communication skills and techniques
- Provide role models who express anger appropriately
- Confront patient about impaired judgment, when appropriate
- Request and expect verbal communication
- Give positive feedback when patient reaches out to others
- Encourage patient to change environment, such as going outside for walks or to movies
- Facilitate patient input and planning of future activities
- Encourage small group planning for special activities
- Explore strengths and weaknesses of current network of relationships

1st edition 1992; revised 2000, 2004, 2008

Background Readings:

Frisch, N. (2006). Group therapy. In N. Frisch & L. Frisch (Eds.), *Psychiatric mental health nursing* (pp. 756–769). Albany, NY: Delmar.

Hawkins, J., Kosterman, R., Catalano, R., Hill, K., & Abbott, R. (2005). Promoting positive adult functioning through social development intervention in childhood. *Archives of Pediatric and Adolescent Medicine, 159*(1), 25–32.

Kopelowicz, A. & Liberman, R. (2003). Integrating treatment with rehabilitation for persons with major mental illnesses. *Psychiatric Services, 54*(11), 1491–1498.

Resnick, B. & Fleishell, A. (2002). Developing a restorative care program. *American Journal of Nursing, 102*(7), 91–95.

Swanson, E. & Drury, J. (2001). Sensory/perceptual alterations. In M. Maas, K. Buckwalter, M. Hardy, T. Tripp-Reimer, M. Titler, & J. Specht (Eds.), *Nursing care of older adults: Diagnoses, outcomes, and interventions* (pp. 476–491). St. Louis: Mosby.

Varcarolis, E. (2006). Mood disorders/depression. In E. Varcarolis, V. Carson, & N. Shoemaker (Eds.), *Foundations of psychiatric/mental health nursing: A clinical approach* (pp. 326–358). Philadelphia: Saunders Elsevier.

Waterman, J., Blegen, M., Clinton, P., & Specht, J. (2001). Social isolation. In M. Maas, K. Buckwalter, M. Hardy, T. Tripp-Reimer, M. Titler, & J. Specht (Eds.), *Nursing care of older adults: Diagnoses, outcomes, and interventions* (pp. 651–663). St. Louis: Mosby.

Weiss, S. (2004). Children. In C. Kneisl, H. Wilson, & E. Trigoboff (Eds.), *Contemporary psychiatric-mental health nursing* (pp. 589–614). Upper Saddle River, NJ: Prentice Hall.

Specimen Management 7820

Definition: Obtaining, preparing, and preserving a specimen for a laboratory test

Activities:

- Obtain required sample, according to protocol
- Instruct patient how to collect and preserve specimen, as appropriate
- Provide specimen container required
- Apply special specimen collection devices, as needed, for infants, toddlers, or impaired adults
- Assist with the biopsy of a tissue or organ, as appropriate
- Assist with aspiration of fluid from a body cavity, as appropriate
- Store specimen collected over time, according to protocol
- Seal all specimen containers to prevent leakage or contamination
- Label specimen with appropriate data prior to leaving the patient
- Place specimen in appropriate container for transport
- Arrange transport of the specimen to the laboratory
- Order specimen-related routine laboratory tests, as appropriate

1st edition 1992; revised 2008

Background Readings:

Perry, A. G. & Potter, P. A. (2006). *Clinical nursing skills and techniques* (6th ed.). St. Louis: Mosby.

Potter, A. G. & Perry, P. A. (2005). *Fundamentals of nursing* (6th ed.). St. Louis: Mosby.

Taylor, C., Lillis, C., & LeMone, P. (2007). *Fundamentals of nursing: The art and science of nursing care*. Philadelphia: Lippincott Williams and Wilkins.

Spiritual Growth Facilitation 5426

Definition: Facilitation of growth in patient's capacity to identify, connect with, and call upon the source of meaning, purpose, comfort, strength, and hope in their lives

Activities:

- Demonstrate caring presence and comfort by spending time with patient, patient's family, and significant others
- Encourage conversation that assists the patient in sorting out spiritual concerns
- Model healthy relating and reasoning skills
- Assist patient with identifying barriers and attitudes that hinder growth or self-discovery
- Offer individual and group prayer support, as appropriate
- Encourage participation in devotional services, retreats, and special prayer/study programs
- Promote relationships with others for fellowship and service

- Encourage use of spiritual celebration and rituals
- Encourage patient's examination of his/her spiritual commitment based on beliefs and values
- Provide an environment that fosters a meditative/contemplative attitude for self-reflection
- Assist the patient to explore beliefs as related to healing of body, mind, and spirit
- Refer to support groups, mutual self-help, or other spiritually based programs, as appropriate
- Refer for pastoral care or primary spiritual caregiver as issues warrant
- Refer for additional guidance and support in the body, mind, and spirit connection, as needed

3rd edition 2000

Background Readings:

Carson, V. B. (1993). Spirituality: Generic or Christian. *Journal of Christian Nursing, 10*(1), 24–27.

Craven, R. F. & Hirnle, C. J. (2003). Spiritual health. In *Fundamentals of nursing: Human health and function* (4th ed., pp. 1381–1403). Philadelphia: Lippincott Williams & Wilkins.

Hawks, S., Hull, M., Thalman, R., & Ridhins, P. M. (1995). Review of spiritual health: Definition, role, & intervention strategies in health promotion. *American Journal of Health Promotion, 9*(5), 371–377.

Oldnall, A. (1996). A critical analysis of nursing: Meeting the spiritual needs of patients. *Journal of Advanced Nursing, 23*(1), 138–144.

Reed, P. G. (1991). Preferences for spiritually related nursing interventions among terminally ill and nonterminally ill hospitalized adults and well adults. *Applied Nursing Research, 4*(3), 122–128.

Reed, P. G. (1992). An emerging paradigm for the investigation of spirituality in nursing. *Research in Nursing & Health, 15*(5), 349–357.

Schnorr, M. A. (1990). Spiritual caregiving: A key component of parish nursing. In P. A. Solari-Twadell, A. M. Djupe, & M. A. McDermott (Eds.), *Parish nursing: The developing practice.* Park Ridge, IL: National Parish Nurse Resource Center.

Spiritual Support 5420

Definition: Assisting the patient to feel balance and connection with a greater power

Activities:

- Use therapeutic communications to establish trust and empathetic caring
- Utilize tools to monitor and evaluate spiritual well-being, as appropriate
- Encourage individual to review past life and focus on events and relationships that provided spiritual strength and support
- Treat individual with dignity and respect
- Encourage life review through reminiscence
- Encourage participation in interactions with family members, friends, and others
- Provide privacy and quiet times for spiritual activities
- Encourage participation in support groups
- Teach methods of relaxation, meditation, and guided imagery
- Share own beliefs about meaning and purpose, as appropriate
- Share own spiritual perspective, as appropriate
- Provide opportunities for discussion of various belief systems and world views
- Be open to individual's expressions of concern
- Arrange visits by individual's spiritual advisor
- Pray with the individual
- Provide spiritual music, literature, or radio or television programs to the individual
- Be open to individual's expressions of loneliness and powerlessness
- Encourage chapel service attendance, if desired
- Encourage the use of spiritual resources, if desired
- Provide desired spiritual articles, according to individual preferences
- Refer to spiritual advisor of individual's choice
- Use values clarification techniques to help individual clarify beliefs and values, as appropriate
- Be available to listen to individual's feelings
- Express empathy with individual's feelings
- Facilitate individual's use of meditation, prayer, and other religious traditions and rituals
- Listen carefully to individual's communication, and develop a sense of timing for prayer or spiritual rituals
- Assure individual that nurse will be available to support individual in times of suffering
- Be open to individual's feelings about illness and death
- Assist individual to properly express and relieve anger in appropriate ways

1st edition 1992; revised 2004

Background Readings:

Dossey, B. M. (1998). Attending to holistic care. *American Journal of Nursing, 98*(8), 35–38.

Harvey, S. A. (2001). S.C.A.L.E. - Spiritual care at life's end: A multi-disciplinary approach to end-of-life issues in a hospital setting. *Medical Reference Services Quarterly, 20*(4), 63–71.

Hermann, C. P. (2001). Spiritual needs of dying patients: A qualitative study. *Oncology Nursing Forum, 28*(1), 67–72.

LeMone, P. (2001). Spiritual distress. In M. L. Maas, K. C. Buckwalter, M. D. Hardy, T. Tripp-Reimer, M. G. Titler, & J. P. Specht (Eds.), *Nursing care of older adults: Diagnoses, outcomes, and interventions* (pp. 782–793). St. Louis: Mosby.

Maddox, M. (2002). Spiritual assessments in primary care. *The Nurse Practitioner, 27*(2), 12, 14.

Meraviglia, M. G. (1999). Critical analysis of spirituality and its empirical indicators: Prayer and meaning in life. *Journal of Holistic Nursing, 17*(1), 18–33.

Sumner, C. H. (1998). Recognizing and responding. *American Journal of Nursing, 98*(1), 26–30.

Vandenbrink, R. A. (2001). Spiritual assessment: Comparing the tools. *Journal of Christian Nursing, 18*(3), 24–27.

Van Dover, L. J. & Bacon, J. M. (2001). Spiritual care in nursing practice: A close-up view. *Nursing Forum, 36*(3), 18–30.

S

Splinting 0910

Definition: Stabilization, immobilization, and protection of an injured body part with a supportive appliance

Activities:
- Monitor circulation (e.g., pulse, capillary refill, and sensation) in injured body part
- Monitor movement distal to injury site
- Monitor for bleeding at injury site
- Cover open wound with dressing and control bleeding prior to applying splint
- Minimize movement of patient, especially injured body part
- Identify most appropriate splint material (e.g., rigid, soft, anatomical, or traction)
- Pad rigid splints
- Immobilize joint above and joint below injury site
- Support feet using a footboard
- Place injured hand or wrist in position of function
- Apply splint in position injured body part is found, using hands to support injury site, minimizing movement, and using the assistance of another health care team member when possible
- Apply a sling, as appropriate
- Monitor skin integrity under supportive appliance
- Encourage isometric exercises, as appropriate
- Instruct patient or family on how to care for the splint

1st edition 1992; revised 2013

Background Readings:

Pfeiffer, R. P., Thygerson, A., & Palmieri, N. F. (2009). *Sports first aid and injury prevention* [B.Gulli & E. W. Ossman, Medical Eds.]. Sudbury, MA: Jones and Bartlett.

Schottke, D. (2007). Injuries to muscles and bones. In A. N. Pollack (Ed.), *First responder: Your first response in emergency care* (4th ed., pp. 327–367). Sudbury, MA: Jones and Bartlett.

Thygerson, A. (2005). Splinting extremities. In American Academy of Orthopaedic Surgeons, *First aid, CPR, and AED* (4th ed., pp. 239–254). Sudbury, MA: Jones and Bartlett.

Sports-Injury Prevention: Youth 6648

Definition: Reduce the risk of sports-related injury in young athletes

Activities:
- Encourage general fitness as prerequisite to sport participation
- Encourage modification of game rules according to age and ability of participants
- Inform parents of the differences between recreational and organized competitive sports
- Assist athlete in finding a sport that is a good fit with interests and abilities and will promote the development of lifelong fitness behaviors
- Assist parents and athletes to set realistic goals for participation
- Provide resources for parents, athletes, and coaches concerning the psychosocial aspects of sports involvement
- Encourage appropriate matching of competitors by age, weight, and stage of physical maturation
- Monitor adherence to recommended training guidelines and correct biomechanics
- Monitor compliance with safety rules
- Monitor field of play for safe playing conditions
- Monitor proper use and condition of safety equipment
- Encourage appropriate supervision for training, recreation, and competitive events
- Monitor sports physicals to insure they are complete before participation
- Encourage use of warm up and cool down activities to prevent injuries
- Use certified athletic trainers for competitive sports at the junior and senior high school level
- Ensure medical coverage at competitive sporting events, as appropriate
- Develop an emergency plan in case of serious injury
- Coordinate preseason seminars for athletes, families, and coaches to increase awareness of injury prevention
- Collaborate with other professionals in planning programs related to injury prevention
- Inform parents and athletes of steps they can take to prevent injuries
- Inform parents and athletes of signs and symptoms of overuse injuries, dehydration, heat exhaustion, use of performance enhancing drugs, eating disorders, menstrual dysfunction, and stress
- Collect data on injury type, rate, treatment, and referrals
- Monitor the long-term health of athletes
- Monitor return of injured athletes to participation to prevent reinjury
- Provide emotional support for athletes experiencing injury
- Arrange for coaches to get annual CPR and first aid training
- Communicate with coaches the importance of emphasizing "fun" in sports
- Assure coaches are well informed of normal childhood development and the physical, emotional, and social needs of children
- Communicate information about special health care concerns of individual athletes, as appropriate
- Develop oversight groups to ensure education of school and volunteer coaches
- Inform parents of qualifications and behavior expected of coaches
- Encourage parents to become involved in their children's sports programs
- Monitor athletes for sport-related stress and provide referrals for athletes with emotional/psychosocial concerns
- Teach relaxation techniques and coping strategies to athletes, coaches, and parents
- Advocate for the health of young athletes

3rd edition 2000

S

Background Readings:

American College of Sports Medicine. (1994). The prevention of sport injuries of children and adolescents. *Journal of American Academy of Physician's Assistants, 7*(6), 437–442

Dyment, P. (1991). *Sports medicine: Health care for young athletes.* Elk Grove Village, IL: The American Academy of Pediatrics.

Hutchinson, M. R. (1997). Cheerleading injuries, patterns, prevention, case reports. *The Physician and Sports Medicine, 15*(9), 83–86, 89–91, 96.

Overbaugh, K. & Allen, J. (1994). The adolescent athlete. Part I: Pre-season preparation and examination. *Journal of Pediatric Health Care, 8*(4), 146–151.

Overbaugh, K. & Allen, J. (1994). The adolescent athlete. Part II: Injury patterns and prevention. *Journal of Pediatric Health Care, 8*(5), 203–211.

Petlichkoff, L. M. (1992). Youth sport participation and withdrawal: Is it simply a matter of FUN. *Pediatric Exercise Science, 4*(2), 105–110.

Smeltzer, S. C. & Bare, B. G. (2004). Management of patients with musculoskeletal trauma. In *Brunner & Suddarth's textbook of medical surgical nursing* (Vol. 2) (10th ed., pp. 2075–2111). Philadelphia: Lippincott Williams & Wilkins.

Staff Development   7850

Definition: Developing, maintaining, and monitoring competence of staff

Activities:

- Identify learning needs of staff (e.g., new or change in policy and procedures, new hire to organization, transfer within organization, new job requirements, cross-training, equipment upgrades, emerging trends, skills training)
- Identify learner characteristics (e.g., literacy, language, educational background, previous experience, age, motivation, attitude)
- Identify performance problem(s) (e.g., knowledge deficit, skill deficit, motivational deficit), as needed
- Identify instructional goal(s) (e.g., inform staff of changes, provide knowledge and skills, improve proficiency, improve competence)
- Identify standard(s) of learning achievement (e.g., psychomotor, interpersonal, critical thinking)
- Determine instructional learning objectives
- Identify instructional content
- Identify instructional constraints (e.g., time, cost, equipment availability)
- Identify resources that support instruction (e.g., expert consultation, learning materials, time, fiscal resources)
- Identify appropriate individual(s) to provide instruction
- Organize and develop instructional content
- Design teaching and learning activities
- Design methods of preassessment and postassessment/evaluation
- Provide instructional program (e.g., self-directed learning packets, classroom presentation, small group presentation, on-the-job training)
- Evaluate effectiveness of the instruction
- Provide feedback on results of staff development instruction to appropriate individuals
- Monitor competence of staff skills
- Conduct periodic review of competencies
- Determine needed frequency of staff development instruction in order to maintain competency
- Provide financial assistance and time off to attend educational programs as required by job
- Encourage participation in peer review
- Encourage reading of professional journals
- Encourage participation in professional organizations

3rd edition 2000

Background Readings:

Alspach, J. G. (1995). *The educational process in nursing staff development.* St. Louis: Mosby.

Kelly, K. J. (1992). *Nursing staff development: Current competence, future focus.* Philadelphia: J. B. Lippincott.

Rodriguez, L., Patton, C., Stiesmeyer, J. K., & Teikmanis, M. L. (Eds.). (1996). *Manual of staff development.* St. Louis: Mosby.

S

Staff Supervision   7830

Definition: Facilitating the delivery of high-quality patient care by others

Activities:

- Create a work environment that validates the importance of each employee to the organization
- Acknowledge an employee's area of expertise
- Select a management style appropriate to the work situation and employee characteristics
- Encourage open communication
- Identify opportunities for participation in decision making
- Provide a job description for all new employees
- Provide clear expectations for job performance
- Share evaluation methods used with employee
- Foster teamwork and a sense of purpose for the work group
- Set goals for staff, as appropriate
- Consider employee growth in work assignments
- Share information about the organization and future plans
- Listen to employee concerns and suggestions
- Provide feedback on work performance at regular intervals
- Provide coaching and encouragement
- Reinforce good/excellent performance verbally
- Provide recognition for behavior that supports organizational goals
- Maintain an attitude of trust of others

- Seek advice from employees, as appropriate
- Use informal networks to accomplish goals
- Provide challenges and opportunities for employee growth
- Monitor quality of work performance
- Monitor quality of employee's relationships with other health care providers
- Document strengths and weaknesses of employee
- Counsel, when appropriate
- Facilitate employee opportunities to be "winners"
- Seek information on employee concerns for patient care and the work environment
- Seek feedback from patients concerning care provided
- Encourage staff to solve own problems
- Initiate disciplinary action, as appropriate, following policies and procedures
- Counsel employee on how to improve performance, as appropriate
- Set time frames for needed behavior changes, as appropriate
- Provide reeducation, as needed, to improve performance
- Complete evaluation forms at appropriate time intervals
- Discuss evaluation results privately

2nd edition 1996

Background Readings:

Buccheri, R. C. (1986). Nursing supervision: A new look at an old role. *Nursing Administration Quarterly, 11*(1), 11–25.

Christen, J. W. (1987). The changing nature of first-line supervision. *The Health Care Supervisor, 5*(2), 65–70.

Hersey, P. (1989). *Situational leadership in nursing.* Norwalk, CT: Appleton & Lange.

Hersey, P., Blanchard, K., & Johnson, D. E. (2001). *Management of organizational behavior: Utilizing human resources* (8th ed.). Upper Saddle River, NJ: Prentice Hall.

Swansburg, R. C. (1990). *Management and leadership for nurse managers.* Sudbury, MA: Jones and Bartlett.

Stem Cell Infusion   4266

Definition: Infusion of hematopoietic stem cells and monitoring of the patient's response

Activities:

- Ensure the product to be infused has been prepared, labeled, and classified according to institution protocol
- Explain the procedure and the aim of the infusion of hematopoietic stem cells to patients and caregivers
- Inform the patient and the family about the possible negative effects (e.g., transfusion reaction, volume overload, pulmonary embolism, changes in vital signs, and nausea/vomiting) that may appear during infusion
- Use peppermint oil or hard candy to counteract the offensive smell and taste of preservative
- Prepare infusion equipment without filter and other necessary materials (e.g., physiologic serum 0.9%, venous pressure measurement systems, sphygmomanometer, phonendoscope, thermometer, and pulsometer)
- Verify that the infusion equipment has no filter and no infusion pumps to avoid cellular damage
- Use saline solution to flush the equipment
- Prepare emergency material and drugs to treat serious negative reactions, including anaphylaxis kit, oxygen administration equipment, and suction equipment
- Use gloves during the manipulation of the infusion product
- Ensure aseptic manipulation of equipment, connections, and product
- Administer prehydration solution according to the protocol
- Coordinate immediate administration of the defrosted infusion product
- Administer premedication prescribed according to the protocol of the institution
- Avoid irradiation and any type of mechanical or physical damage to the infusion product
- Make sure that the infusion product is received in optimal isolation and refrigeration conditions (1° to 24° C)
- Verify the labeling and the identification of both the bags and the patient (using patient name and hospital number) immediately prior to infusion
- Administer the infusion through a central venous catheter through the largest lumen available for ease of flow
- Infuse each bag at the rate, sequence, and time established in the protocol guidelines of the institution, and according to the tolerance of the patient
- Monitor for possible adverse reactions (e.g., nausea, vomiting, abdominal cramps, diarrhea, facial flare, arrhythmia, dyspnea) and stop the infusion and call the physician, if necessary
- Irrigate the infusion catheter with saline solution after the infusion of each bag
- Irrigate the intravenous line with saline solution if syringes were used to infuse the product in order to reduce the loss of stem cells that could remain in the lumen of the catheter or infusion system
- Dispose of spare material and hazardous waste according to agency protocol
- Monitor vital signs according to institutional protocol during and after the procedure
- Record volume of stem cells and normal saline administered
- Monitor the elimination of urine, paying attention to volume, color, and osmolality
- Observe for signs and symptoms of circulatory overload
- Record the patient's response (e.g., tolerance and negative effects), according to the protocol of the institution
- Document adverse events, according to agency protocol
- Provide patients and family with emotional support

6th edition 2013

Background Readings:

Bevans, M. & Shelburne, N. (2004). Hematopoietic stem cell transplantation. *Clinical Journal of Oncology Nursing, 8*(5), 541–543.

Foundation for the Accreditation of Cellular Therapy. (2003). *Standards for hematopoietic progenitor cell collection, processing & transplantation* (2nd ed.). Omaha, NE: Author.

Saria, M. G. & Gosselin-Acomb, T. K. (2007). Hematopoietic stem cell transplantation: Implications for critical care nurses. *Clinical Journal of Oncology Nursing, 11*(1), 53–63.

Sauer-Heilborn, A., Kadidlo, D. & McCullough, J. (2004). Patient care during infusion of hematopoietic progenitor cells. *Transfusion, 44*(6), 907–916.

S

Subarachnoid Hemorrhage Precautions   2720

Definition: Reduction of internal and external stimuli or stressors to minimize risk of rebleeding prior to surgery or endovascular procedure to secure ruptured aneurysm

Activities:
- Place patient in a private room
- Bed rest with bedside commode, as appropriate
- Maintain darkened room
- Decrease stimuli in patient's environment
- Restrict television, radio, and other stimulants
- Monitor response to visitors
- Limit visitors, if indicated
- Provide information to patient and family regarding need for environmental modifications and visiting limitations
- Give sedation, as needed
- Administer pain medications PRN
- Monitor neurological status
- Notify physician of neurological deterioration
- Monitor pulse and BP
- Maintain hemodynamic parameters within prescribed limits
- Monitor ICP and CPP, if indicated
- Monitor CSF output and characteristics, if indicated
- Administer stool softeners
- Avoid rectal stimulation
- Instruct patient not to strain or perform Valsalva maneuver
- Implement seizure precautions
- Administer anticonvulsants, as appropriate

1st edition 1992; revised 2008

Background Readings:
Ackerman, L. L. (1992). Interventions related to neurological care. In G. M. Bulechek & J. C. McCloskey (Eds.), Symposium on Nursing Interventions. *Nursing Clinics of North America, 27*(2), 325–346.

Barker, E. (2002). Cranial surgery. In E. Barker (Ed.), *Neuroscience nursing – A spectrum of care* (2nd ed., pp. 303–349). St. Louis: Mosby.

Hickey, J. V. & Buckley, D. M. (2003). Cerebral aneurysms. In J. V. Hickey (Ed.), *The clinical practice of neurological and neurosurgical nursing* (5th ed., pp. 523–548). Philadelphia: Lippincott Williams & Wilkins.

Hickle, J. L., Guanci, M. M., Bowman, L., Hermann, L., McGinty, L. B. & Rose, J. (2004). Cerebrovascular events of the nervous system. In M. K. Bader & L. R. Littlejohns (Eds.), *AANN core curriculum for neuroscience nursing* (4th ed., pp. 536–585). Philadelphia: Saunders.

Lee, K. (1980). Aneurysm precautions: A physiologic basis for minimizing rebleeding. *Heart & Lung, 9*(2), 336–343.

Substance Use Prevention   4500

Definition: Prevention of an alcoholic or drug use lifestyle

Activities:
- Assist individual to tolerate increased levels of stress, as appropriate
- Prepare individual for difficult or painful events
- Reduce irritating or frustrating environmental stress
- Reduce social isolation, as appropriate
- Support measures to regulate the sale and distribution of alcohol to minors
- Lobby for increased drinking age
- Recommend responsible changes in the alcohol and drug curricula for primary grades
- Conduct programs in schools on the avoidance of drugs and alcohol as recreational activities
- Encourage responsible decision making about lifestyle choices
- Recommend media campaigns on substance use issues in the community
- Instruct parents in the importance of example in substance use
- Instruct parents and teachers in the identification of signs and symptoms of addiction
- Assist individual to identify substitute tension-reducing strategies
- Support or organize community groups to reduce injuries associated with alcohol, such as SADD (Students Against Destructive Decisions) and MADD (Mothers Against Drunk Driving)
- Survey students in grades 1 to 12 on the use of alcohol and drugs and alcohol-related behaviors
- Instruct parents to support school policy that prohibits drug and alcohol consumption at extracurricular activities
- Assist in organizing activities for teenagers after such functions as prom and homecoming
- Facilitate coordination of efforts between various community groups concerned with substance use
- Encourage parents to participate in children's activities, beginning in preschool through adolescence

1st edition 1992; revised 2000

Background Readings:
Faltz, B. G. & Wing, R. V. (2005). Substance use disorders. In M. A. Boyd (Ed.), *Psychiatric nursing: Contemporary practice* (3rd ed., pp. 524–564). Philadelphia: Lippincott Williams & Wilkins.

Hagemaster, J. (1999). Substance use prevention. In G. M. Bulechek & J. C. McCloskey (Eds.), *Nursing interventions: Effective nursing treatments* (3rd ed., pp. 482–490). Philadelphia: W. B. Saunders.

Hahn, E. J. (1995). Predicting head start parent involvement in an alcohol and other drug prevention program. *Nursing Research, 44*(1), 45–51.

Solari-Twadell, P. A. (1991). Recreational drugs: Societal and professional issues. *Nursing Clinics of North America, 26*(2), 499–509.

S

Substance Use Treatment 4510

Definition: Care of patient and family members demonstrating dysfunction as a result of substance abuse or dependence

Activities:
- Foster a trusting relationship while setting clear limits (i.e., provide gentle but firm evidence of dysfunction, stay focused on substance abuse or dependency, and inspire hope)
- Consider presence of comorbidity, or cooccurring psychiatric or medical disorder, making changes in treatment accordingly
- Assist patient in understanding disorder as a disease related to several factors (e.g., genetic, psychological, and situational circumstances)
- Inform patient that the volume and frequency of substance use leading to dysfunction varies greatly between people
- Instruct patient on effects of substance used (e.g., physical, psychological, and social)
- Discuss treatment needs for associated medical, psychological, social, vocational, housing, and legal difficulties
- Encourage or praise patient efforts to accept responsibility for substance use-related dysfunction and treatment
- Provide symptom management during the detoxification period
- Administer medications (e.g., disulfiram, acamprosate, methadone, naltrexone, nicotine patches or gum, or buprenorphine), as indicated
- Instruct patient or family about medications used for treatment
- Provide therapy (e.g., cognitive therapy, motivational therapy, counseling, family support, family therapy, or adolescent community reinforcement approach), as indicated
- Establish multidisciplinary programs (e.g., short-term inpatient residential therapy, detoxification program, or residential therapeutic community treatment), if appropriate
- Encourage patient to participate in self-help support program during and after treatment (e.g., 12-step programs, Women for Sobriety, or Rational Recovery)
- Discuss importance of abstaining from substance use, identifying most appropriate treatment goal (e.g., complete abstinence, day-by-day sobriety, or use of substance in moderation)
- Coordinate and facilitate group confrontation strategy to address use of and role defenses play in substance use (e.g., denial)
- Instruct patient on stress management techniques (e.g., exercise, meditation, and relaxation therapy)
- Assist patient in developing healthy, effective coping mechanisms
- Identify and address dysfunctional relationship patterns in patient's familial or other social ties (e.g., codependency and enabling)
- Assist in identifying and facilitating connections with supportive persons
- Assist in resocialization, rebuilding relationships, and decreasing self-centeredness
- Monitor for substance use during treatment (e.g., urine screens and breath analysis)
- Monitor for infectious disease (e.g., HIV/AIDS, hepatitis B and C, and tuberculosis), treating and providing assistance to modify behaviors, if necessary
- Assist patient in developing self-worth, encouraging positive efforts and motivation
- Encourage patient to keep a detailed chart of substance use to evaluate progress
- Assist the patient to evaluate the amount of time spent using the substance and the usual patterns within the day
- Participate in efforts to remain abreast of available programs, resources, and legislation aimed at education, prevention, and treatment of substance use disorders
- Instruct patient on symptoms or behaviors increasing chances of relapse (e.g., exhaustion, depression, dishonesty, and complacency)
- Develop plan for relapse prevention (e.g., contracting, identify resources for various needs in stressful situation, and identify health promoting activities to take place of substance use)
- Instruct family on substance use disorder and related dysfunction and include in treatment planning and activities
- Encourage family to participate in recovery efforts
- Provide referral

1st edition 1992; revised 2013

Background Readings:

Essau, C. A. (Ed.). (2008). *Adolescent addition: Epidemiology, assessment, and treatment.* London: Academic Press.

Jacobson, S. A., Pies, R. W., & Katz, I. R. (2007). Treatment of substance-related disorders. In *Clinical manual of geriatric psychopharmacology* (pp. 403–475). Arlington, VA: American Psychiatric.

Lickteig, M. (2009). Substance use disorders. In W. K. Mohr (Ed.), *Psychiatric-mental health nursing: Evidence-based concepts, skills, and practices* (7th ed., pp. 607–650). Philadelphia: Lippincott Williams & Wilkins.

Trigoboff, E. (2009). Substance-related disorders. In C. R. Kneisl & E. Trigoboff (Eds.), *Contemporary psychiatric-mental health nursing* (2nd ed., pp. 323–369). Upper Saddle River, NJ: Pearson Prentice Hall.

World Health Organization, Department of Mental Health and Substance Abuse. (2009). *Guidelines for the psychosocially assisted pharmacological treatment of opioid dependence.* Geneva, Switzerland: Author.

S

Substance Use Treatment: Alcohol Withdrawal   4512

Definition: Care of the patient experiencing sudden cessation of alcohol consumption

Activities:

- Create a low-stimulation environment for detoxification
- Monitor vital signs during withdrawal
- Monitor for delirium tremens
- Administer anticonvulsants or sedatives, as appropriate
- Medicate to relieve physical discomfort, as needed
- Approach abusive patient behavior in a neutral manner
- Address hallucinations in a therapeutic manner
- Maintain adequate nutrition and fluid intake
- Administer vitamin therapy, as appropriate
- Monitor for covert alcohol consumption during detoxification
- Listen to patient's concerns about alcohol withdrawal
- Provide emotional support to patient/family, as appropriate
- Provide verbal reassurance, as appropriate
- Provide reality orientation, as appropriate
- Reassure patient that depression and fatigue commonly occur during withdrawal

Background Readings:

Faltz, B. G. & Wing, R. V. (2005). Substance use disorders. In M. A. Boyd (Ed.), *Psychiatric nursing: Contemporary practice* (3rd ed., pp. 524–564). Philadelphia: Lippincott Williams & Wilkins.

Joyce, C. (1989). The woman alcoholic. *American Journal of Nursing, 89*(10), 1314–1316.

Powell, A. F. & Minick, M. P. (1988). Alcohol withdrawal syndrome. *American Journal of Nursing, 88*(3), 312–315.

Stuart, G. W. & Jefferson, L. V. (2005). Chemically mediated responses and substance-related disorders. In G. W. Stuart & M. T. Laraia (Eds.), *Principles and practice of psychiatric nursing* (8th ed., pp. 473–516). St. Louis: Mosby.

1st edition 1992; revised 2000

Substance Use Treatment: Drug Withdrawal   4514

Definition: Care of patient experiencing drug detoxification

Activities:

- Monitor vital signs
- Monitor respiratory and cardiac systems (e.g., hypertension, tachycardia, and bradypnea)
- Monitor for changes in level of consciousness
- Monitor intake and output
- Monitor for suicidal tendencies
- Implement precautions for patient at risk for suicide
- Monitor withdrawal symptoms (e.g., fatigue, sensory disturbances, irritability, violence, depression, panic attacks, cravings, insomnia, agitation, muscle pain, appetite changes, yawning, weakness, headache, runny nose, dilated pupils, chills, anxiety, sweating, nausea, vomiting, tremors, psychosis, and ataxia)
- Provide symptom management
- Administer medications (e.g., benzodiazepines, chlorpromazine, diazepam, nicotine replacement, phenobarbital, clonidine, trazodone, methadone, alpha-2 adrenergic agonists, and antipsychotics), remaining aware of cross-tolerance
- Implement precautions for patient at risk for seizures
- Provide adequate nutrition (e.g., small amounts of fluids frequently and high-calorie foods)
- Assist with activities of daily living
- Implement precautions for patient at risk for falling
- Maintain low-stimulation environment (e.g., talk in a low, calm voice; provide reassurance about safety; and ensure a comfortable, darkened, quiet, and nonthreatening environment)
- Reorient patient to reality
- Encourage patient to participate in follow-up support (e.g., peer group therapy, individual or family counseling, and drug recovery educational programs)
- Offer supportive assistance (e.g., provision of food and shelter, structured psychotherapy)
- Provide referral
- Facilitate support by family and significant others
- Provide support to family or significant others, as appropriate
- Instruct patient and family on process of drug use and dependency

1st edition 1992, revised 2013

Background Readings:

Lickteig, M. (2009). Substance use disorders. In W. K. Mohr (Ed.), *Psychiatric-mental health nursing: Evidence-based concepts, skills, and practices* (7th ed., pp. 607–650). Philadelphia: Lippincott Williams & Wilkins.

Trigoboff, E. (2009). Substance-related disorders. In C. R. Kneisl & E. Trigoboff (Eds.), *Contemporary psychiatric-mental health nursing* (2nd ed., pp. 323–369). Upper Saddle River, NJ: Pearson Prentice Hall.

World Health Organization, Department of Mental Health and Substance Abuse. (2009). *Guidelines for the psychosocially assisted pharmacological treatment of opioid dependence.* Geneva, Switzerland: Author.

S

Substance Use Treatment: Overdose   4516

Definition: Care of a patient demonstrating toxic effects as a result of consuming one or more drugs

Activities:
- Create or maintain an open airway
- Monitor respiratory, cardiac, gastrointestinal, renal, and neurological status
- Monitor vital signs
- Place patient in most appropriate position (e.g., semi-Fowler's position if patient is awake, left lateral recumbent position if patient is unresponsive)
- Provide safe environment (i.e., pad side rails, keep bed in lowest position, remove dangerous objects, and position safety officer near patient's room)
- Establish rapport with patient or family (i.e., use nonjudgmental approach, do not reprimand)
- Perform necessary toxicology screening and system function tests (e.g., urine and serum drug screening, arterial blood gases, electrolyte levels, liver enzymes, blood urea nitrogen, and creatinine)
- Contact poison control center for assistance in determining definitive treatment
- Establish intravenous access, administering infusions as prescribed
- Monitor for symptoms specific to drug consumed (e.g., constricted pupils, hypotension, and bradycardia for opiate overdose; nausea, vomiting, diaphoresis, and right upper quadrant pain 48 to 72 hours after acetaminophen overdose; and dilated pupils, tachycardia, seizures, and chest pain for cocaine overdose)
- Administer agents specific to substance consumed and patient symptoms (e.g., antiemetics, naloxone, thiamine, glucose, flumazenil, calcium, vasopressors, antiarrhythmics, and inotropics)
- Administer agents or perform procedures to impair drug absorption and increase drug excretion (e.g., ipecac, activated charcoal, gastric lavage, hemodialysis, cathartics, exchange transfusion, altering urine and serum pH, and whole-bowel irrigation)
- Communicate with patient, providing reassurance, addressing hallucinations or delusions, and conveying understanding of fears or other feelings
- Monitor intake and output
- Treat hyperthermia (i.e., apply ice packs for fever caused by amphetamine or cocaine intoxication)
- Provide emotional support to patient and family
- Monitor for suicidal tendencies
- Provide instruction on proper use of drug
- Assist patient in identifying ways to minimize potential for accidental overdose (e.g., store medications in original container, address issues with confusion or memory, and store medications out of children's reach)
- Instruct family or caregiver on patient's need for follow-up care
- Instruct family or caregiver on aspiration and seizure precautions
- Provide referral (e.g., home health agency, social worker, psychiatry, or drug use treatment program)

1st edition 1992; revised 2013

Background Readings:
Johnson, J. M. (2009). Over-the-counter overdoses: A review of ibuprofen, acetaminophen, and aspirin toxicity in adults. *Advanced Emergency Nursing Journal, 30*(4), 369–78.

Smeltzer, S. C., Bare, B. G., Hinkle, J. L., & Cheever, K. H. (2008). Emergency nursing. In *Brunner & Suddarth's textbook of medical-surgical nursing* (11th ed., pp. 2516–2557). Philadelphia: Lippincott Williams & Wilkins.

Sturt, P. A. (2005). Toxicologic conditions. In J. Fultz & P. A. Sturt (Eds.), *Mosby's emergency nursing reference* (3rd ed., pp. 643–681). St. Louis: Elsevier Mosby.

Suicide Prevention   6340

Definition: Reducing the risk for self-inflicted harm with intent to end life

Activities:
- Determine presence and degree of suicidal risk
- Determine if patient has available means to follow through with suicide plan
- Consider hospitalization of patient who is at serious risk for suicidal behavior
- Treat and manage any psychiatric illness or symptoms that may be placing patient at risk for suicide (e.g., mood disorder, hallucinations, delusions, panic, substance abuse, grief, personality disorder, organic impairment, crisis)
- Administer medications to decrease anxiety, agitation, or psychosis and to stabilize mood, as appropriate
- Advocate for quality of life and pain control issues
- Conduct mouth checks following medication administration to ensure that patient is not "cheeking" the medications for later overdose attempt
- Provide small amounts of prescriptive medications that may be lethal to those at risk to decrease the opportunity for suicide, as appropriate
- Monitor for medication side effects and desired outcomes
- Involve patient in planning his/her own treatment, as appropriate
- Instruct patient in coping strategies (e.g., assertiveness training, impulse control, and progressive muscle relaxation), as appropriate
- Contract (verbally or in writing) with patient for "no self-harm" for a specified period of time, recontracting at specified time intervals, as appropriate
- Implement necessary actions to reduce an individual's immediate distress when negotiating a no-self-harm or safety contract
- Identify immediate safety needs when negotiating a no-self-harm or safety contract
- Assist the individual in discussing his/her feelings about the contract
- Observe individual for signs of incongruence that may indicate lack of commitment to fulfilling the contract
- Take action to prevent individual from harming or killing self, when contract is a no-self-harm or safety contract (e.g., increased observation, removal of objects that may be used to harm self)

- Interact with the patient at regular intervals to convey caring and openness and to provide an opportunity for patient to talk about feelings
- Utilize direct, nonjudgmental approach in discussing suicide
- Encourage patient to seek out care providers to talk as the urge to harm self occurs
- Avoid repeated discussion of past suicide history by keeping discussions oriented in the present and the future
- Discuss plans for dealing with suicidal ideation in the future (e.g., precipitating factors, who to contact, where to go for help, ways to alleviate feelings of self-harm)
- Assist patient to identify network of supportive persons and resources (e.g., clergy, family, providers)
- Initiate suicide precautions (e.g., ongoing observation and monitoring of the patient, provision of a protective environment) for the patient who is at serious risk of suicide
- Place patient in least restrictive environment that allows for necessary level of observation
- Continue regular assessment of suicidal risk (at least daily) in order to adjust suicide precautions appropriately
- Consult with treatment team before modifying suicide precautions
- Search the newly hospitalized patient and personal belongings for weapons/potential weapons during inpatient admission procedure, as appropriate
- Search environment routinely and remove dangerous items to maintain it as hazard free
- Limit access to windows, unless locked and shatterproof, as appropriate
- Limit patient use of potential weapons (e.g., sharps and rope-like objects)
- Monitor patient during use of potential weapons (e.g., razor)
- Utilize protective interventions (e.g., area restrictions, seclusion, physical restraints) if patient lacks the restraint to refrain from harming self, as needed
- Communicate risk and relevant safety issues to other care providers
- Assign hospitalized patient to a room located near nursing station for ease in observation, as appropriate
- Increase surveillance of hospitalized patients at times when staffing is predictably low (e.g., staff meetings, change of shift report, staff mealtimes, nights, weekends, times of chaos on nursing unit)

- Consider strategies to decrease isolation and opportunity to act on harmful thoughts (e.g., use of a sitter)
- Observe, record, and report any change in mood or behavior that may signify increasing suicidal risk and document results of regular surveillance checks
- Explain suicide precautions and relevant safety issues to the patient/family/significant others (e.g., purpose, duration, behavioral expectations, and behavioral consequences)
- Facilitate support of patient by family and friends
- Involve family in discharge planning (e.g., illness/medication teaching, recognition of increasing suicidal risk, patient's plan for dealing with thoughts of harming self, community resources)
- Refer patient to mental health care provider (e.g., psychiatrist or psychiatric/mental health advanced practice nurse) for evaluation and treatment of suicide ideation and behavior, as needed
- Provide information about what community resources and outreach programs are available
- Improve access to mental health services
- Increase the public's awareness that suicide is a preventable health problem

1st edition 1992; revised 2000, 2004

Background Readings:

Conwell, Y. (1997). Management of suicidal behavior in the elderly. *Psychiatric Clinics of North America, 20*(3), 667–683.

Drew, B. L. (2001). Self-harm behavior and no-suicide contracting in psychiatric inpatient settings. *Archives of Psychiatric Nursing, 15*(3), 99–106.

Hirschfeld, R. M. A. & Russel, J. M. (1997). Assessment and treatment of suicidal patients. *New England Journal of Medicine, 337*(13), 910–915.

Potter, M. L., & Dawson, A. M. (2001). From safety contract to safety agreement. *Journal of Psychosocial Nursing, 39*(8), 38–45.

Schultz, J. M., & Videbeck, S. D. (1998). Lippincott's manual of psychiatric nursing care plans. Philadelphia: J. B. Lippincott.

Stuart, G. W. (2005). Self-protective responses and suicidal behavior. In G. W. Stuart & M. T. Laraia (Eds.), *Principles and practice of psychiatric nursing* (8th ed., pp. 364–385). St. Louis: Mosby.

Valente, S. M. & Trainor, D. (1998). Rational suicide among patients who are terminally ill. *Association of Operating Room Nurses Journal, 68*(2), 252–255, 257–258, 260–264.

S

Supply Management   7840

Definition: Ensuring acquisition and maintenance of appropriate items for providing patient care

Activities:
- Identify items commonly used for patient care
- Determine stock level needed for each item
- Add new items to inventory list, as appropriate
- Check items for expiration dates at specific intervals
- Inspect integrity of sterile packages
- Ensure that supply area is cleaned regularly
- Avoid stockpiling expensive items
- Order new or replacement equipment, as necessary
- Ensure that maintenance requirements on special equipment are completed
- Order patient education materials, as appropriate
- Order specialty items for patient, as appropriate

- Charge patient for supplies, as appropriate
- Mark unit/agency equipment for identification, as appropriate
- Review supply budget, as appropriate

2nd edition 1996

Background Readings:

Keller, R. A. (1992). Buying smart . . . purchasing equipment and supplies. *Emergency, 24*(1), 78–80.

Rowland, H. S. & Rowland, B. L. (1997). *Nursing administration handbook* (4th ed.). Sudbury, MA: Jones and Bartlett.

Stasen, L. (1982). *Key business skills for nurse managers.* Philadelphia: J. B. Lippincott.

Support Group 5430

Definition: Use of a group environment to provide emotional support and health-related information for members

Activities:

- Determine level and appropriateness of patient's present support system
- Use a support group during transitional stages to help patient adjust to a new lifestyle
- Determine purpose of the group and nature of the group process
- Determine the most appropriate venue for the group's meeting (e.g., face to face or online)
- Identify faith-based groups as available options for clients, as appropriate
- Create a relaxed, accepting atmosphere
- Clarify early on the goals of the group and the members' and leader's responsibilities
- Use a co-leader, as appropriate
- Use a written contract, if deemed appropriate
- Choose members who can contribute to and benefit from group interaction
- Form a group of optimal size (e.g., 5 to 12 members)
- Address the issue of mandatory attendance
- Address the issue of whether new members can join at any time
- Establish a time and place for the group meeting
- Meet in 1- to 2-hour sessions, as appropriate
- Begin and end on time, and expect participants to remain until the conclusion
- Arrange chairs in a circle in close proximity
- Schedule a limited number of sessions (e.g., 6 to 12), in which the work of the group will be accomplished
- Publicize membership policies to avoid problems that may arise as the group progresses
- Monitor and direct active involvement of group members
- Encourage expression and sharing of experiential knowledge
- Encourage expression of mutual aid
- Encourage appropriate referrals to professionals for information
- Emphasize personal responsibility and control
- Maintain positive pressure for behavior change
- Emphasize the importance of active coping
- Identify topic themes that occur in the group discussion
- Do not allow group to become a nonproductive social gathering
- Assist the group to progress through the stages of group development, from orientation through cohesiveness to termination
- Attend to the needs of the group as a whole, as well as the needs of individual members
- Refer the patient to other specialists, as appropriate

1st edition 1992; revised 2013

Background Readings:

American Psychiatric Nurses Association. (2007). *Psychiatric-mental health nursing: Scope and standards of practice.* Washington, DC: Author.

Cincinnati Children's Hospital Medical Center. (2009). *Best evidence statement (BESt) inpatient support groups for families of children with intractable epilepsy.* Cincinnati, OH: Author.

Dundon, E. (2006). Adolescent depression: A metasynthesis. *Journal of Pediatric Health Care, 20*(6), 384–392.

Kurlowicz, L. & Harvath, T. A. (2008). Depression. In E. Capezuti, D. Zwicker, M. Mezey, & T. Fulmer (Eds.), *Evidence-based geriatric nursing protocols for best practice* (3rd ed., pp. 57–82.). New York: Springer.

McQueen, K., Montgomery, P., Lappan-Gracon, S., Evans, M., & Gunter, J. (2008). Evidence-based recommendations for depressive symptoms in postpartum women. *Journal of Obstetric, Gynecologic and Neonatal Nursing, 37*(2), 127–136.

Percy, C. A., Gibbs, T., Potter, L., & Boardman, S. (2009). Nurse-led peer support group: Experiences of women with polycystic ovary syndrome. *Journal of Advanced Nursing, 65*(10), 2046–2055.

Support System Enhancement 5440

Definition: Facilitation of support to patient by family, friends, and community

Activities:

- Identify psychological response to situation and availability of support system
- Determine adequacy of existing social networks
- Identify degree of family support, financial support, and other resources
- Determine barriers to unused and underused support systems
- Monitor current family situation and the support network
- Encourage the patient to participate in social and community activities
- Encourage relationships with persons who have common interests and goals
- Refer to a self-help group or Internet-based resource, as appropriate
- Identify community resource strengths and weaknesses and advocate for change when appropriate
- Refer to a community-based prevention or treatment program, as appropriate
- Provide services in a caring and supportive manner
- Involve family, significant others, and friends in the care and planning
- Identify available resources for caregiver support
- Explain to concerned others how they can help

1st edition 1992; revised 2013

Background Readings:

Commission on Social Determinants of Health. (2008). *Closing the gap in a generation: Health equity through action on the social determinants of health.* Geneva, Switzerland: World Health Organization.

Dossey, B. M. & Keegan, L. (2009). *Holistic nursing: A handbook for practice* (5th ed.). Sudbury, MA: Jones & Bartlett.

Häggman-Laitila, A., Tanninen, H. M., & Pietilä, A. M. (2010). Effectiveness of resource-enhancing family-oriented intervention. *Journal of Clinical Nursing, 19*(17–18), 2500–2510.

Hudson, D. B., Campbell-Grossman C., Keating-Lefler, R., & Cline, P. (2008). New mothers network: The development of an internet-based social support intervention for African American mothers. *Issues in Comprehensive Pediatric Nursing, 31*(1), 23–35.

Stuart, G. W. (2009). Prevention and mental health promotion. In G. W. Stuart (Ed.), *Principles and practice of psychiatric nursing* (9th ed., pp. 172–183). St. Louis: Mosby Elsevier.

Surgical Assistance 2900

Definition: Assisting the surgeon or dentist with operative procedures and care of the surgical patient

Activities:
- Perform surgical hand antisepsis in accordance with the hospital protocol or rules
- Don a sterile gown and gloves using aseptic technique
- Assist the surgical team while they don gown and gloves
- Adopt a position that allows you to keep the surgical field in sight throughout the surgery
- Anticipate and provide needed supplies and instruments throughout the procedure
- Ensure that appropriate instruments, supplies, and equipment are sterile and in good working order
- Transfer the scalpel or dermatographic pencil to the surgeon, as appropriate
- Provide the instruments in an appropriate safe manner
- Grasp tissue, as appropriate
- Dissect tissue, as appropriate
- Irrigate and suction surgical wound, as appropriate
- Protect tissue, as appropriate
- Provide hemostasis, as appropriate
- Maintain the sterility of the surgical field throughout the procedure, disposing of contaminated elements and taking measures to preserve surgical integrity and asepsis
- Remove soiled sponges and deposit them in an appropriate place, replacing them with clean ones
- Clean the incision site and drains of blood, secretions, and residual skin antiseptic
- Assist in the closing of the surgical wound
- Dry the skin at the incision site and drains
- Apply reinforcement bands, dressings, or bandages to the surgical wound
- Assist in estimating blood loss
- Connect the drains to their collection systems, attach them, and keep them in the appropriate position
- Prepare and care for specimens, as appropriate
- Communicate information to the surgical team, as appropriate
- Communicate patient status and progress to family, as appropriate
- Arrange for equipment needed immediately after surgery
- Assist in transferring patient to the cart or bed and transport to appropriate postanesthesia or postoperative area
- Report to the postanesthesia or postoperative nurse pertinent information about the patient and procedure performed
- Document information, as per agency policy

2nd edition 1996, revised 2013

Background Readings:

Association of periOperative Registered Nurses. (2010). *Perioperative standards and recommended practices.* Denver: Author.

Fuller, J. (2008). *Surgical technology: Principles and practice* (4th ed.) Madrid: Panamericana.

Phippen, M., Ulmer, B. C., & Wells, M. M. (2009). *Competency for safe patient care during operative and invasive procedures.* Denver: Competency & Credentialing Institute.

Rothrock, J. C. (2010). *Alexander's care of the patient in surgery* (14th ed.). St. Louis: Elsevier Mosby.

Rothrock, J. C. & Siefert, P. C. (2009). *Assisting in surgery: Patient centered care.* Denver: Competency & Credentialing Institute.

Surgical Instrumentation Management 2910

Definition: Managing the requirements for materials, instruments, equipment, and sterility of the surgical field

Activities:
- Consult surgical schedules, operating room assignments, and obtain information on the surgical procedure and anesthetic technique
- Determine the equipment, instruments, and supplies needed for care of the patient in surgery, and make arrangements for availability
- Assemble equipment, instruments, and supplies for the surgery
- Change into the scrubs, footwear, cap, and mask specific to the surgical area before entering the operating room
- Place tables containing instruments and equipment in the appropriate areas
- Check instruments and arrange in order of use
- Keep sharp and pointed objects (e.g., scalpel blades and needles) separate from other objects in order to avoid injuries during preparation
- Verify the safety and proper operation of the equipment and instruments required for patient care (e.g., surgical table, perfusion pumps, temperature regulating equipment, electric scalpels)

- Prepare supplies, drugs, and solutions for use, as indicated
- Obtain the sterile supplies and materials appropriate to the surgery, observing aseptic technique
- Confirm the integrity of the packages or wrappings, expiration dates, and sterility controls and follow the traceability of the materials in keeping with hospital regulations
- Prepare the consumable clothing and supplies appropriate to the type of surgery
- Turn on and position lights
- Drape the instrument tables, Mayo tables, and auxiliary tables with sterile cloth or impermeable fields, as appropriate
- Establish a safety perimeter around the tables and materials with regard to other professional and nonsterile areas
- Provide towels/pads for the surgical team to dry their hands on
- Secure devices in the surgical field (e.g., cables, circuit cameras, aspirators)
- Remove instruments and supplies from the surgical table once the surgery is finished
- Remove field forceps, aspirator tube, electric scalpel, and other elements from the surgical field following the conclusion of the operation
- Roll up the fields, sheets, and surgical drapes used in the surgery, avoiding the spread and contamination of the air, and dispose of them in an appropriate container
- Remove scalpel blades from their handles, needles, sharp, and pointed objects and deposit them in appropriate containers
- Separate the clean materials and instruments from the dirty or highly contaminated ones to facilitate cleaning, disinfection, and later sterilization
- Coordinate and assist in the cleaning and preparation of the operating room for the next patient (i.e., collect and put away machines, supports, and other supplies)

6th edition 2013

Background Readings:

Association of periOperative Registered Nurses. (2010). *Perioperative standards and recommended practices*. Denver: Author.

Fuller, J. (2008). *Surgical technology: Principles and practice* (4th ed.) Madrid: Panamericana.

Gruendemann, B. J. & Magnun, S. S. (2001). *Infection prevention in surgical settings*. Philadelphia: Saunders.

Phippen, M., Ulmer, B. C., & Wells, M. M. (2009). *Competency for safe patient care during operative and invasive procedures*. Denver: Competency & Credentialing Institute.

Rothrock, J. C. (2010). *Alexander's care of the patient in surgery* (14th ed.). St. Louis: Elsevier Mosby.

Rothrock, J. C. & Siefert, P. C. (2009). *Assisting in surgery: Patient centered care*. Denver: Competency & Credentialing Institute.

Surgical Precautions 2920

Definition: Minimizing the potential for iatrogenic injury to the patient related to a surgical procedure

Activities:
- Check ground isolation monitor
- Arrange the oxygenation and artificial ventilation equipment and material (e.g., laryngoscopes, tubes, aspirator, masks, Magill forceps, stiffening wires, phonendoscope)
- Verify the correct functioning of equipment
- Monitor the accessories specific to the required surgical position (e.g., supports, stirrups, fasteners)
- Check suction for adequate pressure and complete assembly of canisters, tubing, and catheters
- Remove any unsafe equipment
- Verify consent for surgery and other treatments, as appropriate
- Participate in a preoperative briefing with others, as per agency policy
- Welcome the patient, establishing a relationship of trust and offering counsel
- Verify with the patient or appropriate others the procedure and surgical site
- Verify that patient's identification band and blood band are correct
- Ask patient or appropriate other to state patient's name and birth date
- Participate in the preoperative "time out" to verify correct patient, procedure, and site, as per agency policy
- Ensure documentation and communication of any allergies
- Assist in the transfer of the patient to the surgical table while monitoring devices
- Preserve the patient's privacy, avoiding unnecessary exposure or chills
- Count sponges, sharps, and instruments before, during, and after surgery, as per agency policy
- Record results of counts, as per agency policy
- Remove and store prostheses appropriately
- Provide a sterile container for depositing sharp objects
- Provide an electrosurgical unit, grounding pad, and active electrode, as appropriate
- Verify integrity of electrical cords
- Verify proper functioning of electrosurgical unit
- Verify absence of cardiac pacemaker, other electrical implant, or metal prostheses, contraindicating use of electrosurgical cautery
- Verify that the patient is not touching metal
- Inspect the patient's skin at the site of grounding pad
- Apply grounding pad to dry, intact skin with minimal hair, over large muscle mass, and as close to the operative site as possible
- Verify that prep solutions are nonflammable, or that flammable prep agents have evaporated prior to draping
- Remove residual flammable prep agents before the start of surgery
- Evacuate oxygen from under surgical drapes
- Take precautions against ionizing radiation or use protective equipment in situations that require it, before the surgery starts
- Protect grounding pad from prep and irrigation solutions and damage
- Apply and use holster to store active electrode during surgery
- Adjust coagulation and cutting currents, as instructed by physician or agency policy
- Inspect the patient's skin for injury after use of electrosurgery

- Deposit waste materials in the appropriate containers
- Assist in the transfer of the patient, verifying the proper position of tubes, catheters, and drains, and adopting the position appropriate to the surgery performed
- Cover the patient to avoid unnecessary exposure and loss of heat
- Document appropriate information on the operative record
- Participate in a postoperative debriefing, as per agency policy

2nd edition 1996, revised 2013

Background Readings:

Association of periOperative Registered Nurses. (2010). *Perioperative standards and recommended practices.* Denver: Author.

Emergency Care Research Institute (ECRI). (2007). Electrosurgery. *Healthcare Risk Control Risk Analysis* (Vol. 4). Plymouth Meeting, PA: Author.

Fuller, J. (2008). *Surgical technology: Principles and practice* (4th ed.). Madrid: Panamericana.

Gruendemann, B. J. & Magnun, S. S. (2001). *Infection prevention in surgical settings.* Philadelphia: Saunders.

Phippen, M., Ulmer, B. C., & Wells, M. M. (2009). *Competency for safe patient care during operative and invasive procedures.* Denver: Competency & Credentialing Institute.

Rothrock, J. C. (2010). *Alexander's care of the patient in surgery* (14th ed.). St. Louis: Elsevier Mosby.

Rothrock, J. C. & Siefert, P. C. (2009). *Assisting in surgery: Patient centered care.* Denver: Competency & Credentialing Institute.

World Alliance for Patient Safety. (2008). *Surgical safety checklist and implementation manual.* Geneva, Switzerland: World Health Organization.

Surgical Preparation 2930

Definition: Providing care to a patient immediately prior to surgery and verifying required procedures/tests and documentation in the clinical record

Activities:

- Identify patient's level of anxiety/fear concerning the surgical procedure
- Reinforce preoperative teaching information
- Complete preoperative checklist
- Ensure patient is NPO, as appropriate
- Ensure that a completed history and physical is recorded in the chart
- Verify that the surgical consent form is properly signed
- Verify that the required lab and diagnostic test results are in the chart
- Verify that blood transfusions are available, as appropriate
- Verify that an EKG has been completed, as appropriate
- List allergies on the front of the chart
- Communicate special care considerations such as blindness, hearing loss, or handicap to operating room staff, as appropriate
- Determine whether patient's wishes about health care are known (e.g., advance directives, organ donor cards)
- Verify that patient identification band, allergy band, and blood bands are readable and in place
- Remove jewelry and/or tape rings in place, as appropriate
- Remove nail polish, makeup, and hairpins, as appropriate
- Remove dentures, glasses, contacts, or other prostheses, as appropriate
- Ensure that money or valuables are in a safe place, as appropriate
- Administer bowel preparation medications, as appropriate
- Explain preoperative medications that will be used, as appropriate
- Administer and document preoperative medications, as appropriate
- Start IV therapy, as directed
- Send required medications or equipment with patient to the operating room, as appropriate
- Insert NG tube or Foley catheter, as appropriate
- Explain tubing and equipment associated with preparation activities
- Administer surgical shave, scrub, shower, enema, and/or douche as appropriate
- Apply antiembolism stockings, as appropriate
- Apply sequential compression device sleeves, as appropriate
- Instruct patient to void immediately prior to preoperative medications, as appropriate
- Check that patient is in proper attire, based on institutional policy
- Support patient with high anxiety/fear level
- Assist patient onto cart for transport, as appropriate
- Provide time for family members to speak with patient prior to transport
- Encourage parents to accompany child to the operating room, as appropriate
- Provide information to family concerning waiting areas and visiting times for surgical patients
- Support family members, as appropriate
- Prepare room for patient's return postoperative

1st edition 1992; revised 2000

Background Readings:

Kozier, B., Erb, G., Berman, A., & Snyder, S. (2004). Perioperative nursing. In *Fundamentals of nursing: Concepts, processes, and practice* (7th ed., pp. 896–935). Upper Saddle River, NJ: Prentice Hall.

Perry, A. G. & Potter, P. A. (2006). *Clinical nursing skills and techniques* (6th ed.). St. Louis: Mosby.

S

Surveillance 6650

Definition: Purposeful and ongoing acquisition, interpretation, and synthesis of patient data for clinical decision-making

Activities:

- Determine patient's health risks, as appropriate
- Obtain information about normal behavior and routines
- Ask patient for her or his perception of health status
- Select appropriate patient indices for ongoing monitoring, based on patient's condition
- Determine presence of patient trigger areas for immediate response (e.g., change in vital signs, low or elevated heart rate, low or elevated blood pressure, difficulty breathing, low oxygen saturation despite increasing oxygen delivery, change in level of consciousness, repeated or prolonged seizures, chest pain, acute changes in mental status, or when nurse or patient "just feels something is wrong")
- Activate the rapid response team if indicated by presence of trigger areas, per agency protocol
- Ask patient about recent signs, symptoms, or problems
- Establish the frequency of data collection and interpretation, as indicated by status of the patient
- Monitor unstable or critically ill stable patients (e.g., patients who require frequent neurological assessments, patients experiencing cardiac dysrhythmias, patients receiving continuous intravenous infusions of medications such as nitroglycerine or insulin)
- Facilitate acquisition of diagnostic tests, as appropriate
- Interpret results of diagnostic tests, as appropriate
- Retrieve and interpret laboratory data
- Contact physician, as appropriate
- Explain diagnostic test results to patient and families
- Involve patient and family in monitoring activities, as appropriate
- Monitor patient's ability to do self-care activities
- Monitor neurological status
- Monitor behavior patterns
- Monitor cognitive ability
- Monitor emotional state
- Monitor vital signs, as appropriate
- Collaborate with physician to institute invasive hemodynamic monitoring, as appropriate
- Collaborate with physician to institute ICP monitoring, as appropriate
- Monitor comfort level, and take appropriate action
- Monitor coping strategies used by patient and family
- Monitor changes in sleep patterns
- Monitor oxygenation and initiate measures to promote adequate oxygenation of vital organs
- Initiate routine skin surveillance in high-risk patient
- Monitor for signs and symptoms of fluid and electrolyte imbalance
- Monitor tissue perfusion, as appropriate
- Monitor for infection, as appropriate
- Monitor nutritional status, as appropriate
- Monitor gastrointestinal function, as appropriate
- Monitor elimination patterns, as appropriate
- Monitor for bleeding tendencies in high-risk patient
- Note type and amount of drainage from tubes and orifices and notify the physician of significant changes
- Troubleshoot equipment and systems to enhance acquisition of reliable patient data
- Compare current status with previous status to detect improvements and deterioration in patient's condition
- Initiate and/or change medical treatment to maintain patient parameters within the limits ordered by the physician, using established protocols
- Facilitate acquisition of interdisciplinary services (e.g., pastoral services or audiology), as appropriate
- Obtain a physician consult when patient data indicates a needed change in medical therapy
- Institute appropriate treatment, using standing protocols
- Prioritize actions, based on patient status
- Analyze physician orders in conjunction with patient status to ensure safety of the patient
- Obtain consultation from the appropriate health care worker to initiate new treatment or change existing treatments
- Provide proper environment for desirable patient outcomes (e.g., match nurse competency to patient care needs; provide required patient to nurse ratio; provide adequate auxiliary staffing; ensure continuity of care)

1st edition 1992; revised 2004; 2013

Background Readings:

Baird, S. K. & Turbin, L. B. (2011). Condition concern: An innovative response system for enhancing hospitalized patient care and safety. *Journal of Nursing Care Quality, 26*(3), 199–207.

Butner, S. C. (2011). Rapid response team effectiveness. *Dimensions of Critical Care Nursing, 30*(4), 201–205.

Kelly, L. & Vincent, D. (2011). The dimensions of nursing surveillance: A concept analysis. *Journal of Advanced Nursing, 67*(3), 652–661.

Kutney-Lee, A., Lake, E. T., & Aiken, L. H. (2009). Development of the hospital nurse surveillance capacity profile. *Research in Nursing & Health, 32*(2), 217–222.

Mailey, J., Digiovine, B., Baillod, D., Gnam, G., Jordan, J., & Rubinfeld, I., (2006). Reducing hospital standardized mortality rate with early interventions. *Journal of Trauma Nursing, 13*(4), 178–182.

Schmid, A., Hoffman, L., Happ, M. B., Wolf, G. A., & DeVita, M. (2007). Failure to rescue: A literature review. *Journal of Nursing Administration, 37*(4), 188–198.

Shever, L. L. (2011). The impact of nursing surveillance on failure to rescue. *Research & Theory for Nursing Practice, 25*(2), 107–126.

Shever, L. L., Titler, M. G., Kerr, P., Qin, R., Kim, T., & Picone, D. M. (2008). The effect of high nursing surveillance on hospital cost. *Journal of Nursing Scholarship, 40*(2), 161–169.

S

Surveillance: Community   6652

Definition: Purposeful and ongoing acquisition, interpretation, and synthesis of data for decision- making in the community

Activities:
- Identify the purpose, procedure, and reporting mechanisms for required and voluntary health data reporting systems
- Collect data related to health events, such as diseases and injuries to be reported
- Establish frequency of data collection and analysis
- Report data using standard reporting mechanisms
- Collaborate with other agencies in the collection, analysis, and reporting of data
- Follow up on reports to appropriate agencies to ensure accuracy and usefulness of information
- Instruct patients, families, and agencies regarding the importance of follow-up of contagious disease treatment
- Participate in program development (e.g., teaching, policy making, lobbying) as associated with community data collection and reporting
- Use reports to recognize need for additional data collection, analysis, and interpretation

3rd edition 2000

Background Readings:

Block, A. B., Onorato, I. M., Ihle, W. W., Hadler, J. L., Hayden, C. H., & Snider, D. E. (1996). The need for epidemic intelligence. *Public Health Reports, 111*(1), 26–33.

Clemen-Stone, S., McGuire, S., & Eigisti, D. (1997). *Comprehensive community health nursing: Family, aggregate, and community practice.* St. Louis: Mosby.

Harkness, G. (1995). *Epidemiology in nursing practice.* St. Louis: Mosby.

U.S. Department of Health & Human Services. (1991). *Healthy people 2000: National health promotion and disease prevention objectives.* Washington, DC: U.S. Government Printing Service.

U.S. Department of Health & Human Services. (1995). *Healthy people 2000: Midcourse review and 1995 revisions.* Washington, DC: U.S. Government Printing Service.

Valanais, B. (1992). *Epidemiology in nursing and health care* (2nd ed.). Norwalk, CT: Appleton & Lange.

Surveillance: Late Pregnancy   6656

Definition: Purposeful and ongoing acquisition, interpretation, and synthesis of maternal-fetal data for treatment, observation, or admission

Activities:
- Review obstetrical history, if available
- Determine maternal-fetal health risk(s) through client interview
- Establish gestational age by reviewing history or calculating expected date of confinement (EDC) from last menstrual period
- Monitor maternal vital signs
- Monitor behavior of woman and support person
- Implement electronic fetal monitoring
- Inquire about presence and quality of fetal movement
- Monitor for signs of premature labor (e.g., <4 contractions per hour, backache, cramping, show, and pelvic pressure from 20 to 37 weeks of gestation), as appropriate
- Monitor for signs of pregnancy-induced hypertension (e.g., hypertension, headache, blurred vision, nausea, vomiting, visual alterations, hyperreflexia, edema, and proteinuria), as appropriate
- Monitor elimination patterns, as appropriate
- Monitor for signs of urinary tract infection, as appropriate
- Facilitate acquisition of diagnostic tests, as appropriate
- Interpret results of diagnostic tests, as appropriate
- Retrieve and interpret laboratory data; contact physician, as appropriate
- Explain diagnostic test results to patient and family
- Initiate interventions for IV therapy, fluid resuscitation, and medication administration, as ordered
- Monitor comfort level, and take appropriate action
- Monitor nutritional status, as appropriate
- Monitor changes in sleep patterns, as appropriate
- Obtain history of sexually transmitted diseases and frequency of intercourse, as appropriate
- Monitor uterine activity (e.g., frequency, duration, and intensity of contractions)
- Perform Leopold's maneuver to determine fetal position
- Note type, amount, and onset of vaginal drainage
- Perform speculum exam for diagnosis of spontaneous rupture of amniotic membranes, unless there is evidence of frank bleeding
- Test amniotic fluid (e.g., nitrazaine, ferning, and pooling), as appropriate
- Obtain cervical cultures, as appropriate (e.g., history of beta-streptococcal infection, herpes, or prolonged rupture of membranes)
- Examine cervix for dilatation, effacement, softening, position, and station
- Perform ultrasonography to determine fetal presentation or placental position, as appropriate
- Institute appropriate treatment, using standing protocols
- Prioritize actions, based on patient status (e.g., treat, continue to observe, admit, or discharge)

2nd edition 1996

Background Readings:

Angelini, D. J., Zannieri, C. L., Silva, V. B., Fein, E., & Ward, P. J. (1990). Toward a concept of triage for labor and delivery: Staff perceptions and role utilization. *Journal of Perinatal & Neonatal Nursing, 4*(3), 1–11.

Eganhouse, D. J. (1991). A comparative study of variables differentiating false labor from early labor. *Journal of Perinatology, 11*(3), 249–257.

Pillitteri, A. (2007). *Maternal and child health nursing: Care of the childbearing and childrearing family* (5th ed.). Philadelphia: Lippincott Williams & Wilkins.

S

Surveillance: Remote Electronic 6658

Definition: Purposeful and ongoing acquisition of patient data via electronic modalities (telephone, video, conferencing, e-mail) from distant locations, as well as interpretation and synthesis of patient data for clinical decision-making with individuals or populations

Activities:

- Determine that you are interacting with the patient or, if with someone else, that you have the patient's permission to interact with them
- Identify self with name, credentials, organization; let caller know if call is being recorded (e.g., for quality monitoring)
- Inform patient about interaction process and obtain consent
- Determine patient's health risk(s), as appropriate
- Obtain information about usual patient behavior and routines
- Establish the frequency of data collection and interpretation, as indicated by status of the patient
- Monitor incoming data for validity and reliability
- Interpret results of diagnostic indicators such as vital signs, glucose readings, EKGs
- Collaborate/consult with physician resources, as necessary
- Explain test results and interventions to patient and family
- Monitor comfort level, and take appropriate action
- Monitor coping strategies and actions used by patient and family
- Initiate skin surveillance in high-risk patient when high resolution video monitoring is in use
- Monitor for potential problems, based on current status (i.e., infection, fluid and electrolyte balance, tissue perfusion, nutrition, and elimination)
- Troubleshoot all equipment and systems to enhance acquisition of reliable patient data
- Coordinate placement/replacement/setup of equipment/supplies
- Compare current status with previous status to detect improvements and or deterioration in patient's condition
- Initiate and/or change medical treatment to maintain patient parameter with the limits ordered by the physician, using established guidelines
- Facilitate acquisition of interdisciplinary services (e.g., pastoral services), as appropriate
- Prioritize actions based on patient status
- Analyze physician orders in conjunction with patient status to ensure safety of the patient
- Obtain consultation from appropriate health care worker to initiate new treatment or change existing treatments
- Advocate for patient's welfare, as necessary
- Maintain confidentiality, keeping in mind the specific threats to confidentiality implicit in the electronic modality in use
- Determine need and establish time intervals for further intermittent assessment
- Document assessments, advice, instructions, or other information given to patient, according to specified guidelines
- Determine how patient or family member can be reached for future surveillance, as appropriate
- Document permission for return call and identify person(s) able to receive call
- Identify or aggregate data that has programmatic or population implications

3rd edition 2000

Background Readings:

American Academy of Ambulatory Care Nursing & American Nurses Association. (1997). *Nursing in ambulatory care: The future is here.* Washington, DC: American Nurses.

American Academy of Ambulatory Nursing. (1997). *Telephone nursing practice administration and practice standards.* Pitman, NJ: Anthony J. Jannetti.

Wheeler, S. Q. & Windt, J. H. (Eds.). (1993). *Telephone triage: Theory, practice, and protocol development.* Albany, NY: Delmar.

Sustenance Support 7500

Definition: Helping an individual/family in need to locate food, clothing, or shelter

Activities:

- Determine adequacy of patient's financial situation
- Determine adequacy of food supplies in home
- Inform individual/families about how to access local food pantries and free lunch programs
- Inform individual/families about how to access low-rent housing and subsidy programs
- Inform about rental laws and protections
- Inform individual/families of available emergency housing shelter programs
- Arrange transportation to emergency housing shelter
- Discuss with the individual/families available job service agencies
- Arrange for individual/families transportation to job services, if necessary
- Inform individual/families of agency providing clothing assistance
- Arrange transportation to agency providing clothing assistance, as necessary
- Inform individual/families of agency programs for support, such as Red Cross and Salvation Army, as appropriate
- Discuss with the individual/families financial aid support available
- Assist individual/families to complete forms for assistance, such as housing and financial aid
- Inform individual/families of available free health clinics
- Assist individual/families to reach free health clinics
- Inform individual/families of eligibility requirements for food stamps
- Inform individual/families of available schools and/or day care centers, as appropriate

1st edition 1992; revised 2001, 2008

Background Readings:

Brush, B. L. & Powers, E. M. (2001). Health and service utilization patterns among homeless men in transition: Exploring the need for on-site, shelter-based nursing care. *Scholarly Inquiry in Nursing Practice, 15*(2), 143–154.

Green, D. M. (2005). History, discussion and review of a best practices model for service delivery for the homeless. *Social Work in Mental Health, 3*(4), 1–16

Mulroy, E. A. (2004). A user-friendly approach to program evaluation and effective community interventions for families at risk of homelessness. *Social Work, 49*(4), 573–586.

Strehlow, A. J. & Amos-Jones, T. (1999). The homeless as a vulnerable population. *Nursing Clinics of North America, 34*(2), 261–274.

Suturing   3620

Definition: Approximating edges of a wound using sterile suture material and a needle

Activities:
- Identify patient allergies to anesthetics, tape, and/or providone-iodine or other topical solutions
- Identify history of keloid formation, as appropriate
- Refer deep, facial, joint, or potentially infected wounds to a physician
- Immobilize a frightened child or confused adult, as appropriate
- Shave hair from the immediate wound site
- Cleanse the surrounding skin with soap and water or other mild antiseptic solution
- Use sterile technique
- Administer a topical or injectable anesthetic to the area, as appropriate
- Allow sufficient time for the anesthetic to numb the area
- Select an appropriate gauge suture material
- Determine method of suturing (continuous or interrupted) most appropriate for the wound
- Position the needle so that it enters and exits perpendicular to the skin surface
- Pull the needle through, following the line or curve of the needle itself
- Pull the suture tight enough to not buckle the skin
- Secure the suture line with square knots
- Cleanse the area before applying an antiseptic or dressing
- Apply a dressing, as appropriate
- Instruct patient on how to care for the suture line, including signs and symptoms of infection
- Instruct patient when sutures should be removed
- Remove sutures, as indicated
- Schedule return visit, as appropriate

1st edition 1992; revised 1996

Background Readings:

Meeker, M. H. & Rothrock, J. C. (1998). *Alexander's care of the patient in surgery* (11th ed.). St. Louis: Mosby.

Perry, A. G. & Potter, P. A. (2006). *Clinical nursing skills and techniques* (6th ed.). St. Louis: Mosby.

Swallowing Therapy   1860

Definition: Facilitating swallowing and preventing complications of impaired swallowing

Activities:
- Collaborate with other members of health care team (i.e., occupational therapist, speech pathologist, and dietician) to provide continuity in patient's rehabilitative plan
- Determine patient's ability to focus attention on learning/performing eating and swallowing tasks
- Remove distractions from environment prior to working with patient on swallowing
- Provide privacy for patient, as desired or indicated
- Position self so that patient can see and hear you speak
- Explain rationale of swallowing regimen to patient/family
- Collaborate with speech therapist to instruct patient's family about swallowing exercise regimen
- Provide/use assistive devices, as appropriate
- Avoid use of drinking straws
- Assist patient to sit in an erect position (as close to 90 degrees as possible) for feeding/exercise
- Assist patient to position head in forward flexion in preparation for swallowing ("chin tuck")
- Assist to maintain sitting position for 30 minutes after completing meal
- Instruct patient to open and close mouth in preparation for food manipulation
- Instruct patient not to talk during eating, if appropriate
- Guide patient in phonating staccato "ahs" to promote soft palate elevation, if appropriate
- Provide a lollipop for patient to suck on to enhance tongue strength, if appropriate
- Assist hemiplegic patient to sit with affected arm forward on table
- Assist patient to place food at back of mouth and on unaffected side
- Monitor for signs and symptoms of aspiration
- Monitor patient's tongue movements while eating
- Monitor for sealing of lips during eating, drinking, and swallowing

S

- Monitor for signs of fatigue during eating, drinking, and swallowing
- Provide rest period before eating/exercise to prevent excessive fatigue
- Check mouth for pocketing of food after eating
- Instruct patient to reach for particles of food on lips or chin with tongue
- Assist patient to remove food particles from lips and chin, if patient is unable to extend tongue
- Instruct family/caregiver how to position, feed, and monitor patient
- Instruct patient/caregiver on nutritional requirements and dietary modifications, in collaboration with dietician
- Instruct patient/caregiver on emergency measures for choking
- Instruct patient/caregiver how to check for pocketed food after eating
- Provide written instructions, as appropriate
- Provide scheduled practice sessions for family/caregiver, as needed
- Provide/monitor consistency of food/liquid based on findings of swallowing study
- Consult with therapist and/or physician to gradually advance consistency of patient's food
- Assist to maintain adequate caloric and fluid intake
- Monitor body weight
- Monitor body hydration (e.g., intake, output, skin turgor, mucous membranes)
- Provide mouth care as needed

1st edition 1992; revised 2000

Background Readings:

Baker, D. M. (1993). Assessment and management of impairments in swallowing. *Nursing Clinics of North America, 28*(4), 793–806.

Davies, P. (1993). *Steps to follow: A guide to the treatment of adult hemiplegia based on the concept of K & B Bobath.* Berlin, Germany: Springer-Verlag.

Emick-Herring, B. & Wood, P. (1990). A team approach to neurologically based swallowing disorders. *Rehabilitation Nursing, 15*(3), 126–132.

Glick, O. J. (1992). Interventions related to activity and movement. In G. M. Bulechek & J. C. McCloskey (Eds.), Symposium on nursing interventions. *Nursing Clinics of North America, 27*(2), 541–568.

Killen, J. M. (1996). Understanding dysphagia: Interventions for care. *MEDSURG Nursing, 5*(2), 99–105.

Maat, M. T. & Tandy, L. (1991). Impaired swallowing. In M. Maas, K. Buckwalter, & M. Hardy (Eds.), *Nursing diagnoses and interventions for the elderly* (pp. 106–116). Redwood City, CA: Addison-Wesley.

McHale, J. M., Phipps, M. A., Horvath, K., & Schmelz, J. (1998). Expert nursing knowledge in the care of patients at risk for impaired swallowing. *Image: Journal of Nursing Scholarship, 30*(2), 137–141.

Perry, A. G. & Potter, P. A. (2006). *Clinical nursing skills and techniques* (6th ed.). St. Louis: Mosby.

S

Teaching: Disease Process   5602

Definition: Assisting the patient to understand information related to a specific disease process

Activities:
- Appraise the patient's current level of knowledge related to specific disease process
- Explain the pathophysiology of the disease and how it relates to the anatomy and physiology, as appropriate
- Review patient's knowledge about condition
- Acknowledge patient's knowledge about condition
- Describe common signs and symptoms of the disease, as appropriate
- Explore with patient what she/he has already done to manage the symptoms
- Describe the disease process, as appropriate
- Identify possible etiologies, as appropriate
- Provide information to the patient about condition, as appropriate
- Identify changes in physical condition for patient
- Avoid empty reassurances
- Provide reassurance about patient's condition, as appropriate
- Provide the family/significant other(s) with information about the patient's progress, as appropriate
- Provide information about available diagnostic measures, as appropriate
- Discuss lifestyle changes that may be required to prevent future complications and/or control the disease process
- Discuss therapy/treatment options
- Describe rationale behind management/therapy/treatment recommendations
- Encourage the patient to explore options/get a second opinion, as appropriate or indicated
- Describe possible chronic complications, as appropriate
- Instruct the patient on measures to prevent/minimize side effects of treatment for the disease, as appropriate
- Instruct the patient on measures to control/minimize symptoms, as appropriate
- Explore possible resources/support, as appropriate
- Refer the patient to local community agencies/support groups, as appropriate
- Instruct the patient on which signs and symptoms to report to the health care provider, as appropriate
- Provide the phone number(s) to call if complications occur
- Reinforce information provided by other health care team members, as appropriate

1st edition 1992; revised 2000, 2004

Background Readings:
Kozier, B., Erb, G., Berman, A., & Snyder, S. (2004). Teaching. In *Fundamentals of nursing: Concepts, processes, and practice* (7th ed., pp. 445–468). Upper Saddle River, NJ: Prentice Hall.
Rakel, B. A. (1992). Interventions related to patient teaching. In G. M. Bulechek & J. C. McCloskey (Eds.), Symposium on nursing interventions. *Nursing Clinics of North America, 27*(2), 397–424.

Teaching: Foot Care   5603

Definition: Preparing a patient at risk and/or significant other to provide preventive foot care

Activities:
- Determine current level of knowledge and skills related to foot care
- Determine current foot care practices
- Provide information related to the level of risk for injury
- Recommend toe nail and callus trimming by a specialist, as appropriate
- Provide written foot care guidelines
- Assist in developing a plan for daily foot assessment and care at home
- Determine capacity to carry out foot care, (i.e., visual acuity, physical mobility, and judgment)
- Recommend assistance of a significant other with foot care if vision is impaired or if there are problems with mobility
- Recommend daily foot inspection over all surfaces and between the toes looking for redness, swelling, warmth, dryness, maceration, tenderness, or open areas
- Instruct to use a mirror or the assistance of another to carry out foot inspection, as needed
- Recommend daily washing of feet using warm water and mild soap
- Recommend thoroughly drying feet after washing them, especially between the toes
- Instruct to hydrate the skin daily by brief soaking or bathing in room temperature water followed by application of an emollient
- Provide information regarding the relationship between neuropathy, injury, and vascular disease and the risk for ulceration and lower extremity amputation in persons with diabetes
- Advise regarding when it is appropriate to contact a health professional, including the presence of a nonhealing or infected lesion
- Advise regarding appropriate self-care measures for minor foot problems
- Caution about potential sources of injury to the feet, (e.g., heat, cold, cutting corns or calluses, chemicals, use of strong antiseptics or astringents, use of adhesive tape, and going barefoot or wearing thongs or open-toe shoes)
- Instruct on proper technique for toenail trimming, (i.e., cutting relatively straight across, following the contour of the toe, and filing sharp edges with an emery board)
- Instruct on care of soft calluses, including gentle buffing with a towel or pumice stone after a bath

T

- Recommend specialist care for thick fungal or ingrown toenails, corns, or calluses, as indicated
- Describe appropriate shoes, (i.e., low heeled with a shoe shape that matches foot shape; adequate depth of toe box; soles made of material that will absorb shock; adjustable fit by lace or straps; uppers made of breathable, soft, and flexible materials; changes made for gait and limb-length disorders; and potential for modification, if necessary)
- Describe appropriate socks, (i.e., absorbent material and non-constricting)
- Recommend guidelines to be followed when purchasing new shoes, including having feet properly measured and fitted at the time of purchase
- Recommend wearing new shoes only for a few hours at a time for the first two weeks
- Instruct to inspect inside shoes daily for foreign objects, nail points, torn linings, and rough areas
- Instruct to change shoes two times, (e.g., 12 noon and 5 pm) each day to avoid local repetitive pressure
- Explain the necessity for prescriptive footwear or orthotics, as appropriate
- Caution about activities that cause pressure on nerves and blood vessels, including elastic bands on socks or crossing legs
- Advise to stop smoking, as appropriate
- Include the family/significant others in instruction, as appropriate
- Reinforce information provided by other health professionals, as appropriate

4th edition 2004

Background Readings:

American Diabetes Association. (1998). Preventive foot care in people with diabetes. *Diabetes, 21*(12), 2178–2179.

Collier, J. H., Kinion, E. S., & Brodbeck, C. A. (1996). Evolving role of CNSs in developing risk-anchored preventive interventions. *Clinical Nurse Specialist, 10*(3), 131–136, 143.

Culleton, J. L. (1999). Preventing diabetic foot complications. *Postgraduate Medicine, 106*(1), 78–84.

Kozier, B., Erb, G., Berman, A., & Snyder, S. (2004). Hygiene. In *Fundamentals of nursing: Concepts, processes, and practice* (7th ed., pp. 679–755). Upper Saddle River, NJ: Prentice Hall.

Kruger, S., & Guthrie, D. (1992). Foot care: Knowledge, retention, and self-care practices. *The Diabetes Educator, 18*(6), 487–490.

Litzelman, D. K., Slemenda, C. W., Langefeld, C. D., Hays, L. M., Welch, M. A., Bild, D. E., et al. (1993). Reduction of lower extremity clinical abnormalities in patients with non-insulin-dependent diabetes. A randomized controlled trial. *Annals of Internal Medicine, 119*(1), 36–41.

Mayfield, J. A., Reiber, G. E., Sanders, L. J., Janise, D., & Pogach, L. M. (1998). Preventive foot care in people with diabetes. *Diabetes Care, 21*(12), 2161–2177.

Plummer, E. S., & Albert, S. G. (1995). Foot care assessment in patients with diabetes: A screening algorithm for patient education and referral. *The Diabetic Educator, 21*(1), 47–51.

Reiber, G. E., Pecoraro, R. E., & Koepsell, T. D. (1992). Risk factors for amputation in patient with diabetes mellitus. A case control study. *Annuals of Internal Medicine, 117*(2), 97–105.

Teaching: Group 5604

Definition: Development, implementation, and evaluation of a patient teaching program for a group of individuals experiencing the same health condition

Activities:

- Provide an environment conducive to learning
- Include the family/significant others, as appropriate
- Establish the need for a program
- Determine administrative support
- Determine budget
- Coordinate resources within the facility to form a planning/advisory committee that can contribute to positive outcomes for the program and provide a forum for ensuring commitment to the program
- Utilize community resources, as appropriate
- Define potential target population(s)
- Write program goals
- Outline major content area(s)
- Write learning objectives
- Write a job description for a coordinator responsible for patient education
- Select a coordinator
- Preview available educational materials
- Develop new educational materials, as appropriate
- List possible teaching strategies, educational materials, and learning activities
- Train the teaching personnel, as appropriate
- Educate the staff about the patient teaching program, as appropriate
- Provide a written schedule, including dates, times, and places of the teaching sessions/classes, to the staff and/or patient(s), as appropriate
- Determine appropriate days/times to reach maximum number of patients
- Prepare announcements/memos to publicize outcomes, as appropriate
- Control the size and competencies of the group, as appropriate
- Orient patient(s)/significant others to educational program and the objectives it is designed to accomplish
- Provide for special needs of learners (i.e., handicap access, portable oxygen), as appropriate
- Adapt the educational methods/materials to the group's learning needs/characteristics, as appropriate
- Provide group instruction
- Evaluate the patient's progress in the program and mastery of content
- Document the patient's progress on the permanent medical record
- Revise teaching strategies/learning activities, if necessary, to increase learning

T

- Provide forms for the patient to evaluate the program
- Provide for further individual instruction as appropriate
- Evaluate the extent to which program goals were attained
- Communicate the program's goal attainment evaluation to the planning/advisory committee
- Hold summative evaluation sessions for the planning/advisory committee to revamp the program, as appropriate
- Document the number of patients who have attained the learning objectives
- Refer the patient to other specialists/agencies to meet the learning objectives, as appropriate

1st edition 1992; revised 2000

Background Readings:

Bastable, S. B. (1997). *Nurse as educator: Principles of teaching and learning* (pp. 264–266). Sudbury, MA: Jones & Bartlett.

Kozier, B., Erb, G., Berman, A., & Snyder, S. (2004). Teaching. In *Fundamentals of nursing: Concepts, processes, and practice* (7th ed., pp. 446–468). Upper Saddle River, NJ: Prentice Hall.

Rakel, B. A. (1992). Interventions related to patient teaching. In G. M. Bulechek & J. C. McCloskey (Eds.), Symposium on nursing interventions. *Nursing Clinics of North America, 27*(2), 397–424.

Redman, B. K. (1997). Teaching: Theory, and interpersonal techniques. In B. K. Redman (Ed.), *The process of patient education* (8th ed.). St. Louis: Mosby.

Teaching: Individual   5606

Definition: Planning, implementation, and evaluation of a teaching program designed to address a patient's particular needs

Activities:
- Establish rapport
- Establish teacher credibility, as appropriate
- Determine the patient's learning needs
- Determine patient readiness to learn
- Appraise the patient's current level of knowledge and understanding of content
- Appraise the patient's educational level
- Appraise the patient's cognitive, psychomotor, and affective abilities or disabilities
- Determine the patient's ability to learn specific information (i.e., developmental level, physiological status, orientation, pain, fatigue, unfulfilled basic needs, emotional state, and adaptation to illness)
- Determine the patient's motivation to learn specific information (i.e., health beliefs, past noncompliance, bad experiences with health care or learning, and conflicting goals)
- Enhance the patient's readiness to learn, as appropriate
- Set mutual, realistic learning goals with the patient
- Identify learning objectives necessary to reach goals
- Determine the sequence for presenting the information
- Appraise the patient's learning style
- Select appropriate teaching methods and strategies
- Select appropriate educational materials
- Provide instructional pamphlets, videos, and online resources, when appropriate
- Tailor the content to the patient's cognitive, psychomotor, and affective abilities or disabilities
- Adjust instruction to facilitate learning, as appropriate
- Provide an environment conducive to learning
- Instruct the patient, when appropriate
- Evaluate the patient's achievement of the stated objectives
- Reinforce behavior, as appropriate
- Correct information misinterpretations, as appropriate
- Provide time for the patient to ask questions and discuss concerns
- Select new teaching methods or strategies, if previous ones were ineffective
- Refer the patient to other specialists or agencies to meet the learning objectives, as appropriate
- Document the content presented, the written materials provided, and the patient's receptivity to and understanding of the information or patient behaviors that indicate learning, on the permanent medical record
- Include the family, as appropriate

1st edition 1992; revised 2013

Background Readings:

Falvo, D. R. (2011). *Effective patient education: A guide to increased adherence.* Sudbury, MA: Jones & Bartlett.

Friedman, A. J., Cosby, R., Boyko, S., Hatton-Bauer, J., & Turnbull, G. (2011). Effective teaching strategies and methods of delivery for patient education: A systematic review and practice guideline recommendations. *Journal of Cancer Education, 26*(1), 12–21.

Garvey, N., & Noonan, B. (2011). Providing individualized education to patients post myocardial infarction: A literature review. *British Journal of Cardiac Nursing, 6*(2), 73–79.

Potter, P. A., & Perry, A. C. (2009). *Fundamentals of nursing* (7th ed.). St. Louis: Mosby .

T

Teaching: Infant Nutrition 0-3 Months 5640

Definition: Instruction on nutrition and feeding practices through the first three months of life

Activities:

- Provide parents with written materials appropriate to identified knowledge needs
- Instruct parent/caregiver to feed only breast milk or formula for first year (no solids before 4 months)
- Instruct parent/caregiver to always hold infant when giving bottle
- Instruct parent/caregiver to never prop bottle or give bottle in bed
- Instruct parent/caregiver to avoid putting cereal in bottle (only formula or breast milk)
- Instruct parent/caregiver to limit water intake to ½ oz to 1 oz at a time, 4 oz daily
- Instruct parent/caregiver to avoid use of honey or corn syrup
- Instruct parent/caregiver to allow nonnutritive sucking
- Instruct parent/caregiver to discard leftover formula and clean bottle after every feeding

5th edition 2008

Background Readings:

Barnes, L. A. (Ed.). (1993). *Pediatric nutrition handbook* (3rd ed.). Elk Grove Village, IL: American Academy of Pediatrics.

California Department of Health Services WIC Supplemental Nutrition Branch. (1998). *Feeding your baby birth to 8 months* [Brochure]. Sacramento, CA: Author.

Formon, S. J. (1993). *Nutrition of normal infants.* St. Louis: Mosby.

Hockenberry, M. J. (2005). *Wong's essentials of pediatric nursing* (7th ed.). St. Louis: Mosby.

Hockenberry, M. J. (2006). *Wong's nursing care for infants and children* (8th ed.). St. Louis: Mosby.

Pillitteri, A. (2007). *Maternal and child health nursing: Care of the childbearing and childrearing family* (5th ed.). Philadelphia: Lippincott Williams & Wilkins.

Satter, E., & Sharkey, P. B. (1997). *Ellyn Satter's nutrition and feeding for infants and children: Handout masters.* Madison, WI: Author.

Teaching: Infant Nutrition 4-6 Months 5641

Definition: Instruction on nutrition and feeding practices from the fourth month through the sixth month of life

Activities:

- Provide parents with written materials appropriate to identified knowledge needs
- Instruct parent/caregiver to introduce solids (pureed) without added salt or sugar
- Instruct parent/caregiver to introduce iron-fortified infant cereal
- Instruct parent/caregiver to introduce one new food at a time
- Instruct parent/caregiver to avoid giving juice or sweetened drinks
- Instruct parent/caregiver to feed from a spoon only

5th edition 2008

Formon, S. J. (1993). *Nutrition of normal infants.* St. Louis: Mosby.

Hockenberry, M. J. (2005). *Wong's essentials of pediatric nursing* (7th ed.). St. Louis: Mosby.

Hockenberry, M. J. (2006). *Wong's nursing care for infants and children* (8th ed.). St. Louis: Mosby.

Pillitteri, A. (2007). *Maternal and child health nursing: Care of the childbearing and childrearing family* (5th ed.). Philadelphia: Lippincott Williams & Wilkins.

Satter, E., & Sharkey, P. B. (1997). *Ellyn Satter's nutrition and feeding for infants and children: Handout masters.* Madison, WI: Author.

T

Background Readings:

Barnes, L. A. (Ed.). (1993). *Pediatric nutrition handbook* (3rd ed.). Elk Grove Village, IL: American Academy of Pediatrics.

California Department of Health Services WIC Supplemental Nutrition Branch. (1998). *Feeding your baby birth to 8 months* [Brochure]. Sacramento, CA: Author.

Teaching: Infant Nutrition 7-9 Months   5642

Definition: Instruction on nutrition and feeding practices from the seventh month through the ninth month of life

Activities:

- Provide parents with written materials appropriate to identified knowledge needs
- Instruct parent/caregiver to introduce finger foods when infant can sit up
- Instruct parent/caregiver to introduce cup when infant can sit up
- Instruct parent/caregiver to have infant join family at meal times
- Instruct parent/caregiver to let infant begin self-feedings and observe to avoid choking
- Instruct parent/caregiver to offer fluids after solids
- Instruct parent/caregiver to avoid sugary desserts and soda
- Instruct parent/caregiver to offer a variety of foods, according to the food pyramid
- Instruct parent/caregiver to introduce limited amounts of diluted juice in a cup

5th edition 2008

Background Readings:

Barnes, L. A. (Ed.). (1993). *Pediatric nutrition handbook* (3rd ed.). Elk Grove Village, IL: American Academy of Pediatrics.

California Department of Health Services WIC Supplemental Nutrition Branch. (1998a). *Feeding your baby 6–12 months* [Brochure]. Sacramento, CA: Author.

California Department of Health Services WIC Supplemental Nutrition Branch. (1998b). *Feeding your baby birth to 8 months* [Brochure]. Sacramento, CA: Author.

Formon, S. J. (1993). *Nutrition of normal infants*. St. Louis: Mosby.

Hockenberry, M. J. (2005). *Wong's essentials of pediatric nursing* (7th ed.). St. Louis: Mosby.

Hockenberry, M. J. (2006). *Wong's nursing care for infants and children* (8th ed.). St. Louis: Mosby.

Pillitteri, A. (2007). *Maternal and child health nursing: Care of the childbearing and childrearing family* (5th ed.). Philadelphia: Lippincott Williams & Wilkins.

Satter, E., & Sharkey, P. B. (1997). *Ellyn Satter's nutrition and feeding for infants and children: Handout masters*. Madison, WI: Author.

Teaching: Infant Nutrition 10-12 Months   5643

Definition: Instruction on nutrition and feeding practices from the tenth month through the twelfth month of life

Activities:

- Provide parents with written materials appropriate to identified knowledge needs
- Instruct parent/caregiver to offer three meals and healthy snacks
- Instruct parent/caregiver to begin to wean from bottle
- Instruct parent/caregiver to avoid fruit drinks and flavored milk
- Instruct parent/caregiver to begin table foods
- Instruct parent/caregiver to allow infant to feed self with a spoon

5th edition 2008

Formon, S. J. (1993). *Nutrition of normal infants*. St. Louis: Mosby.

Hockenberry, M. J. (2005). *Wong's essentials of pediatric nursing* (7th ed.). St. Louis: Mosby.

Hockenberry, M. J. (2006). *Wong's nursing care for infants and children* (8th ed.). St. Louis: Mosby.

Pillitteri, A. (2007). *Maternal and child health nursing: Care of the childbearing and childrearing family* (5th ed.). Philadelphia: Lippincott Williams & Wilkins.

Satter, E., & Sharkey, P. B. (1997). *Ellyn Satter's nutrition and feeding for infants and children: Handout masters*. Madison, WI: Author.

Background Readings:

Barnes, L. A. (Ed.). (1993). *Pediatric nutrition handbook* (3rd ed.). Elk Grove Village, IL: American Academy of Pediatrics.

California Department of Health Services WIC Supplemental Nutrition Branch. (1998). *Feeding your baby 6–12 months* [Brochure]. Sacramento, CA: Author.

T

Teaching: Infant Safety 0-3 Months   5645

Definition: Instruction on safety through the first three months of life

Activities:

- Provide parents with written materials appropriate to identified knowledge needs
- Instruct parent/caregiver to install and use car seat according to manufacturer's recommendations
- Instruct parent/caregiver to place infant on back to sleep and keep loose bedding, pillows, and toys out of crib
- Instruct parent/caregiver to use only cribs that are safe
- Instruct parent/caregiver to avoid use of jewelry or cords/chains on infant
- Instruct parent/caregiver to use and maintain all equipment properly (e.g., swings, strollers, playpens, port-a-cribs)
- Instruct parent/caregiver to avoid holding infant while drinking hot liquids or smoking

- Instruct parent/caregiver to hold infant when feeding, avoid propping of bottle, and test formula temperature
- Instruct parent/caregiver to monitor experienced/trained child-care providers
- Instruct parent/caregiver how to prevent falls
- Instruct parent/caregiver to test water temperature of bath
- Instruct parent/caregiver to keep pets a safe distance from infant
- Instruct parent/caregiver to never to shake, toss, or swing infant in the air

5th edition 2008

Background Readings:

American Academy of Pediatrics. (1994). *Birth to 6 months: Safety for your child* [Brochure]. Elk Grove Village, IL: Author.

California Center for Childhood Injury Prevention. (1997). *Safe home assessment program*. San Diego, CA: Author.

California Department of Health Services Childhood Lead Poisoning Prevention Branch. (1994). *Lead: Simple things that you can do to prevent childhood lead poisoning* [Brochure]. Sacramento, CA: Author.

Hockenberry, M. J. (2005). *Wong's essentials of pediatric nursing* (7th ed.). St. Louis: Mosby.

Hockenberry, M. J. (2006). *Wong's nursing care for infants and children* (8th ed.). St. Louis: Mosby.

Pillitteri, A. (2007). *Maternal and child health nursing: Care of the childbearing and childrearing family* (5th ed.). Philadelphia: Lippincott Williams & Wilkins.

Teaching: Infant Safety 4-6 Months

5646

Definition: Instruction on safety from the fourth month through the sixth month of life

Activities:

- Provide parents with written materials appropriate to identified knowledge needs
- Instruct parent/caregiver to avoid use of walkers or jumpers due to danger of injury and detrimental effects on muscle development
- Instruct parent/caregiver never to leave infant unattended in the bath, grocery cart, high chair, on sofa, etc.
- Instruct parent/caregiver to evaluate hanging crib toys
- Instruct parent/caregiver to use a safe high chair when infant is able to sit
- Instruct parent/caregiver to feed only soft or mashed foods
- Instruct parent/caregiver to remove small objects from infant's reach

5th edition 2008

Background Readings:

American Academy of Pediatrics. (1994a). *6 to 12 months: Safety for your child* [Brochure]. Elk Grove Village, IL: Author.

American Academy of Pediatrics. (1994b). *Birth to 6 months: Safety for your child* [Brochure]. Elk Grove Village, IL: Author.

California Center for Childhood Injury Prevention. (1997). *Safe home assessment program*. San Diego, CA: Author.

California Department of Health Services Childhood Lead Poisoning Prevention Branch. (1994). *Lead: Simple things that you can do to prevent childhood lead poisoning* [Brochure]. Sacramento, CA: Author.

Hockenberry, M. J. (2005). *Wong's essentials of pediatric nursing* (7th ed.). St. Louis: Mosby.

Hockenberry, M. J. (2006). *Wong's nursing care for infants and children* (8th ed.). St. Louis: Mosby.

Pillitteri, A. (2007). *Maternal and child health nursing: Care of the childbearing and childrearing family* (5th ed.). Philadelphia: Lippincott Williams & Wilkins.

Teaching: Infant Safety 7-9 Months

5647

Definition: Instruction on safety from the seventh month through the ninth month of life

Activities:

- Provide parents with written materials appropriate to identified knowledge needs
- Instruct parent/caregiver to avoid sources of lead poisoning
- Instruct parent/caregiver to keep dangerous items out of infant's reach
- Instruct parent/caregiver to provide barriers to dangerous areas
- Instruct parent/caregiver to supervise infant's activity at all times

5th edition 2008

Background Readings:

American Academy of Pediatrics. (1994). *6 to 12 months: Safety for your child* [Brochure]. Elk Grove Village, IL: Author.

California Center for Childhood Injury Prevention. (1997). *Safe home assessment program*. San Diego, CA: Author.

California Department of Health Services Childhood Lead Poisoning Prevention Branch. (1994). *Lead: Simple things that you can do to prevent childhood lead poisoning* [Brochure]. Sacramento, CA: Author.

Hockenberry, M. J. (2005). *Wong's essentials of pediatric nursing* (7th ed.). St. Louis: Mosby.

Hockenberry, M. J. (2006). *Wong's nursing care for infants and children* (8th ed.). St. Louis: Mosby.

Pillitteri, A. (2007). *Maternal and child health nursing: Care of the childbearing and childrearing family* (5th ed.). Philadelphia: Lippincott Williams & Wilkins.

Teaching: Infant Safety 10-12 Months   5648

Definition: Instruction on safety from the tenth month through the twelfth month of life

Activities:
- Provide parents with written materials appropriate to identified knowledge needs
- Instruct parent/caregiver to provide protection from glass furniture, sharp edges, unstable furniture, and appliances
- Instruct parent/caregiver to store all cleaning supplies, medications, and personal care products out of infant's reach
- Instruct parent/caregiver to use childproof latches on cupboards
- Instruct parent/caregiver to prevent infant's access to upper story windows, balconies, and stairs
- Instruct parent/caregiver to keep infant away from ponds, pools, toilets, and all containers with liquid to prevent drowning
- Instruct parent/caregiver to select toys according to manufacturer's age recommendations
- Instruct parent/caregiver to ensure multiple barriers to pool/hot tub area

5th edition 2008

Background Readings:
American Academy of Pediatrics. (1994a). *1 to 2 years: Safety for your child* [Brochure]. Elk Grove Village, IL: Author.
American Academy of Pediatrics. (1994b). *6 to 12 months: Safety for your child* [Brochure]. Elk Grove Village, IL: Author.
California Center for Childhood Injury Prevention. (1997). *Safe home assessment program.* San Diego, CA: Author.
California Department of Health Services Childhood Lead Poisoning Prevention Branch. (1994). *Lead: Simple things that you can do to prevent childhood lead poisoning* [Brochure]. Sacramento, CA: Author.
Hockenberry, M. J. (2005). *Wong's essentials of pediatric nursing* (7th ed.). St. Louis: Mosby.
Hockenberry, M. J. (2006). *Wong's nursing care for infants and children* (8th ed.). St. Louis: Mosby.
Pillitteri, A. (2007). *Maternal and child health nursing: Care of the childbearing and childrearing family* (5th ed.). Philadelphia: Lippincott Williams & Wilkins.

Teaching: Infant Stimulation 0-4 Months   5655

Definition: Teaching parents and caregivers to provide developmentally appropriate sensory activities to promote development and movement through the first four months of life

Activities:
- Describe normal infant development
- Assist parents to identify infant readiness cues and responses to stimulation
- Protect infant from overstimulation
- Assist parents to set up routine for infant stimulation
- Instruct parents/caregivers to perform activities that encourage movement and/or provide sensory stimulation
- Have parents demonstrate techniques learned during teaching
- Instruct parents to promote face-to-face interaction with infant
- Instruct parents to talk, sing, and smile at infant while giving care
- Instruct parents to praise infant for all efforts to respond to stimulation
- Instruct parents to tell infant his/her name frequently
- Instruct parents to whisper to baby
- Instruct parents to encourage touching and hugging infant frequently
- Instruct parents to respond to crying by holding, rocking, singing, talking, walking, repositioning, rubbing/massaging back, and wrapping, as appropriate
- Instruct parents to rock infant in either an upright position or cradle position
- Instruct parents to sponge or tub bathe using various massaging strokes with a soft wash cloth or sponge and pat dry with soft towel
- Instruct parents to massage infant by rubbing lotion in gentle but firm strokes
- Instruct parents to rub soft toys on infant's body
- Instruct parents to encourage infant to feel different textures and identify them for infant
- Instruct parents to blow air in circles on alert infant's arms, legs, and tummy
- Instruct parents to encourage infant to grasp soft toys or caregiver's fingers
- Instruct parents to promote shaking of rattles, encouraging auditory following
- Instruct parents to provide opportunities for infant to reach for objects
- Instruct parents to encourage visual following of objects
- Instruct parents to reposition infant every hour unless sleeping, placing in infant seat, swing, stroller, as appropriate
- Instruct parents to place infant on tummy while awake to encourage head lifting
- Instruct parents to position infant on back under cradle gym
- Instruct parents to play peek-a-boo with infant
- Instruct parents to encourage infant to look in mirror

5th edition 2008

Background Readings:
Broussard, A. B., & Kidman, S. (1990). Incorporating infant stimulation concepts into prenatal classes. *Journal of Obstetric, Gynecologic, and Neonatal Nursing, 19*(5), 381–387.
Harrison, L. L. (1985). Effects of early supplemental stimulation programs for premature infants: Review of the literature. *Maternal-Child Nursing Journal, 14*(2), 125.
Hockenberry, M. J. (2005). *Wong's essentials of pediatric nursing* (7th ed.). St. Louis: Mosby.
Hockenberry, M. J. (2006). *Wong's nursing care for infants and children* (8th ed.). St. Louis: Mosby.
Korner, A. F. (1990). Infant stimulation: Issues of theory and research. *Clinics in Perinatology, 17*(1), 173–184.
Pillitteri, A. (2007). *Maternal and child health nursing: Care of the childbearing and childrearing family* (5th ed.). Philadelphia: Lippincott Williams & Wilkins.

T

Teaching: Infant Stimulation 5-8 Months   5656

Definition: Teaching parents and caregivers to provide developmentally appropriate sensory activities to promote development and movement from the fifth month through the eighth month of life

Activities:

- Describe normal infant development
- Assist parents to identify infant readiness cues and responses to stimulation
- Protect infant from overstimulation
- Assist parents to set up routine for infant stimulation
- Instruct parents/caregivers to perform activities that encourage movement and/or provide sensory stimulation
- Have parents demonstrate techniques learned during teaching
- Instruct parents to place infant on tummy, putting caregiver's palms on soles of infant's feet and pushing gently forward
- Instruct parents to stand infant on caregiver's lap, swaying side to side
- Instruct parents to encourage infant to lay on back and kick with feet
- Instruct parents to lay infant on back or tummy and help to roll over
- Instruct parents to provide opportunity for infant to explore cloth or soft plastic books
- Instruct parents to introduce infant to body parts
- Instruct parents to encourage infant to use toys for teething
- Instruct parents to play pat-a-cake with infant
- Instruct parents to play hide and seek with infant
- Instruct parents to encourage infant to bang toys together
- Instruct parents to encourage hand transfer of toys
- Instruct parents to place infant in high chair, encouraging infant to feel food and feed self
- Instruct parents to dance with infant while holding infant upright

5th edition 2008

Background Readings:

Broussard, A. B., & Kidman, S. (1990). Incorporating infant stimulation concepts into prenatal classes. *Journal of Obstetric, Gynecologic, and Neonatal Nursing, 19*(5), 381-387.

Harrison, L. L. (1985). Effects of early supplemental stimulation programs for premature infants: Review of the literature. *Maternal-Child Nursing Journal, 14*(2), 125.

Hockenberry, M. J. (2005). *Wong's essentials of pediatric nursing* (7th ed.). St. Louis: Mosby.

Hockenberry, M. J. (2006). *Wong's nursing care for infants and children* (8th ed.). St. Louis: Mosby.

Korner, A. F. (1990). Infant stimulation: Issues of theory and research. *Clinics in Perinatology, 17*(1), 173–184.

Pillitteri, A. (2007). *Maternal and child health nursing: Care of the childbearing and childrearing family* (5th ed.). Philadelphia: Lippincott Williams & Wilkins.

Teaching: Infant Stimulation 9-12 Months   5657

Definition: Teaching parents and caregivers to provide developmentally appropriate sensory activities to promote development and movement from the ninth month through the twelfth month of life

Activities:

- Describe normal infant development
- Assist parents to identify infant readiness cues and responses to stimulation
- Protect infant from overstimulation
- Assist parents to set up routine for infant stimulation
- Instruct parents/caregivers to perform activities that encourage movement and/or provide sensory stimulation
- Have parents demonstrate techniques learned during teaching
- Instruct parents to pull infant to standing, holding onto hands for stabilization
- Instruct parents to guide infant to walk, holding infant by hands/wrists with arms above head
- Instruct parents to encourage ball play (e.g., rolling, grasping, stopping, retrieving)
- Instruct parents to introduce use of cup at meal times, assisting infant to grasp and put to mouth
- Instruct parents to wave bye-bye to infant while encouraging infant to imitate
- Instruct parents to take infant on a house tour, identifying objects and rooms
- Instruct parents to play follow the leader, practicing imitation of infant noises, animals, or songs
- Instruct parents to say words to infant, encouraging infant to say them back
- Instruct parents to demonstrate how to remove and replace objects from a container
- Instruct parents to demonstrate stacking objects

5th edition 2008

Background Readings:

Broussard, A. B., & Kidman, S. (1990). Incorporating infant stimulation concepts into prenatal classes. *Journal of Obstetric, Gynecologic, and Neonatal Nursing, 19*(5), 381–387.

Harrison, L. L. (1985). Effects of early supplemental stimulation programs for premature infants: Review of the literature. *Maternal-Child Nursing Journal, 14*(2), 125.

Hockenberry, M. J. (2005). *Wong's essentials of pediatric nursing* (7th ed.). St. Louis: Mosby.

Hockenberry, M. J. (2006). *Wong's nursing care for infants and children* (8th ed.). St. Louis: Mosby.

Korner, A. F. (1990). Infant stimulation: Issues of theory and research. *Clinics in Perinatology, 17*(1), 173–184.

Pillitteri, A. (2007). *Maternal and child health nursing: Care of the childbearing and childrearing family* (5th ed.). Philadelphia: Lippincott Williams & Wilkins.

T

Teaching: Preoperative 5610

Definition: Assisting a patient to understand and mentally prepare for surgery and the postoperative recovery period

Activities:

- Inform the patient and family of the scheduled date, time, and location of surgery
- Inform the patient and family how long the surgery is expected to last
- Determine the patient's previous surgical experiences, background, culture, and level of knowledge related to surgery
- Appraise the patient's and family's anxiety relating to surgery
- Provide time for the patient to ask questions and discuss concerns
- Describe the preoperative routines (e.g., anesthesia, diet, bowel preparation, tests/labs, voiding, skin preparation, IV therapy, clothing, family waiting area, transportation to operating room), as appropriate
- Describe any preoperative medications, the effects these will have on the patient, and the rationale for using them
- Inform the family of the location to wait for the results of the surgery, as appropriate
- Conduct a tour of the postsurgical unit and waiting area, as appropriate
- Introduce the patient to the staff who will be involved in the surgery and postoperative care, as appropriate
- Reinforce the patient's confidence in the staff involved, as appropriate
- Provide information on what will be heard, smelled, seen, tasted, or felt during the event
- Discuss possible pain control measures
- Explain the purpose of frequent postoperative assessments
- Describe the postoperative routines and equipment (e.g., medications, respiratory treatments, tubes, machines, support hose, surgical dressings, ambulation, diet, family visitation) and explain their purpose
- Instruct the patient on the technique of getting out of bed, as appropriate
- Evaluate the patient's ability to demonstrate getting out of bed, as appropriate
- Instruct the patient on the technique of splinting, coughing, and deep breathing
- Evaluate the patient's ability to demonstrate splinting incision, coughing, and deep breathing

- Instruct the patient on how to use the incentive spirometer
- Evaluate the patient's ability to demonstrate proper use of the incentive spirometer
- Instruct the patient on the technique of leg exercises
- Evaluate the patient's ability to demonstrate leg exercises
- Stress the importance of early ambulation and pulmonary care
- Inform the patient how to assist in recuperation
- Reinforce information provided by other health care team members, as appropriate
- Determine the patient's expectations of the surgery
- Correct unrealistic expectations of the surgery, as appropriate
- Provide time for the patient to rehearse events that will happen, as appropriate
- Instruct the patient to use coping techniques directed at controlling specific aspects of the experience (e.g., relaxation, imagery), as appropriate
- Instruct patient in regard to smoking cessation, as appropriate
- Instruct in a way that matches the patient's style of learning, including the use of holistic approaches and educational materials, as appropriate
- Document teaching, including patient's response to teaching

1st edition 1992; revised 2013

Background Readings:

deWit, S. C. (2009). *Medical-surgical nursing: Concepts and practice.* St. Louis: Saunders.

Kruzik, N. (2009). Benefits of preoperative education for adult elective surgery patients. *AORN Journal, 90*(3), 381–387.

Lewis, S. L., Dirksen, S. R., Heitkemper, M. M., Bucher, L., & Camera, I. M. (2011). *Medical surgical nursing: Assessment and management of clinical problems* (8th ed.). St. Louis: Elsevier Mosby.

Potter, P. A., Perry, A. C., Stockert, P. A., & Hall, A. M. (2013). *Fundamentals of nursing* (8th ed.). St. Louis: Elsevier Mosby.

Selimen, D., & Andsoy, I. I. (2011). The importance of a holistic approach during the perioperative period. *AORN Journal, 93*(4), 482–490.

Teaching: Prescribed Diet 5614

Definition: Preparing a patient to correctly follow a prescribed diet

Activities:

- Appraise the patient's current level of knowledge about prescribed diet
- Appraise the patient's current and past eating patterns, as well as preferred foods and current eating habits
- Determine the patient's and family's perspectives, cultural backgrounds, and other factors that may affect the patient's willingness to follow prescribed diet
- Determine any financial limitations that may affect food purchases
- Instruct the patient on the proper name of the prescribed diet
- Explain the purpose of diet adherence to overall health
- Inform the patient about how long the diet should be followed

- Instruct the patient about how to keep a food diary, as appropriate
- Instruct the patient on allowed and prohibited foods
- Inform the patient of possible drug and food interactions, as appropriate
- Assist the patient to accommodate food preferences into the prescribed diet
- Assist the patient in substituting ingredients to conform favorite recipes to the prescribed diet
- Instruct the patient about how to read labels and select appropriate foods
- Observe the patient's selection of foods appropriate to prescribed diet

- Instruct the patient about how to plan appropriate meals
- Provide written meal plans, as appropriate
- Recommend a cookbook that includes recipes consistent with the diet, as appropriate
- Reinforce information provided by other health care team members, as appropriate
- Reinforce the importance of continued monitoring and changing needs that may require further alteration of dietary plan of care
- Refer patient to dietitian, as appropriate
- Include the family, as appropriate

1st edition 1992; revised 2013

Background Readings:

deWit, S. C. (2009). *Medical-surgical nursing: Concepts and practice*. St. Louis: Saunders.

Dossey, B. M., & Keegan, L. (2009). *Holistic nursing* (5th ed.). Sudbury, MA: Jones & Bartlett.

Dudek, S. G. (2007). *Nutrition essentials for nursing practice* (5th rev ed.). Philadelphia: Lippincott Williams & Wilkins.

Lewis, S. L., Dirksen, S. R., Heitkemper, M. M., Bucher, L. & Camera, I. M. (2011). *Medical surgical nursing: Assessment and management of clinical problems* (8th ed.). St. Louis: Elsevier Mosby.

Potter, P. A., Perry, A. C., Stockert, P. A., & Hall, A. M. (2013). *Fundamentals of nursing* (8th ed.). St. Louis: Elsevier Mosby.

Teaching: Prescribed Exercise   5612

Definition: Preparing a patient to achieve or maintain a prescribed level of exercise

Activities:

- Appraise the patient's current level of exercise and knowledge of prescribed exercise
- Monitor the patient for physiological and psychological limitations, as well as background and culture
- Inform the patient of the purpose for, and the benefits of, the prescribed exercise
- Assist the patient in setting goals for slow, steady increase in exercise
- Instruct patient regarding use of pain medication and alternative methods of pain control prior to exercise, as needed
- Instruct the patient how to perform the prescribed exercise
- Instruct the patient how to monitor tolerance of the exercise
- Instruct the patient how to keep an exercise diary, as appropriate
- Inform the patient what activities are appropriate based on physical condition
- Caution the patient on the dangers of overestimating capabilities, as appropriate
- Warn the patient of the effects of extreme heat and cold, as appropriate
- Instruct the patient on methods to conserve energy, as appropriate
- Instruct the patient about how to properly stretch before and after exercise and the rationale for doing so, as appropriate
- Instruct the patient how to warm up and cool down before and after exercise and the importance of doing so, as appropriate
- Instruct the patient on good posture and body mechanics, as appropriate
- Instruct patient to report signs of possible problems, (e.g., pain, dizziness, and swelling) to health care provider
- Observe the patient perform the prescribed exercise
- Provide information on available assistive devices that may be used to facilitate performance of the required skill, as appropriate
- Instruct the patient on the assembly, use, and maintenance of assistive devices, as appropriate
- Assist the patient to incorporate exercise regimen into daily routine
- Assist the patient to properly alternate periods of rest and activity
- Refer the patient to physical therapist, occupational therapist, or exercise physiologist, as appropriate
- Reinforce information provided by other health care team members, as appropriate
- Provide written information or diagrams for continued reference
- Provide frequent feedback to prevent bad habits from forming
- Include the family, as appropriate
- Provide information on available community resources and support groups to increase the patient's compliance with exercise, as appropriate
- Refer the patient to a rehabilitation center, as appropriate

1st edition 1992, revised 2013

Background Readings:

Berman, A., Snyder, S., Kozier, B., & Erb, G. (2008). Activity and exercise. In *Kozier & Erb's fundamentals of nursing: Concepts, processes, and practice*. (8th ed., pp. 1104–1162). Upper Saddle River, NJ: Prentice Hall.

deWit, S. C. (2009). *Medical-surgical nursing: Concepts and practice*. St. Louis: Saunders.

Perme, C., & Chandrashekar, R. (2009). Early mobility and walking program for patients in intensive care units: Creating a standard of care. *American Journal of Critical Care, 18*(3), 212–221.

Potter, P. A., Perry, A. C., Stockert, P. A., & Hall, A. M. (2013). *Fundamentals of nursing* (8th ed.). St. Louis: Elsevier Mosby.

Pryor, J. (2009). Coaching patients to self-care: A primary responsibility of nursing. *International Journal of Older People Nursing, 4*(2), 79–88.

T

Teaching: Prescribed Medication   5616

Definition: Preparing a patient to safely take prescribed medications and monitor for their effects

Activities:

- Instruct the patient to recognize distinctive characteristics of the medication(s), as appropriate
- Inform the patient of both the generic and brand names of each medication
- Instruct the patient on the purpose and action of each medication
- Explain how health care providers choose the most appropriate medication
- Instruct the patient on the dosage, route, and duration of each medication
- Instruct the patient on the proper administration/application of each medication
- Review patient's knowledge of medications
- Acknowledge patient's knowledge of medications
- Evaluate the patient's ability to self-administer medications
- Instruct the patient to perform needed procedures before taking a medication (e.g., check pulse, glucose), as appropriate
- Inform the patient what to do if a dose of medication is missed
- Instruct the patient on which criteria to use when deciding to alter the medication dosage/schedule, as appropriate
- Inform the patient of consequences of not taking or abruptly discontinuing medication(s), as appropriate
- Instruct the patient on specific precautions to observe when taking medication(s) (e.g., no driving/using power tools), as appropriate
- Instruct the patient on possible adverse side effects of each medication
- Instruct the patient how to relieve and/or prevent certain side effects, as appropriate
- Instruct the patient on appropriate actions to take if side effects occur
- Instruct the patient on the signs and symptoms of overdosage/underdosage
- Inform the patient of possible drug/food interactions, as appropriate
- Instruct the patient how to properly store the medication(s)
- Instruct the patient on the proper care of devices used for administration
- Instruct patients on proper disposal of needles and syringes at home, as appropriate, and where to dispose of the sharps container in their community
- Provide the patient with written information about the action, purpose, side effects, etc. of medications
- Assist the patient to develop a written medication schedule
- Instruct the patient to carry documentation of his/her prescribed medication regimen
- Instruct the patient how to fill his/her prescription(s), as appropriate
- Inform the patient of possible changes in appearance and/or dosage when filling generic medication prescription(s)
- Warn the patient of the risks associated with taking expired medication
- Caution the patient against giving prescribed medication to others
- Determine the patient's ability to obtain required medications
- Provide information on medication reimbursement, as appropriate
- Provide information on cost savings programs/organizations to obtain medications and devices, as appropriate
- Provide information on medication alert devices and how to obtain them
- Reinforce information provided by other health care team members, as appropriate
- Include the family/significant others, as appropriate

1st edition 1992; revised 1996, 2004

Background Readings:

Aschenbrenner, D. S., & Venable, S. J. (2006). *Drug therapy in nursing* (2nd ed.). Philadelphia: Lippincott Williams & Wilkins.

Devine, E. C., & Reifschneider, E. (1995). A meta-analysis of the effects of psychoeducational care in adults with hypertension. *Nursing Research*, 44(4), 237–245.

Doak, C. C. (1996). *Teaching patients with low literary skills* (2nd ed.). Philadelphia: Lippincott.

Hayes, K. S. (1998). Randomized trial of geragogy-based medication instruction in the emergency department. *Nursing Research*, 47(4), 211–218.

Kleoppel, J. W., & Henry, D. W. (1987). Teaching patients, families, and communities about their medications. In C. E. Smith (Ed.), *Patient education: Nurses in partnership with other health professionals* (pp. 271–296). Philadelphia: Saunders.

Kozier, B., Erb, G., Berman, A., & Snyder, S. (2004). Teaching. In *Fundamentals of nursing: Concepts, processes, and practice* (7th ed., pp. 445–468). Upper Saddle River, NJ: Prentice Hall.

Proos, M., Reiler, P., Eagan, J., Stengrevices, S., Castile, J., & Arian, D. (1992). A study of the effects of self-medication on patient's knowledge of and compliance with their medication regimen. *Journal of Nursing Care Quality*, *(special report)*, 18–26.

Rakel, B. A. (1992). Interventions related to patient teaching. In G. M. Bulechek & J. C. McCloskey (Eds.), Symposium on nursing interventions. *Nursing Clinics of North America*, 27(2), 397–424.

T

Teaching: Procedure/Treatment 5618

Definition: Preparing a patient to understand and mentally prepare for a prescribed procedure or treatment

Activities:

- Inform the patient/significant other(s) about when and where the procedure/treatment will take place, as appropriate
- Inform the patient/significant other(s) about how long the procedure/treatment is expected to last
- Inform the patient/significant other(s) about who will be performing the procedure/treatment
- Reinforce the patient's confidence in the staff involved, as appropriate
- Determine the patient's previous experience(s) and level of knowledge related to procedure/treatment
- Explain the purpose of the procedure/treatment
- Describe the preprocedure/treatment activities
- Explain the procedure/treatment
- Obtain witness/patient's informed consent for the procedure/treatment according to agency policy, as appropriate
- Instruct the patient on how to cooperate/participate during the procedure/treatment, as appropriate
- Involve child in procedure (hold bandage) but don't give a choice about completing procedure
- Conduct a tour of the procedure/treatment room and waiting area, as appropriate
- Introduce the patient to the staff who will be involved in the procedure/treatment, as appropriate
- Explain the need for certain equipment (e.g., monitoring devices) and their function
- Discuss the need for special measures during the procedure/treatment, as appropriate
- Provide information on what will be heard, smelled, seen, tasted, or felt during the event
- Describe the postprocedure/posttreatment assessments/activities and the rationale for them
- Inform patients on how they can aid in recuperation
- Reinforce information provided by other health care team members, as appropriate
- Provide time for the patient to rehearse events that will happen, as appropriate
- Instruct the patient to use coping techniques directed at controlling specific aspects of the experience (e.g., relaxation and imagery), as appropriate
- Provide distraction for a child patient that will divert attention away from procedure
- Provide information on when and where results will be available and who will explain them
- Determine the patient's expectations of the procedure/treatment
- Correct unrealistic expectations of the procedure/treatment, as appropriate
- Discuss alternative treatments, as appropriate
- Provide time for the patient to ask questions and discuss concerns
- Include the family/significant others, as appropriate

1st edition 1992; revised 2000

Background Readings:

Kozier, B., Erb, G., Berman, A., & Snyder, S. (2004). Teaching. In *Fundamentals of nursing: Concepts, processes, and practice* (7th ed., pp. 445–468). Upper Saddle River, NJ: Prentice Hall.

Monroe, D. (1989). Patient teaching for x-ray and other diagnostics. *RN*, 52(12), 36–40.

Rakel, B. A. (1992). Interventions related to patient teaching. In G. M. Bulechek & J. C. McCloskey (Eds.), Symposium on nursing interventions. *Nursing Clinics of North America*, 27(2), 397–424.

Teaching: Psychomotor Skill 5620

Definition: Preparing a patient to perform a psychomotor skill

Activities:

- Establish rapport
- Establish teacher credibility, as appropriate
- Determine the patient's learning needs
- Determine patient readiness to learn
- Establish level of patient ability in performing skill
- Adjust teaching methodology to accommodate patient age and ability, as needed
- Demonstrate the skill for the patient
- Give clear, step-by-step directions
- Instruct the patient to perform the skill one step at a time
- Inform the patient of the rationale for performing the skill in the specified manner
- Guide patients' bodies so that they can experience the physical sensations that accompany the correct motions, as appropriate
- Provide written information or diagrams, as appropriate
- Provide practice sessions (spaced to avoid fatigue, but often enough to prevent excessive forgetting), as appropriate
- Provide adequate time for task mastery
- Observe patient demonstrate the skill
- Provide frequent feedback to patients on what they are doing correctly and incorrectly, so that bad habits are not formed
- Provide information on available assistive devices that may be used to facilitate performance of the required skill, as appropriate
- Instruct the patient on the assembly, use, and maintenance of assistive devices, as appropriate
- Include the family, as appropriate

1st edition 1992; revised 2013

Background Readings:

Falvo, D.R. (2011). *Effective patient education: A guide to increased adherence.* Sudbury, MA: Jones and Bartlett.

Friedman, A. J., Cosby, R., Boyko, S., Hatton-Bauer, J., & Turnbull, G. (2011). Effective teaching strategies and methods of delivery for patient education: A systematic review and practice guideline recommendations. *Journal of Cancer Education, 26*(1), 12–21.

Potter, P. A., Perry, A. C., Stockert, P. A., & Hall, A. M. (2013). *Fundamentals of nursing* (8th ed.). St. Louis: Elsevier Mosby.

Teaching: Safe Sex   5622

Definition: Providing instruction concerning protection during sexual activity

Activities:
- Obtain sexual history, including number of past sexual partners, frequency of intercourse, and past occurrences of and treatments for sexually transmitted infections (STIs)
- Instruct patient on anatomy and physiology of human reproduction
- Instruct patient on STI and conception, as necessary
- Instruct patient on factors that increase risk of STI (e.g., unprotected sexual intercourse, increased genital mucosal surface area, increased number of sexual contacts, presence of genital sores, advanced illness, and sexual intercourse during menstruation)
- Discuss patient's knowledge, understanding, motivation, and commitment level regarding various sexual protection methods
- Discuss methods of sexual protection for sexual intercourse and oral sex (e.g., medication-free, barrier, vaccination, hormonal, intrauterine device, abstinence, and sterilization) including effectiveness, side effects, contraindications, and signs and symptoms that warrant reporting to a health care professional
- Discuss religious, cultural, developmental, socioeconomical, and individual considerations pertaining to sexual protection choice
- Provide accurate information pertaining to the implications of having multiple sexual partners
- Instruct patient on low-risk sexual practices, such as those which avoid bodily penetration or the exchange of body fluids
- Instruct patient on the importance of good hygiene, using a water-soluble lubricant, and voiding after intercourse to decrease the susceptibility to infections
- Instruct patient on proper use of condoms (e.g., how to choose, keep intact, apply, and remove)
- Provide patient with sexual protection products (e.g., condoms and dental dams)
- Encourage patient to obtain routine examinations and report signs and symptoms of STIs to a health care provider
- Encourage patient to discuss sexual histories and safe sex practices with partner
- Discuss with patient importance of sexual partner notification when diagnosed with STI
- Consider population-based factors affecting safe sex education (e.g., culturally-tailored interventions, ethnically matched providers)
- Use social networks (e.g., internet, phone) to reach marginalized or geographically isolated populations

1st edition 1992; revised 2013

Background Readings:

Paranjape, A., Bernstein, L., St. George, D. M., Doyle, J., Henderson, S., & Corbie-Smith, G. (2006). Effect of relationship factors on safer sex decisions in older inner-city women. *Journal of Women's Health, 15*(1), 90–97.

Vergidis, P. I., & Falagas, M. E. (2009). Meta-analyses on behavioral interventions to reduce the risk of transmission of HIV. *Infectious Disease Clinics of North America, 23*(2), 309-314.

Ward, S. L., & Hisley, S. M. (2009). *Maternal-child nursing care: Optimizing outcomes for mothers, children, & families.* Philadelphia: F. A. Davis.

Wilson, T. E., Hogben, M., Malka, E. S., Liddon, N., McCormack, W. M., Rubin, S.R., & Augenbraun, M. A. (2009). A randomized controlled trial for reducing risks for sexually transmitted infections through enhanced patient-based partner notification. *American Journal of Public Health, 99*(Suppl. 1), S104–S110.

Teaching: Sexuality   5624

Definition: Assisting individuals to understand physical and psychosocial dimensions of sexual growth and development

Activities:
- Create an accepting, nonjudgmental atmosphere
- Explain human anatomy and physiology of the male and female body
- Explain the anatomy and physiology of human reproduction
- Discuss signs of fertility (related to ovulation and menstrual cycle)
- Explain emotional development during childhood and adolescence
- Facilitate communication between the child, adolescent, and parent
- Support parents' role as the primary sexuality educator of their children
- Educate parents on sexual growth and development through the life span
- Provide parents with a bibliography of sexuality education materials
- Discuss what values are, how we obtain them, and their effect on our choices in life
- Facilitate the child's and adolescent's awareness of family, peer, societal, and media influence on values
- Use appropriate questions to assist the child and adolescent to reflect on what is important personally
- Discuss peer and social pressures to sexual activity
- Explore the meaning of sexual roles
- Discuss sexual behavior and appropriate ways to express one's feelings and needs
- Inform children and adolescents of the benefits to postponing sexual activity
- Educate children and adolescents on the negative consequences of early childbearing (e.g., poverty and loss of education and career opportunities)
- Teach children and adolescents about sexually transmitted diseases and AIDS
- Promote responsibility for sexual behavior
- Discuss benefits of abstinence
- Inform children and adolescents about effective contraceptives

T

- Instruct accessibility of contraceptives and how to obtain them
- Assist adolescents in choosing an appropriate contraceptive, as appropriate
- Facilitate role playing where decision making and assertive communication skills may be practiced to resist peer and social pressures of sexual activity
- Enhance self-esteem through peer role modeling and role playing

2nd edition 1996

Background Readings:

Howard, M., & McCabe, J. (1990). Helping teenagers postpone sexual involvement. *Family Planning Perspectives, 22*(1), 21–26.

Kirby, D., Barth, R., Leland, N., & Fetro, J. (1991). Reducing the risk: Impact of a new curriculum on sexual risk-taking. *Family Planning Perspectives, 23*(6), 253–263.

Pillitteri, A. (2007). Reproductive and sexual health. In *Maternal and child health nursing: Care of the childbearing and childrearing family* (5th ed., pp. 65–101). Philadelphia: Lippincott Williams & Wilkins.

Roth, B. (1993). Fertility awareness as a component of sexuality education. *Nurse Practitioner, 18*(3), 40–53.

Smith, M. (1993). Pediatric sexuality: Promoting normal sexual development in children. *Nurse Practitioner, 18*(8), 37–44.

Stevens-Simon, C. (1993). Clinical applications of adolescent female sexual development. *Nurse Practitioner, 18*(12), 18–29.

Vincent, M. L., Clearie, A. F., & Schluchter, M. D. (1987). Reducing adolescent pregnancy through school and community-based education. *Journal of American Medical Association, 257*(24), 3382–3385.

Teaching: Toddler Nutrition 13-18 Months   5660

Definition: Instruction on nutrition and feeding practices from the thirteenth month through the eighteenth month of life

Activities:

- Provide parents with written materials appropriate to identified knowledge needs
- Instruct parent/caregiver to discontinue bottle feeding
- Instruct parent/caregiver to offer textured solids
- Instruct parent/caregiver to continue use of spoon and self-feeding
- Instruct parent/caregiver to introduce dairy products
- Instruct parent/caregiver to provide healthy snacks
- Instruct parent/caregiver to offer small portions and frequent feedings
- Instruct parent/caregiver to avoid "diet" food/drinks (e.g., nonfat milk, diet soda)
- Instruct parent/caregiver to avoid forcefeeding as there is decreased appetite

5th edition 2008

Background Readings:

Barnes, L. A. (Ed.). (1993). *Pediatric nutrition handbook* (3rd ed.). Elk Grove Village, IL: American Academy of Pediatrics.

California Department of Health Services WIC Supplemental Nutrition Branch. (1998). *Feeding your baby 1–3 years old* [Brochure]. Sacramento, CA: Author.

Formon, S. J. (1993). *Nutrition of normal infants.* St. Louis: Mosby.

Hockenberry, M. J. (2005). *Wong's essentials of pediatric nursing* (7th ed.). St. Louis: Mosby.

Hockenberry, M. J. (2006). *Wong's nursing care of infants and children* (8th ed.). St. Louis: Mosby.

Pillitteri, A. (2007). *Maternal and child health nursing: Care of the childbearing and childrearing family* (5th ed.). Philadelphia: Lippincott Williams & Wilkins.

Satter, E., & Sharkey, P. B. (1997). *Ellyn Satter's nutrition and feeding for infants and children: Handout masters.* Madison, WI: Author.

Teaching: Toddler Nutrition 19-24 Months   5661

Definition: Instruction on nutrition and feeding practices from the nineteenth month through the twenty-fourth month of life

Activities:

- Provide parents with written materials appropriate to identified knowledge needs
- Instruct parent/caregiver to encourage drinking water for thirst
- Instruct parent/caregiver to limit fluids before meals
- Instruct parent/caregiver to offer high iron and protein foods
- Instruct parent/caregiver to have regular mealtimes and eat as a family
- Instruct parent/caregiver to increase or decrease foods, as appropriate
- Instruct parent/caregiver to avoid fruit drinks and flavored milk
- Instruct parent/caregiver to read the labels for nutritive content
- Instruct parent/caregiver to discontinue bottle feeding

5th edition 2008

Background Readings:

Barnes, L. A. (Ed.). (1993). *Pediatric nutrition handbook* (3rd ed.). Elk Grove Village, IL: American Academy of Pediatrics.

California Department of Health Services WIC Supplemental Nutrition Branch. (1998). *Feeding your baby 1–3 years old* [Brochure]. Sacramento, CA: Author.

Formon, S. J. (1993). *Nutrition of normal infants.* St. Louis: Mosby.

Hockenberry, M. J. (2005). *Wong's essentials of pediatric nursing* (7th ed.). St. Louis: Mosby.

Hockenberry, M. J. (2006). *Wong's nursing care of infants and children* (8th ed.). St. Louis: Mosby.

Pillitteri, A. (2007). *Maternal and child health nursing: Care of the childbearing and childrearing family* (5th ed.). Philadelphia: Lippincott Williams & Wilkins.

Satter, E., & Sharkey, P. B. (1997). *Ellyn Satter's nutrition and feeding for infants and children: Handout masters.* Madison, WI: Author.

Teaching: Toddler Nutrition 25-36 Months   5662

Definition: Instruction on nutrition and feeding practices from the twenty-fifth month through the thirty-sixth month of life

Activities:
- Provide parents with written materials appropriate to identified knowledge needs
- Instruct parent/caregiver to give child healthy food choices
- Instruct parent/caregiver to encourage raw/cooked vegetables
- Instruct parent/caregiver to provide healthy snacks between meals
- Instruct parent/caregiver to be creative in food preparation for picky eater
- Instruct parent/caregiver to offer small portions of food
- Instruct parent/caregiver to limit fat content in foods
- Instruct parent/caregiver to have child participate in food preparation
- Instruct parent/caregiver to offer iron-fortified cereals, avoiding high-sugar cereals
- Instruct parent/caregiver to increase protein foods
- Instruct parent/caregiver to include all food groups
- Instruct parent/caregiver to avoid use of food as rewards

Background Readings:
Barnes, L. A. (Ed.). (1993). *Pediatric nutrition handbook* (3rd ed.). Elk Grove Village, IL: American Academy of Pediatrics.
California Department of Health Services WIC Supplemental Nutrition Branch. (1998). *Feeding your baby 1–3 years old* [Brochure]. Sacramento, CA: Author.
Formon, S. J. (1993). *Nutrition of normal infants.* St. Louis: Mosby.
Hockenberry, M. J. (2005). *Wong's essentials of pediatric nursing* (7th ed.). St. Louis: Mosby.
Hockenberry, M. J. (2006). *Wong's nursing care for infants and children* (8th ed.). St. Louis: Mosby.
Pillitteri, A. (2007). *Maternal and child health nursing: Care of the childbearing and childrearing family* (5th ed.). Philadelphia: Lippincott Williams & Wilkins.
Satter, E., & Sharkey, P. B. (1997). *Ellyn Satter's nutrition and feeding for infants and children: Handout masters.* Madison, WI: Author.

5th edition 2008

Teaching: Toddler Safety 13-18 Months   5665

Definition: Instruction on safety from the thirteenth month through the eighteenth month of life

Activities:
- Provide parents with written materials appropriate to identified knowledge needs
- Instruct parent/caregiver to supervise child outdoors
- Instruct parent/caregiver to educate child about dangers of throwing and hitting
- Instruct parent/caregiver to prevent access to electrical outlets, cords, and electrical equipment/appliances/tools
- Instruct parent/caregiver to store weapons and weapon-like items under lock and key
- Instruct parent/caregiver to educate child about safe ways of interacting with pets
- Instruct parent/caregiver to secure doors/gates to prevent child's access to dangerous areas (e.g., street, driveway, pool)
- Instruct parent/caregiver to dispose of and/or remove the doors to unused refrigerators, ice chests, and other air-tight containers
- Instruct parent/caregiver to use back burners of the stove, install knob covers, and/or restrict child's access to kitchen
- Instruct parent/caregiver to set home water heater temperature to between 120 degrees and 130 degrees Fahrenheit

Background Readings:
American Academy of Pediatrics. (1994a). *1 to 2 years: Safety for your child* [Brochure]. Elk Grove, IL: Author.
American Academy of Pediatrics. (1994b). *2 to 4 years: Safety for your child* [Brochure]. Elk Grove, IL: Author.
California Center for Childhood Injury Prevention. (1997). *Safe home assessment program.* San Diego, CA: Author.
California Department of Health Services Childhood Lead Poisoning Prevention Branch. (1994). *Lead: Simple things that you can do to prevent childhood lead poisoning* [Brochure]. Sacramento, CA: Author.
Hockenberry, M. J. (2005). *Wong's essentials of pediatric nursing* (7th ed.). St. Louis: Mosby.
Hockenberry, M. J. (2006). *Wong's nursing care for infants and children* (8th ed.). St. Louis: Mosby.
Pillitteri, A. (2007). *Maternal and child health nursing: Care of the childbearing and childrearing family* (5th ed.). Philadelphia: Lippincott Williams & Wilkins.

5th edition 2008

T

Teaching: Toddler Safety 19-24 Months   5666

Definition: Instruction on safety from the nineteenth month through the twenty-fourth month of life

Activities:

- Provide parents with written materials appropriate to identified knowledge needs
- Instruct parent/caregiver to install car seat and use it according to manufacturer's recommendations
- Instruct parent/caregiver to store sharp objects, appliances, and kitchen items out of child's reach
- Instruct parent/caregiver to instruct child on dangers of the street
- Instruct parent/caregiver to store all cleaning supplies, medications, and personal care products out of child's reach
- Instruct parent/caregiver to ensure multiple barriers to pool/hot tub area

5th edition 2008

Background Readings:

American Academy of Pediatrics. (1994a). *1 to 2 years: Safety for your child* [Brochure]. Elk Grove, IL: Author.

American Academy of Pediatrics. (1994b). *2 to 4 years: Safety for your child* [Brochure]. Elk Grove, IL: Author.

California Center for Childhood Injury Prevention. (1997). *Safe home assessment program.* San Diego, CA: Author.

California Department of Health Services Childhood Lead Poisoning Prevention Branch. (1994). *Lead: Simple things that you can do to prevent childhood lead poisoning* [Brochure]. Sacramento, CA: Author.

Hockenberry, M. J. (2005). *Wong's essentials of pediatric nursing* (7th ed.). St. Louis: Mosby.

Hockenberry, M. J. (2006). *Wong's nursing care for infants and children* (8th ed.). St. Louis: Mosby.

Pillitteri, A. (2007). *Maternal and child health nursing: Care of the childbearing and childrearing family* (5th ed.). Philadelphia: Lippincott Williams & Wilkins.

Teaching: Toddler Safety 25-36 Months   5667

Definition: Instruction on safety from the twenty-fifth month through the thirty-sixth month of life

Activities:

- Provide parents with written materials appropriate to identified knowledge needs
- Instruct parent/caregiver to instruct child on dangers of weapons
- Instruct parent/caregiver to select toys according to manufacturer's age recommendations
- Instruct parent/caregiver to provide supervision and instruct about safe use of large climbing and riding toys
- Instruct parent/caregiver to store matches/lighters out of child's reach and instruct child the dangers of fire and fire starters
- Instruct parent/caregiver to always supervise child around swimming pools, ponds, hot tubs
- Instruct parent/caregiver to instruct child about stranger danger and good touch/bad touch
- Instruct parent/caregiver to provide an approved helmet for bike riding and instruct child to always wear it
- Instruct parent/caregiver to prevent child's access to upper story windows, balconies, and stairs
- Instruct parent/caregiver to closely supervise child when out in public settings
- Instruct parent/caregiver to instruct child how to get adult help when he/she feels scared or in danger

5th edition 2008

Background Readings:

American Academy of Pediatrics. (1994). *2 to 4 years: Safety for your child* [Brochure]. Elk Grove, IL: Author.

California Center for Childhood Injury Prevention. (1997). *Safe home assessment program.* San Diego, CA: Author.

California Department of Health Services Childhood Lead Poisoning Prevention Branch. (1994). *Lead: Simple things that you can do to prevent childhood lead poisoning* [Brochure]. Sacramento, CA: Author.

Hockenberry, M. J. (2005). *Wong's essentials of pediatric nursing* (7th ed.). St. Louis: Mosby.

Hockenberry, M. J. (2006). *Wong's nursing care for infants and children* (8th ed.). St. Louis: Mosby.

Pillitteri, A. (2007). *Maternal and child health nursing: Care of the childbearing and childrearing family* (5th ed.). Philadelphia: Lippincott Williams & Wilkins.

T

Teaching: Toilet Training 5634

Definition: Instruction on determining the child's readiness and strategies to assist the child to learn independent toileting skills

Activities:
- Instruct parent about how to determine the child's physical readiness for toilet training (e.g., child is at least 18 to 24 months of age; evidence of being able to hold urine before void; recognizes urge to go or that he/she has just voided or defecated; shows some regularity in elimination patterns; ability to navigate to the toilet/potty, sit on it, and get off when completed; ability to remove and replace clothing before and after elimination; ability to wipe self and wash hands after elimination)
- Instruct parent about how to determine the child's psychosocial readiness for toilet training (e.g., child expresses interest in and desire to participate/cooperate in toileting; has vocabulary to communicate need to eliminate; is anxious to please parents; imitates the behaviors of others)
- Instruct parent about how to determine parental/family readiness for toilet training: (e.g., parent has knowledge and time to devote to training process; parent/family is experiencing no major transitions during or shortly after the process such as change of job or residence, divorce, birth of another child; has realistic expectations about child development and the time and energy needed to successfully complete the process; understands child may regress during times of stress or illness)
- Provide information on strategies to promote toilet training
- Provide information on how to dress the child in loose, easy-to-remove clothing
- Provide information on how to agree on vocabulary to be used during training process
- Provide information on opportunities for child to observe others during the toileting process
- Provide information on how to take the child to the potty to introduce him/her to the equipment and process
- Provide information on how to take the child to the potty on a regular basis and encourage him/her to sit
- Provide information on how to reinforce the child's success with any part of the process
- Provide information on how to consider the child's temperament or behavior style when planning strategies
- Provide information on how to expect and ignore accidents
- Provide information on how to communicate strategies, expectations, and progress to other care providers
- Support parents throughout this process
- Encourage parents to be flexible and creative in developing and implementing training strategies
- Provide additional information, as requested or needed

4th edition 2004; revised 2008

Background Readings:

Brazelton, T. B., Christophersen, E. R., Frauman, A. C., Gorski, P. A., Poole, J. M., Stradtler, A. C., & Wright, C. D. (1999). Instruction, timelines, and medical influences affecting toilet training. *Pediatrics, 103*(6), 1353–1358.

Doran, J., & Lister, A. (1998). Toilet training: Meeting the needs of children and parents. *Community Practitioner, 71*(5), 179–180.

Hockenberry, M. J. (2005). *Wong's essentials of pediatric nursing* (7th ed.). St. Louis: Mosby.

Hockenberry, M. J. (2006). *Wong's nursing care for infants and children* (8th ed.). St. Louis: Mosby.

Kinservik, M. A., & Friedhoff, M. M. (2000). Control issues in toilet training. *Pediatric Nursing, 26*(3), 267–274.

Pillitteri, A. (2007). *Maternal and child health nursing: Care of the childbearing and childrearing family* (5th ed.). Philadelphia: Lippincott Williams & Wilkins.

Stadtler, A. C., Gorski, P. A., & Brazelton, T. B. (1999). Toilet training methods, clinical interventions, and recommendations. *Pediatrics, 103*(6), 1359–1361.

Technology Management 7880

Definition: Use of technical equipment and devices to monitor patient condition or sustain life

Activities:
- Change or replace patient care equipment, per protocol
- Provide standby equipment, as appropriate
- Maintain equipment in good working order
- Correct malfunctioning equipment
- Zero and calibrate equipment, as appropriate
- Keep emergency equipment in an appropriate and readily accessible place
- Ensure proper grounding of electronic equipment
- Plug equipment into electrical outlets connected to an emergency power source
- Have equipment periodically checked by bioengineering, as appropriate
- Recharge batteries in portable patient care equipment
- Set alarm limits on equipment, as appropriate
- Respond to equipment alarms appropriately
- Consult with other health care team members, and recommend equipment or devices for patient use
- Use alterations in machine-derived data as an impetus for reassessing the patient
- Verify patient data downloaded from biomedical devices to electronic health record
- Integrate clinical decision support to notify and remind caregiver of clinical abnormal and potential risks
- Display clinical summaries and trend analysis of pertinent patient-related data
- Calculate scores from valid and reliable health care assessment instruments
- Compare machine-derived data with nurse's perception of patient's condition

T

- Explain potential risks and benefits of using this technology
- Facilitate obtaining informed consent, as appropriate
- Place bedside equipment strategically to maximize patient access and prevent tripping over tubes and cords
- Become knowledgeable of the equipment and proficient in using it
- Instruct patient and family how to operate equipment, as appropriate
- Inform the patient and family of the expected patient outcomes and side effects associated with using the equipment
- Facilitate ethical decision making related to use of life-sustaining and life-support technologies, as appropriate
- Demonstrate to family members how to communicate with patient on life-support equipment
- Facilitate interaction between family members and patient who is receiving life-support therapy
- Monitor the effect of equipment use on the physiological, psychological, and social functioning of the patient and family
- Monitor effectiveness of the technology on patient outcomes

1st edition 1992; revised 2013

Background Readings:

Brokel, J. M., Schwichtenberg, T. J., Wakefield, D. S., Ward, M. M., Shaw, M. G., & Kramer, J. M. (2011). Evaluating clinical decision support rules as an intervention in clinician workflows with technology. CIN. *Computers, Informatics, Nursing, 29*(1), 36–42.

Dorr, D. A., Wilcox, A. B., Brunker, C.P., Burdon, R.E., & Donnelly, S.M. (2008). The effect of technology-supported, multidisease care management on the mortality and hospitalization of seniors. *The American Geriatrics Society, 56*(12), 2195–2220.

Gibson, F., Aldiss, S., Taylor, R. M., Maguire, R., McCann, L., Sage, M., & Kearney, N. (2010). Utilization of the medical research council evaluation framework in the development of technology for symptom management. *Cancer Nursing, 33*(5), 343–352.

Mahlmeister, L. R. Human factors and error in perinatal care: The interplay between nurses, machines, and the work environment. *Journal of Perinatal & Neonatal Nursing, 24*(1), 12–21.

Telephone Consultation 8180

Definition: Eliciting patient's concerns, listening, and providing support, information, or teaching in response to patient's stated concerns, over the telephone

Activities:

- Identify self with name and credentials, organization; let caller know if call is being recorded (e.g., for quality monitoring), using voice to create therapeutic relationship
- Inform patient about call process and obtain consent
- Consider cultural and socioeconomic barriers to patient's response
- Obtain information about purpose of the call (e.g., medical diagnoses, if any, past health history, and current treatment regimen)
- Identify concerns about health status
- Establish level of caller's knowledge and source of that knowledge
- Determine patient's ability to understand telephone teaching/instructions (e.g., hearing deficits, confusion, language barriers)
- Provide means of overcoming any identified barrier to learning or use of support system(s)
- Identify degree of family support and involvement in care
- Inquire about related complaints/symptoms, according to standard protocol, if available
- Obtain data related to effectiveness of current treatment(s), if any, by consulting and citing approved references as sources (e.g., "American Red Cross suggests . . . ")
- Determine psychological response to situation and availability of support system(s)
- Determine safety risk to caller and/others
- Determine whether concerns require further evaluation (use standard protocol)
- Provide clear instruction on how to access needed care, if concerns are acute
- Provide information about treatment regimen and resultant self-care responsibilities, as necessary, according to scope of practice and established guidelines
- Provide information about prescribed therapies and medications, as appropriate
- Provide information about health promotion/health education, as appropriate
- Identify actual/potential problems related to implementation of self-care regimen
- Make recommendations about regimen changes, as appropriate (using established guidelines, if available)
- Consult with physician/primary care provider about changes in the treatment regimen, as necessary
- Provide information about community resources, educational programs, support groups, and self-help groups, as indicated
- Provide services in a caring and supportive manner
- Involve family/significant others in the care and planning
- Answer questions
- Determine caller's understanding of information provided
- Maintain confidentiality, as indicated
- Document any assessments, advice, instructions, or other information given to patient, according to specified guidelines
- Follow guidelines for investigating or reporting suspected child, geriatric, or spousal abuse situations
- Follow up to determine disposition; document disposition and patient's intended action(s)
- Determine need, and establish time intervals for further intermittent assessment, as appropriate
- Determine how patient or family member can be reached for a return telephone call, as appropriate.

- Document permission for return call and identify persons able to receive call information
- Discuss and resolve problem calls with supervisory/collegial help

2nd edition 1996; revised 2000

Background Readings:

American Academy of Ambulatory Nursing. (1997). *Telephone nursing practice administration and practice standards*. Pitman, NJ: Anthony J. Jannetti.

Anderson, K., Qiu, Y., Whittaker, A. R., & Lucas, M. (2001). Breath sounds, asthma, and the mobile phone. *Lancet, 358*(9290), 1343–1344.

Haas, S. A., & Androwich, I. A. (1999). Telephone consultation. In G. M. Bulechek & J. C. McCloskey (Eds.), *Nursing interventions: Effective nursing treatments* (3rd ed., pp. 670–685). Philadelphia: Saunders.

Hagan, L., Morin, D., & Lepine, R. (2000). Evaluation of telenursing outcomes: Satisfaction, self-care practices, and cost savings. *Public Health Nursing, 17*(4), 305–313.

Larson-Dahn, M. L. (2001). Tel-eNurse practice: Quality of care and patient outcomes. *Journal of Nursing Administration, 31*(3), 145–152.

Poole, S. G., Schmitt, B. D., Carruth, T., Peterson-Smith, A. A., & Slusarski, M. (1993). After-hours telephone coverage: The application of an area-wide telephone triage and advice system for pediatric practices. *Pediatrics, 92*(5), 670–679.

Wheeler, S., & Siebelt, B. (1997). Calling all nurses: How to perform telephone triage. *Nursing, 97*(7), 37–41.

Telephone Follow-Up   8190

Definition: Providing results of testing or evaluating patient's response and determining potential for problems as a result of previous treatment, examination, or testing, over the telephone

Activities:

- Determine that you are actually speaking to the patient or, if someone else, that you have the patient's permission to give information to that person
- Identify self with name and credentials, organization; let caller know if call is being recorded (e.g., for quality monitoring)
- Inform patient about call process and obtain consent
- Notify patient of test results, as indicated (positive results with significant health implications, such as biopsy results, should not be given over the phone by the nurse)
- Use intermediary services such as language relay services, TTY/TDD (teletypewriter/telecommunications device for the deaf), or emerging telecommunication technologies such as computer networks or visual displays, as appropriate
- Assist with prescription refills, according to established guidelines
- Solicit and answer questions
- Provide information about community resources, educational programs, support groups, and self-help groups, as indicated
- Establish a date and time for follow-up care or referral appointment
- Provide information about treatment regimen and resultant self-care responsibilities, as necessary according to scope of practice and established guidelines
- Maintain confidentiality
- Do not leave follow-up messages on answering machines or voicemail to ensure confidentiality
- Document any assessments, advice, instructions, or other information given to patient, according to specified guidelines
- Determine how patient or family member can be reached for a return telephone call, as appropriate
- Document permission for return call and identify persons able to receive call

3rd edition 2000

Background Readings:

American Academy of Ambulatory Care Nursing & American Nurses Association. (1997). *Nursing in ambulatory care: The future is here*. Washington, DC: Author.

American Academy of Ambulatory Nursing. (1997). *Telephone nursing practice administration and practice standards*. Pitman, NJ: Anthony J. Jannetti.

Anderson, K., Oiu, Y., Whittaker, A. R., & Lucas, M. (2001). Breath sounds, asthma, and the mobile phone. *Lancet, 358*(9290), 1343–1344.

Hagan, L., Morin, D., & Lepine, R. (2000). Evaluation of telenursing outcomes: Satisfaction, self-care practices, and cost savings. *Public Health Nursing, 17*(4), 305–313.

Larson-Dahn, M. L. (2001). Tel-eNurse practice: Quality of care and patient outcomes. *Journal of Nursing Administration, 31*(3), 145–152.

Pidd, H., McGrory, K. J., & Payne, S. R. (2000). Telephone follow-up after urological surgery. *Professional Nurse, 15*(7), 449–451.

Weaver, L. A., & Doran, K. A. (2001). Telephone follow-up after cardiac surgery. *American Journal of Nursing, 101*(5), 24OO, 24QQ, 24SS–24UU.

T

Temperature Regulation 3900

Definition: Attaining or maintaining body temperature within a normal range

Activities:

- Monitor temperature at least every 2 hours, as appropriate
- Monitor newborn's temperature until stabilized
- Institute a continuous core temperature monitoring device, as appropriate
- Monitor blood pressure, pulse, and respiration, as appropriate
- Monitor skin color and temperature
- Monitor for and report signs and symptoms of hypothermia and hyperthermia
- Promote adequate fluid and nutritional intake
- Wrap infant immediately after birth to prevent heat loss
- Wrap a low birthweight infant in plastic (e.g., polyethylene, polyurethane) immediately after birth while still covered with amniotic fluid, as appropriate and according to agency protocol
- Apply stockinette cap to prevent heat loss of newborn
- Place newborn in isolette or under warmer, as needed
- Maintain humidity at 50% or greater in incubator to reduce evaporative heat loss
- Prewarm items (e.g., blankets, snugglies) placed next to infant in incubator
- Instruct patient how to prevent heat exhaustion and heat stroke
- Discuss importance of thermoregulation and possible negative effects of excess chilling, as appropriate
- Instruct patient, particularly elderly patients, about actions to prevent hypothermia from cold exposure
- Inform patient of indications of heat exhaustion and appropriate emergency treatment, as appropriate
- Inform about indications of hypothermia and appropriate emergency treatment, as appropriate
- Use a warming mattress, warm blankets, and warm ambient environment to raise body temperature, as appropriate
- Use a cooling mattress, water circulating blankets, tepid baths, ice pack or gel pad application, and intravascular cooling catheterization to lower body temperature, as appropriate
- Adjust environmental temperature to patient needs
- Give appropriate medication to prevent or control shivering
- Administer antipyretic medication, as appropriate
- Preserve normothermia in newly deceased patients who are organ donors by increasing temperature of ambient air; use of infrared warming lights, warm air, or water blanket; or instillation of warmed IV fluids, as appropriate

1st edition 1992, revised 2013

Background Readings:

Bassin , S. L., Bleck, T. P., & Nathan, B. D. (2008). Intravascular temperature control system to maintain normothermia in organ donors. *Neurocritical Care, 8*(1), 31–35.

Knobel, R., & Holditch-Davis, D. (2010). Thermoregulation and health loss prevention after birth and during neonatal intensive-care unit stabilization of extremely low-birthweight infants. *Advances in Neonatal Care, 10*(5 Suppl. 5), S7–S14.

Kozier, B., Erb, G., Berman, A., & Snyder, S. (2004). *Fundamentals of nursing: Concepts, processes, and practice* (7th ed.). Upper Saddle River, NJ: Prentice Hall.

Pillitteri, A. (2007). *Maternal and child health nursing: Care of the childbearing and childrearing family* (5th ed.). Philadelphia: Lippincott Williams & Wilkins.

Potter, P. A., & Perry, A. G. (2006). *Fundamentals of nursing* (6th ed.). St. Louis: Mosby.

Thompson, H. J., Kirkness, C. J., & Mitchell, P. H. (2007). Fever management practices of neuroscience nurses: National and regional perspective. *Journal of Neuroscience Nursing, 39*(3), 151–162.

Temperature Regulation: Perioperative 3902

Definition: Attaining and maintaining desired body temperature throughout the surgical event

Activities:

- Identify and discuss type of anesthesia planned for patient with surgical team
- Identify patient risk factors for experiencing abnormalities in body temperature (e.g., general or major regional anesthesia, age, major trauma, patients with burns, low body weight, personal or familial risk for malignant hyperthermia)
- Prewarm the patient with active warming device (e.g., forced-air warming) for at least 15 minutes before start of anesthesia, as appropriate
- Transport patient using warming device (e.g., heated isolette), as appropriate
- Apply and regulate active warming device (e.g., forced-air warming)
- Adjust ambient room temperature to minimize the risk of hypothermia (i.e., in addition to forced-air warming, when large surface areas are exposed, maintain room temperature at or above 73.4° F or 23° C)
- Minimize exposure of patient during surgical prepping and procedure, when possible
- Provide warm or cool irrigating solutions, as appropriate
- Monitor the temperature of irrigating solutions
- Warm or cool intravenous fluids, as appropriate
- Provide and regulate blood warmer
- Provide or assist in provision of heated, humidified anesthetic gases, as appropriate
- Provide heated intraperitoneal gases (e.g., carbon dioxide) for laparoscopy
- Discontinue active warming activities (e.g., forced air warming), when appropriate
- Monitor vital signs, including continuous core body temperature
- Monitor for abnormal or unintentional increases or decreases in body temperature
- Monitor electrocardiography results
- Monitor expired carbon dioxide (capnography)

- Monitor laboratory results (e.g., arterial blood gases, electrolytes)
- Ensure active warming equipment and supplies are in place and in good working order
- Maintain emergency equipment and supplies for malignant hyperthermia, per protocol, including dantrolene sodium, in perioperative and perianesthesia areas
- Initiate malignant hyperthermia protocol, as appropriate
- Prepare or administer dantrolene sodium
- Provide handoff communication regarding patient risk of abnormalities in temperature (e.g., personal or familial risk for malignant hyperthermia)
- Ensure proper body temperature until patient is awake and alert

2nd edition 1996; revised 2013

Background Readings:

Association of PeriOperative Registered Nurses. (2011). Recommended practices for the prevention of unplanned perioperative hypothermia. In *Perioperative standards and recommended practices for inpatient and ambulatory settings* (pp. 307–320). Denver, CO: Author.

Hooper, V. D., Chard, R., Clifford, T., Fetzer, S., Fossum, S., Godden, B., et al. (2009). ASPAN's evidence-based clinical practice guideline for the promotion of perioperative normothermia. *Journal of PeriAnesthesia Nursing, 24*(5), 271–287.

Hopkins, P. M. (2011). Malignant hyperthermia: Pharmacology of triggering. *British Journal of Anaesthesia, 107*(1), 48–56.

Malignant Hyperthermia Association. (2010). *Transfer of care guidelines.* Sherburne, NY: Author.

Sessler, D. I. (2008). Temperature monitoring and perioperative thermoregulation. *Anesthesiology, 109*(2), 318–338.

Therapeutic Play   4430

Definition: Purposeful and directive use of toys or other materials to assist children in communicating their perception and knowledge of their world and to help in gaining mastery of their environment

Activities:

- Provide a quiet environment that is free from interruptions
- Provide sufficient time to allow for effective play
- Structure play session to facilitate desired outcome
- Communicate the purpose of play session to child and parent
- Discuss play activities with family
- Set limits for therapeutic play session
- Provide safe play equipment
- Provide developmentally appropriate play equipment
- Provide play equipment that stimulates creative, expressive play
- Provide play equipment that stimulates role playing
- Provide real or simulated hospital operating room medical equipment to encourage expression of knowledge and feelings about hospitalization, treatments, or illness
- Supervise therapeutic play sessions
- Encourage child to manipulate play equipment
- Encourage child to share feelings, knowledge, and perceptions
- Validate child's feelings expressed during the play session
- Communicate acceptance of feelings, both positive and negative, expressed through play
- Observe the child's use of play equipment
- Monitor child's reactions and anxiety level throughout play session
- Identify child's misconceptions or fears through comments made during (hospital role) play session
- Continue play sessions on a regular basis to establish trust and reduce fear of unfamiliar equipment or treatments, as appropriate
- Record observations made during play session

1st edition 1992; revised 2000

Background Readings:

Hart, R., Powell, M. A., Mather, P. L., & Slack, J. L. (1992). *Therapeutic play activities for hospitalized children.* St. Louis: Mosby.

Raphel, S., & Bennett, C. F. (2005). Child psychiatric nursing. In G. W. Stuart & M. T. Laraia (Eds.), *Principles and practice of psychiatric nursing* (8th ed., pp. 728–752). St. Louis: Mosby.

Snyder, M. (1992). Play. In M. Snyder (Ed.), *Independent nursing interventions* (2nd ed., pp. 287–293). Albany, NY: Delmar.

Tiedeman, M. E., Simon, K. A., & Clatworthy, S. (1990). Communication through therapeutic play. In M. J. Craft & J. A. Denehy (Eds.), *Nursing interventions for infants and children* (pp. 93–110). Philadelphia: Saunders.

Vessey, J. A., & Mahon, M. M. (1990). Therapeutic play and the hospitalized child. *Journal of Pediatric Nursing, 5*(5), 328–333.

T

Therapeutic Touch 5465

Definition: Attuning to the universal energy field by seeking to act as a healing influence using the natural sensitivity of hands and passing them over the body to gently focus, direct, and modulate the human energy field

Activities:
- Create a comfortable environment without distractions
- Determine willingness to experience the intervention
- Identify mutual goals for the session
- Advise the patient to ask questions whenever they arise
- Place patient in either a comfortable sitting or supine position
- Center self by focusing awareness on the inner self
- Focus on the intention to facilitate wholeness and healing at all levels of consciousness
- Place hands with palms facing the patient 3 to 5 inches from their body
- Begin the one to two minute assessment by moving the hands slowly and steadily over as much of the patient as possible, from head to toe and front to back
- Move the hands in very gentle downward movements through the patient's energy field, thinking of the patient as a unitary whole and facilitating an open and balanced energy flow
- Note the overall pattern of the energy flow, especially any areas of disturbance such as congestion or unevenness, which may be perceived through very subtle cues in the hands, for example, temperature change, tingling, or other subtle feelings of movement
- Focus intention on facilitating symmetry and healing in disturbed areas
- Continue the treatment by very gently facilitating the flow of healing energy into areas of disturbance
- Finish when it is judged that the appropriate amount of change has taken place (i.e., for an infant, 1 to 2 minutes; for an adult, 5-10 minutes), keeping in mind the importance of gentleness
- Encourage the patient to rest for 20 minutes or more after treatment
- Note whether the patient has experienced a relaxation response and any related changes

1st edition 1992; revised 2000, 2013

Background Readings:

Coakley, A. B., & Duffy, M. E. (2010). The effect of therapeutic touch on postoperative patients. *Journal of Holistic Nursing, 28*(3), 193–200.

Engle, V. F., & Graney, M. J. (2000). Biobehavioral effects of therapeutic touch. *Journal of Nursing Scholarship, 32*(3), 287–293.

Krieger, D. (1993). *The personal practice of therapeutic touch: Accepting your power to heal.* Santa Fe, NM: Bear & Company.

Krieger, D. (2002). *Therapeutic touch: As transpersonal healing.* Brooklyn, NY: Lantern Books.

Monroe, C. M. (2009). The effects of therapeutic touch on pain. *Journal of Holistic Nursing, 27*(2), 85–92.

O'Mathuna, D. P. (2000). Evidence-based practice and reviews of therapeutic touch. *Journal of Nursing Scholarship, 32*(3), 279–285.

Peters, R. M. (1999). The effectiveness of therapeutic touch: A meta-analytic review. *Nursing Science Quarterly, 12*(1), 52–61.

Sayre-Adams, J., & Wright, S. (1995). The essentials of practice. In J. Sayre-Adams & S. Wright (Eds.), *The theory and practice of therapeutic touch* (pp. 75–110). Edinburgh: Churchill Livingstone.

Winstead-Fry P., & Kijek, J. (1999). An integrative review and meta-analysis of therapeutic touch research. *Alternative Therapies in Health & Medicine, 5(6),* 58–67.

Therapy Group 5450

Definition: Application of psychotherapeutic techniques to a group, including the utilization of interactions between members of the group

Activities:
- Determine the purpose of the group (e.g., maintenance of reality testing, facilitation of communication, examination of interpersonal skills, and support) and the nature of the group process
- Form a group of optimal size: 5 to 12 members
- Choose group members who are willing to participate actively and take responsibility for own problems
- Determine whether level of motivation is high enough to benefit from group therapy
- Use a coleader, as appropriate
- Address the issue of mandatory attendance
- Address the issue of whether new members can join at any time
- Establish a time and place for the group meeting
- Meet in 1 to 2 hour sessions, as appropriate
- Begin and end on time and expect participants to remain until the conclusion
- Arrange chairs in a circle in close proximity
- Move the group to the working stage as quickly as possible
- Assist the group in forming therapeutic norms
- Help the group to work through their resistance to change
- Give the group a sense of direction that enables them to identify and resolve each step of development
- Use the technique of "process illumination" to encourage exploration of the significant meaning of the message
- Encourage self-disclosure and discussion of the past only as it relates to the function and goals of the group
- Use the technique of "here and now activation" to move the focus from the generic to the personal, from the abstract to the specific
- Encourage members to share things they have in common with each other
- Encourage members to share their anger, sadness, humor, mistrust, and other feelings with each other
- Assist members in the process of exploration and acceptance of any anger felt toward the group leader and others
- Confront behaviors that threaten group cohesion (e.g., tardiness, absences, disruptive extragroup socialization, subgrouping, and scapegoating)

T

- Provide social reinforcement (e.g., verbal and nonverbal) for desired behaviors/responses
- Provide structured group exercises, as appropriate, to promote group function and insight
- Use role playing and problem solving, as appropriate
- Help members provide feedback to each other, so that they develop insights into their own behavior
- Incorporate leaderless sessions, when appropriate to the goals and function of the group
- Conclude session with a summary of the proceedings
- Meet individually with the member who desires premature termination to examine rationale for this
- Assist member to terminate from the group, if appropriate
- Assist group to review the past history and a member's relationship with the group when someone leaves
- Recruit new members, as appropriate, to maintain the integrity of the group
- Provide an individualized orientation session for each new member of the group before first group session

1st edition 1992; revised 1996

Background Readings:

Boyd, M. A. (2005). Interventions with groups. In M. A. Boyd (Ed.), *Psychiatric nursing: Contemporary practice* (3rd ed., pp. 233–242). Philadelphia: Lippincott Williams & Wilkins.

LaSalle, P. M., & LaSalle, A. J. (2005). Therapeutic groups. In G. W. Stuart & M. T. Laraia (Eds.), *Principles and practice of psychiatric nursing* (8th ed., pp. 668–681). St. Louis: Mosby.

Lassiter, P. G. (1992). Working with groups in the community. In M. Stanhope & J. Lancaster (Eds.), *Community health nursing* (3rd ed., pp. 277–291). St. Louis: Mosby.

Snyder, M. (1992). Groups. In M. Snyder (Ed.), *Independent nursing interventions* (2nd ed., pp. 244–255). Albany, NY: Delmar.

Wieland, V., & Cummings, S. (1992). Group psychotherapy. In G. M. Bulechek & J. C. McCloskey (Eds.), *Nursing interventions: Essential nursing treatments* (2nd ed., pp. 340–351). Philadelphia: Saunders.

Yalom, I. D. (1985). *The theory and practice of group psychotherapy* (3rd ed.). New York: Basic Books.

Thrombolytic Therapy Management　　4270

Definition: Collection and analysis of patient data to expedite safe, appropriate provision of an agent that dissolves a thrombus

Activities:
- Verify patient's identity
- Obtain history of present illness and medical history
- Perform physical examination (e.g., general appearance, heart rate, blood pressure, respiratory rate, temperature, pain level, height, and weight)
- Explain all procedures to the patient and significant other
- Allow significant other at patient's bedside, if possible
- Obtain pulse oximetry and apply oxygen, as appropriate
- Perform targeted assessment of the system that is indicated by the history of present illness
- Obtain 12-lead EKG, as appropriate
- Initiate intravenous line and obtain blood samples for laboratory tests
- Obtain stat computerized tomography head scan, as appropriate
- Obtain V/Q scan, as appropriate
- Consider guidelines for candidacy (e.g., therapy inclusion and exclusion criteria)
- Determine if the patient will receive the therapy
- Obtain informed consent
- Prepare for thrombolytic therapy, if indicated
- Obtain additional intravenous access site
- Avoid arterial sampling to prevent bleeding complications
- Prepare thrombolytic agents, per facility protocol
- Administer thrombolytic agents according to specific guidelines for administration

- Administer additional medications as ordered
- Continually monitor cardiac rhythm, vital signs, level of pain, heart and lung sounds, level of consciousness, peripheral perfusion, intake and output, change in neurological status, and for resolution of symptoms, as indicated
- Observe for signs of bleeding
- Obtain additional radiological tests, as indicated (e.g., chest x-ray)
- Prepare to initiate basic and advanced life support measures, if indicated
- Prepare to transfer for definitive care (e.g., cardiac catheterization lab, ICU)

5th edition 2008

Background Readings:

Emergency Nursing Association. (1997). *Standards of emergency nursing practice* (4th ed.). Des Plaines, IL: Author.

Emergency Nursing Association. (2000). *Emergency nursing core curriculum* (5th ed.). Philadelphia: Saunders.

Hazinski, M. F., Cummins, R. O., & Field, J. M. (Eds.). (2002). *2000 handbook of emergency cardiovascular care for healthcare providers*. Dallas, TX: American Heart Association.

Lacy, C. F., Armstrong, L. L., Goldman, M. P., & Lance, L. L. (2005). *Drug information handbook* (13th ed.). Hudson, OH: Lexi-Comp.

T

Total Parenteral Nutrition (TPN) Administration 1200

Definition: Delivery of nutrients intravenously and monitoring of patient response

Activities:
- Assure placement of proper intravenous line related to duration of nutrients to be infused (e.g., centrally placed line preferred; peripheral lines only in well-nourished individuals expecting to need TPN for less than 2 weeks)
- Use central lines only for infusion of high caloric nutrients or hyperosmolar solutions (e.g., 10% dextrose, 2% amino acids with standard additives)
- Assure TPN solutions infused in a noncentral catheter are limited to osmolarity less than 900 mOsm/L
- Insert peripheral intravenous central catheter, per agency protocol
- Ascertain correct placement of intravenous central catheter by x-ray examination
- Maintain central line patency and dressing, per agency protocol
- Monitor for infiltration, infection, and metabolic complications (e.g., hyperlipidemia, elevated triglycerides, thrombocytopenia, platelet dysfunction)
- Check the TPN solution to ensure that correct nutrients are included, as ordered
- Maintain sterile technique when preparing and hanging TPN solutions
- Provide regular, aseptic, and meticulous care of the central venous catheter, particularly the catheter exit site, to assure prolonged, safe and complication-free use
- Avoid use of the catheter for purposes other than delivery of TPN (e.g., blood transfusions and blood sampling)
- Use an infusion pump for delivery of TPN solutions
- Maintain a constant flow rate of TPN solution
- Avoid rapid replacement of TPN solution when interrupted for supplemental infusions
- Monitor daily weight
- Monitor intake and output
- Monitor serum albumin, total protein, electrolyte, lipid profiles, glucose levels, and chemistry profile
- Monitor vital signs, as indicated
- Monitor urine glucose for glycosuria, acetone, and protein
- Maintain a small oral nutritional intake during TPN, whenever possible
- Encourage a gradual transition from parenteral to enteral feeding, if indicated
- Administer insulin, as ordered, to maintain serum glucose level in the designated range, as appropriate
- Report abnormal signs and symptoms associated with TPN to the physician, and modify care accordingly
- Maintain universal precautions
- Instruct patient and family care of and indications for TPN
- Assure patient and family comprehension and competency prior to discharge home with ongoing TPN

1st edition 1992; revised 2013

Background Readings:

American Society for Parenteral and Enteral Nutrition (A.S.P.E.N.) Board of Directors. (2009). Clinical guidelines for the use of parenteral and enteral nutrition in adult and pediatric patients. *Journal of Parenteral & Enteral Nutrition, 33*(3), 255–259.

Kerner, J. A. Jr., Hurwitz, M., Duggan, C., Watkins, J., & Walker, W. A. (2008). Parenteral nutrition. In C. Duggan, J. Watkins, & W. A. Walker (Eds.), *Nutrition in pediatrics: Basic science & clinical applications* (4th ed., pp. 777–793). Hamilton, Ontario: BC Decker.

Pittiruti, M., Hamilton, H., Biffi, R., MacFie, J., & Pertkiewicz, M. (2009). ESPEN guidelines on parenteral nutrition: Central venous catheters. *Clinical Nutrition, 28*(4), 365–377.

Touch 5460

Definition: Providing comfort and communication through purposeful tactile contact

Activities:
- Evaluate one's own personal comfort in using touch with patients and family members
- Evaluate the readiness of the patient when offering touch
- Evaluate the environmental context before offering touch
- Determine which body part is best to touch and the length of touch that produces the most positive responses in the recipient
- Observe cultural taboos about touch
- Hug reassuringly, when appropriate
- Put arm around patient's shoulders, as appropriate
- Hold patient's hand to provide emotional support
- Apply gentle pressure at wrist, hand, or shoulder of seriously ill patient
- Rub back in synchrony with patient's breathing, as appropriate
- Stroke body part in slow, rhythmical fashion, as appropriate
- Massage around painful area, as appropriate
- Elicit from parents common actions used to soothe and calm their child
- Hold infant or child firmly and snugly
- Encourage parents to touch newborn or ill child
- Surround premature infant with blanket rolls (nesting)
- Swaddle infant snugly in a blanket to keep arms and legs close to the body
- Place infant on mother's body immediately after birth
- Encourage mother to hold, touch, and examine the infant while umbilical cord is being severed
- Encourage parents to hold infant
- Encourage parents to massage infant
- Demonstrate quieting techniques for infants
- Provide appropriate pacifier for nonnutritive sucking in newborns
- Provide oral stimulation exercises before tube feedings in premature infants
- Evaluate the effect when using touch

1st edition 1992; revised 2008

Background Readings:

Gleeson, M., & Timmins, F. (2005). A review of the use and clinical effectiveness of touch as a nursing intervention. *Clinical Effectiveness in Nursing, 9*(1-2), 69–77.

Molsberry, D., & Shogan, M. G. (1990). Communicating through touch. In M. J. Craft & J. A. Denehy (Eds.), *Nursing interventions for infants and children* (pp. 127–150). Philadelphia: Saunders.

Rombalski, J. J. (2003). A personal journey in understanding physical touch as a nursing intervention. *Journal of Holistic Nursing, 21*(1), 73–80.

Snyder, M., & Nojima, Y. (1998). Purposeful touch. In M. Snyder & R. Lindquist (Eds.), *Complementary/alternative therapies in nursing* (3rd ed., pp. 149–158). New York: Springer.

Weiss, S. J. (1988). Touch. In J. Fitzpatrick, R. Taunton, & J. Benoliel (Eds.), *Annual Review of Nursing Research,* 6, 3–27.

Weiss, S. J. (1992). The tactile environment of caregiving: Implications for health science and health care. *The Science of Caring, 3*(2), 33–40.

Traction/Immobilization Care 0940

Definition: Management of a patient who has traction and/or a stabilizing device to immobilize and stabilize a body part

Activities:

- Position in proper body alignment
- Maintain proper position in bed to enhance traction
- Ensure that proper weights are being applied
- Ensure that the ropes and pulleys hang freely
- Ensure that the pull of ropes and weights remains along the axis of the fractured bone
- Brace traction weights while moving patient
- Maintain traction at all times
- Monitor self-care ability while in traction
- Monitor external fixation device
- Monitor pin insertion sites
- Monitor skin and bony prominences for signs of skin breakdown
- Monitor circulation, movement, and sensation of affected extremity
- Monitor for complications of immobility
- Perform pin insertion site care
- Administer appropriate skin care at friction points
- Provide trapeze for movement in bed, as appropriate
- Instruct on bracing device care, as needed
- Instruct on external fixation device care, as needed
- Instruct on pin site care, as needed
- Instruct in importance of adequate nutrition for bone healing

1st edition 1992; revised 1996

Background Readings:

F. A. Davis. (1989). *Taber's cyclopedic medical dictionary* (16th ed.). Philadelphia: Author.

Mourad, L. A. (1991). *Orthopedic disorders: Mosby's clinical nursing series.* St. Louis: Mosby.

Phipps, W. J., Long, B. C., & Woods, N. F. (1998). *Medical-surgical nursing: Concepts and clinical practice* (6th ed.). St. Louis: Mosby.

Smeltzer, S. C., & Bare, B. G. (2004). Musculoskeletal care modalities. In *Brunner & Suddarth's textbook of medical surgical nursing* (Vol. 2) (10th ed., pp. 2017–2045). Philadelphia: Lippincott Williams & Wilkins.

Transcutaneous Electrical Nerve Stimulation (TENS) 1540

Definition: Stimulation of skin and underlying tissue with controlled, low-voltage electrical pulses

Activities:

- Discuss the rationale for and limits and potential problems of TENS with the patient and family
- Determine whether a recommendation for TENS is appropriate
- Do not use TENS if the patient has a pacemaker
- Discuss therapy with provider and obtain prescription for TENS, if appropriate
- Verify that the TENS unit has full battery charge
- Inspect the wires for first signs of wear, replacing wires as needed
- Select stimulation site, considering alternate sites when direct application is not possible (e.g., adjacent to, distal to, bracketing the site, between affected areas and the brain, and contralateral to the pain)
- Apply disposable or reusable electrodes to the site of stimulation
- Apply wires to electrodes and TENS unit, making sure wires are securely plugged into connections
- Determine therapeutic amplitude, rate, and pulse width
- Adjust the amplitude, rate, and pulse width to predetermined settings indicated
- Maintain stimulation for predetermined interval (e.g., continuous or intermittent)
- Secure TENS unit to the patient (e.g., on patient's belt or waistband of pants) if continuous application is necessary
- Discontinue use when sensation is strong yet tolerable
- Adjust the site and settings to achieve the desired response based on individual tolerance
- Inspect sites of electrodes for possible skin irritation at every application or at least every 12 hours
- Provide verbal and written instruction on the use of TENS and its operation
- Use TENS alone or in conjunction with other measures, as appropriate
- Document the effectiveness of TENS

1st edition 1992; revised 2013

Background Readings:

DeSantana, J. M., Walsh, D. M., Vance, C., Rakel, B. A., & Sluka, K. A. (2008). Effectiveness of transcutaneous electrical nerve stimulation for treatment of hyperalgesia and pain. *Current Rheumatology Reports, 10*(6), 492–499.

Herr, K. A., & Kwekkeboom, K. L. (2003). Assisting older clients with pain management in the home. *Home Health Care Management and Practice, 15*(3), 237–250.

Lynn, P. (2011). *Taylor's clinical nursing skills: A nursing process approach* (3rd ed.). Philadelphia: Lippincott Williams & Wilkins.

Sluka, K. S. & Walsh, D. M. (2003). Transcutaneous nerve stimulation: Basic science mechanisms and clinical effectiveness. *Journal of Pain, 4*(3), 109–121.

T

Transfer 0970

Definition: Moving a patient with limitation of independent movement

Activities:

- Review chart for activity orders
- Determine mobility level and limitations of movement
- Determine level of consciousness and ability to cooperate
- Plan type and method of move
- Determine amount and type of assistance needed
- Make sure equipment works before using it
- Discuss need for relocation with patient and/or family
- Discuss with patient and helpers how the move will be done
- Assist patient in receiving all necessary care (e.g., personal hygiene, gathering belongings) before performing the transfer, as appropriate
- Provide privacy, avoid drafts, and preserve the patient's modesty
- Make sure the new location of the patient is ready
- Adjust equipment as needed to working heights and lock all wheels
- Raise side rail on opposite side of nurse to prevent patient from falling out of bed
- Use proper body mechanics during movements
- Keep patient body in proper alignment during movements
- Raise and move patient with hydraulic lift, as necessary
- Move patient using transfer board, as necessary
- Transfer patient from a bed to stretcher, or vice versa, using a turning sheet, as appropriate
- Use a belt to assist a patient who can stand with assistance, as appropriate
- Use an incubator, stretcher, or bed to move a weak, injured, or surgical patient from one area to another
- Use a wheelchair to move a patient unable to walk
- Cradle and carry an infant or small child
- Assist patient to ambulate using your body as a human crutch, as appropriate
- Maintain traction devices during move, as appropriate
- Evaluate patient at end of transfer for proper body alignment, nonocclusion of tubes, wrinkle-free linens, unnecessarily exposed skin, adequate patient level of comfort, raised side rails, and call bell within reach

5th edition 2008

Background Readings:

Craven, R. (2006). *Fundamentals of nursing* (5th ed.). Philadelphia: Lippincott Williams & Wilkins.

Perry, A. G., & Potter, P. A. (2004). *Fundamentals of nursing* (6th ed.). St. Louis: Mosby.

Perry, A. G., & Potter, P. A. (2006). *Clinical nursing skills and techniques* (6th ed.). St. Louis: Mosby.

Stabl, L. (1996). How to transfer patients to other units. *American Journal of Nursing, 96*(8), 57–58.

Transport: Interfacility 7890

Definition: Moving a patient from one facility to another

Activities:

- Assure that a medical screening examination has been performed and documented
- Assure that the patient has been stabilized within the capabilities of the transferring facility or has met the conditions under which unstable patients may be transferred under the Emergency Treatment and Labor Act (EMTALA)
- Determine need for transfer of patient, ensuring that the patient requires treatment at the receiving facility and the benefits of the transfer outweigh the risks
- Obtain written order from physician to transport patient
- Identify preference of patient or significant others for receiving facility and physician, as appropriate
- Document that the receiving facility will accept the patient and has the necessary equipment and staff to handle the clinical situation
- Obtain written consent for transfer from patient or significant others
- Obtain written consent for transfer of minors, as appropriate
- Obtain written consent for release of patient information to receiving facility
- Facilitate the contact of receiving physician by attending physician, as indicated per EMTALA laws, and document this contact
- Arrange for required type of transport
- Provide a nurse-to-nurse clinical report about the patient to the receiving facility and document this contact
- Mobilize and provide necessary personnel, transfer equipment, and pharmaceuticals
- Copy medical records for receiving facility, including current record of events
- Assure that the medical records accompany the patient to the receiving facility
- Complete the certification for transfer that is signed, timed, and dated by the physician
- Document the medical reason for transfer as well as the medical benefits and risks of the transfer, as indicated per EMTALA laws
- Document all information pertaining to patients refusing transfer
- Attempt to secure written statement of refusal to transfer from patient, if indicated
- Continue to treat patients refusing transfer within the capability of the facility

5th edition 2008

Background Readings:

Bowen, S. L. (2004). Neonatal transport. In M. T. Verklan & M. Walden (Eds.), *Core curriculum for neonatal intensive care nursing.* (Chap. 21). Philadelphia: Saunders.

Casaubon, D. (2001). EMTALA: Practical application with an algorithm. *Journal of Emergency Nursing, 27*(4), 364–368.

Gilstrap, L. C., Oh, W., Greene, M. F., & Lemons, J. A. (Eds.). (2002). Inter-hospital care of the Perinatal patient. In *Guidelines for perinatal care* (5th ed., pp. 57–71). Elk Grove Village, IL: American Academy of Pediatrics & American College of Obstetricians and Gynecologists.

Glass, D. L., Rebstock, J., & Handberg, E. (2004). Emergency Treatment and Labor Act (EMTALA): Avoiding the pitfalls. *Journal of Perinatal and Neonatal Nursing, 18*(2), 103–114.

Society of Critical Care Medicine. (1993). Guidelines for the transfer of critically ill patients. *Critical Care Medicine, 21*(6), 931–937.

Warren, J., Fromm, R. E., Orr, R. A., Rotello, L. C., & Horst, H. M. (2004). Guidelines for the inter- and intra-hospital transport of critically ill patients. *Critical Care Medicine, 32*(1), 256–262.

Transport: Intrafacility   7892

Definition: Moving a patient from one area of a facility to another

Activities:
- Facilitate pretransport coordination and communication
- Obtain physician order prior to transport, as appropriate
- Determine amount and type of assistance needed
- Provide appropriate personnel to assist in transport
- Provide appropriate equipment to assist in transport
- Discuss need for relocation with patient and significant others
- Assist patient in receiving all necessary care (e.g., personal hygiene, gathering belongings) before performing the transfer, as appropriate
- Make sure the new location for the patient is ready
- Move patient using required equipment, as necessary
- Use an incubator, stretcher, or bed to move a weak, injured, or surgical patient from one area to another
- Use a wheelchair to move a patient unable to walk
- Cradle and carry an infant or small child
- Assist patient to ambulate using your body as a human crutch, as appropriate
- Provide escort during transport, as needed
- Monitor as appropriate during transport
- Provide a clinical report about patient to the receiving location, as appropriate
- Document pertinent information related to transport
- Evacuate patients in emergencies such as fire, hurricane, or tornado, according to agency disaster plan

5th edition 2008

Background Readings:

Craven, R. F., & Hirnle, C. J. (2004). *Fundamentals of nursing: Human health and function* (4th ed.). Philadelphia: Lippincott Williams & Wilkins.

Perry, A. G., & Potter, P. A. (2001). *Fundamentals of nursing* (5th ed.). St. Louis: Mosby.

Perry, A. G., & Potter, P. A. (2006). *Clinical nursing skills and techniques* (6th ed.). St. Louis: Mosby.

Stabl, L. (1996). How to transfer patients to other units. *American Journal of Nursing, 96*(8), 57–58.

Warren, J., Fromm, R. E., Orr, R. A., Rotello, L. C., & Horst, H. M. (2004). Guidelines for the inter- and intra-hospital transport of critically ill patients. *Critical Care Medicine, 32*(1), 256–262.

Trauma Therapy: Child   5410

Definition: Use of an interactive helping process to resolve a trauma experienced by a child

Activities:
- Teach specific stress management techniques before trauma exploration to restore a sense of control over thoughts and feelings
- Explore the trauma and its meaning to the child
- Use developmentally appropriate language to ask about the trauma
- Use relaxation and desensitization procedures to assist the child to describe the event
- Establish trust, safety, and the right to gain access to carefully guarded trauma material by monitoring reactions to the disclosure
- Proceed with therapy at the child's own pace
- Establish a signal the child can give if the trauma-focused work becomes overwhelming
- Focus therapy on self-regulation and rebuilding a sense of security
- Use art and play to promote expression
- Involve the parents or appropriate caretakers in therapy, as appropriate
- Educate the parents about their child's response to the trauma and to the process of therapy
- Assist parents in resolving their own emotional distress about the trauma
- Assist appropriate others to provide support
- Avoid involving parents or caretakers if they are the cause of the trauma
- Assist the child to reconsider assumptions made about the traumatic event with step-by-step analysis of any perceptive and cognitive distortions
- Explore and correct inaccurate attributions regarding the trauma, including omen formation and survivor's guilt
- Help identify and cope with feelings

T

- Explain the grief process to the child and parent(s), as appropriate
- Assist the child to examine any distorted assumptions and conclusions
- Assist child in reestablishing a sense of security and predictability in his/her life
- Assist child to integrate the restructured trauma events into history and life experience
- Address posttrauma role functioning in family life, peer relationships, and school performance

4th edition 2004

Background Readings:

Boyd, M. R. (2005). Caring for abused persons. In M. A. Boyd (Ed.), *Psychiatric nursing: Contemporary practice* (3rd ed., pp. 823–856). Philadelphia: Lippincott Williams & Wilkins.

Clark, C. C. (1997). Posttraumatic stress disorder: How to support healing. *American Journal of Nursing, 97*(8), 27–33.

DiPalma, L. M. (1997). Integrating trauma theory into nursing practice and education. *Clinical Nurse Specialist, 11*(3), 102–107.

Pifferbaum, B. (1997). Posttraumatic stress disorder in children: A review of the last 10 years. *Journal of the American Academy of Child and Adolescent Psychiatry, 36*(11), 1503–1511.

Triage: Disaster 6362

Definition: Establishing priorities of patient care for urgent treatment while allocating scarce resources

Activities:
- Ready an area and equipment for triage
- Acquire information about the nature of the problem, emergency, accident, or disaster
- Consider the resources that are available
- Contact appropriate personnel
- Evaluate critical patients from the field first
- Evacuate injured as appropriate
- Participate in prioritization of patients for treatment
- Monitor for and treat life-threatening injuries or acute needs
- Identify the patient's chief complaint
- Obtain information about the patient's past medical history
- Check for medical alert tags, as appropriate
- Conduct a primary survey of all body systems, as appropriate
- Initiate appropriate emergency measures, as indicated
- Perform a secondary body system survey, as appropriate
- Attach appropriate identification, as indicated by patient's status
- Assist with performance of diagnostic tests, as indicated by the patient's condition

3rd edition 2000

Background Readings:

Mezza, I. (1992). Triage: Setting priorities for health care. *Nursing Forum, 27*(2), 15–19.

Pepe, P. E. (1988). Whom to resuscitate. In J. M. Civetta, R. W. Taylor, & R. K. Kirby (Eds.), *Critical care*. Philadelphia: Lippincott.

Smeltzer, S. C., & Bare, B. G. (2004). Terrorism, mass casualty, and disaster nursing. In *Brunner & Suddarth's textbook of medical surgical nursing* (Vol. 2, 10th ed., pp. 2183–2198). Philadelphia: Lippincott Williams & Wilkins.

Triage: Emergency Center 6364

Definition: Establishing priorities and initiating treatment for patients in an emergency center

Activities:
- Monitor breathing and circulation
- Perform crisis intervention, as appropriate
- Diffuse escalating violence, as appropriate
- Take patients requiring urgent care to treatment area immediately
- Evaluate and transfer mothers in labor
- Explain the triage process to those presenting for service
- Monitor vital signs
- Perform a physical examination relevant to chief complaint
- Obtain a pertinent medical history
- Identify current medications
- Classify according to acuity of condition
- Refer nonurgent patients to clinics, other primary care providers, or health department
- Contact poison control resource and initiate treatment, as appropriate
- Splint possibly fractured extremities, as appropriate
- Perform initial burn care, as appropriate
- Control bleeding
- Dress wounds
- Preserve amputated parts
- Initiate treatment protocols
- Order diagnostic tests, as appropriate
- Assign patients to physicians and/or treatment teams
- Provide information to receiving caregiver
- Monitor patients waiting to be seen
- Serve as liaison between health care team and persons in waiting area
- Answer questions from patients and families
- Reassure patients and families
- Perform grief counseling
- Take phone calls from persons requesting information
- Control traffic flow of visitors and patients

3rd edition 2000

Background Readings:
Donatelli, N. S., Flaherty, L., Greenberg, L., Larson, L., & Newberry, L. (Eds.). (1995). *Standards of emergency nursing practice* (3rd ed.). St. Louis: Mosby.
Emergency Nurses Association. (1996). *Standards of emergency nursing practice*. Chicago: Author.

Smeltzer, S. C., & Bare, B. G. (2004). Emergency nursing. In *Brunner & Suddarth's textbook of medical surgical nursing* (Vol. 2, 10th ed., pp. 2147–2182). Philadelphia: Lippincott Williams & Wilkins.

Triage: Telephone 6366

Definition: Determining the nature and urgency of a problem(s) and providing directions for the level of care required, over the telephone

Activities:
- Identify self with name and credentials, organization; let caller know if call is being recorded (e.g., for quality monitoring)
- Display willingness to help (e.g., "How may I help?")
- Obtain information about purpose of the call (e.g., nature of crisis, symptoms, medical diagnosis, past health history, and current treatment regimen)
- Consider cultural and socioeconomic barriers to patient's response
- Identify patient's concerns about health status
- Speak directly to the patient, whenever possible
- Direct, facilitate, and calm caller by giving simple instructions for action, as needed
- Inquire about related complaint/symptoms (according to standard guidelines, if available)
- Use standardized symptom-based guidelines to identify and evaluate significant data and classify urgency of symptoms, as available
- Prioritize reported symptoms, determining those with highest possible risk first
- Obtain data related to effectiveness of current treatment(s), if any
- Determine whether concerns require further evaluation (use standard guidelines, if available)
- Provide first aid instructions or emergency directions for crises (e.g., CPR instructions or birthing), using standard guidelines
- Stay on the line while contacting emergency services, according to organization's protocol
- Provide clear directions for transport to the hospital, as needed
- Advise patient on options for referral and/or intervention
- Provide information about treatment regimen and resultant self-care responsibilities as necessary, according to scope of practice and established guidelines
- Confirm patient's understanding of advice or directions through verbalization
- Determine need, and establish time intervals for further intermittent assessment
- Document any assessments, advice, instructions, or other information given to patient, according to specified guidelines
- Determine how patient or family member can be reached for return telephone calls, as appropriate
- Document permission for return call and identify persons able to receive call information
- Follow up, as necessary, to determine disposition; document disposition and patient's intended action
- Maintain confidentiality, as indicated
- Discuss and resolve problem calls with supervisory/collegial help

3rd edition 2000

Background Readings:
American Academy of Ambulatory Nursing. (1997). *Telephone nursing practice administration and practice standards*. Pitman, NJ: Anthony J. Jannetti.
Janowski, M. (1995). Is telephone triage calling you. *American Journal of Nursing, 95*(1), 59–62.
Katz, H. P. (1990). *Telephone medicine, triage and training: A handbook for primary care health professionals*. Philadelphia: F. A. Davis.
Smeltzer, S. C., & Bare, B. G. (2004). Emergency nursing. In *Brunner & Suddarth's textbook of medical surgical nursing* (Vol. 2, 10th ed., pp. 2147–2182). Philadelphia: Lippincott Williams & Wilkins.
Stock, C. M. (1995). Standardization of telephone triage: Is it time. *Journal of Nursing Law, 2*(2), 19–25.
Wheeler, S., & Siebelt, B. (1997). Calling all nurses: How to perform telephone triage. *Nursing, 97*(7), 37–41.

T

Truth Telling 5470

Definition: Use of whole truth, partial truth, or decision delay to promote the patient's self-determination and well-being

Activities:

- Clarify own values about the particular situation
- Clarify the values of the patient, family, health care team, and institution about the particular situation
- Clarify own knowledge base and communication skills about the situation
- Determine patient's desire and preference for truth in the situation
- Consult with the patient's family before telling the truth, as culturally appropriate
- Point out discrepancies between the patient's expressed beliefs and behaviors, as appropriate
- Collaborate with other health care providers about the choice of options (i.e., whole truth, partial truth, or decision delay) and their needed participation in the options
- Determine risks to patient and self associated with each option
- Choose one of the options, based on the ethics of the situation and leaning more favorably toward the use of truth or partial truth
- Establish a trusting relationship
- Deliver the truth with sensitivity, warmth, and directness
- Make time to deal with the consequences of the truth
- Refer to another if that person has better rapport, better knowledge and skills to deliver the truth, or more time and ability to deal with the consequences of telling the truth
- Prepare the patient for truth telling by encouraging them to invite family/significant other to be present
- Remain with the patient to whom you have told the truth and be prepared to clarify, support, and receive feedback
- Be physically present to communicate caring and support, if decision to withhold information has been made
- Choose decision delay when there is missing information, lack of knowledge, and lack of rapport
- Attend to verbal and nonverbal cues during the communication process
- Monitor the patient's and family's responses to the interaction, including alterations in pain, restlessness, anxiety, mood change, involvement in care, ability to synthesize new information, ability to verbalize feelings, and reported satisfaction with care, as appropriate
- Document the patient's responses at various stages of the intervention

1st edition 1992; revised 2008

Background Readings:

Collis, S. P. (2006). The importance of truth-telling in health care. *Nursing Standard, 20*(17), 41–45.

Glass, E., & Cluxton, D. (2004). Truth-telling: Ethical issues in clinical practice. *Journal of Hospice and Palliative Nursing, 6*(4), 232–242.

Hertogh, C. M., The, B. A., Miesen, B. M., & Eefsting, J. A. (2004). Truth telling and truthfulness in the care for patients with advanced dementia: An ethnographic study in Dutch nursing homes. *Social Science & Medicine, 59*(8), 1685–1693.

Jotkowitz, A. B., Clarifield, A. M., & Glick, S. (2005). The care of patients with dementia: A modern Jewish ethical perspective. *Journal of the American Geriatrics Society, 53*(5), 881–884.

Tuckett, A. G. (2004). Truth-telling in clinical practice and the arguments for and against: A review of the literature. *Nursing Ethics, 11*(5), 500–513.

Williamson, C. B., & Livingston, D. J. (1992). Truth telling. In G. M. Bulechek & J. C. McCloskey (Eds.), *Nursing interventions: Essential nursing treatments* (2nd ed., pp. 151–167). Philadelphia: Saunders.

Wros, P. L., Doutrich, D., & Izumi, S. (2004). Ethical concerns: Comparison of values from two cultures. *Nursing & Health Sciences, 6*(2), 131–140.

Tube Care 1870

Definition: Management of a patient with an external drainage device exiting the body

Activities:

- Determine indication for the indwelling tube or catheter
- Use automatic stop orders and reminders to request an order to remove the device when the indication is resolved
- Maintain proper hand hygiene before, during, and after tube insertion or manipulation
- Maintain patency of tube, as indicated by tube type and manufacturer directions
- Keep the drainage container at the proper level
- Provide sufficiently long tubing to allow freedom of movement, as appropriate
- Secure tubing to prevent pressure and accidental removal
- Monitor patency of catheter and tube drainage device or system, noting any difficulty in drainage
- Monitor amount, color, and consistency of drainage from tube
- Empty the collection appliance, according to organizational policy, patient condition, and manufacturer instructions
- Ensure proper placement of the tube
- Assure functioning of tube and associated equipment
- Connect tube to suction or proper drainage device, as appropriate
- Check tube patency, as appropriate
- Irrigate tube to ensure patency, according to organizational policy, patient condition, and manufacturer instructions
- Change tube routinely, as indicated by agency protocol
- Inspect the area around the tube insertion site for redness and skin breakdown, as appropriate
- Administer skin care and dressing changes at the tube insertion site, as appropriate
- Assist the patient in securing tube(s) and drainage devices while walking, sitting, and standing, as appropriate
- Encourage periods of increased activity, as appropriate
- Clamp tubing, if appropriate, to facilitate ambulation
- Monitor patient's and family members' responses to presence of external drainage devices

- Instruct patient and family the purpose of the tube and how to care for it
- Provide emotional support to deal with long-term use of tubes and external drainage devices, as appropriate

1st edition 1992; revised 2013

Background Readings:

Best, C., & Hitchings, H. (2010). Enteral tube feeding: From hospital to home. *British Journal of Nursing, 19*(3), 174–179.

Briggs, D. (2010). Nursing care and management of patients with intrapleural drains. *Nursing Standard, 24*(21), 47–56.

Foxley, S. (2011). Indwelling urinary catheters: Accurate monitoring of urine output. *British Journal of Nursing, 20*(9), 564–569.

Herter, R., & Kazer, M. (2010). Best practices in urinary catheter care. *Home Healthcare Nurse, 28*(6), 342–349.

Mongardon, N., Tremey, B., & Marty. J. (2010). Thoracentesis and chest tube management in critical care medicine: A multicenter survey of current practice. *CHEST, 138(6),* 1524–1525.

Nazarko L. (2010). Effective evidence-based catheter management: An update. *British Journal of Nursing, 19*(15), 948–955.

Omorogieva, O. (2010). Managing patients on enteral feeding tubes in the community. *British Journal of Community Nursing, 15*(Suppl.11) S6–S13.

Tube Care: Chest   1872

Definition: Management of a patient with an external device exiting the chest cavity

Activities:

- Determine indication for the indwelling chest tube (e.g., pneumothorax versus drainage of fluids)
- Maintain proper hand hygiene before, during, and after chest tube insertion or manipulation
- Monitor for audible air leaks after insertion (i.e., indicates improper insertion of tube requiring additional sutures or repositioning)
- Assure familiarity with chest valve device (e.g., water-seal drainage, drainage valve, or flutter valve) and drainage equipment
- Follow manufacturer recommendations for care of chest valve device and drainage equipment
- Monitor for proper functioning of device, correct placement in the pleural space, and tube patency (i.e., respiratory swing or fluid oscillating as patient breathes, either in tube or at the fluid meniscus)
- Note presence of continuous bubbling during inspiration and expiration, indicating either potential worsening of patient condition or a breach in the closed drainage system
- Monitor for signs and symptoms of pneumothorax
- Monitor for symptoms of resolving pneumothorax (e.g., decrease in bubbling, respiratory swinging, or tidaling in underwater drainage seal device and tubing)
- Assess patient experiencing sudden changes in swinging, tidaling, or bubbling for emergent conditions
- Ensure that all tubing connections are securely attached and taped
- Assure use of one-way drainage device, usually an underwater seal drainage bottle
- Adhere to the recommended water seal level indicated on the underwater seal drainage bottle (i.e., too little water leads to pneumothorax, too much water results in ineffective drainage or ineffective resolution of pneumothorax)
- Keep the external water seal drainage container below chest level
- Clamp chest tubes whenever external water seal drainage container is positioned above chest level for extended periods, assuring clamps are in place for as brief a time as possible
- Use only nontraumatic chest tube clamps
- Assure nontraumatic chest tube clamps are available for any accidental disconnection or damage to the drainage system or to the tubes (e.g., tape spare set of nontraumatic clamps to head of bed or to wall behind head board)
- Provide sufficiently long tubing to allow freedom of movement, as appropriate
- Anchor the tubing securely
- Assure use of multi-chamber underwater seal drain devices that provide separate chambers for drainage, water seal, and suction, when indicated by patient condition
- Monitor x-ray reports for tube position
- Document chest tube tidaling, output, and air leaks
- Document bubbling of the suction chamber of the chest tube drainage system and tidaling in water-seal chamber
- Perform stripping and milking of tube only when indicated by the patient condition (e.g., patient symptomatic and tube occluded), or as ordered by the physician
- Monitor for crepitus around chest tube site
- Observe for signs of intrapleural fluid accumulation
- Observe volume, shade, color, and consistency of drainage from lung, and record appropriately
- Observe for signs of infection
- Send questionable tube drainage for culture and sensitivity (e.g., cloudy or purulent drainage or patient with high temperature)
- Assist patient to cough, deep breathe, and turn every 2 hours
- Document patient response to cough, deep breath, and turn, including swinging, tidaling, and bubbling in chest tube and drainage system
- Clean around the tube insertion site, per agency protocol
- Change dressing around chest tube every 48 to 72 hours and as needed, per agency protocol
- Use petroleum jelly gauze for dressing change
- Ensure that chest tube drainage device is maintained in an upright position
- Change chest tube drainage bottles or multi-chamber drain devices, as needed to avoid overfilling or for infection control purposes
- Avoid occluding the drainage bottle or device when still attached to the patient, when changing the bottles or devices
- Instruct patient and family about proper chest tube care

1st edition 1992; revised 2013

Background Readings:

Briggs, D. (2010). Nursing care and management of patients with intrapleural drains. *Nursing Standard, 24*(21), 47–56.

Halm, M.A. (2007). To strip or not to strip? Physiological effects of chest tube manipulation. *American Journal of Critical Care, 16*(6), 609–612.

Mongardon, N., Tremey, B., & Marty. J. (2010). Thoracentesis and chest tube management in critical care medicine: A multicenter survey of current practice. *CHEST, 138(6)*, 1524–1525.

Taubert, J., Bungay, S., Banaglorioso, C., Adams., A., Mathew, J., & Magana, E. (2008). An evidence-based approach in education of nurses and their role in care of the oncology patient with a chest tube. *Oncology Nursing Forum, 35*(3), 531–532.

Tube Care: Gastrointestinal 1874

Definition: Management of a patient with a gastrointestinal tube

Activities:

- Monitor for correct placement of the tube, per agency protocol
- Verify placement with x-ray, per agency protocol
- Connect tube to suction, if indicated
- Secure tube to appropriate body part with consideration for patient comfort and skin integrity
- Irrigate tube, per agency protocol
- Monitor for sensations of fullness, nausea, and vomiting
- Monitor bowel sounds
- Monitor for diarrhea
- Monitor fluid and electrolyte status
- Monitor amount, color, and consistency of nasogastric output
- Replace the amount of gastrointestinal output with the appropriate IV solution, as ordered
- Provide nose and mouth care three to four times daily, or as needed
- Provide hard candy or chewing gum to moisten mouth, as appropriate
- Initiate and monitor delivery of enteral tube feedings, per agency protocol
- Teach patient and family how to care for tube, when indicated
- Provide skin care around tube insertion site
- Remove tube when indicated

1st edition 1992; revised 2000

Background Readings:

Bowers, S. (1996). Tubes: A nurses' guide to enteral feeding devices. *MedSurg Nursing, 5*(5), 313–326.

Craven, R. F., & Hirnle, C. J. (2003). Nutrition. In *Fundamentals of nursing: Human health and function* (4th ed., pp. 941–981). Philadelphia: Lippincott Williams & Wilkins.

Perry, A. G., & Potter, P. A. (1998). *Clinical nursing skills and techniques.* St. Louis: Mosby.

Thompson, J. M., McFarland, G. K., Hirsch, J. E., & Tucker, S. M. (1998). *Mosby's clinical nursing* (4th ed.). St. Louis: Mosby.

Tube Care: Umbilical Line 1875

Definition: Management of a newborn with an umbilical catheter

Activities:

- Assist with or insert umbilical catheter in appropriate neonates (e.g., birthweight of <1500 g, or shock)
- Check position of catheter with x-ray examination
- Infuse medication and nutrients, as ordered or per protocol
- Obtain venous or arterial pressures, as appropriate
- Apply antiseptic medication to umbilical stump, per protocol
- Flush catheter with heparinized solution, as appropriate
- Change stopcock daily and as needed
- Secure connections with tape, as needed, to keep line intact
- Cleanse outer surface with alcohol, as needed
- Stabilize catheter with tape
- Restrain ankles and wrists
- Document infant response to restraints, per protocol
- Provide frequent range of motion to restrained limbs
- Cleanse umbilical stump with alcohol, as needed
- Position infant on back
- Document appearance of umbilical site and nurse actions
- Observe for signs requiring catheter removal (e.g., pulseless leg, darkening of toes, hypertension, redness around umbilicus, and visible clots in catheter)
- Remove catheter, as appropriate per order or protocol, by withdrawing catheter slowly over 5 minutes
- Apply pressure to umbilicus or clamp vessel with hemostat
- Leave umbilicus uncovered
- Observe for hemorrhage

2nd edition 1996

Background Readings:

Merenstein, G. B., & Gardner, S. L. (1993). *Handbook of neonatal intensive care.* St. Louis: Mosby.

Pernoll, M. L., Benda, G. I., & Babson, S. G. (1986). *Diagnosis and management of the fetus and neonate at risk: A guide for team care.* St. Louis: Mosby.

Pillitteri, A. (2007). Nursing care of high-risk newborn and family. In *Maternal and child health nursing: Care of the childbearing and childrearing family* (5th ed., pp. 747–795). Philadelphia: Lippincott Williams & Wilkins.

T

Tube Care: Urinary   1876

Definition: Management of a patient with urinary drainage equipment

Activities:

- Determine indication for the indwelling urinary catheter
- Use automatic stop orders and reminders to request an order to remove the device when the indication is resolved
- Maintain proper hand hygiene before, during, and after catheter insertion or manipulation
- Maintain a closed, sterile, and unobstructed urinary drainage system
- Assure placement of drainage bag below level of bladder
- Avoid tilting urine bags or meters to empty or measure urine output (i.e., preventative measure for ascending contamination)
- Use urine bags or meters with emptying devices located at the bottom of the device
- Maintain patency of urinary catheter system
- Irrigate urinary catheter system using sterile technique, as appropriate
- Perform routine meatal care with soap and water during daily bathing
- Clean the urinary catheter externally at the meatus
- Cleanse surrounding skin area at regular intervals
- Change the urinary catheter at regular intervals, as indicated and per agency protocol
- Change the urinary drainage apparatus at regular intervals, as indicated and per agency protocol
- Note urinary drainage characteristics
- Clamp suprapubic or retention catheter, as ordered
- Position patient and urinary drainage system to promote urinary drainage (i.e., assure drainage bag is below level of bladder)
- Use a catheter securement device
- Empty urinary drainage apparatus at regular and specified intervals
- Empty the drainage bag before all patient transports
- Avoid placing the drainage bag between the patient's legs during transport
- Disconnect leg bag at night and connect to bedside drainage bag
- Check leg bag straps for constriction at regular intervals
- Maintain meticulous skin care for patients with a leg bag
- Cleanse urinary drainage equipment, per agency protocol
- Obtain urine specimen through closed urinary drainage system's port
- Monitor for bladder distention
- Assure catheter removal as soon as indicated by patient condition
- Explore elimination options to prevent reinsertion (e.g., bladder scanner, bedside commode, urinal, moisture wicking underpads, nursing rounds)
- Instruct patient and family about proper catheter care

1st edition 1992; revised 2000, 2013

Background Readings:

Foxley, S. (2011). Indwelling urinary catheters: Accurate monitoring of urine output. *British Journal of Nursing, 20*(9), 564–569.

Herter, R., & Kazer, M. (2010). Best practices in urinary catheter care. *Home Healthcare Nurse, 28*(6), 342–349.

Hung, A., Giesbrecht, N., Pelingon, P., & Bissonnette, R. (2010). Sterile water versus antiseptic agents as a cleansing agent during periurethral catheterizations. *NENA Outlook, 33*(2), 18–21.

Makic, M. B., VonRueden, K. T., Rauen, C. A., & Chadwick, J. (2011). Evidence-based practice habits: Putting more sacred cows out to pasture. *Critical Care Nurse, 31*(2), 38–62.

Nazarko L. (2010). Effective evidence-based catheter management: An update. *British Journal of Nursing, 19*(15), 948–955.

Newman, D. K., Willson, M. M. (2011). Review of intermittent catheterization and current best practices. *Urologic Nursing, 31*(1), 12–19.

Tube Care: Ventriculostomy/Lumbar Drain   1878

Definition: Management of a patient with an external cerebrospinal fluid drainage system

Activities:

- Monitor drainage trends
- Monitor amount and rate of cerebrospinal fluid (CSF) drainage
- Monitor CSF drainage characteristics: color, clarity, and consistency
- Record CSF drainage
- Change or empty drainage bag, as needed
- Administer antibiotics, as appropriate
- Monitor insertion site for infection
- Reinforce an insertion site dressing, as needed
- Restrain patient, as needed
- Explain and reinforce mobility restrictions to patient
- Monitor for CSF rhinorrhea and otorrhea
- Relevel the drainage apparatus as needed

1st edition 1992; revised 2013

Background Readings:

Arabi, Y., Memish, Z. A., Balkhy, H. H., Francis, C., Ferayanm, A., Shimemeri, A. A., & Almuneef, M. A. (2005). Ventriculostomy-associated infections: Incidence and risk factors. *American Journal of Infection Control, 33*(3), 137–143.

Arbour, R. (2004). Intracranial hypertension: Monitoring and nursing assessment. *Critical Care Nurse, 24*(5), 19–34.

Chi, H., Chang, K., Chang, H., Chiu, N., Huang, F. (2010). Infections associated with indwelling ventriculostomy catheters in a teaching hospital. *International Journal of Infectious Diseases, 14*(3), e216–e219.

Overstreet, M. (2003). How do I manage a lumbar drain? *Nursing 2003, 33*(3), 74.

Robinet, K. (1985). Increased intracranial pressure: Management with an intraventricular catheter. *Journal of Neurosurgical Nursing, 17*(2), 95–104.

T

Ultrasonography: Limited Obstetric   6982

Definition: Performance of ultrasound (U/S) exams to determine ovarian, uterine, or fetal status

Activities:
- Determine indication for ultrasound (U/S) imaging
- Set up equipment
- Instruct patient and family about exam indication(s) and procedure
- Prepare patient physically and emotionally for procedure
- Place transducer on abdomen or in vagina, as appropriate
- Obtain clear picture of anatomic structures on the monitor
- Identify uterine position, size, and endometrial thickness, as appropriate
- Identify ovarian location and size, as appropriate
- Monitor follicular growth throughout ovulation, as appropriate
- Monitor gestational sac growth and location
- Monitor fetal parameters, including number, size, cardiac activity, presentation, and position
- Identify placental location
- Observe for placental abnormalities, as appropriate
- Measure amniotic fluid indexes
- Monitor fetal breathing movements, gross movements, and tone
- Identify fetal structures to parents, as appropriate
- Provide picture of fetus(es), as appropriate
- Discuss test(s) results with primary practitioner, consultants, and patient, as appropriate
- Schedule additional tests or procedures, as necessary
- Clean equipment
- Document findings

2nd edition 1996

Background Readings:

Association of Women's Health, Obstetric, and Neonatal Nurses (1993). *Nursing practice competencies and educational guidelines for limited ultrasound examinations in obstetric and gynecologic/infertility settings.* Washington, DC: Author.

Kohn, C. L., Nelson, A., & Weiner, S. (1980). Gravidas' responses to realtime ultrasound fetal images. *Journal of Obstetric, Gynecologic & Neonatal Nursing, 9*(2), 77–80.

Lumley, J. (1990). Through a glass darkly: Ultrasound and prenatal bonding. *Birth, 17*(4), 214–217.

Milne, L. S., & Rich, O. J. (1981). Cognitive and affective aspects of the response of pregnant women to sonography. *Maternal-Child Nursing Journal, 10*(1), 15–39.

Nurses Association of the American College of Obstetricians and Gynecologists. (1991). *NAACOG committee opinion: The nurse's role in ultrasound.* Washington, DC: Author.

Pillitteri, A. (2007). *Maternal and child health nursing: Care of the childbearing and childrearing family* (5th ed.). Philadelphia: Lippincott Williams & Wilkins.

Unilateral Neglect Management   2760

Definition: Protecting and safely reintegrating the affected part of the body while helping the patient adapt to disturbed perceptual abilities

Activities:
- Monitor for abnormal responses to three primary types of stimuli: sensory, visual, and auditory
- Evaluate baseline mental status, comprehension, motor function, sensory function, attention span, and affective responses
- Provide realistic feedback about patient's perceptual deficit
- Perform personal care in a consistent manner with thorough explanation
- Ensure that affected extremities are properly and safely positioned
- Adapt the environment to the deficit by focusing on the unaffected side during the acute period
- Supervise and/or assist in transferring and ambulating
- Touch unaffected shoulder when initiating conversation
- Place food and beverages within field of vision and turn plate, as necessary
- Rearrange the environment to use the right or left visual field, such as positioning personal items, television, or reading materials within view on unaffected side
- Give frequent reminders to redirect the patient's attention, cueing the patient to the environment
- Avoid rapid movement in the room
- Avoid moving objects in the environment
- Position bed in room so that individuals approach and care for patient on unaffected side
- Keep side rail up on affected side, as appropriate
- Instruct patient to scan from left to right
- Provide range of motion and massage to affected side
- Encourage patient to touch and use affected body part
- Consult with occupational and physical therapists concerning timing and strategies to facilitate reintegration of neglected body parts and function
- Gradually focus patient's attention to the affected side, as patient demonstrates an ability to compensate for neglect
- Gradually move personal items and activity to affected side, as patient demonstrates an ability to compensate for neglect
- Stand on affected side when ambulating with patient, as patient demonstrates an ability to compensate for neglect
- Assist patient with activities of daily living from affected side, as patient demonstrates an ability to compensate for neglect
- Assist patient to bathe and groom affected side first, as patient demonstrates an ability to compensate for neglect

- Focus tactile and verbal stimuli on affected side, as patient demonstrates an ability to compensate for neglect
- Instruct caregivers on the cause, mechanisms, and treatment of unilateral neglect
- Include family in rehabilitation process to support the patient's efforts and assist with care, as appropriate

2nd edition 1996

Background Readings:

Kalbach, L. R. (1991). Unilateral neglect: Mechanisms and nursing care. *Journal of Neuroscience Nursing, 23*(2), 125–129.

Matteson, M. A., & McConnell, E. S. (1988). *Gerontological nursing: Concepts and practice.* Philadelphia, PA: Saunders.

Weitzel, E. A. (2001). Unilateral Neglect. In M. L. Maas, K. C. Buckwalter, M. D. Hardy, T. Tripp-Reimer, M. G. Titler, & J. P. Specht (Eds.), *Nursing care of older adults: Diagnoses, outcomes, & interventions* (pp. 492–502). St. Louis: Mosby.

Urinary Bladder Training   0570

Definition: Improving bladder function for those with urge incontinence by increasing the bladder's ability to hold urine and the patient's ability to suppress urination

Activities:

- Determine ability to recognize urge to void
- Encourage patient to keep a voiding diary
- Keep a continence specification record for 3 days to establish voiding pattern
- Assist patient to identify patterns of incontinence
- Review voiding diary with patient
- Establish interval of initial toileting schedule, based on voiding pattern
- Establish beginning and ending time for toileting schedule, if not for 24 hours
- Establish interval for toileting of not less than 1 hour and preferably not less than 2 hours
- Toilet patient or remind patient to void at prescribed intervals
- Provide privacy for toileting
- Use power of suggestion (e.g., running water or flushing toilet) to assist patient to void
- Avoid leaving patient on toilet for more than 5 minutes
- Reduce toileting interval by one half hour if more than three incontinence episodes occur in 24 hours
- Maintain toileting interval if three or less incontinence episodes occur in 24 hours
- Increase toileting interval by one half hour if patient is unable to void at two or more scheduled toileting times

- Increase the toileting interval by 1 hour if patient has no incontinence episodes for 3 days, until optimal 4-hour interval is achieved
- Express confidence that incontinence can be improved
- Teach the patient to consciously hold urine until the scheduled toileting time
- Discuss daily record of continence with patient to provide reinforcement

2nd edition 1996; revised 2004

Background Readings:

Craven, R. F., & Hirnle, C. J. (2003). Urinary elimination. In *Fundamentals of nursing: Human health and function* (4th ed., pp. 1063–1100). Philadelphia: Lippincott Williams & Wilkins.

Smith, D. A., & Newman, D. K. (1990). Urinary incontinence: A problem not often assessed or treated. *Focus on Geriatric Care and Rehabilitation, 3*(10), 1–9.

Specht, J. P., & Maas, M. L. (2001). Urinary incontinence: Functional, iatrogenic, overflow, reflex, stress, total, and urge. In M. L. Maas, K. C. Buckwalter, M. D. Hardy, T. Tripp-Reimer, M. G. Titler, & J. Specht (Eds.), *Nursing care of older adults: Diagnoses, outcomes & interventions* (pp. 252–278). St. Louis: Mosby.

Urinary Catheterization   0580

Definition: Insertion of a catheter into the bladder for temporary or permanent drainage of urine

Activities:

- Explain procedure and rationale for catheterization
- Assemble appropriate equipment
- Ensure privacy and proper draping of patient for modesty (i.e., only expose genitalia)
- Ensure correct lighting for proper visualization of anatomy
- Prefill catheter bulb to check patency and size
- Maintain strict aseptic technique
- Maintain proper hand hygiene before, during, and after catheter insertion or manipulation

- Position patient appropriately (e.g., female on back with legs apart or on side with upper leg flexed at hip and knee; male on back)
- Cleanse area around urethral meatus with antibacterial solution, sterile saline, or sterile water, per agency protocol
- Insert straight or retention catheter into the bladder, as appropriate
- Use smallest size catheter, as appropriate
- Assure that catheter is inserted far enough into bladder to prevent trauma to urethral tissues with inflation of balloon

- Fill catheter bulb for indwelling catheter, adhering to age and body size manufacturer recommendations (e.g., 10 cc adult, 5 cc child)
- Connect retention catheter to a bedside drainage bag or leg bag
- Secure catheter to skin, as appropriate
- Place drainage bag below level of bladder
- Maintain a closed and unobstructed urinary drainage system
- Monitor intake and output
- Perform or teach patient clean intermittent catheterization, when appropriate
- Perform postvoid residual catheterization, as needed
- Document care including catheter size, type, and bulb fill amount
- Assure catheter removal as soon as indicated by patient condition
- Teach patient and family proper catheter care

1st edition 1992; revised 2013

Background Readings:

Foxley, S. (2011). Indwelling urinary catheters: Accurate monitoring of urine output. *British Journal of Nursing, 20*(9), 564–569.

Herter, R., & Kazer, M. (2010). Best practices in urinary catheter care. *Home Healthcare Nurse, 28*(6), 342–349.

Hung, A., Giesbrecht, N., Pelingon, P., & Bissonnette, R. (2010). Sterile water versus antiseptic agents as a cleansing agent during periurethral catheterizations. *NENA Outlook, 33*(2), 18–21.

Nazarko, L. (2010). Effective evidence-based catheter management: An update. *British Journal of Nursing, 19*(15), 948–955.

Newman, D. K., & Willson, M. M. (2011). Review of intermittent catheterization and current best practices. *Urologic Nursing, 31*(1), 12–19.

Pellatt, G. C. (2007). Urinary elimination: Part 2—retention, incontinence and catheterization. *British Journal of Nursing, 16*(8), 480–482, 484–485.

Pomfret, I. (2007). Urinary catheterization: Selection and clinical management. *British Journal of Community Nursing, 12*(8), 348, 350, 352–354.

Wilson, M. C. (2008). Clean intermittent catheterization and self-catheterization. *British Journal of Nursing, 17*(18), 1140–1146.

Urinary Catheterization: Intermittent 0582

Definition: Regular periodic use of a catheter to empty the bladder

Activities:

- Perform a comprehensive urinary assessment focusing on causes of incontinence (e.g., urinary output, urinary voiding pattern, cognitive function, preexistent urinary problems)
- Teach patient/family purpose, supplies, method, and rationale of intermittent catheterization
- Teach patient/family clean intermittent catheterization technique
- Monitor technique of staff who perform intermittent catheterization in daycare/school settings and document as required by state regulations
- Determine child's readiness and willingness to perform intermittent self-catheterization
- Instruct designated staff how to monitor and support child performing self-catheterization at school
- Provide quiet private room for procedure
- Provide child a private place at school to store catheterization supplies in a school bag or other carrying case that is acceptable to child
- Monitor child performing self catheterization on a regular basis and provide continued instruction and support as needed
- Demonstrate procedure and have a return demonstration, as appropriate
- Assemble appropriate catheterization equipment
- Use clean or sterile technique for catheterization
- Determine catheterization schedule based on a comprehensive urinary assessment
- Adjust frequency of catheterization to maintain output of 300 cc or less for adults
- Maintain patient on prophylactic antibacterial therapy for 2 to 3 weeks at initiation of intermittent catheterization, as appropriate
- Complete a urinalysis about every 2 weeks to 1 month
- Establish a catheterization schedule based on individual needs
- Maintain a detailed record of catheterization schedule, fluid intake, and output
- Teach patient/family signs and symptoms of urinary tract infection
- Monitor color, odor, and clarity of urine

1st edition 1992; revised 1996, 2000

Background Readings:

Craven, R. F., & Hirnle, C. J. (2003). Urinary elimination. In *Fundamentals of nursing: Human health and function* (4th ed., pp. 1063–1100). Philadelphia: Lippincott Williams & Wilkins.

Kozier, B., Erb, G., Berman, A., & Snyder, S. (2004). Urinary elimination. In *Fundamentals of nursing: Concepts, processes, and practice* (7th ed., pp. 1254–1290). Upper Saddle River, NJ: Prentice Hall.

Smigielski, P. A., & Mapel, J. R. (1990). Bowel and bladder maintenance. In M. J. Craft & J. A. Denehy (Eds.), *Nursing interventions for infants and children* (pp. 355–377). Philadelphia: Saunders.

Specht, J. P., Maas, M. L., Willett, S., & Myers, N. (1992). Intermittent catheterization. In G. M. Bulechek & J. C. McCloskey (Eds.), *Nursing interventions: Essential nursing treatments* (2nd ed., pp. 61–72). Philadelphia: Saunders.

Urinary Elimination Management   0590

Definition: Maintenance of an optimum urinary elimination pattern

Activities:
- Monitor urinary elimination including frequency, consistency, odor, volume, and color, as appropriate
- Monitor for signs and symptoms of urinary retention
- Identify factors that contribute to incontinence episodes
- Teach patient signs and symptoms of urinary tract infection
- Note time of last urinary elimination, as appropriate
- Instruct patient/family to record urinary output, as appropriate
- Insert urethral suppository, as appropriate
- Obtain midstream voided specimen for urinalysis, as appropriate
- Refer to physician if signs and symptoms of urinary tract infection occur
- Teach patient to obtain midstream urine specimens at first sign of return of infection signs and symptoms
- Instruct to respond immediately to urge to void, as appropriate
- Teach patient to drink 8 ounces of liquid with meals, between meals, and in early evening
- Assist patient with development of toileting routine, as appropriate
- Instruct patient to empty bladder prior to relevant procedures
- Record time of first voiding following procedure, as appropriate
- Restrict fluids, as needed
- Instruct patient to monitor for signs and symptoms of urinary tract infection

1st edition 1992; revised 2000, 2004

Background Readings:
Craven, R. F., & Hirnle, C. J. (2003). Urinary elimination. In *Fundamentals of nursing: Human health and function* (4th ed., pp. 1063–1100). Philadelphia: Lippincott Williams & Wilkins.
Kozier, B., Erb, G., Berman, A., & Snyder, S. (2004). Urinary elimination. In *Fundamentals of nursing: Concepts, processes, and practice.* (7th ed., pp. 1254–1290). Upper Saddle River, NJ: Prentice Hall.
Smigielski, P. A., & Mapel, J. R. (1990). Bowel and bladder maintenance. In M. J. Craft & J. A. Denehy (Eds.), *Nursing interventions for infants and children.* (pp. 355–377). Philadelphia: Saunders.
Specht, J. P., & Maas, M. L. (2001). Urinary incontinence: Functional, iatrogenic, overflow, reflex, stress, total, and urge. In M. L. Maas, K. C. Buckwalter, M. D. Hardy, T. Tripp-Reimer, M. G. Titler, & J. Specht (Eds.), *Nursing care of older adults: Diagnoses, outcomes & interventions* (pp. 252–278). St. Louis: Mosby.

Urinary Habit Training   0600

Definition: Establishing a predictable pattern of bladder emptying to prevent incontinence for persons with limited cognitive ability who have urge, stress, or functional incontinence

Activities:
- Keep a continence specification record for 3 days to establish voiding pattern
- Establish interval of initial toileting schedule, based on voiding pattern and usual routine (e.g., eating, rising, and retiring)
- Establish beginning and ending time for the toileting schedule, if not for 24 hours
- Establish interval for toileting of preferably not less than 2 hours
- Assist patient to toilet and prompt to void at prescribed intervals
- Provide privacy for toileting
- Use power of suggestion (e.g., running water or flushing toilet) to assist patient to void
- Avoid leaving patient on toilet for more than 5 minutes
- Reduce toileting interval by one half hour if there are more than two incontinence episodes in 24 hours
- Maintain toileting interval if there are two or less incontinence episodes in 24 hours
- Increase the toileting interval by one half hour if patient has no incontinence episodes in 48 hours, until optimal 4-hour interval is achieved
- Discuss daily record of continence with staff to provide reinforcement and encourage compliance with toileting schedule
- Maintain scheduled toileting to assist in establishing and maintaining voiding habit
- Give positive feedback or positive reinforcement (e.g., 5 minutes of social conversation) to patient when he or she voids at scheduled toileting times, and make no comment when patient is incontinent

2nd edition 1996

Background Readings:
Craven, R. F., & Hirnle, C. J. (2003). Urinary elimination. In *Fundamentals of nursing: Human health and function* (4th ed., pp. 1063–1100). Philadelphia: Lippincott Williams & Wilkins.
Kozier, B., Erb, G., Berman, A., & Snyder, S. (2004). Urinary elimination. In *Fundamentals of nursing: Concepts, processes, and practice.* (7th ed., pp. 1254–1290). Upper Saddle River, NJ: Prentice Hall.
Specht, J. P., & Maas, M. L. (2001). Urinary incontinence: Functional, iatrogenic, overflow, reflex, stress, total, and urge. In M. L. Maas, K. C. Buckwalter, M. D. Hardy, T. Tripp-Reimer, M. G. Titler, & J. Specht (Eds.), *Nursing care of older adults: Diagnoses, outcomes & interventions* (pp. 252–278). St. Louis: Mosby.

U

Urinary Incontinence Care

0610

Definition: Assistance in promoting continence and maintaining perineal skin integrity

Activities:

- Identify multifactorial causes of incontinence (e.g., urinary output, voiding pattern, cognitive function, preexistent urinary problems, post-void residual, and medications)
- Provide privacy for elimination
- Explain etiology of problem and rationale for actions
- Monitor urinary elimination, including frequency, consistency, odor, volume, and color
- Discuss procedures and expected outcomes with patient
- Assist to develop/maintain a sense of hope
- Modify clothing and environment to provide easy access to toilet
- Assist to select appropriate incontinence garment/pad for short-term management while more definitive treatment is designed
- Provide protective garments, as needed
- Cleanse genital skin area at regular intervals
- Provide positive feedback for any decrease in episodes of incontinence
- Limit fluids for 2 to 3 hours before bedtime, as appropriate
- Schedule diuretic administration to have least impact on lifestyle
- Instruct patient/family to record urinary output and pattern, as appropriate
- Instruct patient to drink a minimum of 1500 cc fluids a day
- Instruct in ways to avoid constipation or stool impaction
- Limit ingestion of bladder irritants (e.g., colas, coffee, tea, and chocolate)
- Obtain urine for culture and sensitivity testing, as needed
- Monitor effectiveness of surgical, medical, pharmacological, and self-prescribed treatments
- Monitor bowel habits
- Refer to urinary continence specialist, as appropriate

1st edition 1992; revised 1996

Background Readings:

Craven, R. F., & Hirnle, C. J. (2003). Urinary elimination. In *Fundamentals of nursing: Human health and function* (4th ed., pp. 1063–1100). Philadelphia: Lippincott Williams & Wilkins.

Kozier, B., Erb, G., Berman, A., & Snyder, S. (2004). Urinary elimination. In *Fundamentals of nursing: Concepts, processes, and practice.* (7th ed., pp. 1254–1290). Upper Saddle River, NJ: Prentice Hall.

McCormick, K. A., & Palmer, M. N. (1992). Urinary incontinence in older adults. In J. J. Fitzpatrick, R. L. Taunton, & A. K. Jacox (Eds.), *Annual Review of Nursing Research, 10,* 25–53.

McCormick, K. A., Scheve, A. A. S., & Leahy, E. (1988). Nursing management of urinary incontinence in geriatric inpatients. *Nursing Clinics of North America, 23*(1), 231–264.

National Institutes of Health. (1988). Urinary incontinence in adults *Consensus Department Conference Statement 7*(5). Bethesda, MD: Author.

Specht, J. P., & Maas, M. L. (2001). Urinary incontinence: Functional, iatrogenic, overflow, reflex, stress, total, and urge. In M. L. Maas, K. C. Buckwalter, M. D. Hardy, T. Tripp-Reimer, M. G. Titler, & J. Specht (Eds.), *Nursing care of older adults: Diagnoses, outcomes & interventions* (pp. 252–278). St. Louis: Mosby.

Urinary Incontinence Care: Enuresis

0612

Definition: Promotion of urinary continence in children

Activities:

- Assist with diagnostic evaluation (e.g., physical exam, cystogram, cystoscopy, and lab tests to rule out physical causation)
- Interview parent to obtain data about toilet-training history, voiding pattern, urinary tract infections, and food sensitivities
- Determine frequency, duration, and circumstances of enuresis
- Discuss effective and ineffective methods of prior treatment
- Monitor family's and child's level of frustration and stress
- Perform physical exam
- Discuss techniques to use in reducing enuresis (e.g., night light, restricted fluid intake, scheduling nocturnal bathroom trips, and use of alarm system)
- Encourage child to verbalize feelings
- Emphasize child's strengths
- Encourage parents to demonstrate love and acceptance at home to counteract peer ridicule
- Discuss psychosocial dynamics of enuresis with parents (e.g., familial patterns, family disruption, self-esteem issues, and self-limiting characteristic)
- Administer medications as appropriate for short-term control

2nd edition 1996

Background Readings:

Pillitteri, A. (2007). *Maternal and child health nursing: Care of the childbearing and childrearing family* (5th ed.). Philadelphia: Lippincott Williams & Wilkins.

Wong, D. L. (2005). *Wong's essentials of pediatric nursing* (7th ed.). St. Louis: Mosby.

U

Urinary Retention Care   0620

Definition: Assistance in relieving bladder distention

Activities:

- Perform a comprehensive urinary assessment focusing on incontinence (e.g., urinary output, urinary voiding pattern, cognitive function, and preexistent urinary problems)
- Monitor use of nonprescription agents with anticholinergic or alpha-agonist properties
- Monitor effects of prescribed pharmaceuticals, such as calcium channel blockers and anticholinergics
- Provide privacy for elimination
- Use the power of suggestion by running water or flushing the toilet
- Stimulate the reflex bladder by applying cold to the abdomen, stroking the inner thigh, or running water
- Provide enough time for bladder emptying (10 minutes)
- Use spirits of wintergreen in bedpan or urinal
- Provide Credé maneuver, as necessary
- Use double-voiding technique
- Insert urinary catheter, as appropriate
- Instruct patient/family to record urinary output, as appropriate
- Instruct in ways to avoid constipation or stool impaction
- Monitor intake and output
- Monitor degree of bladder distention by palpation and percussion
- Assist with toileting at regular intervals, as appropriate
- Catheterize for residual, as appropriate
- Implement intermittent catheterization, as appropriate
- Refer to urinary continence specialist, as appropriate

1st edition 1992; revised 1996

Background Readings:

Craven, R. F., & Hirnle, C. J. (2003). Urinary elimination. In *Fundamentals of nursing: Human health and function* (4th ed., pp. 1063–1100). Philadelphia: Lippincott Williams & Wilkins.

Kozier, B., Erb, G., Berman, A., & Snyder, S. (2004). Urinary elimination. In *Fundamentals of nursing: Concepts, processes, and practice* (7th ed., pp. 1254–1290). Upper Saddle River, NJ: Prentice Hall.

Potter, P. A., & Perry, A. G. (2006). *Fundamentals of nursing* (6th ed.). St. Louis: Mosby.

U

Validation Therapy   6670

Definition: Use of a method of therapeutic communication with elderly persons with dementia that focuses on emotional rather than factual content

Activities:
- Determine the patient's stage of cognitive impairment (e.g., malo-rientation, time confusion, repetitive-motions, or vegetation)
- Avoid using validation strategies when the confusion is due to acute, reversible causes, or in the vegetation stage of confusion
- Listen with empathy
- Refrain from correcting or contradicting the patient's perceptions and experiences
- Accept the client's reality
- Avoid using "feeling" words
- Ask nonthreatening factual questions (e.g., Who? What? Where? When? How?)
- Avoid asking "Why?"
- Rephrase statements, repeating their key words, while picking up their tempo
- Maintain eye contact while reflecting the look in the patient's eyes
- Match and express the client's emotion (e.g., love, fear, grief)
- Sing and interact using music familiar to the patient
- Observe and mirror body movements
- Use supportive touch (gentle touch to cheek, shoulder, arm, or hand)
- Speak the client's language by listening carefully to the verbs the client uses, and use their preferred sense (auditory, visual, kinesthetic)
- Link behavior to needs such as love, safety, activity, and usefulness
- Reminisce with the patient by reviewing the past
- Help the person find a familiar coping method

5th edition 2008

Background Readings:

Day, C. R. (1997). Validation therapy: A review of the literature. *Journal of Gerontological Nursing, 23*(4), 29–34.

Feil, N. (2002). *The validation breakthrough: Simple techniques for communicating with people with Alzheimer's type dementia* (2nd ed.). Baltimore: Health Professions Press.

Taft, L. B. (1998). Validation therapy. In M. Synder & R. Lindquist (Eds.), *Complementary/alternative therapies in nursing* (3rd ed., pp. 231–242). New York: Springer.

Warner, M. (2000). Designs for validation therapy. *Nursing homes: Long term care management, 49*(6), 25–28, 82–83.

Values Clarification   5480

Definition: Assisting another to clarify her/his own values in order to facilitate effective decision-making

Activities:
- Consider the ethical and legal aspects of free choice, given the particular situation before beginning the intervention
- Create an accepting, nonjudgmental atmosphere
- Encourage consideration of issues
- Encourage consideration of values underlying choices and consequences of the choice
- Use appropriate questions to assist the patient in reflecting on the situation and what is important personally
- Assist patient to prioritize values
- Use a value sheet clarifying technique (written situation and questions), as appropriate
- Pose reflective, clarifying questions that give the patient something to think about
- Avoid use of cross-examining questions
- Encourage patient to make a list of what is important and not important in life and the time spent on each
- Encourage patient to list values that guide behavior in various settings and types of situations
- Develop and implement a plan with the patient to try out choices
- Evaluate the effectiveness of the plan with the patient
- Provide reinforcement for actions in the plan that support the patient's values
- Help patient define alternatives and their advantages and disadvantages
- Help patient to evaluate how values are in agreement with or conflict with those of family members/significant others
- Support the patient in communicating own values to others
- Avoid use of the intervention with persons with serious emotional problems

1st edition 1992; revised 2008

Background Readings:

Clark, C. C. (1996). *Wellness practitioner: Concepts, research and strategies* (2nd ed.). New York: Springer.

Craven, R. F., & Hirnle, C. J. (2007). *Fundamentals of nursing: Human health and functioning* (5th ed.). Philadelphia: Lippincott Williams & Wilkins.

Seroka, A. M. (1994). Values clarification and ethical decision making. *Seminars for Nurse Managers, 2*(1), 8–15.

Wilberding, J. Z. (1992). Values clarification. In G. M. Bulechek & J. C. McCloskey (Eds.), *Nursing interventions: Essential nursing treatments* (2nd ed., pp. 315–325). Philadelphia: Saunders.

V

Vehicle Safety Promotion 9050

Definition: Assisting individuals, families, and communities to increase awareness of measures to reduce unintentional injuries in motorized and nonmotorized vehicle

Activities:
- Determine current awareness of vehicular safety, as appropriate
- Identify the safety needs of target audience
- Identify individuals and groups at high risk for vehicular injury
- Identify safety hazards in environment
- Eliminate safety hazards in the environment, when possible
- Give information about risks associated with motorized or nonmotorized vehicle use, as indicated
- Teach high-risk populations about vehicular hazards and risks (e.g., drinking, risk-taking behaviors, noncompliance with laws)
- Collaborate with community agencies in educational efforts to promote vehicle safety (e.g., schools, police, local health department, child safety coalitions)
- Provide literature about importance and methods to increase vehicle safety
- Educate about rules of the road for drivers of motorized and nonmotorized vehicles
- Educate about the importance of proper and regular use of protective devices to decrease risk of injury (e.g., car seats, seat belts, helmets)
- Emphasize importance of always wearing seat belts
- Encourage drivers not to start automobile until all passengers are restrained
- Encourage adults to role-model the use of seat belts and safe driving practices
- Provide information about proper adjustment so seat belts are comfortable and safe
- Monitor parents' use of approved child safety seats and seat belts
- Educate about proper installation of child safety seats
- Instruct parents to secure infants in child safety seats and children under 13 years of age in the back seat of automobile
- Encourage parents to take child safety seats when traveling (e.g., airplane, train, bus)
- Demonstrate strategies parents can use to keep children occupied while restrained in seat belts or child safety seats
- Praise children and families for proper and regular use of safe practices in vehicles
- Make child safety seats available to all families through community service agencies
- Inform parents of the importance of selecting a bicycle that fits child properly and adjusting it periodically as the child grows
- Encourage use adaptive devices to increase vehicle safety (e.g., mirrors, horns, reflective devices, lights)
- Stress importance of always wearing helmets and bright or reflective clothing on bicycles, motorcycles, and other motorized vehicles (e.g., all terrain vehicles, snow mobiles)
- Emphasize importance of wearing shoes and protective clothing while on motorized and nonmotorized vehicles
- Monitor community injury rates to determine further educational need
- Support legislative initiatives that promote and enforce vehicular safety

3rd edition 2000

Background Readings:

Arneson, S. (2001). Environmental management: Automobile safety. In M. Craft-Rosenberg & J. Denehy (Eds.), *Nursing interventions for infants, children, and families* (pp. 509–520). Thousand Oaks, CA: Sage.

Duchossois, G., & Vanore, M. L. (2002). The development and evolution of a hospital-based child safety seat program. *Journal of Trauma Nursing, 9*(4), 103–110.

Morrison, D. S., Petticrew, M., & Thomson, H. (2003). What are the most effective ways of improving population health through transport interventions? Evidence from systematic reviews. *Journal of Epidemiology & Community Health, 57*(5), 327–333.

Otis, J., Lesage, D., Godin, G., Brown, B., Farley, C., & Lambert, J. (1992). Predicting and reinforcing children's intentions to wear protective helmets while bicycling. *Public Health Reports, 107*(3), 283–289.

Solis, G. R. (1991). Evaluation of a children's safety fair. *Pediatric Nursing, 17*(3), 255–258.

Watts, D., O'Shea, N., Ile, A., Flynn, E., Trask, A., & Kelleher, D. (1997). Effect of a bicycle safety program and free bicycle safety program and free bicycle helmet distribution on the use of bicycle helmets by elementary school children. *Journal of Emergency Nursing, 23*(5), 417–419.

Ventilation Assistance 3390

Definition: Promotion of an optimal spontaneous breathing pattern that maximizes oxygen and carbon dioxide exchange in the lungs

Activities:
- Maintain a patent airway
- Position to alleviate dyspnea
- Position to facilitate ventilation/perfusion matching ("good lung down"), as appropriate
- Assist with frequent position changes, as appropriate
- Position to minimize respiratory efforts (e.g., elevate the head of the bed and provide overbed table for patient to lean on)
- Monitor the effects of position change on oxygenation: ABG, SaO_2, SvO_2, end-tidal CO_2, Qsp/Qt, $A\text{-}aDO_2$ levels
- Encourage slow deep breathing, turning, and coughing
- Use fun techniques to encourage deep breathing for children (e.g., blow bubbles with bubble blower; blow on pinwheel, whistle, harmonica, balloons, party blowers; have blowing contest using ping-pong balls, feathers, etc.)
- Assist with incentive spirometer, as appropriate

- Auscultate breath sounds, noting areas of decreased or absent ventilation, and presence of adventitious sounds
- Monitor for respiratory muscle fatigue
- Initiate and maintain supplemental oxygen, as prescribed
- Administer appropriate pain medication to prevent hypoventilation
- Ambulate three to four times per day, as appropriate
- Monitor respiratory and oxygenation status
- Administer medications (e.g., bronchodilators and inhalers) that promote airway patency and gas exchange
- Teach pursed-lip breathing techniques, as appropriate
- Teach breathing techniques, as appropriate
- Initiate a program of respiratory muscle strength and/or endurance training, as appropriate
- Initiate resuscitation efforts, as appropriate

1st edition 1992; revised 2000

Background Readings:

Carrol, P. (1986). Caring for ventilator patients. *Nursing 86, 16*(2), 34–39.

Craven, R. F., & Hirnle, C. J. (2003). Oxygenation: Respiratory function. In *Fundamentals of nursing: Human health and function* (4th ed., pp. 809–864). Philadelphia: Lippincott Williams & Wilkins.

Glennon, S. (1993). Mechanical support of ventilation. In M. R. Kinney, D. R. Backa, & S. B. Dunbar (Eds.), *AACN's clinical reference for critical-care nursing* (pp. 828–840). St. Louis: Mosby.

Lane, G. H. (1990). Pulmonary therapeutic management. In L. A. Thelan, J. K. Davie, & L. D. Urden (Eds.), *Textbook of critical care nursing* (pp. 444–471). St. Louis: Mosby.

Nelson, D. M. (1992). Interventions related to respiratory care. In G. M. Bulechek & J. C. McCloskey (Eds.), Symposium on nursing interventions. *Nursing Clinics of North America, 27*(2), 301–324.

Pillitteri, A. (2007). *Maternal and child health nursing: Care of the childbearing and childrearing family* (5th ed.). Philadelphia: Lippincott Williams & Wilkins.

Visitation Facilitation 7560

Definition: Promoting beneficial visits by family and friends

Activities:
- Determine patient's preferences for visitation and release of information
- Consider legal/ethical implications regarding patient and family visitation and information rights
- Determine need for limited visitation, such as too many visitors, patient being impatient or tired, or physical status
- Determine need for more visits from family and friends
- Identify specific problems with visits, if any
- Establish flexible, patient-centered visiting policies, as appropriate
- Prepare the environment for visitation
- Discuss visiting policy with family members/significant others
- Discuss policy for overnight stay of family members/significant others
- Discuss family's understanding of patient's condition
- Negotiate family's/significant others' responsibilities and activities to assist patient, such as feeding
- Establish optimal times for family/significant others to visit patient
- Provide rationale for limited visiting time
- Evaluate periodically with both the family and the patient whether visitation practices are meeting the needs of the patient/family, and revise accordingly
- Inform visitors, including children, what they may expect to see and hear before their first hospital visitation, as appropriate
- Explain procedure being done
- Encourage the family member to use touch, as well as verbal communication, as appropriate
- Provide a chair at the bedside
- Be flexible with visitation while facilitating periods of rest
- Monitor patient's response to family visitation
- Note patient's verbal and nonverbal cues regarding visitation
- Facilitate visitation of children, as appropriate
- Encourage use of the telephone to maintain contact with significant others, as appropriate
- Screen visitors, especially children, for communicable diseases before visitation
- Clarify the meaning of what the family member perceived during the visit
- Provide support and care for family members after visitation, as needed
- Provide family with unit telephone number to call when they go home
- Inform family that a nurse will call at home if significant change in patient status occurs
- Provide sleeping arrangements for relatives close to the unit, as appropriate
- Assist family members to find adequate lodging and meals
- Inform family of legislation that they may have the right to 12 weeks unpaid leave of absence from work
- Answer questions and give explanations of care in terms that visitors can understand
- Convey feelings of acceptance to the visitors
- Facilitate meeting/consultation with physician and other providers
- Debrief visitors, including children, after the visit
- Assist parents to plan for ongoing support of children after the visit
- Arrange animal visitation as appropriate

1st edition 1992; revised 2000

Background Readings:

Daly, J. M. (1999). Visitation facilitation. In G. M. Bulecheck, & J. C. McCloskey (Eds.), *Nursing interventions: Effective nursing treatments.* Philadelphia: Saunders.

Halm, M. (1990). The effect of support groups on anxiety of family members during critical illness. *Heart & Lung, 19*(1), 62–71.

Kleiber, C., Davenport, T., & Freyenberger, B. (2006). Open bedside rounds for families with children in pediatric intensive care units. *American Journal of Critical Care, 15*(5), 492–496.

V

Kleiber, C., Montgomery, L. A., & Craft-Rosenberg, M. (1995). Information needs of the siblings of critically ill children. *Children's Health Care, 24,* 47–60.

Krapohl, G. L. (1995). Visiting hours in the adult intensive care unit: Using research to develop a system that works. *Dimensions of Critical Care Nursing, 14*(5), 245–258.

Lazure, L. L. A. (1997). Strategies to increase patient control of visiting. *Dimensions of Critical Care Nursing, 16*(1), 11–19.

Montgomery, L. A., Kleiber, C., Nicholson, A., & Craft-Rosenberg, M. (1997). A research-based sibling visitation program for the neonatal ICU. *Critical Care Nurse, 17*(2), 29–40.

Sims, J. M., & Miracle, V. A. (2006). A look at critical care visitation: The case for flexible visitation. *Dimensions in Critical Care Nursing, 25*(4), 175–181.

Titler, M. G., Cohen, M. Z., & Craft, M. J. (1991). Impact of critical hospitalization: Perceptions of patients, spouses, children, and nurses. *Heart & Lung, 20*(2), 174–181.

Vital Signs Monitoring   6680

Definition: Collection and analysis of cardiovascular, respiratory, and body temperature data to determine and prevent complications

Activities:

- Monitor blood pressure, pulse, temperature, and respiratory status, as appropriate
- Note trends and wide fluctuations in blood pressure
- Monitor blood pressure while patient is lying, sitting, and standing before and after position change, as appropriate
- Monitor blood pressure after patient has taken medications, if possible
- Auscultate blood pressures in both arms and compare, as appropriate
- Monitor blood pressure, pulse, and respirations before, during, and after activity, as appropriate
- Initiate and maintain a continuous temperature monitoring device, as appropriate
- Monitor for and report signs and symptoms of hypothermia and hyperthermia
- Monitor presence and quality of pulses
- Take apical and radial pulses simultaneously and note the difference, as appropriate
- Monitor for pulsus paradoxus
- Monitor for pulsus alternans
- Monitor for a widening or narrowing pulse pressure
- Monitor cardiac rhythm and rate
- Monitor heart tones
- Monitor respiratory rate and rhythm (e.g., depth and symmetry)
- Monitor lung sounds
- Monitor pulse oximetry
- Monitor for abnormal respiratory patterns (e.g., Cheyne-Stokes, Kussmaul, Biot, apneustic, ataxic, and excessive sighing)
- Monitor skin color, temperature, and moistness
- Monitor for central and peripheral cyanosis
- Monitor for clubbing of nail beds
- Monitor for presence of Cushing triad (e.g., wide pulse pressure, bradycardia, and increase in systolic BP)
- Identify possible causes of changes in vital signs
- Check periodically the accuracy of instruments used for acquisition of patient data

1st edition 1992; revised 2004

Background Readings:

Craven, R. F., & Hirnle, C. J. (2003). Vital sign assessment. In *Fundamentals of nursing: Human health and function* (4th ed., pp. 443–476). Philadelphia: Lippincott Williams & Wilkins.

Erickson, R. S., & Yount, S. J. (1991). Comparison of tympanic and oral temperatures in surgical patients. *Nursing Research, 40*(2), 90–93.

Thelan, L. A., & Urden, L. D. (1998). *Critical care nursing: Diagnosis and management* (3rd ed.). St. Louis: Mosby.

Titler, M. G. (1992). Interventions related to surveillance. In G. M. Bulechek & J. C. McCloskey (Eds.), Symposium on nursing interventions. *Nursing Clinics of North America, 27*(2), 495–516.

Vomiting Management   1570

Definition: Prevention and alleviation of vomiting

Activities:

- Assess emesis for color, consistency, blood, timing, and extent to which it is forceful
- Measure or estimate emesis volume
- Suggest carrying plastic bag for emesis containment
- Determine vomiting frequency and duration, using such scales as Duke Descriptive Scales, and Rhodes Index of Nausea and Vomiting (INV) Form 2
- Obtain a complete pretreatment history
- Obtain dietary history containing the person's likes, dislikes, and cultural food preferences
- Identify factors (e.g., medication and procedures) that may cause or contribute to vomiting
- Ensure effective antiemetic drugs are given to prevent vomiting, when possible
- Control environmental factors that may evoke vomiting (e.g., aversive smells, sound, and unpleasant visual stimulation)
- Reduce or eliminate personal factors that precipitate or increase the vomiting (anxiety, fear, and lack of knowledge)
- Position to prevent aspiration
- Maintain oral airway

- Provide physical support during vomiting (such as assisting person to bend over or support the person's head)
- Provide comfort (such as cool cloth to forehead, sponging face, or providing clean dry clothes) during the vomiting episode
- Demonstrate acceptance of vomiting and collaborate with the person when selecting a vomiting control strategy
- Use oral hygiene to clean mouth and nose
- Clean up after the vomiting episode with special attention to removing odors
- Wait at least 30 minutes after vomiting episode before offering more fluids to patient (assuming normal gastrointestinal tract and normal peristalsis)
- Begin fluids that are clear and free of carbonation
- Gradually increase fluids if no vomiting occurs over a 30-minute period
- Monitor for damage to esophagus and posterior pharynx if vomiting and retching are prolonged
- Monitor fluid and electrolyte balance
- Encourage rest
- Utilize nutritional supplements, if necessary, to maintain body weight
- Weigh regularly
- Teach the use of nonpharmacological techniques (e.g., biofeedback, hypnosis, relaxation, guided imagery, music therapy, distraction, acupressure) to manage vomiting
- Encourage the use of nonpharmacological techniques along with other vomiting control measures
- Inform other health care professionals and family members of any nonpharmacological strategies being used by the person
- Assist person and family to seek and provide support for themselves
- Monitor effects of vomiting management throughout

3rd edition 2000

Background Readings:

Fessele, K. S. (1996). Managing the multiple causes of nausea and vomiting in the patient with cancer. *Oncology Nursing Forum, 23*(9), 1409–1417.

Hogan, C. M. (1990). Advances in the management of nausea and vomiting. *Nursing Clinics of North America, 25*(2), 475–497.

Larson, P., Halliburton, P., & DiJulio, J. (1993). Nausea, vomiting, and retching. In V. Carrier-Kohlman, A. M. Lindsey, & C. M. West (Eds.), *Pathophysiological phenomena in nursing human responses to illness.* Philadelphia: Saunders.

Rhodes, V. A. (1990). Nausea, vomiting, and retching. *Nursing Clinics of North America, 25*(4), 885–900.

Smeltzer, S. C., & Bare, B. G. (2004). Oncology: Nursing management in cancer care. In *Brunner & Suddarth's textbook of medical surgical nursing* (Vol. 1) (10th ed., pp. 315–368). Philadelphia: Lippincott Williams & Wilkins.

V

Weight Gain Assistance   1240

Definition: Facilitating gain of body weight

Activities:
- Refer for diagnostic work-up to determine cause of being underweight, as appropriate
- Weigh patient at specified intervals, as appropriate
- Discuss possible causes of low body weight
- Monitor for nausea and vomiting
- Determine cause of nausea and/or vomiting, and treat appropriately
- Administer medications to reduce nausea and pain before eating, as appropriate
- Monitor daily calories consumed
- Monitor serum albumin, lymphocyte, and electrolyte levels
- Encourage increased calorie intake
- Instruct on how to increase calorie intake
- Provide a variety of high-calorie nutritious foods from which to select
- Consider patient's food preferences, as governed by personal choices and cultural and religious preferences
- Provide oral care before meals, as needed
- Provide rest periods, as needed
- Ensure that patient is in a sitting position before eating or feeding
- Assist with eating or feed patient, as appropriate
- Provide foods appropriate for patient: general diet, mechanical soft, blenderized or commercial formula via nasogastric or gastrostomy tube, or total parental nutrition, as ordered by physician
- Create a pleasant, relaxing environment at mealtime
- Serve food in a pleasant, attractive manner
- Discuss with patient and family socioeconomic factors contributing to inadequate nutrition
- Discuss with patient and family perceptions or factors interfering with ability or desire to eat
- Refer to community agencies that can assist in acquiring food, as appropriate
- Teach patient and family meal planning, as appropriate
- Recognize that weight loss may be part of the natural progression of a terminal illness (e.g., cancer)
- Instruct patient and family members on realistic expected outcomes regarding illness and the potential for weight gain
- Determine patient's food preferences regarding favorite foods, seasonings, and temperature
- Provide dietary supplements, as appropriate
- Create a social setting for food consumption, as appropriate
- Teach patient and family how to buy low-cost, nutritious foods, as appropriate
- Reward patient for weight gain
- Chart weight gain progress and post in a strategic location
- Encourage attendance at support groups, as appropriate

1st edition 1992; revised 2004

Background Readings:

Cluskey, M., & Dunton, N. (1999). Serving meals of reduced portion size did not improve appetite among elderly in a personal-care section of a long-term-care community. *Journal of the American Dietetic Association, 99*(6), 733–735.

Ferguson, M., Cook, A., Bender, S., Rimmasch, H., & Voss, A. (2001). Diagnosing and treating involuntary weight loss. *MEDSURG Nursing, 10*(4), 165–175.

Seligman, P. A., Fink, R., & Massey-Seligman, E. J. (1998). Approach to the seriously ill or terminal cancer patient who has a poor appetite. *Seminars in Oncology, 25*(2, Suppl. 6), 33-34.

Thelan, L. A., & Urden, L. D. (1998). *Critical care nursing: Diagnosis and management* (3rd ed.). St. Louis: Mosby.

Wakefield, B. (2001). Altered nutrition: Less than body requirements. In M. L. Maas, K. C. Buckwalter, M. D. Hardy, T. Tripp-Reimer, M. G. Titler, & J. Specht (Eds.), *Nursing care of older adults: Diagnoses, outcomes and interventions* (pp. 145–157). St. Louis: Mosby.

Weight Management   1260

Definition: Facilitating maintenance of optimal body weight and percent body fat

Activities:
- Discuss with individual the relationship between food intake, exercise, weight gain, and weight loss
- Discuss with individual the medical conditions that may affect weight
- Discuss with individual the habits and customs and cultural and heredity factors that influence weight
- Discuss risks associated with being overweight and underweight
- Determine individual motivation for changing eating habits
- Determine individual's ideal body weight
- Determine individual's ideal percent body fat
- Develop with the individual a method to keep a daily record of intake, exercise sessions, and/or changes in body weight
- Encourage individual to write down realistic weekly goals for food intake and exercise and to display them in a location where they can be reviewed daily
- Encourage individual to chart weekly weights, as appropriate
- Encourage individual to consume adequate amounts of water daily
- Plan rewards with the individual to celebrate reaching short-term and long-term goals
- Inform individual about whether support groups are available for assistance
- Assist in developing well-balanced meal plans consistent with level of energy expenditure

1st edition 1992; revised 2004

Background Readings:

National Institutes of Health. (2000). *The practical guide: Identification, evaluation, and treatment of overweight and obesity in adults* (NIH Publication Number 00-4084). Washington, DC: U.S. Department of Health and Human Services.

Thelan, L. A., & Urden, L. D. (1998). *Critical care nursing: Diagnosis and management* (3rd ed.). St. Louis: Mosby.

Whitney, E. N., & Cataldo, C. B. (1991). *Understanding normal and clinical nutrition* (3rd ed.). St. Paul, MN: West Publishing.

W

Weight Reduction Assistance 1280

Definition: Facilitating loss of weight and/or body fat

Activities:

- Determine patient's desire and motivation to reduce weight or body fat
- Determine with the patient the amount of weight loss desired
- Use the terms "weight" or "excess" rather than "obesity", "fatness", and "excess fat"
- Set a realistic weekly goal for weight loss
- Post the weekly goal in a strategic location
- Weigh patient weekly
- Chart progress of reaching final goal, and post in a strategic location
- Discuss setbacks to help patient overcome challenges and be more successful
- Reward patient when attaining goals
- Encourage use of internal reward systems when goals are accomplished
- Set a realistic plan with the patient to include reduced food intake and increased energy expenditure
- Encourage self-monitoring of dietary intake and exercise by having patients keep a paper or handheld electronic diary
- Assist patient to identify motivation for eating and internal and external cues associated with eating
- Encourage substitution of undesirable habits with favorable habits
- Post reminder and encouragement signs to do health-promotion behaviors, rather than eating
- Assist with adjusting diets to lifestyle and activity level
- Facilitate patient participation in at least one energy-expending activity three times a week
- Provide information about amount of energy expended with specific physical activities
- Assist in selection of activities according to amount of desired energy expenditure
- Plan an exercise program, taking into consideration the patient's limitations
- Advise to be active at home while doing household chores and find ways to move during day-to-day activities
- Administer medications for weight loss (e.g., sibutramine, orlistat), as prescribed
- Develop a daily meal plan with a well-balanced diet, reduced calories, and reduced fat, as appropriate
- Encourage the patient to emphasize fruits, vegetables, whole grains, fat-free or low fat milk and milk products, lean meats, fish, beans, and eggs
- Encourage use of sugar substitute, as appropriate
- Recommend adoption of diets that will lead to achievement of long-range goals for weight loss
- Encourage attendance at support groups for weight loss (e.g., Take Off Pounds Sensibly (TOPS),Weight Watchers)
- Refer to a community weight control program, as appropriate
- Refer to an online weight loss program (e.g., Weight-Control Information Network), as appropriate
- Instruct on how to read labels when purchasing food, to control amount of fat and calorie density of food obtained
- Instruct on how to calculate percentage of fat in food products
- Instruct on food selection, in restaurants and social gatherings, that are consistent with planned calorie and nutrient intake
- Discuss with patient and family the influence of alcohol consumption on food ingestion

1st edition 1992, revised 2013

Background Readings:

Kanekar, A., & Sharma, M. (2010). Pharmacological approaches for management of child and adolescent obesity. *Journal of Clinical Medicine Research*, *2*(3), 105–111.

National Institute of Diabetes and Digestive and Kidney Diseases, National Institute of Health. (2007). *Talking with patients about weight loss: Tips for primary care professionals.* (NIH Publication No. 07-5634). Washington, DC: U.S. Department of Health and Human Services.

National Institute of Diabetes and Digestive and Kidney Diseases, National Institute of Health. (2009). *Weight loss for life.* (NIH Publications No. 04-3700). Washington, DC: U.S. Department of Health and Human Services.

National Institute of Diabetes and Digestive and Kidney Diseases, National Institute of Health. (2010). *Active at any size.* (NIH Publication No. 10-4352). Washington, DC: U.S. Department of Health and Human Services.

Shay, L. (2008). Self-monitoring and weight management. *Online Journal of Nursing Informatics, 12*(1).

Whitlock, E.P., OConnor, E. A., Williams, S.B., Beil, T.L., Lutz, K.W. (2008). *Effectiveness of weight management programs in children and adolescents.* Evidence Report/Technology Assessment No. 170 (Publication No. 08-E014). Rockville, MD: Agency for Healthcare Research and Quality.

Wound Care 3660

Definition: Prevention of wound complications and promotion of wound healing

W

Activities:

- Remove dressing and adhesive tape
- Shave the hair surrounding the affected area, as needed
- Monitor characteristics of the wound, including drainage, color, size, and odor
- Measure the wound bed, as appropriate
- Remove embedded material (e.g., splinter, tick, glass, gravel, metal), as needed
- Cleanse with normal saline or a nontoxic cleanser, as appropriate
- Place affected area in a whirlpool bath, as appropriate
- Provide incision site care, as needed
- Administer skin ulcer care, as needed
- Apply an appropriate ointment to the skin/lesion, as appropriate
- Apply a dressing, appropriate for wound type
- Reinforce the dressing, as needed
- Maintain sterile dressing technique when doing wound care, as appropriate
- Change dressing according to amount of exudate and drainage

- Inspect the wound with each dressing change
- Regularly compare and record any changes in the wound
- Position to avoid placing tension on the wound, as appropriate
- Reposition patient at least every 2 hours, as appropriate
- Encourage fluids, as appropriate
- Refer to wound ostomy clinician, as appropriate
- Refer to dietitian, as appropriate
- Apply TENS (transcutaneous electrical nerve stimulation) unit for wound healing enhancement, as appropriate
- Place pressure-relieving devices (i.e., lowair-loss, foam, or gel mattresses; heel or elbow pads; chair cushion), as appropriate
- Assist patient and family to obtain supplies
- Instruct patient and family on storage and disposal of dressings and supplies
- Instruct patient or family member(s) on wound care procedures
- Instruct patient and family on signs and symptoms of infection
- Document wound location, size, and appearance

1st edition 1992; revised 2000, 2004

Background Readings:

Bryant, R. A. (2000). *Acute and chronic wounds: Nursing management.* St. Louis: Mosby.

Dwyer, F. M., & Keeler, D. (1997). Protocols for wound management. *Nursing Management, 28*(7), 45–49.

Hall, P., & Schumann, L. (2001). Wound care: Meeting the challenge. *Journal of the American Academy of Nurse Practitioners, 13*(6), 258–266.

Thompson, J. (2000). A practical guide to wound care. *RN, 63*(1), 48–52.

Wound Care: Burns   3661

Definition: Prevention of wound complications due to burns and facilitation of wound healing

Activities:

- Cool the burn with warm water (20° C) or saline solution at the time of injury, if possible
- Wash chemical wounds continuously for 30 minutes or longer to ensure the elimination of all burn agent
- Determine the area of entrance and exit of electrical burns to evaluate which organs might be involved
- Obtain an electrocardiogram (ECG) in all electrical burns
- Raise the temperature of the patient who has burns due to cold
- Keep the airway open to ensure ventilation
- Monitor the level of consciousness in patients with large burns
- Evaluate the mouth and nasal fossae of the patient to identify any possible lesion due to inhalation
- Evaluate the wound, examining its depth, extension, localization, pain, causative agent, exudation, granulation or necrotic tissue, epithelization, and signs of infection
- Administer tetanus toxoid, as appropriate
- Use physical isolation measures to prevent infection (e.g., mask, gown, sterile gloves, cap, and foot coverings)
- Inform the patient of the procedure to be followed to dress the wound
- Provide comfort measures prior to dressing change
- Set up a sterile field and maintain maximum asepsis throughout the whole process
- Take off outside bandage/dressing by cutting it and soaking with saline solution or water
- Perform debridement of wound, as appropriate
- Apply topical agents to the wound, as needed
- Place an occlusive dressing without exerting compression
- Position to preserve functionality of limbs and joints to avoid retraction
- Provide adequate pain control with pharmacological and non-pharmacological measures
- Provide skin care to donor and graft sites
- Ensure adequate nutritional and fluid intake
- Administer gamma-globulin to avoid fluid shifts, as needed
- Help the patient determine the true extent of the physical and functional changes
- Offer the patient cosmetic correction options
- Recommend methods to protect affected part
- Help the patient accept the physical changes and adapt to their lifestyle (e.g., sexual, family, employment, and social relations)
- Provide acceptance and emotional support throughout care

5th edition 2008

Background Readings:

Badger, J. M. (2001). Burns: the psychological aspects. *American Journal of Nursing, 101*(11), 38–42.

DeSanti, L. (2005). Pathophysiology and current management of burn injury. *Advances in Skin and Wound Care, 18*(6), 323–324.

Flynn, M. B. (2004). Nutritional support for the burn-injured patient. *Critical Care Nursing Clinics of North America, 16*(1), 139-144.

Kavanagh, S., & de Jong, A. (2004). Care of burn patients in the hospital. *Burns, 30*(Suppl. 8), A2–A6.

Pérez, M., Lara, J., Ibáñez, J., Cagigal, L., & León, C. M. (2006). *Guía de Actuación ante el paciente quemado.* Málaga Málaga, España: Complejo Hospitalario Carlos Haya, Unidad de Enfermería de Quemados, Dirección de Enfermería (in Spanish).

Smeltzer, S. C., & Bare, B. G. (2004). *Brunner & Suddarth's textbook of medical-surgical nursing* (10th ed.). Philadelphia: Lippincott Williams & Wilkins.

Thompson, J. T., Meredith, J. W., & Molnar, J. A. (2002). The effect of burn nursing units on burn wound infections. *Journal of Burn Care & Rehabilitation, 23*(4), 281–286.

Weddell, R. (2004). Improving pain management for patients in a hospital burns unit. *Nursing Times, 100*(11), 38–40.

W

Wound Care: Closed Drainage   3662

Definition: Maintenance of a pressure drainage system at the wound site

Activities:
- Gather necessary equipment and supplies at bedside (e.g., calibrated specimen cup, absorbent pad, and gloves)
- Assist patient to comfortable position
- Avoid transfer of microorganisms (i.e., wash hands and don clean disposable gloves)
- Expose catheter insertion site and tubing, placing drainage system on absorbent pad
- Check pump and catheter for patency, seal, and stability, being careful to avoid inadvertent removal of sutures, if present
- Monitor for signs of infection, inflammation, and discomfort around drain
- Notify appropriate health care provider of occluded catheter, signs of infection or discomfort, dislodged tubing, and full drainage system
- Remove plug or disconnect tubing, depending on drainage system type (e.g., Hemovac or Jackson-Pratt)
- Empty drainage into specimen cup, avoiding contamination of drainage spout
- Clean drainage spout using antiseptic swab
- Compress drainage system and hold tightly while reinserting plug or connecting tubing
- Position system appropriately (i.e., avoid kinking of tubing and secure to patient's clothing or bedding, as appropriate)
- Record the volume and characteristics of the drainage (e.g., color, consistency, and odor)
- Compress system to provide suction at regular time intervals, according to institutional policy
- Number the collection devices, if more than one exist
- Discard soiled items in an appropriate manner

1st edition; revised 2013

Background Readings:
Craven, R. F. & Hirnle, C. J. (2009). Skin integrity and wound healing. In *Fundamentals of nursing: Human health and function* (6th ed., pp. 989–1032). Philadelphia: Lippincott Williams & Wilkins.

Smith, S. F., Duell, D. J., & Martin, B. C. (2008). Wound care and dressings. In *Clinical nursing skills: Basic to advanced skills.* (7th ed., pp. 874–938). Upper Saddle River, NJ: Pearson Prentice Hall.

Wound Care: Nonhealing   3664

Definition: Palliative care and prevention of complications of a malignant or other wound that is not expected to heal

Activities:
- Provide adequate pain control (e.g., relaxation, distraction, analgesic therapy to be administered before and after dressing)
- Agree to take breaks while carrying out procedures on the ulcer
- Soak dressing pads in saline solution before removal, when appropriate
- Describe the characteristics of the ulcer, noting the size, location, discharge, color, bleeding, pain, odor, and any edema
- Record changes observed in the evolution of the ulcer
- Note signs and symptoms of wound infection
- Note signs of dermatitis in peri-ulcerous skin, using barrier creams, where appropriate
- Irrigate the ulcer with water or saline solution, avoiding excessive pressure
- Avoid wiping when cleansing
- Avoid the use of antiseptics
- Clean the ulcer, starting with the cleanest zone moving towards the dirtiest
- Gently pat the peri-ulcerous skin dry
- Avoid chemical or mechanical tissue removal
- Apply topical medication (cytostatic, antibiotic, analgesic) as required
- Use activated carbon dressings, if appropriate
- Use highly absorbent dressings in cases of abundant discharge
- Install a drainage device, as needed
- Apply manual pressure on bleeding points or potential bleeding zones
- Discuss with the patient the most worrying aspect of the ulcer
- Ascertain the impact the ulcer is having on the patient's quality of life (e.g., sleep, appetite, activity, humor, relationships)
- Demonstrate to the patient or family members the procedure for caring for the ulcer, as appropriate
- Instruct the patient and family about the signs of infection
- Help the patient and family to obtain the necessary dressing materials
- Demonstrate to the patient and family how to dispose of used dressings
- Demonstrate methods for protecting the wound from blows, pressure, and friction (e.g., use of pillows, cushions, pads)
- Encourage the patient to engage in social activities, exercise, and relaxation, as appropriate
- Encourage the patient to look at the body part that has undergone the change
- Provide the patient and family caregiver with emotional support
- Identify methods of reducing the impact caused by any disfigurement through the use of clothing, if appropriate
- Help the patient to take greater responsibility with self-care, to the extent possible
- Encourage the patient and family to play an active role in treatment and rehabilitation, as appropriate

6th edition 2013

Background Readings:
Carroll, M. C., Fleming, M., Chitambar, C. R., & Neuburg, M. (2002). Diagnosis workup and prognosis of cutaneous metastases of unknown primary origin. *Dermatologic Surgery, 28*(6), 533–535.

Cormio, G., Capotorto, M., Vagno, G., Cazzolla, A., Carriero, C., & Selvaggi, L. (2003). Skin metastases in ovarian carcinoma: A report of nine cases and a review of the literature. *Gynecologic Oncology, 90*(3), 682–685.

W

Emmons, K. R., & Lachman, V. D. (2010). Palliative wound care: A concept analysis. *Journal of Wound, Ostomy, and Continence Nursing, 37*(6), 639–644.

Ferris, F. D., Khateib, A., Fromanin, I., Hoplamazian, L., Hurd, T., Krasner, D., et al. (2007). Palliative wound care: Managing chronic wounds across life's continuum: A consensus statement from the International Palliative Wound Care Initiative. *Journal of Palliative Medicine, 10*(1), 37–39.

Langemo, D. K., Anderson, J., Hanson, D., Thompson, P., & Hunter, S. (2007). Understanding palliative wound care. *Nursing 2007, 37*(1), 65–66.

Lookingbill, D. P., Spangler, N., & Helm, K. F. (1993). Cutaneous metastases in patients with metastatic carcinoma: A retrospective study of 4020 patients. *Journal of the American Academy of Dermatology, 29*(2 Pt 1), 228–236.

Lund-Nielsen, B., Müller, K., & Adamsen, L. (2005). Malignant wounds in women with breast cancer: Feminine and sexual perspectives. *Journal of Clinical Nursing, 14*(1), 56–64.

Seaman, S. (2006). Management of malignant fungating wounds in advanced cancer. *Seminars in Oncology Nursing, 22*(3), 185–193.

Wound Irrigation 3680

Definition: Rinsing or washing out wound with solution

Activities:
- Gather necessary equipment and supplies at bedside (e.g., sterile irrigation set, waterproof pad, sterile basin, sterile irrigating solution, sterile gloves, and equipment for dressing change)
- Identify any allergies related to products used
- Explain the procedure to the patient
- Provide analgesics prior to wound care, as needed
- Assist patient to comfortable position, being sure solution will flow by gravity from least to most contaminated area into collection basin
- Place waterproof pad and bath blankets under patient
- Perform hand hygiene
- Don mask, goggles, and gown, if needed
- Remove dressing and inspect wound and surrounding tissue, reporting abnormalities to appropriate health care provider (e.g., infection and necrosis)
- Pour prescribed irrigating solution into sterile irrigation container, being sure to warm solution to body temperature
- Don sterile gloves
- Open irrigating syringe and place into container with solution
- Place sterile basin at distal end of wound
- Fill irrigating syringe with solution
- Avoid aspirating the solution back into the syringe
- Flush wound gently with solution until solution in bin runs clear, being sure to hold syringe tip 1 inch above wound and rinsing from least to most contaminated area
- Attach sterile latex or silicone catheter to filled syringe, when necessary (e.g., to irrigate deep wounds)
- Avoid forcing the catheter into an abdominal wound, to prevent perforation of the intestine
- Refill irrigation syringe with solution, maintaining sterility (i.e., when using catheter, disconnect catheter, fill syringe, and reconnect catheter)
- Open commercial cleaning solution package if using for irrigation and use according to instructions
- Cleanse and dry surrounding skin after procedure
- Institute appropriate care of wound or burn
- Apply sterile dressing
- Pack the wound with the appropriate type of sterile dressing
- Monitor patient's pain, tolerance, comfort, and anxiety levels during procedure
- Maintain a sterile field during procedure, as appropriate (e.g., use assistants to prevent child from moving and contaminating wound or sterile field and instruct child not to touch wound)
- Instruct patient or family performing procedure at home on appropriate technique and necessary modifications (e.g., stress importance of washing hands before and after irrigation when sterile technique is not used)
- Discard items in an appropriate manner

1st edition 1992; revised 2013

Background Readings:
Craven, R. F. & Hirnle, C. J. (2009). Skin integrity and wound healing. In *Fundamentals of nursing: Human health and function* (6th ed., pp. 989–1032). Philadelphia: Lippincott Williams & Wilkins.

Smith, S. F., Duell, D. J., & Martin, B. C. (2008). Wound care and dressings. In *Clinical nursing skills: Basic to advanced skills* (7th ed., pp. 874–938). Upper Saddle River, NJ: Pearson Prentice Hall.

W

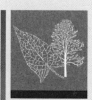

PART FOUR

Core Interventions for Nursing Specialty Areas

Core Interventions for Nursing Specialty Areas

In this section, we list alphabetically the core interventions for 49 specialty areas. Core interventions are defined as a limited, central set of interventions that define the nature of the specialty. A person reading the list of core interventions would be able to determine the area of specialty practice. The core set of interventions does not include all the interventions used by nurses in the specialty; rather, the set includes those interventions used frequently or predominately by nurses in the specialty, or those that are critical to the role of the specialty nurse.

This list of specialty core interventions initially resulted from a survey in 1995 and 1996; the research and an initial list of core interventions for 39 specialty areas were published in the third edition of *Nursing Interventions Classification (NIC)*. The results of the survey were also published in an article: McCloskey, J. C., Bulechek, G., & Donahue, W. (1998). Nursing interventions core to specialty practice, *Nursing Outlook, 46*(2), 67-76. New specialties as well as updates of new interventions were added in the fourth and fifth editions.

For this edition, interventions new to the sixth edition and five new specialties were added: Diabetes Nursing, HIV/AIDS Nursing, Home Health Nursing, Plastic Surgery Nursing, and Transplant Nursing. In addition Chemical Dependency Nursing and Addictions Nursing were combined into one specialty area. Parish Nursing was renamed Faith Community Nursing. The entire list of 49 specialties for which core interventions are identified follows:

1. Ambulatory Nursing
2. Anesthesia Nursing
3. Chemical Dependency and Addictions Nursing
4. Child and Adolescent Psychiatric Nursing
5. College Health Nursing
6. Community Public Health Nursing
7. Correctional Nursing
8. Critical Care Nursing
9. Dermatology Nursing
10. Developmental Disability Nursing
11. Diabetes Nursing
12. Emergency Nursing
13. End of Life Care Nursing
14. Faith Community Nursing
15. Flight Nursing
16. Forensic Nursing
17. Gastroenterological Nursing
18. Genetics Nursing
19. Gerontological Nursing
20. HIV/AIDS Nursing
21. Holistic Nursing
22. Home Health Nursing
23. Infection Control and Epidemiological Nursing
24. Intravenous Nursing
25. Medical-Surgical Nursing
26. Midwifery Nursing
27. Neonatal Nursing
28. Nephrology Nursing
29. Neuroscience Nursing
30. Obstetric Nursing
31. Occupational Health Nursing
32. Oncology Nursing
33. Ophthalmic Nursing
34. Orthopedic Nursing
35. Otorhinolaryngology and Head/Neck Nursing
36. Pain Management Nursing
37. Pediatric Nursing
38. Pediatric Oncology Nursing
39. Perioperative Nursing
40. Plastic Surgery Nursing
41. Psychiatric/Mental Health Nursing
42. Radiological Nursing
43. Rehabilitation Nursing
44. School Nursing
45. Spinal Cord Injury Nursing
46. Transplant Nursing
47. Urologic Nursing
48. Vascular Nursing
49. Women's Health Nursing

The identification of core interventions by specialty is an initial step to communicate the nature of nursing in different practice areas. The listing of core interventions by specialty areas of practice is very useful in the development of nursing information systems, staff education programs, nurse competency evaluations, referral networks, certification/licensing examinations, nursing school curricula, and research and theory construction. We encourage members of specialty organizations who are interested in building clinical databases to use the interventions contained in NIC so that nurses can achieve the benefits inherent in a standardized language. We welcome the submission of new interventions as users see the need.

Ambulatory Nursing

- Anxiety Reduction
- Bedside Laboratory Testing
- Behavior Modification
- Capillary Blood Sample
- Coping Enhancement
- Decision-Making Support
- Delegation
- Documentation
- Emotional Support
- Examination Assistance
- Health Education
- Health Literacy Enhancement
- Health Screening
- Health System Guidance
- Immunization/Vaccination Management
- Medication Administration: Intradermal
- Medication Administration: Intramuscular (IM)
- Medication Administration: Intravenous (IV)
- Medication Administration: Oral
- Medication Management
- Medication Prescribing
- Nutritional Counseling
- Physician Support
- Prescribing: Diagnostic Testing
- Prescribing: Non-Pharmacologic Treatment
- Referral
- Risk Identification
- Staff Supervision
- Teaching: Disease Process
- Teaching: Individual
- Teaching: Prescribed Diet
- Teaching: Prescribed Medication
- Teaching: Procedure/Treatment
- Telephone Follow-Up
- Transport: Interfacility
- Triage: Emergency Center
- Triage: Telephone
- Vital Signs Monitoring

Anesthesia Nursing

- Acid-Base Management
- Acid-Base Management: Metabolic Acidosis
- Acid-Base Management: Metabolic Alkalosis
- Acid-Base Management: Respiratory Acidosis
- Acid-Base Management: Respiratory Alkalosis
- Acid-Base Monitoring
- Airway Insertion and Stabilization
- Airway Management
- Airway Suctioning
- Analgesic Administration
- Analgesic Administration: Intraspinal
- Anaphylaxis Management
- Anesthesia Administration
- Artificial Airway Management
- Autotransfusion
- Blood Products Administration
- Circulatory Care: Mechanical Assist Device
- Code Management
- Controlled Substance Checking
- Defibrillator Management: External
- Defibrillator Management: Internal
- Documentation
- Dysrhythmia Management
- Electrolyte Management
- Electrolyte Management: Hypercalcemia
- Electrolyte Management: Hyperkalemia
- Electrolyte Management: Hypermagnesemia
- Electrolyte Management: Hypernatremia
- Electrolyte Management: Hyperphosphatemia
- Electrolyte Management: Hypocalcemia
- Electrolyte Management: Hypokalemia
- Electrolyte Management: Hypomagnesemia
- Electrolyte Management: Hyponatremia
- Electrolyte Management: Hypophosphatemia
- Electrolyte Monitoring
- Emergency Care
- Endotracheal Extubation
- Eye Care
- Fluid Management
- Fluid Monitoring
- Fluid Resuscitation
- Hyperglycemia Management
- Hypervolemia Management
- Hypoglycemia Management
- Hypothermia Induction Therapy
- Hypothermia Treatment
- Hypovolemia Management
- Incident Reporting
- Infection Control: Intraoperative
- Intracranial Pressure (ICP) Monitoring
- Intravenous (IV) Insertion
- Laboratory Data Interpretation
- Laser Precautions
- Latex Precautions
- Learning Facilitation
- Malignant Hyperthermia Precautions
- Mechanical Ventilation Management: Invasive
- Medication Administration
- Medication Administration: Intramuscular (IM)
- Medication Administration: Intraspinal
- Medication Administration: Intravenous (IV)
- Medication Administration: Oral
- Medication Management
- Medication Prescribing
- Nausea Management
- Oxygen Therapy
- Pacemaker Management: Permanent
- Pacemaker Management: Temporary
- Pain Management
- Patient-Controlled Analgesia (PCA) Assistance
- Patient Identification
- Peripherally Inserted Central Catheter (PICC) Care

- Phlebotomy: Arterial Blood Sample
- Phlebotomy: Blood Unit Acquisition
- Phlebotomy: Cannulated Vessel
- Phlebotomy: Venous Blood Sample
- Physician Support
- Pneumatic Tourniquet Precautions
- Positioning: Intraoperative
- Postanesthesia Care
- Preoperative Coordination
- Prescribing: Diagnostic Testing
- Quality Monitoring
- Referral
- Respiratory Monitoring
- Resuscitation
- Resuscitation: Fetus
- Resuscitation: Neonate
- Sedation Management
- Shock Management
- Shock Management: Cardiac
- Shock Management: Vasogenic
- Shock Management: Volume
- Surgical Precautions
- Surgical Preparation
- Teaching: Preoperative
- Technology Management
- Transcutaneous Electrical Nerve Stimulation (TENS)
- Triage: Emergency Center
- Ventilation Assistance
- Vital Signs Monitoring

Chemical Dependency and Addictions Nursing

- Active Listening
- Anger Control Assistance
- Anticipatory Guidance
- Assertiveness Training
- Behavior Management
- Behavior Modification: Social Skills
- Capillary Blood Sample
- Chemical Restraint
- Commendation
- Conflict Mediation
- Coping Enhancement
- Counseling
- Delirium Management
- Discharge Planning
- Eating Disorders Management
- Elopement Precautions
- Environmental Management: Safety
- Family Therapy
- Fluid/Electrolyte Management
- Forgiveness Facilitation
- Guilt Work Facilitation
- Health Education
- Health Screening
- Hope Inspiration
- Impulse Control Training
- Journaling
- Life Skills Enhancement
- Limit Setting
- Medication Administration
- Medication Management
- Nutrition Management
- Patient Contracting
- Recreation Therapy
- Referral
- Risk Identification
- Self-Awareness Enhancement
- Self-Esteem Enhancement
- Self-Responsibility Facilitation
- Smoking Cessation Assistance
- Socialization Enhancement
- Spiritual Support
- Substance Use Prevention
- Substance Use Treatment
- Substance Use Treatment: Alcohol Withdrawal
- Substance Use Treatment: Drug Withdrawal
- Substance Use Treatment: Overdose
- Support Group
- Teaching: Disease Process
- Teaching: Group
- Teaching: Safe Sex
- Therapy Group
- Vital Signs Monitoring

Child and Adolescent Psychiatric Nursing

- Abuse Protection Support: Child
- Activity Therapy
- Art Therapy
- Behavior Management: Overactivity/Inattention
- Behavior Management: Self-Harm
- Behavior Management: Sexual
- Behavior Modification: Social Skills
- Bowel Incontinence Care: Encopresis
- Case Management
- Complex Relationship Building
- Conflict Mediation
- Delusion Management
- Developmental Enhancement: Adolescent
- Developmental Enhancement: Child
- Elopement Precautions
- Environmental Management: Community
- Family Involvement Promotion
- Family Mobilization
- Family Process Maintenance
- Family Therapy
- Health Education
- Health Literacy Enhancement

- Impulse Control Training
- Life Skills Enhancement
- Medication Management
- Medication Prescribing
- Mood Management
- Multidisciplinary Care Conference
- Normalization Promotion
- Parenting Promotion
- Resiliency Promotion
- Staff Supervision
- Teaching: Prescribed Medication
- Telephone Consultation
- Trauma Therapy: Child
- Urinary Incontinence Care: Enuresis

College Health Nursing

- Active Listening
- Anxiety Reduction
- Asthma Management
- Communicable Disease Management
- Coping Enhancement
- Counseling
- Crisis Intervention
- Decision-Making Support
- Eating Disorders Management
- Emotional Support
- First Aid
- Health Education
- Health Screening
- Health System Guidance
- Immunization/Vaccination Management
- Medication Administration: Subcutaneous
- Medication Management
- Medication Prescribing
- Nutrition Management
- Prescribing: Diagnostic Testing
- Prescribing: Non-Pharmacologic Treatment
- Rape-Trauma Treatment
- Referral
- Self-Esteem Enhancement
- Sexual Counseling
- Sleep Enhancement
- Smoking Cessation Assistance
- Sports-Injury Prevention: Youth
- Substance Use Prevention
- Suicide Prevention
- Teaching: Individual
- Teaching: Safe Sex
- Teaching: Sexuality
- Vehicle Safety Promotion
- Weight Management

Community Public Health Nursing

- Abuse Protection Support
- Bioterrorism Preparedness
- Case Management
- Community Disaster Preparedness
- Community Health Development
- Consultation
- Culture Brokerage
- Environmental Management: Community
- Environmental Management: Home Preparation
- Environmental Management: Worker Safety
- Environmental Risk Protection
- Family Planning: Contraception
- Fiscal Resource Management
- Health Care Information Exchange
- Health Education
- Health Literacy Enhancement
- Health Policy Monitoring
- Health Screening
- Health System Guidance
- Home Maintenance Assistance
- Immunization/Vaccination Management
- Medication Administration: Subcutaneous
- Parenting Promotion
- Program Development
- Referral
- Risk Identification
- Social Marketing
- Surveillance: Community
- Sustenance Support
- Teaching: Group
- Teaching: Infant Nutrition 0-3 Months
- Teaching: Infant Nutrition 4-6 Months
- Teaching: Infant Nutrition 7-9 Months
- Teaching: Infant Nutrition 10-12 Months
- Teaching: Infant Safety 0-3 Months
- Teaching: Infant Safety 4-6 Months
- Teaching: Infant Safety 7-9 Months
- Teaching: Infant Safety 10-12 Months
- Teaching: Safe Sex
- Teaching: Toddler Nutrition 13-18 Months
- Teaching: Toddler Nutrition 19-24 Months
- Teaching: Toddler Nutrition 25-36 Months
- Teaching: Toddler Safety 13-18 Months
- Teaching: Toddler Safety 19-24 Months
- Teaching: Toddler Safety 25-36 Months
- Vehicle Safety Promotion

Correctional Nursing

- Active Listening
- Anger Control Assistance
- Area Restriction
- Commendation
- Complex Relationship Building
- Coping Enhancement
- Counseling
- Culture Brokerage
- Emergency Care
- Emotional Support
- Environmental Management: Violence Prevention
- Environmental Risk Protection
- Family Integrity Promotion
- First Aid
- Forgiveness Facilitation
- Health Care Information Exchange
- Health Policy Monitoring
- Health Screening
- Hope Inspiration
- Humor
- Life Skills Enhancement
- Limit Setting
- Medication Administration
- Medication Management
- Nutrition Management
- Patient Contracting
- Presence
- Program Development
- Referral
- Skin Surveillance
- Substance Use Prevention
- Substance Use Treatment
- Substance Use Treatment: Alcohol Withdrawal
- Substance Use Treatment: Drug Withdrawal
- Substance Use Treatment: Overdose
- Suicide Prevention
- Surveillance
- Teaching: Group
- Teaching: Individual
- Teaching: Prescribed Medication
- Teaching: Safe Sex
- Wound Care

Critical Care Nursing

- Acid-Base Monitoring
- Airway Management
- Airway Suctioning
- Analgesic Administration
- Anxiety Reduction
- Artificial Airway Management
- Cardiac Care: Acute
- Cardiac Risk Management
- Caregiver Support
- Central Venous Access Device Management
- Circulatory Care: Mechanical Assist Device
- Code Management
- Decision-Making Support
- Defibrillator Management: External
- Defibrillator Management: Internal
- Delegation
- Discharge Planning
- Documentation
- Electrolyte Management
- Electrolyte Monitoring
- Emotional Support
- Family Involvement Promotion
- Family Presence Facilitation
- Fluid/Electrolyte Management
- Fluid Management
- Fluid Monitoring
- Hemodynamic Regulation
- Intracranial Pressure (ICP) Monitoring
- Intravenous (IV) Therapy
- Invasive Hemodynamic Monitoring
- Mechanical Ventilation Management: Invasive
- Mechanical Ventilation Management: Noninvasive
- Mechanical Ventilation Management: Pneumonia Prevention
- Mechanical Ventilatory Weaning
- Medication Administration
- Medication Administration: Intravenous (IV)
- Multidisciplinary Care Conference
- Nausea Management
- Neurologic Monitoring
- Oxygen Therapy
- Pacemaker Management: Permanent
- Pacemaker Management: Temporary
- Pain Management
- Patient Rights Protection
- Physician Support
- Positioning
- Respiratory Monitoring
- Sedation Management
- Shock Management
- Teaching: Procedure/Treatment
- Technology Management
- Temperature Regulation
- Thrombolytic Therapy Management
- Transport: Interfacility
- Transport: Intrafacility
- Visitation Facilitation
- Vital Signs Monitoring
- Vomiting Management

Dermatology Nursing

- Behavior Modification
- Body Image Enhancement
- Coping Enhancement
- Decision-Making Support
- Documentation
- Emotional Support
- Environmental Management: Community
- Examination Assistance
- Health Education
- Health Screening
- Incision Site Care
- Infection Control
- Laser Precautions
- Learning Facilitation
- Medication Administration: Skin
- Physician Support
- Pressure Ulcer Care
- Pruritus Management
- Self-Responsibility Facilitation
- Skin Care: Donor Site
- Skin Care: Graft Site
- Skin Care: Topical Treatments
- Skin Surveillance
- Support System Enhancement
- Surgical Assistance
- Teaching: Disease Process
- Teaching: Prescribed Medication
- Teaching: Procedure/Treatment
- Telephone Consultation
- Wound Care
- Wound Irrigation

Developmental Disability Nursing

- Abuse Protection Support
- Anxiety Reduction
- Aspiration Precautions
- Behavior Management
- Behavior Management: Self-Harm
- Behavior Modification: Social Skills
- Bowel Management
- Case Management
- Communication Enhancement: Hearing Deficit
- Communication Enhancement: Speech Deficit
- Communication Enhancement: Visual Deficit
- Developmental Enhancement: Adolescent
- Developmental Enhancement: Child
- Developmental Enhancement: Infant
- Documentation
- Environmental Management: Safety
- Family Involvement Promotion
- Financial Resource Assistance
- Health Education
- Health Literacy Enhancement
- Health Screening
- Incident Reporting
- Infection Control
- Life Skills Enhancement
- Medication Administration
- Medication Management
- Multidisciplinary Care Conference
- Normalization Promotion
- Nutrition Management
- Patient Rights Protection
- Relocation Stress Reduction
- Risk Identification: Genetic
- Seizure Management
- Seizure Precautions
- Self-Care Assistance
- Self-Care Assistance: IADL
- Staff Supervision
- Teaching: Prescribed Medication
- Teaching: Safe Sex
- Telephone Consultation
- Telephone Follow-Up
- Weight Management

Diabetes Nursing

- Amputation Care
- Caregiver Support
- Case Management
- Decision-Making Support
- Exercise Promotion
- Family Involvement Promotion
- Financial Resource Assistance
- Foot Care
- Health Education
- Health Screening
- Health System Guidance
- Hyperglycemia Management
- Hypoglycemia Management
- Infection Control
- Lower Extremity Monitoring
- Medication Management
- Multidisciplinary Care Conference
- Mutual Goal Setting
- Nutrition Management
- Nutritional Counseling
- Nutritional Monitoring
- Patient Contracting
- Pressure Ulcer Care
- Pressure Ulcer Prevention
- Risk Identification
- Skin Surveillance
- Smoking Cessation Assistance
- Support Group

- Teaching: Disease Process
- Teaching: Foot Care
- Teaching: Prescribed Diet
- Teaching: Prescribed Medication
- Teaching: Procedure/Treatment

- Telephone Consultation
- Telephone Follow-Up
- Weight Management
- Weight Reduction Assistance
- Wound Care: Nonhealing

Emergency Nursing

- Abuse Protection Support: Child
- Abuse Protection Support: Domestic Partner
- Airway Management
- Anaphylaxis Management
- Bioterrorism Preparedness
- Blood Products Administration
- Cardiac Care: Acute
- Circulatory Care: Arterial Insufficiency
- Circulatory Care: Venous Insufficiency
- Code Management
- Crisis Intervention
- Defibrillator Management: External
- Defibrillator Management: Internal
- Documentation
- Dysrhythmia Management
- Electrolyte Management
- Emergency Care
- Family Presence Facilitation
- First Aid
- Fluid/Electrolyte Management
- Fluid Resuscitation
- Forensic Data Collection
- Hyperthermia Treatment
- Hypovolemia Management

- Intravenous (IV) Insertion
- Intravenous (IV) Therapy
- Mechanical Ventilation Management: Noninvasive
- Medication Administration
- Neurologic Monitoring
- Oxygen Therapy
- Pacemaker Management: Temporary
- Pain Management
- Patient Identification
- Phlebotomy: Venous Blood Sample
- Prescribing: Diagnostic Testing
- Rape-Trauma Treatment
- Respiratory Monitoring
- Resuscitation
- Seizure Management
- Shock Management
- Teaching: Individual
- Thrombolytic Therapy Management
- Transport: Interfacility
- Transport: Intrafacility
- Triage: Emergency Center
- Triage: Telephone
- Vital Signs Monitoring
- Wound Care

End of Life Care Nursing

- Active Listening
- Analgesic Administration
- Anticipatory Guidance
- Anxiety Reduction
- Bed Rest Care
- Bowel Management
- Caregiver Support
- Case Management
- Constipation/Impaction Management
- Coping Enhancement
- Decision-Making Support
- Delirium Management
- Dying Care
- Emotional Support
- Energy Management
- Environmental Management
- Family Integrity Promotion
- Family Involvement Promotion
- Financial Resource Assistance
- Fluid/Electrolyte Management
- Forgiveness Facilitation
- Grief Work Facilitation
- Healing Touch
- Health Care Information Exchange

- Health System Guidance
- Medication Management
- Multidisciplinary Care Conference
- Neurologic Monitoring
- Nutrition Management
- Pain Management
- Patient Rights Protection
- Positioning
- Presence
- Pressure Management
- Religious Ritual Enhancement
- Reminiscence Therapy
- Respiratory Monitoring
- Respite Care
- Self-Care Assistance
- Skin Surveillance
- Sleep Enhancement
- Spiritual Support
- Support System Enhancement
- Telephone Consultation
- Touch
- Urinary Elimination Management
- Values Clarification
- Visitation Facilitation

Faith Community Nursing

- Abuse Protection Support
- Active Listening
- Anticipatory Guidance
- Caregiver Support
- Coping Enhancement
- Crisis Intervention
- Culture Brokerage
- Decision-Making Support
- Emotional Support
- Environmental Management: Community
- Family Integrity Promotion
- Family Support
- Forgiveness Facilitation
- Grief Work Facilitation
- Guilt Work Facilitation
- Health Care Information Exchange
- Health Education
- Health Literacy Enhancement
- Health System Guidance
- Hope Inspiration
- Humor
- Listening Visits
- Medication Management
- Presence
- Referral
- Religious Addiction Prevention
- Religious Ritual Enhancement
- Relocation Stress Reduction
- Self-Care Assistance: IADL
- Socialization Enhancement
- Spiritual Growth Facilitation
- Spiritual Support
- Surveillance
- Sustenance Support
- Teaching: Group
- Teaching: Individual
- Telephone Consultation
- Touch
- Values Clarification

Flight Nursing

- Anaphylaxis Management
- Artificial Airway Management
- Bleeding Reduction
- Blood Products Administration
- Cardiac Care: Acute
- Caregiver Support
- Code Management
- Defibrillator Management: External
- Defibrillator Management: Internal
- Emergency Care
- Family Presence Facilitation
- Hypovolemia Management
- Infant Care: Preterm
- Intravenous (IV) Insertion
- Intravenous (IV) Therapy
- Invasive Hemodynamic Monitoring
- Laboratory Data Interpretation
- Mechanical Ventilation Management: Invasive
- Mechanical Ventilation Management: Noninvasive
- Medication Administration
- Oxygen Therapy
- Patient Identification
- Respiratory Monitoring
- Resuscitation
- Sedation Management
- Shock Management
- Shock Management: Cardiac
- Shock Management: Vasogenic
- Shock Management: Volume
- Shock Prevention
- Technology Management
- Telephone Consultation
- Thrombolytic Therapy Management
- Transport: Interfacility
- Triage: Disaster
- Ventilation Assistance
- Vital Signs Monitoring
- Wound Care

Forensic Nursing

- Abuse Protection Support
- Anxiety Reduction
- Calming Technique
- Communicable Disease Management
- Consultation
- Counseling
- Crisis Intervention
- Deposition/Testimony
- Documentation
- Emergency Care
- Emotional Support
- Environmental Management: Violence Prevention
- Examination Assistance
- Family Integrity Promotion
- Forensic Data Collection
- Grief Work Facilitation
- Health Care Information Exchange
- Health Screening
- Health System Guidance
- Incident Reporting

- Laboratory Data Interpretation
- Patient Identification
- Patient Rights Protection
- Postmortem Care
- Rape-Trauma Treatment

- Referral
- Risk Identification
- Specimen Management
- Substance Use Prevention

Gastroenterological Nursing

- Airway Management
- Airway Suctioning
- Anesthesia Administration
- Aspiration Precautions
- Bowel Incontinence Care: Encopresis
- Bowel Management
- Calming Technique
- Constipation/Impaction Management
- Diarrhea Management
- Diet Staging: Weight Loss Surgery
- Distraction
- Emotional Support
- Enema Administration
- Flatulence Reduction
- Gastrointestinal Intubation
- Infection Control

- Intravenous (IV) Insertion
- Medication Administration: Intramuscular (IM)
- Medication Administration: Intravenous (IV)
- Medication Administration: Oral
- Medication Administration: Rectal
- Nausea Management
- Nutritional Counseling
- Ostomy Care
- Sedation Management
- Self-Efficacy Enhancement
- Specimen Management
- Surveillance
- Technology Management
- Tube Care: Gastrointestinal
- Vital Signs Monitoring
- Vomiting Management

Genetics Nursing

- Active Listening
- Anticipatory Guidance
- Anxiety Reduction
- Coping Enhancement
- Counseling
- Crisis Intervention
- Documentation
- Emotional Support
- Environmental Management: Community
- Environmental Risk Protection
- Family Integrity Promotion
- Family Mobilization
- Family Support
- Genetic Counseling
- Grief Work Facilitation
- Health Care Information Exchange
- Health Literacy Enhancement

- Health Policy Monitoring
- Health Screening
- Laboratory Data Interpretation
- Multidisciplinary Care Conference
- Normalization Promotion
- Parent Education: Childrearing Family
- Parent Education: Infant
- Patient Rights Protection
- Preconception Counseling
- Pregnancy Termination Care
- Referral
- Risk Identification: Genetic
- Self-Efficacy Enhancement
- Support Group
- Teaching: Disease Process
- Values Clarification

Gerontological Nursing

- Abuse Protection Support: Elder
- Active Listening
- Activity Therapy
- Behavior Management
- Bibliotherapy
- Bowel Incontinence Care
- Bowel Training
- Caregiver Support

- Case Management
- Communication Enhancement: Hearing Deficit
- Constipation/Impaction Management
- Coping Enhancement
- Delirium Management
- Dementia Management
- Dementia Management: Bathing
- Dementia Management: Wandering

- Dressing
- Dying Care
- Emotional Support
- Enema Administration
- Environmental Management: Comfort
- Environmental Management: Home Preparation
- Exercise Promotion
- Exercise Therapy: Ambulation
- Family Involvement Promotion
- Financial Resource Assistance
- Fluid/Electrolyte Management
- Foot Care
- Grief Work Facilitation
- Hair and Scalp Care
- Health Literacy Enhancement
- Insurance Authorization
- Lower Extremity Monitoring
- Medication Administration
- Medication Prescribing
- Medication Reconciliation
- Nutrition Management
- Patient Rights Protection
- Positioning
- Prescribing: Diagnostic Testing
- Prescribing: Non-Pharmacologic Treatment
- Pressure Management
- Prompted Voiding
- Rectal Prolapse Management
- Relocation Stress Reduction
- Reminiscence Therapy
- Respite Care
- Self-Care Assistance
- Self-Care Assistance: IADL
- Self-Efficacy Enhancement
- Telephone Follow-Up
- Urinary Habit Training
- Urinary Incontinence Care
- Validation Therapy
- Wound Care: Nonhealing

HIV/AIDS Nursing

- Acid-Base Management
- Anxiety Reduction
- Bed Rest Care
- Caregiver Support
- Case Management
- Cognitive Restructuring
- Communicable Disease Management
- Coping Enhancement
- Counseling
- Decision-Making Support
- Diarrhea Management
- Dying Care
- Electrolyte Management
- Electrolyte Monitoring
- Emotional Support
- Energy Management
- Exercise Promotion
- Family Integrity Promotion
- Family Involvement Promotion
- Family Support
- Fever Treatment
- Financial Resource Assistance
- Fluid Management
- Fluid Monitoring
- Health Education
- Health Screening
- Health System Guidance
- Infection Control
- Infection Protection
- Insurance Authorization
- Medication Administration
- Medication Management
- Medication Reconciliation
- Memory Training
- Mood Management
- Multidisciplinary Care Conference
- Nausea Management
- Patient Rights Protection
- Self-Care Assistance
- Teaching: Disease Process
- Teaching: Individual
- Teaching: Prescribed Medication
- Teaching: Procedure/Treatment
- Values Clarification
- Vital Signs Monitoring
- Wound Care

Holistic Nursing

- Active Listening
- Acupressure
- Animal-Assisted Therapy
- Anticipatory Guidance
- Anxiety Reduction
- Aromatherapy
- Art Therapy
- Autogenic Training
- Bibliotherapy
- Biofeedback
- Body Image Enhancement
- Calming Technique
- Caregiver Support
- Cognitive Restructuring
- Coping Enhancement
- Counseling
- Decision-Making Support
- Emotional Support
- Energy Management
- Environmental Management
- Exercise Promotion
- Family Involvement Promotion

- Guided Imagery
- Healing Touch
- Health Education
- Health Screening
- Hope Inspiration
- Humor
- Journaling
- Massage
- Meditation Facilitation
- Music Therapy
- Mutual Goal Setting
- Nutritional Counseling
- Presence
- Progressive Muscle Relaxation
- Reiki
- Relaxation Therapy
- Self-Awareness Enhancement
- Self-Efficacy Enhancement
- Self-Esteem Enhancement
- Self-Modification Assistance
- Self-Responsibility Facilitation
- Spiritual Growth Facilitation
- Spiritual Support
- Teaching: Group
- Teaching: Individual
- Therapeutic Touch
- Touch
- Truth Telling
- Values Clarification

Home Health Nursing

- Bathing
- Bed Rest Care
- Bowel Management
- Caregiver Support
- Dementia Management: Wandering
- Developmental Enhancement: Infant
- Dressing
- Dying Care
- Emotional Support
- Environmental Management: Comfort
- Environmental Management: Home Preparation
- Fall Prevention
- Family Involvement Promotion
- Hair and Scalp Care
- Health Education
- Home Maintenance Assistance
- Lactation Counseling
- Medication Management
- Ostomy Care
- Pain Management
- Parent Education: Childrearing Family
- Parent Education: Infant
- Parenting Promotion
- Prescribing: Non-Pharmacologic Treatment
- Referral
- Risk Identification
- Security Enhancement
- Self-Care Assistance: Bathing/Hygiene
- Self-Care Assistance: Dressing/Grooming
- Self-Care Assistance: IADL
- Self-Care Assistance: Toileting
- Sibling Support
- Smoking Cessation Assistance
- Surveillance: Remote Electronic
- Teaching: Individual
- Teaching: Infant Nutrition 0-3 Months
- Teaching: Infant Safety 0-3 Months
- Teaching: Prescribed Diet
- Teaching: Prescribed Medication
- Teaching: Procedure/Treatment
- Urinary Catheterization
- Vital Signs Monitoring

Infection Control and Epidemiological Nursing

- Bioterrorism Preparedness
- Communicable Disease Management
- Environmental Management: Safety
- Environmental Risk Protection
- Health Education
- Health Policy Monitoring
- Immunization/Vaccination Management
- Infection Control
- Infection Control: Intraoperative
- Infection Protection
- Latex Precautions
- Learning Facilitation
- Product Evaluation
- Program Development
- Quality Monitoring
- Research Data Collection
- Risk Identification
- Surveillance
- Teaching: Safe Sex

Intravenous Nursing

- Acid-Base Management
- Acid-Base Management: Metabolic Acidosis
- Acid-Base Management: Metabolic Alkalosis
- Acid-Base Management: Respiratory Acidosis
- Acid-Base Management: Respiratory Alkalosis
- Acid-Base Monitoring
- Allergy Management
- Analgesic Administration: Intraspinal
- Blood Products Administration
- Capillary Blood Sample
- Caregiver Support
- Central Venous Access Device Management
- Chemotherapy Management
- Dialysis Access Maintenance
- Electrolyte Management
- Electrolyte Management: Hypercalcemia
- Electrolyte Management: Hyperkalemia
- Electrolyte Management: Hypermagnesemia
- Electrolyte Management: Hypernatremia
- Electrolyte Management: Hyperphosphatemia
- Electrolyte Management: Hypocalcemia
- Electrolyte Management: Hypokalemia
- Electrolyte Management: Hypomagnesemia
- Electrolyte Management: Hyponatremia
- Electrolyte Management: Hypophosphatemia
- Electrolyte Monitoring
- Environmental Management: Safety
- Fluid/Electrolyte Management
- Fluid Management
- Fluid Monitoring
- Health Care Information Exchange
- Health Education
- Hyperglycemia Management
- Hypervolemia Management
- Hypothermia Treatment
- Hypovolemia Management
- Incident Reporting
- Infection Control
- Infection Protection
- Intravenous (IV) Insertion
- Intravenous (IV) Therapy
- Invasive Hemodynamic Monitoring
- Laboratory Data Interpretation
- Medication Administration: Intraosseous
- Medication Administration: Intraspinal
- Medication Administration: Intravenous (IV)
- Medication Administration: Ventricular Reservoir
- Nutrition Management
- Nutrition Therapy
- Nutritional Monitoring
- Pain Management
- Patient-Controlled Analgesia (PCA) Assistance
- Peripherally Inserted Central Catheter (PICC) Care
- Peritoneal Dialysis Therapy
- Phlebotomy: Arterial Blood Sample
- Phlebotomy: Blood Unit Acquisition
- Phlebotomy: Cannulated Vessel
- Phlebotomy: Venous Blood Sample
- Product Evaluation
- Quality Monitoring
- Risk Identification
- Supply Management
- Teaching: Prescribed Medication
- Teaching: Procedure/Treatment
- Technology Management
- Thrombolytic Therapy Management
- Total Parenteral Nutrition (TPN) Administration
- Tube Care: Umbilical Line
- Tube Care: Ventriculostomy/Lumbar Drain

Medical-Surgical Nursing

- Acid-Base Management
- Airway Suctioning
- Artificial Airway Management
- Aspiration Precautions
- Asthma Management
- Bed Rest Care
- Bleeding Reduction: Gastrointestinal
- Blood Products Administration
- Bowel Incontinence Care
- Bowel Training
- Capillary Blood Sample
- Central Venous Access Device Management
- Chemical Restraint
- Chemotherapy Management
- Circulatory Care: Arterial Insufficiency
- Circulatory Care: Venous Insufficiency
- Code Management
- Critical Path Development
- Diet Staging
- Discharge Planning
- Documentation
- Electrolyte Management
- Emotional Support
- Enema Administration
- Enteral Tube Feeding
- Fall Prevention
- Family Involvement Promotion
- Family Presence Facilitation
- Fluid/Electrolyte Management
- Gastrointestinal Intubation
- Health Literacy Enhancement
- Hyperglycemia Management
- Hypoglycemia Management
- Incision Site Care
- Infection Control
- Intravenous (IV) Insertion
- Intravenous (IV) Therapy
- Laboratory Data Interpretation
- Mechanical Ventilation Management: Noninvasive
- Medication Administration
- Medication Management
- Medication Reconciliation

- Multidisciplinary Care Conference
- Nausea Management
- Neurologic Monitoring
- Nutrition Management
- Ostomy Care
- Oxygen Therapy
- Pacemaker Management: Permanent
- Pain Management
- Patient-Controlled Analgesia (PCA) Assistance
- Patient Identification
- Patient Rights Protection
- Physical Restraint
- Postmortem Care
- Pressure Management
- Pressure Ulcer Care
- Pressure Ulcer Prevention
- Quality Monitoring
- Respiratory Monitoring
- Seizure Management
- Seizure Precautions
- Self-Care Assistance
- Shock Management
- Shock Prevention
- Skin Surveillance
- Staff Supervision
- Teaching: Disease Process
- Teaching: Individual
- Teaching: Prescribed Medication
- Teaching: Procedure/Treatment
- Total Parenteral Nutrition (TPN) Administration
- Traction/Immobilization Care
- Tube Care: Chest
- Tube Care: Gastrointestinal
- Tube Care: Urinary
- Urinary Elimination Management
- Urinary Incontinence Care
- Vital Signs Monitoring
- Vomiting Management
- Wound Care
- Wound Care: Nonhealing

Midwifery Nursing

- Abuse Protection Support
- Active Listening
- Admission Care
- Amnioinfusion
- Anticipatory Guidance
- Attachment Promotion
- Birthing
- Breast Examination
- Childbirth Preparation
- Decision-Making Support
- Delegation
- Discharge Planning
- Documentation
- Emotional Support
- Environmental Management
- Family Integrity Promotion: Childbearing Family
- Family Planning: Contraception
- Family Planning: Unplanned Pregnancy
- Fertility Preservation
- Health Education
- Health Screening
- High-Risk Pregnancy Care
- Hormone Replacement Therapy
- Infant Care: Newborn
- Infant Care: Preterm
- Intrapartal Care
- Lactation Counseling
- Lactation Suppression
- Medication Administration: Intraspinal
- Medication Management
- Medication Prescribing
- Nutritional Counseling
- Pain Management
- Parent Education: Infant
- Physician Support
- Postpartal Care
- Premenstrual Syndrome (PMS) Management
- Prescribing: Diagnostic Testing
- Referral
- Risk Identification: Childbearing Family
- Self-Efficacy Enhancement
- Sexual Counseling
- Suturing
- Teaching: Individual
- Telephone Consultation

Neonatal Nursing

- Acid-Base Management
- Airway Insertion and Stabilization
- Airway Management
- Airway Suctioning
- Analgesic Administration
- Artificial Airway Management
- Attachment Promotion
- Blood Products Administration
- Bottle Feeding
- Caregiver Support
- Central Venous Access Device Management
- Circumcision Care
- Critical Path Development
- Discharge Planning
- Documentation
- Electrolyte Management
- Electrolyte Management: Hypercalcemia
- Electrolyte Management: Hyperkalemia
- Electrolyte Management: Hypermagnesemia
- Electrolyte Management: Hypernatremia

- Electrolyte Management: Hyperphosphatemia
- Electrolyte Management: Hypocalcemia
- Electrolyte Management: Hypokalemia
- Electrolyte Management: Hypomagnesemia
- Electrolyte Management: Hyponatremia
- Electrolyte Management: Hypophosphatemia
- Endotracheal Extubation
- Enteral Tube Feeding
- Environmental Management
- Environmental Management: Comfort
- Eye Care
- Family Involvement Promotion
- Family Support
- Feeding
- Fluid Management
- Fluid Monitoring
- Health Care Information Exchange
- Hypovolemia Management
- Infant Care
- Infant Care: Newborn
- Infant Care: Preterm
- Infection Protection
- Intravenous (IV) Insertion
- Intravenous (IV) Therapy
- Kangaroo Care
- Laboratory Data Interpretation
- Lactation Counseling
- Mechanical Ventilation Management: Invasive
- Mechanical Ventilation Management: Noninvasive
- Mechanical Ventilatory Weaning
- Medication Administration
- Medication Administration: Enteral
- Medication Administration: Eye
- Medication Administration: Intramuscular (IM)
- Medication Administration: Intravenous (IV)
- Medication Administration: Oral
- Medication Management

- Multidisciplinary Care Conference
- Nonnutritive Sucking
- Nutrition Management
- Nutrition Therapy
- Nutritional Monitoring
- Ostomy Care
- Oxygen Therapy
- Pain Management
- Parent Education: Infant
- Patient Identification
- Phototherapy: Neonate
- Positioning
- Respiratory Monitoring
- Resuscitation
- Resuscitation: Neonate
- Shock Management: Volume
- Sibling Support
- Skin Care: Topical Treatments
- Skin Surveillance
- Sleep Enhancement
- Surveillance
- Technology Management
- Temperature Regulation
- Total Parenteral Nutrition (TPN) Administration
- Transport: Interfacility
- Transport: Intrafacility
- Tube Care: Chest
- Tube Care: Gastrointestinal
- Tube Care: Umbilical Line
- Tube Care: Urinary
- Urinary Catheterization
- Urinary Catheterization: Intermittent
- Ventilation Assistance
- Visitation Facilitation
- Vital Signs Monitoring
- Wound Care

Nephrology Nursing

- Acid-Base Management
- Bedside Laboratory Testing
- Bleeding Reduction: Wound
- Capillary Blood Sample
- Case Management
- Constipation/Impaction Management
- Culture Brokerage
- Decision-Making Support
- Delegation
- Dialyses Access Maintenance
- Electrolyte Management
- Electrolyte Monitoring
- Emotional Support
- Environmental Management: Comfort
- Environmental Management: Safety
- Family Involvement Promotion
- Financial Resource Assistance
- Fluid/Electrolyte Management
- Fluid Management
- Fluid Monitoring
- Health Literacy Enhancement

- Hemodialysis Therapy
- Hyperglycemia Management
- Hypervolemia Management
- Hypoglycemia Management
- Hypovolemia Management
- Infection Control
- Infection Protection
- Laboratory Data Interpretation
- Medication Administration
- Medication Management
- Multidisciplinary Care Conference
- Nausea Management
- Nutritional Monitoring
- Organ Procurement
- Peritoneal Dialysis Therapy
- Phlebotomy: Cannulated Vessel
- Physician Support
- Pruritus Management
- Self-Efficacy Enhancement
- Specimen Management
- Teaching: Disease Process

- Teaching: Individual
- Teaching: Prescribed Medication
- Teaching: Procedure/Treatment
- Teaching: Psychomotor Skill
- Technology Management

- Telephone Consultation
- Values Clarification
- Vital Signs Monitoring
- Vomiting Management

Neuroscience Nursing

- Airway Management
- Anxiety Reduction
- Behavior Management
- Body Image Enhancement
- Bowel Management
- Cerebral Edema Management
- Cerebral Perfusion Promotion
- Chemical Restraint
- Cognitive Stimulation
- Communication Enhancement: Speech Deficit
- Communication Enhancement: Visual Deficit
- Delirium Management
- Delusion Management
- Dementia Management
- Dementia Management: Wandering
- Dysreflexia Management
- Energy Management
- Environmental Management: Safety
- Fall Prevention
- Hypothermia Induction Therapy

- Intracranial Pressure (ICP) Monitoring
- Medication Administration
- Medication Management
- Neurologic Monitoring
- Pain Management
- Positioning: Neurologic
- Seizure Management
- Seizure Precautions
- Self-Efficacy Enhancement
- Sleep Enhancement
- Subarachnoid Hemorrhage Precautions
- Surveillance
- Swallowing Therapy
- Temperature Regulation
- Thrombolytic Therapy Management
- Tube Care: Ventriculostomy/Lumbar Drain
- Unilateral Neglect Management
- Urinary Catheterization: Intermittent
- Urinary Elimination Management
- Vehicle Safety Promotion

Obstetric Nursing

- Attachment Promotion
- Birthing
- Bleeding Reduction: Antepartum Uterus
- Bleeding Reduction: Postpartum Uterus
- Bottle Feeding
- Cesarean Birth Care
- Childbirth Preparation
- Circumcision Care
- Electronic Fetal Monitoring: Antepartum
- Electronic Fetal Monitoring: Intrapartum
- Family Integrity Promotion: Childbearing Family
- Family Planning: Contraception
- Grief Work Facilitation: Perinatal Death
- Health Literacy Enhancement
- High-Risk Pregnancy Care
- Infant Care
- Infant Care: Newborn
- Intrapartal Care

- Intrapartal Care: High-Risk Delivery
- Invasive Hemodynamic Monitoring
- Labor Induction
- Labor Suppression
- Lactation Counseling
- Medication Administration
- Medication Administration: Intraspinal
- Pain Management
- Parent Education: Infant
- Parenting Promotion
- Postpartal Care
- Pregnancy Termination Care
- Prenatal Care
- Resuscitation: Fetus
- Resuscitation: Neonate
- Risk Identification: Childbearing Family
- Substance Use Treatment
- Surveillance: Late Pregnancy

Occupational Health Nursing

- Active Listening
- Allergy Management
- Anticipatory Guidance
- Anxiety Reduction
- Asthma Management
- Bioterrorism Preparedness
- Cardiac Care: Rehabilitative
- Case Management
- Communicable Disease Management
- Counseling
- Crisis Intervention
- Decision-Making Support
- Defibrillator Management: External
- Ear Care
- Emergency Care
- Emotional Support
- Environmental Management: Community
- Environmental Management: Safety
- Environmental Management: Violence Prevention
- Environmental Management: Worker Safety
- Environmental Risk Protection
- Exercise Promotion
- Fall Prevention
- Family Support
- Health Education
- Health Literacy Enhancement
- Health Screening
- Health System Guidance
- Immunization/Vaccination Management
- Infection Protection
- Insurance Authorization
- Nutritional Counseling
- Parent Education: Adolescent
- Parent Education: Childrearing Family
- Prenatal Care
- Referral
- Respiratory Monitoring
- Risk Identification
- Smoking Cessation Assistance
- Social Marketing
- Substance Use Prevention
- Substance Use Treatment
- Teaching: Group
- Teaching: Individual
- Technology Management
- Telephone Consultation
- Telephone Follow-Up
- Triage: Disaster
- Vehicle Safety Promotion
- Weight Management
- Weight Reduction Assistance
- Wound Care

Oncology Nursing

- Analgesic Administration
- Anxiety Reduction
- Bleeding Precautions
- Bowel Management
- Caregiver Support
- Central Venous Access Device Management
- Chemotherapy Management
- Coping Enhancement
- Dying Care
- Energy Management
- Environmental Management: Comfort
- Family Involvement Promotion
- Fever Treatment
- Financial Resource Assistance
- Fluid Management
- Healing Touch
- Hope Inspiration
- Infection Control
- Infection Protection
- Intravenous (IV) Insertion
- Laboratory Data Interpretation
- Medication Administration
- Medication Management
- Nausea Management
- Nutrition Management
- Nutritional Monitoring
- Pain Management
- Peripheral Sensation Management
- Phlebotomy: Cannulated Vessel
- Preparatory Sensory Information
- Radiation Therapy Management
- Reiki
- Self-Efficacy Enhancement
- Spiritual Support
- Stem Cell Infusion
- Support Group
- Teaching: Disease Process
- Teaching: Procedure/Treatment
- Telephone Follow-Up
- Therapeutic Touch
- Urinary Elimination Management
- Vomiting Management
- Wound Care: Nonhealing

Ophthalmic Nursing

- Active Listening
- Communication Enhancement: Visual Deficit
- Consultation
- Contact Lens Care
- Discharge Planning
- Dry Eye Prevention
- Emotional Support
- Eye Care
- Fall Prevention
- Family Involvement Promotion
- Hypoglycemia Management
- Incision Site Care
- Infection Control
- Infection Control: Intraoperative
- Intravenous (IV) Insertion
- Intravenous (IV) Therapy
- Laser Precautions
- Medication Administration
- Medication Administration: Eye
- Medication Administration: Intramuscular (IM)
- Medication Administration: Oral
- Preoperative Coordination
- Sedation Management
- Self-Care Assistance: IADL
- Surgical Assistance
- Surgical Preparation
- Surveillance
- Teaching: Disease Process
- Teaching: Individual
- Teaching: Preoperative
- Teaching: Prescribed Medication
- Teaching: Procedure/Treatment
- Teaching: Psychomotor Skill
- Telephone Follow-Up
- Vital Signs Monitoring

Orthopedic Nursing

- Amputation Care
- Analgesic Administration
- Autotransfusion
- Bathing
- Bed Rest Care
- Blood Products Administration
- Cast Care: Maintenance
- Cast Care: Wet
- Constipation/Impaction Management
- Controlled Substance Checking
- Cough Enhancement
- Critical Path Development
- Delirium Management
- Discharge Planning
- Embolus Care: Peripheral
- Exercise Promotion
- Exercise Therapy: Ambulation
- Exercise Therapy: Joint Mobility
- Fall Prevention
- Heat/Cold Application
- Incision Site Care
- Infection Control
- Intravenous (IV) Insertion
- Intravenous (IV) Therapy
- Lower Extremity Monitoring
- Medication Administration
- Medication Administration: Intramuscular (IM)
- Medication Administration: Intravenous (IV)
- Medication Administration: Oral
- Pain Management
- Patient-Controlled Analgesia (PCA) Assistance
- Physical Restraint
- Positioning
- Positioning: Wheelchair
- Preparatory Sensory Information
- Pressure Management
- Self-Care Assistance
- Self-Care Assistance: IADL
- Self-Care Assistance: Transfer
- Skin Care: Topical Treatments
- Skin Surveillance
- Splinting
- Teaching: Individual
- Teaching: Preoperative
- Teaching: Prescribed Exercise
- Teaching: Prescribed Medication
- Teaching: Procedure/Treatment
- Traction/Immobilization Care
- Tube Care: Urinary
- Urinary Retention Care
- Wound Care
- Wound Care: Closed Drainage

Otorhinolaryngology and Head/Neck Nursing

- Airway Insertion and Stabilization
- Airway Management
- Airway Suctioning
- Allergy Management
- Analgesic Administration
- Anxiety Reduction
- Artificial Airway Management
- Aspiration Precautions
- Asthma Management
- Bleeding Reduction: Nasal
- Body Image Enhancement
- Chemotherapy Management
- Communication Enhancement: Hearing Deficit
- Communication Enhancement: Speech Deficit
- Critical Path Development
- Discharge Planning
- Ear Care
- Exercise Therapy: Balance
- Infection Control: Intraoperative
- Intracranial Pressure (ICP) Monitoring
- Mechanical Ventilation Management: Noninvasive
- Medication Administration
- Medication Administration: Inhalation
- Medication Administration: Nasal
- Nasal Irrigation
- Oral Health Maintenance
- Oral Health Promotion
- Oral Health Restoration
- Pain Management
- Positioning: Intraoperative
- Postanesthesia Care
- Preoperative Coordination
- Radiation Therapy Management
- Self-Efficacy Enhancement
- Smoking Cessation Assistance
- Surgical Assistance
- Surgical Precautions
- Surgical Preparation
- Swallowing Therapy
- Teaching: Preoperative
- Teaching: Prescribed Diet
- Teaching: Prescribed Exercise
- Teaching: Prescribed Medication
- Teaching: Procedure/Treatment
- Telephone Consultation
- Tube Care
- Wound Care

Pain Management Nursing

- Analgesic Administration
- Analgesic Administration: Intraspinal
- Biofeedback
- Case Management
- Central Venous Access Device Management
- Controlled Substance Checking
- Coping Enhancement
- Decision-Making Support
- Discharge Planning
- Distraction
- Dying Care
- Energy Management
- Environmental Management: Comfort
- Exercise Promotion
- Guided Imagery
- Healing Touch
- Health Care Information Exchange
- Health Education
- Health Policy Monitoring
- Heat/Cold Application
- Humor
- Infection Control
- Insurance Authorization
- Massage
- Medication Administration
- Medication Management
- Medication Reconciliation
- Meditation Facilitation
- Multidisciplinary Care Conference
- Music Therapy
- Mutual Goal Setting
- Pain Management
- Patient Contracting
- Patient-Controlled Analgesia (PCA) Assistance
- Physician Support
- Product Evaluation
- Progressive Muscle Relaxation
- Quality Monitoring
- Referral
- Reiki
- Relaxation Therapy
- Research Data Collection
- Sedation Management
- Self-Efficacy Enhancement
- Self-Esteem Enhancement
- Spiritual Support
- Support Group
- Surgical Assistance
- Surgical Preparation
- Surveillance
- Teaching: Prescribed Medication
- Teaching: Procedure/Treatment
- Therapeutic Touch
- Touch
- Transcutaneous Electrical Nerve Stimulation (TENS)

Pediatric Nursing

- Abuse Protection Support: Child
- Asthma Management
- Caregiver Support
- Developmental Enhancement: Child
- Developmental Enhancement: Infant
- Discharge Planning
- Documentation
- Emotional Support
- Environmental Management: Safety
- Family Involvement Promotion
- Family Presence Facilitation
- Feeding
- Fever Treatment
- Fluid/Electrolyte Management
- Health Education
- Immunization/Vaccination Management
- Infant Care
- Infant Care: Newborn
- Infant Care: Preterm
- Intravenous (IV) Therapy
- Medication Administration
- Multidisciplinary Care Conference
- Normalization Promotion
- Nutrition Management
- Oxygen Therapy
- Pain Management
- Parent Education: Adolescent
- Parent Education: Childrearing Family
- Parent Education: Infant
- Parenting Promotion
- Respiratory Monitoring
- Risk Identification
- Risk Identification: Genetic
- Sports-Injury Prevention: Youth
- Surveillance
- Teaching: Infant Nutrition 0-3 Months
- Teaching: Infant Nutrition 4-6 Months
- Teaching: Infant Nutrition 7-9 Months
- Teaching: Infant Nutrition 10-12 Months
- Teaching: Infant Safety 0-3 Months
- Teaching: Infant Safety 4-6 Months
- Teaching: Infant Safety 7-9 Months
- Teaching: Infant Safety 10-12 Months
- Teaching: Infant Stimulation 0-4 Months
- Teaching: Infant Stimulation 5-8 Months
- Teaching: Infant Stimulation 9-12 Months
- Teaching: Toddler Nutrition 13-18 Months
- Teaching: Toddler Nutrition 19-24 Months
- Teaching: Toddler Nutrition 25-36 Months
- Teaching: Toddler Safety 13-18 Months
- Teaching: Toddler Safety 19-24 Months
- Teaching: Toddler Safety 25-36 Months
- Teaching: Toilet Training
- Technology Management
- Therapeutic Play
- Total Parenteral Nutrition (TPN) Administration
- Trauma Therapy: Child
- Vehicle Safety Promotion
- Vital Signs Monitoring

Pediatric Oncology Nursing

- Active Listening
- Analgesic Administration
- Anxiety Reduction
- Bleeding Precautions
- Blood Products Administration
- Calming Technique
- Caregiver Support
- Case Management
- Central Venous Access Device Management
- Chemotherapy Management
- Coping Enhancement
- Decision-Making Support
- Developmental Enhancement: Child
- Dying Care
- Family Integrity Promotion
- Family Involvement Promotion
- Family Mobilization
- Family Presence Facilitation
- Family Process Maintenance
- Fever Treatment
- Fluid/Electrolyte Management
- Grief Work Facilitation
- Hope Inspiration
- Infection Protection
- Medication Administration: Intramuscular (IM)
- Medication Administration: Intravenous (IV)
- Medication Administration: Oral
- Multidisciplinary Care Conference
- Nausea Management
- Normalization Promotion
- Pain Management
- Parent Education: Childrearing Family
- Radiation Therapy Management
- Sedation Management
- Sibling Support
- Stem Cell Infusion
- Teaching: Disease Process
- Teaching: Prescribed Medication
- Therapeutic Play
- Total Parenteral Nutrition (TPN) Administration
- Trauma Therapy: Child
- Vomiting Management

Perioperative Nursing

- Active Listening
- Anaphylaxis Management
- Anxiety Reduction
- Autotransfusion
- Blood Products Administration
- Critical Path Development
- Delegation
- Discharge Planning
- Documentation
- Electrolyte Management
- Emotional Support
- Environmental Management: Comfort
- Environmental Management: Safety
- Environmental Management: Worker Safety
- Fluid Monitoring
- Hypothermia Induction Therapy
- Infection Control: Intraoperative
- Laser Precautions
- Latex Precautions
- Malignant Hyperthermia Precautions
- Oxygen Therapy
- Pain Management
- Patient Identification
- Patient Rights Protection
- Physician Support
- Pneumatic Tourniquet Precautions
- Positioning: Intraoperative
- Postanesthesia Care
- Preceptor: Employee
- Preoperative Coordination
- Presence
- Pressure Management
- Product Evaluation
- Quality Monitoring
- Sedation Management
- Self-Care Assistance: Transfer
- Skin Care: Donor Site
- Skin Care: Graft Site
- Skin Surveillance
- Specimen Management
- Supply Management
- Surgical Assistance
- Surgical Instrumentation Management
- Surgical Precautions
- Surgical Preparation
- Suturing
- Teaching: Preoperative
- Technology Management
- Temperature Regulation: Perioperative
- Touch
- Transport: Intrafacility
- Vital Signs Monitoring
- Wound Care

Plastic Surgery Nursing

- Analgesic Administration
- Bleeding Precautions
- Body Image Enhancement
- Counseling
- Decision-Making Support
- Emotional Support
- Guided Imagery
- Heat/Cold Application
- Incision Site Care
- Infection Control
- Infection Protection
- Insurance Authorization
- Intravenous (IV) Therapy
- Journaling
- Laser Precautions
- Medication Administration
- Pain Management
- Patient-Controlled Analgesic (PCA) Assistance
- Patient Identification
- Preoperative Coordination
- Preparatory Sensory Information
- Pruritus Management
- Sedation Management
- Self-Care Assistance
- Skin Care: Donor Site
- Skin Care: Graft Site
- Skin Care: Topical Treatments
- Skin Surveillance
- Sleep Enhancement
- Surgical Instrumentation Management
- Teaching: Individual
- Teaching: Preoperative
- Values Clarification
- Vital Signs Monitoring
- Wound Care

Psychiatric/Mental Health Nursing

- Abuse Protection Support
- Active Listening
- Anger Control Assistance
- Anxiety Reduction
- Area Restriction
- Assertiveness Training
- Behavior Management: Overactivity/Inattention
- Behavior Management: Self-Harm
- Behavior Management: Sexual
- Behavior Modification
- Behavior Modification: Social Skills
- Bibliotherapy
- Body Image Enhancement
- Calming Technique
- Case Management
- Chemical Restraint
- Cognitive Restructuring
- Complex Relationship Building
- Consultation
- Coping Enhancement
- Counseling
- Crisis Intervention
- Delusion Management
- Dementia Management
- Dementia Management: Bathing
- Dementia Management: Wandering
- Eating Disorders Management
- Electroconvulsive Therapy (ECT) Management
- Elopement Precautions
- Environmental Management: Violence Prevention
- Family Involvement Promotion
- Family Therapy
- Fire-Setting Precautions
- Grief Work Facilitation
- Guilt Work Facilitation
- Hallucination Management
- Health Literacy Enhancement
- Impulse Control Training
- Journaling
- Life Skills Enhancement
- Limit Setting
- Listening Visits
- Medication Administration
- Medication Management
- Medication Prescribing
- Milieu Therapy
- Mood Management
- Pass Facilitation
- Phototherapy: Mood/Sleep Regulation
- Physical Restraint
- Prescribing: Diagnostic Testing
- Reality Orientation
- Reminiscence Therapy
- Seclusion
- Self-Awareness Enhancement
- Self-Care Assistance: IADL
- Self-Esteem Enhancement
- Substance Use Prevention
- Substance Use Treatment: Alcohol Withdrawal
- Substance Use Treatment: Drug Withdrawal
- Suicide Prevention
- Support Group
- Therapeutic Play
- Therapy Group

Radiological Nursing

- Airway Management
- Airway Suctioning
- Allergy Management
- Analgesic Administration
- Anxiety Reduction
- Aspiration Precautions
- Bleeding Precautions
- Bleeding Reduction
- Blood Products Administration
- Calming Technique
- Cardiac Risk Management
- Cerebral Perfusion Promotion
- Circulatory Precautions
- Code Management
- Discharge Planning
- Dysrhythmia Management
- Embolus Care: Peripheral
- Embolus Care: Pulmonary
- Embolus Precautions
- Emergency Care
- Emotional Support
- Environmental Management: Safety
- Examination Assistance
- Fluid/Electrolyte Management
- Fluid Management
- Fluid Monitoring
- Fluid Resuscitation
- Health Care Information Exchange
- Health Screening
- Incident Reporting
- Infection Control
- Infection Protection
- Intravenous (IV) Insertion
- Intravenous (IV) Therapy
- Laser Precautions
- Latex Precautions
- Medication Administration
- Medication Administration: Intravenous (IV)
- Neurologic Monitoring
- Oxygen Therapy
- Pacemaker Management: Permanent
- Pain Management
- Preparatory Sensory Information
- Quality Monitoring
- Radiation Therapy Management
- Referral
- Relaxation Therapy
- Research Data Collection

- Respiratory Monitoring
- Resuscitation
- Security Enhancement
- Sedation Management
- Shock Prevention
- Smoking Cessation Assistance
- Staff Supervision
- Teaching: Individual
- Teaching: Procedure/Treatment
- Technology Management

- Telephone Consultation
- Touch
- Tube Care
- Tube Care: Chest
- Tube Care: Gastrointestinal
- Tube Care: Urinary
- Urinary Catheterization
- Ventilation Assistance
- Vital Signs Monitoring

Rehabilitation Nursing

- Amputation Care
- Behavior Management
- Body Image Enhancement
- Body Mechanics Promotion
- Bowel Management
- Case Management
- Communication Enhancement: Speech Deficit
- Coping Enhancement
- Decision-Making Support
- Discharge Planning
- Dressing
- Embolus Precautions
- Emotional Support
- Energy Management
- Environmental Management: Home Preparation
- Environmental Management: Safety
- Exercise Promotion: Strength Training
- Family Involvement Promotion
- Family Support
- Financial Resource Assistance
- Health Education
- Hope Inspiration
- Learning Facilitation

- Life Skills Enhancement
- Medication Management
- Memory Training
- Multidisciplinary Care Conference
- Mutual Goal Setting
- Normalization Promotion
- Nutrition Management
- Pain Management
- Positioning
- Positioning: Wheelchair
- Pressure Ulcer Care
- Pressure Ulcer Prevention
- Relocation Stress Reduction
- Self-Care Assistance
- Self-Care Assistance: IADL
- Self-Efficacy Enhancement
- Self-Responsibility Facilitation
- Socialization Enhancement
- Swallowing Therapy
- Teaching: Individual
- Unilateral Neglect Management
- Urinary Elimination Management
- Wound Care: Nonhealing

School Nursing

- Abuse Protection Support: Child
- Active Listening
- Allergy Management
- Analgesic Administration
- Anger Control Assistance
- Anticipatory Guidance
- Anxiety Reduction
- Asthma Management
- Bleeding Reduction
- Bleeding Reduction: Wound
- Calming Technique
- Caregiver Support
- Commendation
- Contact Lens Care
- Coping Enhancement
- Counseling
- Crisis Intervention
- Decision-Making Support
- Delegation
- Documentation
- Emergency Care

- Emotional Support
- Eye Care
- Family Integrity Promotion
- Family Involvement Promotion
- Family Support
- Fever Treatment
- First Aid
- Grief Work Facilitation
- Health Care Information Exchange
- Health Education
- Health Literacy Enhancement
- Health Screening
- Health System Guidance
- Heat/Cold Application
- Humor
- Infection Control
- Learning Facilitation
- Learning Readiness Enhancement
- Medication Administration: Oral
- Medication Management
- Multidisciplinary Care Conference

- Nutritional Counseling
- Pain Management
- Parent Education: Adolescent
- Parent Education: Childrearing Family
- Patient Rights Protection
- Referral
- Resiliency Promotion
- Self-Efficacy Enhancement
- Self-Esteem Enhancement
- Skin Surveillance
- Socialization Enhancement
- Social Marketing

- Spiritual Support
- Sports-Injury Prevention: Youth
- Substance Use Prevention
- Suicide Prevention
- Support Group
- Teaching: Individual
- Telephone Consultation
- Touch
- Values Clarification
- Vehicle Safety Promotion
- Vital Signs Monitoring
- Wound Care

Spinal Cord Injury Nursing

- Active Listening
- Airway Suctioning
- Artificial Airway Management
- Behavior Management
- Body Image Enhancement
- Bowel Management
- Bowel Training
- Caregiver Support
- Case Management
- Chest Physiotherapy
- Circulatory Precautions
- Coping Enhancement
- Discharge Planning
- Dysreflexia Management
- Emotional Support
- Family Involvement Promotion
- Financial Resource Assistance
- Fluid Management
- Health Care Information Exchange
- Hope Inspiration
- Infection Protection
- Lower Extremity Monitoring
- Mechanical Ventilation Management: Invasive
- Mechanical Ventilation Management: Noninvasive
- Mechanical Ventilation Management: Pneumonia Prevention
- Medication Management
- Multidisciplinary Care Conference
- Mutual Goal Setting

- Nutrition Management
- Pain Management
- Pass Facilitation
- Peripheral Sensation Management
- Positioning
- Positioning: Wheelchair
- Pressure Ulcer Care
- Pressure Ulcer Prevention
- Relocation Stress Reduction
- Self-Care Assistance: Bathing/Hygiene
- Self-Care Assistance: Dressing/Grooming
- Self-Care Assistance: Feeding
- Self-Care Assistance: IADL
- Self-Care Assistance: Toileting
- Self-Care Assistance: Transfer
- Teaching: Disease Process
- Teaching: Group
- Teaching: Individual
- Teaching: Prescribed Medication
- Teaching: Psychomotor Skill
- Traction/Immobilization Care
- Transfer
- Tube Care: Urinary
- Urinary Bladder Training
- Urinary Catheterization
- Urinary Catheterization: Intermittent
- Wound Care: Nonhealing

Transplant Nursing

- Acid-Base Management
- Case Management
- Coping Enhancement
- Counseling
- Decision-Making Support
- Electrolyte Management
- Electrolyte Monitoring
- Emotional Support
- Family Integrity Promotion
- Family Involvement Promotion
- Family Support

- Financial Resource Assistance
- Fluid Management
- Fluid Monitoring
- Hyperglycemia Management
- Hypoglycemia Management
- Infection Control
- Infection Protection
- Insurance Authorization
- Laboratory Data Interpretation
- Medication Administration
- Medication Management

- Medication Reconciliation
- Multidisciplinary Care Conference
- Organ Procurement
- Patient Identification
- Patient Rights Protection
- Stem Cell Infusion
- Support Group
- Surveillance

- Teaching: Disease Process
- Teaching: Individual
- Teaching: Prescribed Medication
- Teaching: Procedure/Treatment
- Values Clarification
- Vital Signs Monitoring
- Wound Care

Urologic Nursing

- Active Listening
- Analgesic Administration
- Behavior Modification
- Biofeedback
- Bladder Irrigation
- Body Image Enhancement
- Caregiver Support
- Case Management
- Chemotherapy Management
- Dialysis Access Maintenance
- Fluid/Electrolyte Management
- Infection Control: Intraoperative
- Intravenous (IV) Therapy
- Latex Precautions
- Medication Administration
- Medication Management
- Ostomy Care
- Pelvic Muscle Exercise
- Pessary Management
- Positioning: Intraoperative
- Preoperative Coordination
- Preparatory Sensory Information

- Prompted Voiding
- Radiation Therapy Management
- Specimen Management
- Surgical Assistance
- Surgical Precautions
- Surgical Preparation
- Teaching: Disease Process
- Teaching: Individual
- Teaching: Preoperative
- Teaching: Prescribed Medication
- Teaching: Procedure/Treatment
- Temperature Regulation: Perioperative
- Tube Care
- Tube Care: Urinary
- Urinary Bladder Training
- Urinary Catheterization
- Urinary Catheterization: Intermittent
- Urinary Elimination Management
- Urinary Habit Training
- Urinary Incontinence Care
- Urinary Retention Care
- Wound Care

Vascular Nursing

- Amputation Care
- Circulatory Care: Arterial Insufficiency
- Circulatory Care: Venous Insufficiency
- Circulatory Precautions
- Discharge Planning
- Embolus Care: Peripheral
- Embolus Care: Pulmonary
- Embolus Precautions
- Exercise Promotion: Strength Training
- Exercise Therapy: Ambulation
- Exercise Therapy: Joint Mobility
- Exercise Therapy: Muscle Control
- Foot Care
- Grief Work Facilitation
- Health Screening
- Incision Site Care
- Infection Protection
- Leech Therapy
- Lower Extremity Monitoring

- Medication Management
- Nail Care
- Nutrition Management
- Pain Management
- Peripheral Sensation Management
- Pressure Ulcer Care
- Pressure Ulcer Prevention
- Risk Identification
- Self-Care Assistance
- Skin Care: Donor Site
- Skin Care: Graft Site
- Skin Care: Topical Treatments
- Smoking Cessation Assistance
- Teaching: Foot Care
- Teaching: Individual
- Teaching: Prescribed Exercise
- Unilateral Neglect Management
- Wound Care
- Wound Care: Nonhealing

Women's Health Nursing

- Abuse Protection Support
- Abuse Protection Support: Domestic Partner
- Anticipatory Guidance
- Behavior Modification
- Body Image Enhancement
- Breast Examination
- Coping Enhancement
- Counseling
- Decision-Making Support
- Emotional Support
- Exercise Promotion
- Family Planning: Contraception
- Family Planning: Infertility
- Family Planning: Unplanned Pregnancy
- Fertility Preservation
- Health Education
- Health Literacy Enhancement
- Health Screening
- Health System Guidance
- Hormone Replacement Therapy
- Listening Visits
- Medication Management
- Nutritional Counseling
- Pelvic Muscle Exercise
- Pessary Management
- Preconception Counseling
- Pregnancy Termination Care
- Premenstrual Syndrome (PMS) Management
- Risk Identification
- Self-Efficacy Enhancement
- Teaching: Disease Process
- Teaching: Individual
- Teaching: Safe Sex
- Telephone Consultation
- Urinary Bladder Training
- Weight Management
- Weight Reduction Assistance

PART FIVE

Estimated Time and Education Level Necessary to Perform NIC Interventions

Estimated Time and Education Level Necessary to Perform NIC Interventions

In this section we list the estimated time to perform, and type of personnel to deliver, each of the 554 interventions in this edition of the Classification. The estimates were derived in the following manner:

Step One: The 433 interventions included in the second edition of NIC were rated in 1999 in response to a request from a user who was incorporating NIC into a coding/reimbursement manual.[1] Small groups of research team members rated selected interventions in their area of expertise on: (1) education needed for each intervention, and (2) time needed for each intervention. Rating group members referred to the NIC second edition[4] for intervention definitions and activities. Each group of raters returned their work to the principal investigators who, with two other members of the research team, reviewed all the ratings for all interventions for overall consistency.

Step Two: In Fall 2000, ratings were done using the same methodology for the 53 interventions new to the third edition of NIC published in 2000.[5] Changes in interventions from the second to third edition were also examined for their impact on the ratings. Following this, all 486 intervention ratings were reviewed together and a few of these modified to be consistent with others in the same class. This information was published in a monograph entitled, "Estimated Time and Educational Requirements to Perform 486 Nursing Interventions,"[2] produced by the Center for Nursing Classification and Clinical Effectiveness at the College of Nursing, The University of Iowa. Portions of the monograph were published in Nursing Economic$ ("Determining Cost of Nursing Interventions: A Beginning").[3]

Step Three and Ongoing: Since 2002, for each of the new editions of the classification, we estimated the time and education for each of the new interventions using the same criteria.

Education needed is defined as the minimal educational level necessary to perform the intervention in most cases in most states, and rated as: (1) nursing assistant/LPN/LVN/technician; (2) RN (basic education, whether baccalaureate, AD, or diploma); or (3) RN with post-basic education or certification. Post-basic education is defined as specialized education or training beyond the RN basic education, including a master's degree with or without certification or short course leading to certificate or certification. These categories were arrived at after thorough discussion. They were chosen over other possibilities because it was felt that the categories allow raters to discriminate among them but are not so fine that raters could not be consistent. The basic types of RN preparation were grouped in one category because this reflects the reality of the practice situation that does not usually differentiate job responsibilities by educational preparation of the RN.

Time needed is defined as the average time needed to perform the intervention. This is an average time that can be used to determine reimbursement rates, long enough that the intervention can be done but not so long that it would price the intervention unreasonably high for insurance or client payment. Time estimates are grouped into five categories: (1) 15 minutes or less; (2) 16 to 30 minutes; (3) 31 to 45 minutes; (4) 46 to 60 minutes; and (5) more than 1 hour.

It is emphasized that the estimates are based on judgments of those who are familiar with the intervention and the specialty practice area. The ratings included here may differ by practice facility and provider. The estimates provide a starting point for estimating time required, level of provider needed, and cost of nursing care.

References

1. Alternative Link, Inc. (2001). *CAM and nursing coding manual.* Las Cruces, NM: Author.
2. Center for Nursing Classification. (2001). *Estimated time and educational requirements to perform 486 nursing interventions.* Iowa City, IA: Author.
3. Iowa Intervention Project. (2001). Determining cost of nursing interventions: A beginning. *Nursing Economic$, 19*(4), 146–160.
4. McCloskey, J. C. & Bulechek, G. M. (Eds.). (1996). *Nursing interventions classification (NIC)* (2nd ed.). St. Louis: Mosby.
5. McCloskey, J. C. & Bulechek, G. M. (Eds.). (2000). *Nursing interventions classification (NIC)*(3rd ed.). St. Louis: Mosby.

Table 1	TIME & EDUCATION FOR 554 NIC INTERVENTIONS LISTED ALPHABETICALLY		
Intervention	Code No.	Educational Level	Time Required
Abuse Protection Support	6400	RN basic	More than 1 hr
Abuse Protection Support: Child	6402	RN basic	More than 1 hr
Abuse Protection Support: Domestic Partner	6403	RN basic	More than 1 hr
Abuse Protection Support: Elder	6404	RN basic	More than 1 hr
Abuse Protection Support: Religious	6408	RN basic	More than 1 hr
Acid-Base Management	1910	RN basic	More than 1 hr
Acid-Base Management: Metabolic Acidosis	1911	RN basic	31-45 min
Acid-Base Management: Metabolic Alkalosis	1912	RN basic	31-45 min
Acid-Base Management: Respiratory Acidosis	1913	RN basic	31-45 min
Acid-Base Management: Respiratory Alkalosis	1914	RN basic	31-45 min
Acid-Base Monitoring	1920	RN basic	15 min or less
Active Listening	4920	RN basic	16-30 min
Activity Therapy	4310	RN basic	46-60 min
Acupressure	1320	RN post basic	16-30 min
Admission Care	7310	RN basic	16-30 min
Airway Insertion and Stabilization	3120	RN basic	16-30 min
Airway Management	3140	RN basic	16-30 min
Airway Suctioning	3160	RN basic	15 min or less
Allergy Management	6410	RN basic	31-45 min
Amnioinfusion	6700	RN post basic	31-45 min
Amputation Care	3420	RN basic	31-45 min
Analgesic Administration	2210	RN basic	16-30 min
Analgesic Administration: Intraspinal	2214	RN post basic	16-30 min
Anaphylaxis Management	6412	RN basic	46-60 min
Anesthesia Administration	2840	RN post basic	More than 1 hr
Anger Control Assistance	4640	RN post basic	16-30 min
Animal-Assisted Therapy	4320	Nursing assistant	16-30 min
Anticipatory Guidance	5210	RN basic	31-45 min
Anxiety Reduction	5820	Nursing assistant	31-45 min
Area Restriction	6420	Nursing assistant	More than 1 hr
Aromatherapy	1330	RN basic	15 min or less
Art Therapy	4330	RN post basic	46-60 min
Artificial Airway Management	3180	RN basic	15 min or less
Aspiration Precautions	3200	Nursing assistant	15 min or less
Assertiveness Training	4340	RN basic	46-60 min
Asthma Management	3210	RN basic	16-30 min
Attachment Promotion	6710	RN basic	More than 1 hr
Autogenic Training	5840	RN post basic	46-60 min
Autotransfusion	2860	RN basic	46-60 min
Bathing	1610	Nursing assistant	16-30 min
Bed Rest Care	0740	Nursing assistant	16-30 min
Bedside Laboratory Testing	7610	Nursing assistant	15 min or less
Behavior Management	4350	RN basic	46-60 min
Behavior Management: Overactivity/Inattention	4352	RN basic	31-45 min
Behavior Management: Self-Harm	4354	RN basic	31-45 min
Behavior Management: Sexual	4356	RN basic	31-45 min
Behavior Modification	4360	RN basic	More than 1 hr
Behavior Modification: Social Skills	4362	RN basic	More than 1 hr
Bibliotherapy	4680	RN post basic	46-60 min
Biofeedback	5860	RN post basic	46-60 min
Bioterrorism Preparedness	8810	RN post basic	More than 1 hr
Birthing	6720	RN post basic	More than 1 hr
Bladder Irrigation	0550	RN basic	16-30 min
Bleeding Precautions	4010	RN basic	31-45 min

Continued

| Table 1 | TIME & EDUCATION FOR 554 NIC INTERVENTIONS LISTED ALPHABETICALLY—CONT'D | | |

Intervention	Code No.	Educational Level	Time Required
Bleeding Reduction	4020	RN basic	46-60 min
Bleeding Reduction: Antepartum Uterus	4021	RN basic	46-60 min
Bleeding Reduction: Gastrointestinal	4022	RN basic	46-60 min
Bleeding Reduction: Nasal	4024	RN basic	16-30 min
Bleeding Reduction: Postpartum Uterus	4026	RN basic	46-60 min
Bleeding Reduction: Wound	4028	RN basic	46-60 min
Blood Products Administration	4030	RN basic	More than 1 hr
Body Image Enhancement	5220	RN basic	31-45 min
Body Mechanics Promotion	0140	RN basic	16-30 min
Bottle Feeding	1052	Nursing assistant	31-45 min
Bowel Incontinence Care	0410	RN basic	16-30 min
Bowel Incontinence Care: Encopresis	0412	RN basic	16-30 min
Bowel Management	0430	RN basic	31-45 min
Bowel Training	0440	RN basic	16-30 min
Breast Examination	6522	RN basic	15 min or less
Calming Technique	5880	Nursing assistant	31-45 min
Capillary Blood Sample	4035	RN basic	15 min or less
Cardiac Care	4040	RN basic	31-45 min
Cardiac Care: Acute	4044	RN basic	31-45 min
Cardiac Care: Rehabilitative	4046	RN basic	More than 1 hr
Cardiac Risk Management	4050	RN basic	31-45 min
Caregiver Support	7040	RN basic	More than 1 hr
Case Management	7320	RN post basic	More than 1 hr
Cast Care: Maintenance	0762	Nursing assistant	15 min or less
Cast Care: Wet	0764	RN basic	16-30 min
Central Venous Access Device Management	4054	RN post basic	31-45 min
Cerebral Edema Management	2540	RN basic	More than 1 hr
Cerebral Perfusion Promotion	2550	RN basic	31-45 min
Cesarean Birth Care	6750	RN basic	31-45 min
Chemical Restraint	6430	RN basic	15 min or less
Chemotherapy Management	2240	RN post basic	46-60 min
Chest Physiotherapy	3230	RN basic	16-30 min
Childbirth Preparation	6760	RN basic	More than 1 hr
Circulatory Care: Arterial Insufficiency	4062	RN basic	15 min or less
Circulatory Care: Mechanical Assist Device	4064	RN basic	31-45 min
Circulatory Care: Venous Insufficiency	4066	RN basic	15 min or less
Circulatory Precautions	4070	RN basic	16-30 min
Circumcision Care	3000	RN basic	46-60 min
Code Management	6140	RN basic	31-45 min
Cognitive Restructuring	4700	RN post basic	16-30 min
Cognitive Stimulation	4720	RN post basic	16-30 min
Commendation	4364	Nursing assistant	15 min or less
Communicable Disease Management	8820	RN basic	46-60 min
Communication Enhancement: Hearing Deficit	4974	Nursing assistant	16-30 min
Communication Enhancement: Speech Deficit	4976	RN basic	31-45 min
Communication Enhancement: Visual Deficit	4978	Nursing assistant	16-30 min
Community Disaster Preparedness	8840	RN basic	More than 1 hr
Community Health Development	8500	RN basic	More than 1 hr
Complex Relationship Building	5000	RN basic	More than 1 hr
Conflict Mediation	5020	RN post basic	46-60 min
Constipation/Impaction Management	0450	RN basic	16-30 min
Consultation	7910	RN basic	46-60 min
Contact Lens Care	1620	Nursing assistant	15 min or less
Controlled Substance Checking	7620	RN basic	15 min or less

Table 1	TIME & EDUCATION FOR 554 NIC INTERVENTIONS LISTED ALPHABETICALLY—CONT'D		
Intervention	**Code No.**	**Educational Level**	**Time Required**
Coping Enhancement	5230	RN basic	31-45 min
Cost Containment	7630	RN basic	31-45 min
Cough Enhancement	3250	Nursing assistant	15 min or less
Counseling	5240	RN post basic	46-60 min
Crisis Intervention	6160	RN post basic	46-60 min
Critical Path Development	7640	RN basic	More than 1 hr
Culture Brokerage	7330	RN basic	16-30 min
Cup Feeding: Newborn	8240	Nursing assistant	31-45 min
Cutaneous Stimulation	1340	RN basic	16-30 min
Decision-Making Support	5250	RN basic	16-30 min
Defibrillator Management: External	4095	RN basic	31-45 min
Defibrillator Management: Internal	4096	RN basic	31-45 min
Delegation	7650	RN basic	15 min or less
Delirium Management	6440	RN basic	More than 1 hr
Delusion Management	6450	RN basic	More than 1 hr
Dementia Management	6460	RN basic	More than 1 hr
Dementia Management: Bathing	6462	Nursing assistant	31-45 min
Dementia Management: Wandering	6466	Nursing assistant	More than 1 hr
Deposition/Testimony	7930	RN basic	More than 1 hr
Developmental Enhancement: Adolescent	8272	RN basic	46-60 min
Developmental Enhancement: Child	8274	RN basic	46-60 min
Developmental Enhancement: Infant	8278	RN basic	46-60 min
Dialysis Access Maintenance	4240	RN basic	15 min or less
Diarrhea Management	0460	RN basic	15 min or less
Diet Staging	1020	RN basic	15 min or less
Diet Staging: Weight Loss Surgery	1024	RN post basic	31-45 min
Discharge Planning	7370	RN basic	46-60 min
Distraction	5900	Nursing assistant	31-45 min
Documentation	7920	RN basic	15 min or less
Dressing	1630	Nursing assistant	15 min or less
Dry Eye Prevention	1350	RN basic	16-30 min
Dying Care	5260	RN basic	16-30 min
Dysreflexia Management	2560	RN basic	16-30 min
Dysrhythmia Management	4090	RN basic	16-30 min
Ear Care	1640	RN basic	16-30 min
Eating Disorders Management	1030	RN post basic	31-45 min
Electroconvulsive Therapy (ECT) Management	2570	RN basic	More than 1 hr
Electrolyte Management	2000	RN basic	31-45 min
Electrolyte Management: Hypercalcemia	2001	RN basic	16-30 min
Electrolyte Management: Hyperkalemia	2002	RN basic	16-30 min
Electrolyte Management: Hypermagnesemia	2003	RN basic	16-30 min
Electrolyte Management: Hypernatremia	2004	RN basic	16-30 min
Electrolyte Management: Hyperphosphatemia	2005	RN basic	16-30 min
Electrolyte Management: Hypocalcemia	2006	RN basic	16-30 min
Electrolyte Management: Hypokalemia	2007	RN basic	16-30 min
Electrolyte Management: Hypomagnesemia	2008	RN basic	16-30 min
Electrolyte Management: Hyponatremia	2009	RN basic	16-30 min
Electrolyte Management: Hypophosphatemia	2010	RN basic	16-30 min
Electrolyte Monitoring	2020	RN basic	15 min or less
Electronic Fetal Monitoring: Antepartum	6771	RN post basic	More than 1 hr
Electronic Fetal Monitoring: Intrapartum	6772	RN post basic	More than 1 hr
Elopement Precautions	6470	Nursing assistant	More than 1 hr
Embolus Care: Peripheral	4104	RN basic	16-30 min
Embolus Care: Pulmonary	4106	RN basic	16-30 min

Continued

| Table 1 | TIME & EDUCATION FOR 554 NIC INTERVENTIONS LISTED ALPHABETICALLY—CONT'D | | |

Intervention	Code No.	Educational Level	Time Required
Embolus Precautions	4110	RN basic	16-30 min
Emergency Care	6200	Nursing assistant	16-30 min
Emergency Cart Checking	7660	Nursing assistant	15 min or less
Emotional Support	5270	RN basic	16-30 min
Endotracheal Extubation	3270	RN basic	15 min or less
Enema Administration	0466	Nursing assistant	16-30 min
Energy Management	0180	RN basic	16-30 min
Enteral Tube Feeding	1056	RN basic	16-30 min
Environmental Management	6480	Nursing assistant	31-45 min
Environmental Management: Comfort	6482	Nursing assistant	15 min or less
Environmental Management: Community	6484	RN basic	More than 1 hr
Environmental Management: Home Preparation	6485	RN basic	More than 1 hr
Environmental Management: Safety	6486	RN basic	31-45 min
Environmental Management: Violence Prevention	6487	Nursing assistant	More than 1 hr
Environmental Management: Worker Safety	6489	RN basic	More than 1 hr
Environmental Risk Protection	8880	RN basic	46-60 min
Examination Assistance	7680	Nursing assistant	16-30 min
Exercise Promotion	0200	RN basic	31-45 min
Exercise Promotion: Strength Training	0201	RN basic	31-45 min
Exercise Promotion: Stretching	0202	RN basic	31-45 min
Exercise Therapy: Ambulation	0221	Nursing assistant	15 min or less
Exercise Therapy: Balance	0222	RN basic	16-30 min
Exercise Therapy: Joint Mobility	0224	RN basic	16-30 min
Exercise Therapy: Muscle Control	0226	RN post basic	16-30 min
Eye Care	1650	RN basic	15 min or less
Fall Prevention	6490	RN basic	More than 1 hr
Family Integrity Promotion	7100	RN basic	More than 1 hr
Family Integrity Promotion: Childbearing Family	7104	RN basic	More than 1 hr
Family Involvement Promotion	7110	RN basic	More than 1 hr
Family Mobilization	7120	RN basic	More than 1 hr
Family Planning: Contraception	6784	RN basic	31-45 min
Family Planning: Infertility	6786	RN post basic	46-60 min
Family Planning: Unplanned Pregnancy	6788	RN basic	46-60 min
Family Presence Facilitation	7170	RN basic	More than 1 hr
Family Process Maintenance	7130	RN basic	More than 1 hr
Family Support	7140	RN basic	More than 1 hr
Family Therapy	7150	RN post basic	More than 1 hr
Feeding	1050	Nursing assistant	16-30 min
Fertility Preservation	7160	RN post basic	31-45 min
Fever Treatment	3740	RN basic	16-30 min
Financial Resource Assistance	7380	RN basic	46-60 min
Fire-Setting Precautions	6500	Nursing assistant	More than 1 hr
First Aid	6240	Nursing assistant	16-30 min
Fiscal Resource Management	8550	RN post basic	More than 1 hr
Flatulence Reduction	0470	RN basic	15 min or less
Fluid/Electrolyte Management	2080	RN basic	15 min or less
Fluid Management	4120	RN basic	31-45 min
Fluid Monitoring	4130	RN basic	16-30 min
Fluid Resuscitation	4140	RN basic	15 min or less
Foot Care	1660	RN basic	16-30 min
Forensic Data Collection	7940	RN post basic	More than 1 hr
Forgiveness Facilitation	5280	RN basic	16-30 min
Gastrointestinal Intubation	1080	RN basic	15 min or less
Genetic Counseling	5242	RN post basic	46-60 min

| Table 1 | TIME & EDUCATION FOR 554 NIC INTERVENTIONS LISTED ALPHABETICALLY—CONT'D |

Intervention	Code No.	Educational Level	Time Required
Grief Work Facilitation	5290	RN basic	31-45 min
Grief Work Facilitation: Perinatal Death	5294	RN basic	31-45 min
Guided Imagery	6000	RN basic	31-45 min
Guilt Work Facilitation	5300	RN basic	31-45 min
Hair and Scalp Care	1670	Nursing assistant	16-30 min
Hallucination Management	6510	RN basic	More than 1 hr
Healing Touch	1390	RN post basic	46-60 min
Health Care Information Exchange	7960	RN basic	15 min or less
Health Education	5510	RN basic	16-30 min
Health Literacy Enhancement	5515	RN basic	16-30 min
Health Policy Monitoring	7970	RN basic	More than 1 hr
Health Screening	6520	RN basic	46-60 min
Health System Guidance	7400	RN basic	16-30 min
Heat/Cold Application	1380	RN basic	15 min or less
Hemodialysis Therapy	2100	RN post basic	More than 1 hr
Hemodynamic Regulation	4150	RN basic	16-30 min
Hemofiltration Therapy	2110	RN basic	More than 1 hr
High-Risk Pregnancy Care	6800	RN post basic	More than 1 hr
Home Maintenance Assistance	7180	RN basic	31-45 min
Hope Inspiration	5310	RN basic	16-30 min
Hormone Replacement Therapy	2280	RN post basic	16-30 min
Humor	5320	Nursing assistant	15 min or less
Hyperglycemia Management	2120	RN basic	More than 1 hr
Hyperthermia Treatment	3786	RN basic	16-30 min
Hypervolemia Management	4170	RN basic	16-30 min
Hypnosis	5920	RN post basic	46-60 min
Hypoglycemia Management	2130	RN basic	More than 1 hr
Hypothermia Induction Therapy	3790	RN basic	More that 1 hr
Hypothermia Treatment	3800	RN basic	More than 1 hr
Hypovolemia Management	4180	RN basic	16-30 min
Immunization/Vaccination Management	6530	RN basic	16-30 min
Impulse Control Training	4370	RN post basic	More than 1 hr
Incident Reporting	7980	RN basic	16-30 min
Incision Site Care	3440	RN basic	31-45 min
Infant Care	6820	RN basic	More than 1 hr
Infant Care: Newborn	6824	RN basic	More than 1 hr
Infant Care: Preterm	6826	RN post basic	More than 1 hr
Infection Control	6540	RN basic	31-45 min
Infection Control: Intraoperative	6545	RN basic	More than 1 hr
Infection Protection	6550	RN basic	31-45 min
Insurance Authorization	7410	RN basic	16-30 min
Intracranial Pressure (ICP) Monitoring	2590	RN basic	More than 1 hr
Intrapartal Care	6830	RN basic	More than 1 hr
Intrapartal Care: High-Risk Delivery	6834	RN post basic	More than 1 hr
Intravenous (IV) Insertion	4190	RN basic	15 min or less
Intravenous (IV) Therapy	4200	RN basic	15 min or less
Invasive Hemodynamic Monitoring	4210	RN basic	46-60 min
Journaling	4740	RN basic	46-60 min
Kangaroo Care	6840	RN basic	46-60 min
Labor Induction	6850	RN post basic	More than 1 hr
Labor Suppression	6860	RN post basic	More than 1 hr
Laboratory Data Interpretation	7690	RN basic	15 min or less
Lactation Counseling	5244	RN basic	31-45 min
Lactation Suppression	6870	RN basic	16-30 min

Continued

| Table 1 | TIME & EDUCATION FOR 554 NIC INTERVENTIONS LISTED ALPHABETICALLY—CONT'D | | |

Intervention	Code No.	Educational Level	Time Required
Laser Precautions	6560	RN post basic	31-45 min
Latex Precautions	6570	RN basic	31-45 min
Learning Facilitation	5520	RN basic	16-30 min
Learning Readiness Enhancement	5540	RN basic	15 min or less
Leech Therapy	3460	RN basic	46-60 min
Life Skills Enhancement	5326	RN post basic	46-60 min
Limit Setting	4380	RN basic	16-30 min
Listening Visits	5328	RN basic	46-60 min
Lower Extremity Monitoring	3480	RN basic	15 min or less
Malignant Hyperthermia Precautions	3840	RN basic	More than 1 hr
Massage	1480	RN basic	15 min or less
Mechanical Ventilation Management: Invasive	3300	RN basic	More than 1 hr
Mechanical Ventilation Management: Noninvasive	3302	RN basic	More than 1 hr
Mechanical Ventilation Management: Pneumonia Prevention	3304	RN basic	More than 1 hr
Mechanical Ventilatory Weaning	3310	RN basic	More than 1 hr
Medication Administration	2300	RN basic	15 min or less
Medication Administration: Ear	2308	Nursing assistant	15 min or less
Medication Administration: Enteral	2301	Nursing assistant	15 min or less
Medication Administration: Eye	2310	Nursing assistant	15 min or less
Medication Administration: Inhalation	2311	Nursing assistant	15 min or less
Medication Administration: Interpleural	2302	RN post basic	15 min or less
Medication Administration: Intradermal	2312	RN basic	15 min or less
Medication Administration: Intramuscular (IM)	2313	RN basic	15 min or less
Medication Administration: Intraosseous	2303	RN post basic	15 min or less
Medication Administration: Intraspinal	2319	RN basic	15 min or less
Medication Administration: Intravenous (IV)	2314	RN basic	15 min or less
Medication Administration: Nasal	2320	Nursing assistant	15 min or less
Medication Administration: Oral	2304	Nursing assistant	15 min or less
Medication Administration: Rectal	2315	Nursing assistant	15 min or less
Medication Administration: Skin	2316	Nursing assistant	15 min or less
Medication Administration: Subcutaneous	2317	RN basic	15 min or less
Medication Administration: Vaginal	2318	Nursing assistant	15 min or less
Medication Administration: Ventricular Reservoir	2307	RN post basic	15 min or less
Medication Management	2380	RN basic	16-30 min
Medication Prescribing	2390	RN post basic	15 min or less
Medication Reconciliation	2395	RN basic	16-30 min
Meditation Facilitation	5960	RN basic	16-30 min
Memory Training	4760	RN post basic	31-45 min
Milieu Therapy	4390	RN basic	More than 1 hr
Mood Management	5330	RN basic	31-45 min
Multidisciplinary Care Conference	8020	RN basic	More than 1 hr
Music Therapy	4400	RN basic	15 min or less
Mutual Goal Setting	4410	RN basic	46-60 min
Nail Care	1680	Nursing assistant	16-30 min
Nasal Irrigation	3316	RN basic	15 min or less
Nausea Management	1450	RN basic	16-30 min
Neurologic Monitoring	2620	RN basic	16-30 min
Nonnutritive Sucking	6900	Nursing assistant	16-30 min
Normalization Promotion	7200	RN basic	More than 1 hr
Nutrition Management	1100	RN post basic	31-45 min
Nutrition Therapy	1120	RN basic	16-30 min
Nutritional Counseling	5246	RN basic	16-30 min
Nutritional Monitoring	1160	RN basic	15 min or less
Oral Health Maintenance	1710	RN basic	15 min or less

Table 1	TIME & EDUCATION FOR 554 NIC INTERVENTIONS LISTED ALPHABETICALLY—CONT'D		
Intervention	**Code No.**	**Educational Level**	**Time Required**
Oral Health Promotion	1720	RN basic	15 min or less
Oral Health Restoration	1730	RN basic	15 min or less
Order Transcription	8060	RN basic	15 min or less
Organ Procurement	6260	RN basic	46-60 min
Ostomy Care	0480	RN post basic	16-30 min
Oxygen Therapy	3320	RN basic	15 min or less
Pacemaker Management: Permanent	4091	RN basic	31-45 min
Pacemaker Management: Temporary	4092	RN basic	31-45 min
Pain Management	1400	RN basic	More than 1 hr
Parent Education: Adolescent	5562	RN basic	16-30 min
Parent Education: Childrearing Family	5566	RN basic	16-30 min
Parent Education: Infant	5568	RN basic	31-45 min
Parenting Promotion	8300	RN basic	31-45 min
Pass Facilitation	7440	RN basic	15 min or less
Patient Contracting	4420	RN basic	46-60 min
Patient-Controlled Analgesia (PCA) Assistance	2400	RN basic	16-30 min
Patient Identification	6574	RN basic	15 min or less
Patient Rights Protection	7460	Nursing assistant	15 min or less
Peer Review	7700	RN basic	More than 1 hr
Pelvic Muscle Exercise	0560	RN post basic	16-30 min
Perineal Care	1750	Nursing assistant	15 min or less
Peripheral Sensation Management	2660	RN basic	15 min or less
Peripherally Inserted Central Catheter (PICC) Care	4220	RN post basic	16-30 min
Peritoneal Dialysis Therapy	2150	RN basic	More than 1 hr
Pessary Management	0630	RN basic	16-30 min
Phlebotomy: Arterial Blood Sample	4232	RN basic	15 min or less
Phlebotomy: Blood Unit Acquisition	4234	RN basic	More than 1 hr
Phlebotomy: Cannulated Vessel	4235	RN basic	15 min or less
Phlebotomy: Venous Blood Sample	4238	RN basic	15 min or less
Phototherapy: Mood/Sleep Regulation	6926	RN basic	31-45 min
Phototherapy: Neonate	6924	RN basic	More than 1 hr
Physical Restraint	6580	RN basic	15 min or less
Physician Support	7710	RN basic	16-30 min
Pneumatic Tourniquet Precautions	6590	RN post basic	More than 1 hr
Positioning	0840	Nursing assistant	16-30 min
Positioning: Intraoperative	0842	RN basic	16-30 min
Positioning: Neurologic	0844	Nursing assistant	16-30 min
Positioning: Wheelchair	0846	RN basic	15 min or less
Postanesthesia Care	2870	RN basic	46-60 min
Postmortem Care	1770	Nursing assistant	16-30 min
Postpartal Care	6930	RN basic	More than 1 hr
Preceptor: Employee	7722	RN basic	More than 1 hr
Preceptor: Student	7726	RN basic	More than 1 hr
Preconception Counseling	5247	RN post basic	More than 1 hr
Pregnancy Termination Care	6950	RN post basic	More than 1 hr
Premenstrual Syndrome (PMS) Management	1440	RN post basic	16-30 min
Prenatal Care	6960	RN basic	More than 1 hr
Preoperative Coordination	2880	RN basic	31-45 min
Preparatory Sensory Information	5580	RN basic	31-45 min
Prescribing: Diagnostic Testing	8080	RN post basic	16-30 min
Prescribing: Non-Pharmacologic Treatment	8086	RN post basic	16-30 min
Presence	5340	Nursing assistant	16-30 min
Pressure Management	3500	RN basic	16-30 min
Pressure Ulcer Care	3520	Nursing assistant	16-30 min

Continued

Table 1	**TIME & EDUCATION FOR 554 NIC INTERVENTIONS LISTED ALPHABETICALLY—CONT'D**		

Intervention	Code No.	Educational Level	Time Required
Pressure Ulcer Prevention	3540	RN basic	16-30 min
Product Evaluation	7760	RN basic	More than 1 hr
Program Development	8700	RN post basic	More than 1 hr
Progressive Muscle Relaxation	1460	RN post basic	16-30 min
Prompted Voiding	0640	Nursing assistant	15 min or less
Pruritus Management	3550	RN basic	16-30 min
Quality Monitoring	7800	RN basic	More than 1 hr
Radiation Therapy Management	6600	RN basic	46-60 min
Rape-Trauma Treatment	6300	RN basic	More than 1 hr
Reality Orientation	4820	Nursing assistant	15 min or less
Recreation Therapy	5360	Nursing assistant	16-30 min
Rectal Prolapse Management	0490	RN post basic	16-30 min
Referral	8100	RN basic	16-30 min
Reiki	1520	RN post basic	46-60 min
Relaxation Therapy	6040	RN basic	31-45 min
Religious Addiction Prevention	5422	RN basic	46-60 min
Religious Ritual Enhancement	5424	RN basic	31-45 min
Relocation Stress Reduction	5350	RN basic	16-30 min
Reminiscence Therapy	4860	RN post basic	46-60 min
Reproductive Technology Management	7886	RN post basic	More than 1 hr
Research Data Collection	8120	RN basic	16-30 min
Resiliency Promotion	8340	RN basic	More than 1 hr
Respiratory Monitoring	3350	RN basic	15 min or less
Respite Care	7260	RN basic	More than 1 hr
Resuscitation	6320	RN basic	16-30 min
Resuscitation: Fetus	6972	RN post basic	More than 1 hr
Resuscitation: Neonate	6974	RN post basic	46-60 min
Risk Identification	6610	RN basic	46-60 min
Risk Identification: Childbearing Family	6612	RN basic	More than 1 hr
Risk Identification: Genetic	6614	RN post basic	More than 1 hr
Role Enhancement	5370	RN basic	16-30 min
Seclusion	6630	RN basic	More than 1 hr
Security Enhancement	5380	RN basic	16-30 min
Sedation Management	2260	RN post basic	More than 1 hr
Seizure Management	2680	RN basic	16-30 min
Seizure Precautions	2690	RN basic	15 min or less
Self-Awareness Enhancement	5390	RN basic	16-30 min
Self-Care Assistance	1800	Nursing assistant	16-30 min
Self-Care Assistance: Bathing/Hygiene	1801	Nursing assistant	15 min or less
Self-Care Assistance: Dressing/Grooming	1802	Nursing assistant	15 min or less
Self-Care Assistance: Feeding	1803	Nursing assistant	16-30 min
Self-Care Assistance: IADL	1805	RN basic	46-60 min
Self-Care Assistance: Toileting	1804	Nursing assistant	15 min or less
Self-Care Assistance: Transfer	1806	Nursing assistant	15 min or less
Self-Efficacy Enhancement	5395	RN basic	31-45 min
Self-Esteem Enhancement	5400	RN basic	16-30 min
Self-Hypnosis Facilitation	5922	RN post basic	46-60 min
Self-Modification Assistance	4470	RN basic	46-60 min
Self-Responsibility Facilitation	4480	RN basic	46-60 min
Sexual Counseling	5248	RN post basic	46-60 min
Shift Report	8140	RN basic	31-45 min
Shock Management	4250	RN basic	16-30 min
Shock Management: Cardiac	4254	RN basic	16-30 min
Shock Management: Vasogenic	4256	RN basic	31-45 min

Table 1	TIME & EDUCATION FOR 554 NIC INTERVENTIONS LISTED ALPHABETICALLY—CONT'D		
Intervention	**Code No.**	**Educational Level**	**Time Required**
Shock Management: Volume	4258	RN basic	31-45 min
Shock Prevention	4260	RN basic	16-30 min
Sibling Support	7280	RN basic	16-30 min
Skin Care: Donor Site	3582	RN basic	16-30 min
Skin Care: Graft Site	3583	RN basic	16-30 min
Skin Care: Topical Treatments	3584	RN basic	16-30 min
Skin Surveillance	3590	RN basic	16-30 min
Sleep Enhancement	1850	RN basic	16-30 min
Smoking Cessation Assistance	4490	RN basic	46-60 min
Social Marketing	8750	RN post basic	More than 1 hr
Socialization Enhancement	5100	RN basic	31-45 min
Specimen Management	7820	Nursing assistant	15 min or less
Spiritual Growth Facilitation	5426	RN basic	31-45 min
Spiritual Support	5420	RN basic	16-30 min
Splinting	0910	RN basic	15 min or less
Sports-Injury Prevention: Youth	6648	RN basic	46-60 min
Staff Development	7850	RN basic	More than 1 hr
Staff Supervision	7830	RN basic	More than 1 hr
Stem Cell Infusion	4266	RN post basic	More than 1 hr
Subarachnoid Hemorrhage Precautions	2720	RN basic	15 min or less
Substance Use Prevention	4500	RN basic	46-60 min
Substance Use Treatment	4510	RN basic	46-60 min
Substance Use Treatment: Alcohol Withdrawal	4512	RN post basic	More than 1 hr
Substance Use Treatment: Drug Withdrawal	4514	RN post basic	More than 1 hr
Substance Use Treatment: Overdose	4516	RN post basic	More than 1 hr
Suicide Prevention	6340	RN basic	More than 1 hr
Supply Management	7840	Nursing assistant	16-30 min
Support Group	5430	RN post basic	46-60 min
Support System Enhancement	5440	RN basic	31-45 min
Surgical Assistance	2900	RN basic	More than 1 hr
Surgical Instrumentation Management	2910	RN basic	More than 1 hr
Surgical Precautions	2920	RN basic	More than 1 hr
Surgical Preparation	2930	RN basic	46-60 min
Surveillance	6650	RN basic	More than 1 hr
Surveillance: Community	6652	RN basic	More than 1 hr
Surveillance: Late Pregnancy	6656	RN post basic	More than 1 hr
Surveillance: Remote Electronic	6658	RN basic	31-45 min
Sustenance Support	7500	RN basic	31-45 min
Suturing	3620	RN basic	16-30 min
Swallowing Therapy	1860	RN basic	31-45 min
Teaching: Disease Process	5602	RN basic	16-30 min
Teaching: Foot Care	5603	RN basic	16-30 min
Teaching: Group	5604	RN basic	More than 1 hr
Teaching: Individual	5606	RN basic	31-45 min
Teaching: Infant Nutrition 0-3 Months	5640	RN basic	16-30 min
Teaching: Infant Nutrition 4-6 Months	5641	RN basic	16-30 min
Teaching: Infant Nutrition 7-9 Months	5642	RN basic	16-30 min
Teaching: Infant Nutrition 10-12 Months	5643	RN basic	16-30 min
Teaching: Infant Safety 0-3 Months	5645	RN basic	16-30 min
Teaching: Infant Safety 4-6 Months	5646	RN basic	16-30 min
Teaching: Infant Safety 7-9 Months	5647	RN basic	16-30 min
Teaching: Infant Safety 10-12 Months	5648	RN basic	16-30 min
Teaching: Infant Stimulation 0-4 Months	5655	RN basic	16-30 min
Teaching: Infant Stimulation 5-8 Months	5656	RN basic	16-30 min

Continued

| Table 1 | TIME & EDUCATION FOR 554 NIC INTERVENTIONS LISTED ALPHABETICALLY—CONT'D | | |

Intervention	Code No.	Educational Level	Time Required
Teaching: Infant Stimulation 9-12 Months	5657	RN basic	16-30 min
Teaching: Preoperative	5610	RN basic	16-30 min
Teaching: Prescribed Diet	5614	RN basic	16-30 min
Teaching: Prescribed Exercise	5612	RN basic	16-30 min
Teaching: Prescribed Medication	5616	RN basic	16-30 min
Teaching: Procedure/Treatment	5618	RN basic	16-30 min
Teaching: Psychomotor Skill	5620	RN basic	16-30 min
Teaching: Safe Sex	5622	RN basic	16-30 min
Teaching: Sexuality	5624	RN basic	16-30 min
Teaching: Toddler Nutrition 13-18 Months	5660	RN basic	16-30 min
Teaching: Toddler Nutrition 19-24 Months	5661	RN basic	16-30 min
Teaching: Toddler Nutrition 25-36 Months	5662	RN basic	16-30 min
Teaching: Toddler Safety 13-18 Months	5665	RN basic	16-30 min
Teaching: Toddler Safety 19-24 Months	5666	RN basic	16-30 min
Teaching: Toddler Safety 25-36 Months	5667	RN basic	16-30 min
Teaching: Toilet Training	5634	RN basic	16-30 min
Technology Management	7880	RN basic	15 min or less
Telephone Consultation	8180	RN basic	16-30 min
Telephone Follow-Up	8190	RN basic	15 min or less
Temperature Regulation	3900	RN basic	31-45 min
Temperature Regulation: Perioperative	3902	RN basic	More than 1 hr
Therapeutic Play	4430	RN basic	46-60 min
Therapeutic Touch	5465	RN post basic	46-60 min
Therapy Group	5450	RN post basic	46-60 min
Thrombolytic Therapy Management	4270	RN basic	More than 1 hr
Total Parenteral Nutrition (TPN) Administration	1200	RN basic	16-30 min
Touch	5460	Nursing assistant	15 min or less
Traction/Immobilization Care	0940	RN basic	15 min or less
Transcutaneous Electrical Nerve Stimulation (TENS)	1540	RN post basic	16-30 min
Transfer	0970	Nursing assistant	15 min or less
Transport: Interfacility	7890	RN basic	16-30 min
Transport: Intrafacility	7892	RN basic	31-45 min
Trauma Therapy: Child	5410	RN post basic	46-60 min
Triage: Disaster	6362	RN basic	15 min or less
Triage: Emergency Center	6364	RN basic	15 min or less
Triage: Telephone	6366	RN basic	15 min or less
Truth Telling	5470	RN basic	16-30 min
Tube Care	1870	Nursing assistant	15 min or less
Tube Care: Chest	1872	RN basic	15 min or less
Tube Care: Gastrointestinal	1874	RN basic	15 min or less
Tube Care: Umbilical Line	1875	RN post basic	46-60 min
Tube Care: Urinary	1876	Nursing assistant	15 min or less
Tube Care: Ventriculostomy/Lumbar Drain	1878	RN basic	15 min or less
Ultrasonography: Limited Obstetric	6982	RN post basic	31-45 min
Unilateral Neglect Management	2760	RN basic	31-45 min
Urinary Bladder Training	0570	RN post basic	16-30 min
Urinary Catheterization	0580	Nursing assistant	15 min or less
Urinary Catheterization: Intermittent	0582	Nursing assistant	15 min or less
Urinary Elimination Management	0590	RN post basic	31-45 min
Urinary Habit Training	0600	RN post basic	31-45 min
Urinary Incontinence Care	0610	RN basic	31-45 min
Urinary Incontinence Care: Enuresis	0612	RN basic	16-30 min
Urinary Retention Care	0620	RN basic	15 min or less
Validation Therapy	6670	RN post basic	46-60 min

| Table 1 | TIME & EDUCATION FOR 554 NIC INTERVENTIONS LISTED ALPHABETICALLY—CONT'D | | |

Intervention	Code No.	Educational Level	Time Required
Values Clarification	5480	RN basic	16-30 min
Vehicle Safety Promotion	9050	RN basic	More than 1 hr
Ventilation Assistance	3390	RN basic	15 min or less
Visitation Facilitation	7560	Nursing assistant	15 min or less
Vital Signs Monitoring	6680	RN basic	15 min or less
Vomiting Management	1570	RN basic	16-30 min
Weight Gain Assistance	1240	RN basic	16-30 min
Weight Management	1260	RN basic	31-45 min
Weight Reduction Assistance	1280	RN basic	16-30 min
Wound Care	3660	RN basic	31-45 min
Wound Care: Burns	3661	RN basic	More than 1 hr
Wound Care: Closed Drainage	3662	RN basic	31-45 min
Wound Care: Nonhealing	3664	RN basic	31-45 min
Wound Irrigation	3680	RN basic	31-45 min

PART SIX

NIC Interventions Linked to NANDA-I Diagnoses

INTRODUCTION TO LINKAGES WITH NANDA-I

This section of the book provides linkages between NANDA-I diagnoses and the Nursing Interventions Classification (NIC) interventions. The 554 NIC interventions included in this edition are linked to the NANDA-I 2012-2014 edition.[1] A *linkage* is defined as a relationship or association between a nursing diagnosis and a nursing intervention that causes them to occur together in order to obtain an outcome or the resolution of a patient's problem. Linkages facilitate the diagnostic reasoning and clinical decision-making of the nurse by identifying nursing interventions that are treatment options for resolution of a nursing diagnosis. They can also assist those who are designing clinical nursing information systems to structure their databases.

The included lists of nursing interventions for each nursing diagnosis are comprehensive, including multiple interventions. The following three levels of interventions are provided for each diagnosis:

1st level: Priority Interventions: These are the most likely/ most obvious intervention(s) to resolve the diagnosis and are in color in the listing of suggested interventions. They were selected because of a good match with the diagnosis' etiology and/or the defining characteristics, have more activities that will resolve the problem, can be used in more settings and are better known from research and clinical use to address the diagnosis.

2nd level: Suggested Interventions: These are interventions that are likely to address the diagnosis but not as likely as the priority interventions for the majority of patients with the diagnosis. These are sometimes mentioned in the literature as addressing the diagnosis, but are not mentioned as often and they may address only selected etiologies or characteristics.

3rd level: Additional Optional: These are interventions that apply only to some patients with the diagnosis, allowing a nurse to further tailor the plan of care to the individual.

The listing of three levels of interventions provides a comprehensive list of interventions for each diagnosis. The list assists the nurse in the selection of interventions, but is not prescriptive. The nurse uses clinical reasoning and judgment

with each individual patient, family, or group to determine the appropriate choice of interventions.

The following steps are suggested when using the linkage list:

1. Review the priority nursing interventions for first consideration as the treatment of choice for resolution of a nursing diagnosis.
2. Review other interventions in the suggested list because these are considered most essential for resolution of the diagnosis.
3. Review the additional suggestions for interventions that may also be used for resolution of the nursing diagnosis.

The second edition of NIC described in detail the methods that were initially used to develop this linkage list. For subsequent editions, the previous linkages were updated by the editors, who added the new diagnoses and interventions and their appropriate linkages. We also included some feedback from users who indicated some additions and deletions.

NANDA-I and the NIC linkages have been incorporated into the NNN linkage work by the Iowa group to link the NANDA-I, NOC, and NIC Classifications. This work has produced a book, now in the third edition.[2,3,4] The provision of links among the three Classifications will facilitate the use of standardized languages in clinical practice and documentation systems, as well as in education.

References

1. *Nursing Diagnoses—Definitions and Classification 2012-2014.* Copyright © 2012, 1994-2012 by NANDA International. Used by arrangement with Blackwell Publishing Limited, a company of John Wiley and Sons, Inc.
2. Johnson, M., Bulechek, G., Butcher, H., Dochterman, J., Maas, M., Moorhead, S., & Swanson, E. (2006). *NANDA, NOC, and NIC Linkages: Nursing diagnoses, outcomes, & interventions.* St. Louis, MO: Mosby.
3. Johnson, M., Bulechek, G., Dochterman, J. M., Maas, M., & Moorhead, S. (2001). *Nursing diagnoses, outcomes, and interventions: NANDA, NOC, and NIC linkages.* St. Louis, MO: Mosby.
4. Johnson, M., Moorhead, S. Bulechek, G., Butcher, H., Dochterman, J., Maas, M., & Swanson, E. (2012). *NOC, and NIC Linkages to NANDA-I and clinical conditions: Supporting critical reasoning and quality care.* Maryland Heights, MO: Mosby.

Activity Intolerance

Definition: Insufficient physiological or psychological energy to endure or complete required or desired daily activities

Suggested Nursing Interventions for Problem Resolution:
Activity Therapy
Body Mechanics Promotion
Cardiac Care: Rehabilitative
Energy Management
Environmental Management
Exercise Promotion: Strength Training
Home Maintenance Assistance
Mood Management
Self-Care Assistance
Self-Care Assistance: IADL
Self-Care Assistance: Transfer
Sleep Enhancement
Teaching: Prescribed Exercise

Additional Optional Interventions:
Animal-Assisted Therapy
Dysrhythmia Management
Environmental Management: Comfort

Exercise Promotion
Exercise Promotion: Stretching
Exercise Therapy: Ambulation
Exercise Therapy: Balance
Exercise Therapy: Joint Mobility
Exercise Therapy: Muscle Control
Family Involvement Promotion
Medication Management
Meditation Facilitation
Music Therapy
Mutual Goal Setting
Nutrition Management
Oxygen Therapy
Pain Management
Progressive Muscle Relaxation
Smoking Cessation Assistance
Spiritual Support
Visitation Facilitation
Weight Management

Activity Intolerance, Risk for

Definition: At risk for experiencing insufficient physiological or psychological energy to endure or complete required or desired daily activities

Suggested Nursing Interventions for Problem Resolution:
Asthma Management
Cardiac Care: Rehabilitative
Cardiac Risk Management
Energy Management
Exercise Promotion
Exercise Promotion: Strength Training
Exercise Promotion: Stretching
Exercise Therapy: Ambulation
Exercise Therapy: Balance
Exercise Therapy: Joint Mobility
Exercise Therapy: Muscle Control
Nutrition Management
Oxygen Therapy
Pacemaker Management: Permanent
Pain Management
Respiratory Monitoring

Risk Identification
Self-Care Assistance: IADL
Sleep Enhancement
Teaching: Prescribed Exercise

Additional Optional Interventions:
Family Mobilization
Hope Inspiration
Medication Management
Mutual Goal Setting
Positioning
Security Enhancement
Self-Esteem Enhancement
Smoking Cessation Assistance
Surveillance
Vital Signs Monitoring
Weight Management

Activity Planning, Ineffective

Definition: Inability to prepare for a set of actions fixed in time and under certain conditions

Suggested Nursing Interventions for Problem Resolution:
Anxiety Reduction
Calming Technique
Coping Enhancement
Decision-Making Support
Life Skills Enhancement
Mutual Goal Setting
Self-Efficacy Enhancement
Self-Responsibility Facilitation

Additional Optional Interventions:
Behavior Modification
Family Involvement Promotion

Financial Resource Assistance
Guided Imagery
Learning Facilitation
Relaxation Therapy
Security Enhancement
Support System Enhancement
Teaching: Individual
Values Clarification

Activity Planning, Risk for Ineffective

Definition: At risk for an inability to prepare for a set of actions fixed in time and under certain conditions

Suggested Nursing Interventions for Problem Resolution:
Activity Therapy
Anticipatory Guidance
Behavior Management
Decision-Making Support
Learning Facilitation
Life Skills Enhancement
Risk Identification
Self-Efficacy Enhancement
Self-Responsibility Facilitation
Support System Enhancement

Additional Associated Outcomes:
Anxiety Reduction
Coping Enhancement
Impulse Control Training
Self-Awareness Enhancement
Self-Esteem Enhancement
Values Clarification

Adverse Reaction to Iodinated Contrast Media, Risk for

Definition: At risk for any noxious or unintended reaction associated with the use of iodinated contrast media that can occur within seven (7) days after contrast agent injection

Suggested Nursing Interventions for Problem Resolution:
Allergy Management
Anxiety Reduction
Fluid Management
Medication Management
Respiratory Monitoring
Risk Identification
Surveillance

Teaching: Prescribed Medication
Vital Signs Monitoring

Additional Associated Outcomes:
Airway Management
Anaphylaxis Management
Environmental Management
Ventilation Assistance

Airway Clearance, Ineffective

Definition: Inability to clear secretions or obstructions from the respiratory tract to maintain a clear airway

Suggested Nursing Interventions for Problem Resolution:
Airway Insertion and Stabilization
Airway Management
Airway Suctioning
Anxiety Reduction
Artificial Airway Management
Aspiration Precautions
Asthma Management
Chest Physiotherapy
Cough Enhancement
Mechanical Ventilation Management: Invasive
Mechanical Ventilation Management: Noninvasive
Mechanical Ventilatory Weaning
Medication Administration: Inhalation
Oxygen Therapy
Positioning
Respiratory Monitoring
Resuscitation: Neonate
Surveillance
Ventilation Assistance
Vital Signs Monitoring

Additional Optional Interventions:
Acid-Base Management
Acid-Base Management: Respiratory Acidosis
Acid-Base Management: Respiratory Alkalosis
Allergy Management
Anaphylaxis Management
Calming Technique
Dysrhythmia Management
Emergency Care
Emotional Support
Endotracheal Extubation
Energy Management
Fluid Management
Fluid Monitoring
Infection Control
Infection Protection
Intravenous (IV) Insertion
Intravenous (IV) Therapy
Phlebotomy: Arterial Blood Sample
Smoking Cessation Assistance
Tube Care: Chest

Allergy Response, Risk for

Definition: Risk of an exaggerated immune response or reaction to substances

Suggested Nursing Interventions for Problem Resolution:
Allergy Management
Asthma Management
Medication Administration
Medication Administration: Intradermal
Medication Administration: Nasal
Medication Administration: Oral
Medication Administration: Skin
Medication Management
Nutrition Management
Respiratory Monitoring
Risk Identification

Surveillance
Teaching: Prescribed Diet
Teaching: Prescribed Medication
Vital Signs Monitoring

Additional Optional Interventions:
Airway Management
Anaphylaxis Management
Environmental Management
Immunization/Vaccination Management
Ventilation Assistance

Anxiety

Definition: Vague uneasy feeling of discomfort or dread accompanied by an autonomic response (the source is often nonspecific or unknown to the individual); a feeling of apprehension caused by anticipation of danger. It is an alerting signal that warns of impending danger and enables the individual to take measures to deal with a threat

Suggested Nursing Interventions for Problem Resolution:
Anticipatory Guidance
Anxiety Reduction
Calming Technique
Coping Enhancement
Dementia Management
Dementia Management: Bathing
Dementia Management: Wandering

Examination Assistance
Presence
Relaxation Therapy
Relocation Stress Reduction
Security Enhancement
Substance Use Treatment
Validation Therapy

Additional Optional Interventions:
Allergy Management
Anger Control Assistance
Animal-Assisted Therapy
Art Therapy
Asthma Management
Autogenic Training
Behavior Management: Self-Harm
Biofeedback
Childbirth Preparation
Counseling
Crisis Intervention
Distraction
Elopement Precautions
Emotional Support
Energy Management
Environmental Management
Exercise Promotion
Genetic Counseling
Grief Work Facilitation
Guided Imagery

High-Risk Pregnancy Care
Hypnosis
Medication Prescribing
Meditation Facilitation
Music Therapy
Premenstrual Syndrome (PMS) Management
Progressive Muscle Relaxation
Reminiscence Therapy
Reproductive Technology Management
Self-Hypnosis Facilitation
Support Group
Teaching: Individual
Teaching: Preoperative
Teaching: Prescribed Medication
Teaching: Procedure/Treatment
Telephone Consultation
Trauma Therapy: Child
Urinary Incontinence Care: Enuresis
Visitation Facilitation
Vital Signs Monitoring

Aspiration, Risk for

Definition: At risk for entry of gastrointestinal secretions, oropharyngeal secretions, solids, or fluids into tracheobronchial passages

Suggested Nursing Interventions for Problem Resolution:
Airway Management
Airway Suctioning
Artificial Airway Management
Aspiration Precautions
Chest Physiotherapy
Cough Enhancement
Neurologic Monitoring
Positioning
Postanesthesia Care
Respiratory Monitoring
Resuscitation: Neonate
Sedation Management
Surveillance
Swallowing Therapy
Vomiting Management

Additional Optional Interventions:
Asthma Management
Dementia Management
Enteral Tube Feeding
Feeding
Gastrointestinal Intubation
Mechanical Ventilation Management: Invasive
Mechanical Ventilation Management: Noninvasive
Mechanical Ventilation Management: Pneumonia Prevention
Mechanical Ventilatory Weaning
Medication Administration: Enteral
Medication Administration: Oral
Risk Identification
Seizure Management
Self-Care Assistance: Feeding
Tube Care: Gastrointestinal
Vital Signs Monitoring

Attachment, Risk for Impaired

Definition: At risk of disruption of the interactive process between parent/significant other and child that fosters the development of a protective and nurturing reciprocal relationship

Suggested Nursing Interventions for Problem Resolution:
Anticipatory Guidance
Anxiety Reduction
Attachment Promotion
Childbirth Preparation
Coping Enhancement
Developmental Enhancement: Child

Family Integrity Promotion: Childbearing Family
Infant Care
Infant Care: Preterm
Normalization Promotion
Parent Education: Childrearing Family
Parent Education: Infant
Parenting Promotion

Risk Identification: Childbearing Family
Role Enhancement
Self-Awareness Enhancement
Self-Esteem Enhancement
Self-Responsibility Facilitation
Socialization Enhancement
Substance Use Prevention
Substance Use Treatment
Support System Enhancement

Additional Optional Interventions:
Behavior Management: Overactivity/Inattention
Behavior Modification
Family Involvement Promotion
Family Mobilization
Family Process Maintenance

Family Support
Family Therapy
Sibling Support
Support Group
Teaching: Infant Nutrition 0-3 Months
Teaching: Infant Nutrition 4-6 Months
Teaching: Infant Nutrition 7-9 Months
Teaching: Infant Nutrition 10-12 Months
Teaching: Infant Safety 0-3 Months
Teaching: Infant Safety 4-6 Months
Teaching: Infant Safety 7-9 Months
Teaching: Infant Safety 10-12 Months
Teaching: Infant Stimulation 0-4 Months
Teaching: Infant Stimulation 5-8 Months
Teaching: Infant Stimulation 9-12 Months
Trauma Therapy: Child

Autonomic Dysreflexia

Definition: Life-threatening, uninhibited sympathetic response of the nervous system to a noxious stimulus after a spinal cord injury at T7 or above

Suggested Nursing Interventions for Problem Resolution:
Airway Management
Anxiety Reduction
Bowel Management
Dysreflexia Management
Fluid Management
Fluid Monitoring
Positioning
Temperature Regulation
Urinary Elimination Management
Vital Signs Monitoring

Additional Optional Interventions:
Cough Enhancement
Infection Control

Infection Protection
Intravenous (IV) Insertion
Intravenous (IV) Therapy
Medication Administration
Medication Management
Neurologic Monitoring
Nutrition Management
Pain Management
Skin Surveillance
Surveillance
Urinary Catheterization
Urinary Catheterization: Intermittent

Autonomic Dysreflexia, Risk for

Definition: At risk for life-threatening, uninhibited response of the sympathetic nervous system, postspinal shock, in an individual with spinal cord injury or lesion at T6 or above (has been demonstrated in patients with injuries at T7 and T8)

Suggested Nursing Interventions for Problem Resolution:
Airway Management
Anxiety Reduction
Bowel Management
Constipation/Impaction Management
Dysreflexia Management
Embolus Care: Peripheral
Fluid Management
Fluid Monitoring
Medication Management
Pain Management
Positioning
Pressure Management

Pressure Ulcer Prevention
Risk Identification
Skin Surveillance
Temperature Regulation
Wound Care
Urinary Elimination Management
Vital Signs Monitoring

Additional Optional Interventions:
Bowel Training
Circulatory Precautions
Cough Enhancement
Exercise Therapy: Joint Mobility

Exercise Therapy: Muscle Control
Flatulence Reduction
High-Risk Pregnancy Care
Infection Control
Infection Protection
Intrapartal Care: High-Risk Delivery
Intravenous (IV) Insertion
Intravenous (IV) Therapy
Medication Administration
Neurologic Monitoring

Nutrition Management
Premenstrual Syndrome (PMS) Management
Pressure Ulcer Care
Sexual Counseling
Substance Use Treatment: Drug Withdrawal
Surveillance
Surveillance: Late Pregnancy
Urinary Catheterization
Urinary Catheterization: Intermittent

Bleeding, Risk for

Definition: At risk for a decrease in blood volume that may compromise health

Suggested Nursing Interventions for Problem Resolution:
Bleeding Precautions
Bleeding Reduction
Bleeding Reduction: Antepartum Uterus
Bleeding Reduction: Gastrointestinal
Bleeding Reduction: Nasal
Bleeding Reduction: Postpartum Uterus
Bleeding Reduction: Wound
Chemotherapy Management
Medication Management
Postpartal Care
Risk Identification
Surveillance
Teaching: Prescribed Medication

Teaching: Procedure/Treatment
Thrombolytic Therapy Management

Additional Optional Interventions:
Central Venous Access Device Management
Circumcision Care
Dialysis Access Maintenance
Environmental Management: Safety
Fall Prevention
Incision Site Care
Prenatal Care
Shock Prevention
Sports Injury Prevention: Youth
Vehicle Safety Promotion

Blood Glucose Level, Risk for Unstable

Definition: At risk for variation of blood glucose/sugar levels from the normal range that may compromise health

Suggested Nursing Interventions for Problem Resolution:
Hyperglycemia Management
Hypoglycemia Management
Medication Management
Self-Efficacy Enhancement
Teaching: Disease Process
Teaching: Prescribed Diet
Teaching: Prescribed Exercise
Teaching: Prescribed Medication
Teaching: Procedure/Treatment

Additional Optional Interventions:
Behavior Modification
Family Involvement Promotion

Health Education
Health Literacy Enhancement
High-Risk Pregnancy Care
Learning Readiness Enhancement
Nutritional Counseling
Nutritional Monitoring
Risk Identification
Self-Responsibility Facilitation
Surveillance
Technology Management
Weight Management

Body Image, Disturbed

Definition: Confusion in mental picture of one's physical self

Suggested Nursing Interventions for Problem Resolution:
Active Listening
Anxiety Reduction
Body Image Enhancement
Coping Enhancement
Counseling
Developmental Enhancement: Adolescent
Developmental Enhancement: Child
Emotional Support
Grief Work Facilitation
Pain Management
Parent Education: Childrearing Family

Presence
Self-Awareness Enhancement
Self-Care Assistance
Self-Esteem Enhancement
Socialization Enhancement
Support Group
Support System Enhancement
Therapy Group
Values Clarification
Weight Management
Wound Care
Wound Care: Burns

Additional Optional Interventions:
Amputation Care
Anticipatory Guidance
Bowel Incontinence Care: Encopresis
Calming Technique
Childbirth Preparation
Cognitive Restructuring
Decision-Making Support
Lactation Counseling

Mutual Goal Setting
Ostomy Care
Patient Contracting
Prenatal Care
Suicide Prevention
Teaching: Sexuality
Truth Telling
Unilateral Neglect Management
Urinary Incontinence Care: Enuresis

Body Temperature, Risk for Imbalanced

Definition: At risk for failure to maintain body temperature within normal range

Suggested Nursing Interventions for Problem Resolution:
Cerebral Edema Management
Environmental Management
Environmental Management: Comfort
Fever Treatment
Fluid Management
Fluid Monitoring
Malignant Hyperthermia Precautions
Medication Management
Postanesthesia Care
Temperature Regulation
Temperature Regulation: Perioperative
Vital Signs Monitoring

Fluid Resuscitation
Heat/Cold Application
Hemodynamic Regulation
Infection Control
Infection Protection
Kangaroo Care
Nutrition Management
Resuscitation: Neonate
Risk Identification
Sedation Management
Surveillance
Weight Management
Wound Care: Burns

Additional Optional Interventions:
Bathing
Energy Management

Bowel Incontinence

Definition: Change in normal bowel habits, characterized by involuntary passage of stool

Suggested Nursing Interventions for Problem Resolution:
Bowel Incontinence Care
Bowel Incontinence Care: Encopresis
Bowel Management
Bowel Training
Diarrhea Management
Perineal Care
Rectal Prolapse Management
Self-Care Assistance: Toileting
Skin Surveillance
Teaching: Toilet Training

Additional Optional Interventions:
Bathing
Dementia Management
Emotional Support
Environmental Management
Exercise Promotion
Exercise Therapy: Ambulation
Nutrition Management

Breast Milk, Insufficient

Definition: Low production of maternal breast milk

Suggested Nursing Interventions for Problem Resolution:
Bottle Feeding
Cup Feeding: Newborn
Fluid/Electrolyte Management
Intravenous (IV) Insertion
Intravenous (IV) Therapy
Lactation Counseling
Nutrition Therapy
Nutritional Monitoring

Additional Optional Interventions:
Enteral Tube Feeding
Infant Care
Medication Management
Substance Use Treatment
Teaching: Infant Nutrition 0-3 Months
Teaching: Infant Nutrition 4-6 Months
Teaching: Infant Nutrition 7-9 Months
Teaching: Infant Nutrition 10-12 Months
Weight Gain Assistance

Breastfeeding, Ineffective

Definition: Dissatisfaction or difficulty a mother, infant, or child experiences with the breastfeeding process

Suggested Nursing Interventions for Problem Resolution:
Anxiety Reduction
Attachment Promotion
Emotional Support
Kangaroo Care
Lactation Counseling
Lactation Suppression
Nutrition Management
Parent Education: Infant
Skin Surveillance
Teaching: Individual
Teaching: Infant Nutrition 0-3 Months

Teaching: Infant Nutrition 4-6 Months
Teaching: Infant Nutrition 7-9 Months
Teaching: Infant Nutrition 10-12 Months
Telephone Consultation

Additional Optional Interventions:
Bottle Feeding
Pain Management
Patient Rights Protection
Sleep Enhancement
Support Group
Weight Management

Breastfeeding, Interrupted

Definition: Break in the continuity of the breastfeeding process as a result of inability or inadvisability to put baby to breast for feeding

Suggested Nursing Interventions for Problem Resolution:
Anticipatory Guidance
Attachment Promotion
Bottle Feeding
Coping Enhancement
Cup Feeding: Newborn
Emotional Support
Lactation Counseling
Lactation Suppression
Nonnutritive Sucking
Parent Education: Infant
Teaching: Individual
Teaching: Infant Nutrition 0-3 Months
Teaching: Infant Nutrition 4-6 Months
Teaching: Infant Nutrition 7-9 Months
Teaching: Infant Nutrition 10-12 Months

Additional Optional Interventions:
Active Listening
Anxiety Reduction
Behavior Modification
Body Image Enhancement
Discharge Planning
Health System Guidance
Nutritional Counseling
Referral
Relaxation Therapy
Support Group
Wound Care

Breastfeeding, Readiness for Enhanced

Definition: A pattern of proficiency and satisfaction of the mother-infant dyad that is sufficient to support the breastfeeding process and can be strengthened

Suggested Nursing Interventions for Problem Resolution:
Anticipatory Guidance
Attachment Promotion
Commendation
Lactation Counseling
Parent Education: Infant
Self-Efficacy Enhancement
Teaching: Individual

Additional Optional Interventions:
Infant Care
Lactation Suppression

Nutrition Therapy
Support Group
Teaching: Infant Nutrition 0-3 Months
Teaching: Infant Nutrition 4-6 Months
Teaching: Infant Nutrition 7-9 Months
Teaching: Infant Nutrition 10-12 Months
Weight Management

Breathing Pattern, Ineffective

Definition: Inspiration and/or expiration that does not provide adequate ventilation

Suggested Nursing Interventions for Problem Resolution:
Airway Management
Airway Suctioning
Allergy Management
Anaphylaxis Management
Anxiety Reduction
Artificial Airway Management
Asthma Management
Cough Enhancement
Mechanical Ventilation Management: Invasive
Mechanical Ventilation Management: Noninvasive
Mechanical Ventilation Management: Pneumonia Prevention
Mechanical Ventilatory Weaning
Medication Administration
Medication Administration: Nasal
Oxygen Therapy
Respiratory Monitoring
Surveillance
Ventilation Assistance
Vital Signs Monitoring

Additional Optional Interventions:
Acid-Base Monitoring
Airway Insertion and Stabilization
Analgesic Administration
Aspiration Precautions
Chest Physiotherapy
Emergency Care
Emotional Support
Endotracheal Extubation
Energy Management
Fluid Monitoring
Medication Management
Neurologic Monitoring
Pain Management
Phlebotomy: Arterial Blood Sample
Phlebotomy: Venous Blood Sample
Positioning
Presence
Progressive Muscle Relaxation
Resuscitation
Smoking Cessation Assistance
Tube Care: Chest

Cardiac Output, Decreased

Definition: Inadequate blood pumped by the heart to meet the metabolic demands of the body

Suggested Nursing Interventions for Problem Resolution:
Acid-Base Management
Acid-Base Management: Metabolic Acidosis
Acid-Base Management: Metabolic Alkalosis
Acid-Base Management: Respiratory Acidosis
Acid-Base Management: Respiratory Alkalosis
Acid-Base Monitoring
Airway Management
Cardiac Care
Cardiac Care: Acute
Cardiac Care: Rehabilitative
Circulatory Care: Arterial Insufficiency
Circulatory Care: Mechanical Assist Device
Circulatory Care: Venous Insufficiency
Code Management
Electrolyte Management
Electrolyte Management: Hypercalcemia
Electrolyte Management: Hyperkalemia
Electrolyte Management: Hypermagnesemia
Electrolyte Management: Hypernatremia
Electrolyte Management: Hyperphosphatemia
Electrolyte Management: Hypocalcemia
Electrolyte Management: Hypokalemia
Electrolyte Management: Hypomagnesemia
Electrolyte Management: Hyponatremia
Electrolyte Management: Hypophosphatemia
Electrolyte Monitoring
Energy Management
Fluid/Electrolyte Management
Fluid Management
Fluid Monitoring
Hemodialysis Therapy
Hemodynamic Regulation
Invasive Hemodynamic Monitoring
Medication Administration
Medication Management
Neurologic Monitoring
Oxygen Therapy
Respiratory Monitoring
Resuscitation
Resuscitation: Fetus

Resuscitation: Neonate
Shock Management
Shock Management: Cardiac
Shock Management: Volume
Shock Prevention
Vital Signs Monitoring

Additional Optional Interventions:
Anxiety Reduction
Bleeding Precautions
Bleeding Reduction
Bleeding Reduction: Antepartum Uterus
Bleeding Reduction: Gastrointestinal
Bleeding Reduction: Nasal
Bleeding Reduction: Postpartum Uterus
Bleeding Reduction: Wound
Blood Products Administration
Cardiac Risk Management
Cerebral Perfusion Promotion
Dying Care
Dysrhythmia Management
Embolus Care: Pulmonary
Emergency Care
Intravenous (IV) Insertion
Intravenous (IV) Therapy
Lower Extremity Monitoring
Nutrition Management
Pacemaker Management: Permanent
Pacemaker Management: Temporary
Pain Management
Patient Rights Protection
Peripherally Inserted Central Catheter (PICC) Care
Peritoneal Dialysis Therapy
Phlebotomy: Arterial Blood Sample
Phlebotomy: Cannulated Vessel
Phlebotomy: Venous Blood Sample
Positioning
Skin Surveillance
Sleep Enhancement
Surveillance
Visitation Facilitation

Caregiver Role Strain

Definition: Difficulty in performing family/significant other caregiver role

Suggested Nursing Interventions for Problem Resolution:
Abuse Protection Support: Child
Abuse Protection Support: Domestic Partner
Abuse Protection Support: Elder
Anticipatory Guidance
Attachment Promotion
Caregiver Support
Coping Enhancement
Decision-Making Support

Energy Management
Financial Resource Management
Health System Guidance
Home Maintenance Assistance
Nutrition Management
Parent Education: Adolescent
Parent Education: Childrearing Family
Parent Education: Infant
Parenting Promotion

Respite Care
Role Enhancement
Teaching: Disease Process
Teaching: Individual
Teaching: Prescribed Diet
Teaching: Prescribed Medication

Additional Optional Interventions:
Behavior Management: Overactivity/Inattention
Case Management
Consultation
Counseling
Family Integrity Promotion
Family Involvement Promotion
Family Mobilization
Family Process Maintenance
Family Support
Family Therapy
Grief Work Facilitation
Guilt Work Facilitation
Kangaroo Care
Presence

Referral
Substance Use Treatment
Support Group
Support System Enhancement
Teaching: Infant Nutrition 0-3 Months
Teaching: Infant Nutrition 4-6 Months
Teaching: Infant Nutrition 7-9 Months
Teaching: Infant Nutrition 10-12 Months
Teaching: Infant Safety 0-3 Months
Teaching: Infant Safety 4-6 Months
Teaching: Infant Safety 7-9 Months
Teaching: Infant Safety 10-12 Months
Teaching: Infant Stimulation 0-4 Months
Teaching: Infant Stimulation 5-8 Months
Teaching: Infant Stimulation 9-12 Months
Teaching: Toddler Nutrition 13-18 Months
Teaching: Toddler Nutrition 19-24 Months
Teaching: Toddler Nutrition 25-36 Months
Teaching: Toddler Safety 13-18 Months
Teaching: Toddler Safety 19-24 Months
Teaching: Toddler Safety 25-36 Months
Teaching: Toilet Training

Caregiver Role Strain, Risk for

Definition: At risk for caregiver vulnerability for difficulty felt in performing the family caregiver role

Suggested Nursing Interventions for Problem Resolution:
Anger Control Assistance
Anticipatory Guidance
Behavior Management
Caregiver Support
Coping Enhancement
Energy Management
Family Support
Financial Resource Assistance
Health System Guidance
Home Maintenance Assistance
Mood Management
Normalization Promotion
Parent Education: Adolescent
Parent Education: Childrearing Family
Parent Education: Infant
Parenting Promotion
Resiliency Promotion
Respite Care
Risk Identification
Role Enhancement
Substance Use Prevention
Support Group
Support System Enhancement
Teaching: Disease Process
Teaching: Individual
Teaching: Prescribed Diet
Teaching: Prescribed Exercise
Teaching: Prescribed Medication
Teaching: Procedure/Treatment
Teaching: Psychomotor Skill

Additional Optional Interventions:
Abuse Protection Support
Behavior Management: Overactivity/Inattention
Cognitive Stimulation

Counseling
Family Integrity Promotion
Family Integrity Promotion: Childbearing Family
Family Involvement Promotion
Family Mobilization
Family Process Maintenance
Family Therapy
Grief Work Facilitation
Guilt Work Facilitation
Infant Care
Kangaroo Care
Reality Orientation
Recreation Therapy
Referral
Socialization Enhancement
Substance Use Treatment
Substance Use Treatment: Drug Withdrawal
Teaching: Infant Nutrition 0-3 Months
Teaching: Infant Nutrition 4-6 Months
Teaching: Infant Nutrition 7-9 Months
Teaching: Infant Nutrition 10-12 Months
Teaching: Infant Safety 0-3 Months
Teaching: Infant Safety 4-6 Months
Teaching: Infant Safety 7-9 Months
Teaching: Infant Safety 10-12 Months
Teaching: Infant Stimulation 0-4 Months
Teaching: Infant Stimulation 5-8 Months
Teaching: Infant Stimulation 9-12 Months
Teaching: Toddler Nutrition 13-18 Months
Teaching: Toddler Nutrition 19-24 Months
Teaching: Toddler Nutrition 25-36 Months
Teaching: Toddler Safety 13-18 Months
Teaching: Toddler Safety 19-24 Months
Teaching: Toddler Safety 25-36 Months
Teaching: Toilet Training

Childbearing Process, Ineffective

Definition: Pregnancy and childbirth process and care of the newborn that does not match the environmental context, norms, and expectations

Suggested Nursing Interventions for Problem Resolution:
Attachment Promotion
Birthing
Childbirth Preparation
Family Involvement Promotion
Family Mobilization
Intrapartal Care
Lactation Counseling
Parent Education: Infant
Parenting Promotion
Postpartal Care
Prenatal Care
Risk Identification: Childbearing Family
Support System Enhancement
Surveillance: Late Pregnancy

Additional Optional Interventions:
Anticipatory Guidance
Caregiver Support

Developmental Enhancement: Infant
Infant Care: Newborn
Role Enhancement
Teaching: Infant Nutrition 0-3 Months
Teaching: Infant Nutrition 4-6 Months
Teaching: Infant Nutrition 7-9 Months
Teaching: Infant Nutrition 10-12 Months
Teaching: Infant Safety 0-3 Months
Teaching: Infant Safety 4-6 Months
Teaching: Infant Safety 7-9 Months
Teaching: Infant Safety 10-12 Months
Teaching: Infant Stimulation 0-4 Months
Teaching: Infant Stimulation 5-8 Months
Teaching: Infant Stimulation 9-12 Months

Childbearing Process, Readiness for Enhanced

Definition: A pattern of preparing for and maintaining a healthy pregnancy, childbirth process, and care of the newborn that is sufficient for ensuring well-being and can be strengthened

Suggested Nursing Interventions for Problem Resolution:
Attachment Promotion
Birthing
Childbirth Preparation
Family Integrity Promotion: Childbearing Family
Intrapartal Care
Lactation Counseling
Parent Education: Infant
Postpartal Care

Preconception Counseling
Prenatal Care

Additional Optional Interventions:
Family Process Maintenance
Family Support
Infant Care: Newborn
Infant Care: Preterm
Risk Identification: Childbearing Family

Childbearing Process, Risk for Ineffective

Definition: Risk for a pregnancy and childbirth process and care of the newborn that does not match the environmental context, norms, and expectations

Suggested Nursing Interventions for Problem Resolution:
Abuse Protection Support
Childbirth Preparation
Family Involvement Promotion
Family Mobilization
Nutritional Counseling
Nutritional Monitoring
Prenatal Care

Risk Identification: Childbearing Family
Role Enhancement
Self-Esteem Enhancement
Substance Use Treatment
Support System Enhancement
Surveillance: Late Pregnancy

Additional Optional Interventions:
Anticipatory Guidance
Decision-Making Support
Learning Facilitation
Parent Education: Infant

Teaching: Infant Nutrition 0-3 Months
Teaching: Infant Safety 0-3 Months
Teaching: Infant Stimulation 0-4 Months
Ultrasonography: Limited Obstetric
Values Clarification

Comfort, Impaired

Definition: Perceived lack of ease, relief, and transcendence in physical, psychospiritual, environmental, cultural, and social dimensions

Suggested Nursing Interventions for Problem Resolution:
Anxiety Reduction
Calming Technique
Culture Brokerage
Dementia Management
Dementia Management: Bathing
Environmental Management: Comfort
Medication Administration
Pain Management
Positioning
Relaxation Therapy
Security Enhancement
Self-Efficacy Enhancement
Self-Modification Assistance

Spiritual Support
Support System Enhancement

Additional Optional Interventions:
Chemotherapy Management
Medication Management
Pruritus Management
Radiation Therapy Management
Sleep Enhancement
Support Group

Comfort, Readiness for Enhanced

Definition: A pattern of ease, relief, and transcendence in physical, psychospiritual, environmental, and/or social dimensions that is sufficient for well-being and can be strengthened

Suggested Nursing Interventions for Problem Resolution:
Assertiveness Training
Coping Enhancement
Decision-Making Support
Emotional Support
Environmental Management
Forgiveness Facilitation
Grief Work Facilitation
Guilt Work Facilitation
Health Education
Hope Inspiration
Pain Management
Self-Awareness Enhancement
Self-Efficacy Enhancement
Self-Esteem Enhancement
Self-Modification Assistance
Socialization Enhancement

Spiritual Growth Facilitation
Spiritual Support
Values Clarification

Additional Optional Interventions:
Anticipatory Guidance
Anxiety Reduction
Counseling
Environmental Management: Comfort
Guided Imagery
Humor
Mood Management
Progressive Muscle Relaxation
Recreation Therapy
Relaxation Therapy
Support Group
Therapy Group

Communication, Impaired Verbal

Definition: Decreased, delayed, or absent ability to receive, process, transmit, and/or use a system of symbols

Suggested Nursing Interventions for Problem Resolution:
Active Listening
Anxiety Reduction
Communication Enhancement: Hearing Deficit
Communication Enhancement: Speech Deficit
Communication Enhancement: Visual Deficit
Culture Brokerage
Decision-Making Support
Dementia Management
Environmental Management
Medication Management
Memory Training
Presence

Touch
Validation Therapy

Additional Optional Interventions:
Art Therapy
Ear Care
Energy Management
Learning Facilitation
Referral
Relocation Stress Reduction
Self-Care Assistance: IADL
Support System Enhancement

Communication, Readiness for Enhanced

Definition: A pattern of exchanging information and ideas with others that is sufficient for meeting one's needs and life's goals, and can be strengthened

Suggested Nursing Interventions for Problem Resolution:
Active Listening
Anxiety Reduction
Assertiveness Training
Commendation
Communication Enhancement: Hearing Deficit
Communication Enhancement: Speech Deficit
Complex Relationship Building
Conflict Mediation
Reality Orientation
Reminiscence Therapy
Socialization Enhancement

Additional Optional Interventions:
Art Therapy
Bibliotherapy
Communication Enhancement: Visual Deficit
Culture Brokerage
Decision-Making Support
Journaling
Music Therapy
Recreation Therapy

Community Coping, Ineffective

Definition: A pattern of community activities for adaptation and problem-solving that is unsatisfactory for meeting the demands or needs of the community

Suggested Nursing Interventions for Problem Resolution:
Bioterrorism Preparedness
Communicable Disease Management
Community Disaster Preparedness
Community Health Development
Environmental Management: Community
Environmental Management: Safety
Environmental Management: Violence Prevention
Environmental Risk Protection
Fiscal Resource Management
Health Education
Health Policy Monitoring
Health Screening
Immunization/Vaccination Management

Program Development
Risk Identification
Surveillance: Community

Additional Optional Interventions:
Case Management
Documentation
Infection Control
Multidisciplinary Care Conference
Referral
Resiliency Promotion
Sustenance Support
Triage: Disaster
Vehicle Safety Promotion

Community Coping, Readiness for Enhanced

Definition: A pattern of community activities for adaptation and problem-solving that is sufficient for meeting the demands or needs of the community for the management of current future problems/stressors and can be strengthened

Suggested Nursing Interventions for Problem Resolution:
Bioterrorism Preparedness
Community Disaster Preparedness
Environmental Management: Community
Environmental Management: Violence Prevention
Environmental Management: Worker Safety
Environmental Risk Protection
Fiscal Resource Management
Health Education
Health Policy Monitoring
Program Development
Surveillance: Community
Vehicle Safety Promotion

Additional Optional Interventions:
Anticipatory Guidance
Communicable Disease Management
Community Health Development
Health Screening
Immunization/Vaccination Management
Resiliency Promotion
Risk Identification

Community Health, Deficient

Definition: Presence of one or more health problems or factors that deter wellness or increase the risk of health problems experienced by an aggregate

Suggested Nursing Interventions for Problem Resolution:
Communicable Disease Management
Community Health Development
Environmental Management: Community
Environmental Risk Protection
Fiscal Resource Management
Health Screening
Program Development
Social Marketing
Surveillance: Community

Additional Optional Interventions:
Bioterrorism Preparedness
Community Disaster Preparedness
Environmental Management: Worker Safety
Health Education
Health Literacy Enhancement
Health Policy Monitoring
Immunization/Vaccination Management
Risk Identification

Confusion, Acute

Definition: Abrupt onset of reversible disturbances of consciousness, attention, cognition, and perception that develop over a short period of time

Suggested Nursing Interventions for Problem Resolution:
Anxiety Reduction
Cognitive Stimulation
Delirium Management
Delusion Management
Environmental Management: Safety
Fall Prevention
Hallucination Management
Medication Administration
Medication Management
Neurologic Monitoring
Pain Management
Physical Restraint
Reality Orientation
Seclusion

Sleep Enhancement
Substance Use Treatment
Substance Use Treatment: Alcohol Withdrawal
Substance Use Treatment: Drug Withdrawal
Vital Signs Monitoring

Additional Optional Interventions:
Acid-Base Management
Analgesic Administration
Calming Technique
Cerebral Perfusion Promotion
Memory Training
Presence
Self-Care Assistance
Touch

Confusion, Chronic

Definition: Irreversible, longstanding, and/or progressive deterioration of intellect and personality characterized by decreased ability to interpret environmental stimuli and decreased capacity for intellectual thought processes, and manifested by disturbances of memory, orientation, and behavior

Suggested Nursing Interventions for Problem Resolution:
Anxiety Reduction
Area Restriction
Calming Technique
Cognitive Stimulation
Delusion Management
Dementia Management
Dementia Management: Bathing
Dementia Management: Wandering
Emotional Support
Energy Management
Environmental Management
Environmental Management: Safety
Family Involvement Promotion
Family Support
Humor
Memory Training
Milieu Therapy
Mood Management
Music Therapy
Presence
Reality Orientation

Reminiscence Therapy
Risk Identification
Sleep Enhancement
Surveillance
Validation Therapy

Additional Optional Interventions:
Activity Therapy
Animal-Assisted Therapy
Art Therapy
Chemical Restraint
Cognitive Restructuring
Decision-Making Support
Exercise Promotion
Fall Prevention
Hallucination Management
Health System Guidance
Medication Management
Patient Rights Protection
Physical Restraint
Recreation Therapy
Relocation Stress Reduction

Confusion, Risk for Acute

Definition: At risk for reversible disturbances of consciousness, attention, cognition, and perception that develop over a short period of time

Suggested Nursing Interventions for Problem Resolution:
Acid-Base Management
Exercise Promotion
Fluid/Electrolyte Management
Fluid Management
Fluid Monitoring
Infection Protection
Medication Administration
Medication Management
Neurologic Monitoring
Pain Management
Postanesthesia Care
Reality Orientation
Risk Identification
Sleep Enhancement

Substance Use Treatment
Substance Use Treatment: Alcohol Withdrawal
Substance Use Treatment: Drug Withdrawal
Substance Use Treatment: Overdose
Surveillance
Urinary Retention Care

Additional Optional Interventions:
Delirium Management
Delusion Management
Environmental Management: Safety
Fall Prevention
Hallucination Management
Vital Signs Monitoring

Constipation

Definition: Decrease in normal frequency of defecation, accompanied by difficult or incomplete passage of stool and/or passage of excessively hard, dry stool

Suggested Nursing Interventions for Problem Resolution:
Bowel Management
Bowel Training
Constipation/Impaction Management
Diet Staging
Enema Administration
Fluid/Electrolyte Management
Fluid Management
Fluid Monitoring
Medication Prescribing
Nutrition Management
Rectal Prolapse Management

Additional Optional Interventions:
Anxiety Reduction
Exercise Promotion

Exercise Therapy: Ambulation
Exercise Therapy: Joint Mobility
Flatulence Reduction
Gastrointestinal Intubation
Medication Administration: Oral
Medication Administration: Rectal
Medication Management
Ostomy Care
Pain Management
Postpartal Care
Prenatal Care
Relaxation Therapy
Self-Care Assistance: Toileting
Skin Surveillance
Teaching: Toilet Training
Tube Care: Gastrointestinal

Constipation, Perceived

Definition: Self-diagnosis of constipation combined with abuse of laxatives, enemas, and/or suppositories to ensure a daily bowel movement

Suggested Nursing Interventions for Problem Resolution:
Active Listening
Bowel Management
Counseling
Fluid Management
Fluid Monitoring
Health Education
Medication Management
Teaching: Individual

Additional Optional Interventions:
Culture Brokerage
Distraction
Exercise Promotion
Nutrition Management
Relaxation Therapy
Self-Modification Assistance
Teaching: Toilet Training

Constipation, Risk for

Definition: At risk for a decrease in normal frequency of defecation, accompanied by difficult or incomplete passage of stool and/or passage of excessively hard, dry stool

Suggested Nursing Interventions for Problem Resolution:
Bowel Management
Bowel Training
Constipation/Impaction Management
Diet Staging
Exercise Promotion
Fluid Management
Fluid Monitoring
Medication Management
Medication Prescribing
Nutrition Management

Additional Optional Interventions:
Anxiety Reduction
Electrolyte Management
Exercise Therapy: Ambulation
Exercise Therapy: Joint Mobility
Flatulence Reduction
Medication Administration: Oral
Mood Management
Nutritional Counseling
Nutritional Monitoring
Oral Health Promotion

Ostomy Care
Pain Management
Prenatal Care
Reality Orientation
Rectal Prolapse Management
Relaxation Therapy
Risk Identification

Self-Care Assistance: Toileting
Surveillance
Teaching: Prescribed Diet
Teaching: Prescribed Medication
Teaching: Toilet Training
Weight Reduction Assistance

Contamination

Definition: Exposure to environmental contaminants in doses sufficient to cause adverse health effects

Suggested Nursing Interventions for Problem Resolution:
Bioterrorism Preparedness
Case Management
Chemotherapy Management
Community Disaster Preparedness
Environmental Management: Safety
Environmental Management: Worker Safety
Environmental Risk Protection
Health Screening
Neurologic Monitoring
Radiation Therapy Management
Respiratory Monitoring
Risk Identification
Skin Care: Topical Treatments
Skin Surveillance
Triage: Disaster
Triage: Emergency Center
Ventilation Assistance

Additional Optional Interventions:
Anaphylaxis Management
Energy Management
Fluid/Electrolyte Management
Fluid Management
Infection Control
Infection Protection
Laser Precautions
Nutrition Therapy
Risk Identification: Genetic
Specimen Management
Surveillance
Sustenance Support
Vital Signs Monitoring
Wound Care

Contamination, Risk for

Definition: Accentuated risk of exposure to environmental contaminants in doses sufficient to cause adverse health effects

Suggested Nursing Interventions for Problem Resolution:
Bioterrorism Preparedness
Community Disaster Preparedness
Environmental Management: Community
Environmental Management: Safety
Environmental Management: Worker Safety
Environmental Risk Protection
Health Policy Monitoring
Infection Control
Infection Protection
Surveillance: Community

Additional Optional Interventions:
Health Education
Health Screening

Nutritional Counseling
Prenatal Care
Program Development
Risk Identification
Smoking Cessation Assistance
Social Marketing
Sustenance Support
Teaching: Infant Safety 0-3 Months
Teaching: Infant Safety 4-6 Months
Teaching: Infant Safety 7-9 Months
Teaching: Infant Safety 10-12 Months
Teaching: Toddler Safety 13-18 Months
Teaching: Toddler Safety 19-24 Months
Teaching: Toddler Safety 25-36 Months

Coping, Defensive

Definition: Repeated projection of falsely positive self-evaluation based on a self-protective pattern that defends against underlying perceived threats to positive self-regard

Suggested Nursing Interventions for Problem Resolution:
Body Image Enhancement
Complex Relationship Building
Coping Enhancement
Patient Contracting
Resiliency Promotion
Self-Awareness Enhancement
Self-Efficacy Enhancement
Self-Esteem Enhancement
Socialization Enhancement
Support System Enhancement
Values Clarification

Additional Optional Interventions:
Behavior Modification
Behavior Modification: Social Skills
Cognitive Restructuring
Counseling
Emotional Support
Environmental Management
Forgiveness Facilitation
Reminiscence Therapy
Self-Responsibility Facilitation
Therapy Group
Truth Telling

Coping, Ineffective

Definition: Inability to form a valid appraisal of the stressors, inadequate choices of practiced responses, and/or inability to use available resources

Suggested Nursing Interventions for Problem Resolution:
Anger Control Assistance
Anticipatory Guidance
Anxiety Reduction
Behavior Management: Self-Harm
Behavior Management: Sexual
Behavior Modification
Calming Technique
Complex Relationship Building
Coping Enhancement
Counseling
Crisis Intervention
Decision-Making Support
Delusion Management
Dementia Management
Distraction
Emotional Support
Environmental Management
Fire-Setting Precautions
Forgiveness Facilitation
Impulse Control Training
Life Skills Enhancement
Meditation Facilitation
Mood Management
Presence
Progressive Muscle Relaxation
Reminiscence Therapy
Role Enhancement
Sleep Enhancement
Substance Use Prevention
Support Group
Support System Enhancement
Teaching: Individual
Therapy Group

Additional Optional Interventions:
Abuse Protection Support
Activity Therapy
Animal-Assisted Therapy
Art Therapy
Autogenic Training
Behavior Management
Biofeedback
Cognitive Restructuring
Environmental Management: Violence Prevention
Family Therapy
Health System Guidance
Hypnosis
Learning Facilitation
Learning Readiness Enhancement
Limit Setting
Medication Administration
Medication Management
Mutual Goal Setting
Patient Contracting
Seclusion
Self-Esteem Enhancement
Self-Modification Assistance
Self-Responsibility Facilitation
Substance Use Treatment
Substance Use Treatment: Alcohol Withdrawal
Substance Use Treatment: Drug Withdrawal
Substance Use Treatment: Overdose
Sustenance Support

Coping, Readiness for Enhanced

Definition: A pattern of cognitive and behavioral efforts to manage demands that is sufficient for well-being and can be strengthened

Suggested Nursing Interventions for Problem Resolution:
Anticipatory Guidance
Commendation
Coping Enhancement
Counseling
Decision-Making Support
Emotional Support
Environmental Management
Journaling
Mood Management
Mutual Goal Setting
Patient Contracting
Progressive Muscle Relaxation
Role Enhancement
Self-Awareness Enhancement
Self-Efficacy Enhancement
Self-Esteem Enhancement

Self-Modification Assistance
Self-Responsibility Facilitation
Support Group
Support System Enhancement

Additional Optional Interventions:
Anger Control Assistance
Anxiety Reduction
Impulse Control Training
Learning Facilitation
Medication Management
Meditation Facilitation
Reminiscence Therapy
Resiliency Promotion
Substance Use Prevention
Substance Use Treatment

Death Anxiety

Definition: Vague uneasy feeling of discomfort or dread generated by perceptions of a real or imagined threat to one's existence

Suggested Nursing Interventions for Problem Resolution:
Anxiety Reduction
Caregiver Support
Coping Enhancement
Decision-Making Support
Dying Care
Emotional Support
Forgiveness Facilitation
Grief Work Facilitation
Guided Imagery
Hope Inspiration
Medication Management
Mutual Goal Setting
Pain Management
Patient-Controlled Analgesia (PCA) Assistance
Presence
Referral
Relaxation Therapy
Religious Ritual Enhancement
Spiritual Growth Facilitation

Spiritual Support
Values Clarification

Additional Optional Interventions:
Active Listening
Animal-Assisted Therapy
Bibliotherapy
Calming Technique
Culture Brokerage
Family Integrity Promotion
Family Process Maintenance
Family Support
Mood Management
Music Therapy
Patient Rights Protection
Reminiscence Therapy
Visitation Facilitation

Decision-Making, Readiness for Enhanced

Definition: A pattern of choosing a course of action that is sufficient for meeting short- and long-term health-related goals and can be strengthened

Suggested Nursing Interventions for Problem Resolution:
Commendation
Coping Enhancement
Counseling
Decision-Making Support
Health System Guidance
Mutual Goal Setting
Patient Contracting
Preconception Counseling
Self-Efficacy Enhancement
Self-Modification Assistance
Self-Responsibility Facilitation

Support System Enhancement
Values Clarification

Additional Optional Interventions:
Emotional Support
Family Involvement Promotion
Family Mobilization
Health Education
Health Literacy Enhancement
Learning Facilitation

Decisional Conflict

Definition: Uncertainty about the course of action to be taken when the choice among competing actions involves risk, loss, or challenge to values and beliefs

Suggested Nursing Interventions for Problem Resolution:
Assertiveness Training
Coping Enhancement
Counseling
Decision-Making Support
Health Education
Health Literacy Enhancement
Health System Guidance
Learning Facilitation
Mutual Goal Setting
Preconception Counseling
Self-Awareness Enhancement
Support System Enhancement
Teaching: Individual
Values Clarification

Additional Optional Interventions:
Active Listening
Anticipatory Guidance
Anxiety Reduction
Culture Brokerage
Guided Imagery
Journaling
Meditation Facilitation
Music Therapy
Patient Contracting
Preparatory Sensory Information
Relaxation Therapy
Reminiscence Therapy
Spiritual Support

Denial, Ineffective

Definition: Conscious or unconscious attempt to disavow the knowledge or meaning of an event to reduce anxiety and/or fear, but leading to the detriment of health

Suggested Nursing Interventions for Problem Resolution:
Anxiety Reduction
Complex Relationship Building
Coping Enhancement
Counseling
Emotional Support
Family Mobilization
Reality Orientation
Self-Awareness Enhancement
Self-Efficacy Enhancement
Self-Modification Assistance
Self-Responsibility Facilitation
Support System Enhancement
Truth Telling

Additional Optional Interventions:
Calming Technique
Cognitive Restructuring
Decision-Making Support
Dying Care
Family Therapy
Milieu Therapy
Mutual Goal Setting
Reminiscence Therapy
Security Enhancement
Spiritual Support
Teaching: Disease Process
Therapeutic Play
Therapy Group

Dentition, Impaired

Definition: Disruption in tooth development/eruption patterns or structural integrity of individual teeth

Suggested Nursing Interventions for Problem Resolution:
Medication Management
Nutrition Management
Oral Health Maintenance
Oral Health Restoration
Pain Management
Referral

Additional Optional Interventions:
Health System Guidance
Insurance Authorization
Teaching: Psychomotor Skill

Development, Risk for Delayed

Definition: At risk for delay of 25% or more in one or more of the areas of social or self-regulatory behavior, or in cognitive, language, gross motor, or fine motor skills

Suggested Nursing Interventions for Problem Resolution:
Anticipatory Guidance
Attachment Promotion
Behavior Management
Behavior Management: Overactivity/Inattention
Behavior Modification
Behavior Modification: Social Skills
Bowel Incontinence Care: Encopresis
Caregiver Support
Counseling
Developmental Enhancement: Adolescent
Developmental Enhancement: Child
Developmental Enhancement: Infant
Family Therapy
Genetic Counseling
Health Screening
High-Risk Pregnancy Care
Infection Protection
Intrapartal Care
Intrapartal Care: High-Risk Delivery
Parent Education: Childrearing Family
Parenting Promotion
Preconception Counseling
Prenatal Care
Risk Identification: Genetic
Self-Responsibility Facilitation
Substance Use Treatment
Support Group
Support System Enhancement
Urinary Incontinence Care: Enuresis

Additional Optional Interventions:
Abuse Protection Support: Child
Coping Enhancement
Decision-Making Support
Electronic Fetal Monitoring: Antepartum
Electronic Fetal Monitoring: Intrapartum
Family Planning: Contraception
Family Planning: Unplanned Pregnancy
Impulse Control Training
Infant Care: Newborn
Infant Care: Preterm
Mood Management
Respite Care
Teaching: Infant Nutrition 0-3 Months
Teaching: Infant Nutrition 4-6 Months
Teaching: Infant Nutrition 7-9 Months
Teaching: Infant Nutrition 10-12 Months
Teaching: Infant Safety 0-3 Months
Teaching: Infant Safety 4-6 Months
Teaching: Infant Safety 7-9 Months
Teaching: Infant Safety 10-12 Months
Teaching: Infant Stimulation 0-4 Months
Teaching: Infant Stimulation 5-8 Months
Teaching: Infant Stimulation 9-12 Months
Teaching: Toddler Nutrition 13-18 Months
Teaching: Toddler Nutrition 19-24 Months
Teaching: Toddler Nutrition 25-36 Months
Teaching: Toddler Safety 13-18 Months
Teaching: Toddler Safety 19-24 Months
Teaching: Toddler Safety 25-36 Months
Teaching: Toilet Training

Diarrhea

Definition: Passage of loose, unformed stools

Suggested Nursing Interventions for Problem Resolution:
Bowel Management
Diarrhea Management
Electrolyte Monitoring
Fluid/Electrolyte Management
Fluid Management
Fluid Monitoring
Medication Management
Medication Prescribing
Nutrition Management
Ostomy Care
Perineal Care
Skin Surveillance

Additional Optional Interventions:
Anxiety Reduction
Chemotherapy Management

Enteral Tube Feeding
Environmental Management
Infection Control
Intravenous (IV) Insertion
Intravenous (IV) Therapy
Peripherally Inserted Central Catheter (PICC) Care
Radiation Therapy Management
Self-Care Assistance: Toileting
Skin Care: Topical Treatment
Substance Use Treatment
Total Parenteral Nutrition (TPN) Administration
Tube Care: Gastrointestinal
Weight Management

Disuse Syndrome, Risk for

Definition: At risk for deterioration of body systems as the result of prescribed or unavoidable musculoskeletal inactivity

Suggested Nursing Interventions for Problem Resolution:
Analgesic Administration
Bed Rest Care
Bowel Management
Cast Care: Maintenance
Cerebral Edema Management
Cerebral Perfusion Promotion
Energy Management
Environmental Management
Exercise Promotion: Stretching
Exercise Therapy: Joint Mobility
Exercise Therapy: Muscle Control
Fluid Management
Fluid Monitoring
Intracranial Pressure (ICP) Monitoring
Medication Administration
Medication Management
Pain Management
Positioning
Positioning: Intraoperative
Pressure Management
Skin Surveillance

Additional Optional Interventions:
Exercise Promotion
Exercise Promotion: Strength Training
Nutrition Management
Physical Restraint
Pneumatic Tourniquet Precautions
Positioning: Wheelchair
Progressive Muscle Relaxation
Reality Orientation
Relaxation Therapy
Risk Identification
Splinting
Surveillance
Traction/Immobilization Care
Transfer
Unilateral Neglect Management
Vital Signs Monitoring

Diversional Activity, Deficient

Definition: Decreased stimulation from (or interest or engagement in) recreational or leisure activities

Suggested Nursing Interventions for Problem Resolution:
Activity Therapy
Animal-Assisted Therapy
Art Therapy
Milieu Therapy
Music Therapy
Mutual Goal Setting
Recreation Therapy
Reminiscence Therapy
Self-Esteem Enhancement
Self-Responsibility Facilitation
Socialization Enhancement
Therapeutic Play
Visitation Facilitation

Additional Optional Interventions:
Energy Management
Environmental Management
Exercise Promotion
Family Process Maintenance
Pain Management
Pass Facilitation
Patient Contracting
Self-Modification Assistance
Support Group
Teaching: Individual

Dry Eye, Risk for

Definition: At risk for eye discomfort or damage to the cornea and conjunctiva due to reduced quantity or quality of tears to moisten the eye

Suggested Nursing Interventions for Problem Resolution:
Contact Lens Care
Dry Eye Prevention
Environmental Management: Comfort
Eye Care
Medication Administration: Eye
Medication Management

Additional Optional Interventions:
Allergy Management
Nutrition Management
Smoking Cessation Assistance

Electrolyte, Risk for Imbalance

Definition: At risk for change in serum electrolyte levels that may compromise health

Suggested Nursing Interventions for Problem Resolution:
Diarrhea Management
Eating Disorders Management
Electrolyte Management
Electrolyte Monitoring
Fluid/Electrolyte Management
Fluid Management
Fluid Monitoring
Fluid Resuscitation
Medication Management
Nausea Management

Risk Identification
Surveillance
Vomiting Management

Additional Optional Interventions:
Hemodialysis Therapy
Medication Reconciliation
Peritoneal Dialysis Therapy
Wound Care: Burns
Wound Care: Closed Drainage

Energy Field, Disturbed

Definition: Disruption of the flow of energy surrounding a person's being that results in disharmony of the body, mind, and/or spirit

Suggested Nursing Interventions for Problem Resolution:
Acupressure
Anxiety Reduction
Energy Management
Grief Work Facilitation
Guided Imagery
Healing Touch
Meditation Facilitation
Pain Management
Reiki
Spiritual Support
Therapeutic Touch
Vital Signs Monitoring

Additional Optional Interventions:
Aromatherapy
Body Image Enhancement

Communication Enhancement: Hearing Deficit
Communication Enhancement: Visual Deficit
Environmental Management
Fever Treatment
Hope Inspiration
Massage
Milieu Therapy
Music Therapy
Postanesthesia Care
Presence
Self-Awareness Enhancement
Self-Esteem Enhancement
Spiritual Growth Facilitation
Temperature Regulation

Environmental Interpretation Syndrome, Impaired

Definition: Consistent lack of orientation to person, place, time, or circumstances over more than 3-6 months, necessitating a protective environment

Suggested Nursing Interventions for Problem Resolution:
Anxiety Reduction
Communication Enhancement: Speech Deficit
Dementia Management
Dementia Management: Bathing
Dementia Management: Wandering
Elopement Precautions
Emotional Support
Energy Management
Environmental Management
Environmental Management: Safety
Fall Prevention
Memory Training
Milieu Therapy
Mood Management
Music Therapy
Reality Orientation
Reminiscence Therapy
Risk Identification
Security Enhancement

Sleep Enhancement
Surveillance
Validation Therapy

Additional Optional Interventions:
Animal-Assisted Therapy
Area Restriction
Behavior Management
Calming Technique
Cognitive Stimulation
Feeding
Medication Management
Patient Rights Protection
Self-Care Assistance
Self-Care Assistance: Bathing/Hygiene
Self-Care Assistance: Dressing/Grooming
Self-Care Assistance: Feeding
Self-Care Assistance: Toileting
Therapeutic Play
Touch

Failure to Thrive, Adult

Definition: Progressive functional deterioration of a physical and cognitive nature. The individual's ability to live with multisystem diseases, cope with ensuing problems, and manage his or her care is remarkably diminished

Suggested Nursing Interventions for Problem Resolution:
Caregiver Support
Case Management
Cognitive Simulation
Coping Enhancement
Decision-Making Support
Diet Staging
Energy Management
Environmental Management: Comfort
Feeding
Financial Resource Assistance
Fluid Monitoring
Hope Inspiration
Medication Management
Mood Management
Nutrition Management
Nutrition Therapy
Nutritional Monitoring
Patient Rights Protection
Relocation Stress Reduction
Self-Care Assistance
Self-Care Assistance: Bathing/Hygiene

Self-Care Assistance: Dressing/Grooming
Self-Care Assistance: Feeding
Self-Care Assistance: IADL
Self-Care Assistance: Toileting
Spiritual Support
Weight Gain Assistance

Additional Optional Interventions:
Animal-Assisted Therapy
Bathing
Dementia Management
Dressing
Dying Care
Family Involvement Promotion
Family Mobilization
Family Process Maintenance
Foot Care
Hair and Scalp Care
Home Maintenance Assistance
Nail Care
Resiliency Promotion
Suicide Prevention

Falls, Risk for

Definition: At risk for increased susceptibility to falling that may cause physical harm

Suggested Nursing Interventions for Problem Resolution:
Area Restriction
Body Mechanics Promotion
Dementia Management
Dementia Management: Bathing
Environmental Management: Safety
Exercise Therapy: Balance
Exercise Therapy: Muscle Control
Fall Prevention
Medication Management
Positioning
Positioning: Wheelchair
Risk Identification
Seizure Precautions
Self-Care Assistance: Toileting
Self-Care Assistance: Transfer
Teaching: Infant Safety 0-3 Months
Teaching: Infant Safety 4-6 Months
Teaching: Infant Safety 7-9 Months
Teaching: Infant Safety 10-12 Months
Teaching: Toddler Safety 13-18 Months
Teaching: Toddler Safety 19-24 Months
Teaching: Toddler Safety 25-36 Months

Transfer
Urinary Elimination Management
Vital Signs Monitoring

Additional Optional Interventions:
Bowel Management
Circulatory Care: Arterial Insufficiency
Circulatory Care: Venous Insufficiency
Cognitive Stimulation
Communication Enhancement: Hearing Deficit
Communication Enhancement: Visual Deficit
Delirium Management
Diarrhea Management
Exercise Promotion
Exercise Promotion: Strength Training
Exercise Promotion: Stretching
Exercise Therapy: Ambulation
Exercise Therapy: Joint Mobility
Hypoglycemia Management
Pain Management
Self-Care Assistance
Sleep Enhancement

Family Coping, Compromised

Definition: An usually supportive primary person (family member, significant other, or close friend) who provides insufficient, ineffective, or compromised support, comfort, assistance, or encouragement that may be needed by the client to manage or master adaptive tasks related to his or her health challenge

Suggested Nursing Interventions for Problem Resolution:
Abuse Protection Support: Child
Abuse Protection Support: Domestic Partner
Abuse Protection Support: Elder
Caregiver Support
Complex Relationship Building
Coping Enhancement
Emotional Support
Family Integrity Promotion
Family Involvement Promotion
Family Mobilization
Family Presence Facilitation
Family Process Maintenance
Family Support
Grief Work Facilitation: Perinatal Death
Health System Guidance
Learning Facilitation
Normalization Promotion
Respite Care
Spiritual Support
Support Group

Support System Enhancement
Sustenance Support

Additional Optional Interventions:
Abuse Protection Support
Anger Control Assistance
Anxiety Reduction
Behavior Management: Overactivity/Inattention
Calming Technique
Counseling
Crisis Intervention
Decision-Making Support
Environmental Management: Comfort
Environmental Management: Violence Prevention
Family Therapy
Mutual Goal Setting
Relocation Stress Reduction
Reminiscence Therapy
Role Enhancement
Sibling Support
Trauma Therapy: Child

Family Coping, Disabled

Definition: Behavior of primary person (family member, significant other, or close friend) that disables his or her capacities and the client's capacities to effectively address tasks essential to either person's adaptation to the health challenge

Suggested Nursing Interventions for Problem Resolution:
Abuse Protection Support: Child
Abuse Protection Support: Domestic Partner
Abuse Protection Support: Elder
Caregiver Support
Complex Relationship Building
Coping Enhancement
Counseling
Family Integrity Promotion
Family Involvement Promotion
Family Mobilization
Family Process Maintenance
Family Support
Family Therapy
Health System Guidance
Learning Facilitation
Normalization Promotion

Respite Care
Spiritual Support
Sustenance Support

Additional Optional Interventions:
Abuse Protection Support
Anger Control Assistance
Anxiety Reduction
Calming Technique
Crisis Intervention
Decision-Making Support
Environmental Management: Comfort
Environmental Management: Home Preparation
Environmental Management: Violence Prevention
Mutual Goal Setting
Relocation Stress Reduction
Trauma Therapy: Child

Family Coping, Readiness for Enhanced

Definition: A pattern of management of adaptive tasks by primary person (family member, significant other, or close friend) involved with the client's health challenge that is sufficient for health and growth, in regard to self and in relation to the client, and can be strengthened

Suggested Nursing Interventions for Problem Resolution:
Anticipatory Guidance
Caregiver Support
Coping Enhancement
Counseling
Developmental Enhancement: Adolescent
Developmental Enhancement: Child
Family Involvement Promotion
Family Mobilization
Family Support
Health Education
High-Risk Pregnancy Care
Learning Facilitation
Normalization Promotion
Parent Education: Adolescent
Parent Education: Childrearing Family
Parent Education: Infant
Pass Facilitation
Preconception Counseling
Resiliency Promotion
Respite Care
Self-Modification Assistance
Sibling Support

Additional Optional Interventions:
Family Integrity Promotion
Family Planning: Contraception

Family Therapy
Grief Work Facilitation: Perinatal Death
Mutual Goal Setting
Prenatal Care
Reproductive Technology Management
Risk Identification: Genetic
Role Enhancement
Teaching: Individual
Teaching: Infant Nutrition 0-3 Months
Teaching: Infant Nutrition 4-6 Months
Teaching: Infant Nutrition 7-9 Months
Teaching: Infant Nutrition 10-12 Months
Teaching: Infant Safety 0-3 Months
Teaching: Infant Safety 4-6 Months
Teaching: Infant Safety 7-9 Months
Teaching: Infant Safety 10-12 Months
Teaching: Infant Stimulation 0-4 Months
Teaching: Infant Stimulation 5-8 Months
Teaching: Infant Stimulation 9-12 Months
Teaching: Toddler Nutrition 13-18 Months
Teaching: Toddler Nutrition 19-24 Months
Teaching: Toddler Nutrition 25-36 Months
Teaching: Toddler Safety 13-18 Months
Teaching: Toddler Safety 19-24 Months
Teaching: Toddler Safety 25-36 Months
Teaching: Toilet Training

Family Processes, Dysfunctional

Definition: Psychosocial, spiritual, and physiological functions of the family unit are chronically disorganized, which leads to conflict, denial of problems, resistance to change, ineffective problem-solving, and a series of self-perpetuating crises

Suggested Nursing Interventions for Problem Resolution:
Abuse Protection Support
Abuse Protection Support: Child
Abuse Protection Support: Domestic Partner
Abuse Protection Support: Elder
Anger Control Assistance
Anxiety Reduction
Behavior Management
Conflict Mediation
Coping Enhancement
Counseling
Crisis Intervention
Decision-Making Support
Emotional Support
Family Integrity Promotion
Family Integrity Promotion: Childbearing Family
Family Process Maintenance
Family Support
Family Therapy
Impulse Control Training

Limit Setting
Mutual Goal Setting
Normalization Promotion
Resiliency Promotion
Self-Awareness Enhancement
Self-Responsibility Facilitation
Spiritual Support
Substance Use Prevention
Substance Use Treatment
Support Group
Therapy Group

Additional Optional Interventions:
Behavior Modification
Body Image Enhancement
Calming Technique
Parenting Promotion
Referral
Role Enhancement
Teaching: Disease Process

Family Processes, Interrupted

Definition: Change in family relationships and/or functioning

Suggested Nursing Interventions for Problem Resolution:
Coping Enhancement
Counseling
Crisis Intervention
Developmental Enhancement: Adolescent
Developmental Enhancement: Child
Emotional Support
Family Integrity Promotion
Family Integrity Promotion: Childbearing Family
Family Involvement Promotion
Family Mobilization
Family Presence Facilitation
Family Process Maintenance
Family Support
Family Therapy
Financial Resource Assistance
Health System Guidance
Normalization Promotion
Resiliency Promotion
Role Enhancement
Support System Enhancement

Additional Optional Interventions:
Assertiveness Training
Attachment Promotion

Behavior Management
Behavior Modification
Caregiver Support
Conflict Mediation
Decision-Making Support
Dementia Management
Family Planning: Contraception
Family Planning: Infertility
Family Planning: Unplanned Pregnancy
Grief Work Facilitation
Guilt Work Facilitation
Home Maintenance Assistance
Infant Care: Newborn
Infant Care: Preterm
Labor Suppression
Mutual Goal Setting
Parent Education: Adolescent
Parent Education: Childrearing Family
Parent Education: Infant
Prenatal Care
Reproductive Technology Management
Respite Care
Self-Esteem Enhancement
Support Group
Visitation Facilitation

Family Processes, Readiness for Enhanced

Definition: A pattern of family functioning that is sufficient to support the well-being of family members and can be strengthened

Suggested Nursing Interventions for Problem Resolution:
Coping Enhancement
Counseling
Decision-Making Support
Developmental Enhancement: Adolescent
Developmental Enhancement: Child
Emotional Support
Family Integrity Promotion
Family Integrity Promotion: Childbearing Family
Family Involvement Promotion
Family Mobilization
Family Process Maintenance
Family Support
Health Education
Health Screening
Health System Guidance
Normalization Promotion
Parent Education: Adolescent

Parent Education: Childrearing Family
Parent Education: Infant
Resiliency Promotion
Role Enhancement
Support System Enhancement

Additional Optional Interventions:
Caregiver Support
Conflict Mediation
Family Planning: Contraception
Family Planning: Infertility
Family Planning: Unplanned Pregnancy
Family Therapy
Financial Resource Assistance
Grief Work Facilitation
Guilt Work Facilitation
Support Group

Family Therapeutic Regimen Management, Ineffective

Definition: A pattern of regulating and integrating into family processes a program for the treatment of illness and its sequelae that is unsatisfactory for meeting specific health goals

Suggested Nursing Interventions for Problem Resolution:
Caregiver Support
Case Management
Conflict Mediation
Counseling
Decision-Making Support
Family Integrity Promotion
Family Involvement Promotion
Family Mobilization
Family Process Maintenance
Family Support
Family Therapy
Financial Resource Assistance
Health System Guidance
Normalization Promotion
Risk Identification
Role Enhancement

Sibling Support
Sustenance Support
Teaching: Disease Process
Teaching: Procedure/Treatment

Additional Optional Interventions:
Abuse Protection Support
Coping Enhancement
Culture Brokerage
Home Maintenance Assistance
Referral
Relocation Stress Reduction
Resiliency Promotion
Respite Care
Self-Efficacy Enhancement
Support Group
Support System Enhancement

Fatigue

Definition: An overwhelming sustained sense of exhaustion and decreased capacity for physical and mental work at the usual level

Suggested Nursing Interventions for Problem Resolution:
Energy Management
Environmental Management
Exercise Promotion
Mood Management
Mutual Goal Setting
Nutrition Management
Sleep Enhancement

Additional Optional Interventions:
Activity Therapy
Anxiety Reduction
Asthma Management

Chemotherapy Management
Coping Enhancement
Decision-Making Support
Dementia Management
Exercise Promotion: Strength Training
Exercise Promotion: Stretching
Exercise Therapy: Ambulation
Exercise Therapy: Balance
Exercise Therapy: Joint Mobility
Exercise Therapy: Muscle Control
Medication Management
Relaxation Therapy
Support System Enhancement

Fear

Definition: Response to a perceived threat that is consciously recognized as a danger

Suggested Nursing Interventions for Problem Resolution:
Anxiety Reduction
Calming Technique
Cognitive Restructuring
Coping Enhancement
Counseling
Crisis Intervention
Decision-Making Support

Emotional Support
Environmental Management
Examination Assistance
Preparatory Sensory Information
Presence
Security Enhancement
Support System Enhancement
Touch

Additional Optional Interventions:
Anger Control Assistance
Art Therapy
Autogenic Training
Biofeedback
Childbirth Preparation
Communication Enhancement: Hearing Deficit
Communication Enhancement: Visual Deficit
Family Presence Facilitation
Grief Work Facilitation: Perinatal Death
Guided Imagery
High-Risk Pregnancy Care
Hypnosis

Labor Suppression
Meditation Facilitation
Progressive Muscle Relaxation
Relaxation Therapy
Reminiscence Therapy
Self-Esteem Enhancement
Spiritual Support
Support Group
Teaching: Preoperative
Teaching: Procedure/Treatment
Therapy Group
Vital Signs Monitoring

Fluid Balance, Readiness for Enhanced

Definition: A pattern of equilibrium between the fluid volume and chemical composition of body fluids that is sufficient for meeting physical needs and can be strengthened

Suggested Nursing Interventions for Problem Resolution:
Electrolyte Management
Fluid/Electrolyte Management
Fluid Management
Fluid Monitoring
Medication Management
Self-Efficacy Enhancement
Vital Signs Monitoring

Additional Optional Interventions:
Fever Treatment
Hypovolemia Management
Intravenous (IV) Insertion
Intravenous (IV) Therapy
Nutrition Management
Teaching: Individual

Fluid Volume, Deficient

Definition: Decreased intravascular, interstitial, and/or intracellular fluid. This refers to dehydration, water loss alone without change in sodium

Suggested Nursing Interventions for Problem Resolution:
Bleeding Precautions
Bleeding Reduction
Bleeding Reduction: Antepartum Uterus
Bleeding Reduction: Gastrointestinal
Bleeding Reduction: Postpartum Uterus
Bleeding Reduction: Wound
Blood Products Administration
Cardiac Care: Acute
Central Venous Access Device Management
Diarrhea Management
Electrolyte Management
Electrolyte Management: Hypercalcemia
Electrolyte Management: Hyperkalemia
Electrolyte Management: Hypermagnesemia
Electrolyte Management: Hypernatremia
Electrolyte Management: Hyperphosphatemia
Electrolyte Management: Hypocalcemia
Electrolyte Management: Hypokalemia
Electrolyte Management: Hypomagnesemia
Electrolyte Management: Hyponatremia
Electrolyte Management: Hypophosphatemia
Electrolyte Monitoring

Fever Treatment
Fluid/Electrolyte Management
Fluid Management
Fluid Monitoring
Hypovolemia Management
Intravenous (IV) Insertion
Intravenous (IV) Therapy
Shock Management
Shock Management: Volume
Shock Prevention
Surveillance
Vital Signs Monitoring
Vomiting Management

Additional Optional Interventions:
Bottle Feeding
Capillary Blood Sample
Dysrhythmia Management
Feeding
Gastrointestinal Intubation
Hemodynamic Regulation
Medication Management
Neurologic Monitoring

Nutrition Management
Peripherally Inserted Central Catheter (PICC) Care
Phlebotomy: Arterial Blood Sample
Phlebotomy: Cannulated Vessel
Phlebotomy: Venous Blood Sample
Temperature Regulation
Total Parenteral Nutrition (TPN) Administration

Tube Care: Chest
Tube Care: Gastrointestinal
Urinary Catheterization
Weight Management
Wound Care
Wound Care: Burns

Fluid Volume, Excess

Definition: Increased isotonic fluid retention

Suggested Nursing Interventions for Problem Resolution:
Acid-Base Management
Electrolyte Management
Electrolyte Management: Hypercalcemia
Electrolyte Management: Hyperkalemia
Electrolyte Management: Hypermagnesemia
Electrolyte Management: Hypernatremia
Electrolyte Management: Hyperphosphatemia
Electrolyte Management: Hypocalcemia
Electrolyte Management: Hypokalemia
Electrolyte Management: Hypomagnesemia
Electrolyte Management: Hyponatremia
Electrolyte Management: Hypophosphatemia
Electrolyte Monitoring
Fluid/Electrolyte Management
Fluid Management
Fluid Monitoring
Hypervolemia Management
Intravenous (IV) Insertion
Intravenous (IV) Therapy
Vital Signs Monitoring

Additional Optional Interventions:
Capillary Blood Sample
Cerebral Edema Management

Dialysis Access Maintenance
Dysrhythmia Management
Feeding
Gastrointestinal Intubation
Hemodialysis Therapy
Hemodynamic Regulation
Invasive Hemodynamic Monitoring
Medication Management
Neurologic Monitoring
Nutrition Management
Peripherally Inserted Central Catheter (PICC) Care
Peritoneal Dialysis Therapy
Phlebotomy: Arterial Blood Sample
Phlebotomy: Cannulated Vessel
Phlebotomy: Venous Blood Sample
Positioning
Skin Surveillance
Total Parenteral Nutrition (TPN) Administration
Tube Care: Gastrointestinal
Urinary Catheterization
Weight Management
Wound Care

Fluid Volume, Risk for Deficient

Definition: At risk for experiencing decreased intravascular, interstitial, and/or intracellular fluid. This refers to dehydration, water loss alone without change in sodium

Suggested Nursing Interventions for Problem Resolution:
Autotransfusion
Bleeding Precautions
Bleeding Reduction
Bleeding Reduction: Antepartum Uterus
Bleeding Reduction: Gastrointestinal
Bleeding Reduction: Nasal
Bleeding Reduction: Postpartum Uterus
Bleeding Reduction: Wound
Blood Products Administration
Bottle Feeding
Cardiac Care: Acute
Central Venous Access Device Management
Diarrhea Management

Electrolyte Management
Electrolyte Management: Hypernatremia
Electrolyte Monitoring
Fever Treatment
Fluid/Electrolyte Management
Fluid Management
Fluid Monitoring
Fluid Resuscitation
Hypovolemia Management
Infection Protection
Intravenous (IV) Insertion
Intravenous (IV) Therapy
Shock Management
Shock Management: Volume

Shock Prevention
Surveillance
Vital Signs Monitoring
Vomiting Management

Additional Optional Interventions:
Capillary Blood Sample
Feeding
Gastrointestinal Intubation
Malignant Hyperthermia Precautions
Medication Management
Neurologic Monitoring
Nutrition Management
Peripherally Inserted Central Catheter (PICC) Care

Phlebotomy: Arterial Blood Sample
Phlebotomy: Cannulated Vessel
Phlebotomy: Venous Blood Sample
Risk Identification
Temperature Regulation
Total Parenteral Nutrition (TPN) Administration
Tube Care: Chest
Tube Care: Gastrointestinal
Urinary Catheterization
Weight Management
Wound Care
Wound Care: Burns
Wound Care: Closed Drainage

Fluid Volume, Risk for Imbalanced

Definition: At risk for a decrease, increase, or rapid shift from one to the other of intravascular, interstitial, and/or intracellular fluid that may compromise health. This refers to body fluid loss, gain, or both.

Suggested Nursing Interventions for Problem Resolution:
Autotransfusion
Bleeding Precautions
Bleeding Reduction
Bleeding Reduction: Gastrointestinal
Blood Products Administration
Central Venous Access Device Management
Electrolyte Management
Electrolyte Monitoring
Fever Treatment
Fluid/Electrolyte Management
Fluid Management
Fluid Monitoring
Gastrointestinal Intubation
Hemodynamic Regulation
Hypervolemia Management
Hypovolemia Management
Infection Control
Infection Protection
Intravenous (IV) Insertion
Intravenous (IV) Therapy
Invasive Hemodynamic Monitoring
Risk Identification
Shock Management

Shock Management: Vasogenic
Shock Management: Volume
Shock Prevention
Surveillance
Vital Signs Monitoring
Wound Care: Burns

Additional Optional Interventions:
Capillary Blood Sample
Cerebral Edema Management
Dysrhythmia Management
Medication Management
Neurologic Monitoring
Nutrition Management
Peripherally Inserted Central Catheter (PICC) Care
Phlebotomy: Arterial Blood Sample
Phlebotomy: Cannulated Vessel
Phlebotomy: Venous Blood Sample
Temperature Regulation
Total Parenteral Nutrition (TPN) Administration
Tube Care: Chest
Tube Care: Gastrointestinal
Urinary Catheterization
Wound Care

Gas Exchange, Impaired

Definition: Excess or deficit in oxygenation and/or carbon dioxide elimination at the alveolar-capillary membrane

Suggested Nursing Interventions for Problem Resolution:
Acid-Base Management
Acid-Base Management: Metabolic Acidosis
Acid-Base Management: Metabolic Alkalosis
Acid-Base Management: Respiratory Acidosis
Acid-Base Management: Respiratory Alkalosis
Acid-Base Monitoring
Airway Management
Bedside Laboratory Testing
Cough Enhancement
Exercise Promotion
Laboratory Data Interpretation
Mechanical Ventilation Management: Invasive
Mechanical Ventilation Management: Noninvasive
Oxygen Therapy
Postanesthesia Care
Respiratory Monitoring
Resuscitation: Neonate
Vital Signs Monitoring

Additional Optional Interventions:
Airway Suctioning
Allergy Management
Anxiety Reduction
Artificial Airway Management
Aspiration Precautions
Asthma Management

Chest Physiotherapy
Coping Enhancement
Dysrhythmia Management
Embolus Care: Pulmonary
Energy Management
Exercise Therapy: Ambulation
Fluid Management
Fluid Monitoring
Hemodynamic Regulation
Intravenous (IV) Insertion
Intravenous (IV) Therapy
Invasive Hemodynamic Monitoring
Malignant Hyperthermia Precautions
Mechanical Ventilatory Weaning
Nutrition Management
Pain Management
Peripherally Inserted Central Catheter (PICC) Care
Phlebotomy: Arterial Blood Sample
Positioning
Resuscitation
Shock Management
Smoking Cessation Assistance
Surveillance
Total Parenteral Nutrition (TPN) Administration
Tube Care: Chest
Ventilation Assistance

Gastrointestinal Motility, Dysfunctional

Definition: Increased, decreased, ineffective, or lack of peristaltic activity within the gastrointestinal system

Suggested Nursing Interventions for Problem Resolution:
Bowel Management
Diarrhea Management
Diet Staging
Flatulence Reduction
Gastrointestinal Intubation
Medication Administration
Medication Management
Nausea Management
Tube Care: Gastrointestinal
Vomiting Management

Additional Optional Interventions:
Allergy Management
Bowel Incontinence Care
Bowel Training
Constipation/Impaction Management
Enema Administration
Enteral Tube Feeding
Nutritional Counseling
Nutritional Monitoring
Ostomy Care

Gastrointestinal Motility, Risk for Dysfunctional

Definition: At risk for increased, decreased, ineffective, or lack of peristaltic activity within the gastrointestinal system

Suggested Nursing Interventions for Problem Resolution:
Anxiety Reduction
Diet Staging
Exercise Promotion
Exercise Therapy: Ambulation
Infection Control
Infection Protection
Medication Management
Nutrition Management
Nutrition Therapy
Nutritional Counseling

Nutritional Monitoring
Risk Identification
Surveillance
Teaching: Disease Process
Teaching: Prescribed Diet
Teaching: Prescribed Medication

Additional Optional Interventions:
Gastrointestinal Intubation
Ostomy Care
Tube Care: Gastrointestinal

Gastrointestinal Perfusion, Risk for Ineffective

Definition: At risk for decrease in gastrointestinal circulation that may compromise health

Suggested Nursing Interventions for Problem Resolution:
Bleeding Precautions
Bleeding Reduction
Bleeding Reduction: Gastrointestinal
Cardiac Care
Cardiac Care: Acute
Circulatory Care: Arterial Insufficiency
Circulatory Care: Venous Insufficiency
Fluid Management
Hemodynamic Regulation
Medication Management
Nutritional Counseling
Nutrition Therapy
Pacemaker Management: Permanent
Pacemaker Management: Temporary

Risk Identification
Smoking Cessation Assistance
Substance Use Treatment
Surveillance
Teaching: Disease Process
Teaching: Prescribed Diet
Teaching: Prescribed Medication
Teaching: Procedure/Treatment
Thrombolytic Therapy Management

Additional Optional Interventions:
Gastrointestinal Intubation
Tube Care: Gastrointestinal
Vital Signs Monitoring

Grieving

Definition: A normal complex process that includes emotional, physical, spiritual, social, and intellectual responses and behaviors by which individuals, families, and communities incorporate an actual, anticipated, or perceived loss in their daily lives

Suggested Nursing Interventions for Problem Resolution:
Active Listening
Anger Control Assistance
Anticipatory Guidance
Coping Enhancement
Counseling
Dying Care
Emotional Support
Family Integrity Promotion
Family Process Maintenance
Family Support
Grief Work Facilitation
Grief Work Facilitation: Perinatal Death
Hope Inspiration
Journaling
Presence
Reminiscence Therapy
Sleep Enhancement
Support System Enhancement

Touch
Truth Telling

Additional Optional Interventions:
Bioterrorism Preparedness
Community Disaster Preparedness
Environmental Management
Environmental Management: Comfort
Family Presence Facilitation
Family Therapy
Mood Management
Normalization Promotion
Organ Procurement
Reproductive Technology Management
Spiritual Growth Facilitation
Spiritual Support
Substance Use Prevention
Support Group

Grieving, Complicated

Definition: A disorder that occurs after the death of a significant other, in which the experience of distress accompanying bereavement fails to follow normative expectations and manifests in functional impairment

Suggested Nursing Interventions for Problem Resolution:
Active Listening
Anger Control Assistance
Anxiety Reduction
Coping Enhancement
Counseling
Crisis Intervention
Culture Brokerage
Emotional Support
Family Integrity Promotion
Family Mobilization
Family Support
Family Therapy
Forgiveness Facilitation
Grief Work Facilitation
Grief Work Facilitation: Perinatal Death
Journaling
Mood Management
Presence

Role Enhancement
Self-Awareness Enhancement
Sleep Enhancement
Spiritual Support

Additional Optional Interventions:
Art Therapy
Guilt Work Facilitation
Hope Inspiration
Mutual Goal Setting
Normalization Promotion
Nutrition Management
Relaxation Therapy
Reminiscence Therapy
Substance Use Prevention
Suicide Prevention
Support Group
Support System Enhancement
Values Clarification

Grieving, Complicated, Risk for

Definition: At risk for a disorder that occurs after the death of a significant other, in which the experience of distress accompanying bereavement fails to follow normative expectations and manifests in functional impairment

Suggested Nursing Interventions for Problem Resolution:
Active Listening
Anger Control Assistance
Coping Enhancement
Counseling
Crisis Intervention
Culture Brokerage
Emotional Support
Family Integrity Promotion
Family Mobilization
Family Support
Family Therapy
Forgiveness Facilitation
Grief Work Facilitation
Grief Work Facilitation: Perinatal Death
Journaling
Mood Management
Presence
Sleep Enhancement
Spiritual Growth Facilitation

Spiritual Support
Support Group
Support System Enhancement

Additional Optional Interventions:
Anxiety Reduction
Art Therapy
Guilt Work Facilitation
Hope Inspiration
Mutual Goal Setting
Normalization Promotion
Nutrition Management
Relaxation Therapy
Reminiscence Therapy
Resiliency Promotion
Risk Identification
Substance Use Prevention
Surveillance
Values Clarification

Growth and Development, Delayed

Definition: Deviations from age-group norms

Suggested Nursing Interventions for Problem Resolution:
Anticipatory Guidance
Attachment Promotion
Behavior Management
Behavior Management: Overactivity/Inattention
Behavior Modification
Behavior Modification: Social Skills
Body Mechanics Promotion
Bowel Incontinence Care: Encopresis
Caregiver Support
Counseling
Developmental Enhancement: Adolescent
Developmental Enhancement: Child
Developmental Enhancement: Infant
Exercise Promotion
Family Therapy
Health Screening
High-Risk Pregnancy Care
Impulse Control Training
Infant Care: Newborn
Infant Care: Preterm
Nutrition Management
Nutrition Therapy
Nutritional Monitoring
Parent Education: Adolescent
Parent Education: Childrearing Family
Parent Education: Infant
Parenting Promotion
Resiliency Promotion
Risk Identification
Self-Responsibility Facilitation
Support Group

Support System Enhancement
Teaching: Infant Stimulation 0-4 Months
Teaching: Infant Stimulation 5-8 Months
Teaching: Infant Stimulation 9-12 Months
Urinary Incontinence Care: Enuresis

Additional Optional Interventions:
Abuse Protection Support: Child
Behavior Management: Sexual
Coping Enhancement
Decision-Making Support
Fire-Setting Precautions
Presence
Reproductive Technology Management
Respite Care
Teaching: Infant Nutrition 0-3 Months
Teaching: Infant Nutrition 4-6 Months
Teaching: Infant Nutrition 7-9 Months
Teaching: Infant Nutrition 10-12 Months
Teaching: Infant Safety 0-3 Months
Teaching: Infant Safety 4-6 Months
Teaching: Infant Safety 7-9 Months
Teaching: Infant Safety 10-12 Months
Teaching: Toddler Nutrition 13-18 Months
Teaching: Toddler Nutrition 19-24 Months
Teaching: Toddler Nutrition 25-36 Months
Teaching: Toddler Safety 13-18 Months
Teaching: Toddler Safety 19-24 Months
Teaching: Toddler Safety 25-36 Months
Teaching: Toilet Training
Weight Management

Growth, Risk for Disproportionate

Definition: At risk for growth above the 97th percentile or below the 3rd percentile for age, crossing two percentile channels

Suggested Nursing Interventions for Problem Resolution:
Attachment Promotion
Behavior Modification
Bottle Feeding
Caregiver Support
Counseling
Eating Disorders Management
Environmental Management: Community
Environmental Management: Violence Prevention
Family Therapy
Health Education
Health Screening
Infection Control
Kangaroo Care
Lactation Counseling
Learning Facilitation
Nutrition Management
Nutrition Therapy
Nutritional Monitoring
Parent Education: Childrearing Family
Preconception Counseling
Prenatal Care
Risk Identification
Risk Identification: Genetic
Substance Use Prevention
Substance Use Treatment

Teaching: Infant Nutrition 0-3 Months
Teaching: Infant Nutrition 4-6 Months
Teaching: Infant Nutrition 7-9 Months
Teaching: Infant Nutrition 10-12 Months
Teaching: Prescribed Diet
Teaching: Toddler Nutrition 13-18 Months
Teaching: Toddler Nutrition 19-24 Months
Teaching: Toddler Nutrition 25-36 Months
Weight Gain Assistance
Weight Management
Weight Reduction Assistance

Additional Optional Interventions:
Abuse Protection Support: Child
Anger Control Assistance
Coping Enhancement
Enteral Tube Feeding
Financial Resource Assistance
Parent Education: Infant
Sibling Support
Swallowing Therapy
Total Parenteral Nutrition (TPN) Administration

Health Behavior, Risk-Prone

Definition: Impaired ability to modify lifestyle/behaviors in a manner that improves health status

Suggested Nursing Interventions for Problem Resolution:
Behavior Modification
Complex Relationship Building
Coping Enhancement
Decision-Making Support
Financial Resource Assistance
Health System Guidance
Learning Facilitation
Learning Readiness Enhancement
Mutual Goal Setting
Role Enhancement
Self-Efficacy Enhancement
Self-Responsibility Facilitation
Teaching: Disease Process
Values Clarification

Additional Optional Interventions:
Anticipatory Guidance
Anxiety Reduction
Caregiver Support
Counseling
Health Education
Patient Contracting
Risk Identification
Smoking Cessation Assistance
Substance Use Treatment
Support Group
Therapy Group

Health Maintenance, Ineffective

Definition: Inability to identify, manage, and/or seek help to maintain health

Suggested Nursing Interventions for Problem Resolution:
Anticipatory Guidance
Coping Enhancement
Decision-Making Support
Discharge Planning
Exercise Promotion
Family Involvement Promotion
Financial Resource Assistance
Health Education
Health Literacy Enhancement
Health Screening
Health System Guidance
Learning Facilitation
Learning Readiness Enhancement
Mutual Goal Setting
Referral
Risk Identification
Risk Identification: Childbearing Family
Self-Efficacy Enhancement
Self-Responsibility Facilitation
Support System Enhancement
Teaching: Disease Process
Teaching: Individual
Teaching: Procedure/Treatment

Additional Optional Interventions:
Case Management
Cognitive Restructuring
Counseling
Environmental Management: Community
Environmental Management: Worker Safety
Family Mobilization
Family Process Maintenance
Grief Work Facilitation
Medication Management
Nutrition Management
Patient Contracting
Self-Awareness Enhancement
Self-Care Assistance
Self-Modification Assistance
Smoking Cessation Assistance
Spiritual Support
Substance Use Prevention
Support Group
Values Clarification
Weight Management

Home Maintenance, Impaired

Definition: Inability to independently maintain a safe, growth-promoting immediate environment

Suggested Nursing Interventions for Problem Resolution:
Discharge Planning
Family Support
Financial Resource Assistance
Home Maintenance Assistance
Parenting Promotion
Pass Facilitation
Role Enhancement
Self-Care Assistance: IADL
Support System Enhancement
Sustenance Support

Additional Optional Interventions:
Caregiver Support
Counseling
Energy Management
Environmental Management
Environmental Management: Home Preparation
Mutual Goal Setting
Referral
Teaching: Individual

Hope, Readiness for Enhanced

Definition: A pattern of expectations and desires for mobilizing energy on one's own behalf that is sufficient for well-being and can be strengthened

Suggested Nursing Interventions for Problem Resolution:
Decision-Making Support
Emotional Support
Energy Management
Hope Inspiration
Journaling
Mood Management
Mutual Goal Setting
Patient Contracting
Presence
Reminiscence Therapy
Self-Efficacy Enhancement
Self-Esteem Enhancement
Self-Modification Assistance
Self-Responsibility Facilitation

Sleep Enhancement
Socialization Enhancement
Spiritual Growth Facilitation
Support Group
Support System Enhancement

Additional Optional Interventions:
Activity Therapy
Animal-Assisted Therapy
Counseling
Exercise Promotion
Grief Work Facilitation
Music Therapy
Spiritual Support

Hopelessness

Definition: Subjective state in which an individual sees limited or no alternatives or personal choices available and is unable to mobilize energy on his/her own behalf

Suggested Nursing Interventions for Problem Resolution:
Complex Relationship Building
Coping Enhancement
Decision-Making Support
Emotional Support
Energy Management
Hope Inspiration
Mood Management
Presence
Reminiscence Therapy
Sleep Enhancement

Socialization Enhancement
Spiritual Growth Facilitation
Support Group
Support System Enhancement
Values Clarification

Additional Optional Interventions:
Activity Therapy
Anger Control Assistance
Animal-Assisted Therapy
Cognitive Stimulation

Counseling
Crisis Intervention
Distraction
Electroconvulsive Therapy (ECT) Management
Exercise Promotion
Exercise Therapy: Ambulation
Grief Work Facilitation
Grief Work Facilitation: Perinatal Death
Music Therapy

Mutual Goal Setting
Patient Contracting
Phototherapy: Mood/Sleep Regulation
Resiliency Promotion
Self-Care Assistance
Self-Modification Assistance
Spiritual Support
Suicide Prevention
Therapeutic Play

Human Dignity, Risk for Compromised

Definition: At risk for perceived loss of respect and honor

Suggested Nursing Interventions for Problem Resolution:
Anticipatory Guidance
Culture Brokerage
Decision-Making Support
Examination Assistance
Health Care Information Exchange
Health System Guidance
Patient Rights Protection
Presence

Additional Optional Interventions:
Abuse Protection Support
Admission Care
Bowel Incontinence Care
Coping Enhancement
Discharge Planning
Family Involvement Promotion
Financial Resource Assistance
Multidisciplinary Care Conference
Risk Identification

Hyperthermia

Definition: Body temperature elevated above normal range

Suggested Nursing Interventions For Problem Resolution:
Bathing
Environmental Management
Fever Treatment
Fluid Management
Hemodynamic Regulation
Infant Care: Newborn
Infection Control
Infection Protection
Malignant Hyperthermia Precautions
Medication Management
Medication Prescribing
Shock Management

Temperature Regulation
Temperature Regulation: Perioperative
Vital Signs Monitoring

Additional Optional Interventions:
Heat/Cold Application
Nutrition Management
Oxygen Therapy
Peripherally Inserted Central Catheter (PICC) Care
Seizure Management
Seizure Precautions
Skin Surveillance
Total Parenteral Nutrition (TPN) Administration

Hypothermia

Definition: Body temperature below normal range

Suggested Nursing Interventions for Problem Resolution:
Electrolyte Monitoring
Environmental Management
Fluid/Electrolyte Management
Fluid Management
Fluid Monitoring
Hemodynamic Regulation
Hypothermia Induction Therapy
Hypothermia Treatment
Infant Care: Newborn
Oxygen Therapy
Respiratory Monitoring
Shock Management
Shock Prevention

Temperature Regulation
Temperature Regulation: Perioperative
Vital Signs Monitoring

Additional Optional Interventions:
Circulatory Care: Arterial Insufficiency
Circulatory Care: Venous Insufficiency
Heat/Cold Application
Peripherally Inserted Central Catheter (PICC) Care
Shock Management: Cardiac
Shock Management: Vasogenic
Skin Surveillance
Total Parenteral Nutrition (TPN) Administration

Immunization Status, Readiness for Enhanced

Definition: A pattern of conforming to local, national, and/or international standards of immunization to prevent infectious disease(s) that is sufficient to protect a person, family, or community and can be strengthened

Suggested Nursing Interventions for Problem Resolution:
Anticipatory Guidance
Commendation
Community Health Development
Health Education
Health Screening
Health System Guidance
Immunization/Vaccination Management
Medication Administration
Medication Prescribing

Program Development
Risk Identification
Self-Efficacy Enhancement

Additional Optional Interventions:
Documentation
Family Mobilization
Financial Resource Assistance
Health Policy Monitoring
Insurance Authorization

Impulse Control, Ineffective

Definition: A pattern of performing rapid, unplanned reactions to internal or external stimuli without regard for the negative consequences of these reactions to the impulsive individual or to others

Suggested Nursing Interventions for Problem Resolution:
Anger Control Assistance
Behavior Management
Body Image Enhancement
Coping Enhancement
Decision-Making Support
Hope Inspiration
Impulse Control Training
Limit Setting
Milieu Therapy
Mood Management
Self-Awareness Enhancement
Self-Esteem Enhancement

Self-Responsibility Facilitation
Substance Use Treatment
Values Clarification

Additional Optional Interventions:
Behavior Management
Behavior Modification: Social Skills
Energy Management
Environmental Management: Violence Prevention
Smoking Cessation Assistance
Suicide Prevention
Support Group

Infant Behavior, Disorganized

Definition: Disintegrated physiological and neurobehavioral responses of infant to the environment

Suggested Nursing Interventions for Problem Resolution:
Attachment Promotion
Energy Management
Environmental Management
Environmental Management: Comfort
Infant Care
Infant Care: Newborn
Infant Care: Preterm
Kangaroo Care
Lactation Counseling
Neurologic Monitoring
Nonnutritive Sucking
Nutritional Monitoring
Pain Management
Positioning
Respiratory Monitoring

Sleep Enhancement
Temperature Regulation
Vital Signs Monitoring

Additional Optional Interventions:
Bottle Feeding
Circumcision Care
Cutaneous Stimulation
Parent Education: Infant
Risk Identification: Genetic
Teaching: Infant Nutrition 0-3 Months
Teaching: Infant Nutrition 4-6 Months
Teaching: Infant Nutrition 7-9 Months
Teaching: Infant Nutrition 10-12 Months
Teaching: Infant Safety 0-3 Months
Teaching: Infant Safety 4-6 Months

Teaching: Infant Safety 7-9 Months
Teaching: Infant Safety 10-12 Months
Teaching: Infant Stimulation 0-4 Months
Teaching: Infant Stimulation 5-8 Months

Teaching: Infant Stimulation 9-12 Months
Touch
Visitation Facilitation

Infant Behavior, Organized, Readiness for Enhanced

Definition: A pattern of modulation of the physiological and behavioral systems of functioning (i.e., autonomic, motor, state-organization, self-regulatory, and attentional-interactional systems) in an infant that is sufficient for well-being and can be strengthened

Suggested Nursing Interventions for Problem Resolution:
Anticipatory Guidance
Attachment Promotion
Energy Management
Environmental Management
Family Integrity Promotion: Childbearing Family
Family Mobilization
Infant Care
Infant Care: Newborn
Infant Care: Preterm
Kangaroo Care
Nonnutritive Sucking
Pain Management
Parent Education: Infant
Sleep Enhancement
Touch

Additional Optional Interventions:
Circumcision Care
Cutaneous Stimulation

Developmental Enhancement: Child
Lactation Counseling
Music Therapy
Surveillance
Teaching: Infant Nutrition 0-3 Months
Teaching: Infant Nutrition 4-6 Months
Teaching: Infant Nutrition 7-9 Months
Teaching: Infant Nutrition 10-12 Months
Teaching: Infant Safety 0-3 Months
Teaching: Infant Safety 4-6 Months
Teaching: Infant Safety 7-9 Months
Teaching: Infant Safety 10-12 Months
Teaching: Infant Stimulation 0-4 Months
Teaching: Infant Stimulation 5-8 Months
Teaching: Infant Stimulation 9-12 Months
Visitation Facilitation
Vital Signs Monitoring

Infant Behavior, Risk for Disorganized

Definition: At risk for alteration in integrating and modulation of the physiological and behavioral systems of functioning (i.e., autonomic, motor, state-organization, self-regulatory, and attentional-interactional systems)

Suggested Nursing Interventions for Problem Resolution:
Environmental Management
Environmental Management: Comfort
Infant Care
Infant Care: Newborn
Infant Care: Preterm
Kangaroo Care
Lactation Counseling
Neurologic Monitoring
Nonnutritive Sucking
Nutritional Monitoring
Pain Management
Positioning
Respiratory Monitoring
Risk Identification
Surveillance
Vital Signs Monitoring

Additional Optional Interventions:
Bottle Feeding
Circumcision Care
Teaching: Infant Nutrition 0-3 Months
Teaching: Infant Nutrition 4-6 Months
Teaching: Infant Nutrition 7-9 Months
Teaching: Infant Nutrition 10-12 Months
Teaching: Infant Safety 0-3 Months
Teaching: Infant Safety 4-6 Months
Teaching: Infant Safety 7-9 Months
Teaching: Infant Safety 10-12 Months
Teaching: Infant Stimulation 0-4 Months
Teaching: Infant Stimulation 5-8 Months
Teaching: Infant Stimulation 9-12 Months
Temperature Regulation

Infant Feeding Pattern, Ineffective

Definition: Impaired ability of an infant to suck or coordinate the suck/swallow response, resulting in inadequate oral nutrition for metabolic needs

Suggested Nursing Interventions for Problem Resolution:
Aspiration Precautions
Bottle Feeding
Energy Management
Enteral Tube Feeding
Environmental Management
Fluid Management
Fluid Monitoring
Kangaroo Care
Lactation Counseling
Nonnutritive Sucking
Nutrition Management
Nutritional Monitoring
Swallowing Therapy
Tube Care: Umbilical Line
Weight Management

Additional Optional Interventions:
Gastrointestinal Intubation
Infant Care
Parent Education: Infant
Referral
Teaching: Infant Nutrition 0-3 Months
Teaching: Infant Nutrition 4-6 Months
Teaching: Infant Nutrition 7-9 Months
Teaching: Infant Nutrition 10-12 Months
Teaching: Infant Safety 0-3 Months
Teaching: Infant Safety 4-6 Months
Teaching: Infant Safety 7-9 Months
Teaching: Infant Safety 10-12 Months
Teaching: Infant Stimulation 0-4 Months
Teaching: Infant Stimulation 5-8 Months
Teaching: Infant Stimulation 9-12 Months

Infection, Risk for

Definition: At risk for being invaded by pathogenic organisms

Suggested Nursing Interventions for Problem Resolution:
Amnioinfusion
Amputation Care
Circumcision Care
Communicable Disease Management
Cough Enhancement
High-Risk Pregnancy Care
Immunization/Vaccination Management
Incision Site Care
Infection Control
Infection Control: Intraoperative
Infection Protection
Intrapartal Care
Intrapartal Care: High-Risk Delivery
Labor Induction
Medication Management
Medication Prescribing
Nutrition Management
Nutrition Therapy
Nutritional Monitoring
Oral Health Promotion
Oral Health Restoration
Perineal Care
Postpartal Care
Pregnancy Termination Care
Pressure Ulcer Care
Pressure Ulcer Prevention
Risk Identification
Skin Care: Donor Site
Skin Care: Graft Site
Skin Surveillance
Surveillance

Teaching: Safe Sex
Tube Care: Umbilical Line
Wound Care
Wound Care: Burns
Wound Care: Closed Drainage

Additional Optional Interventions:
Airway Management
Bathing
Cesarean Birth Care
Electrolyte Monitoring
Environmental Management
Exercise Promotion
Fertility Preservation
Fluid/Electrolyte Management
Home Maintenance Assistance
Positioning
Pruritus Management
Respiratory Monitoring
Resuscitation: Fetus
Resuscitation: Neonate
Smoking Cessation Assistance
Teaching: Disease Process
Teaching: Sexuality
Tube Care
Tube Care: Chest
Tube Care: Gastrointestinal
Tube Care: Urinary
Tube Care: Ventriculostomy/Lumbar Drain
Vital Signs Monitoring
Wound Care: Nonhealing
Wound Irrigation

Injury, Risk for

Definition: At risk for injury as a result of environmental conditions interacting with the individual's adaptive and defensive resources

Suggested Nursing Interventions for Problem Resolution:
Abuse Protection Support
Abuse Protection Support: Child
Abuse Protection Support: Domestic Partner
Abuse Protection Support: Elder
Allergy Management
Bleeding Precautions
Communicable Disease Management
Delusion Management
Dementia Management
Dementia Management: Bathing
Dementia Management: Wandering
Electronic Fetal Monitoring: Antepartum
Electronic Fetal Monitoring: Intrapartum
Energy Management
Environmental Management: Safety
Environmental Management: Violence Prevention
Exercise Promotion
Exercise Therapy: Ambulation
Fall Prevention
Fire-Setting Precautions
Home Maintenance Assistance
Immunization/Vaccination Management
Impulse Control Training
Infection Control
Intrapartal Care
Intrapartal Care: High-Risk Delivery
Labor Induction
Labor Suppression
Laser Precautions
Latex Precautions
Malignant Hyperthermia Precautions
Medication Management
Nutrition Therapy
Nutritional Monitoring
Parent Education: Adolescent
Parent Education: Childrearing Family
Parent Education: Infant
Physical Restraint
Pneumatic Tourniquet Precautions
Positioning: Intraoperative
Postanesthesia Care

Pressure Management
Pressure Ulcer Care
Pressure Ulcer Prevention
Reality Orientation
Risk Identification
Seclusion
Security Enhancement
Sedation Management
Seizure Management
Seizure Precautions
Sports-Injury Prevention: Youth
Surgical Precautions
Surveillance
Teaching: Infant Safety 0-3 Months
Teaching: Infant Safety 4-6 Months
Teaching: Infant Safety 7-9 Months
Teaching: Infant Safety 10-12 Months
Teaching: Toddler Safety 13-18 Months
Teaching: Toddler Safety 19-24 Months
Teaching: Toddler Safety 25-36 Months
Thrombolytic Therapy Management
Transfer

Additional Optional Interventions:
Airway Management
Airway Suctioning
Anger Control Assistance
Artificial Airway Management
Asthma Management
Cerebral Edema Management
Electroconvulsive Therapy (ECT) Management
Health Education
High-Risk Pregnancy Care
Infection Protection
Medication Administration
Neurologic Monitoring
Presence
Referral
Respite Care
Resuscitation: Fetus
Resuscitation: Neonate

Insomnia

Definition: A disruption in amount and quality of sleep that impairs functioning

Suggested Nursing Interventions for Problem Resolution:
Dementia Management
Energy Management
Environmental Management
Environmental Management: Comfort
Hormone Replacement Therapy
Medication Administration
Medication Management
Medication Prescribing
Mood Management
Pain Management
Phototherapy: Mood/Sleep Regulation
Relaxation Therapy
Security Enhancement
Sleep Enhancement
Touch

Additional Optional Interventions:
Anxiety Reduction
Autogenic Training
Bathing
Calming Technique
Coping Enhancement
Exercise Promotion
Exercise Therapy: Ambulation
Kangaroo Care
Massage
Meditation Facilitation
Music Therapy
Nutrition Management
Positioning
Progressive Muscle Relaxation
Self-Care Assistance: Toileting
Urinary Incontinence Care: Enuresis

Intracranial Adaptive Capacity, Decreased

Definition: Intracranial fluid dynamic mechanisms that normally compensate for increases in intracranial volumes are compromised, resulting in repeated disproportionate increases in intracranial pressure (ICP) in response to a variety of noxious and non-noxious stimuli

Suggested Nursing Interventions for Problem Resolution:
Cerebral Edema Management
Cerebral Perfusion Promotion
Fluid/Electrolyte Management
Fluid Management
Fluid Monitoring
Intracranial Pressure (ICP) Monitoring
Intravenous (IV) Insertion
Intravenous (IV) Therapy
Laboratory Data Interpretation
Medication Administration
Medication Management
Neurologic Monitoring
Peripheral Sensation Management
Positioning: Neurologic

Surveillance
Tube Care: Ventriculostomy/Lumbar Drain
Vital Signs Monitoring

Additional Optional Interventions:
Acid-Base Management
Airway Management
Anxiety Reduction
Infection Protection
Patient Rights Protection
Positioning
Presence
Seizure Management
Seizure Precautions
Touch

Knowledge Deficient

Definition: Absence or deficiency of cognitive information related to a specific topic

Suggested Nursing Interventions for Problem Resolution:
Anticipatory Guidance
Childbirth Preparation
Family Planning: Contraception
Health Education
Health Literacy Enhancement
Health System Guidance
Lactation Counseling
Learning Facilitation
Learning Readiness Enhancement
Parent Education: Adolescent
Parent Education: Childrearing Family
Parent Education: Infant
Patient Rights Protection
Preconception Counseling
Preparatory Sensory Information
Substance Use Prevention
Teaching: Disease Process
Teaching: Foot Care
Teaching: Individual
Teaching: Infant Nutrition 0-3 Months
Teaching: Infant Nutrition 4-6 Months
Teaching: Infant Nutrition 7-9 Months
Teaching: Infant Nutrition 10-12 Months
Teaching: Infant Safety 0-3 Months
Teaching: Infant Safety 4-6 Months
Teaching: Infant Safety 7-9 Months
Teaching: Infant Safety 10-12 Months
Teaching: Infant Stimulation 0-4 Months
Teaching: Infant Stimulation 5-8 Months
Teaching: Infant Stimulation 9-12 Months
Teaching: Preoperative
Teaching: Prescribed Diet
Teaching: Prescribed Exercise
Teaching: Prescribed Medication
Teaching: Procedure/Treatment
Teaching: Psychomotor Skill
Teaching: Safe Sex
Teaching: Sexuality
Teaching: Toddler Nutrition 13-18 Months
Teaching: Toddler Nutrition 19-24 Months
Teaching: Toddler Nutrition 25-36 Months
Teaching: Toddler Safety 13-18 Months
Teaching: Toddler Safety 19-24 Months
Teaching: Toddler Safety 25-36 Months
Teaching: Toilet Training

Additional Optional Interventions:
Admission Care
Allergy Management
Anxiety Reduction
Asthma Management
Behavior Modification
Behavior Modification: Social Skills
Body Mechanics Promotion
Cardiac Risk Management
Circulatory Care: Venous Insufficiency
Counseling
Decision-Making Support
Developmental Enhancement: Child
Discharge Planning
Energy Management
Environmental Management: Safety
Examination Assistance
Fall Prevention
Family Planning: Infertility
Fertility Preservation
Genetic Counseling
Health Screening
Home Maintenance Assistance
Hypervolemia Management
Infection Control
Lactation Counseling
Nutrition Management
Nutritional Counseling
Ostomy Care
Pain Management
Parenting Promotion
Postpartal Care
Prenatal Care
Referral
Risk Identification
Self-Efficacy Enhancement
Self-Modification Assistance
Sexual Counseling
Staff Development
Substance Use Treatment
Support Group
Teaching: Group
Therapeutic Play
Values Clarification
Vehicle Safety Promotion
Weight Management

Knowledge, Readiness for Enhanced

Definition: A pattern of cognitive information related to a specific topic, or its acquisition, that is sufficient for meeting health-related goals and can be strengthened

Suggested Nursing Interventions for Problem Resolution:
Commendation
Decision-Making Support
Health Education
Health System Guidance
Learning Facilitation
Learning Readiness Enhancement
Parenting Promotion
Patient Contracting
Program Development
Self-Efficacy Enhancement
Self-Modification Assistance
Self-Responsibility Facilitation
Social Marketing

Additional Optional Interventions:
Parent Education: Adolescent
Parent Education: Childrearing Family
Parent Education: Infant
Teaching: Disease Process
Teaching: Foot Care
Teaching: Individual
Teaching: Infant Nutrition 0-3 Months
Teaching: Infant Nutrition 4-6 Months

Teaching: Infant Nutrition 7-9 Months
Teaching: Infant Nutrition 10-12 Months
Teaching: Infant Safety 0-3 Months
Teaching: Infant Safety 4-6 Months
Teaching: Infant Safety 7-9 Months
Teaching: Infant Safety 10-12 Months
Teaching: Infant Stimulation 0-4 Months
Teaching: Infant Stimulation 5-8 Months
Teaching: Infant Stimulation 9-12 Months
Teaching: Preoperative
Teaching: Prescribed Diet
Teaching: Prescribed Exercise
Teaching: Prescribed Medication
Teaching: Procedure/Treatment
Teaching: Psychomotor Skill
Teaching: Safe Sex
Teaching: Sexuality
Teaching: Toddler Nutrition 13-18 Months
Teaching: Toddler Nutrition 19-24 Months
Teaching: Toddler Nutrition 25-36 Months
Teaching: Toddler Safety 13-18 Months
Teaching: Toddler Safety 19-24 Months
Teaching: Toddler Safety 25-36 Months
Teaching: Toilet Training

Latex Allergy Response

Definition: A hypersensitive reaction to natural latex rubber products

Suggested Nursing Interventions for Problem Resolution:
Airway Management
Allergy Management
Emergency Care
Environmental Management
Environmental Risk Protection
Latex Precautions
Medication Administration
Medication Administration: Nasal
Medication Administration: Skin
Respiratory Monitoring
Risk Identification

Skin Surveillance
Teaching: Individual
Vital Signs Monitoring

Additional Optional Interventions:
Anaphylaxis Management
Code Management
Fluid Management
Intravenous (IV) Insertion
Intravenous (IV) Therapy
Shock Prevention
Surveillance

Latex Allergy Response, Risk for

Definition: Risk of hypersensitivity to natural latex rubber products that may compromise health

Suggested Nursing Interventions for Problem Resolution:
Allergy Management
Environmental Management
Environmental Risk Protection
Health System Guidance
Latex Precautions
Risk Identification
Teaching: Individual

Additional Optional Interventions:
Environmental Management: Worker Safety
Health Care Information Exchange
Surveillance
Teaching: Prescribed Diet

Lifestyle, Sedentary

Definition: Reports a habit of life that is characterized by a low physical activity level

Suggested Nursing Interventions for Problem Resolution:
Activity Therapy
Exercise Promotion
Exercise Promotion: Strength Training
Exercise Promotion: Stretching
Exercise Therapy: Ambulation
Exercise Therapy: Balance
Exercise Therapy: Joint Mobility
Exercise Therapy: Muscle Control
Self-Modification Assistance

Self-Responsibility Facilitation
Teaching: Prescribed Exercise

Additional Optional Interventions:
Body Mechanics Promotion
Energy Management
Fall Prevention
Recreation Therapy
Therapeutic Play
Weight Management

Liver Function, Risk for Impaired

Definition: At risk for a decrease in liver function that may compromise health

Suggested Nursing Interventions for Problem Resolution:
Infection Control
Infection Protection
Medication Management
Risk Identification
Substance Use Treatment
Substance Use Treatment: Alcohol Withdrawal
Substance Use Treatment: Drug Withdrawal
Substance Use Treatment: Overdose
Surveillance

Teaching: Individual
Teaching: Prescribed Medication

Additional Optional Interventions:
Acid-Base Management
Fluid/Electrolyte Management
Health Screening
Hemodialysis Therapy
Hemofiltration Therapy

Loneliness, Risk for

Definition: At risk of experiencing discomfort associated with a desire or need for more contact with others

Suggested Nursing Interventions for Problem Resolution:
Activity Therapy
Anxiety Reduction
Assertiveness Training
Behavior Modification: Social Skills
Caregiver Support
Complex Relationship Building
Coping Enhancement
Counseling
Emotional Support
Energy Management
Environmental Management
Family Integrity Promotion
Family Integrity Promotion: Childbearing Family
Family Involvement Promotion
Family Mobilization
Family Process Maintenance
Family Support
Grief Work Facilitation
Hope Inspiration
Mood Management

Presence
Relocation Stress Reduction
Self-Awareness Enhancement
Self-Esteem Enhancement
Socialization Enhancement
Support System Enhancement
Visitation Facilitation

Additional Optional Interventions:
Animal-Assisted Therapy
Art Therapy
Body Image Enhancement
Exercise Promotion
Family Therapy
Parenting Promotion
Recreation Therapy
Reminiscence Therapy
Risk Identification
Sibling Support
Support Group
Therapy Group

Maternal-Fetal Dyad, Risk for Disturbed

Definition: At risk for disruption of the symbiotic maternal-fetal dyad as a result of comorbid or pregnancy-related conditions

Suggested Nursing Interventions for Problem Resolution:
Abuse Protection Support: Domestic Partner
Asthma Management
Bleeding Reduction: Antepartum Uterus
Cardiac Care
Cardiac Risk Management
Electronic Fetal Monitoring: Antepartum
High-Risk Pregnancy Care
Medication Management
Nausea Management
Preconception Counseling
Prenatal Care
Respiratory Monitoring
Risk Identification
Seizure Management
Seizure Precautions
Smoking Cessation Assistance
Substance Use Treatment

Substance Use Treatment: Alcohol Withdrawal
Substance Use Treatment: Drug Withdrawal
Surveillance
Surveillance: Late Pregnancy
Teaching: Disease Process
Teaching: Prescribed Diet
Teaching: Prescribed Medication
Ultrasonography: Limited Obstetric
Vital Signs Monitoring
Vomiting Management

Additional Optional Interventions:
Childbirth Preparation
Family Integrity Promotion: Childbearing Family
Labor Induction
Labor Suppression
Support System Enhancement

Memory, Impaired

Definition: Inability to remember or recall bits of information or behavioral skills

Suggested Nursing Interventions for Problem Resolution:
Anxiety Reduction
Cardiac Care
Cerebral Perfusion Promotion
Cognitive Stimulation
Delirium Management
Dementia Management
Electrolyte Monitoring
Environmental Management
Environmental Management: Safety
Fluid/Electrolyte Management
Fluid Management
Fluid Monitoring
Medication Management
Memory Training
Neurologic Monitoring
Oxygen Therapy

Reality Orientation
Surveillance
Validation Therapy

Additional Optional Interventions:
Area Restriction
Calming Technique
Emotional Support
Family Support
Milieu Therapy
Patient Rights Protection
Reminiscence Therapy

Mobility: Bed, Impaired

Definition: Limitation of independent movement from one bed position to another

Suggested Nursing Interventions for Problem Resolution:
Bathing
Bed Rest Care
Body Mechanics Promotion
Dressing
Exercise Promotion: Stretching
Exercise Therapy: Joint Mobility

Exercise Therapy: Muscle Control
Feeding
Foot Care
Hair and Scalp Care
Nail Care
Oral Health Maintenance
Perineal Care

Positioning
Positioning: Neurologic
Teaching: Prescribed Exercise
Transfer

Additional Optional Interventions:
Bowel Management
Fall Prevention
Medication Management
Mutual Goal Setting
Nutrition Management

Pain Management
Self-Care Assistance
Self-Care Assistance: Bathing/Hygiene
Self-Care Assistance: Dressing/Grooming
Self-Care Assistance: Feeding
Self-Care Assistance: IADL
Self-Care Assistance: Toileting
Self-Care Assistance: Transfer
Sleep Enhancement
Traction/Immobilization Care
Urinary Elimination Management

Mobility: Physical, Impaired

Definition: Limitation in independent, purposeful physical movement of the body or of one or more extremities

Suggested Nursing Interventions for Problem Resolution:
Bed Rest Care
Body Mechanics Promotion
Energy Management
Environmental Management
Exercise Promotion
Exercise Promotion: Strength Training
Exercise Promotion: Stretching
Exercise Therapy: Ambulation
Exercise Therapy: Balance
Exercise Therapy: Joint Mobility
Exercise Therapy: Muscle Control
Mood Management
Pain Management
Positioning
Positioning: Neurologic
Positioning: Wheelchair
Self-Care Assistance
Self-Care Assistance: IADL
Self-Care Assistance: Transfer
Teaching: Prescribed Exercise
Traction/Immobilization Care

Additional Optional Interventions:
Activity Therapy
Autogenic Training
Cast Care: Maintenance
Cast Care: Wet
Circulatory Care: Arterial Insufficiency
Circulatory Care: Venous Insufficiency
Circulatory Precautions
Fall Prevention
Foot Care
Massage
Medication Management
Neurologic Monitoring
Nutrition Therapy
Peripheral Sensation Management
Physical Restraint
Pressure Management
Progressive Muscle Relaxation
Skin Surveillance
Splinting
Weight Management

Mobility: Wheelchair, Impaired

Definition: Limitation of independent operation of wheelchair within environment

Suggested Nursing Interventions for Problem Resolution:
Body Mechanics Promotion
Energy Management
Environmental Management
Exercise Promotion
Exercise Promotion: Strength Training
Exercise Promotion: Stretching
Exercise Therapy: Balance
Exercise Therapy: Muscle Control
Positioning
Positioning: Neurologic
Positioning: Wheelchair
Self-Care Assistance
Self-Care Assistance: IADL

Self-Care Assistance: Transfer
Teaching: Prescribed Exercise
Transfer
Transport: Intrafacility

Additional Optional Interventions:
Fall Prevention
Medication Management
Mood Management
Mutual Goal Setting
Nutrition Management
Pain Management
Sleep Enhancement
Weight Management

Moral Distress

Definition: Response to the inability to carry out one's chosen ethical/moral decision/action

Suggested Nursing Interventions for Problem Resolution:
Conflict Mediation
Culture Brokerage
Decision-Making Support
Emotional Support
Health System Guidance
Hope Inspiration
Spiritual Support
Truth Telling
Values Clarification

Additional Optional Interventions:
Anger Control Assistance
Anxiety Reduction
Dying Care
Forgiveness Facilitation
Grief Work Facilitation
Guilt Work Facilitation
Patient Rights Protection
Spiritual Growth Facilitation

Nausea

Definition: A subjective phenomenon of an unpleasant feeling in the back of the throat and stomach that may or may not result in vomiting

Suggested Nursing Interventions for Problem Resolution:
Anxiety Reduction
Calming Technique
Diet Staging
Distraction
Fluid/Electrolyte Management
Fluid Monitoring
Medication Administration
Medication Management
Nausea Management
Nutritional Monitoring
Pain Management
Relaxation Therapy

Additional Optional Interventions:
Acupressure
Aspiration Precautions
Central Venous Access Device Management
Cerebral Edema Management
Gastrointestinal Intubation
Intravenous (IV) Insertion
Intravenous (IV) Therapy
Temperature Regulation
Vomiting Management

Neonatal Jaundice

Definition: The yellow-orange tint of the neonate's skin and mucous membranes that occurs after 24 hours of life as a result of unconjugated bilirubin in the circulation

Suggested Nursing Interventions for Problem Resolution:
Parent Education: Infant
Phlebotomy: Venous Blood Sample
Phototherapy: Neonate
Surveillance
Vital Signs Monitoring

Additional Optional Interventions:
Caregiver Support
Infant Care: Newborn
Intravenous (IV) Insertion
Intravenous (IV) Therapy

Neonatal Jaundice, Risk for

Definition: At risk for the yellow–orange tint of the neonate's skin and mucous membranes that occurs after 24 hours of life as a result of unconjugated bilirubin in the circulation

Suggested Nursing Interventions for Problem Resolution:
Capillary Blood Sample
Fluid Monitoring
Infant Care: Newborn
Infant Care: Preterm
Lactation Counseling
Prescribing: Diagnostic Testing
Prescribing: Nonpharmacologic Treatment

Additional Optional Interventions:
Bottle Feeding
Cup Feeding: Newborn
Intravenous (IV) Therapy
Phototherapy: Neonate
Tube Care: Umbilical Line

Noncompliance

Definition: Behavior of person and/or caregiver that fails to coincide with a health-promoting or therapeutic plan agreed upon by the person (and/or family and/or community) and healthcare professional. In the presence of an agreed upon, health promoting, or therapeutic plan, the person's or caregiver's behavior is fully or partially nonadherent and may lead to clinically ineffective or partially ineffective outcomes.

Suggested Nursing Interventions for Problem Resolution:
Caregiver Support
Coping Enhancement
Counseling
Culture Brokerage
Decision-Making Support
Discharge Planning
Elopement Precautions
Financial Resource Assistance
Health Education
Health System Guidance
Insurance Authorization
Learning Facilitation
Mutual Goal Setting
Nutritional Counseling
Patient Contracting
Patient Rights Protection
Self-Efficacy Enhancement
Self-Modification Assistance
Self-Responsibility Facilitation
Support System Enhancement
Teaching: Disease Process
Teaching: Individual
Teaching: Prescribed Diet
Teaching: Prescribed Exercise
Teaching: Prescribed Medication
Teaching: Procedure/Treatment
Teaching: Psychomotor Skill
Telephone Consultation

Truth Telling
Values Clarification

Additional Optional Interventions:
Case Management
Home Maintenance Assistance
Medication Management
Prenatal Care
Referral
Smoking Cessation Assistance
Support Group
Teaching: Infant Nutrition 0-3 Months
Teaching: Infant Nutrition 4-6 Months
Teaching: Infant Nutrition 7-9 Months
Teaching: Infant Nutrition 10-12 Months
Teaching: Infant Safety 0-3 Months
Teaching: Infant Safety 4-6 Months
Teaching: Infant Safety 7-9 Months
Teaching: Infant Safety 10-12 Months
Teaching: Infant Stimulation 0-4 Months
Teaching: Infant Stimulation 5-8 Months
Teaching: Infant Stimulation 9-12 Months
Teaching: Safe Sex
Teaching: Toddler Nutrition 13-18 Months
Teaching: Toddler Nutrition 19-24 Months
Teaching: Toddler Nutrition 25-36 Months
Teaching: Toddler Safety 13-18 Months
Teaching: Toddler Safety 19-24 Months
Teaching: Toddler Safety 25-36 Months

Nutrition: Imbalanced, Less Than Body Requirements

Definition: Intake of nutrients insufficient to meet metabolic needs

Suggested Nursing Interventions for Problem Resolution:
Diarrhea Management
Diet Staging
Eating Disorders Management
Financial Resource Assistance
Fluid/Electrolyte Management
Fluid Management
Fluid Monitoring
Lactation Counseling
Nutrition Management
Nutrition Therapy
Nutritional Counseling
Nutritional Monitoring
Self-Care Assistance: Feeding
Sustenance Support
Swallowing Therapy
Vital Signs Monitoring

Weight Gain Assistance
Weight Management

Additional Optional Interventions:
Allergy Management
Bottle Feeding
Bowel Management
Central Venous Access Device Management
Chemotherapy Management
Dementia Management
Energy Management
Enteral Tube Feeding
Feeding
Gastrointestinal Intubation
Hyperglycemia Management
Hypoglycemia Management
Infant Care

Intravenous (IV) Insertion
Intravenous (IV) Therapy
Laboratory Data Interpretation
Medication Management
Mutual Goal Setting
Phlebotomy: Venous Blood Sample

Positioning
Radiation Therapy Management
Referral
Teaching: Individual
Teaching: Prescribed Diet
Total Parenteral Nutrition (TPN) Administration

Nutrition: Imbalanced, More Than Body Requirements

Definition: Intake of nutrients that exceeds metabolic needs

Suggested Nursing Interventions for Problem Resolution:
Behavior Modification
Exercise Promotion
Fluid Management
Nutrition Management
Nutritional Counseling
Nutritional Monitoring
Teaching: Prescribed Diet
Weight Management
Weight Reduction Assistance

Additional Optional Interventions:
Anxiety Reduction
Behavior Management
Bottle Feeding
Coping Enhancement
Enteral Tube Feeding

Exercise Therapy: Ambulation
Feeding
Fluid Monitoring
Hyperglycemia Management
Hypoglycemia Management
Infant Care
Limit Setting
Mutual Goal Setting
Nutrition Therapy
Patient Contracting
Referral
Self-Modification Assistance
Self-Responsibility Facilitation
Skin Surveillance
Support Group
Teaching: Individual

Nutrition, Readiness for Enhanced

Definition: A pattern of nutrient intake that is sufficient for meeting metabolic needs and can be strengthened

Suggested Nursing Interventions for Problem Resolution:
Commendation
Health Education
Hyperglycemia Management
Hypoglycemia Management
Mutual Goal Setting
Nutritional Counseling
Patient Contracting
Self-Efficacy Enhancement
Self-Modification Assistance
Self-Responsibility Facilitation
Teaching: Individual
Weight Management

Additional Optional Interventions:
Nutrition Management
Nutritional Monitoring

Self-Care Assistance: Feeding
Teaching: Infant Nutrition 0-3 Months
Teaching: Infant Nutrition 4-6 Months
Teaching: Infant Nutrition 7-9 Months
Teaching: Infant Nutrition 10-12 Months
Teaching: Prescribed Diet
Teaching: Toddler Nutrition 13-18 Months
Teaching: Toddler Nutrition 19-24 Months
Teaching: Toddler Nutrition 25-36 Months
Weight Gain Assistance
Weight Reduction Assistance

Nutrition: Imbalanced, Risk for More Than Body Requirements

Definition: At risk for an intake of nutrients that exceeds metabolic needs

Suggested Nursing Interventions for Problem Resolution:
Anxiety Reduction
Behavior Modification
Exercise Promotion
Nutrition Management
Nutrition Therapy
Nutritional Counseling
Nutritional Monitoring
Risk Identification
Self-Modification Assistance
Teaching: Infant Nutrition 0-3 Months
Teaching: Infant Nutrition 4-6 Months
Teaching: Infant Nutrition 7-9 Months
Teaching: Infant Nutrition 10-12 Months

Teaching: Toddler Nutrition 13-18 Months
Teaching: Toddler Nutrition 19-24 Months
Teaching: Toddler Nutrition 25-36 Months
Weight Management

Additional Optional Interventions:
Bottle Feeding
Enteral Tube Feeding
Infant Care
Mutual Goal Setting
Teaching: Individual
Teaching: Prescribed Diet
Weight Reduction Assistance

Oral Mucous Membrane, Impaired

Definition: Disruptions of the lips and/or soft tissue of the oral cavity

Suggested Nursing Interventions for Problem Resolution:
Fluid Management
Nutrition Management
Oral Health Maintenance
Oral Health Promotion
Oral Health Restoration
Self-Care Assistance

Additional Optional Interventions:
Airway Insertion and Stabilization
Airway Suctioning
Artificial Airway Management

Bleeding Precautions
Chemotherapy Management
Diet Staging
Dying Care
Exercise Therapy: Joint Mobility
Financial Resource Assistance
Medication Management
Pain Management
Substance Use Treatment
Radiation Therapy Management
Wound Care

Pain, Acute

Definition: Unpleasant sensory and emotional experience arising from actual or potential tissue damage or described in terms of such damage (International Association for the Study of Pain); sudden or slow onset of any intensity from mild to severe with an anticipated or predictable end and a duration of < 6 months

Suggested Nursing Interventions for Problem Resolution:
Acupressure
Analgesic Administration
Analgesic Administration: Intraspinal
Anesthesia Administration
Anxiety Reduction
Cutaneous Stimulation
Environmental Management: Comfort
Flatulence Reduction
Heat/Cold Application
Medication Administration
Medication Administration: Intramuscular (IM)
Medication Administration: Intravenous (IV)
Medication Administration: Oral
Medication Management
Medication Prescribing
Pain Management
Patient-Controlled Analgesia (PCA) Assistance
Rectal Prolapse Management
Sedation Management
Transcutaneous Electrical Nerve Stimulation (TENS)

Additional Optional Interventions:
Active Listening
Animal-Assisted Therapy
Autogenic Training
Bathing
Biofeedback
Body Mechanics Promotion
Bowel Management
Coping Enhancement
Distraction
Emotional Support

Energy Management
Environmental Management
Exercise Promotion
Exercise Promotion: Stretching
Exercise Therapy: Ambulation
Exercise Therapy: Balance
Exercise Therapy: Joint Mobility
Exercise Therapy: Muscle Control
Grief Work Facilitation
Guided Imagery
Hope Inspiration
Humor
Hypnosis
Intrapartal Care: High-Risk Delivery
Lactation Suppression
Massage
Meditation Facilitation
Music Therapy
Oral Health Restoration
Oxygen Therapy
Positioning
Postanesthesia Care
Preparatory Sensory Information
Presence
Progressive Muscle Relaxation
Relaxation Therapy
Security Enhancement
Self-Hypnosis Facilitation
Sleep Enhancement
Therapeutic Play
Therapeutic Touch
Touch
Vital Signs Monitoring

Pain, Chronic

Definition: Unpleasant sensory and emotional experience arising from actual or potential tissue damage or described in terms of such damage (International Association for the Study of Pain); sudden or slow onset of any intensity from mild to severe, constant or recurring without an anticipated or predictable end and with a duration of > 6 months

Suggested Nursing Interventions for Problem Resolution:
Acupressure
Analgesic Administration
Analgesic Administration: Intraspinal
Coping Enhancement
Cutaneous Stimulation
Guided Imagery
Heat/Cold Application
Massage
Medication Administration
Medication Management
Medication Prescribing
Mood Management

Pain Management
Patient-Controlled Analgesia (PCA) Assistance
Progressive Muscle Relaxation
Transcutaneous Electrical Nerve Stimulation (TENS)

Additional Optional Interventions:
Active Listening
Animal-Assisted Therapy
Autogenic Training
Biofeedback
Distraction
Environmental Management: Comfort
Exercise Promotion: Stretching

Exercise Therapy: Ambulation
Exercise Therapy: Joint Mobility
Exercise Therapy: Muscle Control
Healing Touch
Humor
Hypnosis
Meditation Facilitation
Music Therapy

Positioning
Reiki
Relaxation Therapy
Self-Hypnosis Facilitation
Sleep Enhancement
Therapeutic Touch
Touch
Vital Signs Monitoring

Parental Role Conflict

Definition: Parent experience of role confusion and conflict in response to crisis

Suggested Nursing Interventions for Problem Resolution:
Abuse Protection Support: Child
Caregiver Support
Childbirth Preparation
Coping Enhancement
Counseling
Crisis Intervention
Decision-Making Support
Discharge Planning
Family Integrity Promotion
Family Integrity Promotion: Childbearing Family
Family Planning: Unplanned Pregnancy
Family Presence Facilitation
Family Process Maintenance
Family Support
Family Therapy
Grief Work Facilitation: Perinatal Death
High-Risk Pregnancy Care

Parenting Promotion
Role Enhancement
Self-Esteem Enhancement
Socialization Enhancement
Teaching: Procedure/Treatment

Additional Optional Interventions:
Attachment Promotion
Developmental Enhancement: Adolescent
Developmental Enhancement: Child
Health System Guidance
Limit Setting
Mutual Goal Setting
Parent Education: Adolescent
Parent Education: Childrearing Family
Respite Care
Trauma Therapy: Child
Values Clarification
Visitation Facilitation

Parenting, Impaired

Definition: Inability of the primary caretaker to create, maintain, or regain an environment that promotes the optimum growth and development of the child

Suggested Nursing Interventions for Problem Resolution:
Abuse Protection Support: Child
Anticipatory Guidance
Anxiety Reduction
Attachment Promotion
Caregiver Support
Coping Enhancement
Counseling
Developmental Enhancement: Adolescent
Developmental Enhancement: Child
Family Integrity Promotion
Family Support
Family Therapy
Guilt Work Facilitation
Mutual Goal Setting
Normalization Promotion
Parenting Promotion
Risk Identification: Childbearing Family

Role Enhancement
Security Enhancement
Self-Esteem Enhancement
Substance Use Treatment
Support Group
Support System Enhancement
Teaching: Individual

Additional Optional Interventions:
Behavior Management: Overactivity/Inattention
Childbirth Preparation
Environmental Management: Safety
Family Integrity Promotion: Childbearing Family
Family Involvement Promotion
Family Planning: Contraception
Family Planning: Unplanned Pregnancy
Family Process Maintenance
Financial Resource Assistance

Health Education
Home Maintenance Assistance
Infant Care
Intrapartal Care
Kangaroo Care
Parent Education: Adolescent
Parent Education: Childrearing Family

Parent Education: Infant
Patient Contracting
Postpartal Care
Prenatal Care
Respite Care
Surveillance

Parenting, Readiness for Enhanced

Definition: A pattern of providing an environment for children or other dependent person(s) that is sufficient to nurture growth and development, and can be strengthened

Suggested Nursing Interventions for Problem Resolution:
Anticipatory Guidance
Attachment Promotion
Caregiver Support
Commendation
Coping Enhancement
Developmental Enhancement: Adolescent
Developmental Enhancement: Child
Family Integrity Promotion
Family Integrity Promotion: Childbearing Family
Parenting Promotion
Role Enhancement
Self-Efficacy Enhancement
Support System Enhancement

Additional Optional Interventions:
Family Involvement Promotion
Financial Resource Assistance
Infant Care
Infant Care: Newborn
Infant Care: Preterm
Normalization Promotion
Parent Education: Adolescent

Parent Education: Childrearing Family
Parent Education: Infant
Self-Esteem Enhancement
Sibling Support
Teaching: Infant Nutrition 0-3 Months
Teaching: Infant Nutrition 4-6 Months
Teaching: Infant Nutrition 7-9 Months
Teaching: Infant Nutrition 10-12 Months
Teaching: Infant Safety 0-3 Months
Teaching: Infant Safety 4-6 Months
Teaching: Infant Safety 7-9 Months
Teaching: Infant Safety 10-12 Months
Teaching: Infant Stimulation 0-4 Months
Teaching: Infant Stimulation 5-8 Months
Teaching: Infant Stimulation 9-12 Months
Teaching: Toddler Nutrition 13-18 Months
Teaching: Toddler Nutrition 19-24 Months
Teaching: Toddler Nutrition 25-36 Months
Teaching: Toddler Safety 13-18 Months
Teaching: Toddler Safety 19-24 Months
Teaching: Toddler Safety 25-36 Months
Teaching: Toilet Training

Parenting, Risk for Impaired

Definition: At risk for inability of the primary caretaker to create, maintain, or regain an environment that promotes the optimum growth and development of the child

Suggested Nursing Interventions for Problem Resolution:
Abuse Protection Support: Child
Anticipatory Guidance
Attachment Promotion
Caregiver Support
Coping Enhancement
Decision-Making Support
Developmental Enhancement: Adolescent
Developmental Enhancement: Child
Family Integrity Promotion
Family Planning: Contraception
Family Planning: Unplanned Pregnancy
Health Literacy Enhancement
High-Risk Pregnancy Care

Learning Facilitation
Learning Readiness Enhancement
Mood Management
Normalization Promotion
Parenting Promotion
Resiliency Promotion
Risk Identification
Role Enhancement
Self-Esteem Enhancement
Sibling Support
Substance Use Prevention
Substance Use Treatment
Support System Enhancement
Teaching: Sexuality

Additional Optional Interventions:
Anger Control Assistance
Anxiety Reduction
Behavior Management: Overactivity/Inattention
Behavior Modification: Social Skills
Childbirth Preparation
Energy Management
Family Integrity Promotion: Childbearing Family
Family Involvement Promotion
Family Process Maintenance
Family Therapy
Financial Resource Assistance

Health Education
Home Maintenance Assistance
Parent Education: Adolescent
Parent Education: Childrearing Family
Parent Education: Infant
Patient Contracting
Postpartal Care
Prenatal Care
Respite Care
Sleep Enhancement
Support Group
Surveillance

Perioperative Positioning Injury, Risk for

Definition: At risk for inadvertent anatomical and physical changes as a result of posture or equipment used during an invasive/surgical procedure

Suggested Nursing Interventions for Problem Resolution:
Aspiration Precautions
Bleeding Reduction: Wound
Cerebral Perfusion Promotion
Circulatory Care: Arterial Insufficiency
Circulatory Care: Venous Insufficiency
Circulatory Precautions
Delirium Management
Embolus Precautions
Fluid Management
Incision Site Care
Peripheral Sensation Management
Positioning: Intraoperative
Pressure Management

Reality Orientation
Risk Identification
Skin Surveillance
Surgical Precautions
Surveillance
Temperature Regulation: Perioperative

Additional Optional Interventions:
Cast Care: Wet
Embolus Care: Peripheral
Embolus Care: Pulmonary
Infection Control: Intraoperative
Nutrition Therapy

Peripheral Neurovascular Dysfunction, Risk for

Definition: At risk for disruption in circulation, sensation, or motion of an extremity

Suggested Nursing Interventions for Problem Resolution:
Cast Care: Maintenance
Cast Care: Wet
Circulatory Care: Arterial Insufficiency
Circulatory Care: Venous Insufficiency
Circulatory Precautions
Cutaneous Stimulation
Embolus Care: Peripheral
Embolus Precautions
Exercise Therapy: Joint Mobility
Lower Extremity Monitoring
Neurologic Monitoring
Peripheral Sensation Management
Physical Restraint
Pneumatic Tourniquet Precautions
Positioning
Positioning: Intraoperative
Positioning: Neurologic
Positioning: Wheelchair
Pressure Management

Pressure Ulcer Prevention
Risk Identification
Skin Surveillance
Splinting
Surveillance
Traction/Immobilization Care

Additional Optional Interventions:
Bed Rest Care
Bleeding Precautions
Body Mechanics Promotion
Cardiac Care
Exercise Promotion
Exercise Therapy: Ambulation
Fluid Management
Heat/Cold Application
Pain Management
Teaching: Prescribed Exercise
Vital Signs Monitoring
Wound Care: Burns

Personal Identity, Disturbed

Definition: Inability to maintain an integrated and complete perception of self

Suggested Nursing Interventions for Problem Resolution:
Anticipatory Guidance
Body Image Enhancement
Counseling
Crisis Intervention
Culture Brokerage
Decision-Making Support
Delusion Management
Dementia Management
Developmental Enhancement: Adolescent
Developmental Enhancement: Child
Hallucination Management
Mood Management
Mutual Goal Setting
Self-Awareness Enhancement
Self-Esteem Enhancement
Self-Responsibility Facilitation
Sexual Counseling
Substance Use Prevention
Teaching: Sexuality

Additional Optional Interventions:
Anxiety Reduction
Art Therapy
Assertiveness Training
Behavior Management: Self-Harm
Bibliotherapy
Calming Technique
Cognitive Restructuring
Complex Relationship Building
Coping Enhancement
Delirium Management
Emotional Support
Life Skills Enhancement
Religious Addiction Prevention
Security Enhancement
Self-Care Assistance
Substance Use Treatment
Substance Use Treatment: Alcohol Withdrawal
Substance Use Treatment: Drug Withdrawal
Substance Use Treatment: Overdose
Therapy Group
Values Clarification

Personal Identity, Risk for Disturbed

Definition: Risk for the inability to maintain an integrated and complete perception of self

Suggested Nursing Interventions for Problem Resolution:
Cognitive Restructuring
Coping Enhancement
Counseling
Family Therapy
Medication Management
Mood Management
Role Enhancement
Self-Awareness Enhancement
Self-Esteem Enhancement
Substance Use Treatment
Support System Enhancement

Additional Optional Interventions:
Complex Relationship Building
Crisis Intervention
Dementia Management
Reality Orientation
Role Enhancement
Socialization Enhancement
Support Group
Therapy Group

Poisoning, Risk for

Definition: At risk of accidental exposure to, or ingestion of, drugs or dangerous products in sufficient doses that may compromise health

Suggested Nursing Interventions for Problem Resolution:
Communication Enhancement: Visual Deficit
Delirium Management
Dementia Management
Environmental Management: Safety
Environmental Management: Worker Safety

Medication Management
Medication Reconciliation
Mood Management
Risk Identification
Substance Use Prevention
Substance Use Treatment

Surveillance
Teaching: Infant Safety 7-9 Months
Teaching: Infant Safety 10-12 Months
Teaching: Prescribed Medication
Teaching: Toddler Safety 13-18 Months
Teaching: Toddler Safety 19-24 Months
Teaching: Toddler Safety 25-36 Months

Additional Optional Interventions:
Bioterrorism Preparedness
Chemotherapy Management
Environmental Risk Protection
First Aid
Fluid/Electrolyte Management
Health Education
Parent Education: Adolescent
Parent Education: Childrearing Family
Parent Education: Infant
Vital Signs Monitoring

Post-Trauma Syndrome

Definition: Sustained maladaptive response to a traumatic, overwhelming event

Suggested Nursing Interventions for Problem Resolution:
Anger Control Assistance
Anxiety Reduction
Behavior Management: Self-Harm
Coping Enhancement
Counseling
Forgiveness Facilitation
Grief Work Facilitation
Guilt Work Facilitation
Hope Inspiration
Impulse Control Training
Life Skills Enhancement
Medication Management
Mood Management
Rape-Trauma Treatment
Relaxation Therapy
Security Enhancement
Substance Use Prevention
Substance Use Treatment

Support System Enhancement
Trauma Therapy: Child

Additional Optional Interventions:
Abuse Protection Support
Environmental Management
Financial Resource Assistance
Journaling
Mutual Goal Setting
Progressive Muscle Relaxation
Reality Orientation
Reminiscence Therapy
Sleep Enhancement
Socialization Enhancement
Suicide Prevention
Support Group
Therapy Group

Post-Trauma Syndrome, Risk for

Definition: A risk for sustained maladaptive response to a traumatic, overwhelming event

Suggested Nursing Interventions for Problem Resolution:
Active Listening
Anxiety Reduction
Coping Enhancement
Counseling
Crisis Intervention
Decision-Making Support
Forgiveness Facilitation
Guilt Work Facilitation
Hope Inspiration
Presence
Rape-Trauma Treatment
Relaxation Therapy
Resiliency Promotion
Risk Identification
Security Enhancement
Self-Esteem Enhancement
Spiritual Support
Support Group

Support System Enhancement
Telephone Follow-Up
Trauma Therapy: Child

Additional Optional Interventions:
Animal-Assisted Therapy
Environmental Management
Family Involvement Promotion
Family Mobilization
Financial Resource Assistance
Life Skills Enhancement
Mutual Goal Setting
Progressive Muscle Relaxation
Reality Orientation
Reminiscence Therapy
Socialization Enhancement
Substance Use Prevention
Suicide Prevention
Surveillance

Power, Readiness for Enhanced

Definition: A pattern of participating knowingly in change that is sufficient for well-being and can be strengthened

Suggested Nursing Interventions for Problem Resolution:
Anticipatory Guidance
Assertiveness Training
Commendation
Decision-Making Support
Emotional Support
Health Education
Health System Guidance
Learning Facilitation
Mutual Goal Setting
Resiliency Promotion
Self-Awareness Enhancement
Self-Efficacy Enhancement
Self-Esteem Enhancement

Self-Modification Assistance
Self-Responsibility Facilitation
Values Clarification

Additional Optional Interventions:
Abuse Protection Support
Anxiety Reduction
Conflict Mediation
Crisis Intervention
Environmental Management
Life Skills Enhancement
Meditation Facilitation

Powerlessness

Definition: The lived experience of lack of control over a situation, including a perception that one's actions do not significantly affect an outcome

Suggested Nursing Interventions for Problem Resolution:
Assertiveness Training
Cognitive Restructuring
Complex Relationship Building
Decision-Making Support
Emotional Support
Financial Resource Assistance
Health System Guidance
Hope Inspiration
Learning Facilitation
Mood Management
Mutual Goal Setting
Patient Rights Protection
Presence
Relocation Stress Reduction
Self-Awareness Enhancement
Self-Efficacy Enhancement
Self-Esteem Enhancement
Self-Responsibility Facilitation
Support System Enhancement
Values Clarification

Additional Optional Interventions:
Abuse Protection Support
Activity Therapy
Animal-Assisted Therapy
Anticipatory Guidance
Anxiety Reduction
Art Therapy
Crisis Intervention
Environmental Management
Family Involvement Promotion
Life Skills Enhancement
Meditation Facilitation
Patient Contracting
Progressive Muscle Relaxation
Rape-Trauma Treatment
Reminiscence Therapy
Self-Care Assistance
Support Group
Teaching: Individual

Powerlessness, Risk for

Definition: At risk for the lived experience of lack of control over a situation, including a perception that one's actions do not significantly affect an outcome

Suggested Nursing Interventions for Problem Resolution:
Anticipatory Guidance
Assertiveness Training
Body Image Enhancement
Coping Enhancement
Crisis Intervention
Decision-Making Support
Dying Care
Emotional Support
Health System Guidance
Hope Inspiration
Learning Facilitation
Mood Management
Mutual Goal Setting
Presence
Relocation Stress Reduction
Resiliency Promotion
Risk Identification
Self-Efficacy Enhancement
Self-Esteem Enhancement

Self-Responsibility Facilitation
Teaching: Disease Process
Teaching: Prescribed Diet
Teaching: Prescribed Medication
Teaching: Procedure/Treatment
Values Clarification

Additional Optional Interventions:
Abuse Protection Support
Activity Therapy
Animal-Assisted Therapy
Anxiety Reduction
Art Therapy
Cognitive Restructuring
Complex Relationship Building
Environmental Management
Family Involvement Promotion
Financial Resource Assistance
Meditation Facilitation
Rape-Trauma Treatment

Protection, Ineffective

Definition: Decrease in the ability to guard self from internal or external threats such as illness or injury

Suggested Nursing Interventions for Problem Resolution:
Bleeding Precautions
Chemotherapy Management
Coping Enhancement
Eating Disorders Management
Emergency Care
Energy Management
Exercise Therapy: Ambulation
Exercise Therapy: Balance
Immunization/Vaccination Management
Incision Site Care
Infection Control
Infection Protection
Latex Precautions
Peripheral Sensation Management
Postanesthesia Care
Pressure Management
Reality Orientation
Respiratory Monitoring
Risk Identification
Self-Care Assistance
Surgical Precautions
Surveillance
Surveillance: Late Pregnancy
Surveillance: Remote Electronic

Ventilation Assistance
Wound Care

Additional Optional Interventions:
Allergy Management
Autotransfusion
Dementia Management
Electronic Fetal Monitoring: Antepartum
Electronic Fetal Monitoring: Intrapartum
Intrapartal Care: High-Risk Delivery
Labor Induction
Nutrition Management
Nutrition Therapy
Nutritional Counseling
Phototherapy: Neonate
Positioning
Pressure Ulcer Prevention
Pruritus Management
Seclusion
Sleep Enhancement
Substance Use Treatment
Support Group
Teaching: Individual
Ultrasonography: Limited Obstetric

Rape-Trauma Syndrome

Definition: Sustained maladaptive response to a forced, violent sexual penetration against the victim's will and consent

Suggested Nursing Interventions for Problem Resolution:
Abuse Protection Support
Abuse Protection Support: Child
Abuse Protection Support: Domestic Partner
Abuse Protection Support: Elder
Anger Control Assistance
Anxiety Reduction
Calming Technique
Counseling
Crisis Intervention
Decision-Making Support
Emotional Support
Hope Inspiration
Presence
Rape-Trauma Treatment
Referral
Self-Esteem Enhancement
Sexual Counseling
Specimen Management
Support Group

Support System Enhancement
Trauma Therapy: Child
Vital Signs Monitoring
Wound Care

Additional Optional Interventions:
Anticipatory Guidance
Art Therapy
Coping Enhancement
Family Planning: Contraception
Forensic Data Collection
Grief Work Facilitation
Health Screening
Pain Management
Risk Identification
Security Enhancement
Spiritual Support
Substance Use Prevention
Therapeutic Play
Therapy Group

Relationship, Ineffective

Definition: A pattern of mutual partnership that is insufficient to provide for each other's needs

Suggested Nursing Interventions for Problem Resolution:
Abuse Protection Support
Conflict Mediation
Counseling
Family Integrity Promotion
Family Therapy
Substance Use Treatment
Support Group
Support System Enhancement

Additional Optional Interventions:
Behavior Modification
Behavior Modification: Social Skills
Cognitive Restructuring
Coping Enhancement
Family Support
Life Skills Enhancement
Resiliency Promotion

Relationship, Readiness for Enhanced

Definition: A pattern of mutual partnership that is sufficient to provide for each other's needs and can be strengthened

Suggested Nursing Interventions for Problem Resolution:
Commendation
Family Integrity Promotion
Family Support
Mutual Goal Setting

Role Enhancement
Values Clarification

Additional Optional Interventions:
Family Integrity Promotion: Childbearing Family
Family Mobilization

Relationship, Risk for Ineffective

Definition: Risk for a pattern of mutual partnership that is insufficient to provide for each other's needs

Suggested Nursing Interventions for Problem Resolution:
Abuse Protection Support
Behavior Modification
Behavior Modification: Social Skills
Coping Enhancement
Counseling
Family Integrity Promotion
Family Therapy
Substance Use Treatment
Support Group

Additional Optional Interventions:
Family Support
Life Skills Enhancement
Resiliency Promotion
Role Enhancement
Socialization Enhancement
Support System Enhancement

Religiosity, Impaired

Definition: Impaired ability to exercise reliance on beliefs and/or participate in rituals of a particular faith tradition

Suggested Nursing Interventions for Problem Resolution:
Anxiety Reduction
Coping Enhancement
Culture Brokerage
Energy Management
Environmental Management
Family Involvement Promotion
Grief Work Facilitation
Hope Inspiration
Pain Management
Religious Ritual Enhancement
Security Enhancement
Spiritual Growth Facilitation
Spiritual Support

Additional Optional Interventions:
Dying Care
Family Mobilization
Family Process Maintenance
Forgiveness Facilitation
Guilt Work Facilitation
Mood Management
Patient Rights Protection
Relocation Stress Reduction
Reminiscence Therapy

Religiosity, Readiness for Enhanced

Definition: A pattern of reliance on religious beliefs and/or participation in rituals of a particular faith tradition that is sufficient for well-being and can be strengthened

Suggested Nursing Interventions for Problem Resolution:
Conflict Mediation
Coping Enhancement
Forgiveness Facilitation
Guilt Work Facilitation
Hope Inspiration
Religious Addiction Prevention
Religious Ritual Enhancement
Spiritual Growth Facilitation
Spiritual Support

Additional Optional Interventions:
Culture Brokerage
Energy Management
Environmental Management
Family Integrity Promotion
Family Involvement Promotion
Grief Work Facilitation
Pain Management

Religiosity, Risk for Impaired

Definition: At risk for an impaired ability to exercise reliance on religious beliefs and/or participate in rituals of a particular faith tradition

Suggested Nursing Interventions for Problem Resolution:
Anxiety Reduction
Coping Enhancement
Culture Brokerage
Energy Management
Environmental Management
Forgiveness Facilitation
Grief Work Facilitation
Guilt Work Facilitation
Hope Inspiration
Mood Management
Pain Management

Religious Ritual Enhancement
Security Enhancement
Spiritual Growth Facilitation
Spiritual Support
Support System Enhancement

Additional Optional Interventions:
Conflict Mediation
Dying Care
Family Mobilization
Family Process Maintenance
Relocation Stress Reduction
Reminiscence Therapy

Relocation Stress Syndrome

Definition: Physiological and/or psychosocial disturbance following transfer from one environment to another

Suggested Nursing Interventions for Problem Resolution:
Active Listening
Anger Control Assistance
Coping Enhancement
Counseling
Delirium Management
Discharge Planning
Emotional Support
Family Involvement Promotion
Family Mobilization
Family Support
Grief Work Facilitation
Hope Inspiration
Mutual Goal Setting
Patient Rights Protection
Relocation Stress Reduction
Security Enhancement
Self-Responsibility Facilitation
Sleep Enhancement
Socialization Enhancement
Spiritual Support

Support System Enhancement
Visitation Facilitation

Additional Optional Interventions:
Activity Therapy
Admission Care
Animal-Assisted Therapy
Anticipatory Guidance
Anxiety Reduction
Art Therapy
Dementia Management
Humor
Mood Management
Music Therapy
Nutrition Therapy
Nutritional Monitoring
Presence
Recreation Therapy
Reminiscence Therapy
Risk Identification
Touch
Values Clarification

Relocation Stress Syndrome, Risk for

Definition: At risk for physiological and/or psychosocial disturbance following transfer from one environment to another

Suggested Nursing Interventions for Problem Resolution:
Active Listening
Anger Control Assistance
Coping Enhancement
Counseling
Delirium Management
Discharge Planning
Emotional Support
Family Involvement Promotion
Family Mobilization
Family Support
Grief Work Facilitation
Hope Inspiration
Mutual Goal Setting
Patient Rights Protection
Relocation Stress Reduction
Security Enhancement
Self-Efficacy Enhancement
Self-Responsibility Facilitation
Sleep Enhancement
Socialization Enhancement
Spiritual Support

Support System Enhancement
Visitation Facilitation

Additional Optional Interventions:
Activity Therapy
Admission Care
Animal-Assisted Therapy
Anticipatory Guidance
Anxiety Reduction
Art Therapy
Dementia Management
Humor
Music Therapy
Nutrition Therapy
Nutritional Monitoring
Presence
Recreation Therapy
Reminiscence Therapy
Risk Identification
Touch
Transport: Interfacility

Renal Perfusion, Risk for Ineffective

Definition: At risk for a decrease in blood circulation to the kidney that may compromise health

Suggested Nursing Interventions for Problem Resolution:
Acid-Base Monitoring
Bleeding Reduction
Bleeding Reduction: Gastrointestinal
Blood Products Administration
Embolus Care: Peripheral
Embolus Precautions
Fluid Management
Hemodynamic Regulation
Hypovolemia Management
Infection Control
Medication Management
Oxygen Therapy
Risk Identification
Shock Management

Shock Prevention
Smoking Cessation Assistance
Surveillance
Teaching: Disease Process
Teaching: Prescribed Diet
Teaching: Prescribed Medication
Teaching: Procedure/Treatment
Vital Signs Monitoring

Additional Optional Interventions:
Acid-Base Management: Metabolic Acidosis
Acid-Base Management: Metabolic Alkalosis
Chemotherapy Management
Circulatory Care: Arterial Insufficiency
Environmental Management: Safety
Thrombolytic Therapy Management

Resilience, Impaired Individual

Definition: Decreased ability to sustain a pattern of positive responses to an adverse situation or crisis

Suggested Nursing Interventions for Problem Resolution:
Anger Control Assistance
Behavior Management
Coping Enhancement
Guilt Work Facilitation
Mood Management
Resiliency Promotion
Self-Esteem Enhancement
Socialization Enhancement
Substance Use Treatment

Additional Optional Interventions:
Crisis Intervention
Environmental Management: Violence Prevention
Hope Inspiration
Mutual Goal Setting
Self-Responsibility Facilitation
Support Group

Resilience, Readiness for Enhanced

Definition: A pattern of positive responses to an adverse situation or crisis that is sufficient for optimizing human potential and can be strengthened

Suggested Nursing Interventions for Problem Resolution:
Anticipatory Guidance
Commendation
Coping Enhancement
Crisis Intervention
Environmental Management: Violence Prevention
Mutual Goal Setting
Resiliency Promotion
Self-Efficacy Enhancement
Self-Responsibility Facilitation

Additional Optional Interventions:
Self-Esteem Enhancement
Substance Use Prevention
Support Group
Support System Enhancement

Resilience, Risk for Compromised

Definition: At risk for decreased ability to sustain a pattern of positive responses to an adverse situation or crisis

Suggested Nursing Interventions for Problem Resolution:
Anxiety Reduction
Anticipatory Guidance
Behavior Modification
Calming Technique
Coping Enhancement
Crisis Intervention
Grief Work Facilitation
Grief Work Facilitation: Perinatal Death
Guilt Work Facilitation
Hope Inspiration

Resiliency Promotion
Risk Identification
Self-Efficacy Enhancement
Self-Responsibility Facilitation
Substance Use Prevention
Support System Enhancement

Additional Optional Interventions:
Culture Brokerage
Family Planning: Unplanned Pregnancy
Relaxation Therapy
Relocation Stress Reduction
Sustenance Support

Role Performance, Ineffective

Definition: Patterns of behavior and self-expression that do not match the environmental context, norms, and expectations

Suggested Nursing Interventions for Problem Resolution:
Anticipatory Guidance
Caregiver Support
Complex Relationship Building
Conflict Mediation
Coping Enhancement
Energy Management
Life Skills Enhancement
Mood Management
Normalization Promotion
Pain Management
Parent Education: Adolescent
Parent Education: Childrearing Family
Parent Education: Infant
Parenting Promotion
Role Enhancement
Self-Awareness Enhancement
Self-Efficacy Enhancement

Self-Esteem Enhancement
Support System Enhancement

Additional Optional Interventions:
Abuse Protection Support
Body Image Enhancement
Cognitive Stimulation
Counseling
Family Therapy
Hope Inspiration
Labor Suppression
Mutual Goal Setting
Reproductive Technology Management
Substance Use Treatment
Support Group
Teaching: Individual
Teaching: Sexuality
Values Clarification

Self-Care Deficit: Bathing

Definition: Impaired ability to perform or complete bathing activities for self

Suggested Nursing Interventions for Problem Resolution:
Bathing
Contact Lens Care
Dementia Management: Bathing
Ear Care
Eye Care
Foot Care
Hair and Scalp Care
Infant Care
Nail Care
Oral Health Maintenance
Perineal Care
Self-Care Assistance: Bathing/Hygiene
Self-Responsibility Facilitation
Teaching: Individual

Additional Optional Interventions:
Anxiety Reduction
Behavior Management
Behavior Modification

Body Image Enhancement
Decision-Making Support
Discharge Planning
Emotional Support
Energy Management
Exercise Promotion
Exercise Promotion: Stretching
Exercise Therapy: Ambulation
Exercise Therapy: Balance
Exercise Therapy: Joint Mobility
Exercise Therapy: Muscle Control
Fall Prevention
Mutual Goal Setting
Pain Management
Patient Contracting
Positioning
Self-Care Assistance
Self-Care Assistance: IADL
Self-Esteem Enhancement

Self-Care Deficit: Dressing

Definition: Impaired ability to perform or complete dressing activities for self

Suggested Nursing Interventions for Problem Resolution:
Dressing
Energy Management
Environmental Management
Exercise Promotion
Hair and Scalp Care
Nail Care
Self-Care Assistance: Dressing/Grooming

Additional Optional Interventions:
Anxiety Reduction
Body Image Enhancement
Dementia Management

Discharge Planning
Exercise Promotion: Stretching
Exercise Therapy: Ambulation
Exercise Therapy: Balance
Exercise Therapy: Joint Mobility
Exercise Therapy: Muscle Control
Pain Management
Patient Contracting
Self-Care Assistance
Self-Care Assistance: IADL
Skin Surveillance
Teaching: Individual

Self-Care Deficit: Feeding

Definition: Impaired ability to perform or complete self-feeding activities

Suggested Nursing Interventions for Problem Resolution:
Bottle Feeding
Environmental Management
Feeding
Nutrition Management
Nutritional Monitoring
Oral Health Maintenance
Positioning
Self-Care Assistance: Feeding
Swallowing Therapy

Communication Enhancement: Visual Deficit
Discharge Planning
Energy Management
Pain Management
Patient Contracting
Self-Care Assistance
Self-Care Assistance: IADL
Socialization Enhancement
Teaching: Individual

Additional Optional Interventions:
Anxiety Reduction
Communication Enhancement: Hearing Deficit

Self-Care Deficit: Toileting

Definition: Impaired ability to perform or complete toileting activities for self

Suggested Nursing Interventions for Problem Resolution:
Bowel Incontinence Care: Encopresis
Bowel Management
Environmental Management
Fluid Management
Medication Management
Nutrition Management
Patient Contracting
Perineal Care
Self-Care Assistance: Toileting
Self-Care Assistance: Transfer
Teaching: Individual
Urinary Elimination Management

Constipation/Impaction Management
Dementia Management
Enema Administration
Exercise Promotion
Exercise Promotion: Stretching
Exercise Therapy: Ambulation
Exercise Therapy: Balance
Exercise Therapy: Joint Mobility
Exercise Therapy: Muscle Control
Fluid Monitoring
Ostomy Care
Pain Management
Self-Care Assistance
Self-Care Assistance: IADL
Skin Surveillance

Additional Optional Interventions:
Anxiety Reduction
Bathing

Self-Care, Readiness for Enhanced

Definition: A pattern of performing activities for oneself that helps to meet health-related goals and can be strengthened

Suggested Nursing Interventions for Problem Resolution:
Commendation
Discharge Planning
Energy Management
Environmental Management: Home Preparation
Exercise Promotion
Mood Management
Mutual Goal Setting
Pain Management

Self-Care Assistance
Self-Care Assistance: IADL
Self-Efficacy Enhancement
Self-Esteem Enhancement
Self-Modification Assistance
Self-Responsibility Facilitation
Teaching: Individual
Teaching: Prescribed Medication

Additional Optional Interventions:
Exercise Promotion: Strength Training
Exercise Promotion: Stretching
Exercise Therapy: Ambulation
Exercise Therapy: Balance
Exercise Therapy: Joint Mobility

Exercise Therapy: Muscle Control
Self-Care Assistance: Bathing/Hygiene
Self-Care Assistance: Dressing/Grooming
Self-Care Assistance: Feeding
Self-Care Assistance: Toileting
Self-Care Assistance: Transfer

Self-Concept, Readiness for Enhanced

Definition: A pattern of perceptions or ideas about the self that is sufficient for well-being and can be strengthened

Suggested Nursing Interventions for Problem Resolution:
Assertiveness Training
Body Image Enhancement
Commendation
Coping Enhancement
Emotional Support
Mood Management
Role Enhancement
Self-Awareness Enhancement
Self-Efficacy Enhancement
Self-Esteem Enhancement
Self-Modification Assistance
Self-Responsibility Facilitation

Support Group
Weight Management

Additional Optional Interventions:
Counseling
Decision-Making Support
Socialization Enhancement
Substance Use Prevention
Substance Use Treatment
Support System Enhancement
Therapy Group
Values Clarification

Self-Esteem: Chronic Low

Definition: Longstanding negative self-evaluating/feelings about self or self-capabilities

Suggested Nursing Interventions for Problem Resolution:
Assertiveness Training
Body Image Enhancement
Cognitive Restructuring
Counseling
Emotional Support
Hope Inspiration
Mood Management
Self-Esteem Enhancement
Socialization Enhancement
Support System Enhancement

Additional Optional Interventions:
Active Listening
Anxiety Reduction

Complex Relationship Building
Coping Enhancement
Crisis Intervention
Decision-Making Support
Grief Work Facilitation
Guilt Work Facilitation
Mutual Goal Setting
Pain Management
Presence
Role Enhancement
Suicide Prevention
Support Group
Therapy Group
Values Clarification

Self-Esteem: Chronic Low, Risk for

Definition: At risk for longstanding negative self-evaluating/feelings about self or self-capabilities

Suggested Nursing Interventions for Problem Resolution:

Coping Enhancement
Crisis Intervention
Grief Work Facilitation
Guilt Work Facilitation
Hope Inspiration
Mood Management
Self-Esteem Enhancement
Socialization Enhancement
Support Group
Trauma Therapy: Child

Counseling
Emotional Support
Journaling
Music Therapy
Recreation Therapy
Reminiscence Therapy
Role Enhancement
Self-Awareness Enhancement
Substance Use Prevention
Therapy Group

Additional Optional Interventions:
Art Therapy
Bibliotherapy

Self-Esteem: Situational Low

Definition: Development of a negative perception of self-worth in response to a current situation

Suggested Nursing Interventions for Problem Resolution:

Anticipatory Guidance
Assertiveness Training
Body Image Enhancement
Coping Enhancement
Decision-Making Support
Guilt Work Facilitation
Mood Management
Resiliency Promotion
Role Enhancement
Self-Esteem Enhancement
Socialization Enhancement

Art Therapy
Complex Relationship Building
Counseling
Developmental Enhancement: Adolescent
Developmental Enhancement: Child
Emotional Support
Grief Work Facilitation
Grief Work Facilitation: Perinatal Death
Hormone Replacement Therapy
Support System Enhancement

Additional Optional Interventions:
Abuse Protection Support
Animal-Assisted Therapy

Self-Esteem: Situational Low, Risk for

Definition: At risk for developing negative perception of self-worth in response to a current situation

Suggested Nursing Interventions for Problem Resolution:

Abuse Protection Support
Assertiveness Training
Behavior Modification
Body Image Enhancement
Childbirth Preparation
Counseling
Coping Enhancement
Developmental Enhancement: Adolescent
Developmental Enhancement: Child
Emotional Support

Grief Work Facilitation
Grief Work Facilitation: Perinatal Death
Guilt Work Facilitation
Mood Management
Relocation Stress Reduction
Resiliency Promotion
Role Enhancement
Self-Awareness Enhancement
Self-Esteem Enhancement
Self-Responsibility Facilitation
Substance Use Prevention

Substance Use Treatment
Support Group
Therapy Group
Values Clarification
Weight Management

Additional Optional Interventions:
Animal-Assisted Therapy
Art Therapy
Bowel Incontinence Care: Encopresis
Cognitive Restructuring

Complex Relationship Building
Decision-Making Support
Hormone Replacement Therapy
Lactation Counseling
Mutual Goal Setting
Prenatal Care
Reminiscence Therapy
Sustenance Support
Teaching: Sexuality
Urinary Incontinence Care: Enuresis

Self-Health Management, Ineffective

Definition: Pattern of regulating and integrating into daily living a therapeutic regimen for treatment of illness and its sequelae that is unsatisfactory for meeting specific health goals

Suggested Nursing Interventions for Problem Resolution:
Active Listening
Behavior Modification
Cognitive Restructuring
Complex Relationship Building
Coping Enhancement
Counseling
Crisis Intervention
Culture Brokerage
Decision-Making Support
Emotional Support
Family Support
Financial Resource Assistance
Health System Guidance
Learning Facilitation
Medication Management
Mutual Goal Setting
Nutritional Counseling
Patient Contracting
Risk Identification
Self-Awareness Enhancement
Self-Care Assistance
Self-Efficacy Enhancement
Self-Esteem Enhancement
Self-Modification Assistance
Self-Responsibility Facilitation
Substance Use Treatment

Teaching: Disease Process
Teaching: Individual
Teaching: Prescribed Diet
Teaching: Prescribed Exercise
Teaching: Prescribed Medication
Teaching: Procedure/Treatment
Teaching: Psychomotor Skill
Telephone Consultation
Telephone Follow-Up
Values Clarification

Additional Optional Interventions:
Asthma Management
Bibliotherapy
Exercise Promotion
Family Integrity Promotion
Family Mobilization
Humor
Learning Facilitation
Presence
Referral
Smoking Cessation Assistance
Support Group
Support System Enhancement
Truth Telling

Self-Health Management, Readiness for Enhanced

Definition: A pattern of regulating and integrating into daily living a therapeutic regimen for treatment of illness and the sequelae that is sufficient for meeting health-related goals and can be strengthened

Suggested Nursing Interventions for Problem Resolution:
Anticipatory Guidance
Commendation
Decision-Making Support
Health Education
Health Screening
Health System Guidance

Learning Facilitation
Mutual Goal Setting
Risk Identification
Self-Efficacy Enhancement
Self-Modification Assistance
Support Group
Surveillance

Teaching: Individual
Teaching: Procedure/Treatment

Additional Optional Interventions:
Culture Brokerage
Family Involvement Promotion
Financial Resource Assistance

Referral
Self-Esteem Enhancement
Self-Responsibility Facilitation
Support Group
Support System Enhancement
Values Clarification

Self-Mutilation

Definition: Deliberate self-injurious behavior causing tissue damage with the intent of causing nonfatal injury to attain relief of tension

Suggested Nursing Interventions for Problem Resolution:
Abuse Protection Support: Child
Active Listening
Activity Therapy
Anger Control Assistance
Anxiety Reduction
Area Restriction
Behavior Management
Behavior Management: Self-Harm
Behavior Modification
Body Image Enhancement
Calming Technique
Chemical Restraint
Cognitive Restructuring
Counseling
Developmental Enhancement: Adolescent
Environmental Management: Safety
Environmental Management: Violence Prevention
Impulse Control Training
Limit Setting
Mood Management
Mutual Goal Setting
Physical Restraint
Presence
Risk Identification

Seclusion
Self-Awareness Enhancement
Self-Esteem Enhancement
Self-Modification Assistance
Self-Responsibility Facilitation
Socialization Enhancement
Substance Use Treatment
Suicide Prevention
Wound Care

Additional Optional Interventions:
Animal-Assisted Therapy
Anticipatory Guidance
Art Therapy
Assertiveness Training
Bibliotherapy
Emotional Support
Family Therapy
Grief Work Facilitation
Hallucination Management
Medication Administration
Milieu Therapy
Patient Contracting
Security Enhancement
Therapy Group

Self-Mutilation, Risk for

Definition: At risk for deliberate self-injurious behavior causing tissue damage with the intent of causing nonfatal injury to attain relief of tension

Suggested Nursing Interventions for Problem Resolution:
Abuse Protection Support
Abuse Protection Support: Child
Active Listening
Activity Therapy
Anger Control Assistance
Anxiety Reduction
Area Restriction
Behavior Management
Behavior Management: Self-Harm
Behavior Modification
Body Image Enhancement
Calming Technique

Cognitive Restructuring
Coping Enhancement
Counseling
Delusion Management
Developmental Enhancement: Adolescent
Developmental Enhancement: Child
Environmental Management: Safety
Environmental Management: Violence Prevention
Family Integrity Promotion
Guilt Work Facilitation
Limit Setting
Mood Management
Mutual Goal Setting

Risk Identification
Self-Awareness Enhancement
Self-Esteem Enhancement
Self-Modification Assistance
Self-Responsibility Facilitation
Sexual Counseling
Socialization Enhancement
Substance Use Treatment
Suicide Prevention

Additional Optional Interventions:
Animal-Assisted Therapy
Anticipatory Guidance

Art Therapy
Assertiveness Training
Bibliotherapy
Emotional Support
Family Therapy
Grief Work Facilitation
Hallucination Management
Impulse Control Training
Medication Administration
Milieu Therapy
Patient Contracting
Security Enhancement
Therapy Group

Self-Neglect

Definition: A constellation of culturally framed behaviors involving one or more self-care activities in which there is a failure to maintain a socially accepted standard of health and well-being

Suggested Nursing Interventions for Problem Resolution:
Anxiety Reduction
Dementia Management
Mood Management
Oral Health Maintenance
Self-Care Assistance
Self-Care Assistance: Bathing/Hygiene
Self-Care Assistance: Dressing/Grooming
Self-Care Assistance: IADL
Self-Care Assistance: Toileting
Self-Efficacy Enhancement

Additional Optional Interventions:
Coping Enhancement
Environmental Management
Life Skills Enhancement
Medication Management
Self-Esteem Enhancement
Self-Responsibility Facilitation
Substance Use Treatment

Sexual Dysfunction

Definition: The state in which an individual experiences a change in sexual function during the sexual response phases of desire, excitation, and/or orgasm, which is viewed as unsatisfying, unrewarding, or inadequate

Suggested Nursing Interventions for Problem Resolution:
Abuse Protection Support
Anxiety Reduction
Behavior Management: Sexual
Childbirth Preparation
Medication Management
Prenatal Care
Reproductive Technology Management
Role Enhancement
Self-Awareness Enhancement
Self-Esteem Enhancement
Sexual Counseling
Teaching: Safe Sex
Teaching: Sexuality

Additional Optional Interventions:
Circulatory Care: Arterial Insufficiency
Counseling

Decision-Making Support
Energy Management
Family Planning: Contraception
Family Planning: Infertility
Family Process Maintenance
Fertility Preservation
Hormone Replacement Therapy
Pain Management
Postpartal Care
Premenstrual Syndrome (PMS) Management
Relaxation Therapy
Substance Use Treatment
Substance Use Treatment: Alcohol Withdrawal
Teaching: Individual
Therapy Group
Values Clarification

Sexuality Pattern, Ineffective

Definition: Expressions of concern regarding own sexuality

Suggested Nursing Interventions for Problem Resolution:
Anticipatory Guidance
Anxiety Reduction
Body Image Enhancement
Coping Enhancement
Counseling
Family Planning: Contraception
Family Planning: Infertility
Fertility Preservation
Reproductive Technology Management
Self-Awareness Enhancement
Sexual Counseling
Teaching: Safe Sex
Teaching: Sexuality

Additional Optional Interventions:
Abuse Protection Support
Behavior Management: Sexual
Decision-Making Support
Hormone Replacement Therapy
Postpartal Care
Premenstrual Syndrome (PMS) Management
Self-Esteem Enhancement
Support Group
Support System Enhancement

Shock, Risk for

Definition: At risk for an inadequate blood flow to the body's tissues, which may lead to life-threatening cellular dysfunction

Suggested Nursing Interventions for Problem Resolution:
Allergy Management
Bleeding Precautions
Bleeding Reduction
Bleeding Reduction: Antepartum Uterus
Bleeding Reduction: Gastrointestinal
Bleeding Reduction: Nasal
Bleeding Reduction: Postpartum Uterus
Bleeding Reduction: Wound
Blood Products Administration
Fluid Management
Fluid Monitoring
Fluid Resuscitation
Hemodynamic Regulation
Hypovolemia Management
Infection Control
Infection Protection
Oxygen Therapy

Risk Identification
Shock Prevention
Surveillance
Vital Signs Monitoring

Additional Optional Interventions:
Anaphylaxis Management
Cardiac Care
Central Venous Access Device Management
Circulatory Care: Arterial Insufficiency
Circulatory Care: Venous Insufficiency
Embolus Care: Pulmonary
Hypoglycemia Management
Intravenous (IV) Insertion
Intravenous (IV) Therapy
Medication Administration
Respiratory Monitoring

Skin Integrity, Impaired

Definition: Altered epidermis and/or dermis

Suggested Nursing Interventions for Problem Resolution:
Amputation Care
Bathing
Bleeding Reduction
Bleeding Reduction: Wound
Cast Care: Maintenance
Cast Care: Wet
Circulatory Precautions
Electrolyte Monitoring

Exercise Promotion
Fluid/Electrolyte Management
Foot Care
Incision Site Care
Latex Precautions
Lower Extremity Monitoring
Medication Administration: Skin
Medication Management
Ostomy Care

Perineal Care
Positioning
Pressure Management
Pressure Ulcer Care
Pressure Ulcer Prevention
Pruritus Management
Skin Care: Donor Site
Skin Care: Graft Site
Skin Care: Topical Treatments
Skin Surveillance
Splinting
Suturing
Teaching: Foot Care
Traction/Immobilization Care
Wound Care
Wound Care: Burns
Wound Care: Closed Drainage
Wound Care: Nonhealing
Wound Irrigation

Additional Optional Interventions:
Bed Rest Care
Cutaneous Stimulation
Exercise Promotion: Stretching
Exercise Therapy: Ambulation
Exercise Therapy: Balance
Exercise Therapy: Joint Mobility
Exercise Therapy: Muscle Control
Infection Control
Infection Protection
Leech Therapy
Nutrition Management
Nutrition Therapy
Peripherally Inserted Central Catheter (PICC) Care
Surveillance
Total Parenteral Nutrition (TPN) Administration
Transcutaneous Electrical Nerve Stimulation (TENS)
Vital Signs Monitoring

Skin Integrity, Risk for Impaired

Definition: At risk for alteration in epidermis and/or dermis

Suggested Nursing Interventions for Problem Resolution:
Amputation Care
Bathing
Bed Rest Care
Bowel Incontinence Care
Cast Care: Maintenance
Cast Care: Wet
Circulatory Care: Arterial Insufficiency
Circulatory Care: Venous Insufficiency
Circulatory Precautions
Eating Disorders Management
Foot Care
Incision Site Care
Infection Control
Infection Protection
Lactation Counseling
Latex Precautions
Lower Extremity Monitoring
Medication Administration: Skin
Nutrition Management
Nutrition Therapy
Ostomy Care
Perineal Care
Positioning
Positioning: Intraoperative
Pressure Management
Pressure Ulcer Prevention
Pruritus Management
Radiation Therapy Management
Risk Identification
Skin Care: Topical Treatments

Skin Surveillance
Splinting
Surveillance
Teaching: Foot Care
Traction/Immobilization Care
Tube Care: Umbilical Line
Wound Care

Additional Optional Interventions:
Bleeding Precautions
Electrolyte Monitoring
Exercise Promotion
Exercise Promotion: Strength Training
Exercise Promotion: Stretching
Exercise Therapy: Ambulation
Exercise Therapy: Balance
Exercise Therapy: Joint Mobility
Exercise Therapy: Muscle Control
Fluid/Electrolyte Management
Fluid Management
Medication Management
Nail Care
Pneumatic Tourniquet Precautions
Rectal Prolapse Management
Total Parenteral Nutrition (TPN) Administration
Transcutaneous Electrical Nerve Stimulation (TENS)
Vital Signs Monitoring
Weight Gain Assistance
Weight Reduction Assistance

Sleep Deprivation

Definition: Prolonged periods of time without sleep (sustained natural, periodic suspension of relative consciousness)

Suggested Nursing Interventions for Problem Resolution:
Anxiety Reduction
Coping Enhancement
Delirium Management
Dementia Management
Energy Management
Environmental Management: Comfort
Exercise Promotion
Guided Imagery
Medication Management
Meditation Facilitation
Pain Management
Phototherapy: Mood/Sleep Regulation
Progressive Muscle Relaxation
Sleep Enhancement

Additional Optional Interventions:
Animal-Assisted Therapy
Art Therapy
Massage
Music Therapy
Nausea Management
Reality Orientation
Reminiscence Therapy
Sustenance Support
Urinary Incontinence Care: Enuresis
Vomiting Management

Sleep Pattern, Disturbed

Definition: Time-limited interruptions of sleep amount and quality due to external factors

Suggested Nursing Interventions for Problem Resolution:
Caregiver Support
Dementia Management
Environmental Management
Environmental Management: Comfort
Hormone Replacement Therapy
Medication Administration
Medication Management
Medication Prescribing
Phototherapy: Mood/Sleep Regulation
Positioning
Relaxation Therapy
Security Enhancement
Self-Care Assistance: Toileting
Sleep Enhancement

Additional Optional Interventions:
Anxiety Reduction
Autogenic Training
Bathing
Calming Technique
Coping Enhancement
Energy Management
Exercise Promotion
Exercise Therapy: Ambulation
Massage
Meditation Facilitation
Music Therapy
Nutrition Management
Pain Management
Progressive Muscle Relaxation

Sleep, Readiness for Enhanced

Definition: A pattern of natural, periodic suspension of consciousness that provides adequate rest, sustains desired lifestyle, and can be strengthened

Suggested Nursing Interventions for Problem Resolution:
Anxiety Reduction
Coping Enhancement
Energy Management
Environmental Management: Comfort
Exercise Promotion
Medication Management
Positioning
Self-Efficacy Enhancement
Sleep Enhancement

Additional Optional Interventions:
Dementia Management
Guided Imagery
Massage
Music Therapy
Phototherapy: Mood/Sleep Regulation
Progressive Muscle Relaxation

Social Interaction, Impaired

Definition: Insufficient or excessive quantity or ineffective quality of social exchange

Suggested Nursing Interventions for Problem Resolution:
Behavior Management: Overactivity/Inattention
Behavior Management: Sexual
Behavior Modification: Social Skills
Communication Enhancement: Hearing Deficit
Communication Enhancement: Speech Deficit
Communication Enhancement: Visual Deficit
Complex Relationship Building
Dementia Management
Developmental Enhancement: Adolescent
Developmental Enhancement: Child
Life Skills Enhancement
Normalization Promotion
Reminiscence Therapy
Resiliency Promotion
Self-Awareness Enhancement
Self-Esteem Enhancement
Socialization Enhancement
Substance Use Treatment
Support Group
Support System Enhancement
Therapy Group
Values Clarification

Additional Optional Interventions:
Abuse Protection Support
Active Listening
Anger Control Assistance
Animal-Assisted Therapy
Anxiety Reduction
Assertiveness Training
Cognitive Stimulation
Coping Enhancement
Family Integrity Promotion
Family Process Maintenance
Family Support
Family Therapy
Humor
Mutual Goal Setting
Pass Facilitation
Recreation Therapy
Relocation Stress Reduction
Substance Use Treatment: Alcohol Withdrawal
Substance Use Treatment: Drug Withdrawal
Substance Use Treatment: Overdose
Teaching: Individual
Therapeutic Play
Truth Telling

Social Isolation

Definition: Aloneness experienced by the individual and perceived as imposed by others and as a negative or threatening state

Suggested Nursing Interventions for Problem Resolution:
Abuse Protection Support: Child
Abuse Protection Support: Domestic Partner
Abuse Protection Support: Elder
Activity Therapy
Behavior Modification: Social Skills
Body Image Enhancement
Complex Relationship Building
Counseling
Developmental Enhancement: Adolescent
Developmental Enhancement: Child
Emotional Support
Environmental Management
Family Integrity Promotion
Family Involvement Promotion
Hope Inspiration
Normalization Promotion
Presence
Recreation Therapy
Relocation Stress Reduction
Self-Awareness Enhancement
Self-Esteem Enhancement

Socialization Enhancement
Support System Enhancement
Visitation Facilitation

Additional Optional Interventions:
Animal-Assisted Therapy
Art Therapy
Bowel Management
Exercise Promotion
Family Therapy
Grief Work Facilitation
Mood Management
Mutual Goal Setting
Pass Facilitation
Reminiscence Therapy
Support Group
Therapy Group
Urinary Elimination Management
Weight Management

Sorrow: Chronic

Definition: Cyclical, recurring, and potentially progressive pattern of pervasive sadness experienced (by a parent, caregiver, or individual with chronic illness or disability) in response to continual loss throughout the trajectory of an illness or disability

Suggested Nursing Interventions for Problem Resolution:
Caregiver Support
Coping Enhancement
Counseling
Decision-Making Support
Emotional Support
Energy Management
Genetic Counseling
Grief Work Facilitation
Grief Work Facilitation: Perinatal Death
Hope Inspiration
Mood Management
Resiliency Promotion
Respite Care
Socialization Enhancement

Spiritual Growth Facilitation
Spiritual Support
Support Group

Additional Optional Interventions:
Activity Therapy
Anger Control Assistance
Animal-Assisted Therapy
Dying Care
Exercise Promotion
Forgiveness Facilitation
Humor
Music Therapy
Sleep Enhancement
Substance Use Prevention

Spiritual Distress

Definition: Impaired ability to experience and integrate meaning and purpose in life through connectedness with self, others, art, music, literature, nature, and/or a power greater than oneself

Suggested Nursing Interventions for Problem Resolution:
Anticipatory Guidance
Coping Enhancement
Counseling
Crisis Intervention
Decision-Making Support
Dying Care
Emotional Support
Forgiveness Facilitation
Grief Work Facilitation
Guilt Work Facilitation
Hope Inspiration
Pain Management
Presence
Resiliency Promotion
Spiritual Growth Facilitation
Spiritual Support
Support Group
Values Clarification

Additional Optional Interventions:
Abuse Protection Support: Religious
Active Listening
Activity Therapy
Animal-Assisted Therapy
Anxiety Reduction
Art Therapy
Caregiver Support
Distraction
Family Planning: Unplanned Pregnancy
Family Support
Mood Management
Music Therapy
Referral
Religious Addiction Prevention
Reminiscence Therapy
Security Enhancement
Socialization Enhancement
Touch
Truth Telling

Spiritual Distress, Risk for

Definition: At risk for an impaired ability to experience and integrate meaning and purpose in life through connectedness with self, others, art, music, literature, nature, and/or a power greater than oneself

Suggested Nursing Interventions for Problem Resolution:
Active Listening
Anticipatory Guidance
Anxiety Reduction
Behavior Modification: Social Skills

Community Disaster Preparedness
Conflict Mediation
Coping Enhancement
Counseling
Culture Brokerage

Decision-Making Support
Dying Care
Emotional Support
Environmental Management: Comfort
Forgiveness Facilitation
Grief Work Facilitation
Grief Work Facilitation: Perinatal Death
Hope Inspiration
Mood Management
Pain Management
Relocation Stress Reduction
Resiliency Promotion
Risk Identification
Self-Awareness Enhancement
Self-Esteem Enhancement
Spiritual Growth Facilitation
Spiritual Support
Substance Use Treatment

Support Group
Support System Enhancement
Values Clarification

Additional Optional Interventions:
Abuse Protection Support: Religious
Animal-Assisted Therapy
Caregiver Support
Family Support
Music Therapy
Referral
Religious Addiction Prevention
Religious Ritual Enhancement
Reminiscence Therapy
Socialization Enhancement
Truth Telling

Spiritual Well-Being, Readiness for Enhanced

Definition: A pattern of experiencing and integrating meaning and purpose in life through connectedness with self, others, art, music, literature, nature, and/or a power greater than oneself that is sufficient for well-being and can be strengthened

Suggested Nursing Interventions for Problem Resolution:
Bibliotherapy
Commendation
Forgiveness Facilitation
Journaling
Meditation Facilitation
Religious Ritual Enhancement
Resiliency Promotion
Role Enhancement
Self-Awareness Enhancement
Self-Esteem Enhancement
Self-Modification Assistance
Self-Responsibility Facilitation
Spiritual Growth Facilitation
Spiritual Support

Additional Optional Interventions:
Art Therapy
Autogenic Training
Body Image Enhancement
Guided Imagery
Hope Inspiration
Music Therapy
Religious Addiction Prevention
Reminiscence Therapy
Values Clarification

Stress Overload

Definition: Excessive amounts and types of demands that require action

Suggested Nursing Interventions for Problem Resolution:
Anger Control Assistance
Anxiety Reduction
Coping Enhancement
Decision-Making Support
Emotional Support
Financial Resource Assistance
Progressive Muscle Relaxation
Relaxation Therapy
Resiliency Promotion
Substance Use Prevention
Support Group
Support System Enhancement

Additional Optional Interventions:
Abuse Protection Support
Counseling
Crisis Intervention
Environmental Management
Environmental Management: Violence Prevention
Family Process Maintenance
Family Therapy
Life Skills Enhancement
Meditation Facilitation
Sleep Enhancement
Sustenance Support
Therapy Group

Sudden Infant Death Syndrome, Risk for

Definition: At risk for sudden death of an infant under 1 year of age

Suggested Nursing Interventions for Problem Resolution:
Health Screening
Infant Care
Infant Care: Newborn
Infant Care: Preterm
Parent Education: Infant
Prenatal Care
Risk Identification
Risk Identification: Childbearing Family
Smoking Cessation Assistance
Surveillance
Teaching: Infant Safety 0-3 Months
Teaching: Infant Safety 4-6 Months
Teaching: Infant Safety 7-9 Months
Teaching: Infant Safety 10-12 Months
Temperature Regulation

Additional Optional Interventions:
Caregiver Support
Immunization/Vaccination Management
Parenting Promotion
Teaching: Infant Nutrition 0-3 Months
Teaching: Infant Nutrition 4-6 Months
Teaching: Infant Nutrition 7-9 Months
Teaching: Infant Nutrition 10-12 Months
Teaching: Infant Stimulation 0-4 Months
Teaching: Infant Stimulation 5-8 Months
Teaching: Infant Stimulation 9-12 Months
Technology Management

Suffocation, Risk for

Definition: At risk of accidental suffocation (inadequate air available for inhalation)

Suggested Nursing Interventions for Problem Resolution:
Airway Management
Artificial Airway Management
Aspiration Precautions
Asthma Management
Environmental Management: Safety
Postanesthesia Care
Respiratory Monitoring
Risk Identification
Security Enhancement
Surveillance
Swallowing Therapy
Teaching: Infant Safety 0-3 Months
Teaching: Infant Safety 4-6 Months
Teaching: Infant Safety 7-9 Months

Teaching: Infant Safety 10-12 Months
Teaching: Toddler Safety 13-18 Months
Teaching: Toddler Safety 19-24 Months
Teaching: Toddler Safety 25-36 Months
Vital Signs Monitoring

Additional Optional Interventions:
Impulse Control Training
Infant Care
Infant Care: Newborn
Infant Care: Preterm
Parent Education: Infant
Positioning
Substance Use Treatment: Overdose
Suicide Prevention

Suicide, Risk for

Definition: At risk for self-inflicted, life-threatening injury

Suggested Nursing Interventions for Problem Resolution:
Anger Control Assistance
Anxiety Reduction
Area Restriction
Behavior Management: Self-Harm
Behavior Modification
Calming Technique
Coping Enhancement
Counseling
Crisis Intervention
Delusion Management

Environmental Management: Safety
Financial Resource Assistance
Guilt Work Facilitation
Hope Inspiration
Impulse Control Training
Limit Setting
Mood Management
Pain Management
Patient Contracting
Presence
Risk Identification

Substance Use Treatment
Suicide Prevention
Support Group
Teaching: Sexuality
Therapy Group

Additional Optional Interventions:
Abuse Protection Support: Child
Assertiveness Training
Behavior Modification: Social Skills
Cognitive Restructuring
Family Integrity Promotion
Family Involvement Promotion
Family Therapy

Forgiveness Facilitation
Grief Work Facilitation
Hallucination Management
Medication Management
Phototherapy: Mood/Sleep Regulation
Relocation Stress Reduction
Role Enhancement
Self-Awareness Enhancement
Self-Esteem Enhancement
Self-Modification Assistance
Self-Responsibility Facilitation
Socialization Enhancement
Support System Enhancement
Surveillance

Surgical Recovery, Delayed

Definition: Extension of the number of postoperative days required to initiate and perform activities that maintain life, health, and well-being

Suggested Nursing Interventions for Problem Resolution:
Case Management
Diet Staging
Embolus Precautions
Energy Management
Exercise Therapy: Ambulation
Fever Treatment
Fluid/Electrolyte Management
Incision Site Care
Infection Control
Infection Control: Intraoperative
Medication Administration
Medication Management
Nausea Management
Nutrition Management
Nutrition Therapy
Pain Management
Preoperative Coordination
Self-Care Assistance
Sleep Enhancement
Surveillance
Temperature Regulation
Vital Signs Monitoring
Vomiting Management
Wound Care

Additional Optional Interventions:
Airway Management
Bed Rest Care
Bowel Management
Caregiver Support
Cough Enhancement
Discharge Planning
Enteral Tube Feeding
Environmental Management: Home Preparation
Health Care Information Exchange
Health System Guidance
Home Maintenance Assistance
Insurance Authorization
Multidisciplinary Care Conference
Oral Health Maintenance
Positioning
Respiratory Monitoring
Telephone Consultation
Urinary Elimination Management
Wound Care: Closed Drainage
Wound Irrigation

Swallowing, Impaired

Definition: Abnormal functioning of the swallowing mechanism associated with deficits in oral, pharyngeal, or esophageal structure or function

Suggested Nursing Interventions for Problem Resolution:
Airway Suctioning
Aspiration Precautions
Positioning
Progressive Muscle Relaxation
Surveillance
Swallowing Therapy

Additional Optional Interventions:
Anxiety Reduction
Emotional Support
Enteral Tube Feeding
Feeding
Medication Management
Nutrition Management
Referral
Self-Care Assistance: Feeding

Thermal Injury, Risk for

Definition: At risk for damage to skin and mucous membranes due to extreme temperatures

Suggested Nursing Interventions for Problem Resolution:
Area Restriction
Circulatory Precautions
Dementia Management
Environmental Management: Safety
Hyperthermia Treatment
Laser Precautions
Lower Extremity Monitoring
Peripheral Sensation Management
Radiation Therapy Management
Risk Identification
Skin Surveillance
Teaching: Infant Safety 0-3 Months
Teaching: Infant Safety 4-6 Months

Teaching: Infant Safety 7-9 Months
Teaching: Infant Safety 10-12 Months
Teaching: Toddler Safety 13-18 Months
Teaching: Toddler Safety 19-24 Months
Teaching: Toddler Safety 25-36 Months
Unilateral Neglect Management

Additional Optional Interventions:
Fire-Setting Precautions
Smoking Cessation Assistance
Substance Use Treatment
Surgical Precautions
Teaching: Foot Care

Thermoregulation, Ineffective

Definition: Temperature fluctuation between hypothermia and hyperthermia

Suggested Nursing Interventions for Problem Resolution:
Bathing
Environmental Management
Fever Treatment
Fluid Management
Fluid Monitoring
Hemodynamic Regulation
Hyperthermia Treatment
Infant Care: Newborn
Infant Care: Preterm

Temperature Regulation
Temperature Regulation: Perioperative
Vital Signs Monitoring

Additional Optional Interventions:
Anxiety Reduction
Blood Products Administration
Medication Administration
Peripherally Inserted Central Catheter (PICC) Care
Phlebotomy: Arterial Blood Sample

Tissue Integrity, Impaired

Definition: Damage to mucous membrane, corneal, integumentary, or subcutaneous tissues

Suggested Nursing Interventions for Problem Resolution:
Bleeding Reduction: Gastrointestinal
Bleeding Reduction: Nasal
Bleeding Reduction: Postpartum Uterus
Blood Products Administration
Electrolyte Monitoring
Fluid Management
Fluid Monitoring
Incision Site Care
Infection Protection
Latex Precautions
Medication Administration: Ear
Medication Administration: Eye
Medication Administration: Rectal
Medication Administration: Vaginal
Nutrition Management

Nutrition Therapy
Oral Health Maintenance
Oral Health Restoration
Perineal Care
Positioning
Pressure Ulcer Care
Pressure Ulcer Prevention
Rectal Prolapse Management
Skin Care: Donor Site
Skin Care: Graft Site
Skin Care: Topical Treatments
Skin Surveillance
Splinting
Suturing
Traction/Immobilization Care
Urinary Incontinence Care

Wound Care
Wound Care: Burns
Wound Care: Nonhealing
Wound Irrigation

Additional Optional Interventions:
Bathing
Infection Control
Leech Therapy

Lower Extremity Monitoring
Massage
Medication Administration
Medication Management
Ostomy Care
Pressure Management
Teaching: Foot Care
Tube Care: Urinary
Vital Signs Monitoring

Tissue Perfusion: Cardiac, Risk for Decreased

Definition: At risk for decrease in cardiac (coronary) circulation that may compromise health

Suggested Nursing Interventions for Problem Resolution:
Cardiac Risk Management
Exercise Promotion
Fluid Management
Fluid Resuscitation
Health Education
Hyperglycemia Management
Medication Management
Nutritional Counseling
Oxygen Therapy
Risk Identification
Smoking Cessation Assistance
Substance Use Treatment
Teaching: Prescribed Diet

Teaching: Prescribed Medication
Vital Signs Monitoring
Weight Reduction Assistance

Additional Optional Interventions:
Embolus Precautions
Family Planning: Contraception
Health Screening
Phlebotomy: Venous Blood Sample
Surveillance

Tissue Perfusion: Cerebral, Risk for Ineffective

Definition: At risk for decrease in cerebral tissue circulation that may compromise health

Suggested Nursing Interventions for Problem Resolution:
Cardiac Care
Cardiac Care: Acute
Cardiac Risk Management
Cerebral Edema Management
Embolus Care: Peripheral
Embolus Care: Pulmonary
Embolus Precautions
Hemodynamic Regulation
Intracranial Pressure (ICP) Monitoring
Medication Management
Neurologic Monitoring
Risk Identification
Subarachnoid Hemorrhage Precautions
Surveillance
Teaching: Disease Process
Teaching: Prescribed Diet

Teaching: Prescribed Medication
Teaching: Procedure/Treatment
Thrombolytic Therapy Management

Additional Optional Interventions:
Bleeding Precautions
Circulatory Care: Arterial Insufficiency
Circulatory Care: Venous Insufficiency
Defibrillator Management: External
Defibrillator Management: Internal
Infection Control
Pacemaker Management: Permanent
Pacemaker Management: Temporary
Seizure Precautions
Substance Use Treatment
Vital Signs Monitoring

Tissue Perfusion: Peripheral, Ineffective

Definition: Decrease in blood circulation to the periphery that may compromise health

Suggested Nursing Interventions for Problem Resolution:
Acid-Base Management
Acid-Base Monitoring
Bedside Laboratory Testing
Circulatory Care: Arterial Insufficiency
Circulatory Care: Mechanical Assist Device
Circulatory Care: Venous Insufficiency
Circulatory Precautions
Emergency Care
Fluid/Electrolyte Management
Fluid Management
Fluid Monitoring
Foot Care
Hemodynamic Regulation
Hypervolemia Management
Hypovolemia Management
Invasive Hemodynamic Monitoring
Laboratory Data Interpretation
Lower Extremity Monitoring
Neurologic Monitoring
Nutrition Management
Oxygen Therapy
Peripheral Sensation Management
Pneumatic Tourniquet Precautions
Positioning
Pressure Ulcer Prevention
Resuscitation
Resuscitation: Neonate

Shock Management
Shock Management: Cardiac
Shock Management: Vasogenic
Skin Surveillance
Smoking Cessation Assistance
Teaching: Disease Process
Vital Signs Monitoring

Additional Optional Interventions:
Embolus Care: Peripheral
Embolus Precautions
Exercise Promotion
Exercise Therapy: Ambulation
Exercise Therapy: Balance
Exercise Therapy: Joint Mobility
Exercise Therapy: Muscle Control
Intravenous (IV) Insertion
Intravenous (IV) Therapy
Medication Administration
Medication Management
Pain Management
Peripherally Inserted Central Catheter (PICC) Care
Phlebotomy: Arterial Blood Sample
Phlebotomy: Cannulated Vessel
Phlebotomy: Venous Blood Sample
Surveillance
Temperature Regulation
Total Parenteral Nutrition (TPN) Administration

Tissue Perfusion: Peripheral, Risk for Ineffective

Definition: At risk for a decrease in blood circulation to the periphery that may compromise health

Suggested Nursing Interventions for Problem Resolution:
Circulatory Care: Venous Insufficiency
Circulatory Precautions
Embolus Care: Peripheral
Embolus Precautions
Exercise Promotion
Hyperglycemia Management
Hypoglycemia Management
Lower Extremity Monitoring
Skin Surveillance
Smoking Cessation Assistance
Teaching: Disease Process
Teaching: Foot Care
Teaching: Prescribed Diet

Teaching: Prescribed Exercise
Teaching: Prescribed Medication
Weight Reduction Assistance

Additional Optional Interventions:
Bed Rest Care
Laboratory Data Interpretation
Medication Administration
Medication Management
Medication Prescribing
Peripheral Sensation Management
Positioning
Splinting
Vital Signs Monitoring

Transfer Ability, Impaired

Definition: Limitation of independent movement between two nearby surfaces

Suggested Nursing Interventions for Problem Resolution:
Body Mechanics Promotion
Energy Management
Environmental Management: Safety
Exercise Promotion
Exercise Promotion: Strength Training
Exercise Promotion: Stretching
Exercise Therapy: Balance
Exercise Therapy: Muscle Control
Fall Prevention
Positioning
Positioning: Neurologic
Positioning: Wheelchair
Self-Care Assistance: Transfer
Teaching: Prescribed Exercise
Transfer
Transport: Intrafacility

Additional Optional Interventions:
Dementia Management
Medication Management
Mutual Goal Setting
Nutrition Management
Pain Management
Self-Care Assistance
Self-Care Assistance: Bathing/Hygiene
Self-Care Assistance: Dressing/Grooming
Self-Care Assistance: Feeding
Self-Care Assistance: Toileting
Sleep Enhancement
Weight Reduction Assistance

Trauma, Risk for

Definition: Accentuated risk of accidental tissue injury, (e.g., wound, burn, fracture)

Suggested Nursing Interventions for Problem Resolution:
Communication Enhancement: Visual Deficit
Delirium Management
Dementia Management
Elopement Precautions
Environmental Management: Safety
Environmental Management: Violence Prevention
Environmental Management: Worker Safety
Fall Prevention
Health Education
Laser Precautions
Peripheral Sensation Management
Physical Restraint
Positioning
Pressure Management
Radiation Therapy Management
Reality Orientation
Risk Identification
Seizure Precautions
Skin Surveillance
Sports-Injury Prevention: Youth
Surgical Precautions
Surveillance
Teaching: Disease Process
Teaching: Individual

Teaching: Infant Safety 0-3 Months
Teaching: Infant Safety 4-6 Months
Teaching: Infant Safety 7-9 Months
Teaching: Infant Safety 10-12 Months
Teaching: Toddler Safety 13-18 Months
Teaching: Toddler Safety 19-24 Months
Teaching: Toddler Safety 25-36 Months
Vehicle Safety Promotion
Vital Signs Monitoring

Additional Optional Interventions:
Embolus Precautions
Exercise Promotion: Strength Training
Exercise Therapy: Balance
Exercise Therapy: Muscle Control
Parent Education: Adolescent
Parent Education: Childrearing Family
Parent Education: Infant
Positioning: Neurologic
Positioning: Wheelchair
Self-Care Assistance: Transfer
Substance Use Treatment
Substance Use Treatment: Alcohol Withdrawal
Substance Use Treatment: Drug Withdrawal

Unilateral Neglect

Definition: Impairment in sensory and motor response, mental representation, and spatial attention of the body, and the corresponding environment, characterized by inattention to one side and overattention to the opposite side. Left-side neglect is more severe and persistent than right-side neglect

Suggested Nursing Interventions for Problem Resolution:
Body Image Enhancement
Communication Enhancement: Visual Deficit
Coping Enhancement
Environmental Management: Safety
Fall Prevention
Neurologic Monitoring
Positioning
Self-Care Assistance
Touch
Unilateral Neglect Management

Additional Optional Interventions:
Amputation Care
Caregiver Support

Cerebral Perfusion Promotion
Exercise Promotion
Exercise Promotion: Stretching
Exercise Therapy: Ambulation
Exercise Therapy: Balance
Exercise Therapy: Joint Mobility
Exercise Therapy: Muscle Control
Lower Extremity Monitoring
Mutual Goal Setting
Support System Enhancement
Teaching: Individual

Urinary Elimination, Impaired

Definition: Dysfunction in urine elimination

Suggested Nursing Interventions for Problem Resolution:
Bladder Irrigation
Fluid Management
Fluid Monitoring
Medication Management
Medication Prescribing
Pelvic Muscle Exercise
Pessary Management
Prompted Voiding
Urinary Catheterization
Urinary Catheterization: Intermittent
Urinary Elimination Management
Urinary Incontinence Care
Urinary Incontinence Care: Enuresis
Urinary Retention Care

Additional Optional Interventions:
Anxiety Reduction
Hemodialysis Therapy
Infection Control
Infection Protection
Pain Management
Perineal Care
Postpartal Care
Self-Care Assistance: Toileting
Skin Surveillance
Teaching: Toilet Training
Tube Care: Urinary
Weight Management

Urinary Elimination, Readiness for Enhanced

Definition: A pattern of urinary functions that is sufficient for meeting eliminatory needs and can be strengthened

Suggested Nursing Interventions for Problem Resolution:
Commendation
Fluid Management
Fluid Monitoring
Medication Management
Medication Prescribing
Pelvic Muscle Exercise
Pessary Management
Self-Care Assistance: Toileting

Self-Efficacy Enhancement
Self-Esteem Enhancement
Self-Responsibility Facilitation
Teaching: Toilet Training
Urinary Elimination Management

Additional Optional Interventions:
Prompted Voiding
Tube Care: Urinary

Urinary Bladder Training
Urinary Catheterization
Urinary Catheterization: Intermittent
Urinary Habit Training

Urinary Incontinence Care
Urinary Incontinence Care: Enuresis
Urinary Retention Care

Urinary Incontinence: Functional

Definition: Inability of a usually continent person to reach the toilet in time to avoid unintentional loss of urine

Suggested Nursing Interventions for Problem Resolution:
Environmental Management
Pelvic Muscle Exercise
Prompted Voiding
Self-Care Assistance: Toileting
Urinary Elimination Management
Urinary Habit Training
Urinary Incontinence Care

Additional Optional Interventions:
Bathing
Communication Enhancement: Visual Deficit
Dressing
Exercise Promotion
Exercise Therapy: Ambulation
Perineal Care
Self-Awareness Enhancement

Urinary Incontinence: Overflow

Definition: Involuntary loss of urine associated with overdistention of the bladder

Suggested Nursing Interventions for Problem Resolution:
Fluid Management
Medication Management
Teaching: Prescribed Medication
Tube Care: Urinary
Urinary Catheterization
Urinary Catheterization: Intermittent
Urinary Incontinence Care
Urinary Retention Care

Additional Optional Interventions:
Bathing
Perineal Care
Pessary Management
Skin Surveillance
Urinary Elimination Management

Urinary Incontinence: Reflex

Definition: Involuntary loss of urine at somewhat predictable intervals when a specific bladder volume is reached

Suggested Nursing Interventions for Problem Resolution:
Fluid Management
Pelvic Muscle Exercise
Tube Care: Urinary
Urinary Bladder Training
Urinary Catheterization
Urinary Catheterization: Intermittent
Urinary Elimination Management

Urinary Incontinence Care
Urinary Retention Care

Additional Optional Interventions:
Bathing
Perineal Care
Self-Care Assistance: Bathing/Hygiene
Self-Care Assistance: Toileting
Teaching: Procedure/Treatment

Urinary Incontinence: Stress

Definition: Sudden leakage of urine with activities that increase intra-abdominal pressure

Suggested Nursing Interventions for Problem Resolution:
Biofeedback
Medication Management
Pelvic Muscle Exercise
Pessary Management
Teaching: Individual
Teaching: Prescribed Medication
Urinary Elimination Management
Urinary Habit Training

Urinary Incontinence Care
Weight Management

Additional Optional Interventions:
Perineal Care
Respiratory Monitoring
Self-Care Assistance: Toileting

Urinary Incontinence: Urge

Definition: Involuntary passage of urine occurring soon after a strong sense of urgency to void

Suggested Nursing Interventions for Problem Resolution:
Environmental Management
Fluid Management
Fluid Monitoring
Medication Management
Urinary Bladder Training
Urinary Elimination Management
Urinary Habit Training
Urinary Incontinence Care

Additional Optional Interventions:
Bathing
Infection Control
Perineal Care
Self-Care Assistance: Toileting
Teaching: Toilet Training
Tube Care: Urinary
Urinary Catheterization
Urinary Catheterization: Intermittent

Urinary Incontinence: Urge, Risk for

Definition: At risk for involuntary passage of urine occurring soon after a strong sensation of urgency to void

Suggested Nursing Interventions for Problem Resolution:
Environmental Management
Fluid Management
Fluid Monitoring
Infection Control
Medication Management
Self-Care Assistance: Toileting
Substance Use Treatment
Teaching: Prescribed Medication
Urinary Elimination Management
Urinary Habit Training

Additional Optional Interventions:
Exercise Promotion
Pelvic Muscle Exercise
Perineal Care
Pessary Management
Prompted Voiding
Risk Identification
Teaching: Toilet Training
Tube Care: Urinary
Urinary Catheterization
Weight Management

Urinary Retention

Definition: Incomplete emptying of the bladder

Suggested Nursing Interventions for Problem Resolution:
Bladder Irrigation
Fluid Management
Fluid Monitoring
Medication Management
Tube Care: Urinary
Urinary Catheterization
Urinary Catheterization: Intermittent
Urinary Elimination Management
Urinary Retention Care

Additional Optional Interventions:
Distraction
Exercise Promotion
Exercise Therapy: Ambulation
Exercise Therapy: Balance
Exercise Therapy: Joint Mobility
Exercise Therapy: Muscle Control
Massage
Perineal Care
Relaxation Therapy

Vascular Trauma, Risk for

Definition: At risk for damage to a vein and its surrounding tissues related to the presence of a catheter and/or infused solutions

Suggested Nursing Interventions for Problem Resolution:
Allergy Management
Central Venous Access Device Management
Dialysis Access Maintenance
Intravenous (IV) Insertion
Intravenous (IV) Therapy
Invasive Hemodynamic Monitoring
Medication Administration: Intravenous (IV)
Peripherally Inserted Central Catheter (PICC) Care

Phlebotomy: Cannulated Vessel
Risk Identification
Skin Surveillance

Additional Optional Interventions:
Bleeding Precautions
Embolus Precautions
Infection Protection
Pressure Management

Ventilation, Impaired Spontaneous

Definition: Decreased energy reserves resulting in an inability to maintain independent breathing that is adequate to support life

Suggested Nursing Interventions for Problem Resolution:
Acid-Base Management
Acid-Base Management: Respiratory Acidosis
Acid-Base Management: Respiratory Alkalosis
Acid-Base Monitoring
Airway Management
Airway Suctioning
Anxiety Reduction
Artificial Airway Management
Aspiration Precautions
Calming Technique
Chest Physiotherapy
Emotional Support
Energy Management
Environmental Management
Environmental Management: Comfort
Environmental Management: Safety
Fluid/Electrolyte Management
Fluid Management
Fluid Monitoring
Fluid Resuscitation
Infection Control
Infection Protection
Mechanical Ventilation Management: Invasive
Mechanical Ventilation Management: Noninvasive
Mechanical Ventilation Management: Pneumonia Prevention
Mechanical Ventilatory Weaning
Medication Administration
Oral Health Maintenance
Oxygen Therapy
Positioning
Respiratory Monitoring
Resuscitation: Neonate

Skin Surveillance
Ventilation Assistance
Vital Signs Monitoring

Additional Optional Interventions:
Active Listening
Bed Rest Care
Body Image Enhancement
Coping Enhancement
Decision-Making Support
Distraction
Emergency Care
Endotracheal Extubation
Hope Inspiration
Humor
Intravenous (IV) Insertion
Intravenous (IV) Therapy
Patient Rights Protection
Phlebotomy: Arterial Blood Sample
Physical Restraint
Presence
Pressure Management
Pressure Ulcer Prevention
Security Enhancement
Self-Care Assistance
Spiritual Support
Surveillance
Technology Management
Touch
Tube Care
Tube Care: Chest
Tube Care: Gastrointestinal
Tube Care: Urinary

Ventilatory Weaning Response, Dysfunctional

Definition: Inability to adjust to lowered levels of mechanical ventilator support that interrupts and prolongs the weaning process

Suggested Nursing Interventions for Problem Resolution:
Acid-Base Management
Airway Management
Anxiety Reduction
Artificial Airway Management
Aspiration Precautions
Environmental Management: Comfort
Mechanical Ventilation Management: Invasive
Mechanical Ventilation Management: Noninvasive
Mechanical Ventilation Management: Pneumonia Prevention
Mechanical Ventilatory Weaning
Pain Management
Preparatory Sensory Information
Respiratory Monitoring
Ventilation Assistance
Vital Signs Monitoring

Coping Enhancement
Distraction
Emotional Support
Endotracheal Extubation
Energy Management
Environmental Management: Comfort
Hope Inspiration
Phlebotomy: Arterial Blood Sample
Presence
Relaxation Therapy
Sleep Enhancement
Support System Enhancement
Surveillance
Teaching: Procedure/Treatment
Technology Management
Touch

Additional Optional Interventions:
Calming Technique
Communication Enhancement: Speech Deficit

Violence: Other-Directed, Risk for

Definition: At risk for behaviors in which an individual demonstrates that he or she can be physically, emotionally, and/or sexually harmful to others

Suggested Nursing Interventions for Problem Resolution:
Abuse Protection Support
Abuse Protection Support: Child
Abuse Protection Support: Domestic Partner
Abuse Protection Support: Elder
Anger Control Assistance
Anxiety Reduction
Area Restriction
Art Therapy
Behavior Management
Behavior Management: Overactivity/Inattention
Behavior Management: Sexual
Behavior Modification
Calming Technique
Coping Enhancement
Crisis Intervention
Delusion Management
Dementia Management
Dementia Management: Bathing
Distraction
Environmental Management: Violence Prevention
Fire-Setting Precautions
Hallucination Management
Impulse Control Training
Medication Administration
Mood Management
Physical Restraint
Risk Identification
Seclusion

Security Enhancement
Substance Use Prevention
Substance Use Treatment
Substance Use Treatment: Alcohol Withdrawal
Substance Use Treatment: Drug Withdrawal
Suicide Prevention
Support System Enhancement
Surveillance

Additional Optional Interventions:
Animal-Assisted Therapy
Behavior Modification: Social Skills
Family Involvement Promotion
Family Support
Guilt Work Facilitation
Intrapartal Care
Medication Management
Mutual Goal Setting
Neurologic Monitoring
Prenatal Care
Presence
Reality Orientation
Seizure Management
Self-Esteem Enhancement
Support Group
Therapeutic Play
Triage: Emergency Center
Triage: Telephone

Violence: Self-Directed, Risk for

Definition: At risk for behaviors in which an individual demonstrates that he or she can be physically, emotionally, and/or sexually harmful to self

Suggested Nursing Interventions for Problem Resolution:
Anger Control Assistance
Anxiety Reduction
Area Restriction
Behavior Management: Self-Harm
Behavior Modification
Calming Technique
Coping Enhancement
Counseling
Crisis Intervention
Delusion Management
Environmental Management: Safety
Environmental Management: Violence Prevention
Impulse Control Training
Limit Setting
Mood Management
Patient Contracting
Physical Restraint
Risk Identification
Seclusion
Security Enhancement
Self-Awareness Enhancement
Self-Esteem Enhancement
Self-Modification Assistance
Self-Responsibility Facilitation
Substance Use Treatment
Substance Use Treatment: Alcohol Withdrawal

Substance Use Treatment: Drug Withdrawal
Substance Use Treatment: Overdose
Suicide Prevention

Additional Optional Interventions:
Animal-Assisted Therapy
Assertiveness Training
Behavior Modification: Social Skills
Cognitive Restructuring
Conflict Mediation
Dementia Management
Family Integrity Promotion
Family Involvement Promotion
Family Therapy
Grief Work Facilitation
Guilt Work Facilitation
Hallucination Management
Medication Management
Hope Inspiration
Phototherapy: Mood/Sleep Regulation
Recreation Therapy
Socialization Enhancement
Support Group
Support System Enhancement
Teaching: Safe Sex
Therapy Group

Walking, Impaired

Definition: Limitation of independent movement within the environment on foot

Suggested Nursing Interventions for Problem Resolution:
Body Mechanics Promotion
Energy Management
Environmental Management
Exercise Promotion
Exercise Promotion: Strength Training
Exercise Promotion: Stretching
Exercise Therapy: Ambulation
Exercise Therapy: Balance
Exercise Therapy: Joint Mobility
Exercise Therapy: Muscle Control
Fall Prevention
Pain Management

Positioning
Teaching: Prescribed Exercise
Transport: Interfacility
Transport: Intrafacility

Additional Optional Interventions:
Lower Extremity Monitoring
Medication Management
Mutual Goal Setting
Nutrition Management
Sleep Enhancement
Weight Reduction Assistance

Wandering

Definition: Meandering, aimless, or repetitive locomotion that exposes the individual to harm; frequently incongruent with boundaries, limits, or obstacles

Suggested Nursing Interventions for Problem Resolution:
Area Restriction
Behavior Management
Behavior Management: Overactivity/Inattention
Dementia Management
Dementia Management: Wandering
Elopement Precautions
Environmental Management: Safety
Fall Prevention
Limit Setting
Medication Management
Pain Management
Reality Orientation
Self-Care Assistance
Teaching: Toddler Safety 13-18 Months

Teaching: Toddler Safety 19-24 Months
Teaching: Toddler Safety 25-36 Months
Validation Therapy

Additional Optional Interventions:
Anxiety Reduction
Calming Technique
Caregiver Support
Distraction
Family Involvement Promotion
Health System Guidance
Patient Rights Protection
Relocation Stress Reduction
Respite Care
Urinary Elimination Management

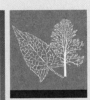

PART SEVEN

Appendixes

Interventions: New, Revised, and Retired Since the Fifth Edition

INTERVENTIONS NEW TO THE SIXTH EDITION (n=23)

Central Venous Access Device Management
Commendation
Cup Feeding: Newborn
Dementia Management: Wandering
Developmental Enhancement: Infant
Diet Staging: Weight Loss Surgery
Dry Eye Prevention
Enema Administration
Healing Touch
Hyperthermia Treatment
Infant Care: Newborn
Infant Care: Preterm

Life Skills Enhancement
Listening Visits
Mechanical Ventilation Management: Pneumonia Prevention
Nasal Irrigation
Patient Identification
Prescribing: Diagnostic Testing
Prescribing: Nonpharmacologic Treatment
Reiki
Stem Cell Infusion
Surgical Instrumentation Management
Wound Care: Nonhealing

INTERVENTIONS REVISED FOR THE SIXTH EDITION

Label Name Changes (n=5)

Cardiac Risk Management (formerly Cardiac Precautions)
Cesarean Birth Care (formerly Cesarean Section Care)
Hair and Scalp Care (formerly Hair Care)

Teaching: Prescribed Exercise (formerly Teaching: Prescribed Activity/Exercise)
Temperature Regulation: Perioperative (formerly Temperature Regulation: Intraoperative)

Substantive Intervention Changes: Major (n=74)

Interventions in this category have substantive changes in definition or addition/revision of multiple activities that further explicate the nursing actions associated with the intervention.

Acid-Base Management
Acid-Base Management: Metabolic Acidosis
Acid-Base Management: Metabolic Alkalosis
Acid-Base Management: Respiratory Acidosis
Acid-Base Management: Respiratory Alkalosis
Acid-Base Monitoring
Activity Therapy
Airway Insertion and Stabilization
Airway Suctioning
Amputation Care
Artificial Airway Management
Aspiration Precautions
Attachment Promotion
Cardiac Care: Acute
Cardiac Risk Management
Cesarean Birth Care
Chest Physiotherapy
Circulatory Precautions
Code Management
Communication Enhancement: Hearing Deficit

Communication Enhancement: Speech Deficit
Communication Enhancement: Visual Deficit
Contact Lens Care
Ear Care
Embolus Care: Peripheral
Embolus Care: Pulmonary
Embolus Precautions
Emergency Care
Family Planning: Contraception
Fever Treatment
First Aid
Fluid/Electrolyte Management
Fluid Monitoring
Hair and Scalp Care
Hemodynamic Regulation
Hypervolemia Management
Hypothermia Treatment
Hypovolemia Management
Infant Care
Intravenous (IV) Insertion

Kangaroo Care
Lactation Counseling
Lactation Suppression
Malignant Hyperthermia Precautions
Medication Administration: Interpleural
Nutrition Management
Nutritional Monitoring
Oral Health Promotion
Oral Health Restoration
Peripherally Inserted Central Catheter (PICC) Care
Positioning: Neurologic
Postmortem Care
Postpartal Care
Prenatal Care
Resuscitation
Risk Identification
Risk Identification: Childbearing Family

Splinting
Substance Use Treatment
Substance Use Treatment: Drug Withdrawal
Substance Use Treatment: Overdose
Surgical Assistance
Surgical Precautions
Teaching: Safe Sex
Temperature Regulation
Temperature Regulation: Perioperative
Therapeutic Touch
Total Parenteral Nutrition (TPN) Administration
Transcutaneous Electrical Nerve Stimulation (TENS)
Tube Care: Chest
Tube Care: Urinary
Urinary Catheterization
Wound Care: Closed Drainage
Wound Irrigation

Substantive Intervention Changes: Minor (n=54)

Interventions in this category have additions or revisions of a few activities that enhance the clinical application of the intervention.

Abuse Protection Support: Child
Abuse Protection Support: Domestic Partner
Abuse Protection Support: Elder
Anticipatory Guidance
Art Therapy
Bed Rest Care
Behavior Modification
Bleeding Reduction
Bowel Incontinence Care
Bowel Training
Calming Technique
Cardiac Care
Cardiac Care: Rehabilitative
Cognitive Stimulation
Coping Enhancement
Cutaneous Stimulation
Delirium Management
Diet Staging
Distraction
Dying Care
Dysrhythmia Management
Environmental Management: Violence Prevention
Heat/Cold Application
Infection Control: Intraoperative
Infection Protection
Learning Facilitation
Medication Administration

Parent Education: Adolescent
Parent Education: Childrearing Family
Patient-Controlled Analgesia (PCA) Assistance
Perineal Care
Peripheral Sensation Management
Positioning: Wheelchair
Referral
Respiratory Monitoring
Respite Care
Seclusion
Seizure Management
Seizure Precautions
Self-Esteem Enhancement
Self-Modification Assistance
Sexual Counseling
Support Group
Support System Enhancement
Surveillance
Teaching: Individual
Teaching: Preoperative
Teaching: Prescribed Diet
Teaching: Prescribed Exercise
Teaching: Psychomotor Skill
Technology Management
Tube Care
Tube Care: Ventriculostomy/Lumbar Drain
Weight Reduction Assistance

INTERVENTIONS IN THE FIFTH EDITION THAT WERE RETIRED IN THIS EDITION (n=11)

Bowel Irrigation changed to Enema Administration

Breastfeeding Assistance subsumed under Lactation Counseling

Developmental Care changed to Infant Care: Preterm

Environmental Management: Attachment Process subsumed under Attachment Promotion

Heat Exposure Treatment changed to Hyperthermia Treatment

Hemorrhage Control subsumed under Bleeding Reduction

Newborn Care changed to Infant Care: Newborn

Newborn Monitoring subsumed under Infant Care: Newborn

Prosthesis Care subsumed under Amputation Care

Surveillance: Safety subsumed under other interventions

Venous Access Device (VAD) Maintenance changed to Central Venous Access Device Management

Guidelines for Submission of a New or Revised Intervention

This appendix contains materials to assist you in preparing an intervention to submit for review or to suggest a change for an existing intervention. It is important that a submitter be familiar with NIC and with the Principles for Intervention Development and Refinement (included in this Appendix) before developing or revising an intervention.

THE MATERIALS NEEDED

All submissions should be submitted in English and formatted in the same style as appears in NIC. Background readings/references should be in APA format. Materials that are too difficult to read or incomplete will be sent back to the submitter without being reviewed.

Each submission of a **proposed new intervention** should include a label, a definition, activities listed in logical order, and a short list of background readings that support the intervention. In addition, a *rationale for inclusion* should also be attached and the submitter should *note how the proposed new intervention differs from existing interventions*. If a new intervention would call for changes in existing interventions, these changes should also be submitted. The Demographic Information Form should be filled out and included for each submitter.

Each submission for a **revised intervention** should indicate how the proposed changes relate to the existing intervention. In most instances, a copy of the intervention from the NIC book with additions, deletions, and modifications made with track changes is the best way to clearly indicate changes. A rationale must also be included. The Demographic Information Form should be filled out and included for each submitter.

THE REVIEW PROCESS

1. Submitted materials for proposed new or revised interventions are assigned to two or three reviewers who have expertise in the content area and who are familiar with NIC.
2. Each reviewer receives a copy of what has been submitted and a review form.
3. Each reviewer is asked to return comments and recommendations within 1 month. The initial submission and the reviewer's comments are then reviewed by the research team and a decision is made.
4. Approximately 2 to 6 months after submission, the submitter will receive a letter stating the outcome of the process. If the decision is for inclusion in NIC, the submitter will be acknowledged in the next edition.

PRINCIPLES FOR INTERVENTION DEVELOPMENT AND REFINEMENT

A set of guiding principles is necessary in forming intervention labels, definitions, and activities. Such principles, used to maintain consistency and cohesion within the Classification, can help the user understand the Classification's language and form.

General Principles for Intervention Labels

Intervention labels are concepts. The following principles should be used when selecting names for concepts:
1. They should be noun statements; no verbs.
2. They should, preferably, be three words or less; no more than five words.
3. When a two-part label is required, use a colon to separate the words (e.g., Bleeding Reduction: Nasal). Guidelines for use of the colon are: (1) avoid unless it is indicated and desired by clinical practice and (2) use to indicate a more specialized area of practice only when there are different activities that require a new intervention.
4. Capitalize each word.
5. Labels will include modifiers to represent the nurse's actions. Choose modifiers to represent the nurse's actions (e.g., Administration, Assistance, Management, Promotion). The modifier should be selected based on its meaning, how it sounds in relationship to the other words in the label, and its acceptability in general practice. Some of the possible modifiers are listed here:
   Administration: directing the movement or behavior of, having charge of; see also Management
   Assistance: helping
   Care: paying close attention, giving protection, being concerned about
   Enhancement: making greater, augmenting, increasing; see also Promotion
   Maintenance: continuing or carrying on, supporting
   Management: directing the movement or behavior of, having charge of; see also Administration
   Monitoring: watching and checking
   Precaution: taking care beforehand against a possible danger; see also Protection
   Promotion: advancing; see also Enhancement
   Protection: shielding from injury; see also Precaution
   Reduction: lessening, diminishing

Restoration: reinstating, bringing back to normal or unimpaired state

Therapy: having a therapeutic nature, healing

NOTE: Some of these terms mean the same thing; a choice of which one to use will depend upon which sounds better in context and whether one is already more familiar and more accepted in practice.

General Principles for Definitions of Interventions

A definition for an intervention label is a phrase that defines the concept. It is a summary of the most distinguishing characteristics. The definition, together with the defining activities, delineates the boundaries of nurse behavior circumscribed by the label. The following principles assist in developing definitions of interventions:

1. Use phrases (not complete sentences) that describe the behavior of the nurse and can stand alone without examples.
2. Avoid using terms for the patient and nurse, but when a term must be used, *patient* or *person* is preferred rather than *client*.
3. For those phrases that begin with a verb form, consider the situation and choose either the -ion form (e.g., limitation) or the -ing form (e.g., limiting).

General Principles for Activities

Activities are actions that a nurse does to implement the intervention. The following principles relate to activities:

1. Begin each activity with a verb. Possible verbs include *assist, administer, explain, avoid, inspect, facilitate, monitor,* and *use.* Use the most active verb that is appropriate for the situation. Use the term *monitor* rather than *assess.* Monitoring is a type of assessment but is done postdiagnosis as part of an intervention rather than as preparation for making a diagnosis. Avoid the terms *observe* and *evaluate.*
2. Keep the activities as generic as possible (e.g., instead of saying, "place on Kinair bed" or "place on circlectric bed," say "place on therapeutic bed"). Eliminate brand names.
3. Avoid combining two different ideas in one activity unless they illustrate the same point.
4. Avoid repeating an idea; when two activities are saying the same thing, even in different words, eliminate one.
5. Focus on the critical activities; do not worry about including all supporting activities. The number of activities depends on the intervention, but, on average, use a one-page list.
6. Word similar activities the same across interventions.
7. Word activities so they are clear without referring to the patient or the nurse. If the patient must be referred to, use the term *patient* or *person* in preference to *client* or other terms. Use the terms *family member(s)* or *significant other(s)* rather than *spouse.*
8. Add the phrase "as appropriate," "as necessary," or "as needed" to the end of those activities that are important but used only on some occasions.
9. Check for consistency between the activities and the label's definition.
10. Arrange the activities in the order in which they are usually carried out, when appropriate.

DEMOGRAPHIC INFORMATION FORM

(Please complete and submit with new/revised intervention[s].)

Please complete the following:

1. Are you currently employed as an RN?
   _____ (1) Yes, _____ (2) No, am an RN but not currently employed as an RN
   _____ (3) No, am studying to be an RN _____ (4) No, am not an RN

2. How long have you practiced as an RN?
   _____ (0) Not Practiced as an RN
   _____ (1) 1 Year or Less
   _____ (2) 1 to 3 Years
   _____ (3) 3 to 5 Years
   _____ (4) 5 to 10 Years
   _____ (5) Over 10 Years

3. Which of the following *best* describes the setting in which you are employed? (Check only *ONE* area.)
   _____ (1) Hospital
   _____ (2) Long-Term Care
   _____ (3) Public/Community Health
   _____ (4) Occupational Health
   _____ (5) Office Nursing
   _____ (6) School Nursing
   _____ (7) Outpatient Setting
   _____ (8) Nursing Education
   _____ (9) Other (specify) _____

4. Which of the following *best* describes the type of unit/specialty area in which you practice? (Check only *ONE* area.)
   _____ (1) General Medicine
   _____ (2) General Surgery
   _____ (3) Intensive Care
   _____ (4) OB/GYN/Pediatrics
   _____ (5) Specialty Medicine
   _____ (6) Specialty Surgery
   _____ (7) Psychiatric (Adult or Child)
   _____ (8) Ambulatory Care/Outpatient
   _____ (9) General Long-Term Care/Rehabilitation
   _____ (10) Other

5. What is your *highest* level of educational preparation?
   _____ (1) Associate Degree
   _____ (2) Diploma
   _____ (3) Baccalaureate
   _____ (4) Master's
   _____ (5) Doctorate

6. Are you currently certified by any professional organizations?
   _____ (1) Yes _____ (2) No

7. How have you used the Classification?
   _____ Clinical Practice
   _____ Teaching
   _____ Research
   _____ Administration

Please elaborate on how you have used the Classification:

General comments about the Classification:

If your suggestions are included in NIC, we would like to acknowledge your help in the next edition. Please sign here if you will permit us to include your name in the recognition list.

Signature: _____

Print your name: _____

Employment title: _____

Place of employment: _____

Street: _____

City, State, and ZIP Code: _____

Telephone: _____

E-mail address: _____

Please mail, email, or fax this form along with your proposed new or revised interventions(s) to:

Center for Nursing Classification and Clinical Effectiveness:
NIC Review
The University of Iowa College of Nursing:
Iowa City, Iowa 52242-1121
Fax: (319) 335-9990
Phone: (319) 335-7051
Email: classification-center@uiowa.edu

Timeline and Highlights for NIC

1985

Nursing Interventions: Treatments for Nursing Diagnoses, edited by Bulechek and McCloskey and published by Saunders, is one of the first two books to define independent nursing interventions.

1987

Intervention research team formed by Joanne McCloskey and Gloria Bulechek at the University of Iowa.

1990

The Iowa Research Team led by Joanne McCloskey and Gloria Bulechek is funded by a research grant from the National Institute of Nursing Research (1990-1993).

First publication about Nursing Interventions Classification (NIC) appears in print in the *Journal of Professional Nursing*.

1991

American Nurses Association (ANA) recognizes NIC.

1992

The first edition of *Nursing Interventions Classification (NIC)* is published by Mosby.

The Nursing Clinics of North America publishes an entire volume (*Nursing Interventions,* 27[2]. Philadelphia: W.B. Saunders) on the initial survey research on the interventions in the fist edition of NIC.

Nursing Interventions: Essential Nursing Treatments, edited by Bulechek and McCloskey, is published by W.B. Saunders.

1993

NIC is added to National Library of Medicine's Unified Medical Language System Metathesaurus.

The second NIC intervention grant funded by NINR (June 1993-1997; extended to 1998) with Joanne McCloskey and Gloria Bulechek as the co-principal investigators.

NIC is included in the International Council of Nurses (ICN) *International Classification for Nursing Practice* (Alpha version).

Publication of *The NIC Letter* begins at the University of Iowa.

1994

Cumulative Index to Nursing and Health Care Literature (CINAHL) and Silver Platter add NIC to their indexes.

The Joint Commission on Accreditation of Health Care Organizations (JCAHO) includes NIC as means to meet standard on uniform data collection.

The National League for Nursing (NLN) makes a video describing the development and testing of NIC.

An institutional effectiveness grant for preparing PhD candidates and postdoctoral students is funded at The University of Iowa, with Joanne McCloskey and Meridean Maas as directors.

The Nursing Classifications Fund is established at The University of Iowa to provide ongoing financial support for the continued development and use of NIC and NOC.

1995

The Center for Nursing Classification (the Center) at the University of Iowa is approved (December 13) by the Iowa Board of Regents (without funding) to facilitate the ongoing research and implementation of NIC and NOC. A fundraising advisory board for the Center is established and members are appointed.

1996

Mosby publishes the second edition of *Nursing Interventions Classification (NIC)*.

The first meeting of the Center's fundraising advisory board is held.

The ANA's Social Policy Statement includes the NIC definition of an intervention.

The first vendor signs licensing agreement for NIC and NOC.

NIC is linked to the Omaha classification and distributed in a monograph published by the Center.

1997

The NIC Letter becomes *The NIC/NOC Letter.*

The first joint international North American Nursing Diagnosis Association (NANDA), NIC, and NOC Conference is held in St. Charles, Illinois.

1998

NIC submits information to American National Standards Institute Health Informatics Standards Board (ANSI HISB) for Inventory of Clinical Information Standards.

The NIC/ NOC Letter is sponsored by Mosby-Year Book.

Multiple translations of NIC are processed (Dutch, Korean, Chinese, French, Japanese, German, and Spanish).

The Center receives 3 years of support from the College of Nursing at The University of Iowa (1998-2001), is given space on the fourth floor of the College of Nursing, and Joanne McCloskey is appointed director.

NIC interventions are linked to NOC outcomes in monograph published by the Center.

1999

The first Institute on Informatics and Classification is held at the University of Iowa.

Nursing Interventions: Effective Nursing Treatments, edited by Bulechek and McCloskey, is published by W.B. Saunders.

2000

Mosby publishes the third edition of *Nursing Interventions Classification (NIC)*.

The NNN Alliance is created, with Dorothy Jones and Joanne Dochterman as co-chairs.

NIC and NOC linked with Resident Assessment Protocols (RAP) and Outcome and Assessment Information Set (OASIS).

The second Institute on Informatics and Classification is held.

2001

The book that links the three languages—*Nursing Diagnoses, Outcomes, Interventions: NANDA, NOC, and NIC Linkages*—is authored by the NIC and NOC principal investigators and published by Mosby.

An NNN Invitational Common Structure Conference is funded by the National Library of Medicine (Joanne Dochterman and Dorothy Jones, principal investigators) and held in Utica, Illinois, in August.

An effectiveness grant is funded (NINR & Agency for Healthcare Research and Quality [AHRQ]) for large database research with the use of NIC (Marita Titler and Joanne Dochterman). This is likely the first such grant to fund nursing effectiveness research in which a clinical database with nursing standardized language is used.

NIC is registered in Health Level7 (HL7).

The third Institute on Informatics and Classification is held.

2002

The NNN Alliance holds an international conference on nursing language, classification, and informatics in Chicago, Illinois. This is a replacement for NANDA's biennial conference. A White Paper on the development of a common structure for NANDA, NIC, and NOC is presented to conference participants.

Systematized Nomenclature of Medicine (SNOMED) licenses NIC for inclusion in its database.

The Center for Nursing Classification expands name to Center for Nursing Classification and Clinical Effectiveness; endowment reaches $600,000.

The fourth Institute on Informatics and Classification is held.

A 4-hour web course on standardized languages, NANDA, NIC, and NOC, is offered by the Center.

A second institutional training grant for PhD candidates and postdoctoral students in effectiveness research is funded at The University Iowa by NINR, with Joanne Dochterman and Martha Craft-Rosenberg as directors.

The position of Center Fellow is established (to assist in the ongoing development of NIC and NOC), and about 30 people are appointed for 3-year terms.

2003

ANA publishes the Common Taxonomy of Nursing Practice in a monograph, *Unifying Nursing Languages: The Harmonization of NANDA, NIC, and NOC* (edited by Joanne Dochterman and Dorothy Jones).

The first meeting of the CNC Fellows is held on April 11th at the University of Iowa College of Nursing.

NANDA, NIC, NOC software program based on the linkage book *Nursing Diagnoses, Outcomes, and Interventions: NANDA, NOC, and NIC Linkages*, CD-ROM is produced by Mosby.

The Center receives the Sigma Theta Tau International Award for Clinical Scholarship.

The fifth Institute on Nursing Informatics and Classification is held.

Elizabeth Swanson and Howard Butcher join the CNC Executive Board.

A Spanish version of the web course *NIC and NOC 101: The Basics*, translated by Patricia Levi, is offered by the Center.

2004

The 4th edition *Nursing Interventions Classification* and the 3rd edition *Nursing Outcomes Classification* are published by Mosby.

The NNN Alliance holds the second international conference on nursing language, classification, and informatics in Chicago Illinois.

Joanne Dochterman retires as Director of the Center and Sue Moorhead is appointed Director, effective July 1.

A monograph, *Guideline for Conducting Effectiveness Research in Nursing and Other Health Care Services*, authored by Marita Titler, Joanne Dochterman, and David Reed is published by the Center.

The Center for Nursing Classification and Clinical Effectiveness endowment reaches $700,000.

2005

NIC and NOC incorporated into selected GNIRC protocols.

The sixth Institute on Nursing Informatics and Classification is held.

Center Fellows reappointed for 3-year term beginning July 1. Additional fellows nominated and appointed.

The Center celebrates its 10th anniversary in December.

The second Annette Scheffel Fundraising event held December 2nd with a reception and a live and silent auction.

2006

The second edition *NANDA, NOC, and NIC Linkages: Nursing Diagnoses, Outcomes, and Interventions* is published by Mosby.

The NNN Alliance holds the third international conference on nursing language, classification, and informatics in Philadelphia, Pennsylvannia.

Five new Center Fellows appointed at the annual meeting in April.

ANA recognition of NIC and NOC is renewed.

2007

The seventh Institute on Nursing Informatics and Classification is held June 11-13.

CNC offers first research grant for $10,000.

2008

The 5th edition *Nursing Interventions Classification* and the 4th edition *Nursing Outcomes Classification* are published by Mosby.

Joanne Dochterman retires from the CNC Executive Board

The eighth Institute on Nursing Informatics and Classification is held June 9-11.

The Center becomes an affiliate member of The Alliance for Nursing Informatics (ANI).

2009

CNC submits materials to ANA for Biennial Recognition process.

CNC offers first postdoctoral fellowship for $10,000.

2010

The Center offers the first teleconference to Ile Ife, Nigeria, March 14-19.

The ninth Institute on Nursing Informatics and Classification is held June 9-11.

Major renovation to the Center is completed with update of electronic equipment to facilitate the upkeep of the classifications.

2011

Cheryl Wagner accepts appointment as NIC editor.

Elseiver creates NIC/NOC Facebook site and a quarterly newsletter.

2012

The third edition *NOC and NIC Linkages to NANDA-I and Clinical Conditions: Supporting Critical Reasoning and Quality Care* is published by Elsevier Mosby.

The 20th anniversary of NIC and the 15th anniversary of NOC are celebrated along with the NANDA International 40th anniversary at the NANDA-I conference in Houston, Texas.

2013

The 6th edition *Nursing Interventions Classification* and the 5th edition *Nursing Outcomes Classification* are published by Elsevier.

In addition to the above events, NIC and NOC have been presented by the editors over the years at numerous national and international conferences in the following countries: Andorra, Australia, Austria, Brazil, Canada, Columbia, Denmark, England, France, Iceland, Ireland, Italy, Japan, Korea, Mexico, Netherlands, Nigeria, Slovenia, Spain, Switzerland, and Turkey. Currently NIC and NOC are being presented globally by colleagues and students from multiple countries.

APPENDIX D

Abbreviations

A-aDO$_2$	Alveolar arterial Oxygen Pressure Difference
ABG	Arterial Blood Gas
ABO	Blood types **A, B, O**
ACLS	Advanced Cardiac Life Support
ADH	AntiDiuretic Hormone
ADL	Activity of Daily Living
AED	Automated External Defibrillator
AICD	Automatic Implantable Cardioverter Defibrillator
AIDS	Acquired Immune Deficiency Syndrome
ARDS	Adult Respiratory Distress Syndrome
AST	ASpartate aminoTransferase
AV	AtrioVentricular
avDO$_2$	arteriovenous Oxygen Difference
BE	Base Excess
BP	Blood Pressure
BUN	Blood Urea Nitrogen
C	Celsius
Ca	Calcium
CBC	Complete Blood Count
cc	cubic centimeter
CI	Cardiac Index
CK	Creatinine Kinase
cm	centimeter
CNS	Central Nervous System
CO	Cardiac Output
CO$_2$	Carbon dioxide
COPD	Chronic Obstructive Pulmonary Disease
CPAP	Continuous Positive Airway Pressure
CPP	Cerebral Perfusion Pressure
CPR	CardioPulmonary Resuscitation
Cr	Creatinine
CSF	CerebroSpinal Fluid
CVAD	Central Venous Access Device
CVP	Central Venous Pressure
D$_5$W	Dextrose 5% in Water
DNA	DeoxyriboNucleic Acid
DVT	Deep Vein Thrombosis
ECG	ElectroCardioGram
ECT	ElectroConvulsive Therapy
EEG	ElectroEncephaloGram
EKG	ElectroKardioGram
EMG	ElectroMyoGram
EOA	Esophageal Obturator Airway
EOM	ExtraOcular Movement
ET	Endotracheal Tube
FEV$_1$	Forced Expiratory Volume in one second
FiO$_2$	Fraction of inspired Oxygen
FVC	Forced Vital Capacity

GI	GastroIntestinal
g, gm	gram
GFR	Glomerular Filtration Rate
HCl	HydroChloric Acid
HCO$_3$	Bicarbonate
Hct	Hematocrit
Hg	Mercury
Hgb	Hemoglobin
HIV	Human Immunodeficiency Virus
HR	Heart Rate
IADL	Instrumental Activities of Daily Living
ICP	IntraCranial Pressure
ICU	Intensive Care Unit
IM	IntraMuscular
I&O	Intake and Output
IV	IntraVenous
JVD	Jugular Venous Distention
K	Potassium
L	Liter
LDH	Lactate DeHydrogenase
mA	milliAmpere
MAP	Mean Arterial Pressure
MAST	Military AntiShock Trousers
mEq	milliEquivalant
mEq/hr	milliEquivalant per hour
mEq/L	milliEquivalant per liter
mg	milligram
mg/dl	milligram per deciliter
min	minute
ml	milliliter
ml/kg/hr	milliliter per kilogram per hour
mm	millimeters
mm Hg	millimeters of mercury
mmol/L	millimoles per Liter
mOsm/L	milliosmoles per Liter
MVV	Maximal Voluntary Volume
Na	Sodium
NG	NasoGastric
NPO	Non Per Os (nothing by mouth)
NSAID	NonSteroidal AntiInflammatory Drug
OSHA	Occupational Safety and Health Administration
oz	ounce
PAP	Pulmonary Artery Pressure
PAWP	Pulmonary Artery Wedge Pressure
PaCO$_2$	Partial arterial Carbon dioxide pressure
PaO$_2$	Partial arterial Oxygen pressure
PCA	Patient-Controlled Analgesia
pCO$_2$	partial Carbon diOxide pressure
PCWP	Pulmonary Capillary Wedge Pressure

PE	Pulmonary Embolus		ROM	Range Of Motion
PEEP	Positive End Expiratory Pressure		RN	Registered Nurse
PEG	Percutaneous Endoscopic Gastrostomy		SaO_2	Saturation (arterial) Oxygen
PERF	Peak Expiratory Flow Rate		SIADH	Syndrome of Inappropriate AntiDiuretic Hormone
PFT	Pulmonary Function Tests			
pH	Hydrogen ion concentration		SpO_2	Saturation (peripheral) Oxygen
PICC	Peripherally Inserted Central Catheter		SQ	Subcutaneous
PO	Per Os (orally)		STI	Sexually Transmitted Infection
PO_4	Phosphate		SvO_2	Saturation (venous) Oxygen
PRN	Pro Re Nata (as often as necessary)		SVR	Systemic Vascular Resistance
PT	Prothrombin Time		S_3	3rd heart sound
PTT	Partial Thromboplastin Time		S_4	4th heart sound
PVC	Premature Ventricular Contraction		TENS	Transcutaneous Electrical Nerve Stimulation
Q_{sp}/Q_t	physiologic blood flow per minute/cardiac output per minute		TPN	Total Parenteral Nutrition
			V_d/V_t	Physiological dead space/Tidal volume
REM	Rapid Eye Movement		V/Q scan	Ventilation-Perfusion scan
Rh	Rhesus antigen		WBC	White Blood Cell/White Blood Count

Previous Editions and Translations

McCloskey, J. C. & Bulechek, G. M. (Eds.). (1992). *Nursing Interventions Classification* (NIC). St. Louis, MO: Mosby. [336 Interventions]
• Translated into French, 1996: Decarie Editeur Inc.

McCloskey, J. C. & Bulechek, G. M. (Eds.). (1996). *Nursing Interventions Classification* (NIC) (2nd ed.). St. Louis, MO: Mosby. [433 Interventions]
• Translated into Chinese, 2000: Farseeing
• Translated into Dutch, 1997: De Tijdstroom, Utrecht
• Translated into French 2000: Masson
• Translated into Japanese 2001: Nankodo
• Translated into Korean, 1998: Hung Moon Sa
• Translated into Spanish 2000: Sintesis

McCloskey, J. C. & Bulechek, G. M. (Eds.). (2000). *Nursing Interventions Classification* (NIC) (3rd ed.). St. Louis, MO: Mosby. [486 Interventions]
• Translated into Dutch, 2002: Elsevier Gezondheidszorg
• Translated into Japanese, 2002: Nankodo
• Translated into Portuguese, 2004: Artis Medicas
• Translated into Spanish, 2001: Edicones Harcourt, S. A.

Dochterman, J. M. & Bulechek, G. M. (Eds.). (2004). *Nursing Interventions Classification* (NIC) (4th ed.). St. Louis, MO: Mosby. [514 Interventions]
• Translated into German, 2012, Hans Huber
• Translated into Italian, 2007: Casa Editrice Ambrosiana
• Translated into Japanese, 2006, Nankodo
• Translated into Norwegian, 2006, Akribe
• Translated into Portuguese, 2008, Artmed

Bulechek, G., Butcher, H., & Dochterman, J. (Eds.). (2008). *Nursing Interventions Classification* (NIC) (5th ed.). St. Louis, MO: Mosby. [542 interventions]
• Translated into Simplified Chinese, 2009: Elsevier
• Translated into Dutch, 2010: Elsevier Gezondheidszorg
• Translated into Japanese, 2009, Nankodo
• Translated into Portuguese, 2010, Elsevier Editora
• Translated into Spanish, 2009, Elsevier España

Index

Surveillance *(Continued)*
  environmental interpretation syndrome, impaired, 489
  fluid volume, 495, 497
  gastrointestinal perfusion, risk for ineffective, 499
  late pregnancy, 367b
    autonomic dysreflexia, 468
    childbearing process, ineffective, 475
  remote electronic, 368b
Sustenance support, 368–369b
  community coping, ineffective, 477
  contamination, 481
  contamination, risk for, 481
  coping, ineffective, 482
  family coping, 491
  family therapeutic regimen management, ineffective, 494
Suturing, 369b
Swallowing
  aspiration precautions, 466, 552
  impaired, 552b
  nursing interventions for, 552
  therapy, 369–370b

T

Technology management, 387–388b, 469
Telephone consultation, 388–389b, 466, 471
Telephone follow-up, 389b
Temperature regulation, 390b
  autonomic dysreflexia, 467
  body temperature, risk for imbalanced, 470
  energy field, disturbed, 488
  fluid volume, 496, 497
  hyperthermia, 505
  hypothermia, 506
  perioperative, 390–391b, 470, 506
  thermoregulation, 553
Therapeutic play, 391b, 485, 487, 489
Therapeutic touch, 392b
Therapy
  activity, 73b
  animal-assisted, 82b
  art, 85b
  exercise as
    activity intolerance, 463
    ambulation, 184b
    balance, 184–185b
    joint mobility, 185b
    muscle control, 186b
  for family, 194b
  hemodialysis, 215b
  hemofiltration, 216b
  hormone replacement, 219b
  leech, 246b
  music, 269b
  nutrition, 275b
  oxygen, 281–282b
  peritoneal dialysis, 295b
  recreation, 319b
  relaxation, 321–322b
  reminiscence, 323–324b
Therapy group, 392–393b
  body image, disturbed, 469
  comfort, enhanced, readiness for, 476
  coping, 482
  denial, ineffective, 485

Therapy group *(Continued)*
  family process, dysfunctional, 492
  fear, 495
Thermal injury
  environmental management, safety, 553
  nursing interventions for, 553
  risk for, 553b
  risk identification, 553
Thermoregulation, 553, 553b
Thrombolytic therapy management, 393b, 469
Tissue integrity
  impaired, 553–554b
  infection protection, 553
  nursing interventions for, 553–554
  skin surveillance, 553
  wound care, 554
Tissue perfusion
  cardiac, 554
    cardiac risk management, 554
    exercise promotion, 554
    nursing interventions for, 554
    risk for decreased, 554b
    smoking cessation assistance, 554
  cerebral
    cerebral edema management, 554
    intracranial pressure monitoring, 554
    nursing interventions for, 554
    risk for ineffective, 554b
  peripheral
    circulatory care, 555
    ineffective, 555b
    nursing interventions for, 555
    peripheral sensation management, 555
    risk for, 555b
    skin surveillance, 555
    teaching, disease process, 555
Toddler
  nutrition
    13-18 months, 384b, 474, 486, 492, 512
    19-24 months, 384b, 474, 486, 492, 512
    25-36 months, 385b, 474, 486, 492, 512
  safety
    13-18 months, 385b, 474, 481, 486, 490, 492, 512, 556
    19-24 months, 386b, 474, 481, 486, 490, 492, 512, 556
    25-36 months, 386b, 474, 481, 486, 490, 492, 512, 556
Toilet/toileting, 539b
  environmental management, 539
  nursing interventions for, 539
  self-care assistance, 337–338b, 539
    bowel incontinence, 470
    constipation, 480, 481
    diarrhea, 486
    environmental interpretation syndrome, impaired, 489
    failure to thrive, adult, 490
    falls, risk for, 490
    self-care deficit, 539
    toileting, 539
  training on, 387b, 512
    bowel incontinence, 470
    caregiver, role strain of, 474
    constipation, 480, 481
    development, risk for delayed, 486
    family coping, readiness for enhanced, 492
    knowledge, 512